HEALTH ASSESSMENT IN NURSING

SECOND EDITION

Patricia Gonce Morton, RN, PhD
Assistant Professor, Graduate Program
in Trauma and Critical Care Nursing,
University of Maryland, Baltimore

Springhouse Corporation
Springhouse, Pennsylvania

STAFF

Executive Director, Editorial
Stanley Loeb

Director of Trade and Textbooks
Minnie B. Rose, RN, BSN, MEd

Art Director
John Hubbard

Drug Information Editor
George J. Blake, RPh, MS

Associate Acquisitions Editor
Betsy Steinmetz

Editors
Nancy Priff (senior editor), Keith de Pinho

Clinical Consultants
Patricia Dillon, RN, MSN; Cindy Tryniszewski, RN, MSN

Designers
Stephanie Peters (associate art director), Lynn Foulk, Anita Curry, Kevin Curry, Janice Engelke, Elaine Ezrow

Illustrators
John Carlance, Will Davidson, Julie Devito-Kruk, Jean Gardner, John Gist, Bob Jackson, Frank Margasak, Bob Neumann, Judy Newhouse, Gary Phillips, Wiley Searles, Michelle Wilcox

Photographer
John Gallagher

Art Production
Robert Perry (manager), Loretta Caruso, Donald Knauss, Kitty Mace, Robert Wieder

Typographers
David Kosten (director), Diane Paluba (manager), Elizabeth Bergman, Joyce Rossi Biletz, Phyllis Marron, Robin Mayer, Valerie L. Rosenberger

Manufacturing
Deborah Meiris (manager), T.A. Landis, Anna Brindisi

Production Coordinator
Caroline Lemoine

The clinical procedures described and recommended in this publication are based on currently accepted clinical theory and practice and on consultation with medical and nursing authorities. Nevertheless, they cannot be considered absolute and universal recommendations. For individual application, recommendations must be considered in light of the patient's clinical condition and, before administration of new or infrequently used drugs, in light of latest package-insert information. The authors and the publisher disclaim responsibility for any adverse effects resulting directly or indirectly from the suggested procedures, from any undetected errors, or from the reader's misunderstanding of the text.

Printed in the United States of America. RTA-031092

Library of Congress Cataloging-in-Publication Data
Health assessment in nursing [edited by] Patricia Gonce Morton
2nd ed.
p. cm.
Includes bibliographical references and index.
1. Nursing assessment. I. Morton, Patricia Gonce, 1952-
[DNLM: 1. Nursing Assessment. WY 100 H4337]
RTA48.M67 1993
610.73–dc20
DNLM/DLC
for Library of Congress 92-49356
ISBN 0-87434-425-5 CIP

Acknowledgments for photographs and equipment

The following lists acknowledge photographs and equipment pictured in this edition. Copyrights for photographs are held by the groups named in boldface type.

Photographs

Artemis
p. 105PG Breasts
Abdomen – linea nigra
p. 107PG Vernix caseosa
Milia
Head
p. 109PG Extremities – adduction
Extremities – abduction
p. 110PG Anus and genitalia
p. 111PG Sucking or rooting
p. 112PG Tonic neck or "fencing"
Palmar grasp
Moro or "startle"

David A. Clark, MD
p. 108PG Chest circumference

Custom-Medical Stock Photo, Inc.
p. 5PG Mongolian spots, National Medical Slide Bank
p. 6PG Thin, wrinkled skin, 1991 Zuber
Senile lentigines, Zuber
p. 21PG Cornea
p. 23PG Red reflex, Paula Ihnat
Retinal structures
p. 24PG Epicanthal folds, 1991
p. 25PG Arcus senilis, National Medical Slide Bank
p. 27PG Xanthlasma
p. 28PG Corneal abrasions, 1991 Dennis R. Cain
Papilledema
Optic disk atrophy, 1991 National Medical Slide Bank
Cupped optic disk, 1990 Science Photo Library
p. 29PG Superficial retinal hemorrhages, 1990 Science Photo Library
Soft exudates, 1991 Paula Ihnat
Lens opacities, Science Photo Library
p. 30PG Tympanic membrane, Chet Childs
p. 33PG Pediatric otoscopic examination, Marka
Red, bulging tympanic membrane, Siu Biomed Comm
External ear canal drainage, Chet Childs

continued on page 660

CONTENTS IN BRIEF

ADVISORY BOARD xxx

CONSULTANTS xxx

CONTRIBUTORS xxxi

FOREWORD xxxii

PREFACE xxxiv

UNIT ONE The Nurse's Role in Assessment

Unit Introduction 1

1 Assessment and the Nursing Process 2

2 Nursing and Medicine: A Collaborative Approach 20

UNIT TWO Learning Assessment Skills

Unit Introduction 33

3 The Health History 34

4 Physical Assessment Skills 71

UNIT THREE Assessing Activity, Sleep, and Nutrition

Unit Introduction 103

5 Activities of Daily Living and Sleep Patterns 104

6 Nutritional Status 123

UNIT FOUR Assessing Body Structures and Systems

Unit Introduction 149

7 Skin, Hair, and Nails 153

8 Head and Neck 182

9 Eyes and Ears 206

10 Respiratory System 243

11 Cardiovascular System 282

12 Female and Male Breasts 334

13 Gastrointestinal System 354

14 Urinary System 385

Photo Gallery 1PG–112PG

15 Female Reproductive System 413

16 Male Reproductive System 442

17 Nervous System 462

18 Musculoskeletal System 510

19 Immune System and Blood 547

20 Endocrine System 586

UNIT FIVE Special Assessments

Unit Introduction 610

21 Complete and Partial Assessments 611

22 Perinatal and Neonatal Assessment 636

APPENDICES 649

INDEX 661

CONTENTS IN DETAIL

ADVISORY BOARD xxx

CONSULTANTS xxx

CONTRIBUTORS xxxi

FOREWORD xxxii

PREFACE xxxiv

UNIT ONE: THE NURSE'S ROLE IN ASSESSMENT

UNIT INTRODUCTION 1

1 Assessment and the Nursing Process 2

Barbara L. Ogden, RN,C, MSN

Objectives, 2
Introduction, 2
Methods and theories, 3
Problem-solving methods, 4
Reflexive, 4
Trial and error, 4
Intuitive, 4
Scientific, 5
Theories guiding the nursing process, 5
Nursing process steps, 6
Assessment, 6
Interview, 7
Observation, 7
Physical assessment, 7
Recording the data, 7
Nursing diagnosis, 8
Errors in formulating a diagnosis, 9
Planning, 9
Determining priorities, 12
Setting goals, 14
Selecting interventions, 15
The nursing care plan, 16
Implementation, 17
Interdependent interventions, 17
Dependent interventions, 17
Independent interventions, 17
Evaluation, 18
Chapter summary, 18
Study questions, 19
Selected references, 19
Nursing research, 19

2 **Nursing and Medicine: A Collaborative Approach** 20

Linda K. Strodtman, RN, MS, CNS, and Jane Willis Schultz, RN, MSN

Objectives, 20
Introduction, 20
The nursing model, 20
Historical overview, 21
Development of nursing diagnoses, 23
The medical model, 25
Historical overview, 25
The nurse-physician relationship, 26
Historical overview, 26
Collaboration, 27
The NJPC study, 27
Strategies for successful collaboration, 27
Communication, 27
Accountability, 28
Competence and trust, 29
ANA position on collaboration, 29
Collaboration and nursing diagnoses, 30
Chapter summary, 31
Study questions, 31
Selected references, 32
Nursing research, 32

UNIT TWO: LEARNING ASSESSMENT SKILLS

UNIT INTRODUCTION 33

3 **The Health History** 34

Karen A. Stinger, RN,C, MS, PNP, and Elizabeth D. Metzgar, RN,C, MPH, FNP

Objectives, 34
Introduction, 34
Understanding the health history, 34
Biographic data, 36
Health and illness patterns, 36
Health promotion and protection patterns, 36
Role and relationship patterns, 36
Summary of health history data, 37
Developing interviewing skills, 37
Nurse-client communication, 37
Therapeutic use of self, 37
Exhibiting empathy, 37
Demonstrating acceptance, 38
Giving recognition, 38
Client's expectations, 38
Behavioral considerations, 38
Cultural and ethnic considerations, 38
Effective interviewing techniques, 39
Offering general leads, 39
Restating, 39
Reflecting, 39

Verbalizing the implied meaning, 39
Focusing the discussion, 39
Placing a problem (or an event) in proper sequence, 39
Encouraging client participation, 39
Encouraging client evaluation, 39
Clarification or consensual validation, 40
Presenting reality, 40
Making observations, 40
Giving information, 40
Using silence, 40
Summarizing, 40
Interviewing techniques to avoid, 40
Asking why or how questions, 40
Using probing, persistent questioning, 40
Using inappropriate language, 41
Giving advice, 41
Giving false reassurance, 41
Changing the subject or interrupting, 41
Using clichés or stereotyped responses, 41
Giving excessive approval or agreement, 41
Jumping to conclusions, 41
Using defensive responses, 41
Making too many literal responses, 41
Asking leading questions, 42
Conducting the interview, 42
Physical and psychological comfort, 42
The interview structure, 42
Introductory phase, 42
Working phase, 43
Termination phase, 43
Time constraints, 43
Types of questions, 44
Obtaining health history data, 44
Biographic data, 44
Client's name, 44
Address, 44
Telephone number, 44
Contact person, 44
Sex, 44
Age and birth date, 44
Social Security number, 44
Place of birth, 44
Race, nationality, and cultural background, 45
Marital status and names of persons living with the client, 45
Education, 45
Religion, 45
Occupation, 45
Health and Illness patterns, 45
Reason for seeking health care, 45
Current health status, 45
Past health status, 45
Family health status, 47
Status of physiologic systems, 47
Developmental considerations, 47

Health promotion and protection patterns, 51
Health beliefs, 51
Personal habits, 52
Sleep and wake patterns, 53
Exercise and activity, 53
Recreation, 53
Nutrition, 53
Stress and coping, 54
Socioeconomic status, 54
Environmental health patterns, 55
Occupational health patterns, 55
Role and relationship patterns, 56
Self-concept, 56
Cultural influences, 57
Spiritual and religious influences, 58
Family role and relationship patterns, 59
Sexuality and reproductive patterns, 59
Social support patterns, 60
Emotional health status, 63
Summary of health history data, 63
Formulating plans with the client, 63
Special considerations, 63
Modifications for pediatric clients, 63
Modifications for pregnant clients, 64
Modifications for elderly clients, 65
Modifications for disabled clients, 65
Documenting the health history, 66
Chapter summary, 69
Study questions, 69
Selected references, 70
Nursing research, 70

4 Physical Assessment Skills **71**

Linda Grabbe, RN, PhD, CCRN, CNRN

Objectives, 71
Introduction, 71
Assessment equipment, 72
Basic assessment equipment, 72
Thermometer, 73
Stethoscope, 73
Sphygmomanometer, 73
Visual acuity charts, 76
Penlight or flashlight, 76
Measuring tape and pocket ruler, 76
Marking pencil, 76
Scale, 76
Other basic assessment equipment, 76
Advanced assessment equipment, 77
Ophthalmoscope, 77
Nasoscope, 77
Otoscope, 77
Tuning fork, 77

Physical assessment techniques, 81
Inspection, 81
Palpation, 83
Percussion, 83
Auscultation, 86
Approach to physical assessment, 86
Special considerations for pediatric clients, 87
Special considerations for pregnant clients, 89
Special considerations for elderly clients, 89
Special considerations for disabled clients, 90
The general survey, 90
Signs of distress, 90
Facial characteristics, 90
Body type, posture, and movements, 90
Speech, 91
Dress, grooming, and personal hygiene, 91
Psychological state, 91
Special considerations for pediatric clients, 92
Special considerations for elderly clients, 92
Special considerations for disabled clients, 92
Cultural and ethnic considerations, 92
Documenting the general survey, 93
Vital signs, 93
General guidelines, 93
Temperature, 94
Normal and abnormal body temperatures, 94
Pulse, 95
Respiration, 97
Blood pressure, 98
Assessing blood pressure, 100
Normal and abnormal blood pressure readings, 100
Documenting vital signs, 101
Height and weight measurements, 101
Chapter summary, 101
Study questions, 102
Selected references, 102
Nursing research, 102

UNIT THREE: ASSESSING ACTIVITY, SLEEP, AND NUTRITION

UNIT INTRODUCTION 103

5 Activities of Daily Living and Sleep Patterns 104

Ann E. Rogers, RN, PhD, ACP, and Patricia Gonce Morton, RN, PhD

Objectives, 104
Introduction, 104
Activities of daily living, 104
Factors affecting ADLs, 105
Age and developmental status, 105
Culture, 105
Physiologic health, 106
Cognitive function, 106

Psychosocial function, 106
Stress level, 106
Biological rhythms, 107
Assessing ADLs, 107
Personal care activities, 107
Family responsibility activities, 108
Work and school activities, 108
Recreational activities, 109
Socialization activities, 110
Developmental considerations, 110
Observations and documentation, 110
Sleep patterns, 111
Sleep stages, 111
Normal sleep patterns, 111
Factors affecting sleep patterns, 112
Age, 112
Exercise, 113
Smoking, 113
Caffeine, 113
Alcohol, 113
Diet, 113
Environment, 113
Emotional factors, 114
Assessing sleep patterns, 114
Sleep-wake patterns, 114
Excessive daytime sleepiness, 116
Insomnia, 117
Developmental considerations, 120
Observations and documentation, 120
Chapter summary, 120
Study questions, 121
Selected references, 121
Nursing research, 122

6 Nutritional Status 123
JoAnn Hungelmann, RN, DNSc

Objectives, 123
Introduction, 123
Physiology review, 125
Ingestion, digestion, absorption, and excretion, 125
Metabolism, 125
Energy, 125
Carbohydrate metabolism, 126
Protein metabolism, 126
Fat metabolism, 126
Vitamins and minerals, 128
Health history, 128
Health and illness patterns, 128
Current health status, 128
Past health status, 129
Family health status, 129

Developmental considerations, 129
Pediatric client, 131
Infant (newborn to age 1), 131
Toddler (age 1 to 3), 131
Preschooler (age 3 to 6), 131
School-age child (age 6 to 12), 131
Adolescent (age 12 to 18), 132
Pregnant client, 132
Breast-feeding client, 132
Elderly client, 132
Health promotion and protection patterns, 133
Health beliefs, 133
Exercise and activity patterns, 133
Nutritional patterns, 133
Stress and coping patterns, 133
Socioeconomic patterns, 136
Role and relationship patterns, 136
Self-concept, 136
Social support patterns, 136
Physical assessment, 137
Inspection, 137
Palpation, 137
Anthropometric measurements, 137
Developmental considerations, 142
Pediatric clients, 142
Elderly clients, 144
Advanced assessment skills, 144
Documentation, 144
Chapter summary, 147
Study questions, 147
Selected references, 147
Nursing research, 148

UNIT FOUR: ASSESSING BODY STRUCTURES AND SYSTEMS

UNIT INTRODUCTION 149

7 Skin, Hair, and Nails 153

Marcia J. Hill, RN, MSN, and Kathryn J. Conrad, RN, MSN, OCN

Objectives, 153
Introduction, 153
Anatomy and physiology review, 154
Functions of the skin, 155
Protection, 155
Sensory perception, 155
Temperature and blood pressure regulation, 155
Vitamin synthesis, 155
Excretion, 155
Developmental considerations, 155
Pediatric clients, 155
Pregnant clients, 155
Elderly clients, 157

Health history, 157
Health and illness patterns, 159
Current health status, 159
Past health status, 160
Family health status, 160
Developmental considerations, 160
Pediatric client, 160
Pregnant client, 161
Elderly client, 161
Health promotion and protection patterns, 163
Role and relationship patterns, 164
Physical assessment, 165
Preparing for skin, hair, and nail assessment, 165
Body weight, fluid balance, general appearance, and related body systems, 165
Inspection, 166
Skin, 166
Color, 166
Vascular changes, 166
Skin lesions, 167
Hair and scalp, 167
Nails, 167
Abnormal findings, 169
Skin, 169
Hair, 170
Nails, 170
Palpation, 171
Skin, 171
Texture and consistency, 171
Temperature, 171
Moisture, 171
Turgor, 171
Lesions, 171
Hair, 171
Nails, 173
Abnormal findings, 173
Cultural considerations, 173
Developmental considerations, 175
Pediatric client, 175
Pregnant client, 177
Elderly client, 177
Documentation, 177
Chapter summary, 180
Study questions, 180
Selected References, 181
Nursing research, 181

8 Head and Neck 182
Karen A. Stinger, RN,C, MS, PNP

Objectives, 182
Introduction, 182
Anatomy and physiology review, 182
Head and face, 183
Nose, sinuses, mouth, and neck, 183

Health history, 187
Health and illness patterns, 187
Developmental considerations, 188
Pediatric client, 188
Elderly client, 188
Health promotion and protection patterns, 190
Role and relationship patterns, 191
Physical assessment, 191
Examining the head and face, 191
Abnormal findings, 193
Examining the nose and sinuses, 193
Abnormal findings, 193
Examining the mouth and oropharynx, 195
Abnormal findings, 199
Examining the neck, 199
Abnormal findings, 200
Developmental considerations, 200
Pediatric clients, 200
Pregnant clients, 201
Elderly clients, 201
Documentation, 201
Chapter summary, 204
Study questions, 204
Selected references, 205
Nursing research, 205

9 Eyes and Ears **206**
Karen A. Stinger, RN,C, MS, PNP

Objectives, 206
Introduction, 206
Anatomy and physiology review: The eye, 207
Extraocular nerves, muscles, and structures, 209
Intraocular structures, 209
Physiology of vision, 209
Health history: The eye, 211
Health and illness patterns, 211
Current health status, 211
Past health status, 212
Family health status, 213
Developmental considerations, 213
Pediatric client, 213
Elderly client, 215
Health promotion and protection patterns, 215
Role and relationship patterns, 216
Physical assessment: The eye, 216
Vision, 216
Distance vision, 216
Near vision, 217
Color perception, 217
Abnormal findings, 217
Extraocular muscle function, 217
Abnormal findings, 217

Peripheral vision, 219
Abnormal findings, 219
Inspection, 219
Eyelids, eyelashes, eyeball, and lacrimal apparatus, 220
Conjunctiva and sclera, 220
Cornea, anterior chamber, and iris, 221
Pupil, 221
Abnormal findings, 222
Palpation, 222
Abnormal findings, 223
Developmental and ethnic considerations, 224
Pediatric client, 224
Elderly client, 224
Ethnic considerations, 225
Advanced assessment skills, 225
Ophthalmoscopic examination, 225
Tonometry, 227
Documentation: The eye, 230
Anatomy and physiology review: The ear, 230
Health history: The ear, 231
Health and illness patterns, 231
Current health status, 231
Past health status, 231
Developmental considerations, 233
Pediatric client, 233
Elderly client, 234
Health promotion and protection patterns, 234
Role and relationship patterns, 234
Physical assessment: The ear, 235
Inspection, 235
Abnormal findings, 235
Palpation, 235
Abnormal findings, 235
Auditory function screening, 235
Gross hearing screening, 236
Weber's test, 236
Rinne test, 236
Developmental and ethnic considerations, 236
Advanced assessment skills, 239
Otoscopic examination, 239
Documentation: The ear, 240
Chapter summary, 240
Study questions, 241
Selected references, 241
Nursing research, 242

10 Respiratory System **243**
Karen A. Landis, RN, MS, CCRN

Objectives, 243
Introduction, 243
Anatomy and physiology review, 245
Respiratory tract, 245
Thoracic cage, 248
Inspiration and expiration, 248
Pulmonary blood flow, 248

External and internal respiration, 248
Ventilation, 248
Nervous system effect, 252
Musculoskeletal system effect, 252
Pulmonary system effect, 252
Pulmonary perfusion, 252
Diffusion, 252
Acid-base balance, 253
Developmental considerations, 253
Health history, 254
Health and illness patterns, 254
Current health status, 254
Past health status, 255
Family health status, 256
Status of physiologic systems, 256
Developmental considerations, 256
Pediatric client, 258
Elderly client, 258
Health promotion and protection patterns, 259
Role and relationship patterns, 259
Physical assessment, 260
Preparation for respiratory assessment, 260
Inspection, 261
Respiration, 261
Anterior thorax, 262
Posterior thorax, 262
Abnormal findings, 262
Palpation, 264
Trachea and anterior thorax, 264
Posterior thorax, 264
Abnormal findings, 265
Percussion, 266
Abnormal findings, 269
Auscultation, 269
Anterior and lateral thorax, 269
Posterior thorax, 269
Abnormal findings, 270
Developmental considerations, 270
Pediatric clients, 270
Pregnant clients, 273
Elderly clients, 273
Advanced assessment skills, 275
Tactile fremitus, 275
Diaphragmatic excursion, 275
Voice resonance, 278
Documentation, 278
Chapter summary, 280
Study questions, 281
Selected references, 281
Nursing research, 281

11 **Cardiovascular System** **282**
Linda S. Baas, RN, PhD, CCRN

Objectives, 282
Introduction, 282
Anatomy and physiology review, 284
The heart, 284
Chambers and valves, 284
Blood circulation, 285
Pulmonary circulation, 285
Systemic circulation, 285
Coronary circulation, 285
Cardiac conduction system, 285
Extrinsic conduction system, 290
Intrinsic conduction system, 290
Cardiac cycle, 290
Developmental considerations, 292
Pediatric clients, 292
Pregnant clients, 292
Elderly clients, 293
Health history, 293
Health and illness patterns, 293
Current health status, 293
Past health status, 295
Family health status, 298
Developmental considerations, 298
Pediatric client, 298
Pregnant client, 300
Elderly client, 300
Health promotion and protection patterns, 301
Personal habits, 301
Sleep and wake patterns, 301
Exercise and activity patterns, 302
Nutritional patterns, 302
Stress and coping patterns, 303
Other health promotion and protection patterns, 303
Role and relationship patterns, 304
Physical assessment, 305
Preparing for cardiovascular assessment, 305
General appearance, body weight, and vital signs, 306
Body weight, 306
Vital signs, 306
Assessing related body structures, 307
Skin, hair, and nails, 307
Eyes, 308
Inspection, 309
Jugular veins, 309
Precordium, 309
Abnormal findings, 309
Palpation, 310
Pulses, 310
Precordium, 311
Abnormal findings, 315
Percussion, 315

Auscultation, 316
Precordium, 316
Arteries, 319
Abnormal findings, 319
Developmental considerations, 319
Pediatric client, 319
Pregnant client, 320
Elderly client, 320
Advanced assessment skills, 323
Inspection of the jugular venous pulse, 323
Auscultation of extra heart sounds, 323
Third heart sound, 323
Fourth heart sound, 324
Third and fourth heart sounds, 324
Auscultation of murmurs, 324
Location and timing, 324
Pitch, pattern, and quality, 324
Intensity, 325
Causes of murmurs, 325
Auscultation of other abnormal heart sounds, 325
Clicks, 325
Snaps, 325
Rubs, 328
Documentation, 328
Chapter summary, 330
Study questions, 332
Selected references, 332
Nursing research, 333

12 **Female and Male Breasts** 334
Ellis Quinn Youngkin, RN,C, PhD, OGNP

Objectives, 334
Introduction, 334
Anatomy and physiology review, 335
Developmental changes, 335
Puberty, 335
Pregnancy and lactation, 335
Maturity, 338
Health history, 338
Health and illness patterns, 339
Current health status, 339
Past health status, 339
Family health status, 341
Developmental considerations, 341
Pediatric client, 341
Pregnant client, 341
Elderly client, 341
Health promotion and protection patterns, 341
Role and relationship patterns, 342
Physical assessment, 343
Inspection, 343
Abnormal findings, 344
Palpation, 344
Abnormal findings, 344

Developmental considerations, 348
Infants, 348
Adolescents, 348
Pregnant and lactating clients, 348
Elderly clients, 348
Documentation, 349
Chapter summary, 352
Study questions, 353
Selected references, 353
Nursing research, 353

13 Gastrointestinal System 354

Margaret Massoni, RN, MSN, CS

Objectives 354
Introduction, 354
Anatomy and physiology review, 354
Digestion and elimination, 355
Accessory organ functions, 358
Abdominal muscles and blood supply, 358
Health history, 359
Health and illness patterns, 359
Current health status, 359
Past health status, 361
Family health status, 361
Developmental considerations, 361
Pediatric client, 361
Pregnant client, 364
Elderly client, 364
Health promotion and protection patterns, 364
Role and relationship patterns, 365
Physical assessment, 365
Inspection, 365
Abnormal findings, 367
Auscultation, 367
Percussion, 368
Abnormal findings, 369
Palpation, 369
Abnormal findings, 370
Developmental considerations, 370
Pediatric client, 370
Pregnant client, 371
Elderly client, 371
Advanced assessment skills, 374
Liver assessment, 374
Rectal examination, 374
Developmental considerations, 377
Techniques to elicit abdominal pain, 377
Developmental considerations, 377
Documentation, 377
Chapter summary, 382
Study questions, 383
Selected references, 384
Nursing research, 384

14 Urinary System 385

Susan Heidenwolf Weaver, RN, MSN, CCRN, CNA

Objectives, 385
Introduction, 385
Anatomy and physiology review, 387
Urine formation, 387
Hormones and the kidneys, 387
Health history, 391
Health and illness patterns, 391
Current health status, 391
Past health status, 393
Family health status, 393
Developmental considerations, 395
Pediatric client, 395
Pregnant client, 396
Elderly client, 396
Health promotion and protection patterns, 396
Role and relationship patterns, 397
Physical assessment, 397
Preparing for urinary system assessment, 397
Body weight, vital signs, and body position, 398
Assessing related body structures, 398
Eyes, 398
Skin, hair, and nails, 399
Inspection, 400
Abdomen, 400
Urethral meatus, 400
Auscultation, 401
Percussion, 401
Palpation, 402
Developmental considerations, 402
Documentation, 405
Chapter summary, 409
Study questions, 412
Selected references, 412
Nursing research, 412

Photo Gallery 1PG-112PG

These 350 photographs provide a visual review of all the body structures and systems in Unit IV, which includes Chapters 7 through 20. In color and black-and-white, the photographs cover anatomy and physiology, physical assessment, ethnic considerations, developmental considerations, and common abnormalities appropriate to these structures and systems; special prenatal and neonatal assessments supplement Chapter 22.

15 Female Reproductive System 413

Ellis Quinn Youngkin, RN,C, PhD, OGNP

Objectives, 413
Introduction, 413
Anatomy and physiology review, 414
Hormonal function and the menstrual cycle, 414
Physiology of menopause, 415

Health history, 418
Health and illness patterns, 419
Current health status, 419
Past health status, 422
Family health status, 423
Developmental considerations, 423
Pediatric client, 423
Adolescent client, 423
Climacteric client, 424
Health promotion and protection patterns, 425
Role and relationship patterns, 425
Physical assessment, 425
Preparing for the assessment, 425
Inspection, 427
Abnormal findings, 428
Developmental considerations, 428
Advanced assessment skills, 428
Abnormal findings, 428
Documentation, 436
Chapter summary, 440
Study questions, 441
Selected references, 441
Nursing research, 441

16 Male Reproductive System 442
Catherine Paradiso, RN, MS, CCRN

Objectives, 442
Introduction, 442
Anatomy and physiology review, 442
Male sexual function, 443
Spermatogenesis, 443
Hormonal control and sexual development, 445
Health history, 446
Health and illness patterns, 447
Current health status, 447
Past health status, 448
Family health status, 448
Developmental considerations, 450
Pediatric client, 450
Adolescent client, 450
Elderly client, 450
Health promotion and protection patterns, 450
Role and relationship patterns, 451
Physical assessment, 452
Preparing for physical assessment, 452
Inspection, 452
Penis, 452
Scrotum, 453
Inguinal area, 453
Abnormal findings, 453

Palpation, 453
Penis, 453
Scrotum, 453
Inguinal area, 454
Abnormal findings, 454
Developmental considerations, 455
Advanced assessment, 458
Documentation, 460
Chapter summary, 460
Study questions, 461
Selected references, 461
Nursing research, 461

17 Nervous System 462

Karen E. Burgess, RN, MSN

Objectives, 462
Introduction, 462
Anatomy and physiology review, 463
Central and peripheral nervous systems, 470
Reflex responses, 470
Health history, 471
Health and illness patterns, 471
Current health status, 471
Past health status, 472
Family health status, 475
Developmental considerations, 475
Pediatric client, 475
Elderly client, 476
Health promotion and protection patterns, 476
Role and relationship patterns, 477
Physical assessment, 477
Preparing for the assessment, 478
Cerebral function, 478
Level of consciousness, 478
Level of arousal, 478
Orientation, 479
Person, 479
Place, 479
Time, 479
Communication, 479
Verbal responsiveness, 479
Mental status, 480
Abnormal findings, 480
Developmental and cultural considerations, 481
Pediatric client, 481
Elderly client, 481
Client with language barrier, 481
Advanced assessment skills, 481
Formal language skill evaluation, 482
Spontaneous speech, 482
Comprehension, 482
Naming, 482
Repetition, 482
Vocabulary, 482
Reading, 482
Writing, 482
Copying figures, 482

Complete mental status assessment, 482
General appearance and behavior, 482
Mood and affect, 482
Cognitive functions, 482
Attention, 482
Memory, 483
Intellectual skills, 483
Abstract reasoning, 483
Judgment, 483
Thought processes and content, 486
Developmental and cultural considerations, 486
Cranial nerves, 486
Abnormal findings, 486
Olfactory nerve (CN I), 486
Optic nerve (CN II), 486
Oculomotor nerve (CN III), 487
Trochlear nerve (CN IV), 487
Trigeminal nerve (CN V), 487
Abducens nerve (CN VI), 487
Facial nerve (CN VII), 487
Acoustic nerve (CN VIII), 487
Glossopharyngeal (CN IX) and vagus (CN X) nerves, 487
Spinal accessory nerve (CN XI), 487
Hypoglossal nerve (CN XII), 487
Developmental considerations, 487
Pediatric client, 490
Elderly client, 490
Motor system and cerebellar function, 490
Motor function, 490
Abnormal findings, 492
Developmental considerations, 492
Pediatric client, 492
Elderly client, 492
Advanced assessment skills, 492
Sensory system, 494
Abnormal findings, 495
Advanced assessment skills, 495
Developmental considerations, 495
Pediatric client, 495
Elderly client, 495
Reflexes, 495
Advanced assessment skills, 495
Abnormal findings, 497
Developmental considerations, 497
Pediatric client, 497
Elderly client, 497
Vital signs, 501
Temperature, 501
Pulse, 501
Respiration, 501
Blood pressure, 502
Documentation, 502
Chapter summary, 505
Study questions, 508
Selected references, 509
Nursing research, 509

18 Musculoskeletal System 510

Julia L. Swager, RN, MSN

Objectives, 510
Introduction, 510
Anatomy and physiology review, 511
Muscles, 511
Tendons, 511
Ligaments, 511
Bones, 511
Bone function, 513
Bone formation, 513
Cartilage, 515
Joints, 515
Bursae, 515
Skeletal movement, 517
Health history, 517
Health and illness patterns, 517
Current health status, 517
Past health status, 518
Family health status, 520
Developmental considerations, 520
Pediatric client, 520
Female client, 520
Pregnant client, 520
Elderly client, 520
Health promotion and protection patterns, 520
Role and relationship patterns, 521
Physical assessment, 521
Preparing for the assessment, 522
Observing posture, gait, and coordination, 522
Posture, 522
Spinal curvature, 522
Knee positioning, 522
Gait, 522
Coordination, 523
Abnormal findings, 523
Developmental considerations, 523
Pediatric client, 523
Pregnant client, 523
Elderly client, 523
Inspecting and palpating muscles, 523
Tone and mass, 524
Strength, 524
Inspecting and palpating joints and bones, 524
Measurements, 525
Cervical spine, 525
Clavicles, 525
Scapulae, 525
Ribs, 536
Shoulders, 536
Elbows, 537
Wrists, 537
Fingers and thumbs, 537
Thoracic and lumbar spine, 537
Hips and pelvis, 537
Knees, 537
Ankles and feet, 537
Toes, 541

Developmental considerations, 541
Pediatric client, 541
Elderly client, 541
Advanced assessment skills, 541
Documentation, 541
Chapter summary, 544
Study questions, 544
Selected references, 546
Nursing research, 546

19 Immune System and Blood **547**

Regina Shannon-Bodnar, RN, MS, MSN, OCN

Objectives, 547
Introduction, 547
Anatomy and physiology review, 549
Origin, 549
Immune system, 549
Protective surface phenomena, 553
General host defenses, 553
Specific immune responses, 554
Humoral immunity, 554
Cell-mediated immunity, 555
Blood, 555
Erythrocytes, 555
Blood group compatibilities, 555
Thrombocytes, 556
Leukocytes, 557
Granulocytes, 557
Agranulocytes, 558
Developmental considerations, 558
Pediatric client, 558
Elderly client, 558
Health history, 559
Health and illness patterns, 559
Current health status, 559
Past health status, 561
Family health status, 564
Developmental considerations, 564
Pediatric client, 564
Elderly client, 564
Health promotion and protection patterns, 565
Role and relationship patterns, 566
Physical assessment, 566
Preparing for immune system and blood assessment, 566
General appearance and vital signs, 566
Assessing related body structures, 567
Skin, hair, and nails, 567
Head and neck, 567
Eyes and ears, 568
Respiratory system, 568
Cardiovascular system, 568
Gastrointestinal system, 569
Urinary system, 569
Nervous system, 569
Musculoskeletal system, 569
Inspection, 569
Palpation, 572
Abnormal findings, 573

Developmental considerations, 573
Pediatric client, 573
Elderly client, 575
Advanced assessment skills, 575
Documentation, 581
Chapter summary, 584
Study questions, 585
Selected references, 585
Nursing research, 585

20 Endocrine System 586

Linda B. Haas, RN, MN, CDE

Objectives, 586
Introduction, 586
Anatomy and physiology review, 586
Glands, 587
Hormones, 590
Hormonal release and transport, 590
Hormonal action, 590
Hormonal regulation, 590
Pituitary-target gland axis, 590
Hypothalamic-pituitary-target gland axis, 590
Chemical regulation, 591
Nervous system regulation, 591
Hormonal imbalance, 592
Health history, 592
Health and illness patterns, 592
Current health status, 592
Past health status, 593
Family health status, 593
Status of physiologic systems, 593
Developmental considerations, 596
Pediatric client, 596
Pregnant client, 596
Health promotion and protection patterns, 596
Role and relationship patterns, 597
Physical assessment, 597
Vital signs, height, and weight, 597
Abnormal findings, 598
Inspection, 598
General appearance, 598
Skin, hair, and nails, 598
Head and neck, 598
Chest, 598
Genitalia, 598
Extremities, 599
Abnormal findings, 599
General appearance, 599
Skin, hair, and nails, 599
Head and neck, 599
Chest, 600
Genitalia, 600
Extremities, 600
Palpation, 600
Auscultation, 601
Developmental considerations, 601

Documentation, 603
Chapter summary, 608
Study questions, 608
Selected references, 609
Nursing research, 609

UNIT FIVE: SPECIAL ASSESSMENTS

UNIT INTRODUCTION **610**

21 **Complete and Partial Assessments** **611**
Roxana Huebscher, RN, PhD, FNP, OGNP

Objectives, 611
Introduction, 611
Complete assessment, 611
Health history, 611
Physical assessment, 612
Preparing for the complete physical assessment, 612
General survey, 612
Height, weight, and vital signs, 613
Body structures and systems, 613
Documentation, 613
Partial assessment, 633
Health history, 633
Physical assessment, 633
General survey and vital signs, 633
Body structures and systems, 634
Documentation, 634
Chapter summary, 634
Study questions, 634
Selected references, 635
Nursing research, 635

22 **Perinatal and Neonatal Assessments** **636**
Joan Corder-Mabe, RN,C, MS, OGNP

Objectives, 636
Introduction, 636
Prenatal assessment, 636
Health history, 637
Health and illness patterns, 637
Current health status, 637
Past health status, 637
Family health status, 638
Health promotion and protection patterns, 638
Role and relationship patterns, 640
Physical assessment, 641
Documentation, 641
Postpartum assessment, 641
Health history, 641
Health and illness patterns, 641
Health promotion and protection patterns, 641
Role and relationship patterns, 643

Physical assessment, 643
Documentation, 643
Neonatal assessment, 643
Behavioral assessment, 646
Physical assessment, 646
Documentation, 646
Chapter summary, 646
Study questions, 647
Selected references, 647
Nursing research, 647

APPENDICES AND INDEX

Appendix 1: Adult client with altered cardiac output 649
Patricia Dillon, RN, MSN

Appendix 2: Adult client with impaired gas exchange 653
Patricia Dillon, RN, MSN

Appendix 3: Pediatric client with altered comfort 656
Patricia Dillon, RN, MSN

Appendix 4: NANDA nursing diagnoses grouped into Gordon's functional health patterns 659

Index 661

ADVISORY BOARD

CONSULTANTS

Catherine Raeside, RN, MS, CNRN, CPNP, Pediatric Nurse Practitioner, Volunteer Well Baby Clinic, Singapore

Mary Faut Rodts, RN, MS, Assistant Professor, Rush College of Nursing, Rush University, Chicago

Kaye Ronsman, RN,C, MSN, Geriatric Nurse Practitioner, College of Nursing Health Clinic, University of Arizona, Tucson

Linda H. Schakenbach, RN, MSN, CCRN, CS, Clinical Specialist, Surgical Nursing, Fairfax Hospital, Falls Church, Va.

Nancy L. Subolish, BS, RPh, Acting Director, Department of Pharmacy, Quakertown (Pa.) Community Hospital

Mona R. Sutnick, EdD, RD, Director, Sutnik Associates; Lecturer in Community and Preventive Medicine, Medical College of Pennsylvania, Philadelphia

Rita Wickham, RN, MS, Assistant Professor, Rush College of Nursing, Rush University; Practitioner-Teacher, Rush-Presbyterian-St. Luke's Medical Center, Chicago

CONTRIBUTORS

Linda S. Baas, RN, PhD, CCRN, Assistant Professor, College of Nursing and Health, University of Cincinnati

Rachel Z. Booth, RN, PhD, Dean, School of Nursing, University of Alabama at Birmingham

Karen E. Burgess, RN, MSN, Clinical Nurse Specialist, Huntington Memorial Hospital, Pasadena, Calif.

Kathryn J. Conrad, RN, MSN, OCN, Clinical Director, Educational Resources and Services, Pittsburgh Cancer Institute, University of Pittsburgh

Joan Corder-Mabe, RN,C, MS, OGNP, Nurse Practitioner, Kaiser Permanente, Springfield, Va.

Patricia Dillon, RN, MSN, Nursing Instructor, Gwynedd Mercy College, Gwynedd Valley, Pa.

Linda Grabbe, RN, PhD, CCRN, CNRN, Research Assistant, School of Nursing, Georgia State University, Atlanta

Linda B. Haas, RN, MN, CDE, Clinical Nurse Specialist, Endocrinology, Department of Veterans' Affairs Medical Center, Seattle

Marcia J. Hill, RN, MSN, Nursing Manager, The Methodist Hospital; Assistant Clinical Professor, Baylor College of Medicine, Houston

Roxana Huebscher, RN, PhD, FNP, OGNP, Adult Nurse Practitioner, Kaiser Permanente-Franklin Internal Medicine Clinic, Denver

JoAnn Hungelmann, RN, DNSc, Associate Professor, Niehoff School of Nursing, Loyola University of Chicago

Karen A. Landis, RN, MS, CCRN, Pulmonary Clinical Nurse Specialist, Lehigh Valley Hospital, Allentown, Pa.

Margaret Massoni, RN, MSN, CS, Assistant Professor, City University of New York at Staten Island

Elizabeth D. Metzgar, RN,C, MPH, FNP, Assistant Professor, College of Nursing, Montana State University at Missoula

Patricia Gonce Morton, RN, PhD, Assistant Professor, Graduate Program in Trauma and Critical Care Nursing, University of Maryland, Baltimore

Barbara L. Ogden, RN,C, MSN, Assistant Professor and Faculty Liaison, University of Florida, Gainesville Veterans' Administration Medical Center

Catherine Paradiso, RN, MS, CCRN, Instructor, College of Nursing, Rutger's—The State University of N.J., Newark; Clinical Specialist, Clinical Care, St. Vincent's Medical Center, Richmond, N.Y.

Ann E. Rogers, RN, PhD, ACP, Assistant Professor, School of Nursing, University of Michigan, Ann Arbor

Jane Willis Schultz, RN, MSN, Director of Diabetic Services, Johnston-Willis Hospital, Richmond, Va.

Regina Shannon-Bodnar, RN, MS, MSN, OCN, Oncology Clinical Nurse Specialist, Homewood Hospital Center, Johns Hopkins Health System, Baltimore

Karen A. Stinger, RN,C, MS, PNP, Director of Nursing Program, Grays Harbor College, Aberdeen, Wash.

Linda K. Strodtman, RN, MS, CNS, Assistant Professor of Nursing, Clinical Nurse Specialist, University of Michigan, Ann Arbor

Julia L. Swager, RN, MSN, Medical-Surgical Clinical Specialist, Memorial Hospitals Association, Modesto, Calif.

Susan Heidenwolf Weaver, RN, MSN, CCRN, CNA, Assistant Director of Nursing, St. Clares-Riverside Medical Center, Denville, N.J.

Ellis Quinn Youngkin, RN,C, PhD, OGNP, Associate Professor, School of Nursing, Virginia Commonwealth University, Richmond

FOREWORD

This Second Edition of *Health Assessment in Nursing* has received a major update through its 112-page Photo Gallery, which visualizes and dramatizes assessment techniques, normal findings, and abnormal findings. This Photo Gallery reinforces the text and its illustrations, and helps validate laboratory and clinical assessment findings. It offers a special value to the learner who prefers self-paced instruction or whose learning style is highly visual. (A Guide to Major Illustrations and Photographs, located on the inside front and back covers, directs the reader to hundreds of visuals depicting nursing activities.)

In addition to its outstanding Photo Gallery and extensive illustrations, this text distinguishes itself in several ways. First, its approach is holistic and firmly grounded in the nursing process. These characteristics encourage its users to be caring, analytical, and systematic. Second, its approach to data gathering extends beyond physical assessment to biological, psychosocial, and cultural factors. These concerns provide its users with insights into all aspects of the client's health. Third, its approach emphasizes the client's and nurse's individual needs, thereby fostering thoughtfulness, self-understanding, and awareness of age- and sex-specific considerations.

The text's comprehensiveness protects its user from having to consult numerous sources of information, thus saving time and simplifying information retrieval. Its chapter pedagogy includes learning objectives, glossary of terms, chapter summary, study questions, and selected references—all of which direct the reader's attention, clarify vital details, assist in review and recall, and provide direction to additional information. To enhance understanding, attractive graphics sort through complex information. Indeed, the text is notable for its clear and straightforward explanations and rationales.

Health Assessment in Nursing, Second Edition serves as an excellent text for the undergraduate or graduate student, a reference for the practicing nurse, and an update or review for the nurse who is returning to practice. Its holistic emphasis and use of the nursing process make the text equally useful whether the nurse works in an office, hospital, or other health care setting.

The text is divided into five units. Each unit introduction presents a brief overview of the chapters in that unit. This gives the user a framework for approaching and understanding specific content. Unit One, The Nurse's Role in Assessment, relates the nursing process to problem solving, the scientific method, and client assessment. It shows how to use assessment findings to formulate appropriate nursing diagnoses based on the categories established by the North American Nursing Diagnosis Association (NANDA). It also explains how to use assessment findings as the basis for writing client goals and developing clients' plans of care. Unit One also investigates the collaborative roles of nursing and medicine in assessment. After providing a brief history of nursing and medicine, it explores the nurse-physician relationship, highlighting the trend toward increased collaboration.

Unit Two, Learning Assessment Skills, focuses on general assessment skills. Its first chapter describes how to interview clients and gather subjective data through the nursing health history, including psychosocial and cultural assessments. Its second chapter shows how to obtain objective data by using physical assessment skills; the chapter illustrates how to use assessment equipment and perform basic assessment techniques, including inspection, palpation, percussion, auscultation, and vital sign measurements.

Unit Three, Assessing Activity, Sleep, and Nutrition, investigates three especially important concepts because any alteration in body functioning can disrupt a client's nutritional status, sleep and wakefulness patterns, and daily activities.

Unit Four, Assessing Body Structures and Systems, focuses on specific areas of assessment. Unlike most other assessment textbooks, *Health Assessment in Nursing, Second Edition* includes chapters on assessing the urinary system, immune system and blood, and endocrine system—systems that affect all body functions.

Each chapter in Unit Four follows a standard organization. To orient the student to the organs or structures being assessed, each chapter begins with a clearly illustrated review of anatomy and physiology. The chapter continues with a health history section of questions and rationales that assess health and illness patterns, health promotion and protection patterns, and role and relationship patterns. The next section, on physical assessment, discusses specific assessment equipment and techniques and provides strategies for preparing the client. It clearly describes each assessment procedure and illustrates many of these procedures step by step. It also describes normal findings, common abnormal findings, and when appropriate, developmental and ethnic considerations related to the assessment. This section includes step-by-step illustrations of advanced assessment skills—skills needed by those who have mastered the basic ones and whose practice requires more advanced skills. Each chapter in this unit concludes with a section of documenting normal and abnormal findings.

Unit Five, Special Assessments, presents the skills, knowledge, and techniques needed to perform complete, partial, perinatal, and neonatal assessments. Its first chapter integrates information from the previous units to provide guidelines for a comprehensive head-to-toe assessment. It merges the information learned from studying specific structures and systems into the complete assessment used in clinical practice. This chapter also includes guidelines for a partial assessment, which is indicated when time is limited or when the client's condition does not warrant a complete assessment. The second chapter in Unit Five describes basic prenatal, postpartal, and neonatal assessments.

The book concludes with four helpful appendices. Three of these contain a case history of a client with a specific abnormality and show how to gather subjective and objective data. Each of these pieces includes rationales for gathering data and illustrates appropriate documentation of findings. These case studies illustrate how to apply to real-life situations the knowledge and skills acquired in the previous 22 chapters. A fourth piece, NANDA Nursing Diagnoses Grouped into Gordon's Functional Health Patterns, clusters the many nursing diagnoses discussed in the text into patterns that many clinicians find logical and useful.

For the instructor using *Health Assessment in Nursing, Second Edition,* additional resources are available. An *Instructor's Resource Manual* includes chapter-for-chapter overviews, suggested lecture topics, suggested critical thinking activities, and answers to study questions that appear in the text. It also provides materials for testing student knowledge, including matching elements, true or false questions, and a test bank of multiple choice questions. The manual includes overhead transparency masters on anatomy, physiology, assessment techniques, and other vital information. For clinical laboratory use, it includes chapter-specific guides to the health history and physical assessment as well as a blank assessment form suitable for photocopying. A companion *Nurse's Clinical Guide to Health Assessment* is available in a handy size for practical use in the clinical laboratory or practice setting.

This text reflects the expertise of nurses who are well-rounded in assessment theory, practice, and experience. It also displays their depth of understanding of educational principles. Every page shows their concern for the reader's needs to understand—and integrate—theory and practice into holistic assessment. In this Second Edition of *Health Assessment in Nursing,* the author and contributors have brought the clinical laboratory to life, presenting a unique perspective on assessment in an educationally sound format. This text copes admirably with the knowledge explosion in the health care field, bringing together all the aspects of health assessment.

Rachel Z. Booth, RN, PhD
Dean and Professor
University of Alabama School of Nursing
University of Alabama at Birmingham

PREFACE

Through the generations, the nurse's role has changed dramatically. It has grown from that of assistant to the physician to respected member of the health care team. Today, nurses are expected to know more than ever before, and to provide expert care for all types of clients in all settings. To help nurses to manage these responsibilities with competence and confidence, *Health Assessment in Nursing, Second Edition* prepares them to perform a complete and thoughtful assessment, the basis of all care.

This Second Edition is written for student nurses in all types of nursing programs who must learn how to perform complete assessments. It also is written for practicing nurses who wish to polish their assessment skills. Because this edition blends theory and principles with the realities of practice, it is ideal to use in the classroom, in the clinical laboratory, and in clinical practice.

The contributors know that the best way to acquire and hone assessment skills is to learn them in a systematic way. Therefore, the book early on explains how to perform components of a *complete* assessment, which includes a detailed health history, full physical assessment, and a review of pertinent laboratory studies. Although it emphasizes normal assessment findings, it provides basic information about common or important abnormal findings.

Health Assessment in Nursing, Second Edition views assessment within several key themes, including:

- Holistic health care. With this health-oriented approach to assessment, the text views the client as an individual with physical as well as emotional, psychological, intellectual, social, cultural, and spiritual needs. It looks at health as the optimal physical, social, and emotional functioning of an individual—not simply the absence of illness.
- Developmentally and culturally appropriate care. Through this focus, the book can show the reader how to assess a client's developmental status and alter assessment techniques to meet the client's needs, which change significantly across the life span. It also can help the nurse understand how a client's cultural or ethnic background may affect normal findings or individual perceptions of health and illness.
- Nursing process application. This theme is vital because assessment is the foundation of—and the first step in—the nursing process. Therefore, all client care depends on how well the nurse performs this step. *Health Assessment in Nursing, Second Edition* gives the nurse the knowledge and tools for gathering and interpreting assessment findings. Specifically, it describes how to gather data through the nursing health history, physical assessment, and laboratory studies; analyze the collected data; formulate appropriate nursing diagnoses; and document the data using the nursing process.
- Expert nursing care. The text is designed to help the reader master the cognitive, affective, and psychomotor skills needed to perform effective assessments. It not only shows how to perform specific techniques, but also explains why—an important component of critical thinking. For the nurse who has mastered the basic skills, the text teaches advanced assessment skills.

Health Assessment in Nursing, Second Edition is organized into five units: The Nurse's Role in Assessment; Learning Assessment Skills; Assessing Activity, Sleep, and Nutrition; Assessing Body Structures and Systems; and Special Assessments. This organization maximizes understanding by presenting information in a systematic way—from learning assessment techniques, to applying them in specific ways, to integrating them into complete assessments.

Unit One provides an overview of nursing assessment and the nursing process and discusses the relationship of nursing care to medical care. Unit Two teaches the basics of any health assessment—the health history and physical assessment. The information in these two units forms the basis for all the chapters in Units Three and Four. After presenting a brief review of pertinent anatomy and physiology, each chapter shows how to obtain specific health history, physical assessment, and laboratory data for the body system, structure, or function covered in the chapter. Then it shows how to document all assessment information and apply the nursing process. The final unit describes the components of complete, partial, perinatal, and neonatal assessments.

To organize material for easy learning and recall, the text includes numerous pedagogical devices. Each chapter contains objectives that guide learning by listing the main points to be learned, a glossary that explains new terms and functions as a ready reference, a chapter summary that reiterates the main points and relates them to each other, and study questions that help the learner apply the chapter information to specific client situations. The updated selected references for each chapter, which usually include landmark publications, contain a separate listing of nursing research articles. These articles underscore the continuing growth and development of nursing and can assist the reader who wants more information on specific aspects of assessment.

Throughout the text, charts and visual materials attract the reader's attention, summarize information for easy recall, and promote deeper understanding. Bulleted lists and tables encourage rapid review, and charts efficiently organize large amounts of information. Important assessment skills and descriptions of anatomy and physiology are illustrated accurately and clearly.

New in this Second Edition, the Photo Gallery provides 112 pages of vivid color and crisp black-and-white photographs. Grouped between Chapters 14 and 15, these pages (numbered 1PG to 112PG) include 350 dramatic photographs. Organized in the same sequence as the chapters in Units Three, Four, and Five, the Photo Gallery presents:

- *Anatomy and physiology* to allow learning or review of each body system's anatomic structures; these photographs typically have overlays that highlight internal structures in relation to an external view.
- *Physical assessment techniques* to demonstrate physical positions, techniques, and actions in sequence, as well as review normal findings.
- *Developmental and ethnic considerations* to aid in identifying human developmental factors as well as some normal variations associated with various ethnic groups.
- *Common abnormalities* to assist in recognizing significant findings that indicate a specific condition or disease.

To help the nurse plan the assessment, interpret findings, and develop an appropriate care plan, the text includes these recurring charts that summarize key information:

- *Adverse drug reactions* lists drugs by class and describes their possible adverse effects on the body system or structure being assessed.
- *Integrating assessment findings* describes signs and symptoms and related assessment findings that may indicate a particular disorder.
- *Common laboratory studies* describes the studies, normal values or findings, and the significance of abnormal findings related to the body structure or system.
- *Applying the nursing process* presents a short case history; assessment data gathered; appropriate nursing diagnoses; and planning, implementation, and evaluation information. It also includes documentation of the nursing process steps using the S.O.A.P.I.E. format.
- *Advanced assessment skills* illustrates equipment, techniques, and actions for the nurse who has mastered basic skills or must perform special assessments. Each skill is presented clearly in step-by-step format.

Three appendices use case studies to illustrate how to assess a client with a specific health problem and apply the nursing process. A fourth appendix integrates the North American Nursing Diagnosis Association (NANDA) nursing diagnoses into Gordon's functional health patterns.

Health Assessment in Nursing, Second Edition was written by practicing nurses with advanced degrees and by nurse academicians. In addition, all chapters were reviewed by pediatric, geriatric, and cultural health specialists. The efforts of these experts have produced a current, accurate, clinically applicable, and academically sound resource that can be used as an assessment guide for clients of all ages in many different clinical settings. By using *Health Assessment in Nursing, Second Edition,* students and clinicians will gain a comprehensive understanding of the factors that influence health and will increase their abilities to perform nursing assessments with confidence.

Patricia Gonce Morton, RN, PhD

UNIT ONE

The Nurse's Role in Assessment

The past 30 years have seen an explosion in clinical information and technology. In response to this, nursing responsibilities have grown, particularly in client assessment. To meet the challenge of decision making in client care, the nurse needs a comprehensive data base—a prerequisite for nursing diagnoses and individualized interventions.

This unit investigates the nurse's role in gathering the needed data. It instructs the nurse in the principles of assessment and its place in the nursing process. It discusses the nurse's expanding role, highlighting assessment and collaboration as the keys to high-quality client care. This information will benefit the nurse in any clinical setting: hospital, public health center, client's home, clinic, or physician's office. Indeed, assessment is a critical part of every nurse's practice: all nursing decisions and actions will be based on initial and ongoing assessments.

Chapter 1
Assessment and the Nursing Process

Chapter 1 explores the nursing process, a systematic and scientific approach to gathering data about a client. It explains the nursing process steps—assessment, diagnosis, planning, implementation, and evaluation—and discusses their relationship to each other and their role in health assessment. The first part of the chapter highlights assessment and describes how to use assessment findings to formulate nursing diagnoses. It provides a list of diagnostic labels that have been approved by the North American Nursing Diagnosis Association and describes how to use them in the PES (problem, etiology, and signs and symptoms) method for developing nursing diagnoses.

Then the chapter describes different problem-solving methods and thinking styles. A nurse using the nursing process applies the science and art of nursing.

Finally, the chapter discusses how to develop a nursing care plan based on assessment data and nursing diagnoses. It shows how a care plan serves as a written guide for a client's nursing care.

Chapter 2
Nursing and Medicine: A Collaborative Approach

Chapter 2 briefly describes how nursing theories have affected—and continue to affect—nursing practice. It focuses on the development of the nurse's role, which has evolved from that of a physician's helper to that of an independent health care professional whose comprehensive client assessments lead to nursing and medical interventions. This chapter compares and contrasts nursing and medicine based on the differences in their goals and philosophies. Then it reviews historical and current nurse-physician relationships.

The chapter discusses nurse-physician collaboration. It summarizes the results of an important study on collaboration, provides strategies for successful collaboration, explains the position of the American Nurses' Association on this topic, and emphasizes independent and interdependent roles for nurses.

1

Assessment and the Nursing Process

Objectives

After reading and studying this chapter, you should be able to:

1. Identify the steps in the nursing process and explain how each relates to problem solving.
2. Explain the nurse's role in the nursing process.
3. Explain how the subjective and objective data gathered during assessment relate to the nursing process.
4. Define the factors that affect nursing assessment data collection and organization.
5. Identify methods of collecting and organizing nursing assessment data.

Introduction

Quality nursing practice today requires that nurses fulfill numerous roles in various health care settings. Several decades ago, nursing usually was practiced in acute care hospitals or community health agencies; in many cases, nursing practice focused only on disease. However, it has evolved beyond those traditional settings and roles and has expanded its focus. Nursing practice now concerns itself with health—a concept meaning more than just the absence of disease. Health means that the client is functioning at the best level possible—emotionally, spiritually, and socially as well as physically.

Nurses care for clients in various ethnic groups and also of various ages: infants, children, adolescents, adults, and elderly clients. Many nurses continue to practice in such traditional settings as hospitals, where the primary concern is the individual client. Increasing numbers of nurses, however, now practice in nonhospital settings where they are the primary providers of health maintenance information to the public. For example, nurses who are family practitioners focus on assessing a family and how its members relate to one another. Nurses in community health agencies may focus assessment on elderly clients; others in industrial health clinics screen clients for work-related health problems, such as hypertension or pulmonary disorders, and teach prevention behaviors, such as weight or stress control. Still others in free-standing emergency departments provide emergency intervention and teach self-care, or in retirement communities, help clients cope with aging.

Adding to nursing's modern challenge is a client population that now demands legal as well as ethical accountability for nursing actions. Increasingly, nurses, as well as physicians, are correspondents in malpractice lawsuits. Thus, the responsible nurse must keep abreast of current legislation related to changes in nursing practice standards and health care policies.

Besides having a legal responsibility, the nurse has an ethical responsibility to clients. Two categories of ethical responsibility are personal and professional. Personal ethics are chosen by the nurse; professional ethics, by the nursing profession. (For a description of the American Nurses' Association code of ethics, see *The code for nurses,* in Chapter 2.)

Personal and professional ethics sometimes conflict. For example, a nurse may believe that assisting at an abortion is morally and ethically wrong. However, a nurse cannot refuse a client care because professional ethics require caring for any client who needs it.

To help the nurse meet these diverse roles and responsibilities, the nursing profession has developed a system to consider all the factors that affect a client's

Glossary

Assessment: first step in the nursing process; collection and organization of data from such sources as the client, the client's family, medical records, and laboratory and diagnostic test results to obtain a client profile.

Evaluation: fifth and final step in the nursing process; refers to the client's status relevant to goals described in the nursing care plan.

General systems theory: science of wholes; study of the interdependent nature of concepts, models, and principles.

Goal: desired outcome of nursing care; guides the selection and implementation of nursing interventions.

Holistic health care: comprehensive health care approach that considers the client's physical, emotional, social, economic, and spiritual needs; the client's response to illness; and the impact of illness on the client's self-care capacity.

Implementation: fourth step in the nursing process; nursing actions that carry out interventions described in the nursing care plan.

Interventions: actions that the nurse uses to implement the care plan; may be independent (those the nurse can carry out alone, using acquired knowledge and skills), interdependent (those that the nurse performs in collaboration with other professionals), or dependent (those requiring a physician's order).

Nursing care plan: written guide to the client's care including the assessment, nursing diagnoses, planning, goals, and interventions from the time the client enters the health care system; the plan is updated and revised periodically.

Nursing diagnosis: second step in the nursing process; the identification of actual or potential client health problems that nursing intervention can help resolve, diminish, or change.

Nursing process: systematic problem-solving method organized into five consecutive parts—assessment, nursing diagnosis, planning, implementation, and evaluation.

Objective data: factual data, related to the client's problem, obtained by inspection, palpation, percussion, auscultation, and diagnostic tests.

Outcome criteria: part of the nursing care plan goal statement that defines the expected, measurable results of client-centered nursing care; used to evaluate goal achievement.

Planning: third step in the nursing process in which the nurse develops goals that focus on desired outcomes for the client; these goals are documented on the care plan and continuously modified.

Sign: objective finding perceived by an examiner, such as a fever or a rash. Many signs can accompany symptoms: for example, a skin rash is one sign that can accompany itching (a symptom).

Subjective data: data obtained from the client's description of the problem and recorded in the client's words.

Symptom: indication of a disease or change in condition as perceived subjectively by the client; some may be confirmed objectively—for example, numbness of a body part may be proved by absence of response to a pinprick.

care. Called the nursing process, it derives from the scientific method of problem solving. Using the nursing process as a guide, the nurse can formulate strategies that respond to a client's current and potential needs. The process involves interactive problem solving between the nurse and the client and forms the basis for nursing actions and decisions. The nursing process has five steps: assessment, nursing diagnosis, planning, implementation, and evaluation.

Assessment, the subject of this book, is the foundation for the other four steps. In nursing, assessment means the ongoing, systematic collection of data from many sources. Besides data related to the client's physical status, assessment includes data on the client's socioeconomic, cultural, developmental, and emotional status as well as spiritual beliefs.

Systematic collection and review of these data allows identification of problems that nursing care can address and assignment of nursing diagnoses. Effectiveness of the remaining steps of the nursing process relies heavily on the accuracy and thoroughness of assessment.

This chapter briefly explains problem-solving methods and how they relate to the nursing process, as well as how the nursing process is guided by theories from nursing and other disciplines. Finally, it discusses each step of the nursing process.

Methods and theories

Through problem-solving methods, the nursing process promotes the use of the nurse's personal strengths and creativity. It allows the nurse to elicit pertinent information, to formulate solutions, and to begin establishing trust with the client. A trusting nurse-client relationship promotes cooperation and makes the client's association with the health care establishment more positive and personal.

At first, the nursing student must learn to use the nursing process systematically—one step at a time. Then, with experience, the student can combine the nursing process steps, integrating thought and actions for all steps. Overall health care improves when the nursing process is used consistently by all nurses caring for a client. For example, if all nurses caring for a client use the same problem identification method, fewer errors and omissions occur.

Successful use of the nursing process requires application of cognitive (knowledge-based), affective (feeling-based), and psychomotor skills. Cognitive skills allow the nurse to interpret and prioritize data; affective skills allow appropriate and empathetic behavior, such as touch; and psychomotor skills allow techniques such as percussion (performed by striking the fingers on the body surface to assess underlying structures). These nursing skills, combined with various problem-solving methods to implement care, enable the nurse to view the client holistically, as an individual with emotional, social, economic, and spiritual needs as well as physical ones.

The nursing process involves several problem-solving methods based on different thinking styles.

Problem-solving methods

Problem solving is basic to all scientific disciplines. Four methods for approaching problems are presented below: reflexive, trial and error, intuitive, and scientfic.

Reflexive. This method is based on ritualistic thinking—thinking that results in an automatic response, without conscious decisions or extensive deliberation, and applies to familiar and previously encountered situations. For example, if a client says, "I feel like I'm going to vomit," the nurse would reflexively provide an emesis basin.

Ritualistic thinking also occurs when the nurse follows standard protocols. For example, a client with a history of diabetes mellitus is admitted to a clinical unit for an electrocardiogram (EKG), and the unit has a standard protocol that all known diabetic clients must have their blood glucose levels monitored three times a day. In this instance—although diabetes has not caused the client to seek medical attention and has not caused any apparent problem—a protocol directs a specific nursing action, which the nurse implements using ritualistic thinking.

Trial and error. The trial-and-error method of random thinking (free association of ideas) requires little or no previous knowledge to test solutions. Outcomes usually are not recorded. Random thinking requires energy, time, guesswork, and choices (selecting methods that work, discarding methods that do not). For example, the nurse may use the trial-and-error method to discover how to operate a new type of electronic thermometer that does not come with instructions.

Random thinking allows the creative solution of problems without the restrictions imposed by rote performance and the need for factual data. It also permits formulation of new ideas and solutions within the boundaries of institutional policies and safe nursing practice. For example, Joe Crick, who has acute lymphocytic leukemia, is on strict protective isolation precautions. However, he has many friends and enjoys socializing. Since he has been in isolation, Mr. Crick has been showing signs of emotional withdrawal from his family and his primary nurse. Hoping to find a solution, the nurse considers all possible ways, no matter how unusual, to alleviate Mr. Crick's isolation. Finally, the nurse suggests to Mr. Crick's physician that the client, properly gloved, gowned, and masked, leave his room for 30 minutes at 11:30 p.m. for a short stroll in the hall. The physician agrees. Although not completely solving the problem, this solution helps the client regain a sense of control and independence and reassures him that he will not be isolated at all times. The solution is creative and individualized and is unlikely to be found on the standardized nursing care plan.

Intuitive. The intuitive method is based on insight related to appreciative thinking—an increased perception or understanding about a client, a client's values and beliefs, or a situation. In intuitive problem solving, the nurse considers objective client characteristics—for example, age and medical diagnosis—as well as emotions or conditions that the nurse senses about the client, such as sadness, fear, or even impending death.

Some nursing researchers are beginning to look at nursing intuition as a valid aspect of the art of nursing. For example, suppose a nurse feels something is "just not right" about a client. The nurse checks the client's vital signs, finds them normal, and leaves the room to document findings on the client's chart. Yet intuition tells the nurse that something is wrong. Relying on this sense, the nurse returns and finds the client grasping the chest in severe pain. By using intuitive problem solving, the nurse may have saved the client's life.

However, intuitive problem solving can create problems if the nurse bases a hunch on inconclusive evidence, erroneous information, or personal experiences that inaccurately reflect the client's situation. For example, an

Asian woman, visiting her husband, may keep her head lowered. If the nurse assumes the couple is experiencing family problems, that assumption may be wrong. Cultural background may better explain the woman's posture.

Scientific. This method, based on critical thinking and a systematic approach to a problem, is used frequently in medicine and the sciences and is the basis of the nursing process. (See *The nursing process and scientific method* for a comparison.)

Problem solving by the scientific method involves a series of systematic steps:
- identifying the general problem
- collecting relevant data from several sources
- formulating hypotheses (tentative assumptions made to test logical consequences)
- planning ways to test the hypothetical solutions
- implementing the tests
- interpreting the results.

If the results show the desired outcome, the process ends unless another problem is identified. If the results do not reflect the desired outcome, the scientific problem-solving method begins again, this time with modifications of the initial hypotheses.

When learning the nursing process, the student should aim for a balance of all four problem-solving methods, determining which is appropriate at any given time. This balance will help ensure individual and client-centered nursing care and initiate interventions to improve the client's condition. Of the four problem-solving methods, however, the scientific method is the most frequently used; it is the basis for the nursing process.

Nursing process flexibility is necessary because of the many variables involved in nursing practice. Many clients seeking medical help have several health problems that affect one another, so that isolating any one problem without wholly considering the others may result in deficient problem solving. Several interrelated problems can lead to numerous variables, making an exact use of the scientific method nearly impossible.

Theories guiding the nursing process

Besides relying on several problem-solving methods, the nursing process is also guided by theories from nursing and other disciplines, such as psychology and sociology.

A theory consists of propositions, each indicating a relationship between variables (quantities or values subject to change) and concepts. A proposition is a statement or premise related to a theory; a concept is a general idea or abstraction taken from related observable events or facts. Researchers or theorists in all scientific disciplines, including nursing, test the validity of concepts, propositions, and, ultimately, theories.

The nursing profession has given rise to many theories about the nature of nursing. (For further discussion of those theories, see Chapter 2, Nursing and Medicine: A Collaborative Approach.)

Other theories not specific to nursing (called grand theories) also affect nursing practice. One of the most common is the *general systems theory,* which explains the function of whole units in terms of the relationships

The nursing process and scientific method

The nursing process incorporates elements of the scientific method, as shown below. The simplified steps of the nursing process provide structure and flexibility and incorporate intuition as well as science to the art of nursing.

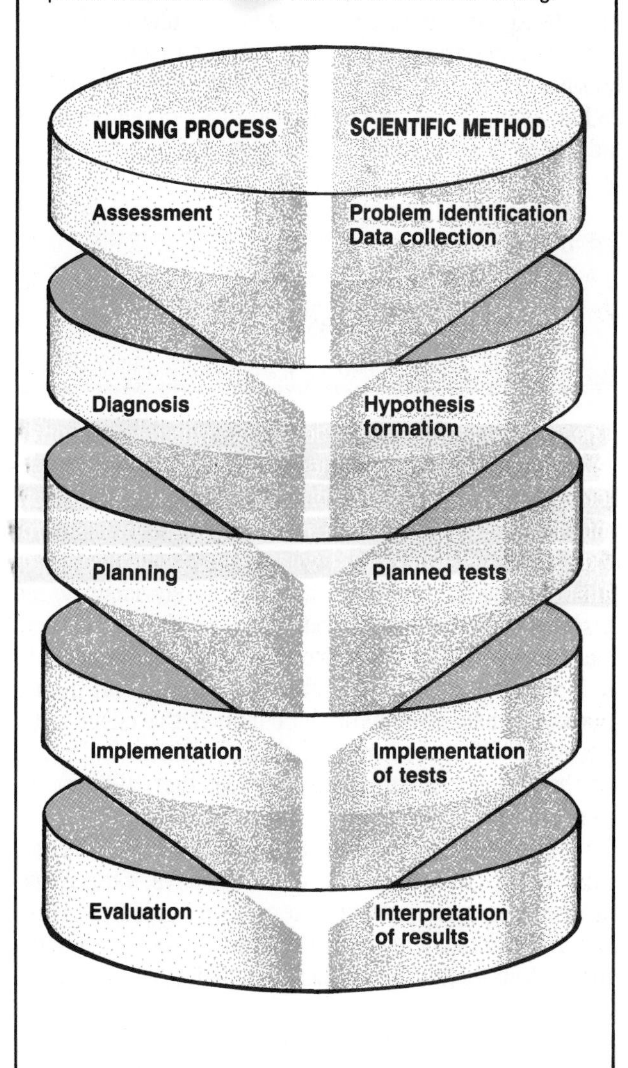

between the whole and its parts. For example, when using the nursing process, the nurse assesses the client's relationship to the total life experience, which includes family and community. Then, the nurse develops a nursing diagnosis, plans and implements care, and evaluates the client outcomes in relationship to the family or community.

Nursing is also affected by *holistic theory*. Holism views the whole being as different from and more than the sum of its parts. According to holistic theory, a person's body, mind, and spirit are interdependent and in dynamic interaction with the environment. Responses to life processes are complex, integrated, and highly individualized. A holistic assessment of a client's health considers growth and development, past experiences, sociocultural influences, and economic factors. According to holistic theory, an illness usually has several causes, with the primary cause commonly identified as nonphysiologic. During the nursing process, the nurse assesses the whole person by asking questions about emotional and spiritual health as well as physical health. What roles does the client have in life: for example, wife, mother? How comfortable is the client with these roles? What feelings does the client express about relationships at home, at work, and in the community?

Nursing process steps

The nursing process helps determine which health problems the nurse can help alleviate, which potential problems the nurse can help prevent, what kind and how much assistance the client requires, who can best provide such assistance, and what desired outcome is realistic. Usually, the client can accurately identify the problems that need attention. However, the nurse's specialized knowledge and current understanding of available resources can help define the client's health care needs for discussion with the client. If the client is incapacitated, assessment can identify deficits and serve as the basis for planning interventions that will improve the situation.

The nursing process is a dynamic activity that begins when the nurse compiles subjective data (information reported by the client) and objective data (information collected through physical assessment techniques and diagnostic studies). The data base grows as the nursing process progresses. New data materialize if the client's condition changes or if the client chooses to reveal more information, which often occurs as the nurse-client relationship grows. For example, a new client with abdominal pain will first talk about the pain. When the pain is relieved, the client may share such other concerns as a recent job loss. By using an organized process to deal with human needs, the nurse can better relate the client's emotional and intellectual characteristics to the health factors that affect the client's life. The process is goal directed and individual, or client, centered. Ideally, the process does not force the client to conform to established solutions. The nursing process invites client participation by respecting the client's individuality and identifying the client's unique characteristics that will direct the way problems are defined and solved.

To get a complete picture of the client's situation, the nurse must perform the five interactive steps of the nursing process—assessment, diagnosis, planning, implementation, and evaluation—systematically. Using the nursing process holistically, the nurse considers all areas of the client's life and body systems, giving problem areas additional consideration. The nursing process steps rarely occur in perfect sequence, nor do the data always lead to a simple and definitive nursing diagnosis. An assessment may reveal several findings that do not fit neatly into a nursing diagnosis, requiring the nurse to plan, implement, and evaluate simultaneously, then plan and implement again, based on the evaluation. The next section of this chapter describes the nursing process steps in detail.

Assessment

The initial phase of the nursing process, assessment takes place during the nurse's first encounter with a new client. However, the process continues throughout the nurse-client association. Simply stated, assessment is the collection of relevant data from various sources (such as the client, the client's spouse or significant other, medical records, and diagnostic test results) to form a complete picture. Depending on the setting, the client may be an individual, a family, or a community. For example, a hospital-based nurse might assess to determine the effect of hospitalization on the client's life. A home-care nurse might assess not only the client but also the family and its ability to participate in the client's care. An occupational health nurse might assess not only the employees but also the plant for safety and the surrounding community for pollution.

In organization and comprehensiveness, the assessment process is similar for all clients. However, the process may differ according to the type of information collected in a given situation. For example, assessment of a client may include much data about dysfunction of a body system, whereas assessment of the family may focus more on family dynamics, cultural mores, and relationships among family members. A community assessment may focus on available community services, the economic status of the population, and the effect of societal factors on the health care of community members rather than on the needs of individuals. The nurse will perform all types of assessment in a given health care setting, seeking help as needed from others on the health care team, and will recognize what type of assessment is needed to construct an accurate client picture.

Collecting appropriate data is the key to accurate and comprehensive assessment. Data are collected from several sources and must be descriptive, relevant, concise, and complete. The data describe the client as a system as well as the problems for which the client seeks health care. For example, a diabetic client seeks health care at the emergency department. Laboratory tests reveal that the client has a low blood glucose level. The low blood glucose level could result from vomiting or from a limited diet caused by lack of money to buy food.

Data are generally categorized in two ways, according to the collection method. *Subjective data*, referred to as symptoms, come directly from the client. These usually are recorded as direct quotations reflecting the client's opinions or feelings about the situation. Examples are "I feel nervous" or "I'm having a lot of pain in my left leg."

Objective data, referred to as signs, are identified through physical assessment techniques and diagnostic studies. These data reflect findings without interpretation. Examples are "pale skin, pulse rate of 140, blood pressure of 90/60 mm Hg." Such statements as "client is in shock" or "client is hypovolemic" are not objective because they interpret the data and reflect the observer's opinion rather than state verifiable facts.

Data also can be grouped according to the informational source. The term *primary source data* refers to data collected directly from the client. These data may be either subjective, such as answers to health history questions, or objective, such as laboratory results. In most cases, information collected from the primary source is the most valuable because usually it reflects the client's situation most accurately.

Other data about a client can be obtained from *secondary sources*. These sources include family members, friends, coworkers, or community service groups; health history and physical assessment reports; and other members of the health care team. Data from secondary sources are valuable because they supply alternative viewpoints to the client's, and they sometimes add data unknown to the client. Many times, because of a client's condition, age, or developmental level, secondary sources are essential to establish a client profile. For example, a child, an elderly client, or a client with profound confusion may be able to answer only the simplest questions. Some clients are inarticulate or speak another language; other clients may be inhibited by anxiety or fear of the health care environment. In any of these cases, a secondary source for assessment data is helpful, even essential.

The initial assessment gathers data to help identify problematic or dysfunctional areas of the client's life. As the nursing process continues, it serves as a baseline against which to compare further assessments. The nurse collects client data in various ways, depending on the client's condition, the nurse's abilities, and the type of information required. The nurse obtains data from the interview, observation, or the physical assessment. Then the nurse records the collected data.

Interview. For the assessment that begins the nursing process, the structured interview is the most common way to collect client data. This interview is goal directed and more formal than a casual social conversation. Talking with the client before conducting a physical assessment allows the nurse to develop a trust relationship before performing potentially threatening procedures. The interview also allows the client to ask questions or voice concerns. (See Chapter 3, The Health History, for a discussion of interview techniques.)

Observation. By looking at the client during the interview, the nurse collects valuable data about the client's emotional state, immediate comfort level, and general physical condition. Observing the client's tone of voice and body language helps the nurse isolate client stress that might require further investigation. (See Chapter 4, Physical Assessment Skills, for a discussion of observation techniques.)

Physical assessment. The nurse performs a physical assessment, collecting objective data, after establishing a rapport with the client during the interview. Although the level of physical assessment depends largely on the health care setting, the nurse must collect basic data on the client's physical condition in any setting. The nursing process, as an ongoing method of problem identification and intervention, requires the nurse to establish a baseline for all assessment areas. (See Chapter 4, Physical Assessment Skills, for a discussion of assessment techniques.)

Recording the data. Data recording follows the baseline assessment. Called documentation, this recording process can be accomplished in several ways. Many health care facilities have standardized admission assessment forms with assessment categories arranged in a checklist. This format saves valuable time and energy by requiring the nurse to write only the information that cannot be checked off; for example, descriptions of coping mechanisms or significant cultural practices.

The nurse should organize the data into body systems (such as respiratory or cardiovascular) or into assessment patterns (such as communicating or valuing) conforming to the currently accepted list of nursing diagnoses. Whatever the organizational pattern, the nurse should record the data systematically, overlooking no details, using appropriate terminology, and referring regularly to the baseline assessment. The nurse also must make sure the documentation is accessible, understandable, complete, and easy to read by all appropriate staff. Legally, these assessment data become a permanent part of the client's medical record, so accuracy and completeness are essential.

Although the primary interview and physical assessment are usually performed as initial admission activities, assessment is ongoing. The nurse collects and records additional information regularly. Assessment can be a deliberate activity, or it can occur incidentally while the nurse administers medications or helps the client with activities of daily living in the home.

Nursing diagnosis

Assigning one or more appropriate nursing diagnoses to a client's situation is the nursing process step that follows the assessment. Usually, the term "diagnosis" is associated with the practice of medicine by physicians, and many health care professionals misunderstand the concept that nurses can and should form nursing diagnoses. One of the most accepted definitions of nursing today comes from the American Nurses' Association, which identifies the nursing profession's function as "the diagnosis and treatment of human responses to actual or potential health problems." The key words are *diagnosis* and *responses.*

Diagnosis means "to investigate the cause or nature of a situation." By this definition, a mechanic makes a diagnosis when fixing a car, and a schoolteacher makes a diagnosis when assessing a student's classroom behavior.

The other key word is *responses.* The nurse's knowledge includes the client's physical and emotional changes during diagnosis and treatment. Unlike the physician, who is largely concerned with the client's illness, the nurse is concerned primarily with the client's responses to physical changes or to prescribed treatments.

For example, Mr. Long's medical diagnosis is squamous cell carcinoma; he will undergo radiation therapy. The physician diagnoses the type of cancer, surgically removes it, and orders pain medication to be administered. The nurse carries out many of the physician's orders. Also, using assessment strategies, the nurse perceives that the prospects of radiation therapy disturb Mr. Long, that he seems progressively unable to perform activities of daily living independently, and that he refuses to take the prescribed pain medication despite demonstrating physical cues that he has pain. All of these data are important to the team caring for Mr. Long. The solutions, or remedies, to the changes in his status may be provided by independent nursing interventions. For example, the nurse can prepare Mr. Long for his radiation therapy by explaining the procedure and alleviating his anxiety. If Mr. Long refuses to take his sleep medication because it makes him feel hung over in the morning, the nurse can speak to the physician about a change. Maybe Mr. Long finds relief with a simple home remedy such as herbal tea. The nurse could arrange that some be brought to him.

Nursing diagnosis, then, is the statement of actual or potential health problems that can be resolved, diminished, or otherwise changed by nursing interventions. The problem areas can be identified by the client, significant others, the nurse, or any combination of the three.

Gradually, the labels assigned to specific nursing diagnoses are being standardized so that all nurses will use the same terminology. The current list of nursing diagnoses (clinically tested and accepted for general use) is published every other year by the North American Nursing Diagnosis Association (NANDA). (See *NANDA taxonomy of nursing diagnoses,* pages 10 and 11.) To maintain the standardized list, NANDA meets biannually to consider new nursing diagnoses submitted by nurses throughout North America.

To assign a nursing diagnosis, the nurse first reviews the assessment data for completeness and accuracy, checking for omissions, inconsistencies, and comprehensiveness, and then supplements areas that require further information.

The next phase involves critical thinking. The nurse reviews and analyzes the assessment data from different perspectives, using standards, established norms, and expectations from other disciplines, such as psychological knowledge to assess the client's self-concept and sociologic knowledge to assess cultural influences. Broad-based nursing knowledge is valuable. If some assessment areas are unfamiliar (for example, sexual function), the nurse can consult current literature or other professionals for help with determining the client's status. Data evaluation methods include asking such questions as: Are the physical assessment data within normal limits for this client? Do specific behaviors or factcrs about this client detract from or contribute to the client's well being? What apparent strengths or weaknesses affect the client's current health status? What resources or demands in the client's environment affect the client's state of health? Is the client satisfied with this state of health?

After critically examining the data, the nurse must decide how the data groups relate to each other. Known as clustering, this process helps establish a broad category of need. (See *Client assessment and the nursing process*, pages 12 and 13, for a description of how to develop a nursing diagnosis.)

After clustering the associated data, the nurse consults the list of accepted nursing diagnoses to find an appropriate label for the client's situation. This label, based on assessment data cues, can reflect actual or potential deficits in the client's situation.

The complete nursing diagnosis statement has three parts: a problem, an etiology, and the signs and symptoms. The first part identifies the problem, for example, "Bowel elimination, altered: constipation." The second part states the etiology (causal or contributing factors), individualizing a particular nursing diagnosis to a specific client. "Bowel elimination, altered: constipation" could be related to such causes as dietary disturbances, immobility, or even medications. By adding an etiologic phrase, such as "related to" or "secondary to," the nurse clarifies the diagnosis and provides direction for the rest of the nursing process. For example, "Skin integrity, impaired: actual, related to prolonged bedrest" and "Comfort, altered: pain related to surgical procedure" are complete nursing statements. The third part of the statement records the signs and symptoms and other subjective and objective data that are essential cues for assigning the diagnosis.

An effective nursing diagnosis is brief and specific to the client.

Errors in formulating a nursing diagnosis

The nursing diagnosis reflects the client's response to illness or potential for illness and should not repeat the assigned medical diagnosis. A way to remember the difference is to consider if the diagnosis is one that a nurse has the legal right and educational preparation to pursue. Statements such as "myocardial infarction" and "cerebral vascular accident" are medical diagnoses, not nursing diagnoses. (See Chapter 2, Nursing and Medicine: A Collaborative Approach, for a discussion of the differences between nursing and medical diagnoses.)

To be effective, the nursing diagnosis assigned to assessment data must be accurate. Although errors occur, they are preventable. A common error is insufficient data leading to an incorrect nursing diagnosis.

After the initial nursing diagnosis is made, additional errors can occur if the nurse overlooks or ignores the need to continue collecting data throughout the nurse-client association.

Continuing assessment requires the nurse to add to the nursing record new subjective data revealed by the client and objective information obtained from diagnostic studies. Then, as data accumulate, the nurse must reevaluate the whole client picture, overlooking no area of client need. The nursing process steps are systematic. They are also cyclical: reevaluation of the client's response to nursing interventions produces new assessment data.

Data misinterpretation is another error that results in incorrect nursing diagnoses. Miscommunication with the client and personal biases also interfere with data interpretation. Psychosocial and cultural data are more often incorrectly interpreted than are concrete physical assessment data, because accurate collection depends on the skills and knowledge of the collector. Also, this type of information tends to be personal to the client. As such, it is less readily available and verifiable than physical assessment data. Nursing conclusions about data that are not validated by the client are common sources of error.

Other errors can occur during documentation of the nursing diagnosis on the client's record. Symptoms, interventions, or medical diagnoses substituted for assigned NANDA nursing diagnoses, which deal with alterations in client functioning, are common sources of errors. The nurse should carefully examine data before making a nursing diagnosis and reevaluate and update the diagnosis as necessary. (For more information, see *The PES method for developing a nursing diagnosis*, page 14.)

(3) Planning

After assessing the client and assigning appropriate nursing diagnoses, the nurse can develop a plan based on the diagnoses that will help the client achieve improved or optimal functioning. A successful plan is tailored to the client, realistic for the nursing practice setting, and appropriate for the client's age and developmental level. It recognizes the client's strengths and weaknesses, relies on client participation, defines achievable goals, and proposes adequate, feasible actions.

Health history information provides a preliminary analysis of the client's strengths and weaknesses and helps determine which of these pose a detriment and

NANDA taxonomy of nursing diagnoses

A taxonomy for classifying nursing diagnoses has evolved over several years. The following list is grouped around nine human response patterns endorsed by the North American Nursing Diagnosis Association, as of summer 1992.

PATTERN 1. Exchanging: A human response pattern involving mutual giving and receiving
1.1.2.1. Altered nutrition: more than body requirements
1.1.2.2. Altered nutrition: less than body requirements
1.1.2.3. Altered nutrition: high risk for more than body requirements
1.2.1.1. High risk for infection
1.2.2.1. High risk for altered body temperature
1.2.2.2. Hypothermia
1.2.2.3. Hyperthermia
1.2.2.4. Ineffective thermoregulation
1.2.3.1. Dysreflexia
1.3.1.1. Constipation
1.3.1.1.1. Perceived constipation
1.3.1.1.2. Colonic constipation
1.3.1.2. Diarrhea
1.3.1.3. Bowel incontinence
1.3.2. Altered urinary elimination
1.3.2.1.1. Stress incontinence
1.3.2.1.2. Reflex incontinence
1.3.2.1.3. Urge incontinence
1.3.2.1.4. Functional incontinence
1.3.2.1.5. Total incontinence
1.3.2.2. Urinary retention
1.4.1.1. Altered (specify type) tissue perfusion (renal, cerebral, cardiopulmonary, gastrointestinal, peripheral)
1.4.1.2.1. Fluid volume excess
1.4.1.2.2.1. Fluid volume deficit
1.4.1.2.2.2. Potential fluid volume deficit
1.4.2.1. Decreased cardiac output
1.5.1.1. Impaired gas exchange
1.5.1.2. Ineffective airway clearance
1.5.1.3. Ineffective breathing pattern
1.5.1.3.1. Inability to sustain spontaneous ventilation
1.5.1.3.2. Dysfunctional ventilatory weaning response
1.6.1. High risk for injury
1.6.1.1. High risk for suffocation
1.6.1.2. High risk for poisoning
1.6.1.3. High risk for trauma
1.6.1.4. High risk for aspiration
1.6.1.5. High risk for disuse syndrome
1.6.2. Altered protection
1.6.2.1. Impaired tissue integrity
1.6.2.1.1. Altered oral mucous membrane
1.6.2.1.2.1. Impaired skin integrity
1.6.2.1.2.2. Potential impaired skin integrity

PATTERN 2. Communicating: A human response pattern involving sending messages
2.1.1.1. Impaired verbal communication

PATTERN 3. Relating: A human response pattern involving establishing bonds
3.1.1. Impaired social interaction
3.1.2. Social isolation
3.2.1. Altered role performance
3.2.1.1.1. Altered parenting
3.2.1.1.2. Potential altered parenting
3.2.1.2.1. Sexual dysfunction
3.2.2. Altered family processes
3.2.3.1. Parental role conflict
3.3. Altered sexuality patterns

PATTERN 4. Valuing: A human response pattern involving the assigning of relative worth
4.1.1. Spiritual distress (distress of the human spirit)

PATTERN 5. Choosing: A human response pattern involving the selection of alternatives
5.1.1.1. Ineffective individual coping
5.1.1.1.1. Impaired adjustment
5.1.1.1.2. Defensive coping
5.1.1.1.3. Ineffective denial
5.1.2.1.1. Ineffective family coping: disabling
5.1.2.1.2. Ineffective family coping: compromised
5.1.2.2. Family coping: potential for growth
5.2.1. Ineffective management of therapeutic regimen (individual)
5.2.1.1. Noncompliance (specify)

5.3.1.1. Decisional conflict (specify)
5.4. Health-seeking behaviors (specify)
PATTERN 6. Moving: A human response pattern involving activity
6.1.1.1. Impaired physical mobility
6.1.1.1.1. High risk for peripheral neurovascular dysfunction
6.1.1.2. Activity intolerance
6.1.1.2.1. Fatigue
6.1.1.3. Potential activity intolerance
6.2.1. Sleep pattern disturbance
6.3.1.1. Diversional activity deficit
6.4.1.1. Impaired home maintenance management
6.4.2. Altered health maintenance
6.5.1. Feeding self-care deficit
6.5.1.1. Impaired swallowing
6.5.1.2. Ineffective breast-feeding
6.5.1.2.1. Interrupted breast-feeding
6.5.1.3. Effective breast-feeding
6.5.1.4. Ineffective infant feeding pattern
6.5.2. Bathing or hygiene self-care deficit
6.5.3. Dressing or grooming self-care deficit
6.5.4. Toileting self-care deficit
6.6. Altered growth and development
6.7. Relocation stress syndrome
PATTERN 7. Perceiving: A human response pattern involving the reception of information
7.1.1. Body image disturbance
7.1.2. Self-esteem disturbance
7.1.2.1. Chronic low self-esteem
7.1.2.2. Situational low self-esteem
7.1.3. Personal identify disturbance
7.2. Sensory-perceptual alterations (specify – visual, auditory, kinesthetic, gustatory, tactile, olfactory)
7.2.1.1. Unilateral neglect
7.3.1. Hopelessness
7.3.2. Powerlessness

PATTERN 8. Knowing: A human response pattern involving the meaning associated with information
8.1.1. Knowledge deficit (specify)
8.3. Altered thought processes
PATTERN 9. Feeling: A human response pattern involving the subjective awareness of information
9.1.1. Pain
9.1.1.1. Chronic pain
9.2.1.1. Dysfunctional grieving
9.2.1.2. Anticipatory grieving
9.2.2. High risk for violence: self-directed or directed at others
9.2.2.1. High risk for self-mutilation
9.2.3. Post-trauma response
9.2.3.1. Rape-trauma syndrome
9.2.3.1.1. Rape-trauma syndrome: compound reaction
9.2.3.1.2. Rape-trauma syndrome: silent reaction
9.3.1. Anxiety
9.3.2. Fear
9.4.1. Caregiver role strain
9.4.2. High risk for caregiver role strain

Client assessment and the nursing process

Shirley Hines, a 34-year-old Black female, has come to the health clinic to have her blood pressure checked. She has a family history of hypertension; one month ago, her brother died at age 40 of a cerebral vascular accident (CVA). The nurse assigned to Ms. Hines conducts a complete interview and performs a physical assessment. After critically reviewing the assessment data, the nurse decides which factors need attention and formulates a care plan using the nursing process. Although the nurse would document all of this information, this chart does not include documentation. Rather, it focuses on data collection and the nursing process.

Assessment data

Dietary recall (24 hour)
Breakfast: orange juice and coffee with cream and sugar, doughnut
Lunch: hamburger with fried onions, 16-ounce soda pop, french fries, chocolate cake
Snack: potato chips
Dinner: breaded fried pork chops, mashed potatoes and gravy, corn, applesauce, white bread (1 slice) and butter, cherry pie, coffee with cream and sugar
Snack: cheese and crackers and milk

Family health status
Mother: CVA at age 54, now partially recovered
Father: hypertension controlled by medication since 1978
Brother: fatal CVA, at age 40
Two children: ages 1 and 2, both alive and well
Husband: in good health

Education: Community college

Mental notes

Ms. Hines has some behaviors (high-caloric and cholesterol intake) that contribute to a potentially serious condition.

Ms. Hines recognizes some current problem areas that she cannot control (family history of hypertension). Also, current research data indicate that Blacks are prone to hypertension.

Ms. Hines has areas of strength that the nurse is careful not to overlook when beginning to cluster data before assigning a nursing diagnosis.

The nursing process

ASSESSMENT	NURSING DIAGNOSES	PLANNING
Subjective (history) data "I'm really worried about my weight and blood pressure.... I want to lose some weight, but I haven't been able to do so." **Objective (physical) data** • B.P. 130/90 mm Hg, pulse 92 and regular, respirations 22 and regular, age 34, weight 202 lb, height 5′2″ • All other physical assessment findings within normal limits.	• Altered nutrition: more than body requirements. • Knowledge deficit: related to dietary requirements. • Disturbance in self-concept, self-esteem: related to obesity.	**Goals** • Client will show weight loss of 2 pounds per week measured by the clinic scale. • Client will achieve a total weight loss of 70 pounds within 9 months, according to the clinic scale. • Client will verbalize correct information related to diet when questioned by nurse. • Client will verbalize three positive characteristics of herself within two weeks of initial weight loss.

which can be used to advantage. Encouraging client participation in developing the plan will help individualize the plan and make it easier to implement.

The plan must help the client maintain current functional levels and prevent new problems from developing. The nurse can accomplish this by working with the client to reduce health risks and improve health and functional levels. The plan also must address consistently decreasing health and functional levels if a permanent solution or complete health restoration cannot be achieved. The nurse must construct a plan for every client, even if the client's dysfunctions are related to terminal illness.

Effective planning includes determining priorities, setting appropriate short- and long-term goals, and selecting interventions to achieve a desired outcome.

a)

Determining priorities

Primary planning involves establishing priorities for and with the client, whenever possible, allowing the client to retain as much control as possible over personal health

Height: 5′2″

Weight: 202 lb.

Pulse: 92 and regular

Respirations: 22 and regular

Blood pressure: 130/90

Assets
- Sought help before symptoms occurred
- Strong family unit
- High education level

Deficits
- Elevated blood pressure
- Poor diet and obesity
- Family and ethnic tendency toward hypertension and cardiovascular disease.
- Two small children (high stress)

Preliminary nursing diagnosis of "Nutrition, altered: more than body requirements, related to poor dietary habits." Ms. Hines agrees that this is a problem area.

IMPLEMENTATION	EVALUATION
• Establish client's baseline weight. • Weigh client at same time on same scale every week. • Schedule appointment with dietitian for dietary instruction. • Counsel family in best ways to support client. • Inform client of local weight-loss support groups. • Monitor client's blood pressure every visit and notify physician of significant changes.	• Client shows 2-pound weight loss per week on clinic scale. • Client has lost 70 pounds in 9 months per clinic scale.

care. When setting priorities, the nurse should help the client realize that resolving one problem before addressing another is unnecessary. Frequently, health problems are approached simultaneously, because they are interrelated by cause and effect.

The nurse should help the client determine priorities by ranking the nursing diagnoses and goals in order of importance. The most frequently used order is psychologist Abraham Maslow's hierarchy of human needs. Briefly, Maslow states that individual survival needs, such as food and water, must be met before other, less life-threatening considerations, such as safety and self-actualization, are fulfilled. For example, a young mother with a fractured leg first requires medical care to repair the leg and nursing care to prevent more problems. However, after meeting the client's priority nursing needs, the nurse must address other needs, such as how the mother's injury affects her role in the family. For example, who will provide child care while the young mother recuperates and the father works?

The PES method for developing a nursing diagnosis

The following summary presents the key elements of the PES method, the most frequently used method for developing a nursing diagnosis.

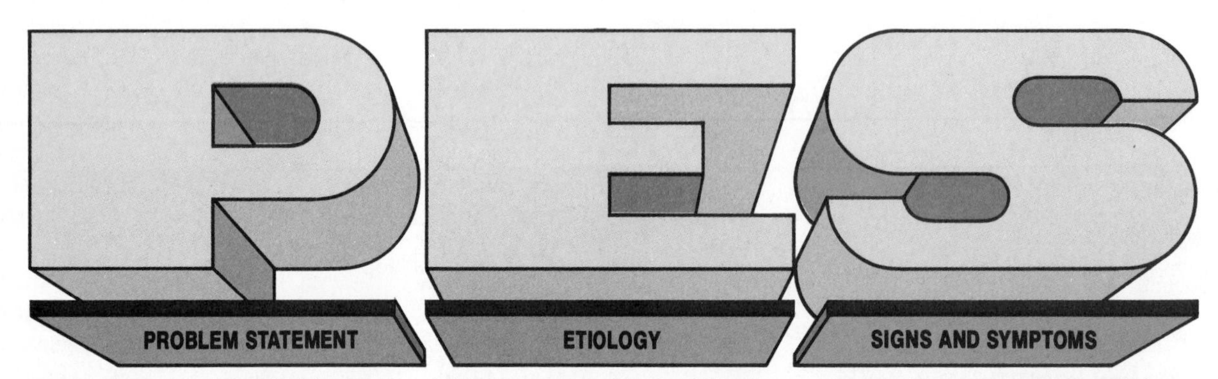

Problem statement: identifies the actual or potential health problem of a client. When choosing a problem statement, the nurse can use the NANDA list of diagnostic labels. The problem statement should fall within nursing's realm, with the nurse writing the problem statement in clear, concise terms.

Etiology: consists of factors related to the developmental or possible cause of the problem. The etiology helps the nurse determine the type of care plan to develop for each nursing diagnosis.

Signs and symptoms or the defining characteristics identify the cluster of cues that define a diagnostic label or problem statement applicable for a particular client. The defining characteristics are a part of the subjective and objective assessment data, which the nurse collects for each client.

Adapted from Gordon, M. *Nursing Diagnosis: Process and Application,* 2nd ed. McGraw-Hill Book Co., 1987. Reprinted with permission from McGraw-Hill Book Co.

The first priority in this situation is to keep the young mother's leg in proper alignment until the physician applies the cast. Problems that may not threaten life but may cause further difficulties are less important. For example, the medical discharge plan after the mother's leg cast is removed should include physical therapy. The nursing discharge plan should show that the physical therapy visits and transportation to and from the health care facility have been coordinated.

Nursing diagnoses that reflect problems concerning relationships or developmental or situational changes should receive a lower priority. For example, helping the young mother learn to accept temporary separation from her children is a low priority. Designating a problem as low priority does not mean it is insignificant, but that it has less nursing care urgency.

When prioritizing problems, the nurse and the client should also consider such related factors as the client's age and health goals, the therapeutic facilities and resources available, and their costs related to the value of the predicted outcome and the client's well-being.

Without physiologic problems requiring urgent care, the client can have greater freedom to establish personal priorities. This enhances client cooperation.

Setting goals

After establishing priorities, the nurse constructs achievable goals for each assigned nursing diagnosis. Several goals may be pertinent in a nursing diagnosis, but only one nursing diagnosis for each goal. A goal, the desired outcome of nursing care, is what the nurse and the client expect to achieve to diminish or remedy a problem or dysfunctional area. Goal setting helps select and implement nursing interventions.

Choosing appropriate and realistic goals is essential. Although nursing plans may require assistance from other health care specialists, the client goals usually require nursing assistance. For example, a client with an assigned nursing diagnosis of "Communication, impaired: verbal, related to aphasia" may have a goal of the client using an alternative communication method (such as a pad and pencil or picture cards) within 3 weeks.

Assuming that the client is capable, this goal is appropriate because the nurse has the expertise to construct or acquire such a device and teach the client to use it. An inappropriate goal would be "the client will be able to speak six full sentences within 3 weeks." This goal is demanding physically and, even if possible, would require a high level of expertise more appropriate to a speech pathologist than to a nurse. Goals can reinforce behavior initiated by other health care professionals, such as ambulation or altered dietary habits.

The nurse must establish client goals that correspond with the physician's medical regimen. As part of a health care team, the nurse cannot encourage the client to establish goals that differ from the physician's. For example, a goal stating that the client will ambulate unassisted twice a day across the room is inappropriate if the physician prescribes strict bed rest.

Written goals on the nursing care plan remind other health team members that a care regimen was selected and is being delivered. Written goals also record the original intent and objective, or intended outcome, of the plan.

Outcome criteria are a simply stated part of the goal statement. Describing client-centered, measureable behaviors, they are used by the client and the nurse to decide whether the goals have been met. Outcome criteria are measured in terms of client, not nursing, achievement. For example, an appropriate statement is "Client will ambulate three times each day for 30 minutes each time"; an inappropriate goal statement would be "Nurse will ambulate client for 30 minutes, three times each day."

The complete goal statement should include a time or deadline. The time signifies short- or long-term goals. The nursing diagnosis for a client's potentially life-threatening (high priority) condition may specify minutes or hours. This type of situation requires establishing a short-term goal to alleviate a potentially dangerous situation. Short-term goals are achievable quickly. Used primarily in acute care settings, intensive care units, and recovery rooms, short-term nursing goals are for clients with rapidly changing or unstable physical conditions. In such cases, a long-term goal may be unrealistic. Short-term goals are also appropriate if the long-term goal is not readily achievable. In such instances, goals act as benchmarks, or progress indicators, for achievement. Often, a series of short-term goals with realistic time limits are set to further long-term goal achievement. For example, for a client who must lose weight, the nurse and the client may set short-term goals as a way to reach the desired outcome of a 65-pound weight loss. The long-term goal may be achievable in 6 months, but related short-term goals, requiring a 1-pound weight loss per week, or 8 to 10 pounds per month, can show the client's progress quickly and positively reinforce adopted, goal-oriented behaviors.

Using the nursing diagnosis as a guide, the nurse should write all long-term goals to reflect the anticipated and possible maximum function level for the client. For a client with a nursing diagnosis of "Bowel elimination, altered: related to incontinence secondary to surgery," an appropriate long-term nursing goal may be to reestablish bowel habits in 2 months.

Some nurses who are unfamiliar with establishing goals for and with clients may consider it the most difficult nursing process phase. Assigning goals and times to activities, when each client functions at an individual pace, is challenging. Knowing how to set specific goals within appropriate time allotments is a skill that comes with experience. Specific nursing diagnosis literature from current professional journals and books helps, too. The nurse should keep in mind that achievement times are as individual as the remaining steps of the nursing process. They can always be revised later if they prove unrealistic.

The complete nursing goal statement is a combination of desired client behavior and predicted outcome, criteria for measurement, time, and conditions (circumstances) under which the behavior will occur. (See *How to write a client goal,* page 16.)

Selecting interventions

After completing the initial planning process phase and setting appropriate goals, the nurse begins the second planning phase—*intervention.* To do this, the nurse first decides what will facilitate long-term and short-term goal achievement. The nursing interventions should be strategies, activities, or actions agreed to by the nurse and the client that help the client reach the goal by diminishing or eliminating the problems defined earlier in the nursing process. The nurse and client then analyze each intervention, and choose one or more that seem likely to achieve the established goals.

The nurse can generate potential nursing actions in several ways, some of which use the alternative thinking styles discussed earlier. Random thinking, or brainstorming, allows potential, safe, and appropriate strategies to be considered until those that are acceptable are generated. This activity frequently produces new ideas for coping with unusual situations. Other, more traditional interventions that either the nurse or the client knows have succeeded previously also may be suggested. For example, Ms. Dearing, a client experiencing sleep disturbances, may know that she sleeps more soundly after drinking warm milk at bedtime. That could be an acceptable intervention to achieve the goal—a complete night's rest. The nurse also may know from experience that a backrub and a linen change at bedtime contribute to a client's undisturbed sleep. This too can be presented as an intervention. Many nurses find helpful information in publications that focus on various potential interventions for established (NANDA) nursing diagnoses.

After compiling the interventions, the nurse, the client, and others involved can review them from several

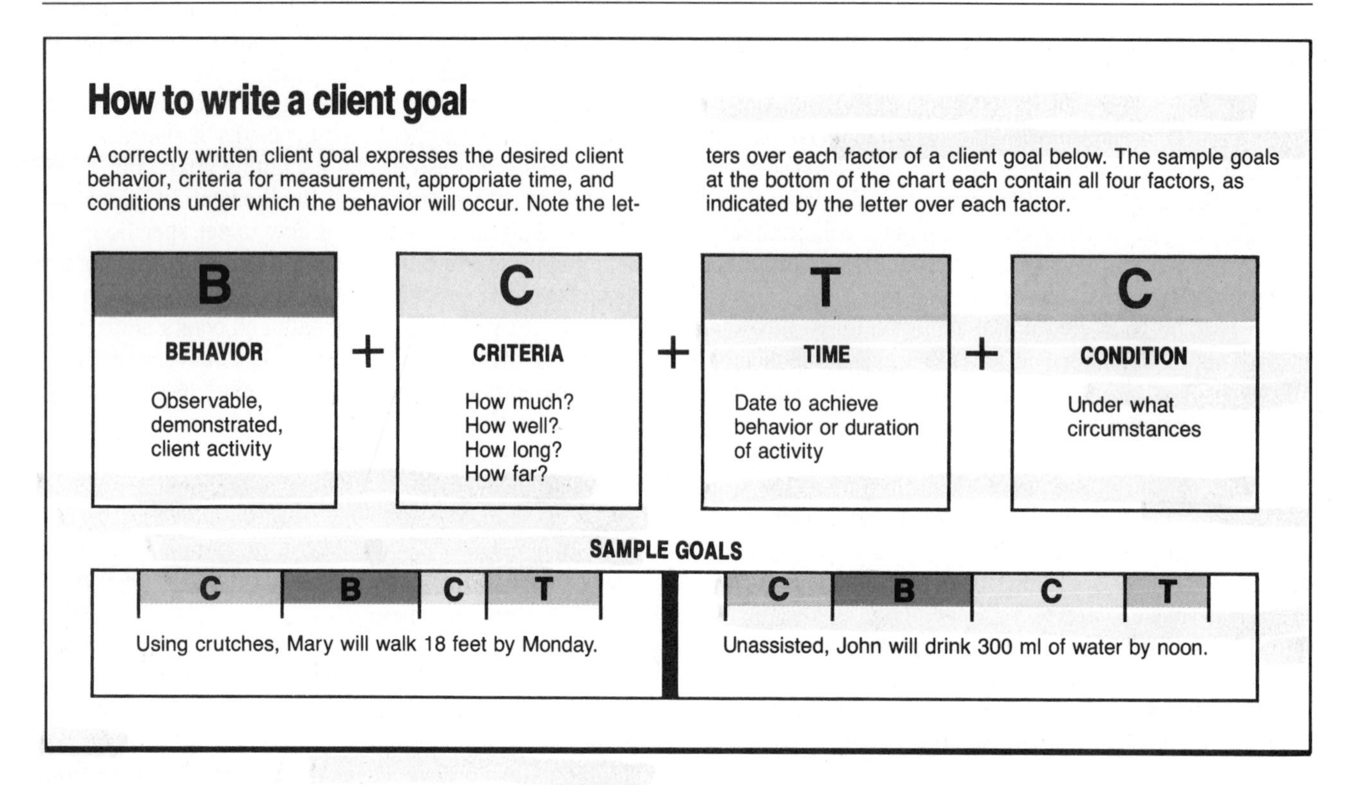

perspectives, including the number of strategies selected for each goal. Usually, three to six choices are sufficient.

The nurse should evaluate with the client the potential effects of each strategy and its probable outcomes, anticipating risks as well as benefits, to prevent problems. Each intervention must provide for client safety, take into account available resources (including supplies and personnel), agree with the client's stated value system, and complement other health care activities required for the client's welfare.

Next, the nurse must consider the rules governing nursing actions and client behaviors in the health care facility. This ensures that the nursing interventions are legally sound and defensible. Finally, the nurse must make sure the interventions are appropriate for the client's age, condition, developmental level, and environment.

The nursing care plan

After the nursing diagnoses are selected, the nurse must choose plans, goals, and interventions and document them in the client's record. Called the nursing care plan, this written guide directs the client's nursing care from admission to discharge. It can be updated and revised as needed.

A standardized care plan may be suitable in a unit or particular setting that houses clients with specific, specialized problems (for example, an oncology or cardiac care unit). Besides incorporating the main aspects of nursing care required by all clients with a similar problem, this type of care plan allows individual differences to be recorded and included.

Nursing care plans also ensure continuity of care for the client. Most clients are seen by many nurses. The care plan allows everyone providing client care to work toward the same goals, using the same measures. It also clearly states priorities for each nursing diagnosis.

Documentation of client progress (or lack of progress) is required by the Joint Commission on Accreditation of Health Care Organizations, and other regulatory groups that monitor health care quality. The nursing care plan identifies which areas of the client's life are under scrutiny and, therefore, need documentation of the progress.

As a management tool, the nursing care plan can be used to determine staffing needs and assignments. A glance at it indicates the level of nursing expertise required to provide complete client care.

The style of the nursing care plan and its location in the client's records depend on the health care facility's procedures. All care plans, however, include written nursing diagnoses, goals, evaluation criteria, and interventions. The nurse should date and sign the initial nursing diagnosis, any revisions, and its resolution; record all pertinent care plan information succinctly, so that little time is required to find the essential points; and use accepted medical abbreviations, but make sure the plan is legible. If specific instructions for nursing interventions or nursing orders are required—for example, for complicated wound care—the nurse lists them in a logical sequence and makes sure they are appropriate. However, these instructions are not included with every nursing activity; instructions for routine skills are in procedure manuals and reference books available in most health care facilities.

Sometimes the care plan includes the client's personal preferences. Cues, such as "prefers to bathe after lunch" or "wife will assist with a.m. care," help improve client care by maintaining continuity and reducing the client's need to repeat requests and desires to each caregiver.

Client discharge plans as well as home health needs and supplies are also written in the nursing care plan to assure that they are being considered from the first nurse-client interaction to the last. Other elements to include in the nursing care plan are the plans and strategies for educating the client and family. (See *Client assessment and the nursing process,* pages 12 and 13, for a sample.) Recording specific teaching strategies and interim goals eliminates the need for repeating the information to other health care professionals.

Implementation

The nurse should implement the nursing care plan as soon as it is established and recorded by working with the client and significant others to perform the designated interventions and by proceeding toward the desired outcome. Interventions usually fall into three categories: interdependent, dependent, and independent.

Interdependent interventions are those the nurse performs in collaboration with other health care professionals to improve the client's knowledge and skills. For example, if a client's communication goals require a speech pathologist's intervention, the nurse will act interdependently by supporting the speech pathologist's strategies. This type of collaboration helps the client achieve goals.

Dependent interventions are activities the nurse performs at the direct request of a physician to help fulfill the medical regimen. This type of activity may include performing an invasive procedure, such as venipuncture or bladder catheterization.

Independent interventions do not require a physician's direction to be implemented, because their execution is suited to the nurse's education and knowledge. Such activities are reflected in and broadly regulated by the nurse practice acts in most states. For example, at a basic level, the community nurse can identify and monitor vital signs, provide skin and mouth care, and instruct the client how to care for a surgical wound after hospitalization. (For further discussion about dependent, independent, and interdependent interventions, see Chapter 2, Nursing and Medicine: A Collaborative Approach.)

Before implementing the care plan, the nurse should quickly reassess the client to ensure that the planned interventions are appropriate. The care plan may call for ambulating the client every 2 hours throughout the day. However, reassessment before ambulation may reveal that the client recently returned from a physical therapy session and is fatigued; therefore, ambulation would be inappropriate despite the established plan. In other words, the plan must be flexible and individualized.

To implement nursing actions effectively, the nurse will need to develop cognitive skills based on behavioral and basic sciences.

Affective skills are as necessary for implementation as they are for assessment. These skills include using verbal and nonverbal communication, such as touching, eye contact, body language, and keeping an appropriate distance. The nurse's empathy in dealing with a client can be particularly effective in achieving a desired outcome. For example, a client with a newly diagnosed terminal illness may accept the diagnosis if the nurse takes the time to sit quietly and listen to the client's concerns and fears.

Besides cognitive and affective skills, implementation requires psychomotor skills. These include such traditional nursing actions as moving clients and equipment safely, changing wound dressings, and administering medications, as well as such techniques as hemodynamic monitoring and dialysis. All require education and experience to be performed safely and effectively. Although manual dexterity is valuable, the nurse's fundamental understanding of the task is more important. The nurse's proficiency will enhance client comfort and security and help to humanize the health care system.

Organizational skills such as counseling, managing, and delegating also will improve care implementation. These develop with time, and grow with experience. They enhance the nursing process by addressing complicated client needs and by organizing client care efficiently.

When implementing nursing interventions, the nurse helps the client learn at the same time. For example, a nurse can perform a "teaching physical assessment" on a newborn with the mother present. During the session, the new mother can learn facts about the new baby such as the purpose and care of the umbilicus, or how to protect the fontanelle. Also, she can listen to the infant's heartbeat.

Evaluation

Although evaluation usually is listed as the final nursing process step, in reality it occurs throughout, particularly during implementation when the nurse should constantly evaluate interventions.

Evaluation is linked to the outcome criteria established for each goal; it can be related to the time established by the outcome criteria, or it can occur at an arbitrary time set by the health care facility for care plan review (every day, every 2 days, and so forth). During evaluation, the nurse collects additional subjective, objective, and physical assessment data relating to the needs identified in the nursing diagnosis; then the nurse assesses these to judge whether the client's goals were met, partially met, or unmet.

If the goals were achieved, the nurse and the client may decide that the nursing diagnosis is no longer valid. In this case, the nurse documents which goals were met and how, and deletes the diagnosis from the nursing care plan according to health care facility procedures. The nurse and the client may judge a goal met, according to the outcome criteria, but decide that the nursing diagnosis remains valid and that interventions are still needed. For example, in the weight-loss example discussed earlier, a short-term goal of a 2-pound weight loss per week may be met, but the long-term goal has yet to be reached. Here, the nursing diagnosis remains valid.

An unmet or partially met goal requires the nurse to reexamine the available data and the complete nursing care plan. Reexamination may uncover an error, omission, or data misinterpretation as the reason the goal was unmet. For example, if the client did not lose 2 pounds as expected, the data review may indicate the client needs more nutritional information (omission), or the client has premenstrual weight gain (misinterpretation).

For an unmet goal, the nurse should analyze the cause and plan a new intervention. After identifying any errors, the nurse can revise the care plan. In some settings, revision is considered the sixth nursing process step. During revision, the nurse clarifies or amends the established data base to reflect any newly discovered information; reexamines and corrects the nursing diagnoses, if necessary; establishes outcome criteria reflecting new information and new or amended nursing strategies; adds this revised nursing care plan and its date to the original document; and then records the rationale for these revisions in the nursing notes.

Even if no errors appear during the care plan review, the nurse should evaluate the client's progress to make sure that nothing was overlooked. In such a case, revisions to the care plan would be minor, perhaps adding newly acquired assessment data.

The completed nursing process should fully portray the client's situation as it relates to nursing practice. A complete assessment is the keystone of the nursing process and structure on which all other nursing activities rely. The general assessment provides an overall picture of the client's situation, whereas an in-depth assessment of the client's physical signs and symptoms as well as situation offers more detail. The initial assessment supplies the foundation for the client's care. Ongoing assessments keep the nursing process dynamic, current, and in step with the client's situation.

Chapter summary

Chapter 1 discusses nursing assessment and the nursing process. The nursing process, a system for making nursing decisions, is an interpretation of the scientific method and is based on theories of nursing and other disciplines.

- The process has five steps: assessment, nursing diagnosis, planning, implementation, and evaluation. The nursing process is dynamic and ongoing; its steps often occur simultaneously.
- The first step, assessment, is the foundation for the other four steps. In assessment, the nurse collects subjective and objective data from various sources. An ongoing activity, assessment begins when the client first enters the health care system.
- The nurse processes the collected data to form the nursing diagnosis (statements of actual or potential health problems) for the nursing care plan, which directs the continuity, completeness, and quality of care the client receives.
- Planning uses goal setting and interventions to help the client attain optimal or improved function.
- Implementation of the nursing care plan relies on interventions, which can be interdependent, dependent, or independent.
- Evaluation reviews the client's status in relation to the established goals.

Study questions

1. Roy Likowski has come to the emergency department complaining of severe chest pain. He states, "It feels as if an elephant is sitting on my chest. I'm having trouble breathing. It's probably just indigestion." You note that Mr. Likowski is pale, diaphoretic (perspiring), and restless. Mrs. Likowski tells you that her husband has been feeling this way for the last 3 hours.

- Which of the above data are considered subjective; which are objective?
- What further data related to Mr. Likowski's condition should you obtain from the primary source and from the secondary source?
- Using the NANDA nursing diagnosis list, which three nursing diagnoses (potential or actual) could be included in Mr. Likowski's care plan?

2. Amy Kline, age 3, was admitted to the pediatric orthopedic unit. Although she has a fractured right femur and severe discomfort, she is alert and oriented. The nursing diagnosis assigned to Amy is "Comfort, altered: pain, related to fracture."

- What data should you obtain immediately from Amy's parents on admission? Give rationales for your choices.
- During which step of the nursing process will you set goals with Amy's parents?
- What additional information do you need to establish goals with Amy's parents?
- What short-term and long-term goals could you construct related to the established nursing diagnosis? (List one of each.)

3. As a home health care nurse, you visit Robert Dunn who has recently been diagnosed with insulin-dependent diabetes mellitus. He is obese and denies knowledge of his correct dietary or medication regimen. The following nursing care plan was established for Mr. Dunn. Unfortunately, multiple errors occur in this plan as written. How would you rewrite this care plan to correct the errors? (Give rationales for your corrections.)

Problem	Goal	Interventions
Diabetes	Client will not have any complications. Client will learn about his disease.	1. Give insulin. 2. Watch for complications. 3. Teach him about diabetes. 4. Teach his wife.

- What assessments should you make to evaluate Mr. Dunn's progress toward the established goals?
- What are correct nursing actions if the identified problems are resolved? If they are unresolved?

4. As a visiting nurse, you are caring for Mr. Jones, who is on bedrest at home after sustaining a closed head injury and bilateral fractured wrists. He tells you his concerns about missing work and his related financial needs. He is the only employed family member.

- What assessments would you make when visiting the Jones family?
- Which nursing diagnoses pertain to Mr. Jones and his family?
- Which factors help you establish priorities among the identified problem areas?

Selected references

Agan, R. (1987). Intuitive knowing as a dimension of nursing. *Advances in Nursing Science,* 10(1), 63-70.

Carpenito, L. (1992). *Nursing diagnosis: Application to clinical practice* (4th ed.). Philadelphia: Lippincott.

Carroll-Johnson, R. (Ed.). (1991). *Classification of nursing diagnoses: Proceedings of the ninth NANDA conference.* Philadelphia: Lippincott.

Gordon, M. (1987). *Nursing diagnosis: Process and application* (2nd ed.). New York: McGraw-Hill.

Mitchell, P. (1981). *Concepts basic to nursing* (3rd ed.). New York: McGraw-Hill.

Von Bertalanffy, L. (1969). *General systems theory.* New York: Braziller.*

Yura, H., and Walsh, M. (1988). *The nursing process* (5th ed.). East Norwalk, CT: Appleton & Lange.

Nursing research

Derdiarian, A. (1990). Effects of using systematic assessment instruments on patient and nurse satisfaction with nursing care. *Oncology Nursing Forum,* 17(1), 95-101.

Martin, P., and York, K. (1986). Relationship among nursing diagnoses and between medical and nursing diagnoses. In *Classification of nursing diagnoses: Proceedings of the sixth conference.* St. Louis: Mosby.

*Landmark publication

2

Nursing and Medicine: A Collaborative Approach

Objectives

After reading and studying this chapter, you should be able to:

1. Explain the historical development of nursing and nursing assessment.

2. Compare how nursing and medicine deliver health care.

3. Explain the elements of collaboration between nurses and physicians.

4. Plan strategies for fostering effective collaboration between nurses and physicians.

Introduction

This chapter compares nursing and medicine, emphasizing historical development, similarities, and differences in health care delivery based on each profession's goals of health care and the effect of collaboration (joint practice) on health promotion. Chapter 2 is designed to help the nurse develop an appreciation of nursing history and the contribution of nursing to health care delivery.

Discussing the nursing approach to health care delivery from a historical perspective, the chapter presents basic nursing theories from Florence Nightingale's famous writings in 1859 to the 1980 policy statement of the American Nurses' Association (ANA) that describes the goal of nursing. This historical introduction describes the roots of nursing and highlights the development of the nursing process, emphasizing assessment. The chapter also discusses the nurse's role in assessment, the need for collaboration, and strategies to meet that need.

Knowledge of the nursing and medical approaches to health care will benefit the nurse in several ways. It should help the nurse clearly identify nursing's unique goals, beliefs, and contributions—an activity that will help define nursing practice. It should provide a better understanding of nursing's and medicine's goals for health care and will give the nurse the basis for dependent, independent, and interdependent nursing practice.

The nursing model

A model is a framework used to describe a profession based on the principles, values, and beliefs that guide the practice of the profession and reflect the profession's goals and philosophies. Theories, which are based on the ideas described in the model, form the basis of many professions. They provide a body of knowledge that can be applied to the profession's practice and that allows practitioners to explain their profession.

Nursing theories, which are derived from nursing models, are composed of several key concepts. Unlike nursing models—which provide an overall perspective of nursing—nursing theories are more specific, because they explain relationships between the key concepts and describe the activities required for the nurse to reach the goals of nursing.

Glossary

Caring: examining and attempting to understand an individual, family, or community to maintain or improve a healthy way of life. Touching, listening, and talking are caring behaviors.

Collaboration: joint communication and decision-making between nurses and physicians designed to meet clients' needs by integrating the care regimens of both professions in one comprehensive approach.

Environment: external conditions that affect life and development, including physical factors, such as clean air and water; social factors, such as relationships with family members and friends; and cultural factors, such as values, beliefs, and lifestyle. A key concept in many nursing models.

Health: optimal physical, social, and emotional functioning of an individual. In health, the individual tries to achieve the maximum potential for a sense of well-being by continually adapting to internal and external stressors. A key concept in many nursing models.

Health problem or concern: anything that impairs or threatens an individual's physical, social, or emotional functioning and that causes or may cause illness or disease. A key concept in many nursing models.

Health promotion: actions taken to develop resources that improve or maintain well-being and self-actualization, or actions taken to protect against health problems. A key concept in many nursing models.

Holism: way of thinking about health that encompasses man (as body, mind, and spirit), environment, family, and community.

Human response: individual's reaction to a health problem. A key concept in many nursing models.

Illness: impairment of an individual's ability to adapt to internal and external environmental stressors. Stressors can be biological, such as bacterial infection; psychological, such as anxiety; or social, such as family problems.

Man or person: individual with biophysical, emotional, psychological, intellectual, social, cultural, and spiritual aspects. A key concept in many nursing models.

Model: framework used to describe a profession based on the principles, values, and beliefs that guide the profession, reflecting the profession's goals and philosophies.

Phenomena: individual or group responses to actual or potential health problems.

Theory: a body of knowledge, based on ideas described in a model, that includes several key concepts, which can be applied to the practice of a profession.

Nursing theories include several key concepts: man or person (individual with biophysical, emotional, psychological, intellectual, social, cultural, and spiritual aspects), environment (external conditions that affect life and development), health (optimal physical, social, and emotional functioning of an individual), and nurse. Many of them also include one or more additional concepts, such as holistic health; health problem or concern; promotion, maintenance, and restoration of health; illness; and human response.

Nursing models and theories help determine nursing's role in health care. As they evolve, nursing models and theories affect the roles of all nurses and reflect changes in men's and women's roles, society's needs and values, economic developments, and technologic advances in health care. Nursing roles will continue to evolve and change to keep pace with changes in health care delivery. (For examples of how the scope of nursing practice has changed, see *The nurse's changing role,* page 22.)

Historical overview

Since the dawn of civilization, individuals have been responsible for their own health care. Even when shamans (witch doctors), priests, physicians, and other specialized members of society assumed health care functions, individuals and families continued to rely on themselves for most of their general health care. Within the family, women traditionally assumed the nursing role as part of the maternal role.

Nursing originated with the spread of Christianity in the 1st century A.D. when nursing was closely associated with religion. Until the late 1800s, nurses received little training. They worked under the direct supervision of physicians and tended to the client's hygiene. They did not actively promote health or teach families to care for the ill.

Historians usually credit Florence Nightingale with the development of the first model for professional nursing in the mid-1800s. After her historic work during the Crimean War, she wrote *Notes on Nursing: What It Is, and What It Is Not.* In this book, Nightingale discussed assessment. She believed that observation (inspection)—the first step in todays assessment process—was essential to every nurse's training. She stressed that observation should be used to save lives and increase health and comfort rather than to accumulate miscellaneous

The nurse's changing role

In the past 50 years, the nurse's role has changed dramatically, and so has the scope of nursing practice. A mirror of the times, the nurse's role has grown from that of a skilled observer in the 1930s to that of a health care professional who performs holistic assessment in the 1990s. The following excerpts from actual nursing notes reflect this change in the nurse's role.

1930s

"Patient admitted to ward in a wheelchair. Stated that he is unable to walk due to pinched nerves of right foot. Patient is crying, says he is homesick. Condition of skin good. Made as comfortable as possible."

This note includes observations only. The nurse's role is limited to that of a skilled observer.

1950s

"25-year-old female admitted ambulatory. Past history of ulcerative colitis. Now in because of abdominal cramps and vomiting x 4 days. Is 8 months pregnant. TPR 99.4, 80, 20. Ht 5'4". Wt 116½. Urine to lab."

This note traces the past and present history of illness as well as observations. The nurse's role has expanded to include interviewing skills that assess the client's past and current health status.

1970s

"12-year-old white female admitted to Room 203 via stretcher from E.R. with leukemia. Parents don't seem to know of diagnosis. TPR 102.8°, 120, 24. Ht 62¼". Wt 100 lb. No known allergies. Has not been eating much for last few days. Appears extremely pale. BP 150/70. No urine obtained. I.V. started. Blood started. Vital signs relatively stable. T 103° when blood started."

This note records intravenous and blood therapy and includes observations as well as information about past illnesses and diet. The nurse's role now includes observation, interviewing, performing procedures (venipuncture), and monitoring.

1990s

"Young, obese Caucasian female states she came here to 'get the sugar out of her blood.' States she found out about her sugar 3 months ago by glucose tolerance test results (in Jan. 1990 miscarried 2-month pregnancy and GTT was part of workup); states she has seen her husband test his blood (fingerstick method) and give himself insulin but has done neither herself; has tried to prepare both 1,800 and 2,200 calorie American Diabetic Association diets as ordered for husband but 'he doesn't stick to it'; has noted increased hunger, increased thirst, increased urination for several months and occasional blurred vision.

"Lives with husband and daughter next door to sister-in-law; husband makes playground equipment; states they are able to 'get by' on his salary, sometimes borrow money and have difficulty paying it back; have Blue Cross/Blue Shield which should pay for this hospitalization; husband has diabetes mellitus (takes insulin), is losing weight but refuses to see doctor—she is concerned about him; states husband will not be able to visit her because of work."

This note records observation and assessment of the client as well as the biophysical, psychosocial, and cultural factors that influence the client's health problem. The nurse's role has grown to include holistic health assessment.

facts. To promote the patient's health, Nightingale recommended changing the environment to provide comfort, quiet, fresh air, and light.

In her 1893 paper, "Sick Nursing and Health Nursing," Nightingale differentiated between nursing that requires training in caring for the sick and nursing that keeps the family healthy. According to Nightingale, the goal of both kinds of nursing was to put people "in the best possible conditions for Nature to restore or to preserve health—to prevent or cure disease or injury."

From Nightingale's time to the 1940s, nursing leaders refined the definition and goal of nursing. They emphasized the importance of using *skilled* observation, distinguishing between subjective and objective findings, and reporting those findings orally and in writing. Nursing leaders also outlined categories of information to observe, which closely resembled those of most modern nursing assessments. As nursing leaders redefined their profession, they began to take a more holistic view of clients and to theorize that nursing was linked to disease prevention and health promotion, which broadened the scope of nursing.

By 1948, Esther Brown, a layperson who headed a national committee to study society's need for nursing, defined nursing as:

> an art and a science which involves the whole patient—body, mind, and spirit; promotes his spiritual, mental, and physical health by teaching and by example; stresses health education and health preservation, as well as ministration to the sick; involves the care of the patient's environment—social and spiritual as well as physical; and gives health service to the family and community as well as to the individual.

Nurses began to propose other definitions, reflecting society's changing needs for nursing. In the 1950s, nurses began to conduct formal nursing research to develop a scientific knowledge base. As they worked, they discovered the need for nursing theories to guide the profession as it evolved. In the 1950s and 1960s, nursing theorists focused on nurse-client relationships and interpersonal communications. They emphasized the philosophy and humanistic aspects of nursing.

Nursing theorist Virginia Henderson (1966) presented a definition of nursing that was subsequently accepted by the International Congress of Nursing:

> The unique function of the nurse is to assist the individual, sick or well, in the performance of those activities contributing to health or its recovery (or to peaceful death) that he would perform unaided if he had the necessary strength, will, or knowledge. And to do this in such a way as to help him gain independence as rapidly as possible.

During the 1970s, theorists focused on the science of nursing, emphasizing technology and introducing such concepts as diagnosis, autonomy, joint practice, and independent practice. In the 1980s, some nursing theorists, such as Jean Watson and Rosemary Parse, returned to the philosophical and humanistic aspects of nursing, incorporating concepts about the art and science of nursing in their theories. (For more information about nursing theories, see *Perspectives on the goal of nursing*, page 24.)

As nurse scholars developed nursing models and theories, the ANA (1980) defined nursing and its scope of practice: "Nursing is the diagnosis and treatment of human responses to actual or potential health problems." To explain the practice of nursing further, the ANA used the following terms: phenomena, theory application, nursing action, and evaluation. *Phenomena* are individual or group responses to actual or potential health problems. Based on assessment findings, the nurse diagnoses the response to the health problem, not the health problem itself. The nurse applies *theories* from nursing and other fields to understand the phenomena. This understanding forms the basis of *nursing actions*, which improve or correct conditions to prevent illness and promote health. The nurse then *evaluates* these actions to determine if they have had beneficial effects.

Widely accepted today, the ANA's definition and terms to describe nursing practice relate to the five steps of the nursing process: assessment, diagnosis, planning, implementation, and evaluation. The nurse assesses the individual or group responses to actual or potential health problems, assigns a nursing diagnosis based on those responses, and uses theories and scientific knowledge to plan the client's care. Implementation of the plan becomes the nursing actions. Then the nurse evaluates the effectiveness of the actions.

Throughout its history, the nursing profession has attempted to define nursing and develop its own body of knowledge. This process has led to the development and use of nursing models, nursing theories, and the nursing process. As a result, the profession has gained a better understanding of the goal of nursing practice and nursing's underlying philosophies.

Development of nursing diagnoses

Today, the nursing process usually includes five components: assessment (data collection), nursing diagnosis, planning, implementation (intervention), and evaluation. (For further information about these components, see Chapter 1, Assessment and the Nursing Process.)

Assessment, in the form of observation described by Nightingale, has long been an important part of nursing activity. For years, however, nurses used observation as a tool primarily to monitor disease status for physicians and secondarily to determine the need for nursing interventions.

Then R. Faye McCain (1965) described a systematic assessment process, "an orderly and precise method of

Perspectives on the goal of nursing

Although nursing theorists differ on the goal of nursing, they agree that the nurse should work *with* the client, not *for* the client. The following chart lists some of the major nursing theorists and describes their perspectives on the goal of nursing.

THEORIST	GOAL OF NURSING
Florence Nightingale (1860s)	To put clients in the best possible conditions for nature to restore or preserve health
Hildegarde Peplau (1950s)	To help move the client's personality and other human processes toward creative, productive, personal, and community living
Virginia Henderson (1960s)	To substitute for what clients lack in physical strength, knowledge, or will to help them become whole or independent
Dorothy Johnson (1960s)	To restore, preserve, or attain a client's behavioral system balance and dynamic stability at the highest possible level
Dorothea Orem (1970s)	To teach and manage continuous self-care to help clients sustain life and health, recover from injury or disease, and cope with their effects; also to move the client toward responsible self-care and family members toward competent decision-making about the client's daily personal care
Martha Rogers (1970s)	To promote harmonious interaction between man and environment, to strengthen the integrity and coherence of the human field (the individual's energy field), and to direct the patterning of human and environmental fields (the environment's energy field) to realize maximum human potential
Sister Callista Roy (1970s)	To promote adaptation in each adaptive mode (physiologic needs, self-concept, role function, and interdependence) to contribute to the client's quality of life, health, and death with dignity
Rosemary Parse (1980s)	To guide the client, family, and society in choosing among the possibilities in the changing health process
Jean Watson (1980s)	To protect, enhance, and preserve humanity through transpersonal human-to-human communications by helping a client find meaning in illness, suffering, pain, and existence; to help a client gain self-knowledge, control, and self-healing and restore a sense of harmony regardless of external circumstances

collecting information about the physiological, psychological, and social behavior of a patient." McCain believed that the nurse should use assessment findings to determine the client's functional abilities and disabilities. For McCain, the primary goal of nursing was to help the client attain and maintain a state of optimum functional ability (dynamic physiological, psychological, and social equilibrium). This goal, on which the modern nursing process is based, differs from the primary goal of medicine, which is to cure and alleviate disease.

McCain proposed that nurses use their traditional tools—observation, inspection, and interview—to make "nursing diagnoses, for planning and evaluating the nursing therapy, and for writing the various nursing orders."

Others objected to the idea of nursing diagnoses, because the word *diagnosis* has a medical connotation: that of diagnosing illnesses, a function belonging solely to physicians. Many nurses preferred the term *need* or *problem.* For years, at national conferences and in publications, nurses debated using nursing diagnoses. Finally, the need for a universal language to define nursing diagnoses became evident, and in 1973, the First National Conference on Classification of Nursing Diagnoses was held. As a result of the conference, nurses today formulate nursing diagnoses of the client's functional abilities in relation to the client's family and environment. (For more information, see *Functional patterns for grouping nursing diagnoses*.) Today, nursing diagnoses—and the nursing process—are widely used and accepted.

In the past, planning and implementation were based on the physician's order. Today, they are based on mutually planned (between client and nurse) goals, with nursing actions individualized for the client, not just for the client's disease. Implementation may involve the client's family or community as well as the client.

Evaluation in the past was based solely on a cure criterion. Now, evaluation is based on client achievement of the mutually set goals.

The nursing process helps delineate the nurse's role by providing a framework for carrying out nursing actions. However, many factors affect the application of the nursing process to nursing practice, including the nurse's education, experience, and competence. Nursing models and theories and the ANA's policy statement provide a framework for nursing practice and guide nursing actions for the profession. Finally, each state's Nurse Practice Act and the ANA Standards of Nursing Practice define the scope of nursing practice, and the ANA Code for Nurses describes the legal and ethical responsibilities of the professional.

Functional patterns for grouping nursing diagnoses

Marjorie Gordon describes the human responses on which the nurse intervenes as functional health patterns. These patterns represent the phenomena that the nurse detects through assessment. Nursing diagnoses serve as labels that describe client responses and as the basis for planning appropriate interventions that the nurse can implement and evaluate.

Today, every nursing diagnosis falls into one of the functional patterns listed below. (See Appendix 4 for a list of NANDA nursing diagnoses grouped under these patterns.)

- Health-perception – health-management pattern
- Nutritional-metabolic pattern
- Elimination pattern
- Activity-exercise pattern
- Sleep-rest pattern
- Cognitive-perceptual pattern
- Self-perception – self-concept pattern
- Role-relationship pattern
- Sexuality-reproductive pattern
- Coping – stress-tolerance pattern
- Value-belief pattern

From Gordon, M. *Manual of Nursing Diagnosis 1991-1992.* New York: McGraw-Hill Book Co., 1991.

The medical model

The medical model reflects the physician's goals of diagnosing and prescribing to cure or alleviate disease, with a focus on body systems.

Historical overview

Because primitive people thought the gods were responsible for all natural phenomena, priests often served as physicians in early civilizations. Their medical knowledge accrued from trial and error as well as customs, traditions, and superstitions. One persistent notion was the doctrine of the four humors. First developed by Empedocles in the 5th century B.C., this doctrine held that the relative distribution of four fluids in the body—blood (fire), bile (air), phlegm (water), and black bile (earth)—determined a person's health and temperament.

Hippocrates, the father of modern medicine, who also lived in the 5th century B.C., opposed this doctrine. He and other ancient Greeks emphasized scientific rationality and the treatment of diseases as natural, rather than divine, phenomena. Nevertheless, the doctrine of the four humors persisted until the 1600s, when William Harvey discovered the circulatory system and explained that the heart is both a muscle and a pump. These discoveries prompted physicians to conduct medicine more rationally and scientifically. Even so, most physicians continued to use the standard medical treatments for the four humors—leeches, purgatives, emetics, and large quantities of alcohol—until the mid-1800s.

During that time, physicians did their best to cure the prevailing diseases caused by poor sanitary conditions in the industrial revolution's burgeoning cities. Physicians aimed their treatment, however, primarily toward alleviating symptoms, rather than correcting underlying diseases. Quack doctors and patent medicines were prevalent. Different branches of medicine developed, such as homeopathy (therapeutic system that uses the smallest drug dose necessary to control symptoms and prescribes only one drug at a time), hydrotherapy (therapeutic system that requires internal or external application of water), and herbalism (therapeutic system that uses herbs).

Finally, in 1847, the medical profession began to organize itself with the founding of the American Medical Association (AMA). In the latter half of the century, major scientific discoveries, such as Louis Pasteur's germ theory in 1865 and Wilhelm Roentgen's rays in 1890, greatly affected medical knowledge and practice. The Johns Hopkins Hospital, Nursing School, and University Medical School became the first center of modern health care in the United States. During this era, medical students trained as apprentices in courses of study that typically lasted for two years or less. Eventually, medical education evolved into a postgraduate, university-based discipline.

Today, as in the past, the medical model for the delivery of health care reflects the primary goal of physicians: the diagnosis (based on the client's chief complaint and physical assessment findings) and treatment of disease, medically or surgically. To achieve that goal, medicine has advanced from a primitive knowledge to a scientific understanding of disease. The medical practice acts of each state define medicine in terms of diagnosing, treating, operating, and prescribing. To protect people from unqualified practitioners, the practice acts usually specify that no one but a qualified physician can practice medicine. In most states, however, the acts allow physicians to delegate some medical tasks to other health care professionals, including nurses.

The nurse-physician relationship

Although the nursing and medical models are similar in some ways, they differ to reflect the manner in which each discipline delivers care and the position each takes on political and social issues surrounding their practices. Similarities between the nursing and medical models spring from their common goal—high-quality client care. Most differences derive from their divergent approaches to meeting the goal of health care: nursing models tend to emphasize *the human response to illness;* medical models tend to emphasize *the cure of diseases*.

The remainder of this chapter describes the history of the nurse-physician relationship, explains how misconceptions may arise, and shows how these professions can complement each other while reaching their common goals.

Historical overview

Nurses and physicians have viewed their relationship differently throughout history. In the early years, most saw the nurse-physician relationship as that of a servant and master. Slowly, this view began to change. Today, nurses and physicians are beginning to collaborate as equal partners in health care.

As early as 1868, the AMA supported nurse training, but it expected physicians to direct the nursing schools. Clara F. Weeks (1891) stated that "a prejudice against the instruction of nurses was entertained at the outset by some of the medical profession, who feared that educated nurses would trench upon their own province" but that the feeling was "fast dying out." She also pointed out, however, that the nurse's first duty to the physician was absolute obedience and that the nurse should be ready to support all of the physician's "efforts with an enthusiasm equal to his own."

During this time, many believed that nursing depended on—and emanated from—the medical profession. By the 1920s, the nurse's relationship to the physician was still that of an assistant who helped perform examinations, tests, treatments, and operations, and who observed and reported the client's condition and response to treatments.

Gradually, however, nurses began to recognize their independent functions. As this occurred, the relationship between nurses and physicians became more strained. In the 1920s, when nursing leaders urged college education for nurses, physicians opposed it, arguing that nurses were already overtrained. In 1929, the AMA opposed the Sheppard-Towner Act (the federal law that funded health education, home visits, and health screening of children and their mothers by public health nurses). The act was not renewed primarily because the AMA felt that nurses "were overstepping their bounds . . . and . . . intruding into the exclusive province of the physician's function" (Rothman, 1978).

Some physicians recognized nurses' independent contributions to client care, but most thought that nurses helped them treat cases and viewed nurses as their handmaidens. A few physicians regarded nurses as their partners. (For other views of nursing and medicine, see *The nurse-physician relationship: 1891 and 1936.*)

Today, nurses and physicans are beginning to view each other as health care professionals who make different—but equally important—contributions to health care. Nurses and physicians need to recognize that both their roles, which are interrelated and complementary, are needed for total client care.

Collaboration

In the 1960s, advanced technology, demands for equal access to health care for all people, and problems related to health insurance forced the U.S. Surgeon General to recognize the need for change in the health care system. He appointed the Consultative Group on Nursing to identify nursing needs and the federal government's role in assuring adequate nursing services. As an outgrowth of the report of this group, the National Commission for the Study of Nursing and Nursing Education in the United States was formed. This commission's final report, the Lysaught Report, eventually led to the establishment in 1972 of a National Joint Practice Commission (NJPC) of medical and nursing experts, with state counterpart committees, to discuss and make recommendations on the roles of physicians and nurses in providing quality health care.

The AMA and ANA established the NJPC as an interprofessional organization for improving health care. From the outset, the commission recognized that nurse-physician collaboration was necessary to meet the goal of better client care. Collaboration refers to joint communication and decision-making between nurses and physicians that is designed to meet clients' needs by integrating the care regimens of both professions in a comprehensive approach. It can occur in any area of practice where the unique expertise of both the nurse and physician will benefit the client.

The NJPC study

Between 1978 and 1981, the NJPC developed a demonstration project that established a model for collaboration in four hospitals. The goals of the project were to increase collaboration between nurses and physicians, to promote better use of nurses, and to improve client care. The commission chose the hospital setting for the study because that is where most nurses and physicians work together to provide client care. It believed that if working relationships changed in hospitals, they would change in other practice settings as well. The commission established guidelines for collaboration, trained the participants, conducted the study, and then measured results.

The study measured the reactions of the principal participants—nurses, physicians, and clients—and revealed that all participants expressed positive reactions when their hospital units were structured according to the NJPC guidelines. Its major conclusions were that clients received improved nursing care and were more satisfied with that care, and that nurses and physicians communicated better, exhibited increased mutual respect and trust, and expressed greater job satisfaction under the NJPC guidelines.

Based on the study results, the NJPC identified five elements that promoted collaboration in hospitals: the use of primary nursing, integrated client records, individual decision-making by nurses, a joint practice committee, and joint care reviews. (For more information, see *The NJPC's elements of collaboration,* page 28.)

The nurse-physician relationship: 1891 and 1936

Between 1891 and 1936, the view of the nurse-physician relationship changed greatly. In 1891, Weeks viewed this relationship as that of a servant and master, stating that the nurse's first duty to the physician was:

1891

"absolute fidelity to his orders, even if the necessary prescribed measures are not apparent to you. You have no responsibility beyond that of faithfully carrying out the directions received."

By 1936, Charles Solomon characterized nurses as physicians' coworkers, stating that the nurse-physician relationship was not that of servant and master but rather that of:

1936

"coequal professional partners engaged upon a single task . . . the maintenance of or the restoration to health of the patient under their mutual care."

Strategies for successful collaboration

Today, some nurses and physicians work in collaborative relationships, but most still work in parallel relationships. To increase collaboration, nurses can use several strategies, including communication, accountability, competence, and trust.

Communication

Of all the strategies for collaboration, communication is the most essential because it promotes understanding

The NJPC's elements of collaboration

According to the National Joint Practice Commission (NJPC) study, five elements foster nurse-physician collaboration and provide the following benefits.

ELEMENT AND DESCRIPTION	BENEFITS
Primary nursing	
Nursing with little or no delegation of nursing tasks to others. One nurse is responsible for a client's comprehensive care	• Direct communication between the primary nurse and physician • Client care coordination by one person • Nursing autonomy • Shared accountability with the physician • Fewer errors in client care • Increased client satisfaction
Integrated client records	
Interdisciplinary client progress notes that combine nurse and physician observations, judgments, and actions and provide a formal means of nurse-physician communication about client care	• Substantive and concise nursing notes • Opportunity for health care professionals to read each others' notes • Less duplication of charted information • Validation of observations and judgments by cosigning of nurse's and physician's notes
Individual decision-making by nurses	
Ability to exercise independent judgment and initiate care based on the judgment. Decisions must lie within the scope of nursing practice	• Greater nursing control of the environment • Greater job satisfaction for nurses
Joint practice committee	
A committee of nurses and physicians that monitors nurse-physician relationships and recommends actions that support collaboration	• Opportunity for nurses and physicians to discuss collaborative practice and work out problems • Improved understanding between nurses and physicians
Joint care reviews	
Monthly review of client charts by a review committee of nurses and physicians to evaluate collaborative care	• Identification of ways to improve client care and collaborative practice

and improves health care. A recent study of client outcomes in the intensive care units of 13 hospitals revealed that mortality was reduced and overall care was improved in the hospitals where physicians and nurses effectively communicated and held each other in high regard (Knaus, 1986). In collaborative practice, the nurse and the physician must clearly understand each other's roles, responsibilities, and care plans.

As quoted in "Joint Practice: A New Dimension in Nurse-Physician Collaboration" (American Journal of Nursing, 1977), Marilyn Fiske and Harold Gardner illustrate the importance of communication with an example from their early days of practice together. "Dr. Gardner would come in and see the patient I was handling . . . . Sometimes he would repeat the taking of the blood pressure . . . this really annoyed me," recalls Fiske. When Fiske asked Gardner why he did this, Gardner replied, "I have to do something when I go into the room. I feel better if I can do something." Fiske notes, "That was interesting, because I had not perceived that as a problem . . . . My perception of the problem was that there was something wrong with me and that he did not trust me. His perception . . . was that he was uncomfortable just standing there with the patient and needed to do something."

Risk-taking is an essential part of communication. The nurse and the physician must be able to put themselves at risk in their interpersonal relations. They need to be able to confront each other and discuss mistakes or concerns openly. Risk-taking in communications will create an atmosphere that fosters growth for both the nurse and the physician, but it requires the nurse to communicate assertively. Assertive communication implies that both the nurse and the physician express themselves with respect for the other's expertise and worth.

Accountability

In nursing, accountability is becoming increasingly important as nurses expand their roles, practice interdependently with physicians and other health care professionals, and become more autonomous.

Accountability requires the nurse to safeguard the client and to practice according to the ANA's Code for Nurses. (For further information, see *The Code for Nurses.*) Sometimes this means questioning institutional rules or challenging a physician's directives when they do not represent the client's best interest.

Accountability also means being autonomous in making judgments and in designing interventions. In the ambulatory care setting especially, this may mean working with the physician to design protocols (mutually determined assessments and interventions). Because protocols are based on standards of care that reflect practice acts and health care professionals' beliefs, they provide a legal and moral mandate to accountability.

Competence and trust

The nurse and the physician must depend on each other's clinical expertise but remain responsible for their own decisions and actions. Therefore, professional competence and trust in each other is absolutely necessary. Trust usually develops after a nurse and physician have worked together for a while. Jean Steel (1981) describes the development of trust as the refinement stage that comes after "a lot of hard work and possibly many hours of negotiation and demonstration. It is a stage . . . in which neither partner must defend his role . . . . The goals of both for improved patient care are consonant . . . and each partner comes to value the contribution to the health care of individuals and families that the other can make."

ANA position on collaboration

Collaboration between the nurse and the physician is vital to meeting the goal of improved client care. The ANA addressed collaboration in its 1980 policy statement and its 1985 Code for Nurses. The ANA policy statement described three basic types of working relationships:

The Code for Nurses

The American Nurses' Association Code for Nurses provides ethical standards of conduct and guidelines for all aspects of nursing practice. Its 11th statement addresses collaboration, and its related interpretive statements (11.1 to 11.3) explain specifically how nurses can meet the public's health needs through collaboration.

1 The nurse provides services with respect for human dignity and the uniqueness of the client, unrestricted by considerations of social or economic status, personal attributes, or the nature of health problems.

2 The nurse safeguards the client's right to privacy by judiciously protecting information of a confidential nature.

3 The nurse acts to safeguard the client and the public when health care and safety are affected by the incompetent, unethical, or illegal practice of any person.

4 The nurse assumes responsibility and accountability for individual nursing judgments and actions.

5 The nurse maintains competence in nursing.

6 The nurse exercises informed judgment and uses individual competence and qualifications as criteria in seeking consultation, accepting responsibilities, and delegating nursing activities to others.

7 The nurse participates in activities that contribute to the ongoing development of the profession's body of knowledge.

8 The nurse participates in the profession's efforts to implement and improve standards of nursing.

9 The nurse participates in the profession's efforts to establish and maintain conditions of employment conducive to high quality nursing care.

10 The nurse participates in the profession's effort to protect the public from misinformation and misrepresentation and to maintain the integrity of nursing.

11 The nurse collaborates with members of the health professions and other citizens in promoting community and national efforts to meet the health needs of the public.

11.1 *Collaboration with Others to Meet Health Needs*
The availability and accessibility of high quality health services to all people require collaborative planning at the local, state, national, and international levels that respects the interdependence of health professionals and clients in health care systems. Nursing care is an integral part of high quality health care, and nurses have an obligation to promote equitable access to nursing and health care for all people.

11.2 *Responsibility to the Public*
The nursing profession is committed to promoting the welfare and safety of all people. The goals and values of nursing are essential to effective delivery of health services. For the benefit of the individual client and the public at large, nursing's goals and commitments need adequate representation. Nurses should ensure this representation by active participation in decision making in institutional and political arenas to assure a just distribution of health care and nursing resources.

11.3 *Relationships with Other Disciplines*
The complexity of health care delivery systems requires a multidisciplinary approach to delivery of services that has the strong support and active participation of all the health professions. Nurses should actively promote the collaborative planning required to ensure the availability and accessibility of high quality health services to all persons whose health needs are unmet.

Code for Nurses with Interpretive Statements. Kansas City, Mo.: American Nurses' Association, 1985.

"The first and most primitive is the one in which one person commands another. The second type can be defined as détente . . . like armed neutrality. The third level is collaboration . . . a relationship based upon recognition that each is richer and more truly real because of the strength and uniqueness of the other."

The 11th statement of the ANA's Code for Nurses addressed collaboration in three ways—cooperation with others to meet health needs, responsibility to the public, and relationships with other disciplines. By following the directives of the code and policy statement, nurses can help improve nurse-physician relationships.

Collaboration and nursing diagnoses

Current nursing models emphasize an independent and collaborative (interdependent) role. In a collaborative relationship, the nurse's and physician's activities sometimes overlap. This overlap is referred to as *collaborative problems, interdependent practice,* or *gray areas of func-*

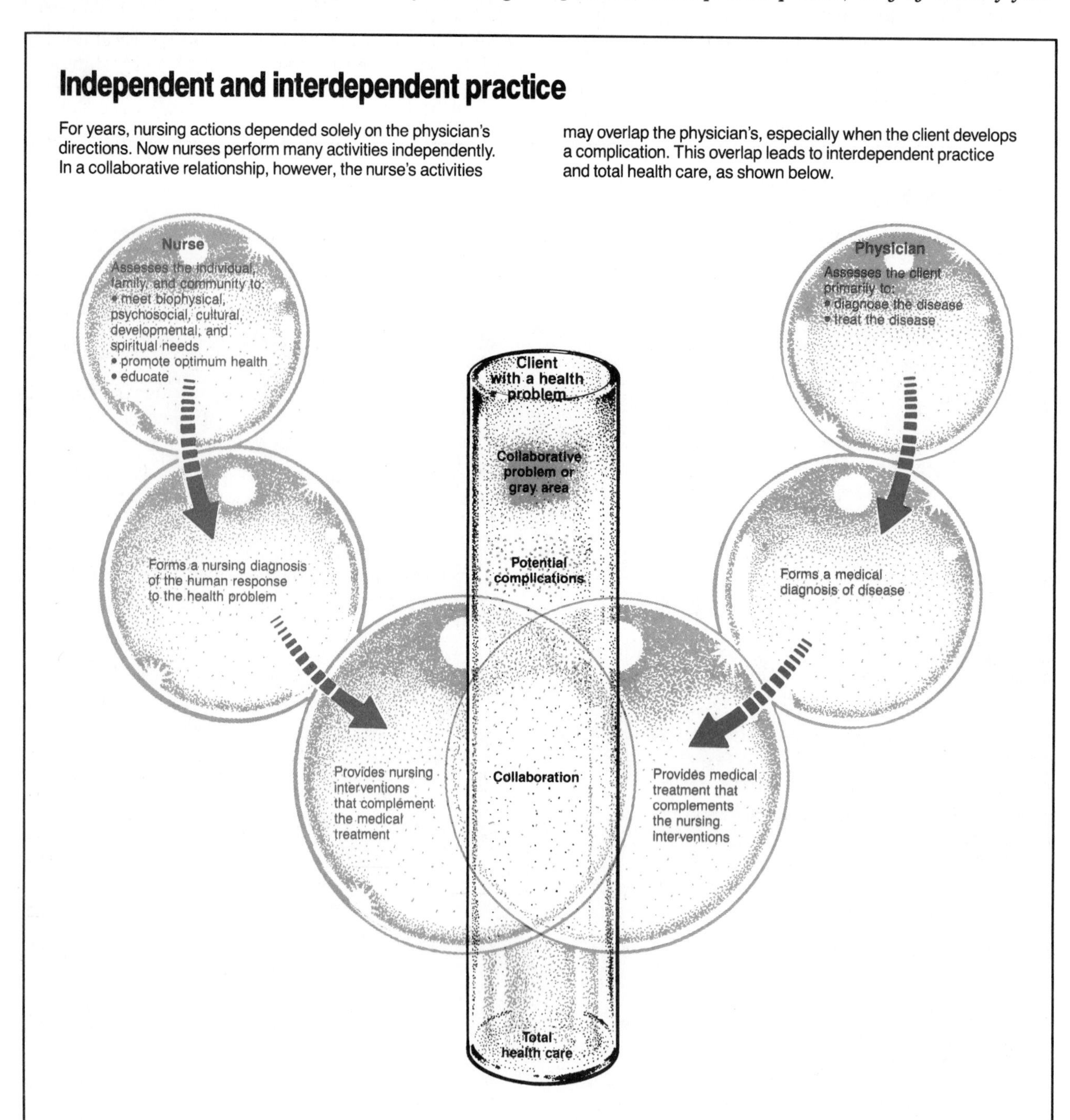

Independent and interdependent practice

For years, nursing actions depended solely on the physician's directions. Now nurses perform many activities independently. In a collaborative relationship, however, the nurse's activities may overlap the physician's, especially when the client develops a complication. This overlap leads to interdependent practice and total health care, as shown below.

tioning. (For an illustration, see *Independent and interdependent practice.*)

Although nursing diagnoses address problems that fall within nursing expertise, many of them have the potential to become collaborative problems, requiring interdependent practice, because most are based on physiologic complications. For example, the nurse may have primary responsibility for airway clearance, but if complications necessitate endotracheal intubation, the problem becomes a collaborative one (Holloway, 1988).

To practice within nursing's legal realm and to avoid misunderstandings with physicians about client care responsibilities, the nurse should foster collaboration. The nurse must also differentiate clearly between nursing diagnoses and independent interventions and potential complications and interdependent interventions.

Chapter summary

Chapter 2 shows how nursing has grown from a woman's occupation that simply served physicians' needs to a profession that makes a unique and independent contribution to health care for individuals, families, and communities. The chapter includes the following points:

- Professional development started in the mid-1800s when Florence Nightingale clearly delineated the nurse's role. This pioneer of professional nursing emphasized skilled observation as part of the nurse's role. Although Nightingale differentiated between sick nursing and health nursing, she believed that their goals were the same: to put people "in the best possible conditions for Nature to restore or to preserve health."
- Nursing leaders of this century developed the rudiments of the nursing process. They also developed many different philosophies and definitions of nursing and focused attention on the nurse's independent functions.
- After much debate about nursing diagnoses, the National Conference on Classification of Nursing Diagnoses was held in 1973. Today, nursing diagnoses are routinely used to describe client responses and to help plan appropriate nursing interventions.
- The professional relationship between nurses and physicians has changed significantly over the years. Nurses and physicians, who are equal professional partners in health care delivery, share the same goal—to provide the best possible client care.
- The National Joint Practice Commission, an interprofessional organization established by the AMA and ANA to improve health care, studied collaboration (joint practice) between nurses and physicians in hospitals. The commission identified five elements that fostered collaboration: primary nursing, integrated client records, individual decision-making by nurses, a joint practice committee, and joint care reviews.
- As nurses become more autonomous in their practice and assume expanded roles, they will need to use several strategies for successful collaboration, including expert communication skills, professional accountability, competence, and trust in the nurse-physician partnership.
- Communication is the most essential strategy because it promotes understanding and improves health care. Accountability requires the nurse to safeguard the client and to practice according to the ANA's Code for Nurses.

Study questions

1. Experts credit the origin of professional nursing to Florence Nightingale in the 1860s. How has the focus of nursing evolved from its original form to its present form? (Include definitions developed by Nightingale, Brown, Henderson, and the American Nurses' Association.)

2. Nightingale described observation as an essential nursing skill. How does observation, as described by Nightingale, relate to today's nursing process?

3. Give an example of a collaborative problem. How does it differ from a nursing diagnosis?

4. What are the elements of collaboration between physicians and nurses?

5. In 1981, the National Joint Practice Commission reported that collaboration between nursing and medicine was necessary to meet the goal of improved client care. What actions can nurses and physicians take to foster effective collaboration?

Selected references

Alfaro, R. (1990). *Application of nursing process: A step-by-step guide to care planning* (2nd ed.). Philadelphia: Lippincott.

Brown, E. (1948). *Nursing for the future.* New York: Russell Sage Foundation.

Carpenito, L. (1989). *Nursing diagnoses: Application to clinical practice* (3rd ed.). Philadelphia: Lippincott.

Code for nurses with interpretive statements. (1985). Kansas City, MO: American Nurses' Association.

Committee on Curriculum of the National League of Nursing Education. (1937). *A curriculum guide for schools of nursing* (2nd ed.). New York: National League of Nursing Education.

Dennis, K., and Prescott, P. (1985). Florence Nightingale – Yesterday, today and tomorrow. *Advances in Nursing Science,* 7(2), 66-81.

Devereux, P. (1981). Does joint practice work? *Journal of Nursing Administration,* 11(6), 39-43.

Devereux, P. (1981). Essential elements of nurse-physician collaboration. *Journal of Nursing Administration,* 11(5), 19-23.

Gordon, M. (1991). *Manual of nursing diagnosis, 1991-1992.* New York: McGraw-Hill.

Gordon, M. (1987). *Nursing diagnosis: Process and application* (2nd ed.). New York: McGraw-Hill.

Henderson, V. (1966). *The nature of nursing.* New York: Macmillan.

Holloway, N. (1988). *Medical-surgical care plans.* Springhouse, PA: Springhouse Corp.

Joint practice: A new dimension in nurse-physician collaboration. (1977). *AJN,* 77(9), 1466-1468.

Kalisch, P., and Kalisch, B. (1986). *The advance of American nursing* (2nd ed.). Boston: Little, Brown.

Knaus, W., Draper, E., Wagner, D., and Zimmerman, D. (1986). An evaluation of outcome from intensive care in major medical centers. *Annals of Internal Medicine,* 104(3), 410-418.

Lysaught, J. (1973). *From abstract into action.* New York: McGraw-Hill.

McCain, R. (1965). Nursing by assessment—not intuition. *AJN,* 65(4), 82-84.

National Joint Practice Commission. (1981). *Guidelines for establishing joint or collaborative practice in hospitals.* Chicago: Neely.

Nightingale, F. (1859). *Notes on nursing: What it is, and what it is not.* London: Harrison.

Nightingale, F. (1954). Sick nursing and health nursing. In L. Seymer (Ed.), *Selected writings of Florence Nightingale.* New York: Macmillan.

Nursing: A social policy statement. (1980). Kansas City, MO: American Nurses' Association.

Nursing Theories Conference Group. (1990). *Nursing theories: The base for professional nursing practice* (3rd ed.). Englewood Cliffs, NJ: Prentice-Hall.

Parse, R. (1981). *Man-living-health: A theory of nursing.* New York: Wiley & Sons.

Paxton, C., and Scoblic, M. (1978). Defining and developing protocols for the nurse practitioner. *Nursing Forum,* 17(3), 269-283.

Pender, N. (1984). Health promotion and illness prevention. In H. Werley and J. Fitzpatrick (Eds.), *Annual review of nursing research.* New York: Springer.

Rothman, S. (1978). *Woman's proper place: A history of changing ideals and practices, 1870 to the present.* New York: Basic Books.

Roy, C. (1984). *Introduction to nursing: An adaptation model* (2nd ed.). Englewood Cliffs, NJ: Prentice-Hall.

Solomon, C. (1936). The role of the nurse in the treatment of disease. *Trained Nurse and Hospital Review,* 97, 236-243.

Standards of Nursing Practice. (1992). Kansas City, MO: American Nurses' Association.

Steel, J. (1981). Putting joint practice into practice. *AJN,* 81, 964-967.

Watson, J. (1985). *Nursing: The philosophy and science of caring.* Niwot, CO: University Press of Colorado.

Weeks, C. (1891). *Textbook of nursing.* New York: Appleton.

Nursing research

Baldwin, A., Welches, L., Walker, D., and Eliastam, M. (1987). Nurses' self-esteem and collaboration with physicians. *Western Journal of Nursing Research,* 19(1), 107-114.

Hodes, J., and Van Crombrugghe, P. (1990). Nurse-physician relationships. *Nursing Management,* 21(7), 73-75.

McLain, B. (1988). Collaborative practice: A critical theory perspective. *Research in Nursing and Health,* 11(6), 391-398.

Note: The dates in this list reflect the historical content of this chapter.

UNIT TWO

Learning Assessment Skills

Unit Two introduces the basic concepts and skills involved in a complete health assessment. It covers the necessary steps in obtaining subjective data (information the client relates during the health history and the cultural and psychosocial assessment) and objective data (information the nurse obtains directly from physical assessment).

Chapter 3 The Health History

After briefly explaining the components of a nursing health history, Chapter 3 discusses important factors affecting the quality of the history, such as the nurse's interviewing skills, the client's beliefs about health care, and sociocultural considerations. Examples of effective and ineffective interviewing techniques are given.

The chapter then presents an in-depth discussion of each component of the history, including biographical data and information about the client's health and illness patterns, health promotion and protection patterns, and role and relationship patterns. Included are examples of questions appropriate to each component.

The chapter also includes strategies for adapting a health history to the client's developmental stage. This technique supports the holistic nursing assessment that views the client as a unique individual.

The chapter concludes with guidelines for documenting health history findings, including sample documentation for a complete history.

Chapter 4 Physical Assessment Skills

Chapter 4 begins with explanations of the equipment used in physical assessment. Equipment is discussed in two sections—that needed to perform a basic assessment and that needed to perform an advanced assessment; this division reflects the two levels of physical assessment. For example, the nurse uses a flashlight to assess pupillary reaction to light (basic assessment) or an ophthalmoscope (advanced assessment).

The chapter then examines the four basic techniques of physical assessment—inspection, palpation, percussion, and auscultation. These techniques require the nurse to develop specific psychomotor skills and to rely on the senses of sight, touch, and hearing.

The chapter concludes with an in-depth discussion of vital signs—temperature, pulse, respirations, and blood pressure—and how to assess them, along with an explanation of how to take anthropometric measurements—height and weight.

3

The Health History

Objectives

After reading and studying this chapter, you should be able to:

1. Explain the purpose and components of a health history.

2. Describe the necessary steps in obtaining an accurate health history.

3. Describe effective and ineffective interviewing techniques.

4. Gather appropriate information for each health history component: biographic data, health and illness patterns, health promotion and protection patterns, role and relationship patterns, and a summary of health history data.

5. Describe modifications needed to accommodate a client's cultural beliefs and developmental differences.

6. Identify personal biases that may prevent you from gathering accurate information.

7. Document a health history correctly.

Introduction

The health history, the major subjective data source about a client's health status, provides insights into actual or potential health problems. A guide to subsequent physical assessment, the health history organizes pertinent physiologic, psychological, cultural, and psychosocial information; it relates to the client's current health status; and accounts for such factors as life-style, family relationships, and cultural influences.

This chapter discusses the essential components of a complete and accurate health history, explains how to communicate effectively with the client, and includes examples of effective and ineffective interviewing techniques. It describes the interview process and suggests appropriate questions; it includes special considerations for pediatric, pregnant, elderly, and disabled clients. Finally, the chapter discusses how to document health history findings. This information emphasizes a broad role for the nurse—one that assumes the nurse will perform independent functions in various settings, such as a health care facility, the home, or a community agency.

Understanding the health history

The health history format provides a logical sequence for the interview and an organized record of the client's responses. Several formats have been developed, causing controversy about whether a nurse should use the traditional medical history format or one that better reflects the nursing process. A good example of the latter, developed by Gordon in 1982, focuses on 11 functional health patterns, including sleep and elimination. (For more information about Gordon's functional health patterns, see Chapter 2, Nursing and Medicine: A Collaborative Approach.)

Glossary

Acculturation: modifications in one or both groups when people from different cultures come in contact with one another.

Acquired role: function or behavior pattern determined by an individual's status in society. An acquired role can be occupational, such as a teacher or nurse, or social, such as a community or church leader.

Affect: outward manifestation of a person's feelings or emotions.

Anxiety: state or feeling of uneasiness, agitation, uncertainty, or fear resulting from the anticipation of some threat or danger, usually of an internal rather than external origin.

Assigned role: function or behavior pattern determined by biological or societal expectations. For example, biological factors determine roles such as brother, sister, father, or mother, whereas society determines sex roles, such as the expectations of what a mother or father does.

Assimilation: loss of cultural identity when an individual becomes part of a different, dominant culture.

Body image: mental picture a person has of the physical self, including appearance and capabilities. Body image is a major component of self-concept.

Clarification: additional information that makes something clear or understandable. A technique used when interviewing a client.

Closed-ended question: question that elicits facts and is structured for a one- or two-word response.

Cognition: mental processes (knowing, learning, thinking, and judging) that make a person aware and provide perception of the world.

Cultural relativism: acknowledgment and application of another person's cultural standards to activities within that culture.

Culture: integrated system of learned behavior patterns that are characteristic of the members of the society and are not biologically inherited. Culture affects beliefs, values, attitudes, and customs.

Development: gradual process of change and differentiation from a simple to a more complex level.

Environment: external conditions that affect life and development.

Ethnic group: societal group within a cultural system. Ethnic groups contain racial, religious, linguistic, and ancestral traits.

Ethnicity: affiliation with a group of people classified according to common racial, national, religious, linguistic, or cultural origin or background.

Ethnocentrism: belief that one's own culture is the best and judgment of all others by one's own cultural standards.

Genogram: chart drawn to illustrate a family's health history and relationship patterns.

Health history: collection of information obtained from a client and other sources that includes psychosocial and cultural concerns as well as physical data. The data provide a base upon which the nurse can make a management plan of the client's diagnosis, treatment, and care.

Holistic health care: system of health care that considers all facets of an individual: physical, psychological, social, and spiritual.

Locus of control: person's perception of who or what controls life events. An individual with an internal locus of control believes that each person has the power to control events; an individual with an external locus of control believes that events occur through the power of others or by chance.

Objective data: information about the client's problems obtained by inspection, palpation, percussion, auscultation, and diagnostic studies.

Open-ended question: question that elicits perceptions and feelings and is structured for a full sentence response.

Reflection: technique of returning a verbal message using the same words in which it was sent.

Religion: organized, codified behaviors, rituals, and practices that reveal a person's faith and beliefs.

Restating: paraphrasing or rewording another's idea without altering its original meaning.

Self-concept: composite of ideas, feelings, and attitudes that a person has about identity, self-worth, capabilities, and limitations.

Self-esteem: confidence and satisfaction an individual has in self. The relationship between an individual's self-image and ideal image determines that person's self-esteem.

Spirituality: set of beliefs that allows a person to define the purpose and meaning of life and provides a philosophy for striving for harmony with the universe.

Subjective data: information obtained when a client describes a problem and an interviewer records the description in the client's words.

Validation: confirmation of information; questioning technique for ensuring the questioner's understanding.

This book presents a comprehensive health history format that emphasizes health, although illness is discussed when appropriate. In practice, the nursing health history differs from the medical history by its holistic focus on the human response to illness. Whereas a physician takes a medical history to guide diagnosis and treatment of illness, a nurse obtains a health history not only to help provide health care, but also to assess the impact of illness on the client and family, to evaluate client health education needs, and to start discharge

Nursing health history

The nursing health history provides subjective data about the client as a person. The list below includes all the components of a comprehensive nursing health history.

Biographic data

Name; address; telephone number; contact person; sex; age and birth date; birthplace; Social Security number; race, nationality, and cultural background; marital status and names of persons living with the client; education; religion; occupation.

Health and illness patterns

- Reason for seeking health care
- Current health status
- Past health status
- Family health status
- Status of physiologic systems
- Developmental considerations

Health promotion and protection patterns

- Health beliefs
- Personal habits
- Sleep and wake patterns
- Exercise and activity patterns
- Recreational patterns
- Nutritional patterns
- Stress and coping patterns
- Socioeconomic patterns
- Environmental health patterns
- Occupational health patterns

Role and relationship patterns

- Self-concept
- Cultural, spiritual, and religious influences
- Family role and relationship patterns
- Sexuality and reproductive patterns
- Social support patterns
- Emotional health status

Summary of health history data

planning. Obviously, both histories have similarities; the differences lie in the rationale for requesting the information and in how the information is used to provide health care.

The nursing health history interview gives the nurse essential data for developing an individualized, mutually established care plan. It also provides an opportunity to teach the client health promotion techniques (wellness strategies). The health history has five major sections: biographic data, health and illness patterns, health promotion and protection patterns, role and relationship patterns, and a summary of health history data. (For details, see *Nursing health history.*)

Biographic data

Biographic data include the client's name, address, telephone number, contact person, sex, age, birth date, birthplace, Social Security number, race, nationality, cultural background, marital status, names of persons living with the client, education, religion, and occupation. This information helps differentiate one client's health record from another's (especially if the names are similar or identical). Biographic data also help the nurse plan the remainder of the interview by providing an overview of potential sociocultural influences.

Besides identifying clients, biographic data are used for epidemiologic comparisons, such as the incidence of a certain health problem in a particular region (for example, parasitic infections in the tropics) or disease prevalence in a specific group (for example, sickle cell anemia in Blacks). Biographic data may also help the nurse assess client reliability. For example, the client who cannot supply accurate information regarding birth date or address may not be able to answer other questions reliably. The nurse may have to seek out a family member to act as a historian and to help the client answer questions.

Health and illness patterns

The health and illness patterns section of the health history has six categories: the client's reason for seeking health care, current health status, past health status, family health status, status of physiologic systems, and developmental considerations. The combined information provides an overview of the client's general health status and helps the nurse anticipate potential health problems.

Health promotion and protection patterns

This health history section allows the nurse to determine the client's perceptions of health, which influence the client's understanding of and compliance with health maintenance practices. This information defines the client's health educational needs and helps cross-check or revise data in other sections of the health history. The major components of health promotion and protection patterns include health beliefs and personal habits, and these eight patterns: sleep and wakefulness, exercise and activity, recreational, nutritional, stress and coping, socioeconomic, environmental health, and occupational health.

Role and relationship patterns

This health history component explores the client's various roles. It helps clarify family and social relationships and how they affect physical and emotional health as well as the client's self-concept. An assessment of client role and relationship patterns includes the following factors: the client's self-concept; cultural, spiritual, and religious influences; family role and relationship, sexuality and reproductive, and social support patterns; and emotional health status.

Summary of health history data

This section of the health history summarizes findings, including normal findings that are pertinent to the assessment. For the well client, the nurse includes a summary of the client's health promotion and protection patterns. This information is written in paragraph form.

Developing interviewing skills

To obtain an accurate health history, the nurse needs a basic knowledge of pathophysiology and psychosocial principles, of interpersonal and communication skills, and of the "therapeutic use of self." The following paragraphs provide guidelines for a successful interview.

Nurse-client communication

Effective health interviews require good communication and interpersonal skills. The interview is a nurse-client dialogue, not a simple question-and-answer session. An effective nursing communication style helps eliminate any mannerisms—the nurse's or the client's—that may hinder candid information exchange. For example, a nurse who constantly gestures while talking may distract the client. The nurse can overcome common barriers to effective communication, including emotional or cultural biases, by developing self-awareness and acceptance of different life-styles. Self-awareness—recognizing and accepting one's feelings, beliefs, and values, including personal biases, strengths, and weaknesses—allows the nurse to communicate more effectively with others who have different values and beliefs. This is important in obtaining accurate, unbiased information.

The nurse's own health experiences and life experiences can influence the therapeutic effectiveness of the nurse-client relationship. For example, the nurse's view of expressing emotions can affect nursing care. A nurse who learned as a child that public displays of emotion are unacceptable may discourage a client or a family member from expressing emotions. The nurse may respond to a weeping client by saying, "Don't worry; everything will be all right." Besides discouraging an open expression of feelings, such a response also denies the client's feelings and may communicate an untrue message.

A nurse who has learned not to express anger may have difficulty accepting a client's anger and may view it as a personal attack. However, a nurse with self-awareness and self-acceptance can respond objectively by encouraging the client to express negative or hostile feelings without taking the anger personally.

The nurse's personal appearance, actions, or stated beliefs may also influence a therapeutic relationship. For example, an elderly client may have a difficult time relating to a nurse who has made disparaging remarks about another elderly client in the client's presence.

Effective interview skills rely on nonverbal as well as verbal communication. The client can manipulate conversation to create a desired impression, but rarely can manipulate nonverbal communication. Also called body language, nonverbal communication is partially unconscious behavior and, therefore, is difficult to conceal or alter. Be aware of such nonverbal communications as eye movements, facial expressions, body gestures, and posture. Disparities between the client's words and actions may provide important insights. For example, a new mother who describes a loving relationship with her infant daughter but who rigidly holds the infant away from her and fails to establish eye contact with or talk to the infant is probably signaling a mother-infant bonding problem.

Therapeutic use of self

Using interpersonal skills in a healing way to help the client is "therapeutic use of self." The concept is sometimes difficult for the beginning nurse to understand and use, partly because it develops with clinical practice and life experiences. Central to the concept is self-awareness, which permits approaching a client with empathy and acceptance and establishes the open, nonthreatening environment needed to obtain a more accurate health history. Three important techniques enhance a nurse's therapeutic use of self: exhibiting empathy, demonstrating acceptance, and giving recognition.

Exhibiting empathy. Empathy, the capacity for understanding another's feelings, helps establish a trust-based relationship and encourages the client to share personal information. To show empathy, use phrases that address the client's feelings; for example, "That must have upset you."

Demonstrating acceptance. Accepting the client's verbal and nonverbal communication is crucial to a successful interview. Acceptance does not signify agreement or disagreement with the client; rather, it demonstrates an effort to remain neutral and nonjudgmental. Neutral statements ("I hear what you are saying," "I see") show acceptance. Nonverbal behaviors, such as nodding or making momentary eye contact, also provide encouragement without indicating agreement or disagreement. However, the "right" words may be useless if the nurse's nonverbal communication, such as rigid posture or an uninterested look, reveals different feelings.

Giving recognition. Put the client at ease during the interview by recognizing the client's communication efforts. To give recognition, listen actively to what the client says, occasionally providing verbal or nonverbal acknowledgment to encourage the client to continue speaking.

Client's expectations

Personal values and previous experiences with the health care system can affect the client's health history expectations.

Although consumer awareness of health-oriented care is increasing, people's basic beliefs about illness and medical treatment have not changed significantly. Many people seek health care only for illness or unfamiliar symptoms. Before they will provide reliable data, some clients may ask why the information is needed. Explain that comprehensive health care starts with a health profile based on a broad range of information. Tell the client that basic health history information is collected once; only updates are needed thereafter. Explain that the health history identifies actual or potential health problems and provides information about the client's health care resources.

Help the client clarify expectations, concerns, and questions. If possible, provide answers that rectify client misconceptions appropriately. A client may be uncomfortable providing personal information; reassure the client that the information is confidential and accessible only to authorized health care professionals. Affirm that, legally, no information can be released to any person or organization without the client's written consent.

Behavioral considerations

Encounters with a hostile or angry client occur occasionally. To maintain control of the interview, do not waste time or energy arguing or feeling insulted. Rather, listen without showing disapproval. Try to relax. Speak in a firm, quiet voice and use short sentences. Avoid abstract ideas or detailed explanations. A composed, unobtrusive, and nonthreatening manner usually soothes the client. However, if this technique fails, postpone the interview and call for assistance, if needed.

If the client appears exceptionally nervous, first make sure your own nervousness is not the cause. Then, with a reassuring approach, comment on the client's anxiety and ask about the cause. Knowing the cause will help you determine the steps to take to relieve the client's anxiety.

Occasionally in interviews, a client may ask direct questions about the nurse's personel life or opinions on a controversial topic. The situation requires a quick decision on how to handle the incident with tact, acceptance, and care. Statements such as, "I appreciate your interest, but we're here to talk about you," or "I'd rather hear what you think," are two suggestions. For the insistent client, a more direct approach usually works: "It's not appropriate for me to answer that question because we are discussing your situation."

Cultural and ethnic considerations

A client's cultural and ethnic background can have a subtle and complex effect on the health history interview. *Culture* refers to an integrated system of learned behavior patterns that are characteristic of members of a society and are not biologically inherited. *Ethnicity* is an affiliation with a group of people classified according to a common racial, national, religious, linguistic, or cultural origin or background.

A person's culture and ethnicity affect beliefs, values, attitudes, and customs. They also help shape educational, occupational, and familial opportunities and expectations. Culture also affects the way a person experiences health and illness. The degree of these effects depends on whether the client has undergone acculturation (modification caused by contact with another culture) or assimilation (loss of cultural identity when an individual becomes part of a different, dominant culture).

The nurse will probably encounter clients from different backgrounds. In North America, major ethnic groups include Asians, Blacks, Caucasians, Hispanics, and Native Americans. Within each group, several cultural distinctions may exist. Cultural influences affect various aspects of the nurse-client relationship—for example, communication. To communicate effectively with clients from different cultural groups, never assume that a client understands English well enough to comprehend all interview questions or medical terms. Speak clearly and carefully, avoiding jargon. If the client's language patterns seem unusual, ask questions to clarify the client's meaning. For example, if a client says that his experience in the nuclear medicine department was "bad," ask a clarifying question, such as "What do you mean by *bad?*" or "How did those tests make you feel?"

If you are not fluent in the client's language, learn the cultural practices and health beliefs of that ethnic group. For example, although a gentle touch usually conveys warmth, concern, and reassurance, some people interpret this nonverbal communication form differently. Be aware of such cultural differences so that no one is misled by your well-meant actions.

Besides being aware of the client's cultural orientation, you need to understand your own attitudes toward clients from different cultures. Because you bring these attitudes and characteristics to the nurse-client relationship, you will need to understand how they have influenced you. Try to avoid ethnocentrism (belief that one's own culture is the best) and judging others by your cultural standards. Instead, develop an attitude of cultural relativism (acknowledgment of another person's cultural standards) and judge a client's actions by his or her own cultural standards.

Avoid stereotyping a client based on cultural background. Although a client may share certain characteristics with others of the same culture, the client will also exhibit individual differences. You should respect cultural factors and individual differences that influence the client's habits, beliefs, and attitudes about health care. Concentrate on developing the client's trust in and rapport with you.

Effective interviewing techniques

To obtain the most benefit from a health history interview, try to make the client feel comfortable, respected, and trusting. Use effective interviewing techniques to help the client identify resources and improve problem-solving abilities. Remember, however, that successful techniques in one situation may not be effective in another, depending on your attitude and the client's interpretation of your questions. Examples of effective interviewing techniques follow.

Offering general leads. General questions give the client an opportunity to speak freely. Such questions as "What brought you here today?" or "Are you concerned about any other things?" direct the client to discuss the most significant concerns. Encourage the client to do most of the talking by providing ample time for reflection and response. Comments like "Please continue," or "What happened next?" facilitate client communication.

Restating. To help clarify what the client means, restate the essence of a client's comments. For example:

CLIENT: The doctor told me to take the heart medicine twice a day.

NURSE: I see, you take digitalis once in the morning and once at night.

CLIENT: No, I take it at 8 a.m. and at noon because he said twice a day.

In this situation, twice a day had a different meaning for the client. Restating the client's words resulted in a client-teaching opportunity to ensure better medication results.

Reflecting. Reflection gives the client an opportunity to reconsider a response. This example invites the client to add information.

CLIENT: I think I've told you all the important things about my meals.

NURSE: Do you think you've covered all the important things about your nutrition?

Verbalizing the implied meaning. Stating what is implied or unspoken sometimes helps interpret a client's statement accurately or yields additional insight into a client's symptoms or concerns. For example:

CLIENT: The demands of being a student complicate my relationship with my children.

NURSE: How do you feel about the amount of time you spend with your children?

Focusing the discussion. To help the client identify significant health concerns, focus on certain discussion points. For example:

NURSE: What do you do for a living?

CLIENT: I'm a coal miner.

NURSE: Are you aware of any health hazards in coal mining?

Placing a problem (or an event) in proper sequence. To identify a problem, determine its course and draw a conclusion. Define the time limits and other factors associated with the problem by asking, "What events led to this?" or "Did this happen before or after (another event)?"

Encouraging client participation. In the health history interview, this technique affirms the client's individual value by encouraging the expression of opinions, concerns, or doubts. For example, questions like "What do you think about the stress-reduction plan we've discussed?" or "You said you couldn't get your breath; what happened after that?" encourage client participation.

Encouraging client evaluation. Promote the client's cooperation in developing a health care action plan by actively encouraging comments on implementation strategies. This technique ensures greater client compliance, leading to a desired outcome. For example:

NURSE: It sounds like you have lots of stress at work and home.

CLIENT: Yes, sometimes I feel overwhelmed.
NURSE: That can be draining; maybe we could work together on a stress-reduction plan.
CLIENT: That sounds great.
NURSE: Have you told your wife how you feel?
CLIENT: Yes, she's trying to help with some things.
NURSE: Have you thought of an exercise program, such as walking, jogging, or bicycling, to reduce stress?
CLIENT: Yes, but I can't find the time.
NURSE: How about half of your lunchtime a couple of times a week?
CLIENT: Well, that might work. I could walk in the park.

Clarification or consensual validation. Because many variables affect the interview and because interpretations of health behaviors or symptoms vary, you may have to clarify meanings. Admitting, for example, "I'm not sure what you mean," or clarifying a particular symptom or concern, for instance, "Was the mole as big as a dime?" prevents misunderstandings.

Presenting reality. When a client makes unrealistic statements or exaggerates, presenting reality usually encourages the client to reevaluate and modify statements. For example:
CLIENT: I never get anything to eat.
NURSE: But Mr. Johnson, when we discussed your eating patterns, you told me that you had three meals a day.
CLIENT: I meant that I never get anything to eat that I like.

Making observations. Observing the client helps you interpret and validate nonverbal behavior. Observations may increase the client's situational awareness and suggest possible alternatives, or open new areas for discussion. For example, the observation, "I notice that you are rubbing your eyes a lot. Do they bother you?" may lead to discussing such health concerns as allergies, vision, or altered sleep patterns.

Giving information. Share information and facts with a client to encourage direct involvement in health care decisions. For example, telling a mother about a new vaccine for *Hemophilus influenzae* in young children will provide her with information to make informed health care choices.

Using silence. Silence sometimes lets the client reorganize thoughts and consider what to say next, while allowing you an opportunity to observe. Although long silences can be awkward, avoid saying something just to reduce anxiety. Using silence effectively is a crucial skill; it can even convey empathy.

Summarizing. To help clarify information and ease the transition between health history sections, provide a brief summary after each major health history component. For example:
NURSE: That completes the family history section. I've noted that your father and grandfather died of heart attacks and your maternal grandmother had a stroke. Everyone else in your immediate family is alive and well, except for your paternal grandmother who has diabetes. Is that correct?
CLIENT: Yes, that's right.
NURSE: Okay, let's review your physiologic status.

Interviewing techniques to avoid

Some interview techniques create communication problems between the nurse and the client. The following paragraphs discuss techniques that may cause such problems.

Avoid
Asking why or how questions. A question that begins with *why* or *how* may be perceived as a threat or a challenge, because it forces the client to justify feelings and thoughts. Some clients feel they should invent an answer if they do not have one. "Why" questions may also be difficult for clients who lack specific knowledge or are unaware of a crucial fact. For example:
CLIENT: I really feel awful today.
NURSE: Why do you feel awful?

Here, a better response would be simple acknowledgment or a question like, "What do you think is making you feel awful?"
CLIENT: I got into a horrible argument with my boyfriend.
NURSE: How do you think that happened?

This question asks for an insight that the client may not have. Instead, encourage a description that the client can supply, for example, "Can you tell me more about what happened?"

Avoid
Using probing, persistent questioning. This style of questioning usually increases client discomfort, creates defensive feelings, and makes the client feel manipulated. One or two attempts to elicit information about a particular topic are sufficient.
NURSE: Can you tell me about any past illnesses?
CLIENT: Well, I had my appendix out, I had scarlet fever, and I was in the hospital for a mental problem.
NURSE: What mental problem?
CLIENT: Manic depression.
NURSE: What was that like?
CLIENT: Oh, I don't know. It was hard and I don't like to think about it.

NURSE: What did you do in your manic phases?

This example, although extreme, illustrates the client's discomfort from probing questions. The questions have little relevance to the client's overall health status, and no further explanations are required after the client names the mental illness.

Using inappropriate language. Do not block communication by using technical jargon or abstract terms that are inappropriate for the client's developmental level, education, or background. Clients may perceive this as an unwillingness to share information or an attempt to hide something from them. Be sure to phrase questions appropriately.

Giving advice. Sharing personal experiences or opinions and giving advice imply that you know what is best for the client—the opposite of collaborating with and encouraging the client to participate in health care decisions. Frequently, a client who asks for advice has already made a decision and wants a sounding board for ideas. For example, if a client asks whether a surgical procedure should be performed, avoid giving advice. Instead, ask, "What would you like to do?" or "What thoughts do you have about it?"

Giving false reassurance. Glib statements and false reassurances, such as "Everything will be fine," devalue a client's feelings and communicate a lack of sensitivity. Avoid offering false reassurance to relieve your anxiety if you are unable to help the client. For example:

CLIENT: My brother looks awful. He's so pale and he's got tubes and wires everywhere. Is he going to die?

NURSE: Don't worry, everything will be fine. Everyone looks like that after that type of surgery.

In this example, a better response would be simply to acknowledge the client's feelings: "It must be frightening for you to see your brother look like this."

Changing the subject or interrupting. Changing the subject or interrupting prevents the client from completing a thought and shifts the conversation's focus. Such behavior indicates a lack of empathy. Also, by interrupting the client's idea flow, you may confuse the client. Wait until the client completes a thought before clarifying a relevant point.

NURSE: What kinds of stress-reduction activities do you enjoy?

CLIENT: I like to jog a lot.

NURSE: Do you know that jogging too much can cause joint damage?

Here, the nurse changed the subject from the client's stress to the harmful effects of jogging. A better response is "Do you do anything else to reduce stress?"

Using clichés or stereotyped responses. Avoid using phrases such as, "You'll feel better in the morning," or "Where there's life there's hope." These phrases may make the client feel uncomfortable or disappointed, and they may discourage the client from expressing genuine feelings. Besides, repeating clichés may convey insensitivity.

Giving excessive approval or agreement. Telling the client that a response is particularly good implies that an opposing response is bad. Similarly, excessive agreement may make the client feel that modifying information is wrong. Also, excessive approval or agreement may be perceived as phoniness, or it may set narrow limits on other client responses by encouraging answers that will gain approval. Of course, the nurse can approve of or agree with a client's statements or thoughts. However, the agreement or approval should be appropriate—not excessive.

Jumping to conclusions. Premature interpretations and hasty conclusions invite inadequate or inaccurate information. For example:

CLIENT: I've had three cans of beer a day for the last 10 years.

NURSE: I'm sure you'll want to quit drinking so much. Quitting will help you feel better and can prevent liver damage.

A negative response to the client's disclosure may make the client withhold additional information in an attempt to regain approval. Do not assume that the client will want to stop doing something because of your opinion. A more productive response would be, "What do you think about that amount of beer?" Better yet, use silence to encourage further client response on the subject.

Using defensive responses. A client may express anger and frustration about a treatment program or health care facility with a verbal attack. Realize that a defensive response from you will imply that the client has no right to express such feelings or opinions, which may increase the client's anger. Consider the following exchange:

CLIENT: The care I received in that hospital was terrible. No one ever answered my call light, and I had to wait hours for a pain pill.

NURSE: I'm sure no one meant to ignore you. Nurses get so busy, sometimes they can't do as much as they'd like.

Instead of defending the nursing profession, show empathy by saying, "That must have been a difficult experience."

Making too many literal responses. A client who cannot state feelings directly may use figurative language with hidden meanings. If you respond literally to such statements, you will lose an opportunity to explore a client's real feelings. To avoid misunderstandings, always base your responses on the client's affect and the conversational context. For example, a client might remark that he is "a real go-getter." This could mean the client sees himself as ambitious and competitive or, if stated ironically, as unsuccessful and a failure.

Asking leading questions. By its phrasing, a leading question suggests the "right" answer. This type of question may force the client to supply a socially acceptable response rather than an honest one. For example, the question "You've never had a venereal disease, have you?" may force the client to answer "No."

Conducting the interview

Physical surroundings, psychological atmosphere, interview structure, and questioning style can all affect the interview flow and outcome. To be an effective interviewer, the nurse should adapt a communication style to fit each client's needs and situation. The following paragraphs provide guidelines for conducting the interview effectively.

Physical and psychological comfort

During the interview, the physical surroundings can directly affect the client's comfort and willingness to provide accurate information. A private room with a door helps ensure freedom from interruptions. An arrangement of comfortable chairs facing but slightly offset from each other creates a friendly feeling. Position the chairs 1 to 4 feet apart to facilitate eye contact and hearing. However, if the client seems to feel this is uncomfortably close, increase the distance.

Besides providing a comfortable physical setting, establish a pleasant atmosphere. Speak in a moderate tone, maintain a calm, unhurried manner, and modify the environment to meet the client's needs. For example, when interviewing a child, stoop or sit in a low chair; when interviewing a bedridden client, minimize feelings of intimidation or powerlessness by sitting in a bedside chair, rather than standing. Prevent distractions for parents accompanied by young children by providing toys and books to occupy the children during the interview. If an elderly client seems to have difficulty hearing the questions, move closer so that the client can observe your facial expressions and lip movements. Also, speak louder, slower, and in a lower pitch to ease communication.

The interview structure

Ideally, the interview includes an introductory phase, a working phase, and a termination phase. Each requires a different communication style to establish the proper tone and provide transition to the next phase.

Introductory phase

In the introductory phase, use nonprobing, client-centered questions and comments to put the client at ease and to explain the health history purpose and desired outcome. Begin by introducing yourself. Show the client where to sit, establish an interview time frame, and ask if the client has any questions about the interview procedure. Spend a few minutes chatting informally before starting the working phase. For example:

NURSE: Good morning, Mrs. Burns. My name is Mary Campo and I am a registered nurse. I'd like to spend about an hour with you this morning to obtain a comprehensive nursing history. Have a seat and I'll explain a little more about that.

CLIENT: Okay.

NURSE: Can I offer you something to drink? I have coffee, tea, and several kinds of juice.

CLIENT: No thanks, I just finished breakfast.

NURSE: I hope that this wasn't an inconvenient appointment time. Did you have to rush to get here?

CLIENT: Oh no, but I was worried about being late. It's raining hard and traffic is slow.

NURSE: Would you like to rest a few minutes or are you ready to get started?

CLIENT: I'm ready.

NURSE: The health history we will complete has several parts. The first is about your current and past health status and your family's illness history. The next is about your life-style, family, job, and daily activities; the last is about nutrition and exercise.

CLIENT: I've never had any medical person ask me about all of those things before.

NURSE: We'll use this information to form your health profile. This is the only time we collect this information, and it will become part of your permanent record. Some of the questions are personal, but all of the information is confidential. Your record will be seen only by other health care professionals and can't be given to anyone without your written permission. Please feel free to tell me if you don't want to answer a question.

CLIENT: I understand, but what do you do with all this information?
NURSE: Basically, I try to identify any potential health problem that you can work on to stay healthy or to improve your health. You and I have our special roles here. My role is to give you information about your health goals and discuss your options. I might refer you to a physician if you seem to have a medical problem. Your role is to identify your health needs and then work with me to achieve them. Does that tell you enough about what we're going to do this morning?
CLIENT: Yes, I think I'm pretty clear about it.
NURSE: Fine then, the interview will take about an hour. Is that all right with you?
CLIENT: Yes, that sounds fine.
NURSE: Do you have any questions to ask me?
CLIENT: Not yet, but I probably will as we go along.
NURSE: Let's start with you telling me what brought you here today and what you expect to happen as a result of your visit.

The preceding script illustrates how to set the proper interview tone, clarify the client's expectations of the interview, construct a time frame, and establish a verbal contract. Experience will show which communication style works best and how to alter it to suit each client's needs.

Working phase

Obtain detailed health history information in the working phase of the interview. Carry a pocket-sized outline of the health history components as a memory helper, if necessary. Temper the natural impulse to take interview notes by recognizing that lengthy note-taking may distract the client, who may wonder if you are listening. If you must take notes, tell the client before the interview starts. Experience will show how to compile pertinent information immediately after the interview and organize the final form later.

Termination phase

The health history ends with the termination phase. Provide a smooth closing by summarizing salient interview points, informing the client about the interview results, explaining how the physical assessment will be conducted, and discussing follow-up plans. These examples illustrate various ways to end an interview.

- Ill or symptomatic client:

NURSE: Well, that pretty much covers the health history. You've given me the information I need. Do you want to add anything?
CLIENT: Not that I can think of.
NURSE: What we'll do next is a head-to-toe physical assessment, which may take 20 to 30 minutes, and laboratory tests. From what you've told me, I need to assess your abdomen carefully. I'm pretty sure I'll need to make a medical referral for you, but we can discuss that later.

- Well client:

NURSE: We've covered all the questions I needed to ask about your health. Can you think of anything you want to add?
CLIENT: No, not right now.
NURSE: All right. Thanks for your cooperation. You've helped me identify some of your health needs. Let's spend some time now discussing them, and then I'll do a physical assessment.

Also, use termination regularly. → I will be here for 5 more weeks, etc (each week).

Time constraints

A client who is ill, in pain, or sedated may have difficulty completing the health history. In such instances, obtain only the information pertaining to the immediate problem. To avoid tiring a seriously ill client, take the history in several sessions or ask a close relative or friend to supply essential information.

For a client who is well or not in discomfort, schedule the necessary time for the health history, usually 45 to 60 minutes. For an elderly client with an extensive health history, it may take more time. Begin the interview by telling the client how much time is allotted. This helps both parties maintain interest and concentrate on the task at hand. Sometimes, the nurse may have too many time constraints to obtain a comprehensive health history in one interview. Again, take the history in several sessions, as necessary.

The completed health history contributes to quality nursing care in several ways.

- The interview process allows the nurse to interact with clients as individuals, which helps minimize their perception of the health care facility as an impersonal place.
- The history data about the client's family and social support system can facilitate discharge planning—an important concern because of the trend toward shorter hospital stays.
- The health promotion section of the history reveals client health education needs as well as health beliefs, which may affect compliance with medication and health care regimens.
- The comprehensive history may uncover overlooked medical or social problems, such as child abuse.

Consider time constraints when planning the interview time frame. To build trust and rapport, do not appear rushed or preoccupied. Adapting and modifying the comprehensive health history to fit a busy health care facility schedule may prove challenging. Here are some time-saving suggestions.

- Take the history in stages while performing such tasks as client baths or dressing changes.
- Ask the client to complete a written form before the interview. Then focus on the most significant or unusual data during the interview.
- Fill in health history information from other sources, such as admission forms or the medical history. This helps avoid duplication of effort and reduces interview time as well.
- Obtain some information from a close relative or friend (either verbally or in writing).

Types of questions

Generally, the health history includes two types of questions: closed-ended, which require only a yes or no response; and open-ended, which permit more subtle and flexible responses. The kinds of questions and the sequence used depends on nurse-client communication styles and personalities.

In terms of quantity and quality, open-ended questions usually result in the most useful information. Also, open-ended questions give clients the feeling they are actively participating in and have some control over the interview.

An inexperienced nurse may prefer closed-ended questions until comfortable with various interview situations. Closed-ended questions help eliminate rambling conversations. They are also useful when the interview requires brevity—for example, when a client reports extreme pain or digresses frequently.

Regardless of the types of questions used, move logically from one history section to the next. Allow the client to concentrate and give complete information on a subject before moving on.

Obtaining health history data

Modify the health history structure to meet the client's current health status. For example, if the client is moderately or acutely ill, collect pertinent medical information first. Do the less-structured, more time-consuming interview parts last, or postpone them until the client feels better.

Health history data include biographic data, health and illness patterns, health promotion and protection patterns, role and relationship patterns, and a summary of health history data.

Biographic data

The first information gathered in a complete health history, biographic data identify the client and provide important sociocultural information.

Client's name. Record the client's full name, including first, middle, and last name and maiden name if the client is a married woman. Some married women prefer to use their maiden names. In such cases, record this along with the spouse's surname. For a pediatric client, verify and record the child's surname as well as the parents' or legal guardians' names.

Some cultures use different methods to indicate family relationships and may have no traditions of maiden names. Some Asians place their surnames first.

Address. Record the client's current address. If the client uses a post office box as the current address, record this as the mailing address but ask for the street address as well. Sometimes, the address reveals socioeconomic information. If the client plans to move soon, list a permanent mailing address, if possible.

Telephone number. Record the client's home and business telephone numbers, if applicable. If the client has no telephone, note this.

Contact person. Record the name, address, and telephone number of a neighbor or relative (besides the spouse) who can act responsibly if the client cannot be reached or if a medical emergency arises. This is especially important for elderly clients who live alone.

Sex. Record the client's sex as male or female.

Age and birth date. Record the client's stated age and compare it to the birth date. For children under age 3, write the age in years and months. For a client who appears confused and cannot supply age information, consider performing a mental status assessment. (For more details, see Chapter 17, Nervous System.) Ask a relative or close friend of the client for information, if necessary.

Social Security number. Often used for identification, the client's Social Security number, Medicare number (if applicable), and health insurance number should be entered in the appropriate place on the client's record.

Place of birth. Record the city, county, and state of birth. Be sure to note whether the client was born in another country, and if so, how long the client has been a resident of this country. The birthplace may correlate with certain environmental risks.

Race, nationality, and cultural background. Identify the client's race, nationality, and culture, because they can affect health status. For example, if unaware that some dark-skinned infants have increased pigmentation on their buttocks and thighs, the nurse could mistake this for bruises, wrongly suspecting a bleeding disorder or child abuse.

A client may also have symptoms of culturally bound syndromes related to cultural practices. For example, a client who believes he or she is under a spell cast by an envious person may engage in some type of folk practice to eliminate the spell.

Marital status and names of persons living with the client. Note whether the client is married. If not, record the most descriptive category: never married, separated, divorced, or widowed. Do not assume that the never-married, separated, divorced, or widowed client lives alone. Ask if anyone lives with the client and note any children or dependents—factors that could affect the client's economic situation.

Education. Record the years of formal schooling, which may affect the client's health knowledge and your phrasing of medical questions. Do not confuse education with intelligence; talking down to the client risks being regarded as condescending. Because learning styles differ, ask clients how they learn best. Some prefer printed materials; others may prefer personal discussions, audiotaped instructions, or videotaped demonstrations. Adjust teaching techniques to suit the client's needs.

Religion. Be tactful when asking about religion. After learning the client's religious preference, ask if the client adheres to any special health care or dietary practices.

Occupation. Record current and previous occupations, because they affect stress and coping patterns and point to potential workplace health hazards. Occupation also provides clues about the client's socioeconomic status and self-concept.

Health and illness patterns

This section of the comprehensive health history includes the client's reason for seeking health care; current, past, and family health history; status of physiologic systems; and developmental considerations.

Reason for seeking health care

Determine why the client is seeking health care by asking, "What brings you here today?" The well client may respond, "I'm here for a routine health check." Then ask what, if any, health needs or concerns the client wants to discuss, and record the response in the client's own words.

If the client has specific symptoms, record that information in the client's own words; for example, "I'm here because I've had stomach pains for the last 2 weeks." Then explore the client's current health status in detail.

Current health status

This component of the health history accompanies the client's reason for seeking health care. Ask the client with a specific symptom or health concern to describe the problem in detail, including any suspected cause. Called a symptom or problem analysis, this technique promotes nurse-client collaboration and helps assess the client's coping ability. (For information on how to determine the scope of a client's symptoms, see *Symptom analysis*, page 46.) For a client who seeks health maintenance assessment, health counseling, or health education, expect to make few notes. Ask the client about recent minor illnesses or health concerns. A good way to begin with the well client is, "How would you describe your health status now?" or "What aspects of your health do you feel good about? What aspects don't you feel good about?" Also, determine the amount and frequency of regularly used nonprescription (over-the-counter) medications and find out whether the client has any communicable disease, such as herpes, hepatitis B, or acquired immunodeficiency syndrome (AIDS). If the client's interest is health promotion or counseling, elicit goal information by asking, "What do you hope to accomplish with health education?"

Past health status

An accurate, holistic client data base includes information about the client's past health, health promotion practices, and previous problems. To build this data base, record childhood and other illnesses, injuries, previous hospitalizations, surgical procedures, immunizations, allergies, and medications taken regularly.

Carefully note childhood diseases, such as measles, mumps, polio, chicken pox, strep throat, scarlet and rheumatic fever, frequent colds, ear infections, and asthma. Abbreviate the childhood illness section for elderly clients, but be sure to note a history of polio, rheumatic fever, and chicken pox (because of its link to herpes zoster—only persons who have had chicken pox can get this illness).

Symptom analysis

When assessing a client with a symptom or health concern, the nurse uses a symptom analysis to help the client describe the problem fully. A method for obtaining a systematic and thorough assessment, the symptom analysis is easy to remember with the mnemonic device, PQRST. The following questions serve as a guide to effective symptom analysis.

P	Q	R	S	T
PROVOCATIVE OR PALLIATIVE	**QUALITY OR QUANTITY**	**REGION OR RADIATION**	**SEVERITY SCALE**	**TIMING**
What causes the symptom? What makes it better or worse? • First occurrence. What were you doing when you first experienced or noticed the symptom? What seems to trigger it: stress? position? certain activities? arguments? (For a physical symptom such as a discharge: What seems to cause it or make it worse? For a psychological symptom: Does the depression occur when you feel rejected?) What relieves the symptom: changing diet? changing position? taking medication? being active? • Aggravation. What makes the symptom worse?	**How does the symptom feel, look, or sound? How much of it are you experiencing now?** • Quality. How would you describe the symptom—how it feels, looks, or sounds? • Quantity. How much are you experiencing now? Is it so much that it prevents you from performing any activities? Is it more or less than you experienced at any other time?	**Where is the symptom located? Does it spread?** • Region. Where does the symptom occur? • Radiation. In the case of pain, does it travel down your back or arms, up your neck, or down your legs?	**How does the symptom rate on a severity scale of 1 to 10, with 10 being the most extreme?** • Severity. How bad is the symptom at its worst? Does it force you to lie down, sit down, or slow down? • Course. Does the symptom seem to be getting better, getting worse, or staying about the same?	**When did the symptom begin? How often does it occur? Is it sudden or gradual?** • Onset. On what date did the symptom first occur? What time did it begin? • Type of onset. How did the symptom start: suddenly? gradually? • Frequency. How often do you experience the symptom: hourly? daily? weekly? monthly? When do you usually experience it: during the day? at night? in the early morning? Does it awaken you? Does it occur before, during, or after meals? Does it occur seasonally? • Duration. How long does an episode of the symptom last?

Also inquire about fractures, head injuries, and other accidents, and note whether the injury resulted in hospitalization. Record the reason for and dates of any hospitalization. Similarly, note any surgical procedures and related complications. Include approximate dates of all illnesses, injuries, surgeries, and hospitalizations.

If the client had a serious illness or was hospitalized, assess the psychological consequences by asking how the experience affected the client and family. Also record whether the client was ever treated for mental illness.

Include the dates and types of immunization in the past health status section. Particularly note childhood vaccinations, including latest tetanus vaccine and, especially for elderly clients, influenza and pneumonia immunizations.

Ask the client to name allergies and list any allergic responses, such as hives, rashes, wheezing, or anaphylaxis. Common allergens include foods, dust, pollen, molds, medications, and animal dander. Specify whether the client has ever received penicillin, other antibiotics, or a blood transfusion; all can cause life-threatening allergic responses.

Ask the client with a chronic disorder about medication and other regimens. For example, if the client has insulin-dependent diabetes, record the type, amount, and time of insulin administrations, as well as dietary restrictions, frequency of blood and urine monitoring, and typical activity patterns.

Also ask about foreign travel and military service to assess potential exposure to such health hazards as malaria or parasitic infections.

Family health status

Health information about the client's relatives also can unmask potential health problems. Some diseases may be genetically linked, such as cardiovascular disease, alcoholism, depression, and cancer. Others, such as hemophilia, cystic fibrosis, sickle-cell anemia, and Tay-Sachs disease, are genetically transmitted.

Determine the general health status of the client's immediate family members, including maternal and paternal grandparents, parents, siblings, aunts, uncles, and children. If any are deceased, record the year and cause of death. As previously discussed, the client's ethnic background may be important.

Begin the family history section by asking about the health of maternal and paternal grandparents. Then proceed through the client's immediate family, noting occurrences of diabetes, cancer, hypertension, obesity, cardiovascular disease, stroke, allergic disorders, genetically transmitted diseases, gout, tuberculosis, hemophilia, mental illness, epilepsy, and mental retardation.

Use a genogram to organize family history data. (For more informatioin, see *Developing a genogram,* page 48.) When developing a client's genogram, include half-siblings—a way to indicate parental divorce and remarriage. As a teaching tool, the genogram can help the client recognize potential health problems and take appropriate preventive action.

Status of physiologic systems

Data about the client's past and current physiologic status are another health history component. A careful assessment helps identify potential or undetected physiologic disorders.

Before beginning the review, prepare the client for specific questions about the past and current function and maintenance of each body system. Remember to perform a symptom analysis for any identified physiologic problem. Also remember to word questions so that they avoid complex technical language. For most clients, conduct the physiologic systems review in head-to-toe sequence.

For an elderly client with a lengthy history, focus on the recent past. Ask, for example, "Have you had problems with your heart in the last year?" Review previous records, if available, to avoid duplicating information already obtained. (For guidelines for questions to ask about each system, see *Assessing physiologic systems,* pages 49 through 51.)

At first, performing the physiologic systems review for a client with a complex medical history can be challenging. You may question which factors are significant or how the factual pieces relate to the whole picture, and you may have difficulty keeping the client with a complex medical history focused on the system being assessed. Assessing each physiologic system just for the presence or absence of specific problems or symptoms is not adequate; determine whether the problems affect the client's ability to carry out activities of daily living, and if so, whether the client can cope effectively with the resulting complications.

Developmental considerations

Human development is the continuous progression from earlier to later stages of maturation. This part of the health history allows the nurse and client to review and record the client's developmental stage and developmental changes. The following principles of normal human development are important for effective assessment.

- Development is patterned, orderly, and predictable with purpose and direction.
- Development is continuous throughout life, although the degree of change in many areas decreases after adolescence.
- Development can occur simultaneously in several areas (such as physically and socially). However, the rate of change in each area varies.
- Development proceeds from simple to complex. For example, an infant cries to gain attention, whereas an older child asks verbally for attention.
- The pace of development varies among individuals.
- Physical and mental stress during periods of critical developmental change, such as puberty, make a person particularly susceptible to outside stressors.

Assessment of the client's developmental status provides an overview of the client's growth, physical abilities and limitations, and cognitive abilities. The length of this section of the health history will vary

Developing a genogram

A genogram provides a visual summary of the health of the client, spouse, children, and parents. To develop a genogram, the nurse first draws the relationship of family members to the client, as shown in the illustration below, then fills in the ages of living members, and notes deceased members and the age at which they died. Also record any diseases that have a familial tendency (such as diabetes mellitus), a genetic tendency (such as Huntington's chorea), or an environmental cause (such as lung cancer from exposure to coal tar).

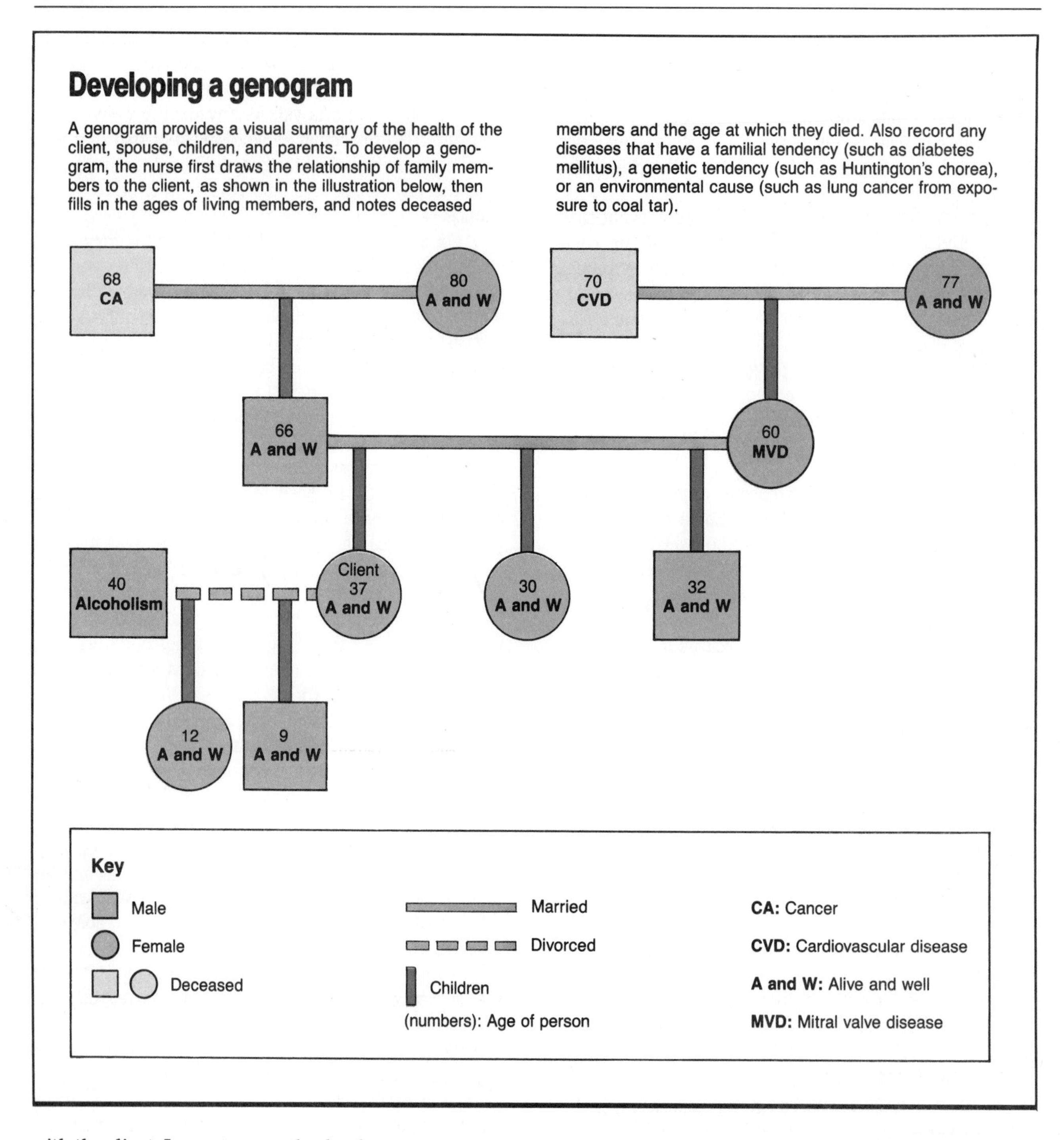

with the client. In most cases, the developmental section of a child's health history will be more detailed than an adult's.

Focus the client's physical development assessment on activities of daily living and the physical capacity to perform them. This is particularly important for elderly clients. (For additional information, see Chapter 5, Activities of Daily Living and Sleep Patterns.)

The assessment of cognitive abilities includes data about the client's thought processes, perceptions, comprehension, and ability to reason.

According to most cognitive developmental theorists, such as Piaget, adults should be able to think as well abstractly as concretely. (For a list of influential developmental theorists and the focus of their theories, see *Summary of cognitive developmental theories,* page 52. When using any of these theories to understand or integrate assessment findings, supplement this informa-

(Text continues on page 51.)

Assessing physiologic systems

When assessing a client's health and illness patterns, the nurse asks selected questions about the function of each body system. Use the phrases below as guidelines for the questions.

General health status

- ☐ Unusual symptoms or problems
- ☐ Excessive fatigue
- ☐ Inability to tolerate exercise
- ☐ Number of colds or other minor illnesses per year
- ☐ Unexplained episodes of fever, weakness, or night sweats
- ☐ Impaired ability to carry out activities of daily living (ADLs)

Skin, hair, and nails

- ☐ Known skin disease, such as psoriasis
- ☐ Itching
- ☐ Skin reaction to hot or cold weather
- ☐ Presence and location of scars, sores, ulcers
- ☐ Presence and location of skin growths such as warts, moles, tumors, or masses
- ☐ Color changes noted in any of the above lesions
- ☐ Changes in amount, texture, or character of hair
- ☐ Presence or development of baldness
- ☐ Hair care practices, including frequency of shampooing, permanent, or hair coloring
- ☐ Changes in nail color or texture
- ☐ Excessive nail splitting, cracking, or breaking

Head and neck

- ☐ Lumps, bumps, or scars from old injuries
- ☐ Headaches (Perform a symptom analysis.)
- ☐ Recent head trauma, injury, or surgery
- ☐ Concussion or unconsciousness from head injury
- ☐ Dizzy spells or fainting
- ☐ Interference with normal range of motion
- ☐ Pain or stiffness (Perform a symptom analysis.)
- ☐ Swelling or masses
- ☐ Enlarged lymph nodes or glands

Nose and sinuses

- ☐ History of frequent nosebleeds
- ☐ History of allergies
- ☐ Postnasal drip
- ☐ Frequent sneezing
- ☐ Frequent nasal drainage (Note color, frequency, and amount.)
- ☐ Impaired ability to smell
- ☐ Pain over the sinuses
- ☐ History of nasal trauma or fracture
- ☐ Difficulty breathing through nostrils
- ☐ History of sinus infection and treatment received

Mouth and throat

- ☐ History of frequent sore throats—especially streptococcal (Perform a symptom analysis.)
- ☐ Current or past mouth lesions, such as abscesses, ulcers, or sores
- ☐ History of oral herpes infections
- ☐ Date and results of last dental examination
- ☐ Overall description of dental health
- ☐ Use of proper dental hygiene, including fluoride toothpaste, where applicable
- ☐ Use of dentures or bridges
- ☐ Bleeding gums
- ☐ History of hoarseness
- ☐ Changes in voice quality
- ☐ Difficulty chewing or swallowing
- ☐ Changes in ability to taste

Eyes

- ☐ Date and results of last vision examination
- ☐ Date and results of last check for glaucoma (for clients over age 50 or with a family history of glaucoma)
- ☐ History of eye infections or eye trauma
- ☐ Use of corrective lenses
- ☐ Itching, tearing, or discharge (Note color, amount, and time of occurrence as well as treatment received.)
- ☐ Eye pain; spots or floaters in visual field
- ☐ History of glaucoma or cataracts
- ☐ Blurred or double vision
- ☐ Unusual sensations, such as twitching
- ☐ Light sensitivity
- ☐ Swelling around eyes or eyelids
- ☐ Visual disturbances, such as rainbows around lights, blind spots, or flashing lights
- ☐ History of retinal detachment
- ☐ History of strabismus or amblyopia

Ears

- ☐ Date and results of last hearing evaluation
- ☐ Abnormal sensitivity to noise
- ☐ Ear pain
- ☐ Ringing or crackling in the ears
- ☐ Recent changes in hearing ability
- ☐ Use of hearing aids
- ☐ History of ear infection
- ☐ History of vertigo
- ☐ Feeling of fullness in the ear
- ☐ Ear care habits, including use of cotton-tipped swabs for ear wax removal
- ☐ Ear wax characteristics
- ☐ Number of ear infections per year (for pediatric clients)

continued

Assessing physiologic systems continued

Respiratory system

- ☐ History of asthma or other breathing problem (Perform a symptom analysis.)
- ☐ Chronic cough (Perform a symptom analysis.)
- ☐ History of coughing up blood
- ☐ Breathing problems after physical exertion
- ☐ Sputum production (Note color, odor, and amount.)
- ☐ Wheezing or noisy respirations
- ☐ History of pneumonia or bronchitis

Cardiovascular system

- ☐ History of chest pain
- ☐ History of palpitations
- ☐ History of heart murmur
- ☐ History of irregular pulses
- ☐ Hypertension
- ☐ Need to sit up to breathe, especially at night
- ☐ Coldness or numbness in extremities
- ☐ Color changes in fingers or toes
- ☐ Swelling or edema in extremities
- ☐ Leg pain when walking; relieved by rest
- ☐ Hair loss on legs

Breasts

- ☐ Date and results of last breast examination (including mammography for women over age 40)
- ☐ Pattern of breast self-examination
- ☐ Breast pain, tenderness, or swelling (Perform a symptom analysis.)
- ☐ History of nipple changes or nipple discharge (Note color, odor, amount, and frequency.)
- ☐ History of breast-feeding

Gastrointestinal system

- ☐ Indigestion or pain associated with eating (Perform a symptom analysis.)
- ☐ History of ulcers
- ☐ History of vomiting blood
- ☐ Burning sensation in esophagus
- ☐ Frequent nausea and vomiting (Perform a symptom analysis.)
- ☐ History of liver disease
- ☐ History of jaundice
- ☐ History of gallbladder disease
- ☐ Abdominal swelling or ascites
- ☐ Changes in bowel elimination pattern
- ☐ Stool characteristics
- ☐ History of diarrhea or constipation
- ☐ History of hemorrhoids
- ☐ Use of digestive aids or laxatives
- ☐ Date and results of last Hemoccult exam (for clients over age 50)

Urinary system

- ☐ Painful urination
- ☐ Characteristics of urine
- ☐ Pattern of urination
- ☐ Hesitancy in starting urine stream
- ☐ Changes in urine stream
- ☐ History of kidney stones
- ☐ History of flank pain
- ☐ Blood in urine
- ☐ History of decreased or excessive urine output
- ☐ Dribbling, incontinence, or stress incontinence
- ☐ Frequent urination at night
- ☐ Difficulty with toilet training (for children)
- ☐ Bed-wetting (for children)
- ☐ History of bladder or kidney infections
- ☐ History of urinary tract infections

Female reproductive system

- ☐ Menstrual history, including age of onset, duration, and amount of flow
- ☐ Date of last menstrual period
- ☐ Painful menstruation
- ☐ History of excessive menstrual bleeding
- ☐ History of missed periods
- ☐ History of bleeding between periods
- ☐ Date and results of last Pap smear
- ☐ Obstetrical history (for women of childbearing age), including number of pregnancies, miscarriages, abortions, live births, and stillbirths
- ☐ Satisfaction with sexual performance
- ☐ History of painful intercourse
- ☐ Contraceptive practices
- ☐ History of sexually transmitted disease
- ☐ Knowledge of how to prevent sexually transmitted disease, including acquired immunodeficiency syndrome (AIDS)
- ☐ Problems with infertility

Male reproductive system

- ☐ Presence of penile lesions
- ☐ Presence of scrotal lesions
- ☐ Prostate problems
- ☐ Pattern of testicular self-examination
- ☐ Satisfaction with sexual performance
- ☐ History of venereal disease
- ☐ Contraceptive practices
- ☐ Knowledge of how to prevent sexually transmitted disease, including AIDS
- ☐ Concern about impotence
- ☐ Concern about sterility

Assessing physiologic systems continued

Nervous system

- ☐ History of fainting or loss of consciousness
- ☐ History of seizures or other nervous system problems; use of medication for seizure control
- ☐ History of cognitive disturbances, including recent or remote memory loss, hallucinations, disorientation, speech and language dysfunction, or inability to concentrate
- ☐ History of sensory disturbances, including tingling, numbness, sensory loss
- ☐ History of motor problems, including problems with gait, balance, coordination, tremor, spasm, or paralysis
- ☐ Interference by cognitive, sensory, or motor symptoms with ADLs

Musculoskeletal system

- ☐ General health status
- ☐ History of fractures
- ☐ Muscle cramping, twitching, pain, or weakness (Perform a symptom analysis.)
- ☐ Limitations on walking, running, or participating in sports
- ☐ Joint swelling, redness, or pain
- ☐ Joint deformity
- ☐ Joint stiffness, including time and duration
- ☐ Noise with joint movement
- ☐ Spinal deformity
- ☐ Chronic back pain (Perform a symptom analysis.)
- ☐ Musculoskeletal-related interference with ADLs

Immune system and blood

- ☐ History of anemia
- ☐ History of bleeding tendencies
- ☐ History of easy bruising
- ☐ History of low platelet count
- ☐ History of becoming easily fatigued
- ☐ History of blood transfusion
- ☐ History of allergies, including eczema, hives, and itching
- ☐ Chronic clear nasal discharge
- ☐ Frequent sneezing
- ☐ Conjunctivitis
- ☐ Interference of allergies with ADLs
- ☐ Usual method for treating allergic symptoms
- ☐ History of frequent unexplained systemic infections
- ☐ Unexplained gland swelling

Endocrine system

- ☐ History of endocrine disease, such as thyroid problems, adrenal problems, or diabetes
- ☐ Unexplained changes in height or weight
- ☐ Increased thirst
- ☐ Increased urinary output
- ☐ Increased food intake
- ☐ Heat or cold intolerance
- ☐ History of goiter
- ☐ Unexplained weakness
- ☐ Previous hormone therapy
- ☐ Changes in hair distribution
- ☐ Changes in skin pigmentation

tion with further reading.) Because adults can develop effective coping strategies and problem-solving skills, obtain additional cognitive development data by assessing the client's mastery of these skills.

Educational background data provide some information about cognitive abilities; the client's communication style and ability to respond verbally provide more information. Certain mental and physical disorders can cause cognitive impairments. If the client's responses suggest cognitive impairment, perform a mental status assessment.

Health promotion and protection patterns

What a client does (or does not do) to stay healthy is affected by such factors as health beliefs, personal habits, sleep and wake patterns, exercise and activity, recreation, nutrition, stress and coping, socioeconomic status, environmental health patterns, and occupational health patterns. To help assess health promotion and protection patterns, ask the client to describe a typical day. The response can provide valuable data on health behaviors and life-style patterns. Actively listen for indications of stress at home or work, and determine whether the client's schedule is reasonable. Although data will overlap, be sure to assess all (or most) elements, depending on the client.

Health beliefs

For the most part, a client's health beliefs are culturally and religiously defined and built on learning and personal experiences with health and illness. Perceptions of health affect comprehension of and compliance with health care recommendations. A client may exhibit various behaviors—not all healthful, such as alcohol or tobacco consumption. The role of the nurse is not to judge or criticize these practices, but rather to inform the client of potential consequences of unhealthful activities and to offer help to change unhealthful habits only if requested.

Ask the following questions to elicit data about a client's health beliefs:

- What are your ideas about health?
- What do you do routinely to stay healthy?

Summary of cognitive developmental theories

Knowledge of the various developmental theories provides the nurse with a framework for cultural and psychosocial assessment. The chart below lists selected developmental theorists and summarizes the focus of their theories.

THEORIST	THEORY FOCUS
Sigmund Freud	Psychosexual. Biological drives influence a person's psychological and personality development.
Erik Erikson	Psychosocial. The human life cycle is composed of eight developmental stages, each containing a developmental crisis to be resolved. Psychosocial strengths emerge with resolution of the crisis.
Abraham Maslow	Self-actualization. People are innately motivated toward psychological growth, self-awareness, and personal freedom. Basic needs must be met before a person can advance to higher needs.
Jean Piaget	Cognitive development. An individual's knowledge comes from the interaction between genetic potential and culturally influenced environmental experiences.
Lawrence Kohlberg	Moral development. Cognitive development and emotional growth affect the individual's ability to make autonomous decisions.
Carol Gilligan	Moral development from a female perspective. Women have moral concern for others based on their innate nurturing instincts. They maintain social rules and the expectations of families, social groups, or culture.
Robert Butler	Life review. Elderly clients spend time reviewing past events and concentrating on past conflicts. This life review correlates with the elderly client's good long-term memory.
Robert Peck	Psychosocial. This theory emphasizes aspects of development from middle age through old age by dividing Erikson's last stage into two parts. There is a developmental crisis to be resolved in each part.
Robert Havighurst	Activity during aging. Elderly clients who stay active and maintain or find substitutes for activities of middle age are more satisfied with life than elderly clients who do not. Diminished activity is equated with increased social isolation and accelerated physical decline.
Elaine Cumming and William Henry	Disengagement during aging. A person naturally gives up roles (a career, for example) and undergoes losses (through death) as aging occurs. As losses occur, a person withdraws from the high activity level of middle age. At the same time, society withdraws from the elderly client to avoid assigning crucial roles to a group with a high death rate. This mutual disengagement helps society and the elderly client prepare for death.
Evelyn Duvall	Family development. Family goes through identifiable stages with tasks to be mastered.

- What are your expectations of health care professionals?
- What are your responsibilities as a health care consumer?
- Can you describe any positive experiences you've had with the health care system?
- Can you describe any negative experiences you've had with the health care system?
- When do you consider yourself to be ill?
- In what ways do you treat your own illnesses?

Personal habits

Assess tobacco use, alcohol consumption, and prescription and nonprescription drug use specifically, because these activities obviously affect healthy functioning.

If the client uses tobacco, inquire about pipes, cigars, cigarettes (filtered or nonfiltered), and chewing tobacco, as well as the amount of tobacco consumed daily and length of time the client has used tobacco. Also assess how stress affects the client's tobacco consumption.

If the client drinks alcohol, determine which type (beer, wine, mixed drinks) and how much (per week or day). Also find out how long (months or years) the client has consumed alcohol. Ask how the client's alcohol intake compares with that of others. Identify any relationship between stress and alcohol intake. Also identify the client's concern about drinking patterns. Find out if the client's drinking pattern has changed over the last 5 years. If so, is the client drinking more or less?

Because caffeine may harm the cardiovascular and other systems, determine how many caffeine-containing products (coffee, tea, cola, chocolate) the client consumes regularly, and how long the client has been consuming them. Ask if the client notices any caffeine-related physiologic effects, such as palpitations, nervousness, or sleeplessness.

While assessing the client's tobacco, alcohol, and caffeine intake, also find out how the client uses drugs. Determine which drugs the client takes—whether prescription, nonprescription, or recreational drugs—and the reasons for taking them. Explore specific nonprescription drug use, especially of aspirin, laxatives, antacids, vitamins, and cold remedies. A client who does not define these as medications may consider them harmless and use them excessively.

Sleep and wake patterns

First, determine the client's ideal sleep and wake pattern; that is, whether the client is a "day" or a "night" person. This reflects the client's circadian rhythm, which is one of several biological rhythms subject to individual differences. (For more information, see Chapter 5, Activities of Daily Living and Sleep Patterns.) Next, ask how much sleep the client needs to feel rested. Then, determine how much sleep the client actually gets, and compare it with the ideal amount.

If the client has difficulty falling or staying asleep, find out what factors the client thinks might be responsible. Inquire about dreams and recurring dreams to reveal clues about the client's psychological health and stress levels.

Defining the client's sleep and wake cycle also helps determine whether the client has a sleep disorder, such as narcolepsy (involuntary attacks of sleep), sleep apnea (airway blockage during sleep), or sleep deprivation. All three conditions impair the client's regular sleep and wake cycle; the first two may be life-threatening, and the third may lead to irritability and, if prolonged, psychosis.

Exercise and activity

Exercise and activity patterns have physiologic and psychological health implications. Physiologic effects include musculoskeletal, cardiovascular, and respiratory fitness along with maintenance of ideal weight. Exercise and activity can reduce stress, especially for workers in sedentary, high-pressure occupations. However, some people who exercise compulsively can increase rather than decrease their stress levels.

First, determine the client's satisfaction with current activity and exercise levels. Ask what activities the client performs and for how long. Find out if the client's physical tolerance is limited by any physiologic conditions, such as angina. Next, record the activity level and frequency. For a client who exercises by walking, for example, record the distance walked, speed of walking, and amount of time spent. Make similar evaluations for other activities. (*Note:* Ask what safety precautions the client uses in potentially hazardous sports. This information helps when planning safety education.)

Recreation

Include recreational pattern assessment in the health history to help evaluate the client's social roles and relationships. Clients with no recreational activities or hobbies are less likely to enjoy social, emotional, and physical health. Conversely, those who spend excessive time with hobbies or recreational activities may be escaping work or family problems. Assess recreational patterns by asking which activities the client prefers for fun and relaxation. Also ask if the client spends as much time as desired on recreational activities. Whether the client participates in recreational activities with others can reveal information about social relationships. (For more information, see Chapter 5, Activities of Daily Living and Sleep Patterns.)

Nutrition

Nutrition affects many body systems, including the integumentary, hematologic, and musculoskeletal systems. It can be affected by physical and psychological disorders. For example, a client with a gastrointestinal disorder that causes nausea may avoid eating; a client with anorexia nervosa may avoid eating because of an overwhelming fear of being fat. (For more information, see Chapter 6, Nutritional Status.)

Perform in-depth nutritional assessments for infants, adolescents, pregnant clients, and elderly clients. First, ask the client about diet, eating habits, use of vitamin and mineral supplements, and satisfaction with body weight. Ask the client to describe meals and snack patterns, and find out which family members buy the groceries and which ones plan and cook the meals. Determine if any health conditions or cultural, ethnic, or religious customs cause the client to alter his or her diet. Finding out whether the client can afford to buy food or can get to the market also is an important consideration in the nutritional assessment.

Ask the client which items are routinely eaten from the five basic food groups: meat, grain, dairy, vegetables, and fruits. Information about the number of servings and the serving size is also important.

Stress and coping

Demands on the body, including emotional, physical, and social demands, cause stress. The amount of stress the client experiences affects physiologic and psychological health. Everyone experiences some stress, whether work-related, health-related, economic, family, social, or interpersonal. A person usually can identify and describe the cause of stress, which may be real or perceived as real. (*Note:* Anxiety differs from stress. It is a less specific response, which the client describes as a sense of threat or dread from an unrecognized source.) Believed to be a causative factor in hypertension, coronary artery disease, and gastrointestinal problems, stress and ineffective coping strategies also affect such social behaviors as domestic violence and substance abuse.

Selye (1956) developed the classic theory for assessing stress when he proposed a three-stage response model called the General Adaptation Syndrome. According to Selye, a stressor—physiologic or psychological—activates immediate neurologic, life-preserving "flight or fight" reactions. This is the *alarm* stage. In the second stage, called the *resistance* stage, the body strives to adapt to the stressor and return to a state of equilibrium. The responses can be functional or dysfunctional and include physiologic signs and symptoms—such as tachycardia (heart rate over 100 beats/minute), nausea, or a stiff neck—or psychological signs and symptoms—such as depression or fatigue. If every response fails despite the body's repeated efforts to adapt to the stressor, the third stage, *exhaustion,* occurs, which can lead to death.

Unusual life experiences, both positive and negative, cause stress and therefore affect health. Holmes and Rahe (1967) demonstrated a relationship between the amount of recent stress in a person's life and the likelihood of that person's becoming ill in the near future. Moreover, the greater the amount of stress, the greater the risk for illness, especially a serious illness. Recent studies indicate that even anticipating a stressful event has the same negative effect. However, other studies show that preventive interventions can help people lessen the negative influence of stress by learning to cope or by alleviating the stressor. The more individuals understand about the causes, characteristics, and effective coping strategies for stress, the more they can minimize its effects.

People manage stress, solve problems, and make decisions by using coping strategies. Usually selected by an individual because of past effectiveness, a coping strategy may be action-oriented or psychologically based. For example, a client who responds to stress by developing headaches may learn to relax and cope by using deep-breathing and temple massage techniques.

The following list provides examples of action-oriented and psychologically based coping strategies:

- using relaxation techniques—meditation, biofeedback, self-hypnosis
- engaging in physical exercise
- participating in an aggressive sport
- developing cognitive problem solving
- identifying and then altering or eliminating the stressor
- talking about the problem with a close friend or relative
- finding humor in the situation
- sharing stressful roles with a significant other
- gathering information
- praying or seeking religious support
- seeking professional help.

Another coping strategy is using defense mechanisms. Defense mechanisms are habitual, automatic avoidance reactions to a threat or a crisis. Traditionally, psychologists considered their use as a negative or non-adaptive coping strategy. However, some experts now think that defense mechanisms, such as denial, may provide short-term protection for a body under life-threatening stress. For example, a person could suffer a myocardial infarction while driving in heavy traffic, but could deny what is happening and drive safely home.

In a crisis, people tend to revert automatically to certain coping strategies that worked in the past. Help the client become aware of these coping strategies by investigating which ones have worked well. Help the client with a high stress level and ineffective coping strategies by introducing various stress-reduction programs. Determine whether stress management is a problem area, and help the client understand how healthy coping contributes to well-being.

The following questions can help assess stress and coping strategies:

- How do you know when you are feeling stressed?
- What situations are stressful to you?
- How do you respond physically to stress? For example, do you sweat, get butterflies in your stomach, develop a headache, or become nauseated?
- What do you do when you are feeling stressed?
- Does stress ever affect your family relationships or your work? If so, how?
- What stresses have you experienced during the past year?
- How did you deal with these stresses?
- Did these stresses cause significant changes for you?
- Do you think stress affects your health?

Socioeconomic status

The client's socioeconomic status can directly affect health behaviors by determining the amount of financial resources available for health care and a healthful lifestyle, including adequate housing, clothing, and nutrition. For example, a client whose insurance plan does not reimburse routine health screening and physical examinations usually seeks health care only for illness. Similarly, a client whose financial resources barely meet basic needs is less likely to use services designed to promote or maintain health.

Assess health-related socioeconomic factors by asking such questions as:

- Do you have health insurance for yourself and your family?
- Does your insurance pay for routine physical or other screening procedures?
- Do you worry about your financial situation?
- Is your income sufficient to pay for food, housing, and clothing?
- Is your income sufficient to pay for extras like recreation and baby-sitting?
- Are you receiving financial aid?

If a client has financial problems, a referral to a community or social service agency for assistance may be indicated.

Environmental health patterns

An assessment of health promotion and protection must investigate ways in which the client's environment affects healthful living. For instance, if the client is exposed to health hazards at home, work, or school, help plan corrective action, if possible, or anticipate potential problems. Assessment questions for a client living in a rural area differ from those for a client from a large city. Potential rural health hazards include polluted water sources, sewers, or septic systems; respiratory disorders caused by grain dust or pesticides; and the lack of nearby health care facilities. Potential urban hazards include air and noise pollution, toxic wastes, limited living space, and poor office lighting and ventilation, among others.

The following questions can help evaluate the client's environmental health risks and concerns:

- Is your total living space adequate?
- Do you have adequate space for personal privacy?
- Does your home have adequate light, heat, water, and ventilation?
- Is the noise level in your home acceptable and comfortable?
- What do you do to avoid safety hazards?
- Are the colors in your home relaxing and aesthetically pleasing?
- How do you view your relationships with those who share your home?
- How would you describe your neighborhood?
- Is your neighborhood adequately lighted?
- How accessible are police, fire, and ambulance services?
- How accessible are grocery stores, drug stores, and health care facilities?
- How accessible is private or public transportation?
- Is the neighborhood aesthetically acceptable?
- Does your community offer senior centers or other resources that help residents meet basic health, social, and ecomonic needs?
- Do you have any special concerns about pollution or other environmental issues? If so, what are they?
- Do you take any steps to reduce environmental risks for yourself, your family, or your community? If so, what do you do?
- What effects do weather and climate have on your respiratory health?
- How does the weather or season affect your mood?

Another environmental health consideration is safety in the home. Find out if the client uses smoke alarms, fire extinguishers, and burglar alarms and if the client practices fire drills. Also, ask about other safety factors in the home. Keep in mind that throw rugs and carelessly placed extension cords pose hazards for pediatric and elderly clients or others with osteoporosis, poor vision, or both. Uncovered electrical outlets and improperly stored cleaning supplies and medications are well-known hazards for children. Also ask if the client uses seat belts or, for a child, a car seat.

Occupational health patterns

The client's occupation may present potential physiologic and psychological health risks. To assess the risks, determine whether the occupation requires safety equipment, such as protective headgear, eyeshields, special clothing, or a respirator. Inquire about the availability of health benefits, such as insurance, sick leave, and vacation benefits. Also assess the amount of job-related stress the client experiences. Be aware of occupations that pose extreme health risks, such as mining, asbestos manufacturing, and production of PCPs, pesticides, solvents, plastics, anesthetics, and other dangerous substances.

The following sample questions can help assess the client's occupational health:

- How would you describe your current job?
- Are you happy with your current job? What do you like and dislike about it?
- How many hours a week do you work?
- How much time does your job allow for meals and rest?
- Are you satisfied with your salary?
- How far do you travel to and from work?

- Are you aware of any health or safety hazards associated with your job? What do you do to reduce or prevent them?
- Does your job involve exposure to radiation, pesticides, heavy metals, asbestos, or dangerous chemicals?
- Do you experience any job-related stresses? If so, how would you describe them?
- How many jobs have you had in the last 5 years?
- How would you describe your ideal job? How does this differ from your current job?

For clients who have retired, list former occupations, note any potential health hazards, and inquire about adjustment to retirement. Ask a homemaker client to describe a typical day. If the homemaker also cares for children, determine whether the schedule includes sufficient time away from them. For a parent who works outside the home, assess stress levels caused by insufficient time spent with the children. For a school-age client, ask about school and activities.

Other tools to help assess client health behaviors include health-risk appraisals and stress-level indicators, such as the Holmes and Rahe inventory.

Role and relationship patterns

A client's role and relationship patterns reflect the client's psychosocial (psychological, emotional, social, spiritual, and sexual) health. To assess role and relationship patterns, investigate the client's self-concept, cultural influences, religious influences, family role and relationship patterns, sexuality and reproductive patterns, social support patterns, and other psychosocial considerations. Each of these patterns can influence the client's health.

Self-concept

Self-concept refers to ideas, feelings, and attitudes that compose a person's identity, worth, capabilities, and limitations. The values and opinions of others, especially those provided during the early childhood years, play an important role in self-concept development.

A client's positive or negative values and perceptions of how others feel about him or her significantly influence behavior. For example, if a client who is age 50 thinks that 50 is "over the hill" and longs to be 30, then the client may feel old and act old. Because of these attitudes and actions, others may see and treat the client as old, and the client may actually age more quickly.

Related to self-concept, locus of control is an individual's perception of what or who controls the events and forces affecting life. Some people feel controlled externally: they think that God, fate, other people, experts, or powerful forces shape their lives. Other people feel controlled internally: they accept primary responsibility for their lives. In turn, this provides them with a feeling of power.

Assess locus of control when helping a client plan for life changes. If the client strongly believes in self-responsibility, providing information about appropriate health care may prove adequate. This allows the client to take charge and to choose the best method for achieving the desired health goals. For example, the nurse can tell the client with high blood pressure to exercise and lose weight; educational materials provided by the nurse can then help the client decide the best way to meet those goals. On the other hand, a client with an external locus of control may need constant urging and encouragement to participate in a program for lowering blood pressure and may need a support group to provide the required external control.

Because self-concept and locus of control affect each client's viewpoint, they can affect health in various ways. For example, a client with a healthy self-concept may form relationships easily, experience fewer problems with depression, and have fewer somatic complaints.

The following questions help assess the client's self-concept:

- How satisfied are you with your current age? What age would you most like to be right now? Why?
- How satisfied are you with your physical appearance?
- What do you like best about your body? What do you like least?
- In relation to other people your age, would you say that you have about the same, more, or less physical stamina and health? How important is this to you?
- In relation to other people your age, would you say that you have about the same, more, or less ability to think and reason well? How important is this to you?
- In relation to other people your age, would you say that you have about the same, more, or less satisfaction in family relationships? How important is this to you?
- Would you say that you are an outgoing person who has many friends and acquaintances, a person who is somewhere between outgoing and shy who has some friends and acquaintances, or a shy, retiring person who has only a few friends and acquaintances? How does this compare with the person you would like to be?
- In relation to other people your age, would you say that you have about the same, more, or less emotional stability?
- What are your strengths and weaknesses?

A client with a healthy self-concept and body image will usually describe more positive personality characteristics than negative ones. However, be wary of responses that contain all negative or all positive characteristics. Further assessment may be needed in this case.

Cultural influences

Culture can profoundly affect a client's views of life and death as well as the client's health beliefs, health habits, roles, relationships, family dynamics, and dietary habits. For example, clients from some cultures resist seeking health care or taking responsibility for changing behaviors that cause health problems because they feel powerless to control their illness, which they may consider punishment for some wrongdoing. Assessment of cultural influences can evaluate these health-related factors as well as identify culturally related strengths, such as a strong family unit.

Assessment of cultural influences is especially useful when the nurse suspects that culture may be affecting the client's health care. For example, a cultural assessment may be invaluable if a client has difficulty understanding English, or if a client has previously sought treatment from a healer, such as shaman or curandero, instead of a health care professional.

To learn how culture affects a client, begin by identifying the client's cultural background. Then ask the questions below to assess the effect of culture on a client's health and to identify potential health problems. Rather than asking all of these questions during every assessment, use the questions as a guide. Vary the depth and number of questions based on the client's answers.

To assess the client's cultural identity, ask these questions:

- To what cultural group do you belong?
- In what country were you born?
- In what country were your parents born?
- If you were raised in North America, were you raised in an ethnic community related to your cultural background?
- How closely do you associate with your ethnic group?
- Is your life-style or belief system different from that of most people in your community? If so, how?

Definitions of health and illness, the selection of health care professionals, and health promotion and protection patterns differ among cultural groups. Clients from some cultural groups believe that another person can wish them ill or that God tests or punishes them with illness. Also, the client's response to physical symptoms varies according to culture, as does the choice of home remedies or the selection of practitioners.

To assess the client's beliefs about health and illness, ask these questions:

- How do you define health?
- How do you define illness?
- What do you believe causes illness?
- What do you believe causes mental illness?
- Do you consider yourself healthy?
- What do you do to stay healthy?
- When do you consider yourself sick?
- What do you do to get better when you are sick?
- What do you do to get better when you are mentally ill?
- Who do you go to when you are sick?
- If you go to a cultural healer, how often do you go?
- Who are the healers in your culture?
- What do the healers tell you to do?

Evaluate the responses to determine the appropriateness of additional questioning. For example, if the client says a healer gave medical advice, ask the client about the advice and its effectiveness. Then ask how the client would feel about trying a treatment prescribed by a physician.

To evaluate the cultural impact on health promotion and protection patterns, ask the client the following questions:

- Does your family follow any special nutritional practices or dietary restrictions?
- What types of food do you usually eat?
- What dietary changes are common in your family during illness? Pregnancy? Old age?

To assess the effects of culture on role and relationship patterns and other psychosocial factors, pose the following questions:

- Who do you consider your family?
- How important to you is your family?
- What are the traditional roles of family members in your culture? Who does what tasks in your family?
- In your family, who takes care of infants and children? Women during childbirth? New mothers? Ill persons? Elderly people? People who are dying?
- How are decisions made in your family?
- What do you believe about marriage?
- What do you believe about child rearing?
- What place do elderly relatives have in your life?
- How important to you is privacy?
- What actions do you take to get privacy when you need it?
- How important to you is your personal property? How important to you is the personal property of others?
- What degree of physical closeness to another person is comfortable for you? How does it differ if the person is a family member, a close friend, a stranger, or a member of the opposite sex?
- What traditions are associated with puberty?
- How do you view a menstruating woman?
- What rules govern sexual activity for a man? For a woman?
- How do you view conception and pregnancy?
- What traditions are associated with childbirth?
- Is the sex of a baby important? Are girl and boy infants treated differently? If so, how?

- How do you view a nursing mother?
- Do you think you should try to control the environment or live in harmony with it?
- What do you think is the meaning of life?
- What do you think about death?
- How important to you is moving up in society?
- What do you think about the past?
- What do you think about the present?
- What do you think about the future?
- How important to you is punctuality?

Make a note of the client's role and relationship patterns. These patterns may be vital to the client's health. For example, a client may not require outside help while recuperating from an illness if members of an extended family are willing to learn to care for the client.

Throughout the cultural assessment, also note any practices that may affect the client's health. Once information about cultural practices is gathered, you have several options:

- If the practice is harmful as based on nursing theory, gently discourage it.
- If the practice is not harmful and the client finds it helpful, encourage the client to continue the practice and suggest ways to incorporate it into the traditional health care plan.
- If the practice is questionable, be cautious about encouraging its continued use, but do not discourage its use.

Spiritual and religious influences

For many people, religion or a spiritual belief system is the most important aspect of life. Spirituality (personal definition of the purpose and meaning of one's life, the world, and the cosmos) may assign meaning to individual and community life, guide daily behavior and life-style, define acceptable health care, and dictate attitudes toward death. A holistic health framework regards an individual as a balance among the components of body, mind, and spirit, all of which act interdependently.

Religion is the component of spirituality that includes a belief in a divine power or being. A religious system usually embraces more specific beliefs, including codified and prescribed behaviors, rituals, or practices that express the person's faith in those beliefs.

A client's health beliefs and practices may be linked closely to religion. For example, a Jehovah's Witness may refuse to accept blood transfusions or blood products for family members, even in life-threatening situations. A Jewish client may want a *mohel* rather than an obstetrician to perform infant circumcision, a Judaic religious rite. Some religions, such as Roman Catholicism, require last rites (anointing the critically ill or injured). Many require baptism of a sick infant. (For more information, see *Beliefs of major world religions,* pages 60 and 61.)

Religious beliefs may affect the health history by determining how comfortable the client feels answering questions on such topics as elimination, sexuality, and family life. The nurse may modify potentially offensive health history sections to promote client cooperation and recognize client sensitivities. Although the beliefs and practices of some religious groups may be difficult to understand, never actively disparage or disregard these beliefs and practices. Instead, try to understand them and, when possible, consider them when conducting the health history interview. Recognize the difficulty of understanding religious beliefs that differ from your own. Awareness of personal values and biases will help you avoid appearing insincere, insensitive, or judgmental.

Keep in mind that a client may not practice any form of organized religion, yet may be spiritual. For example, a client may not believe in a God, but may believe in universal order and the interrelatedness of all living things.

The client may not be aware of how a spiritual assessment relates to health care. Explain that personal views of the individual, health, and illness as well as religious beliefs affect health care practices, and that expressing those views will facilitate their inclusion into a personalized care plan.

Because spiritual and religious beliefs are personal, wait until rapport and a trusting relationship are established with the client before asking too many questions about them. Asking if the client would like to see the facility's chaplain or another clergyperson is always appropriate. If the client expresses an interest, you may ask the following questions to assess spiritual and religious beliefs:

- What relationship do you believe exists between spiritual beliefs and health or illness?
- What do you believe causes ill health?
- What do you believe heals ill health?
- What are your spiritual beliefs about birth, illness, crisis, and death?
- Have any events affected these beliefs? If so, how?
- What are your sources of hope and strength?
- What are your sources of joy?
- What are your sources of peace and harmony?
- Do you belong to a church or follow a particular religion?
- Which spiritual or religious beliefs and practices are of particular importance to you, if any?
- Who is the most important person to help you spiritually?
- Is that person available in a crisis?

- Who else would be helpful in a crisis?
- Would you feel comfortable asking a health care professional for spiritual help?

Family role and relationship patterns

Until the past few decades in North America, the term *family* defined the traditional nuclear family: mother, father, dependent children, and possibly grandparents. Today, however, family structure has changed, making the definition of family much more challenging. For example, a child today could be born into a family with two parents and perhaps a sibling, spend part of his youth in a single-parent family, and a later part in a restructured family with a stepparent and step-siblings. Some couples, married or unmarried, are committed to each other but do not desire children. A homosexual couple also may have a permanent relationship and may care for children. A single mother may raise her children in her parents' home. A useful definition of family, therefore, must be broad. For example, Murray and Zentner (1985) define the family as a primary group consisting of two or more persons who live together and are related by blood, marriage, adoption, or a long-standing agreement. Family members share personal contact, affection, love, harmony, competition, mutual concerns, a continuity of past, present, and future goals, identity, behaviors, and rituals. Within the family, an individual can usually confide thoughts and feelings and be more natural and relaxed than with other people.

When health care focuses on an individual client, the opportunity to assess the family may be limited. Nevertheless, the nurse usually will have to assess the family from the client's perspective. A nurse employed in an institutional or office setting, however, may see family members often enough to gain a broader perspective on the family dynamics and resources that may influence their health and illness. Home health care settings provide a unique opportunity to observe the family's interactions.

Despite its changes in form, the term *family* has endured because it is more a term of function than of structure. According to Friedman (1986), family functions include these five domains:

- Affective—to let family members express emotions, which allows psychological needs to be met.
- Socialization and social placement—to socialize children, making them productive members of society; to confer status on family members.
- Reproductive—to insure family continuity over the generations, and societal survival.
- Economic—to provide sufficient economic resources and to allocate them effectively.
- Health care—to provide life-style practices, such as dietary habits, sleep and rest, exercise and activity, and routine health maintenance, such as immunizations and dental care.

A nursing assessment of the family examines the client's relationships and functions within the family and within other social groups. The assessment also explores the other family members' roles and relationships and studies the family's stressors, coping mechanisms, and values and beliefs about health care. Furthermore, the family assessment explores how an alteration in the client's health affects the family's functioning and it examines the family's ability to meet the basic needs of its members.

Identifying a family's roles will help the nurse discover how a family functions and how the family affects the client. Society creates roles—positions that fulfill certain functions and include certain attitudes and behaviors. Each culture defines particular roles, and each member usually understands the expectations of the other members' roles. Over time, the expected behaviors and attitudes may become specific and rigid.

In some of today's families, roles are relatively flexible. Family members may switch roles or share roles, such as parenting or housekeeping. To perform a role assessment, first identify the family's roles and who performs them. Next, examine how well each individual performs the role, how that individual feels about performing it, and how the family feels about that individual's role.

Although assessing family relationships may be the most important part of the assessment, it can be the most difficult to obtain, especially when relying on the client for all the information. The data are highly subjective and depend on the client's perceived roles in the family and satisfaction with those roles.

Important assessment topics include communication, mutual support, respect, power, sharing, and competition. Different family members may describe these aspects differently. When an individual interview is your only means of obtaining data, word questions carefully and seek clarification to minimize client subjectivity. When assessing family relationships, ask the client to give descriptions or examples. This minimizes defensiveness or the desire to give the "right" answer. Some questions may require further discussion to provide enough information for an adequate assessment. (For sample questions about family functions, roles, and relationships, see *Assessing the family,* page 62.)

Sexuality and reproductive patterns

The client's beliefs and attitudes about sexuality and reproduction directly bear on role and relationship pat-

Beliefs of major world religions

Interwoven with cultural influences are religious or spiritual beliefs that may foster customs and beliefs about health and illness, diet, and family roles.

The chart below provides the nurse with information about major world religions (arranged alphabetically) and their influences on beliefs. This information can help the nurse assess the client's response to health care. Keep in mind, however, that a religion may have many sects, and that members of different sects may have different views of health care. For example, a Seventh Day Adventist may have a very different view of health and illness than an Episcopalian—although members of both sects are Christians.

Buddhism

Beliefs about health and illness
Suffering and illness are a normal part of life. Health is a goal to be worked toward, but is not possible for everyone; it depends on the individual's karma.

Dietary beliefs
Many Buddhists are vegetarians out of respect for animal life. Abstinence from all intoxicants is required.

Beliefs about interpersonal relationships
The Thervada branch believes that individualism is the way to nirvana (transcendent state). The Mahayana branch advocates involvement with others as the right path. Self-disclosure (giving personal information about oneself) is difficult for Buddhists in all branches.

Christianity

Beliefs about health and illness
Suffering and illness are a normal part of life, which is the path to immortality. Some sects view suffering as the will of God—as a necessity for redemption and attainment of heaven. Health is valued because the body is the temple of the soul, but health is not always possible.

Dietary beliefs
Some sects forbid the use of intoxicants or caffeine in tea and coffee. Fasting and meat restriction during Lent are required for some.

Beliefs about interpersonal relationships
Heaven is attained by helping others with life and accepting salvation. Self-disclosure is not difficult.

Confucianism

Beliefs about health and illness
Illness results from failure to live according to prescriptions of Confucius; some believe it is caused by evil spirits. Health is maintained by living according to doctrine and in harmony with earth and nature.

Dietary beliefs
Confucianism has no rigid dietary beliefs or rules.

Beliefs about interpersonal relationships
The family is all-important in the context of family relationships. Self-disclosure is not part of the belief system. Elderly people are respected and revered. Females are considered less valuable than males. Both sexes exhibit little eye contact.

terns. (*Note:* Physiologic reproduction aspects can be assessed while assessing the client's physiologic systems.) A client may feel threatened or embarrassed by discussing sexuality with a nurse who appears uncomfortable with the subject. Approach this topic with sensitivity and consideration for the client's ethnic and religious beliefs. A Muslim client, for example, may be unwilling to discuss sexuality with a health care provider of the opposite sex.

Each developmental stage has its unique concerns regarding sexuality. Adolescents, for example, may be especially aware of their increasing sexual feelings and may be looking for appropriate and acceptable ways to express them. The sexual health history for an older adult should include the perception of aging and its effects on the body and sexual performance. If obtaining data is difficult, at least obtain physiologic and medical information related to sexuality.

Ask the following basic questions to assess sexuality and reproductive patterns:

- Are you sexually active?
- How did you learn about sexuality and reproduction?
- Are you satisfied with your knowledge of sexuality?
- Are you satisfied with your knowledge of birth control?
- How satisfied are you with your sexual role?
- How satisfying do you find your sexual relationship?
- What do you plan to teach your children about sexuality?

Social support patterns

The client's social support systems (outside the family) may consist of friends, co-workers, community agencies, and clergy who provide assistance in times of anxiety

Hinduism

Beliefs about health and illness
Hindus are interested in health and illness only as a guide to reaching infinity. They consider the body a temple.

Dietary beliefs
Many Hindus are vegetarians, but dietary rules are flexible. Many do not eat beef; some will eat other meat.

Beliefs about interpersonal relationships
Believers do not complain or use self-disclosure. They tend to minimize symptoms of illness. Family is an important value.

Islam

Beliefs about health and illness
Believers work to stay healthy. If illness occurs, it is the will of Allah.

Dietary beliefs
Believers do not eat pork or drink intoxicants. They fast during Ramadan.

Beliefs about interpersonal relationships
Moderate self-disclosure is permitted. Family and society are an important part of being Muslim. Women have a lower social status than men.

Judaism

Beliefs about health and illness
Suffering or illness is considered the way to holiness. Believers treat the body as the temple of the soul.

Dietary beliefs
Jews who follow Kosher laws do not eat pork, horse meat, shellfish, or birds of prey. Milk and meat products must not be cooked or eaten together. Fasting is required on some holy days.

Beliefs about interpersonal relationships
Family and society are important. Self-disclosure seldom presents a problem.

Taoism

Beliefs about health and illness
Health will occur if the believer is in balance with nature and the energies of the universe.

Dietary beliefs
Taoists hold flexible dietary beliefs. Some postpartum restrictions exist for cold fluids, fruits, and vegetables.

Beliefs about interpersonal relationships
The family is important to Taoists. Calmness and nondisclosure are considered important.

or crisis. Most clients will report that some, or even most, of their emotional, social, and physical support comes from outside the family. Be concerned, therefore, if a client claims to have no nonfamily support systems. A client who reports no or very limited nonfamily support may also report a sense of isolation, depression, or dissatisfaction with the quality of life.

Social skills (the ability to establish effective, harmonious relationships with one's family, friends, and coworkers) affect health in various ways. Social relationships provide emotional support systems and the impetus to stay well or cope with chronic illnesses. Research studies (Lynch, 1977) indicate that socially isolated people die sooner and have more health problems than socially attached people. Understanding adult developmental stages, such as those proposed by Erik Erikson, can help in your assessment of the client's social capabilities. The data collected in other parts of the roles and relationships section of the health history also provide information about these abilities.

Assess the client's social support systems with the following questions:

- Outside of your family, who can you turn to when you need help with a problem or crisis?
- With what organizations or clubs are you active?
- How would you describe your relationships with your co-workers?
- What kinds of activities do you enjoy with friends?
- How important are these people in your life?
- How satisfied are you with the love, affection, and acceptance they provide?
- Are you satisfied with your knowledge of available community agencies that could provide help?

Assessing the family

Assessment of how and to what extent the client's family fulfills its functions is an important part of the health history. The nurse should assess the family into which the client was born (family of origin) and, if different, the current family.

Use this guide to assess how the client perceives family functions. Because the questions target a nuclear family—that is, mother, father, and children—they may need modification for single-parent families, families that include grandparents, clients who live alone, or unrelated individuals who live as a family.

Affective function

Assessing how family members feel about, and get along with, each other provides important information. In some families, one person performs the "sick role," and the other family members support the illness and keep the member sick. For example, a child whose parents have marital problems may be sick to get attention. The parents may allow the child to be sick so they can focus their attention on the child and avoid dealing with their problems. To assess affective function, ask the following questions:

- How do the members of your family treat each other?
- How do family members regard each other?
- How do the members of your family regard each other's needs and wants?
- How are feelings expressed in your family?
- Can family members safely express both positive and negative feelings?
- What happens in the family when members disagree?
- How do family members deal with conflict?

Socialization and social placement

These questions provide information about the flexibility of family responsibilities, which is helpful for planning a client's discharge. For example, a mother of small children who has just had major surgery may need household help when she goes home, if the husband is not expected to help or does not want to. To assess socialization and social placement, ask the following questions:

- How satisfied are you with your role and your partner's role as a couple?
- How did you decide to have (or not to have) children?
- Do you and your partner agree about how to bring up the children? If not, how do you work out differences?
- Who is responsible for taking care of the children? Is this mutually satisfactory?
- How well do you feel your children are growing up?
- Are family roles negotiable within the limits of age and ability?
- Do you share cultural values and beliefs with the children?

Health care function

This assesssment will uncover many cultural beliefs. Identify the family caregiver and then use that information when planning care. For example, if the client is the caregiver, then the client may need household help when discharged. To assess health care function, ask the following questions:

- Who takes care of family members when they are sick? Who makes doctor appointments?
- Are your children learning skills, such as personal hygiene, healthful eating habits, and the importance of sleep and rest?
- How does your family adjust when a member is ill and unable to fulfill expected roles?

Family and social structures

The client's view of the family and of other social structures affects health care. For example, if the client needing home health care belongs to an ethnic group with a strong sense of family responsibility, then the family probably will care for the client. To assess the importance of family and social structures, ask the following questions:

- How important is your family to you?
- Do you have any friends that you consider family?
- Does anyone other than your immediate family (for example, grandparents) live with you?
- Are you involved in community affairs? Do you enjoy these activities?

Economic function

Financial problems frequently cause family conflict. Ask these questions to explore money issues and how they relate to power roles within the family:

- Does your family income meet the family's basic needs?
- Does money allocation consider family needs in relation to individual needs?
- Who makes decisions about family money allocation?

Emotional health status

To evaluate the client's psychosocial status further, assess the client's emotional health.

The client's self-awareness level and recognition of how personality and feelings affect others are two dimensions of emotional development. Emotional health (integration of feelings and intellect) includes sensitivity to others' feelings and needs as well as responsibility for personal behavior. Use the following questions as guides for assessing a client's emotional health:

- What do you think about your emotional health?
- How do you cope with daily stress? Would you like help?
- How would you describe your usual mood or state of mind?
- How often does your mood change? What things change your mood?
- Do you have feelings of despair?
- Do you have feelings of sadness? Does anything specific make you sad? What do you do when you are sad?

For an elderly client, additional questions include:

- How do you feel about growing older?
- What are the good things about growing older?
- What are the difficult things about growing older?

Summary of health history data

Conclude the health history by summarizing all findings. For the well client, list the client's health promotion strengths and resources along with defined health education needs. If the interview points out a significant health problem, tell the client what it is and what to do about it. For example, suppose that a client's health history reveals physical symptoms (such as indigestion and epigastric pain) and job-related stress, resulting in little time for relaxation. Summarize the data in the following manner:

NURSE: Your health history tells me that you're having frequent attacks of indigestion and stomach pain. You also said you've been under a lot of stress at work. The two seem related. I think we need to look at the relationship between your work stress and the indigestion. Your physical symptoms could be as serious as an ulcer or as minor as too much stomach acid. I recommend a physician referral for some laboratory studies we don't do at the nursing clinic. I'd also like to discuss possible options to reduce your stress level. Then I'll do a complete physical assessment to rule out other problems that might be causing your abdominal pain. Then if I think it is indicated, I will make a physician referral for further evaluation. How do these ideas sound to you?

Formulating plans with the client

In the previous example, the history uncovered a need for stress reduction education. Conduct the health education session immediately, or schedule it for another time. In either case, make sure the client participates in the decision. Occasionally, the client's health history indicates an immediate need for referral to a physician or psychotherapist. Inform the client about any concerns and the reason for them based on the health history. Then make plans with the client about the referral. Offering to set up the appointment for the client increases the likelihood of compliance. Always conclude the interview by giving the client an opportunity to have the last word: "Should we talk about anything else?" or "Do you have any information you want to add or questions you want to ask?"

Special considerations

Modify the health history somewhat for a pediatric, pregnant, elderly, or disabled client, according to the following guidelines.

Modifications for pediatric clients

Although an older child can participate more fully during the health history, even a young child can discuss symptoms to some degree and corroborate a parent's information. Direct as many questions as possible to the child. Base the questions on the child's developmental age so that the child can understand and answer them. Sometimes having the child draw a picture and explain the image will provide information. An adolescent can answer most health history questions, except, perhaps, those dealing with family history and specific details of serious childhood illnesses and hospitalizations. Because an adolescent may be reluctant to reveal thoughts and feelings, interactions can be challenging. A straightforward, uncondescending manner is usually the best approach. To respect the client's right to privacy, ask if the adolescent wants a parent present during the interview. For an adolescent who may be sexually active, conduct the interview without a parent present.

For a young child, however, include a parent to provide the health history. While obtaining it, take the opportunity to assess the parent-child relationship. The interview can provide a nonjudgmental setting for the parent to discuss the satisfactions and frustrations of raising children.

Modifications in the health history for children occur mostly in the following sections: past health status, status of physiologic systems, developmental considerations, and nutritional assessment. Substitute questions about school for occupational information, and assess safety hazards by concentrating on the parent's efforts to prevent accidents. If the child is age 8 or older, ask fewer questions about the perinatal history. If the client is an adolescent, do not obtain data about specific developmental milestones that occurred during the first 2 years of life. (For further modifications, see *Pediatric health history*.)

Focus questions about a child's role and relationship patterns on interactions with parents, siblings, and peers. Ask the parent to describe the child's temperament and ability to get along with siblings and peers, the activities the child performs well, any behavioral problems, and the disciplinary measures that the parent uses. If the parent cannot describe many positive aspects about the child or indicates that the child is overly aggressive, withdrawn, or having school problems, perform an in-depth assessment of family relationship patterns.

Modifications for pregnant clients

Because pregnant clients are usually well, use the same health history format and interview process that you would use for any young adult, but emphasize certain sections during different pregnancy stages. On the client's initial prenatal visit, perform the comprehensive health history and note any obstetric and gynecologic history. If the client has experienced more pregnancies than live births, ask about abortions, miscarriages, and stillbirths. Also discuss infertility, sexually transmitted diseases, and reproductive disorders, such as ovarian cysts. Analyze the client's family history for evidence of genetic diseases, such as cystic fibrosis, Tay-Sachs disease, and metabolic disorders.

Also explore the perinatal history of living children. Significant findings include a history of difficult labor or delivery (including cesarean section); induced labor; forceps delivery; fourth-degree lacerations in the perineum; precipitous or prolonged labor (over 24 hours); and delivery of infants with Apgar scores below 5 after 1 minute, infants who needed resuscitation, or infants who were small or large for gestational age.

Assess for perinatal factors that could put a current pregnancy at risk, such as a maternal history of blood group incompatibilities, diabetes, heart disease, hypertension, kidney disease, or eclampsia. List all medications the client used before and during the pregnancy, including nonprescription drugs. Additional risk factors include exposure to environmental or occupational health hazards, such as radiation or toxic chemicals. Alcohol, recreational drugs, and certain medications can adversely affect the fetus, and some experts recommend that prolonged hot tub use and vigorous high-impact exercises, such as long-distance running or aerobics, should be avoided. Tobacco and caffeine are potential

Pediatric health history

Although the pediatric health history varies somewhat from the one used for adults, it still covers the five basic health history components. Each component includes specific areas the nurse needs to assess for a pediatric client, as shown in the list below. To gain even more information, observe the parent-child interaction and behavior during the interview.

Biographic data

Child's name; parent's name; contact person; address; telephone number; sex; age; birth date; place of birth; race, nationality, and cultural background; religious affiliation

Health and illness patterns

- Current health status
- Prenatal and birth history
- Past health status
- Immunization and screening test history
- Family health status
- Status of physiologic systems
- Developmental milestones and considerations

Health promotion and protection patterns

- Child's or parent's health beliefs
- Personal habits (for adolescents)
- Sleep and wake patterns
- Temperamental assessment
- Behavior and discipline assessment
- Infant and child safety patterns
- Nutritional assessment
- Stress and coping patterns
- Family economic patterns
- Environmental health patterns
- School performance patterns
- Description of a typical day

Role and relationship patterns

- Child's self-concept
- Child's or parent's description of cognitive ability
- Role socialization patterns
- Cultural, spiritual, and religious influences on child's role socialization
- Child's communication patterns
- Sibling relationships
- Child's role in the family
- Child's knowledge of sexuality and reproduction
- Sexuality and sexual relationships (for adolescents)
- Child's peer relationships
- Emotional health status

Summary of health history data

fetal health hazards, as are sexually transmitted diseases such as genital herpes, gonorrhea, syphilis, and AIDS. Viral infections, such as rubella or mononucleosis, in the first trimester can negatively affect fetal development even though maternal risk is minimal.

Determine whether the client receives regular prenatal care, and ask if she has any problems that might interfere with adequate nutrition, such as nausea in the first trimester or heartburn in the last trimester. Perform an in-depth nutritional assessment, noting whether the client uses vitamin and mineral supplements and understands the need for increased caloric intake and a well-balanced diet.

Assessment of role and relationship patterns for a pregnant client focuses on her psychological adjustment to the pregnancy. The following questions help assess these factors:

- Is this a planned pregnancy?
- How do you feel about being pregnant?
- How will your typical day be affected by the baby?
- How will the baby affect other family members' lifestyles?

During the third trimester, assess the effect of the pregnancy on the sleep-wake cycle. The client may experience considerable discomfort when she cannot change positions readily. Her ability to perform daily activities and to exercise adequately are other important concerns. (For more information, see Chapter 22, Perinatal and Neonatal Assessment.)

Modifications for elderly clients

Make health history modifications only when the client shows age-related sensory impairment or a specific physiologic problem, such as aphasia from a stroke (cerebrovascular accident). If the client tires easily or cannot concentrate, try scheduling two or more interview sessions to complete the comprehensive health history.

Although the format for an elderly client remains practically the same as that used for a younger adult, the approach to the health history sections should change slightly. Because of increased age, an elderly client is more likely to have chronic illnesses, causing various symptoms and requiring several medications. Therefore, focus on current problems instead of past ones. Also ask the client to bring in all medications being taken and a dated list of hospitalizations to speed the history taking and clarify or validate information. Do not ask an elderly client about childhood immunizations or an elderly woman about her childbirth experiences. This information is not necessary.

Assess role and relationship patterns thoroughly for an elderly client. The client may experience feelings of loss and social isolation as spouse and friends die or become disabled by illness. Because of changed social roles, an elderly client may have difficulty maintaining a sense of achievement, productivity, and independence.

Some individuals, for example, identify so closely with their occupation that retirement becomes an identity crisis. Some couples who spent little time together before retirement are forced to redefine their relationship and learn how to spend leisure time together.

Other important considerations for an elderly client include assessing health behaviors, safety precautions, and self-concept. For example, how is the client dealing with changes in physical appearance or in the ability to perform activities of daily living? Ask the client to describe a typical day. Inquire about the client's financial status to determine if income is adequate to acquire food, shelter, and health care.

Initiate other modifications if the client appears confused. In such cases, skip over most assessment areas and concentrate on specific, current symptoms (pain, nausea, depression, or impaired sight). Ask a close friend or relative of the client to supply missing information.

Many nurses have skewed perceptions about elderly people from being exposed to sick, dependent, confused, and frail elderly clients in the health care system. Most elderly clients lead active, healthy, and productive lives. Keep this in mind when collecting the health history.

Modifications for disabled clients

Modifications for a disabled client depend on the disability. If the client is severely hearing impaired, or mute, use a written health history questionnaire. After the client completes the questionnaire, concentrate on the identified problem areas. Write any additional questions you need to have answered, and pass notes back and forth with the client. Ask a client with severe vision and hearing impairments to bring a relative or friend to help. For a hearing impaired and mute client, request the services of a sign language interpreter.

Do not modify the health history format for a physically disabled client unless the client cannot tolerate the length of time required to complete the history.

For a mildly or moderately intellectually impaired client, use simple phrases and schedule brief sessions to accommodate a short attention span. A close relative or friend usually is needed to provide information about a severely impaired or intellectually disabled client.

Documenting the health history

The system used to document the health history and other parts of the assessment varies with each health care facility. Some facilities use computerized records that provide standardized formats for documentation. Others use source-oriented records, in which each professional group documents separate data on each client. For example, one part of the record contains physician orders, another contains laboratory data, and another contains nursing data. In a source-oriented record, health care professionals usually document data in narrative (paragraph) form.

Still other health care facilities use problem-oriented records (POR), also known as problem-oriented medical records (POMR). Unlike the source-oriented record system, the POR system focuses on the client's *problems.* With the POR system, data are documented according to the SOAPIE format, which closely follows the nursing process steps. (For a description of problem-oriented documentation, see *Guidelines for SOAPIE documentation.*)

However, regardless of the system used to document the health history, data must be documented according to the following legal guidelines:
- Use the appropriate form and document in ink.
- Be sure the client's name and identification number are on each page.
- Record the date and time of each entry.
- Use standard accepted abbreviations only.
- Document symptoms in the client's own words.
- Be specific; avoid generalizations and vague expressions.
- Write on every line. Do not leave blank spaces.
- If a certain space does not apply to the client, write NA (*not applicable*) in the space.
- Do not backdate or squeeze writing into a previously documented entry.
- Document only work done personally; never document for someone else.
- Do not document value judgments and opinions.
- Sign every entry with your first and last name and title.

The client's record is used by other health care professionals to determine subsequent health needs. Before recording the health history, analyze notes and recollections to formulate a careful assessment of the client-supplied subjective data. (For a sample of a complete health history, see *Documenting the health history,* pages 67 and 68.) Follow the guidelines discussed below when documenting the health history.

Write the history clearly and concisely, omitting information or opinions that might bias the reader. Avoid specific descriptions that label a finding as *normal. Normal* can be interpreted in many ways. If a particular section of the health history has no significant data, note that fact. This is called *recording pertinent negatives,* for example, "Client denies family history of diabetes, heart disease, or cancer."

The written history need not contain full sentences, except where the client's own words are revealing. Use only standardized abbreviations for medical terms. Because the recorded history is a legal document, be sure to date and sign it. Include a written summary of significant health history data at the end. The summary is particularly important as a source for the nursing diagnoses derived from subjective data.

(Text continues on page 69.)

Guidelines for SOAPIE documentation

Many facilities use a problem-oriented record (POR), which employs the SOAPIE method of documentation. The SOAPIE method closely follows the nursing process steps and provides a clear, systematic way to document the client's status and care. (The nurse must use the health care facility's method.) The SOAPIE method uses these components in documentation.

S **subjective (history) data**
What the client reports

O **objective (physical) data**
What the nurse observes, inspects, palpates, percusses, and auscultates

A **assessment**
Nursing diagnosis and a statement of the client's progress or lack of progress

P **plan**
Plan of client care

I **implemention**
Nursing interventions that carry out the plan

E **evaluation**
Review of the results of the implemented plan.

An initial SOAPIE note must include each of the SOAPIE categories, but follow-up notes include only those categories that are appropriate and necessary to document the information.

This textbook uses the SOAPIE method of documentation in the recurring chart, *Applying the nursing process.* For instructive purposes, the final column of the chart contains a sample initial note and follow-up note using the SOAPIE format.

Documenting the health history

This sample illustrates proper documentation of a complete health history.

Biographic data

Name: Carol Doe
Address: 1444 Stony Path Drive, Pineridge, Colorado
Home Phone: 222-555-0302
Work Phone: 222-555-5548
Sex: Female
Age: 37
Birth date: 4/5/52
Social Security number: 173-40-0334
Place of birth: Fairtown, Washington
Race: Caucasian
Nationality: American
Culture: German-American
Marital status: Divorced
Dependents: Mary, age 15; Josh, age 12
Contact person: Sally Jones, sister (104 East Road, Pineridge, Colo.; phone: 222-555-4676)
Religion: Episcopalian
Education: B.S. Chemistry
Occupation: Lab assistant at Acme Chemical Corp.

Health and illness patterns

Reason for seeking health care: "I've been feeling real tired lately, so I wanted a health exam to make sure nothing is wrong."

Current health status: Mrs. Doe says she's been feeling tired for about a month. Denies any other symptoms. Denies loss of appetite or history of anemia or blood loss. States that she has been busier at work than usual and hasn't had enough time to spend with her children because she's going to night school to work on a master's degree. She thinks that the fatigue may be related to a busy schedule rather than a physical problem. She last had a complete physical 4 years ago, including a Pap smear.

Past health status: Had measles, mumps, and chicken pox as a child. Hospitalized at age 6 for tonsillectomy and adenoidectomy and in 1974 and 1977 for births of her children. Had a concussion and a fractured left arm at age 12 from a bike accident. Has had no complications from that. Immunizations are up to date, with last tetanus shot 4 years ago.

Family health status: Maternal and paternal grandfathers are deceased. Both grandmothers are alive and well. Father is alive and well at age 66; mother has mitral valve problems. Her younger brother and younger sister are alive and well. History of cancer and cardiovascular disease. (See genogram.)

Status of physiologic systems:
- General state of health: Complains of fatigue. Has had two head colds in the past year. No other illnesses. Reports good exercise tolerance.
- Skin, hair, and nails: Denies presence of lesions. Hair and nails healthy.
- Head and neck: Denies headaches or other problems. Had a concussion as a child. No history of seizures. Reports no pain or limitation of R.O.M.
- Nose and sinuses: No rhinorrhea, sinus infections, or nosebleeds.
- Mouth and throat: Last dental exam 1 year ago. Has a few fillings. No problems with strep throat or other infections.
- Eyes: Last eye exam 2 years ago. Wears contacts for myopia.
- Ears: Reports no hearing problems. No history of ear infections. Last hearing evaluation 5 years ago.
- Respiratory system: No history of pneumonia, bronchitis, asthma, or dyspnea.
- Cardiovascular system: Denies presence of murmurs and palpitations. No history of heart disease or hypertension.
- Breasts: Reports left slightly larger than right; no masses, no nipple discharge, self-examination twice a year.
- Gastrointestinal system: No history of indigestion, ulcers, or liver disease. Has regular bowel movements 1x a day. Had hemorrhoids with last pregnancy. No problems since.
- Urinary system: No history of kidney stones or infections. Voids clear yellow urine several times a day. Had bladder infection 4 years ago. Took Gantrisin.
- Reproductive system: Has regular periods every 30 days that last 3 to 4 days. Moderate flow, no discomfort. Obstetrical history: Grav 3 para 2, 1 miscarriage at 2 months before oldest child. No complications. No problems with subsequent pregnancies. No hx of S.T.D. Is not currently sexually active. Has taken birth control pills in the past; experienced no adverse reactions. Stated that sexual relationship during marriage was "fine."
- Nervous system: Denies numbness or tingling in extremities.
- Musculoskeletal: Reports no muscle or joint pains or stiffness.
- Immune system and blood: Was anemic during last pregnancy even with iron. No other hx of blood loss or anemia. Reports no lymph gland swelling.
- Endocrine system: No history of thyroid disease. No fainting, polydipsia, polyphagia, or polyuria.

Developmental considerations: Mrs. Doe is in the "young family" stage of development. Has been divorced for 2 years, but has a fairly good relationship with her ex-husband, a recovering alcoholic. Considers her cognitive ability above average. Describes herself as emotionally stable, but does have periods of blueness and loneliness. Says she doesn't have much time to socialize since her divorce. Gets along well with fellow workers.

continued

Documenting the health history continued

Health promotion and protection patterns

Health beliefs: Believes that each person is responsible for leading a life-style conducive to health. Is satisfied with health care providers and previous experiences with health care.

Personal habits: Never smoked. Never used recreational drugs. Takes vitamin and mineral supplements and occasional nonprescription cold medicines. Drinks 1 or 2 glasses of wine a week with dinner. Has 1 or 2 cups of caffeinated coffee in a.m.

Sleep and wake patterns: Describes herself as a morning person. Gets up at 6:30 a.m., goes to bed at 11:30 or 12 p.m. Likes to get about 8 hours of sleep, but rarely does. Needs to study at night after kids are asleep.

Exercise and activity patterns: Jogs 2 miles a week during lunchtime. Says she'd like to be more active but can't find the time.

Recreational patterns: Likes swimming, hiking, and camping. Tries to take children camping at least once each summer. Wishes she had more time for recreation.

Nutritional patterns: 24-hour recall indicates deficit in iron, protein, and calcium. Takes vitamin and mineral supplement. Skips lunch often. Is happy with current weight.

Stress and coping patterns: Says divorce was a real crisis for her. Sought psychotherapy to help with transition. Describes her way of coping as avoiding problems until they get too big. Feels she copes with day-to-day stresses O.K. Mary had school and discipline problems around time of divorce, but is doing better now. Says job is busy and stressful most days. Hasn't figured out how to cope with difficult boss. Is afraid of losing her job.

Socioeconomic patterns: Makes around $18,100 a year, which doesn't allow much for extras. Receives $400 a month for child support. Has health insurance and retirement benefits through job. Ex-husband insures children and pays half of home mortgage.

Environmental health patterns: Is exposed to toxic chemicals at work. Wears gloves and mask when working with dangerous chemicals. No other known environmental hazards. Lives in 3-bedroom house in town.

Occupational health patterns: Works 8 to 9 hours a day with 1 hour for lunch. Gets along well with co-workers. Is having difficulty with new boss who "is always on my case to do more." Doesn't like her job very much and is improving credentials to get a better job. Feels under a lot of pressure at work. Has had present job for 3 years. Before that she was a homemaker.

Role and relationship patterns

Self-concept: Describes herself as fairly attractive with a good sense of humor. Says she still occasionally feels bad about her divorce. Received counseling for 6 months to help with that crisis.

Cultural and religious influences: Says she can't think of any specific important religious or cultural influences. Describes herself as "not very religious" but thinks Sunday school is important for her children.

Family roles and relationships: Says she doesn't get to spend much time with her children. Communicates with ex-husband about child care; describes him as cooperative. He has been helping her financially. Mary and Josh get along well together, but sometimes fight over her time with them. They do a few chores around the house. Says her sister and brother-in-law help her with child care and that she counts on them for moral support. Describes her relationship with her parents as "distant" both geographically and emotionally.

Sexuality and reproductive patterns: Not part of her life at present. Says dating again is difficult.

Social support: Has three close friends who live in her neighborhood. Says she needs to start going out again, but isn't ready at present. Is aware of such community groups as Parents Without Partners.

Other psychosocial considerations: She says she is usually easygoing. Occasionally, she blows up at the kids, usually when she hasn't done anything for herself for a while.

Summary of health history data

Significant findings: Client is a 37-year-old divorced woman who is experiencing a lot of stress from her job and from single parenthood. No significant physical problems identified. Needs physical exam and lab studies to rule out iron deficiency anemia or other physical problems. Answered questions appropriately. Appeared tired and sad.

Chapter summary

This chapter describes the comprehensive health history from the nurse's perspective. It specifies the differences between a nursing health history and a medical history, and supplies psychosocial and cultural information to enhance communication and interviewing skills. Suggested formats and modifications should help the nurse develop personal interviewing approaches.

The health history, a compilation of subjective data, may tell more about a client's health status than a physical assessment. It identifies existing and potential health problems and identifies a client's health promotional and educational needs.

Here are the main points from the chapter:

- The nurse's interpersonal skills and self-awareness level are keys to establishing good client rapport and trust.
- The relationship between the physical, psychosocial, and cultural aspects of an individual are complex, and each affects the client's health status.
- Developmental theories that address an individual's psychosexual, psychosocial, cognitive, and spiritual development are important to the nurse's assessment.
- To avoid creating a stereotype when performing a cultural assessment, the nurse must avoid cultural biases and respect the practices of various cultures.
- Understanding the client's developmental, sociocultural, and religious background also enhances rapport and accurate data collection.
- Physical surroundings and psychological atmosphere affect the client's comfort and willingness to provide accurate information.
- The interview includes three phases: introductory, working, and termination. In the introductory phase, the nurse uses nonprobing questions and comments to put the client at ease and explains the purpose of the interview. In the working phase, the nurse obtains specific health history information. In the termination phase, the nurse summarizes the important points, explains the physical assessment procedure, and discusses follow-up plans.
- The nurse must phrase questions according to the client's level of understanding. Although some questions may seem repetitious, the overlap helps verify and double-check the information.
- During an interview, the nurse should observe the client's verbal and nonverbal behavior while conveying a calm, unhurried, and caring manner.
- The nursing health history contains five components: biographic data; health and illness patterns; health promotion and protection patterns; role and relationship patterns; and a summary of health history data. Each component has several subsections, such as past health status and exercise and activity patterns, that should be addressed, as appropriate.
- A client's religious and spiritual beliefs are an integral part of a holistic health assessment.
- The nurse should record the health history information carefully and concisely. Because the health history is a legal document, it should not contain opinions, biases, or subjective descriptions.
- The health history format and recommendations contained in this chapter are suggestions, not dictums. Obtaining a health history is a process with few absolutes; experience helps the nurse develop an interviewing style. Therapeutic use of self, the single most important variable in successful history taking, will help the nurse develop a collaborative relationship with the client and show interest in and caring for the client as a unique individual.

Study questions

1. What are the five major components of the nursing health history? What information is included in each component?

2. What is the significance of the nursing health history to the overall health assessment process?

3. What are the major factors critical to a nurse's success in obtaining a meaningful and reliable health history?

4. How would you compare effective and ineffective interviewing techniques? Provide sample dialogues that illustrate two effective techniques and two ineffective techniques.

5. How does the content of a health history differ for an elderly client and a pediatric client? How do interviewing techniques differ for these clients?

Selected references

Barry, P., and Ibarra, M. (1990). Multidimensional assessment of the elderly. *Hospital Practice,* 25(4), 117-121, 124, 127-128.

Butler, R. (1963). Life review: An interpretation of reminiscence in the aged. *Psychiatry,* 26, a65.*

Catherman, A. (1990). Biopsychosocial nursing assessment: A way to enhance care plans. *Journal of Psychosocial Nursing and Mental Health Services,* 28(6), 31-35.

Clark, C. (1986). *Wellness nursing: Concepts, theory, research, and practice.* New York: Wiley & Sons.

Clevenger, F. (1990). Interviewing the elderly client. *Advancing Clinical Care,* 5(6), 26-27.

Cummings, E., and Henry, W. (1961). *Growing old: The process of disengagement.* New York: Basic Books.*

Duvall, E. (1984). *Family development* (6th ed.). New York: Harper & Row.

Dychtwald, K. (1986). *Wellness and health promotion for the elderly.* Rockville, MD: Aspen Systems.

Erikson, E. (1964). *Childhood and society.* New York: Norton.*

Freud, S. (1961). *The ego and the id and other works.* London: Hogarth Press and the Institute of Psychoanalysis.*

Friedman, M. (1986). *Family nursing* (2nd ed.). East Norwalk, CT: Appleton & Lange.

Giger, J., and Davidhziar, R. (1990). Contextual care: Religious considerations for culturally appropriate nursing care. *Advancing Clinical Care,* 5(4), 48-51.

Giger, J., and Davidhziar, R. (1990). Transcultural nursing assessment: A method for advancing nursing practice. *International Nursing Review,* 37(1), 199-202.

Gilligan, C. (1982). *In a different voice.* Cambridge, MA: Harvard University Press.*

Havighurst, R. (1963). Successful aging. In R. Williams, et al. (Eds.), *Process of aging* (Vol. 1). New York: Atherton Press.*

Henkle, J., and Kennerly, S. (1990). Cultural diversity: A resource in planning and implementing nursing care. *Public Health Nursing,* 7(3), 145-149.

Hill, L., and Smith, N. (1989). *Self-care nursing: Promotion of health* (2nd ed.). East Norwalk, CT: Appleton & Lange.

Holmes, T., and Rahe, R. (1967). The social readjustment rating scale. *Journal of Psychosomatic Research,* 11(2), 213-218.*

Leininger, M. (1978). *Transcultural nursing: Concepts, theories, and practices.* New York: Wiley & Sons.*

Lynch, J. (1977). *The broken heart: The medical consequences of loneliness.* New York: Basic Books/Harper Colophon Books.*

McFarlane, J. (1986). *The clinical handbook of family nursing.* Albany, NY: Delmar.

Manning, M. (1990). Health assessment of the early adolescent: Challenges and clinical issues. *Nursing Clinics of North America,* 25(4), 823-831.

Maslow, A. (1968). *Toward a psychology of being* (2nd ed.). New York: Van Nostrand Reinhold.*

Murray, R., and Zentner, J. (1985). *Nursing concepts for health promotion* (3rd ed.). East Norwalk, CT: Appleton & Lange.

Peck, R. (1968). Psychological developments in the second half of life. In B. Neugarten (Ed.), *Middle age and aging.* Chicago: University of Chicago Press.*

Pender, N. (1987). *Health promotion in nursing practice* (2nd ed.). East Norwalk, CT: Appleton & Lange.

Piaget, J. (1963). *Origins of intelligence in children.* New York: Norton.*

Pinnell, N., and Meneses, M. (1986). *The nursing process: Theory, application and related processes.* East Norwalk, CT: Appleton & Lange.

Rothenburger, R. (1990). Transcultural nursing: Overcoming obstacles to effective communication. *AORN Journal,* 51(5), 1349-1350, 1352, 1354+.

Scholz, J. (1990). Cultural expressions affecting patient care. *Dimensions in Oncology Nursing,* 4(1), 16-26.

Selye, H. (1956). *The stress of life.* New York: McGraw-Hill.*

Sundeen, S., Stuart G., Rankin, E., and Cohen, S. (1989). *Nurse-client interaction: Implementing the nursing process* (4th ed.). St. Louis: Mosby.

Zimmer, E. (1990). The nursing health history: A powerful tool. *Advancing Clinical Care,* 5(3), 31-32.

Nursing research

Hansen, M., and Resick, L. (1990). Health beliefs, health care, and rural Appalachian subcultures from an ethnographic perspective. *Family and Community Health,* 13(1), 1-10.

McElmurry, B. (1986). Health appraisal of low-income women. In D. Kjervik and I. Martinson (Eds.), *Women in health and illness: Life experiences and crises.* Philadelphia: Saunders.

Roberson, M. (1987). Home remedies: A cultural study. *Home Healthcare Nurse,* 5(1), 35-40.

West, J. (1986). Research in cultural diversity: Unidimensional measures of ethnicity. *Nursing Research,* 8(4), 445-456.

*Landmark publication

4

Physical Assessment Skills

Objectives

After reading and studying this chapter, you should be able to:

1. Discuss the purpose and components of the physical assessment.
2. Describe the equipment required in the physical assessment and its use.
3. Identify the purposes of inspection, palpation, percussion, and auscultation.
4. Demonstrate the techniques of inspection, palpation, percussion, and auscultation.
5. Explain how to approach the physical assessment, including ways to put the client at ease.
6. Describe how to perform a general survey.
7. Demonstrate how to document findings from a general survey.
8. Identify normal vital sign ranges.
9. Demonstrate how to assess and document vital signs.
10. Demonstrate how to measure height and weight properly.

Introduction

Assessment begins with subjective findings, including the health history and review of systems. Then the nurse moves to the physical assessment to obtain objective data about a client.

The physical assessment has four main parts: (4)
• general survey (the nurse's initial observations of the client's general appearance and behavior)
• vital sign measurements (assessment of temperature, pulse and respiration rates, and blood pressure) (4)
• assessment of height and weight
• physical examination (assessment of all structures, organs, and body systems).

This chapter introduces the physical assessment—the objective portion of the complete health assessment. It describes the equipment, basic techniques, and general approach used in the physical assessment, and includes special considerations for pediatric, pregnant, elderly, and disabled clients. Chapter 4 also describes components of the general survey, vital sign measurements, and height and weight measurements. Chapters 7 through 20 describe the physical examination techniques used to assess specific body systems, structures, and functions.

An accurate physical assessment requires use of all of the nurse's senses and an intelligent, systematic approach. The nurse must develop expertise in using special equipment and in performing the four basic assessment techniques: inspection (observing), palpation (feeling body surfaces with the fingers), percussion (striking the fingers against body surfaces), and auscultation (listening to body sounds). (4)

In a complete physical assessment, the nurse uses these techniques to evaluate each body structure, organ, or system in detail. The information obtained completes the client's health picture, substantiating or dispelling the nurse's or client's health concerns and possibly providing new information. Physical assessment findings and the client's history data help the nurse develop nursing diagnoses.

Glossary

Affect: outward manifestation of an individual's feelings or emotions.
Amplitude: width or breadth of range or extent, especially of pulses.
Apical pulse: heart rate auscultated by placing a stethoscope over the apex of the heart.
Auscultation: physical assessment technique in which the examiner listens for sounds in the body to evaluate the condition of the heart, lungs, pleurae, intestines, and other organs or to detect fetal heart sounds. The examiner usually uses a stethoscope to auscultate the frequency, intensity, quality, and duration of these sounds.
Ballottement: palpation technique used to evaluate a floating structure by bouncing it gently and feeling it rebound. It may be used, for example, to check fetal position.
Blood pressure: pressure exerted by the circulating blood volume on arterial walls. Blood pressure depends on myocardial contractile force, blood volume, size and patency of the arterial lumen, and arterial wall elasticity.
Blunt percussion: percussion performed by striking a body surface directly with the fist to elicit tenderness, *not* to create a sound.
Bradycardia: circulatory condition characterized by a slow but regular heart rate below 60 beats per minute.
Bradypnea: abnormally slow respiratory rate (based on an individual's age), which may indicate a pathologic process, such as a central nervous system disturbance.
Diopter: refractive power of a lens with a 1-meter focal distance; for example, an ophthalmoscope has a lens with diopter values from −25 to +40.
Direct (immediate) percussion: percussion performed by striking the fingers directly on the body surface.
Febrile: pertaining to or characterized by fever.
Hyperpnea: deep, rapid, or labored respirations; occurring normally with exercise and abnormally with pain, fever, and metabolic acidosis.
Hyperventilation: ventilation rate that exceeds the rate metabolically required for pulmonary gas exchange. Resulting from increased breathing frequency, increased tidal volume, or both, hyperventilation causes excessive oxygen intake and carbon dioxide elimination.
Hypoventilation: abnormally reduced respiratory rate and depth occurring when alveolar air participating in gas exchange is not sufficient to meet the body's needs. Hypoventilation causes excessive carbon dioxide retention.
Indirect (mediate) percussion: percussion performed by striking a finger of one hand against a finger of the other hand, which is placed over an organ.
Inspection: physical assessment technique in which the examiner uses sight, hearing, and smell to make informed observations.
Orthostatic (postural) hypotension: abnormally low blood pressure occurring when a person stands.
Palpation: physical assessment technique in which the examiner uses the sense of touch to feel pulsations and vibrations or to locate body structures and assess their texture, size, consistency, mobility, and tenderness.
Percussion: physical assessment technique in which the examiner taps on the skin surface with the fingers to assess the size, borders, and consistency of certain internal organs, and to detect and evaluate the amount of fluid in a body cavity.
Perfusion: passage of fluid (blood) through vessels. Perfusion of the pulmonary circulation, for instance, allows for gas diffusion in the alveoli and capillaries.
Pleximeter: mediating device (such as a finger) used to receive light taps during percussion.
Plexor: device (such as a finger) used to tap a mediating device (pleximeter) or to tap the body directly during percussion.
Pulse: rhythmic beating or vibrating movement produced by left ventricular blood ejection.
Tachycardia: circulatory condition characterized by a regular but fast heart rate exceeding 100 beats per minute.
Tachypnea: persistent rapid, shallow breathing that serves as a protective splinting measure against pain (for example, from pleurisy or a fractured rib).

Assessment equipment

For much of the physical assessment, the nurse relies directly on the senses—sight, hearing, smell, and touch—using the eyes, ears, nose, and hands as basic tools. To complete certain assessment steps, however, the nurse must use special equipment.

Basic assessment equipment

Usually, the physical assessment requires a thermometer, stethoscope, sphygmomanometer, visual acuity chart, penlight or flashlight, measuring tape and pocket ruler, marking pencil, and a scale. (For illustrations of some of these items, see *Basic assessment equipment,* pages 74 and 75.)

Thermometer

The nurse uses an oral or rectal thermometer to determine the client's body temperature. Glass-mercury thermometers are available in oral and rectal models. To distinguish between the two, manufacturers make oral thermometers with a blue, long, thin tip; and rectal thermometers with a red, short, round tip.

To move the mercury to zero and thus ensure accurate results, the nurse must shake down the mercury in the thermometer before using it; afterward, it must be cleaned and stored carefully. Also, the glass-mercury thermometer takes longer than an electronic thermometer to register temperature and, in rare cases, may cause rectal perforation.

The electronic thermometer, now preferred in most settings, provides an accurate digital readout in about 30 seconds. It has an unbreakable probe with a disposable, color-coded tip—blue for oral use or red for rectal use. A manual digital thermometer can also provide a rapid temperature readout.

Alternatively, the nurse can measure temperature with a disposable paper-strip thermometer with temperature-sensitive dots. Inexpensive and easy to use, this device prevents contamination between clients. However, it is less accurate than other thermometers.

Thermometers measure temperature in either degrees Fahrenheit (° F.) or degrees centigrade, or Celsius (° C.). Most thermometers measure temperatures between 94° and 106° F. (34.4° and 41.1° C.). However, special hypothermia thermometers have a range of 75° to 104° F. (23.9° to 40° C.).

Stethoscope

The nurse uses a stethoscope to listen to heart, lung, and bowel sounds and to obtain blood pressure and pulse measurements. It consists of a metal chestpiece, single or double tubing connected to binaurals (double ear tubes), and earpieces. Many stethoscopes have a tension bar between the binaurals that helps to hold the earpieces snugly in place and prevent the tubing from kinking.

The nurse may use a stethoscope more often than any other device, and might prefer a high-quality model that improves the accuracy of assessment findings. The earpieces should fit snugly and comfortably. Available in hard plastic or soft rubber, earpieces should occlude the external ear canal to block out extraneous noise and to channel sound waves from the chestpiece to the nurse's ears.

Stethoscope tubing should be made of firm rubber or plastic measuring about 12" to 15" (30.5 to 38.1 cm) long, with an external diameter of 3/8" (1 cm) and an internal lumen of 1/8" (0.32 cm). Longer, lighter tubing conducts sound less effectively.

The chestpiece should have two heads—a diaphragm and a bell. For best results, the chestpiece should weigh about as much as a silver dollar (a lighter chestpiece provides poorer sound transmission). Some stethoscopes have several removable chestpieces, each designed for adult or pediatric use. Others have a chestpiece that can be used on either an adult or a child.

The diaphragm should be rigid, with a diameter of about 1¾" (4.4 cm). When held firmly against the client's chest, it should filter out low-pitched body sounds (such as third and fourth heart sounds) and accentuate normally high-pitched sounds (such as breath and blood pressure sounds).

The bell, on the other hand, should detect low-pitched sounds best. It should be heavy enough to stay in place when held lightly with one finger. The bell should have a diameter that spans an intercostal space (the space between two ribs) and a cup deep enough so that it does not fill with skin when held against a body surface. (For pediatric use, a smaller-diameter bell is available.)

To practice using the stethoscope heads correctly, the nurse should follow these steps. First, assess high-pitched sounds by placing the stethoscope diaphragm head firmly on the client's skin. Next, assess low-pitched sounds by placing the bell head lightly over the appropriate area. *Do not* exert pressure, because this will make the client's chest act as a diaphragm, causing the loss of low-pitched sounds. To switch between the diaphragm and the bell during assessment, grasp the chestpiece between the thumb and index finger and rotate it 180 degrees until it clicks into place.

Sphygmomanometer

The nurse uses a stethoscope and a sphygmomanometer to measure blood pressure. The sphygmomanometer consists of a blood pressure cuff, a hand bulb with a pressure valve, a pressure manometer, and connective tubing. Some models are wall-mounted; others are portable and may be used directly from a box or a wheeled cart.

The blood pressure cuff, typically made of nylon or sturdy cloth, has Velcro strips or metal clips that hold it in place around the client's arm or leg. A rubber bladder inside the cuff inflates when the pressure bulb is squeezed repeatedly.

Cuffs vary in size, with standard sizes available for adults, children, and infants. Special larger cuffs can be used on the thigh or on an obese client. The nurse must select a cuff that fits the client: a too-large cuff

(Text continues on page 76.)

Basic assessment equipment

The basic physical assessment usually requires the nurse to use the following equipment: thermometer, stethoscope, sphygmomanometer, visual acuity charts, and scale.

Thermometer

Several types of thermometers measure body temperature: glass-mercury, chemical dot, digital, and electronic digital. Each type provides accurate readings when used properly.

Glass-mercury thermometer

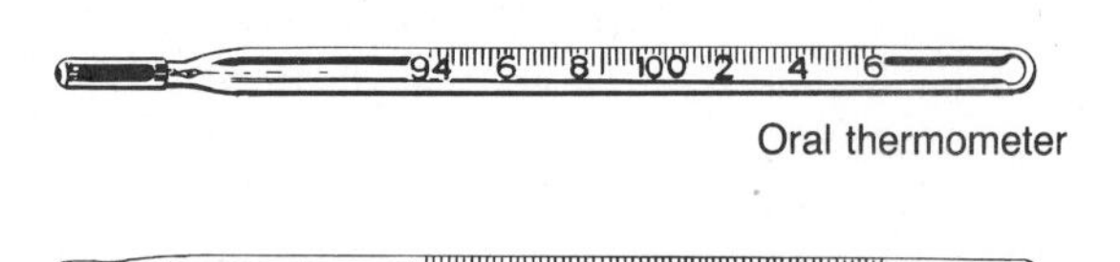

Chemical dot thermometer

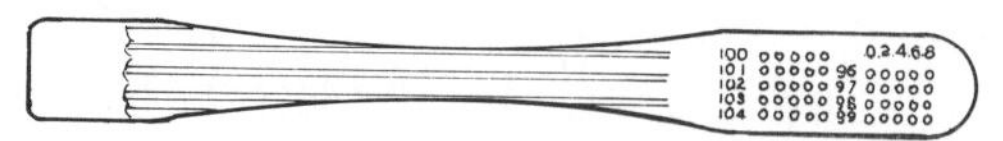

Digital thermometer

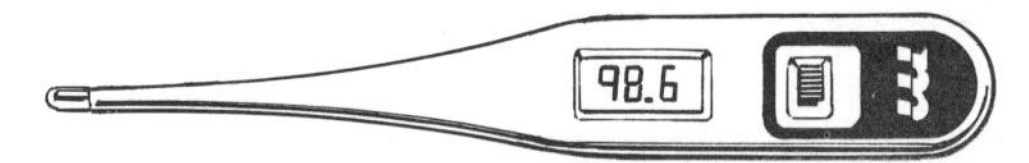

Electronic digital thermometer

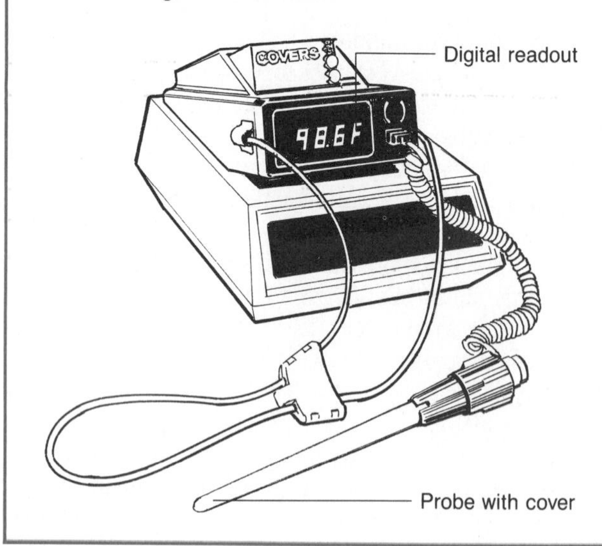

Stethoscope

All stethoscopes have earpieces, binaurals, tubing, and a chestpiece (head). However, some have several removable chestpieces suitable for adult and pediatric clients. Others, designed specifically for use on an adult or a child, have only one chestpiece.

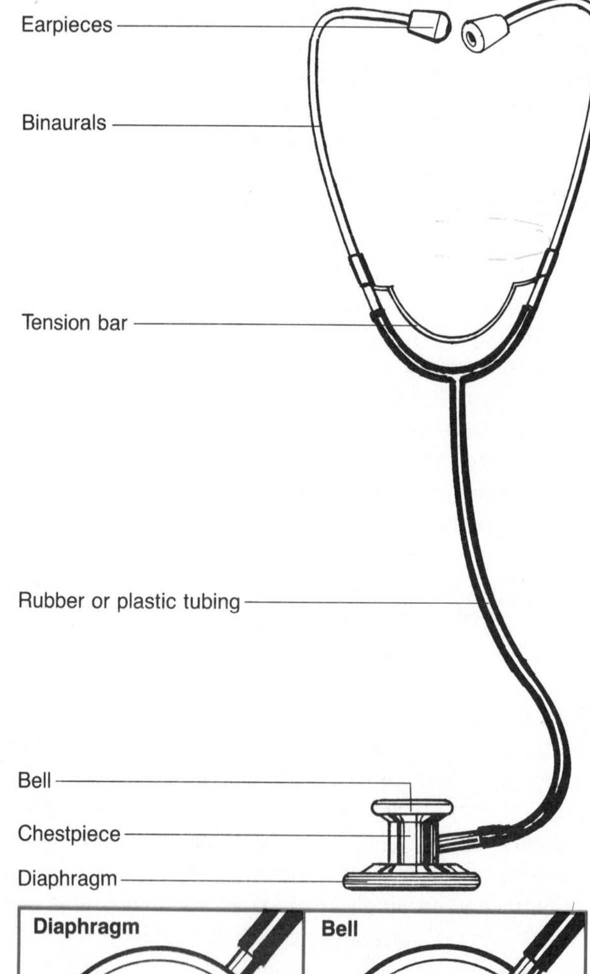

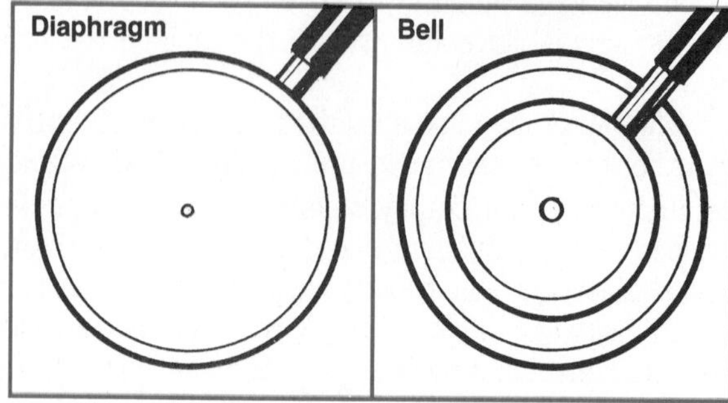

Sphygmomanometer

Most hospitals have sphygmomanometers with a mercury manometer mounted on a wheeled cart or on the wall; others may have an aneroid manometer with a needle gauge that shows the pressure.

Mercury manometer

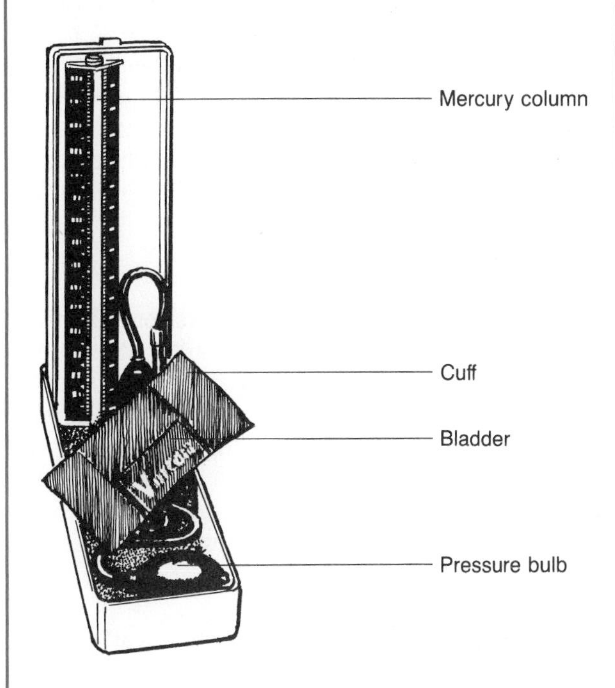

Aneroid manometer

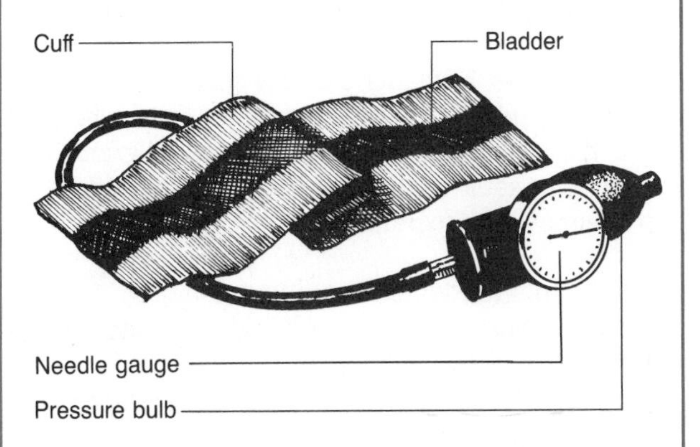

Visual acuity charts

The Snellen alphabet chart consists of 11 lines of letters of graduated size. The Snellen "E" chart uses graduated-sized lines of *E*s facing in different directions.

Snellen alphabet chart

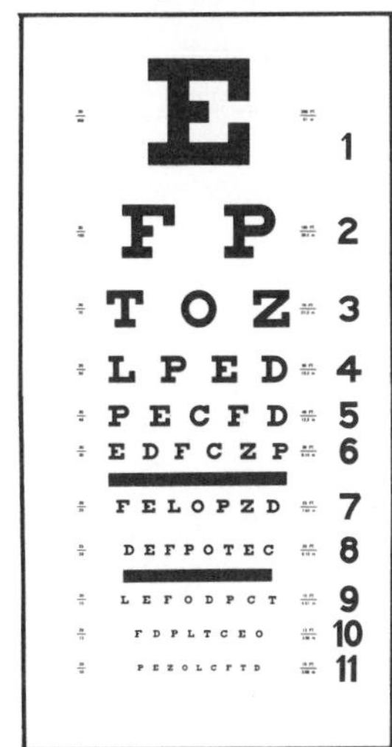

Snellen "E" chart

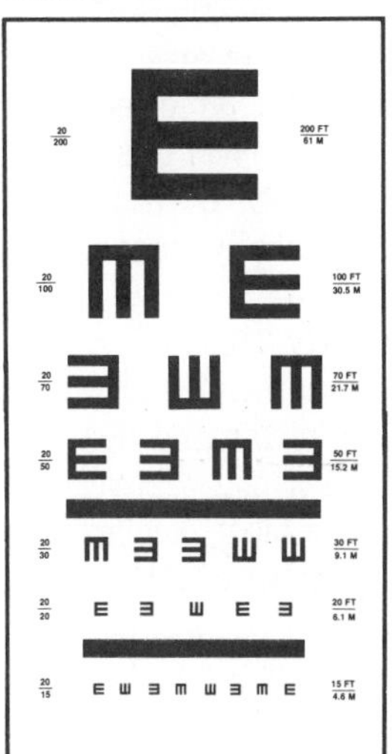

Scale

The scale is one of the first pieces of basic equipment the nurse uses to assess a client. Scales are available for infants and for adults. An infant should be weighed without any clothing. An adult should be weighed lightly dressed and without shoes. The amount of clothing the client wears should be the same at each weigh-in; otherwise the results may vary because clothing can add several pounds to a client's weight.

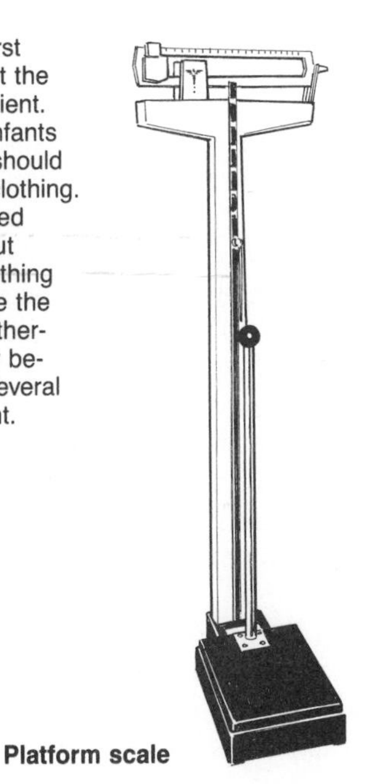

Platform scale

will give a false low reading; a too-small cuff, a false high reading. To determine the proper size, wrap the cuff around the client's arm or leg with the bladder uninflated; the bladder should cover about three quarters of the circumference of the limb.

To measure blood pressure, use a sphygmomanometer and a stethoscope: while listening for blood pressure sounds with the stethoscope, obtain a measurement by watching the manometer. The manometer may be an aneroid model, with a needle gauge, or the more reliable mercury model, with a mercury column. Most aneroid manometer gauges have clips so that the manometer can rest on the table or attach to the cuff.

To obtain an accurate reading, the nurse faces the aneroid manometer directly or views the mercury manometer at eye level to see the meniscus in the mercury column properly. Both manometer types must be calibrated periodically to ensure accuracy.

Visual acuity charts

Various visual acuity charts are used in screening examinations of far and near vision. Mounted on a wall, the far vision chart is read from a distance of 20′ (6 meters). The most commonly used far vision chart, the Snellen alphabet chart, contains 11 lines of various letters of graduated size. Another alphabet chart, the Stycar chart, uses several easily recognized letters, such as X, O, C, and V. The Snellen alphabet chart is appropriate for literate adults and older children; the Stycar chart, for illiterate adults and for prescreening preparation of children over age 2½.

The Snellen "E" chart, used to test young children and illiterate or non–English-speaking clients, consists of eight graduated-sized lines of *E*s facing in various directions. To help a non–English-speaking client understand this chart, the nurse can use hand gestures or ask a family member who understands English or sign language to help explain the examination.

To test near vision, the nurse can use a pocket-sized card containing numbers, letters, and symbols of various sizes. The nurse holds the card about 14″ (35.6 cm) from the client's eyes, and asks the client to identify the various characters; or uses a page from a magazine or newspaper to assess near vision in a literate client. (For more information on using visual acuity charts, see Chapter 9, Eyes and Ears.)

Penlight or flashlight

The nurse uses a penlight or flashlight to evaluate pupillary responses to light during the neurologic assessment and to assess hard-to-see areas, such as oral or nasal structures or the pharynx. Some clinics and hospital units have large flashlights available; however, a personal disposable penlight or a penlight with easily changed batteries is better suited for client assessment.

Measuring tape and pocket ruler

The nurse uses a measuring tape to measure the length, width, and circumference of various body parts and to assess certain gradual anatomic changes, such as arm or leg swelling, a pregnant client's changing fundal height, or an infant's growing head circumference. Disposable paper measuring tapes and retractable tapes made of stronger material are available. (*Note:* The nurse can make a measuring tape by marking a piece of surgical tape in centimeter or inch increments.)

When assessing the thorax and abdomen, the nurse can use a pocket ruler to measure diaphragmatic excursion and liver size. The pocket ruler may also be useful for measuring jugular vein distention height, skin lesion or mass size, and the distance between the apical pulse and sternal border.

Marking pencil

During some parts of the physical assessment, the nurse uses a pencil, such as a wax china marker, to mark the client's skin (for example, to indicate liver size, mark diaphragmatic descent on inspiration, or show peripheral pulse locations when doing repeated assessments—as on a foot with poor circulation). The nurse who uses a marking pencil should be sure that the marks wash off easily and should explain the markings to the client.

Scale

The nurse uses a platform scale with a height attachment to gather height and weight measurements of the client. The nurse begins by balancing the scale at zero, then has the client stand on the platform, measures height by extending the height attachment rod above the client's head, placing the crossbar against the client's crown, and reading the measurement on the height attachment rod. For infants, a smaller platform scale is available. It has curved sides to prevent the infant from falling off while the weight is taken. It measures in grams and ounces; the adult scale measures in pounds, in ¼-lb increments, and kilograms, in ⅒-kg increments.

Other basic assessment equipment

A complete collection of basic physical assessment equipment includes these additional items:

- a wooden tongue depressor to help assess the gag reflex and reveal the pharynx
- safety pins to test how well a client differentiates between dull and sharp pain
- cotton balls to check fine-touch sensitivity

- test tubes filled with hot and cold water to assess temperature sensitivity
- common, easily identified substances, such as ground coffee and vanilla extract, to evaluate smell and taste sensations
- a water-soluble lubricant and disposable latex gloves for rectal and vaginal assessment. (*Note:* The nurse must wear gloves when handling body fluids or touching open lesions or wounds.)

Advanced assessment equipment

Certain steps in the physical assessment may require specialized equipment—ophthalmoscope, nasoscope, otoscope, and tuning fork. Although these devices usually are reserved for nurses with special training and expanded roles, all nurses should be familiar with them and their applications. Other equipment sometimes used in advanced assessment includes the reflex hammer, skin calipers, vaginal speculum, goniometer, and transilluminator. (For more information, see *Advanced assessment equipment,* pages 78 through 81.)

Ophthalmoscope

The nurse uses an ophthalmoscope (a light source and a system of lenses and mirrors) to assess internal eye structures (collectively called the fundus). Light intensity is adjustable, but the nurse should protect the client's comfort by using the lowest intensity possible.

Switching the aperture (ophthalmoscope opening) changes the color or size of the light beam. The large, round aperture proves suitable for most clients; the small, round aperture (sometimes a half circle), for clients with small pupils. To localize and measure fundal lesions, the nurse can use the grid or target aperture; to assess lesion elevation and examine the anterior eye, the slit beam; to assess specific fundal details, the green filter. To identify these apertures, shine the light onto a white piece of paper.

To use the ophthalmoscope, the nurse follows this procedure: hold it in the palm of your hand and place your index finger on the lens selection disk. This disk—a rotating dial on the instrument head—allows you to change the lens to compensate for the client's or your own myopia (nearsightedness) or hyperopia (farsightedness). Lens power is measured in diopters, marked by numbers that appear in an illuminated window as you turn the dial. Diopter values range from about −25 to +40. Positive diopters, numbered in black, show closer structures or compensate for a short, hyperopic eyeball. Negative diopters, numbered in red, help compensate for a longer, myopic eyeball. For positive diopters, turn the dial clockwise; for negative diopters, turn it counterclockwise.

Some ophthalmoscopes must be recharged periodically. To do this, disassemble the handle and plug it into a wall outlet. Also, change batteries and light bulbs as necessary. (For more details on using an ophthalmoscope, see Chapter 9, Eyes and Ears.)

Nasoscope

The nurse uses a nasoscope to assess the nasal interior. The simplest type of nasoscope, the nasal speculum, is a double-bladed metal instrument used with a penlight to assess the lower and middle nasal turbinates and nasal mucosa. Alternatively, assess nasal structures by attaching to the ophthalmoscope handle a short, wide speculum designed especially for the nostrils (nares). The third nasoscope type has a handle similar to an ophthalmoscope handle and a short, narrow head containing a light source. Any of these devices can cause the client discomfort if the nurse is not skilled.

Otoscope

The nurse uses an otoscope to assess the external auditory canal and tympanic membrane. The otoscope head, fixed to the same handle used for the ophthalmoscope, attaches and turns on just as the ophthalmoscope does; it provides light and magnification. Various funnel-like specula, ranging from 1/8" to 3/8" (0.32 to 1 cm) in diameter, fit onto the otoscope head. (For details on using the otoscope, see Chapter 9, Eyes and Ears.)

Tuning fork

The nurse uses a tuning fork to test sound conduction during the auditory assessment and vibratory sensation during the neurologic assessment. Vibrating a specific number of times per second, the tuning fork creates a characteristic sound known as its frequency. Different tuning forks have different frequencies, measured in cycles per second (CPS) or hertz (Hz). A high-frequency (500-Hz to 1,000-Hz) fork helps assess auditory function; a low-frequency (100-Hz to 400-Hz) fork helps assess vibratory sensation.

To use a tuning fork, the nurse follows this procedure: strike it lightly against a firm object, such as a desk top, or against your knee, to activate the vibrations. If the fork tines have knobs, pluck these to activate the vibrations. Then, depending on whether the assessment is for touch or hearing, place the base of the fork on a bony prominence or hold the fork near the client's ear. Do not touch the tines while they vibrate; this dampens the vibrations and interferes with accurate assessment.

(Text continues on page 81.)

Advanced assessment equipment

In the advanced physical assessment, the nurse should expect to use the following equipment: ophthalmoscope, otoscope, nasoscope, tuning forks, reflex hammer, vaginal speculum, skin calipers, transilluminator, and goniometer. The ophthalmoscope comes with various apertures; the otoscope, with specula of various sizes. Nasoscopes, tuning forks, reflex hammers, vaginal specula, skin calipers, transilluminators, and goniometers are available in several types.

Ophthalmoscope

Used to assess the eyes, the ophthalmoscope consists of a handle, which holds batteries, and a head, which twists into place. The head contains a system of mirrors and lenses and a light source. Various apertures fit over the lens.

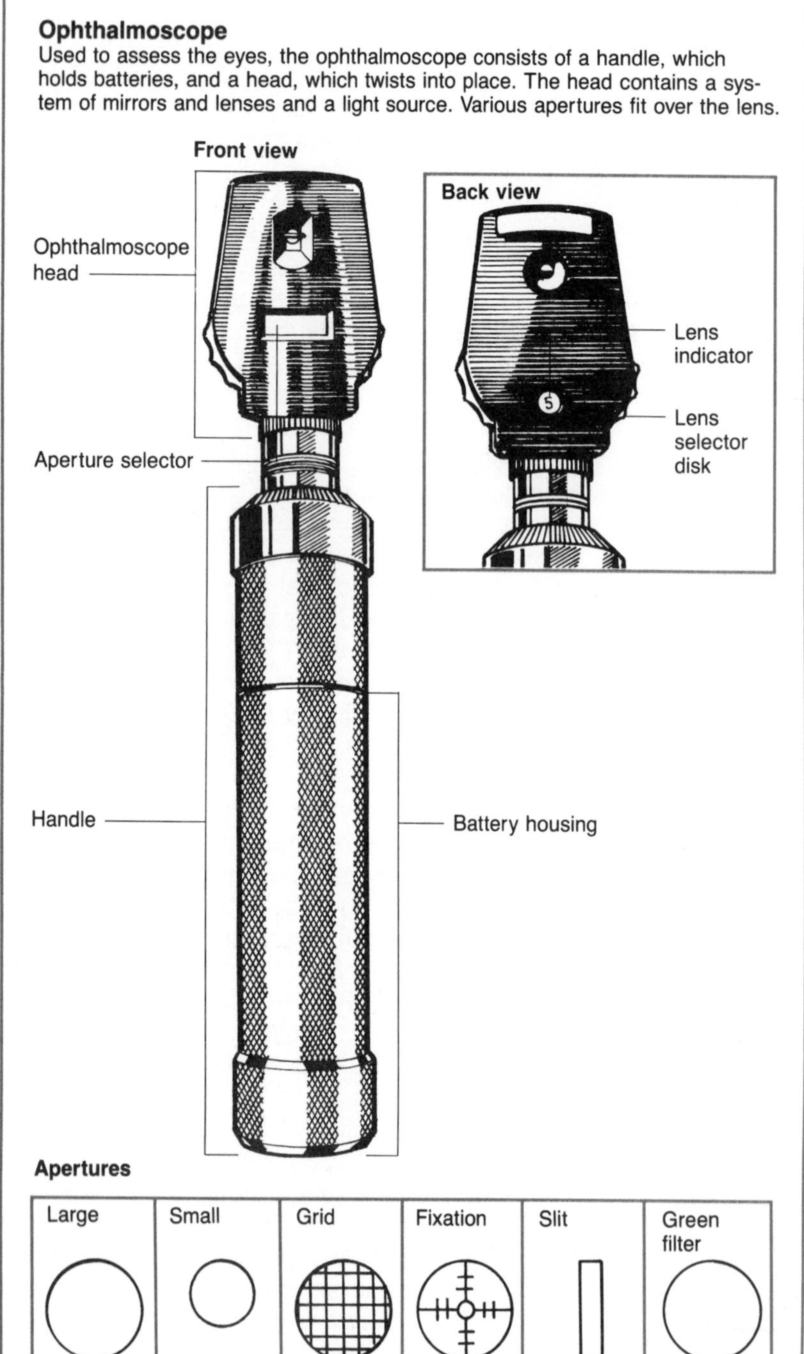

Large	Small	Grid	Fixation	Slit	Green filter

Nasoscope

Used to assess the nostrils, the nasoscope consists of a short, narrow head fitted with a light. A metal nasal speculum used with a penlight, or an ophthalmoscope fitted with a special nasal tip, also may be used to examine the nasal interior.

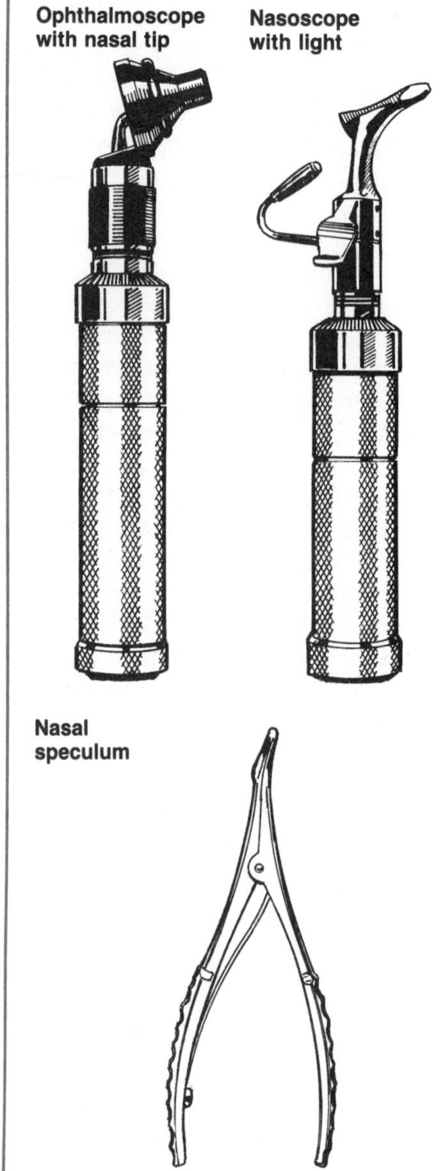

Otoscope

Used to assess the ear, the otoscope consists of a handle and battery housing, a head with light source and magnifying lens, and removable specula of varying sizes.

Magnifying lens

Light source

Speculum

Handle

Battery housing

Various sized specula

Tuning fork

Used to assess touch and hearing, tuning forks produce specific frequencies when struck. A low-frequency fork, such as a 256-Hz, can test vibration sensation; a high-frequency fork, such as a 512-Hz, can test hearing.

256-Hz fork

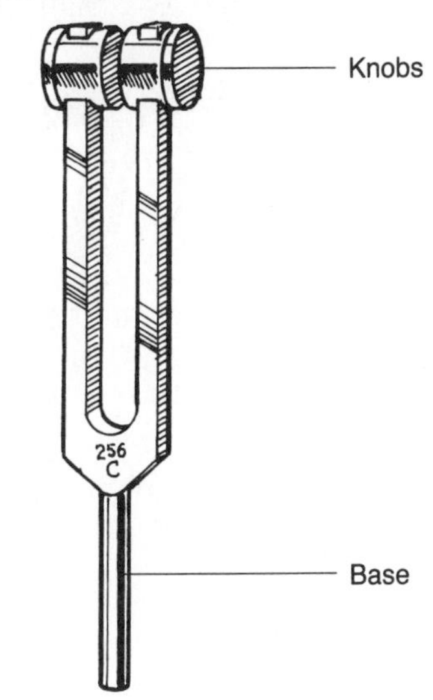

512-Hz fork

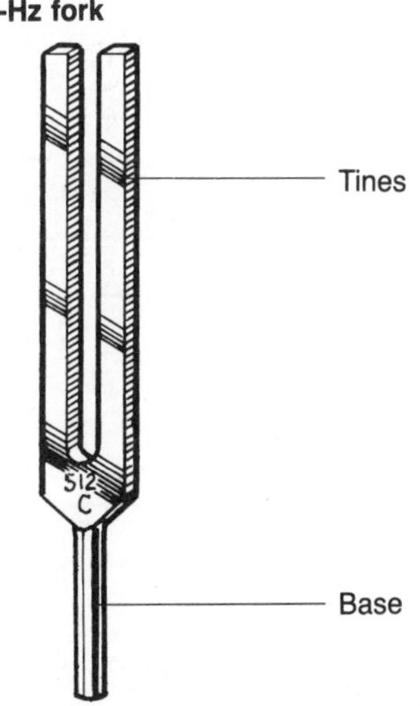

continued

Advanced assessment equipment continued

Reflex hammer
Used to evaluate deep tendon reflexes during the neurologic assessment, this small, rubber-tipped hammer is also called a percussion hammer.

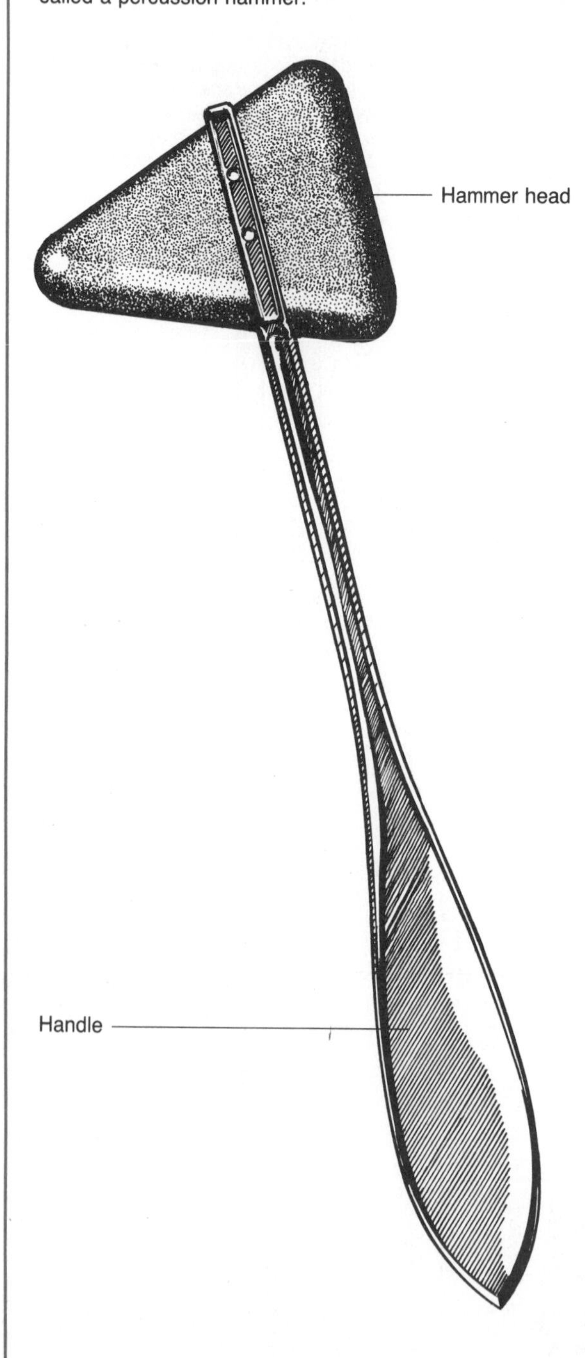

Skin calipers
Used to assess a client's nutritional status, skin calipers measure the thickness in millimeters of subcutaneous tissue.

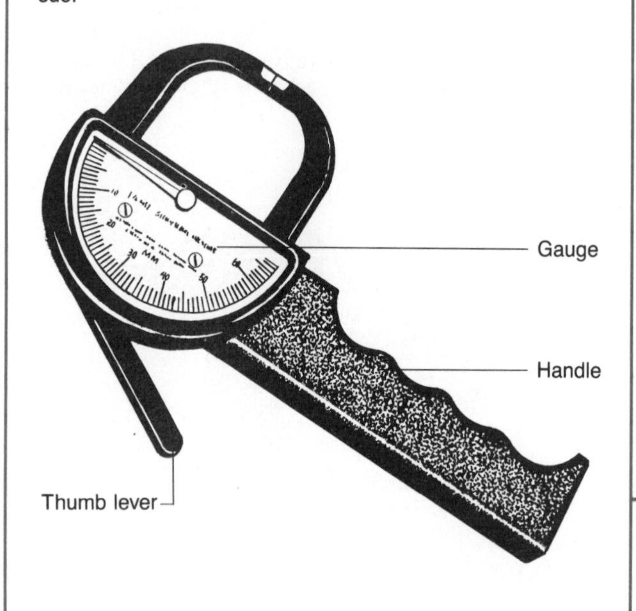

Vaginal speculum
Used to assess the female reproductive system, the vaginal speculum is available in several sizes and in stainless steel or plastic. After applying a water-soluble lubricant, the examiner inserts the speculum into the vaginal canal, then opens it to expose the vaginal walls and the cervix. This allows the examiner to inspect, palpate, and retrieve such specimens as cervical mucus.

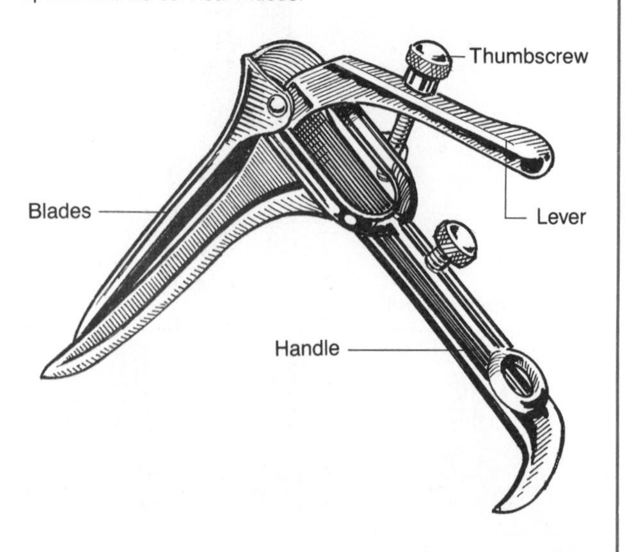

Goniometer
Used to assess joint motion, this device is a protractor with a movable and a fixed arm (axis). The center, or zero point, is placed on the client's joint; the fixed arm is placed perpendicular to the plane of motion. As the client moves the joint, the movable arm indicates the angle in degrees.

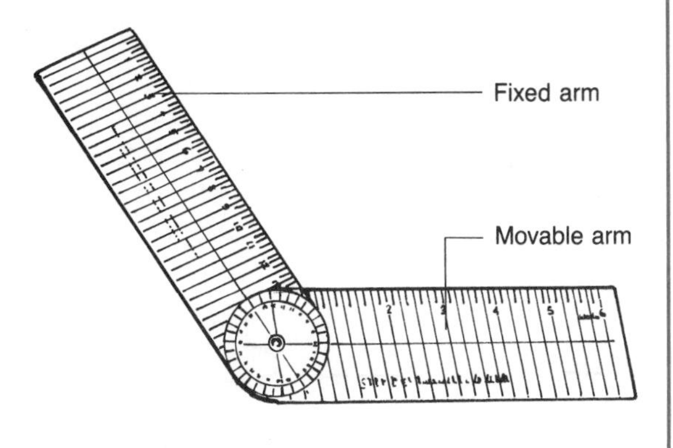

Transilluminator
Used to assess sinus contents, identify hydrocephalus in a child, or detect a scrotal hydrocele, this battery-operated device consists of an ophthalmoscope handle with a transilluminator head (light source with a narrowed light beam). When pressed against the body in a darkened room, the light produces a red glow that can detect air, tissues, or fluid. Electric transilluminators also are available. (*Note:* A flashlight can be converted to a transilluminator by placing a rubber adapter over its lamp.)

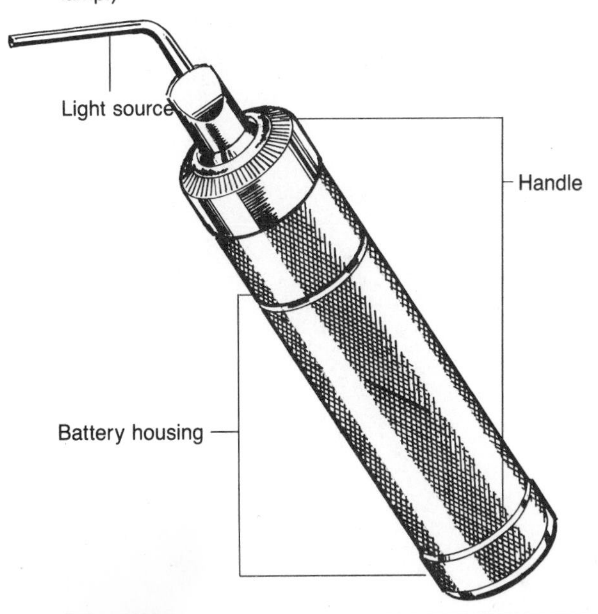

(For more information on using a tuning fork, see Chapter 9, Eyes and Ears, and Chapter 17, Nervous System.)

Physical assessment techniques

To perform the physical assessment, the nurse uses four basic techniques: inspection, palpation, percussion, and auscultation.

Inspection

Critical observation or inspection is the most frequently used assessment technique. Performed correctly, it also reveals more than the other techniques. However, an incomplete or hasty inspection may neglect important details or even yield false or misleading findings. To ensure accurate, useful information, the nurse should approach inspection in a careful, unhurried manner, pay close attention to details, and try to draw logical conclusions from the findings.

Unlike palpation, percussion, and auscultation, inspection is not a single, self-contained assessment step. Instead, it begins on first contact with the client and continues throughout the health history interview, general survey, vital sign measurement, and detailed body systems assessment. With each of these assessment phases, inspection findings enhance and refine the knowledge base.

Inspection can be direct or indirect. During direct inspection, rely totally on sight, hearing, and smell. During indirect inspection, use equipment, such as a nasal or vaginal speculum or an ophthalmoscope, to expose internal tissues or to enhance the view of a specific body area.

As an exercise in inspection, study a tree or shrub for a few minutes with a friend. Then compare observations; they may be quite different. Did you notice leaf shape and color? Did your friend? On close inspection, did you observe bark texture? The nurse must learn to inspect a client holistically, observing the total person as well as probing for minute details.

To inspect a specific body area, first make sure the area is sufficiently exposed and adequately lit. Then, survey the entire area, noting key landmarks and checking the overall condition. Next, focus on specifics—color, shape, texture, size, and movement.

Using the hands in palpation

To enhance palpation technique, the nurse can take advantage of the tactile sensitivity specific to each hand region. The tips and pads of the fingers can best distinguish texture and shape. The back, or dorsal surface, of the hand can best feel for warmth. The ulnar surface, or ball, of the hand (at the base of the fingers on the palmar side) can best feel thrills (fine vibrations over the precordium) and fremitus (tremulous vibrations over the chest wall) as well as vocal vibrations through the chest wall. The thumb and index finger can best assess hair texture, grasp tissues, and feel for lymph node enlargement. The flattened finger pads can best palpate tender tissues, feel for crepitus (crackling) at joints, and lightly probe the abdomen. A single finger or nail tip can best stroke the skin when attempting to elicit the cremasteric (testicular retraction) or abdominal reflexes in the neurologic examination. The whole hand can best test handgrip strength.

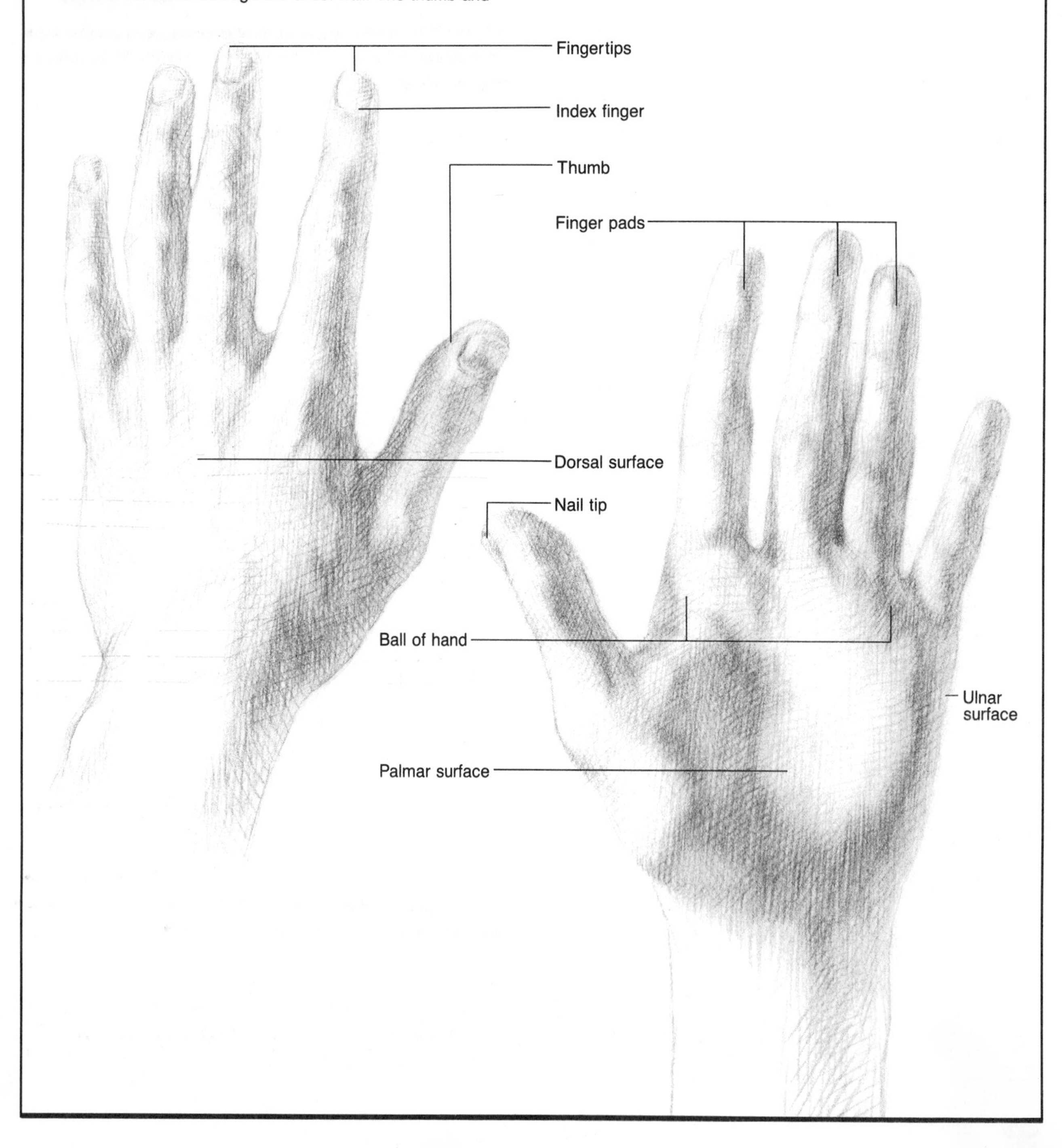

While inspecting the client, always maintain objectivity; do not be misled by preconceived ideas and expectations. Stay alert for unusual and unexpected findings as well as for predictable ones.

Palpation

During palpation, the nurse touches the body to feel pulsations and vibrations, to locate body structures (particularly in the abdomen), and to assess such characteristics as size, texture, warmth, mobility, and tenderness. Palpation allows detection of a pulse, muscle rigidity, enlarged lymph nodes, skin or hair dryness, organ tenderness or breast lumps, and measurement of the chest rising and falling with each respiration.

Usually, palpation follows inspection as the second technique in physical assessment. For example, if a rash is present on inspection, the nurse determines through palpation if the rash has a raised surface or feels tender or warm. However, during an abdominal or urinary system assessment, palpation should come at the end of the examination to avoid causing client discomfort and stimulating peristalsis (smooth muscle contractions that force food through the gastrointestinal tract, bile through the bile duct, and urine through the ureters).

Correct palpation requires a highly developed sense of touch. Learn to use the various parts of the fingers and hands for different purposes; also expect to learn several palpation techniques. (For further information, see *Using the hands in palpation,* and *Palpation techniques,* page 84.)

A client may react to palpation with anxiety, embarrassment, or discomfort. This, in turn, can lead to muscle tension or guarding, possibly interfering with palpation and causing misleading results. To put the client at ease and thus enhance the accuracy of palpation findings, the nurse follows these simple guidelines:

- Warm your hands before beginning.
- Explain what you will do and why, and describe what the client can expect, especially in sensitive areas.
- Encourage the client to relax by taking several deep breaths, concentrating on inhaling and exhaling.
- Stop palpating immediately if the client complains of pain.

Percussion

During percussion, the nurse uses quick, sharp tapping of the fingers or hands against body surfaces (usually the chest and abdomen) to produce sounds, elicit (detect) tenderness, or assess reflexes. Percussing for sound—the most common percussion goal—helps locate organ borders, identify organ shape and position, and determine if an organ is solid or filled with fluid or gas.

Three basic percussion methods include indirect (mediate), direct (immediate), and blunt (fist) percussion. In indirect percussion, the most common method, the examiner taps one finger against an object—usually the middle finger of the other hand—held against the skin surface. Although indirect percussion commonly produces clearer, crisper sounds than direct and blunt percussion, this technique requires practice to achieve good sound quality. (For more information, see *Percussion techniques,* page 85.)

Percussing for sound—perhaps the hardest assessment method to master—requires a skilled touch and an ear trained to detect slight sound variations. Organs and tissues produce sounds of varying loudness, pitch, and duration, depending upon their density. For instance, air-filled cavities, such as the lungs, produce markedly different sounds from those produced by the liver and other dense tissues.

When percussing for sound, the nurse uses quick, light blows to create vibrations that penetrate about 1½" to 2" (4 to 5 cm) under the skin surface. The returning sounds reflect the contents of the percussed body cavity.

Normal percussion sounds over the chest and abdomen include:

- resonance—the long, low, hollow sound heard over an intercostal space lying above healthy lung tissue
- tympany—the loud, high-pitched, drumlike sound heard over a gastric air bubble or gas-filled bowel
- dullness—the soft, high-pitched, thudding sound normally heard over more solid organs, such as the liver and heart. (*Note:* Dullness heard in a normally resonant or tympanic area warrants further investigation.)

Abnormal percussion sounds may be heard over body organs. Consider hyperresonance—a long, loud, low-pitched sound—a classic sign of lung hyperinflation, as in emphysema. Flatness—similar to dullness but shorter in duration and softer in intensity—may also be heard over pleural fluid accumulation or pleural thickening. (For a summary of sounds produced by percussion, see *Percussion sounds,* page 86.)

When percussing, the nurse moves from resonant areas to dull areas to accentuate any sound differences, as in these examples: to identify the lower border of liver dullness, begin percussing over the tympanic abdominal regions, then move up toward the dull liver area. To identify the upper border of liver dullness, begin over the lungs and percuss downward. Compare from side to side, tapping a few times in each area. Except for areas over such organs as the liver, gallbladder, and spleen, percussion findings should be symmetrical.

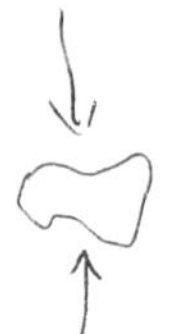

(Text continues on page 86.)

Palpation techniques

To perform thorough assessments, the nurse needs to master the several palpation techniques described here. *Light palpation* involves using the tips and pads of the fingers to apply light pressure to the skin surface. *Ballottement*, a light palpation variation, involves gentle, repetitive bouncing of tissues against the hand (think of bouncing a small ball gently). *Deep palpation* requires use of both hands and heavier pressure.

Light palpation

To perform light palpation, press gently on the skin, indenting it ½″ to ¾″ (1 to 2 cm). Use the lightest touch possible; too much pressure blunts your sensitivity. Close your eyes to concentrate on what your fingers are feeling.

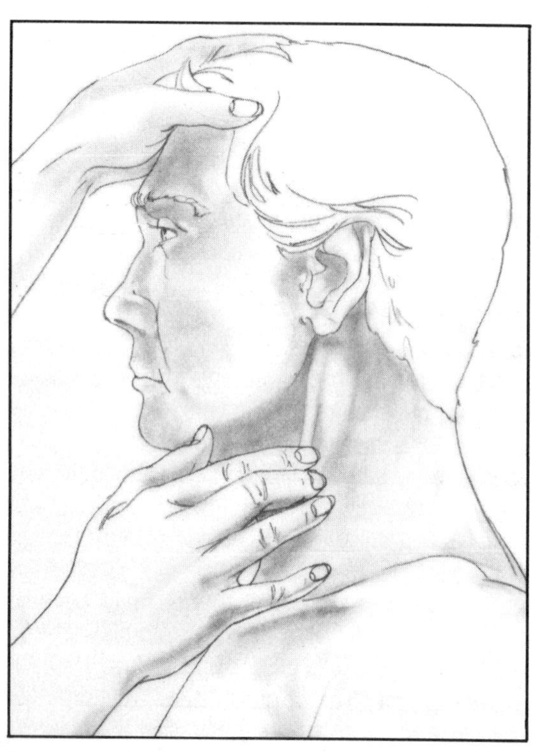

Deep palpation (bimanual palpation)

To perform deep palpation, increase your fingertip pressure, indenting the skin about 1½″ (4 cm). Place your other hand on top of the palpating hand to control and guide your movements. To perform a variation of deep palpation that allows pinpointing an inflamed area, press firmly with one hand, then lift your hand away quickly. If the client complains of increased pain as you release the pressure, you have identified rebound tenderness. (Suspect peritonitis if you elicit rebound tenderness when examining the abdomen.)

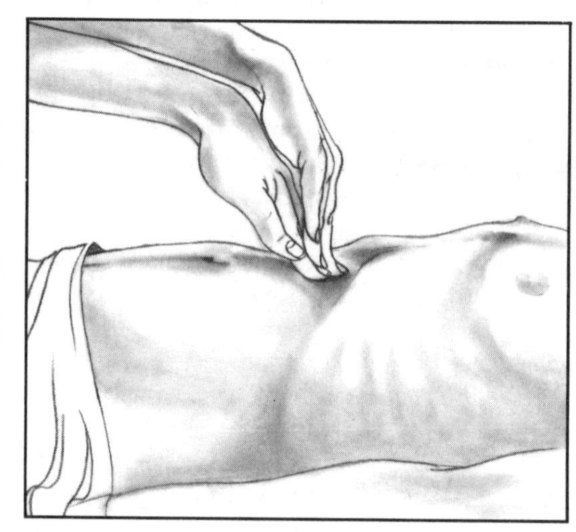

Use both hands (bimanual palpation) to trap a deep, underlying, hard-to-palpate organ (such as the kidney or spleen) or to fix or stabilize an organ (such as the uterus) with one hand and palpate it with the other.

Light ballottement

To perform light ballottement, apply light, rapid pressure from quadrant to quadrant of the client's abdomen. Keep your hand on the skin surface to detect any tissue rebound.

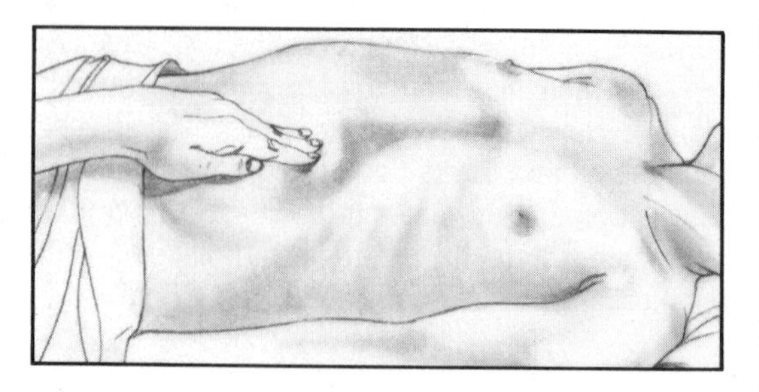

Deep ballottement

To perform deep ballottement, apply abrupt, deep pressure; then release the pressure, but maintain fingertip contact with the skin.

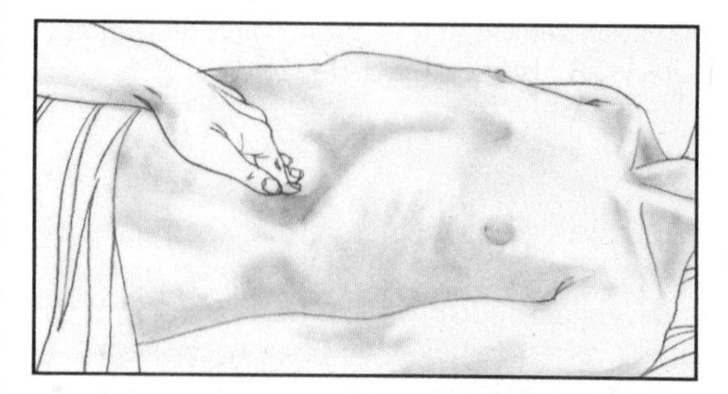

Percussion techniques

To assess clients completely, the nurse needs to be able to perform these three percussion techniques: indirect, direct, and blunt percussion.

Indirect percussion

To perform indirect percussion, use the middle finger of your nondominant hand as the pleximeter (the mediating device used to receive the taps) and the middle finger of your dominant hand as the plexor (the device used to tap the pleximeter). Place the pleximeter finger firmly against a body surface, such as the upper back. With your wrist flexed loosely, use the tip of your plexor finger to deliver a crisp blow just beneath the distal joint of the pleximeter. Be sure to hold the plexor perpendicular to the pleximeter. Tap lightly and quickly, removing the plexor as soon as you have delivered each blow.

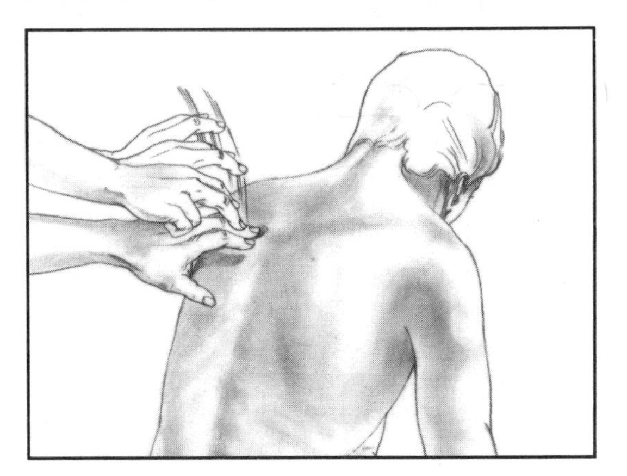

Direct percussion

To perform direct percussion, tap your hand or fingertip directly against the body surface. This method helps assess an adult's sinuses for tenderness or elicit sounds in a child's thorax.

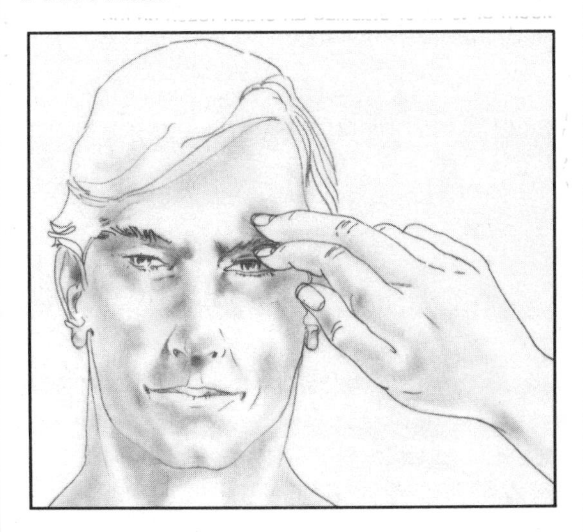

Blunt percussion

To perform blunt percussion, strike the ulnar surface of your fist against the body surface. Alternatively, you may use both hands by placing the palm of one hand over the area to be percussed, then making a fist with the other hand and using it to strike the back of the first hand. Both techniques aim to elicit tenderness—*not* to create a sound—over such organs as the kidneys, gallbladder, or liver. (Another blunt percussion method, used in the neurologic examination, involves tapping a rubber-tipped reflex hammer against a tendon to create a reflexive muscle contraction.)

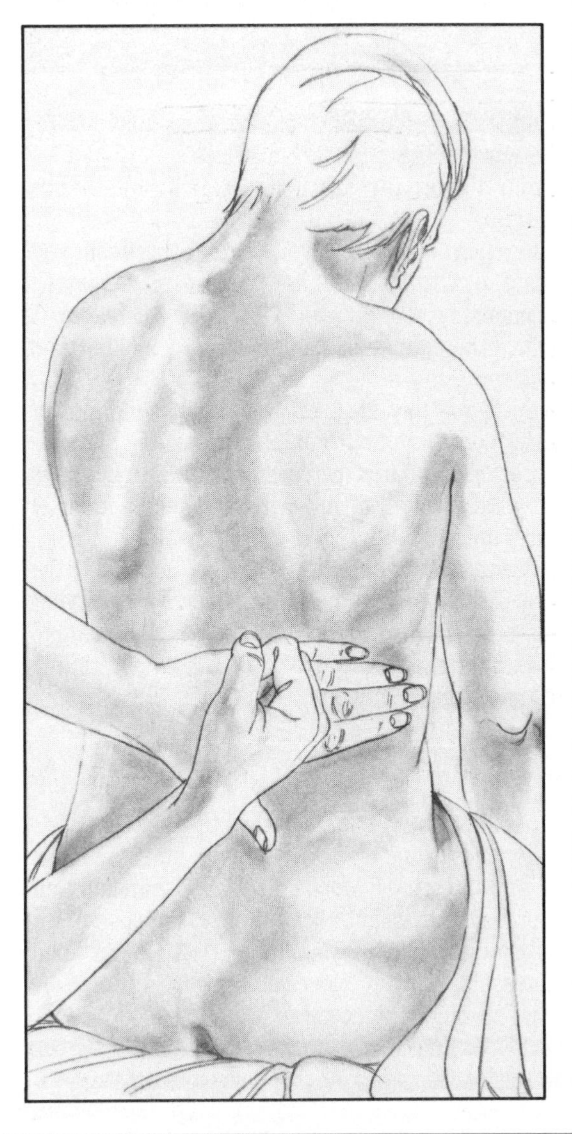

Percussion sounds

Percussion produces sounds that vary according to the tissue being percussed. This chart shows important percussion sounds along with their characteristics and typical locations.

SOUND	INTENSITY	PITCH	DURATION	QUALITY	SOURCE
Resonance	Moderate to loud	Low	Long	Hollow	Normal lung
Tympany	Loud	High	Moderate	Drumlike	Gastric air bubble; intestinal air
Dullness	Soft to moderate	High	Moderate	Thudlike	Liver; full bladder; pregnant uterus
Hyperresonance	Very loud	Very low	Long	Booming	Hyperinflated lung (as in emphysema)
Flatness	Soft	High	Short	Flat	Muscle

To enhance percussion technique and improve results, the nurse follows these guidelines:
• Keep your fingernails short, and warm your hands before starting.
• Have the client void before you begin; otherwise, you could mistake a full bladder for a mass or cause the client discomfort.
• Make sure the examination room or area is quiet and distraction-free.
• Remove any jewelry or other items that could clatter and interfere with the ability to hear returning sounds.
• Before performing blunt percussion, briefly explain to the client what you will do and why. This technique may startle and upset an unprepared client.
• In an obese client, expect percussion sounds to be muffled by a thick subcutaneous fat layer. To help overcome this problem, use the lateral aspect of the thumb as the pleximeter and tap sharply on the last thumb joint with your plexor finger.

Auscultation

During auscultation, the nurse listens to body sounds—particularly those produced by the heart, lungs, vessels, stomach, and intestines. Most auscultated sounds result from air or fluid movement—for example, the rush of air through respiratory pathways, the turbulent flow of blood through vessels, and the movement of gas (agitated by peristalsis) through the bowels.

Usually, the nurse performs auscultation after the other assessment techniques. When examining the abdomen, however, always auscultate second—*after* inspecting but *before* percussing and palpating. That way, bowel sounds are heard before palpation disrupts them.

The nurse can hear body sounds, such as the voice, loud wheezing, or stomach growls, fairly easily, but will need a stethoscope to hear softer ones. An appropriate procedure is this one: Use a high-quality, properly fitting stethoscope, provide a quiet environment, and make sure that the body area to be auscultated is sufficiently exposed. Remember that a gown or bed linens can interfere with sound transmission. Instruct the client to remain quiet and still. Before starting, warm the stethoscope head (diaphragm and bell) in your hand; otherwise, the cold metal may make the client shiver, possibly producing unwanted sounds. Place the diaphragm or bell over the appropriate area. Closing your eyes to help focus your attention, listen intently to individual sounds and try to identify their characteristics. Determine the intensity, pitch, and duration of each sound and check the frequency of recurring sounds.

Approach to physical assessment

The physical assessment may take various forms. A *complete* physical assessment—appropriate for periodic health checks—includes a general survey, vital sign measurements, height and weight measurements, and assessment of all organs and body systems.

However, in the hospital and many other settings, the nurse rarely has the opportunity to perform a complete assessment. In such cases, the nurse may conduct a ***modified*** assessment, using knowledge of the client's history and complaints. For example, if the client has peripheral vascular disease, include skin and peripheral pulse examination in the assessment; if the client has a herniated lumbar disk, test motor function and sensation in the legs and feet.

No matter which type of assessment is performed or where—hospital, clinic, or home—the nurse should keep in mind that the procedure can cause anxiety or fear. The client may worry that the assessment will confirm a suspected illness or uncover an unexpected problem, or may even consider the assessment an invasion of privacy because the nurse must observe and touch sensitive, private, and perhaps painful body areas.

Using the following guidelines can help ensure the correct approach to physical assessment, thereby enhancing the client's and the nurse's comfort. Some guidelines for the nurse serve at all times; others help with a specific type of assessment.

- Begin by introducing yourself. Give your full name. If you wish, explain that you may take longer than a more experienced examiner to complete the assessment. (In many cases, the client appreciates the extra attention.)
- Make sure your grooming, dress, and behavior reflect a professional attitude. This enhances the client's sense of dignity and promotes respect for you. For example, address an adult client by title and last name (such as Mr. Murphy, Mrs. Harper, Rev. Smith, Dr. Jones) unless asked to do otherwise.
- Before starting the assessment, briefly explain what you will do and why; include any position changes that you will ask the client to make. (For more information, see *Client positioning and draping guidelines,* page 88.) As you proceed with the assessment, explain each step in detail. By reassuring the client that the assessment will hold no surprises or unexpected discomfort, you promote trust and cooperation.
- Have all necessary equipment on hand and in working order. Leaving the room to search for equipment could interrupt your concentration and make the client doubt your competence.
- Make sure the examination room is well lighted with natural lighting (preferable) or adequate artificial light.
- To help ensure accurate findings and promote client comfort, ask the client to void before you begin the assessment.
- Respect the client's privacy and modesty. Ask family members and other visitors to leave, then close the door and pull drapes, as appropriate. Let the client undress in privacy, if possible, and provide a gown or sheet to cover up. Drape the client so that you can easily expose body areas for examination. (Allow a modest client to wait until absolutely necessary before removing undergarments.)
- Make the client as comfortable as possible by offering a pillow and making sure that the room and assessment equipment are warm.
- Always warn the client before performing a procedure that may cause discomfort. If posssible, avoid touching tender or painful areas until the end of the assessment.
- Use the same communication skills you applied in the interview. Politely ask the client to follow your instructions. Answer any questions and express thanks for cooperation—but do not let conversation interfere with your concentration. Avoid inappropriate jokes and disparaging comments.
- Be sensitive, unhurried, and reassuring—especially with an elderly client, who may move slowly. If the client seems to be tiring, provide a rest period. Concerned, caring behavior markedly enhances the client's comfort and builds confidence in you.
- Wash your hands before and after the assessment, in the client's presence. Using good hand-washing technique in the client's presence shows that you care for the safety of this client, other clients, and yourself.
- Dress comfortably and minimize position changes during the assessment. When assessing a bedridden client, raise the bed to a level comfortable for you.
- Always use the same systematic approach to assessment, varying it only to accommodate the client's particular needs. This reduces the risk of overlooking a significant finding. For example, develop the habit of working from the same side for all clients so that you assess body regions in the same way each time.
- Avoid negative reactions, such as grimaces or exclamations, to abnormal or unexpected findings and unpleasant odors or sights. Even a seriously ill client may notice your reaction and become anxious, embarrassed, or angry.

Special considerations for pediatric clients

The nurse may perform a pediatric assessment for various purposes, including well-baby visits; routine screenings for eyesight, hearing, and growth and development; and follow-up visits after an illness. Whatever the purpose, use a gentle, patient approach and be sure to assess how well the child has achieved developmental milestones. If possible, also evaluate the parent-child relationship.

Tailor your assessment to the child's age and developmental level. Infants (up to age 1) usually respond and cooperate readily, and rarely mind being undressed

Client positioning and draping guidelines

Requirements for client positioning and draping vary with the body system or region being assessed. These illustrations show the primary positioning and draping arrangements that the nurse uses during a routine assessment.

To examine the head, neck, and anterior and posterior thorax, have the client sit on the edge of the examination table.

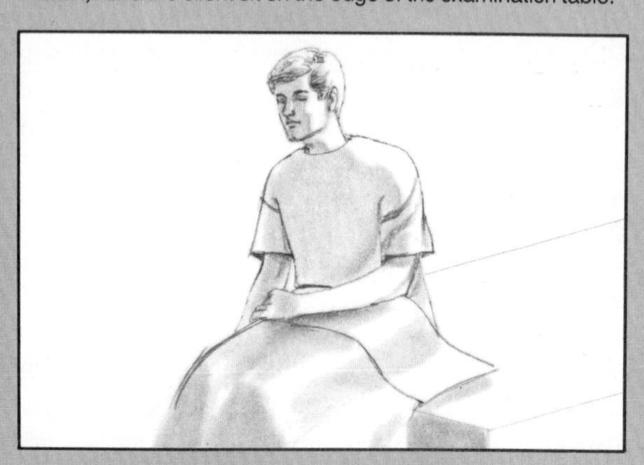

To begin examining the female client's breasts, place her in a seated position. For the second part of the examination, ask her to lie down. When she does, place a small pillow or folded towel beneath her shoulder on the side being examined. To spread her breast more evenly over the chest, ask her to place her arm (on the side being examined) over her head.

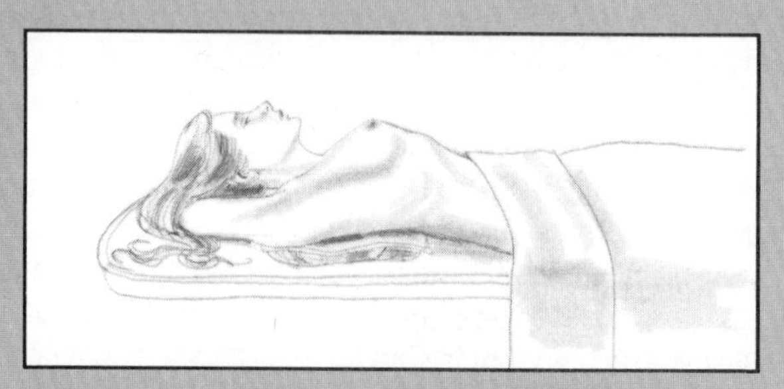

To perform a rectal examination on a male client, have him lean across the examination table. If he cannot stand upright, have him lie on his left side, with his right hip and knee slightly flexed and his buttocks close to the edge of the table.

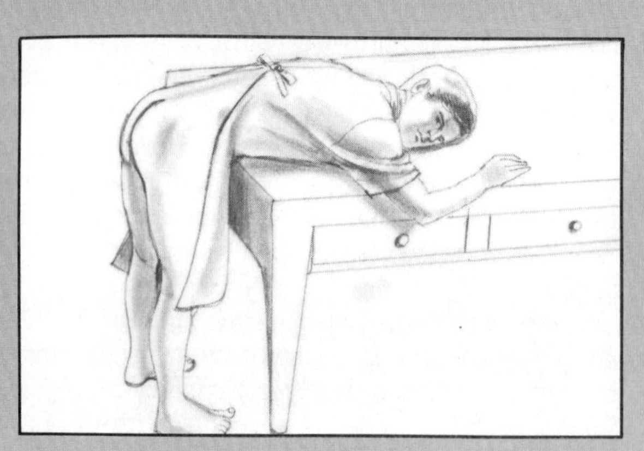

To examine the abdomen and cardiovascular system, place the client supine and stand on the right. For a female client, ensure privacy during abdominal assessment by placing a towel over her breasts and upper thorax. Pull the sheet down as far as her symphysis pubis, but do not expose this area.

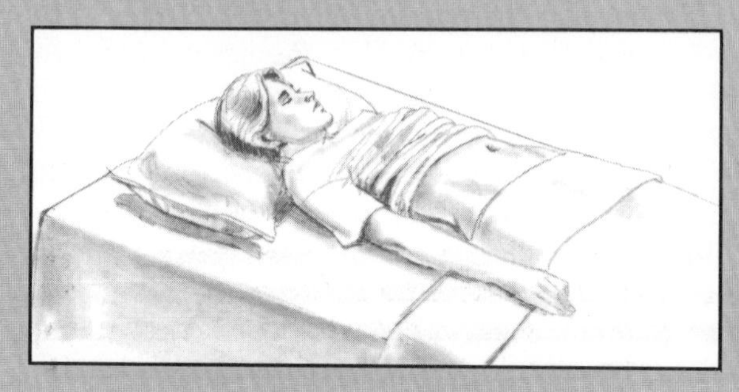

To examine the female client's reproductive system, place her in the lithotomy position. Drape a sheet diagonally over her chest and knees and between her legs. Her buttocks should be at or just past the edge of the table and her feet in the stirrups. The rectal examination may be done in this position, also.

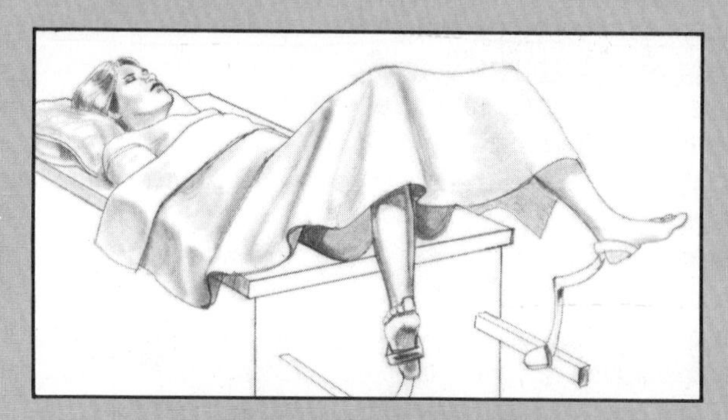

To perform some portions of the neurologic and musculoskeletal examinations, have the client stand (when feasible) or sit.

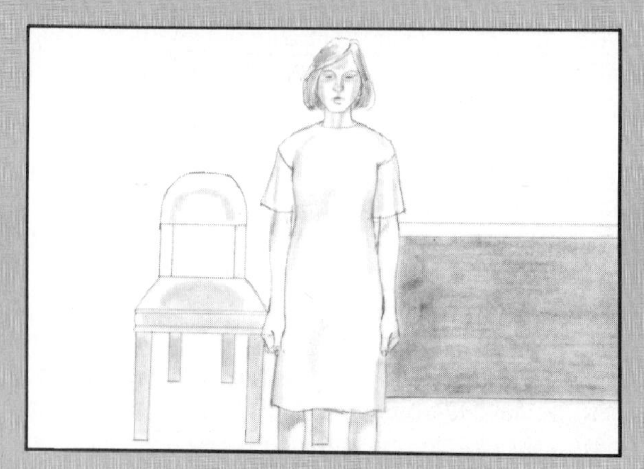

and examined naked. To help the infant relax, coo and smile during the examination. As appropriate, allow the parent to hold the infant. With an infant who breastfeeds during the assessment, assess feeding technique.

A child age 1 to 2 may be more fearful and harder to examine. You may need to calm or distract an upset or uncooperative child with a toy or another diversion, such as funny noises or a game of peek-a-boo. Keep in mind that young children typically find eye, ear, and mouth assessment more distressing than assessment of other body areas. For this reason, examine the head last instead of following the standard head-to-toe format. Hip abduction evaluation also can cause distress, so delay this until late in the examination. Also delay assessment of a crying child, if possible. Crying tenses the muscles, preventing accurate musculoskeletal and neurologic assessment. When accompanied by sobs, crying also can interfere with auscultation of heart sounds.

A child age 2 to 3 may be the most difficult to assess. This child may dislike being undressed and touched and may cling to the parent. To improve the assessment, develop a supportive relationship with the parent and take the time to gain the trust of both parent and child. Encourage the parent to participate, and let the child sit on the parent's lap. Explain each examination instrument and demonstrate its use on the parent. If appropriate, let the child touch the equipment and help with the assessment, such as by holding the stethoscope in place on the chest. When possible, integrate play into the assessment. For example, let the child pretend to listen to your heart or to a doll's heart. These creative touches improve cooperation by developing trust and teaching the child about the body.

By age 4 or 5, a child typically becomes more cooperative and less fearful of the assessment. This child responds especially well when play is incorporated into the assessment, as appropriate.

Compared to a young child, an older child or adolescent proves easier to engage in conversation, follows instructions more willingly, and has a better understanding of the goal of assessment. More independent, this client may ask *not* to have a parent present during the assessment; if so, respect this request. Also, be sensitive to the client's increased sense of modesty. Provide adequate privacy and let the client keep undergarments on until the last minute. Let the adolescent know that you will answer any questions about physical changes related to emerging sexuality—a topic of particular concern at this age.

Special considerations for pregnant clients

Assessment of a pregnant client has a dual focus—the client and her developing fetus. While assessing the maternal and fetal parameters that mark the normal course of pregnancy—fundal height, nutritional status, weight gain, pelvic size, fetal growth, and the changing appearance of the breasts and vagina—the nurse also checks for evidence of pregnancy-related complications. (For detailed assessment steps, see Chapter 22, Perinatal and Neonatal Assessment.)

To help assess a pregnant client properly, the nurse follows these guidelines:

- Be prepared to perform a comprehensive assessment—pregnancy affects a woman's entire body.
- Provide a chair that offers adequate support. A pregnant client in the third trimester usually has trouble getting into and rising from a soft, low chair. Help the client onto the examination table and into position, and drape her appropriately.
- Allow ample time for the assessment so that the client does not feel rushed. Also keep in mind that normal hormonal swings during pregnancy may make the client feel impatient, then embarrassed by her impatience.

Special considerations for elderly clients

When assessing an elderly client, the nurse should be aware that aging normally causes physiologic changes and impairs the body's response to stress, illness, and injury. Specific aging-related changes may include reduced muscle strength and range of motion, vital sign changes, slowed reflexes, impaired sensory perception, and slowed or impaired thought processes. These changes may contribute to the elderly client's increased risk for interrelated and chronic health problems—most notably, cardiovascular and cerebrovascular disease, cancer, dementia, cataracts, diabetes, and lung disease. To complicate matters, an elderly client may take many medications, possibly leading to adverse reactions or unexpected drug interactions that can interfere with interpretation of assessment findings.

During the assessment, address the client respectfully, using the title and last name unless the client requests otherwise. Keep in mind that this client may prefer more formal social conventions than those widely used today and may find an overly casual manner offensive.

Be sure to phrase your instructions simply and slowly, addressing one point at a time. Give the client plenty of time to respond. Because an elderly client may tire easily and have trouble changing positions, allow extra time for each assessment step. However, do not assume that all elderly clients are frail, move slowly, or are hard of hearing. Such preconceptions can interfere with accurate assessment.

Special considerations for disabled clients

The nurse may assess a disabled client during a routine health screening or for a special reason, such as determining eligibility for rehabilitation or setting vocational goals. Whatever the purpose, focus on the client's functional ability and mental capacity. Tailor your assessment to the client's specific needs, assets, and limitations. For example, provide detailed verbal instructions to a blind client; simplify instructions for a developmentally disabled (mentally retarded) client.

A disabled client may reveal beforehand whether the disability limits participation in the assessment. Take the time to learn as much as possible about the client's abilities and impairments before starting the assessment. The client will appreciate this step and may respond with increased cooperation. As with other clients, avoid stereotyping the disabled client; show sensitivity and consideration at all times.

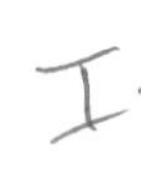

The general survey

As the first step in the physical assessment, the general survey provides vital information about the client's behavior and health status. During this step, the nurse documents initial impressions of the client in a one-paragraph statement—a summary that provides an overall picture guiding subsequent assessment.

The general survey requires skilled, focused observation and a confident, professional approach. The inexperienced nurse may feel self-conscious and may worry about the client's impressions. However, to detect subtle clues from behavior and appearance and derive an accurate client profile, learn to focus all your attention on the client—a skill that comes with practice and experience.

During the first contact with the client, be prepared to receive a steady stream of impressions, mostly visual. The client's sex, race, and approximate age will be obvious. Because some health concerns may relate to these factors, be sure to note them. Also note less obvious factors that may contribute to your overall impression, including signs of distress; facial characteristics; body type, posture, and movements; speech; dress, grooming, and personal hygiene; and psychological state.

(A) Signs of distress

First check for obvious signs of physical or emotional distress. Dyspnea (shortness of breath)—probably the most common sign of distress—suggests a cardiac or respiratory problem. Note any restlessness or wheezing, which may accompany asthma, or shallow, labored respirations, which may signal pneumonia. Determine if dyspnea occurs only with a particular position, such as recumbency; this may indicate cardiac involvement.

Pain, another clue to distress, typically shows in a client's facial expression, body movements, and posture. Check for halting, limited movements and an overly rigid or otherwise odd posture. If the client grimaces, writhes, clutches the abdomen, or shows other obvious signs of pain, stop the assessment and notify a physician.

Be aware that clients express emotional distress in varying ways. One client, for instance, may show distress through jerking hand movements or rapid speech; another may withdraw or sit with the head bowed and arms crossed over the chest.

(B) Facial characteristics

A client's face provides valuable clues to physical, emotional, and psychological well-being. Observe the face for expression, contour, and symmetry. Obvious tension, staring, trembling, a downcast or shifting gaze, or constant blinking suggests a neurologic or psychological problem. Facial trembling, for example, may result from anxiety or a facial nerve problem. A flat expression with no affect (outward manifestation of feelings) commonly accompanies Parkinson's disease (a progressive, degenerative neurologic disorder) and myasthenia gravis (a neuromuscular disorder causing muscle weakness). In some cases, facial trembling may indicate a psychological disturbance.

Abnormal features, such as an enlarged nose and lips, a protruding jaw, and a prominent supraorbital ridge, suggest acromegaly (a chronic metabolic disorder characterized by growth hormone overproduction). Facial asymmetry, with incomplete eye closure and one-sided mouth drooping, may result from the facial nerve paralysis typical of Bell's palsy.

Also, determine whether facial characteristics suggest the client's stated age. Chronic illness can cause dull, sagging, wrinkled skin and other signs of premature aging.

(C) Body type, posture, and movements

Assess the client's general body type, classifying the build as stocky, average, or slender. Check for cachexia (extreme thinness) or obesity. With an obese client, assess for abnormal fat distribution, as in Cushing's syndrome (characterized by truncal obesity and thin limbs). Note any unusual physical features; a rounded barrel chest, for example, may signal chronic lung disease.

While observing the client's overall body structure, pay especially close attention to the hands. Observe the fingers for clubbing (enlargement) or edema (swelling), which may indicate a cardiovascular problem; also check for contractures (abnormally stiff joint positions), suggesting arthritis.

Observe gait and other movements for symmetry, coordination, and smoothness. Note any obvious involuntary movements or deformities—for instance, an amputated limb. Gait problems, such as shuffling, may accompany Parkinson's disease. Limping may stem from previous injury; spasticity, from cerebral palsy. Note any use of assistive devices, such as a cane, walker, brace, or prosthesis (noting this also helps determine whether the client needs assistance with walking). In the hospital, your observations of body movement may take a different focus. For instance, note whether a bedridden client can sit up, turn, and reposition.

Also observe the client's posture—a clue to energy level, psychological status, and skeletal structure. If the client slumps, look for other signs of possible fatigue or depression. A hunched-over posture may mean merely that the client is cold; however, it could reflect guarding (a tense, protective reaction to abdominal pain) or a pulmonary problem. In the classic posture of chronic obstructive lung disease, the client hunches over a bedside table in an attempt to ease breathing.

(D) Speech

Assess the client's speech for tone, clarity, vocal strength, vocabulary, sentence structure, and pace. Hoarseness or softness may indicate laryngitis or cranial nerve paralysis. Inappropriate loudness suggests nervousness. A monotone may reflect depression. Fast, garbled speech may accompany a mental disorder; slow, garbled speech, a cerebrovascular accident (stroke). Note the client's vocabulary and word usage pattern—possible clues to educational level. (This information may help later when you plan the client's care and teaching sessions.)

Listen carefully to the speech pattern. A client with expressive aphasia (a neurologic condition impairing the ability to form words) may speak hesitantly and deliberately. Note whether the client constantly searches for words, repeats your words, or uses rhyming words—possible clues to a psychological disorder. Also identify other obvious speech characteristics, such as stuttering, lisping, or a foreign accent.

(E) Dress, grooming, and personal hygiene

A client's dress, grooming, and personal hygiene may reflect physical and psychological health status. Look for signs of apparent indifference to appearance or inability to perform self-care. Note whether the client's hair looks clean and neat, and evaluate facial and oral hygiene.

Closely observe the client's clothing, and note its appropriateness for the season and situation. Observe how well garments fit and match, and assess their cleanliness and general condition. Clashing colors, for example, could signal mental dysfunction or a visual deficit. However, avoid drawing final conclusions from these observations: although loose hems, holes, or incorrectly buttoned clothing may indicate failing vision or a psychological problem, it could also reflect financial problems.

Note any frank odors, such as alcohol, which may indicate alcoholism; urine, suggesting incontinence or poor hygiene; or excessive perfume or cologne, which may reflect an attempt to mask body odor. However, always consider these findings in context. Not all clients who smell of alcohol are alcoholics; also, certain sociocultural customs may account for specific body odors.

(F) Psychological state

Besides facial expression and posture, other behavioral components can supply important clues to the client's psychological status. For instance, note whether the client cooperates and understands and follows simple instructions, such as "Please sit down." Assess the client's level of awareness, attentiveness, and attention span. Assess the client's orientation to time, place, and person. Note lethargy, drowsiness, or other signs of decreased level of consciousness. (For an explanation of assessing mental status and level of consciousness, See Chapter 17, Nervous System.)

Also note whether the client appears relaxed and comfortable or nervous and fidgety. Extreme anxiety may cause rigidity, trembling, and restlessness; the client may experience abdominal pain and hold the arms against the stomach for relief.

Observe for any bizarre or repeated mannerisms or movements, such as involuntary, spasmodic movements. Check hand position and movement and use of gestures. A client who clasps the hands tightly, uses wildly flailing gestures, or experiences hand trembling may be psychologically disturbed.

If you shake hands, notice whether the client has a firm, steady grasp or a weak one; the latter may signal a neurologic problem or reflect aging-related changes. Also note whether the palm is dry; damp with sweat, as from anxiety; or cold and clammy, as from shock. Watch to see if the client bites the fingernails or constantly plays with an object, such as a tie or purse strap.

Special considerations for pediatric clients

When conducting a general survey of an infant or child, expect certain behaviors to vary according to the child's age. A newborn usually lies quietly in the parent's arms or cries softly when uncomfortable or disturbed. A child age 6 months to 2 years usually clings to the parent and may be scared or uncooperative. Expect a preschooler to show more confidence and curiosity and, after initial shyness, to cooperate with the assessment. A school-age child typically has a longer attention span and follows instructions better.

Evaluate the same details as for an adult, focusing on signs of distress, facial characteristics, posture, activity level, motor coordination, language function, maturity level, and ability to understand and cooperate with the assessment.

Keep in mind that a child may be more spontaneous and restless than an adult, may stare with frank curiosity, and may express emotion readily. Look for signs of anxiety, including thumb sucking, nail biting, and rocking. If a parent is present, observe how the parent and child interact. Note the amount and quality of physical contact and verbal communication, and assess how well the parent responds to the child's needs and copes with any crying or uncooperative behavior.

Special considerations for elderly clients

The general survey of an elderly client resembles that of any adult, but focuses more intensely on certain areas. For example, when observing the client's skin, gait, and posture, expect the normal physiologic changes of aging—loose, wrinkled, dry skin; a stiff, slow gait resulting from bone mineral loss; and a bent, stooped posture and knee flexion from kyphosis (increased thoracic spine curvature). Stay alert for clues to reduced self-care capacity, such as missing buttons or a misbuttoned shirt. Learn to identify key signs of aging-related disorders, such as the flat affect and shuffling gait of Parkinson's disease.

Although many elderly clients remain alert, independent, and active, some are at risk for special problems, including chronic disease, depression, and confusion. Most have endured numerous losses and have grieved for these losses in a healthy manner. However, some react with prolonged depression, anxiety, or other maladaptive responses. Early signs of depression include a short attention span, emotional lability (instability), and inattention to personal dress or hygiene.

Confusion, another finding in some elderly clients, can result from adverse drug reactions or interactions, dehydration, infection, nutritional problems, organic brain changes, and other factors. Unfamiliar surroundings and routines, such as during hospitalization or a stay in an extended-care facility, can contribute to confusion.

While assessing the elderly client, be aware that your attitudes toward aging and elderly persons can color your interpretation of the client's appearance and functional ability. For instance, if you respect the experience and wisdom that come with advanced age, you are more likely to assess a client's abilities in a positive light. If, on the other hand, you view most elderly persons as impaired or helpless, you may diminish the client's abilities.

Special considerations for disabled clients

When assessing the client with a disability, deficit, or deformity that impairs functioning, be sure to address special areas of client concern. Note any obvious signs of disability, such as use of a wheelchair or seeing-eye dog. Assess the client's functional ability, independence level, and attitude toward the disability and the assessment. As always, avoid stereotyping the client, and take a caring, sensitive approach.

Cultural and ethnic considerations

Caring for clients of diverse cultural and ethnic backgrounds is commonplace for the nurse. A client's lifestyle, values, beliefs, and cultural and ethnic customs can play a key role in appearance, behavior, and attitude toward health and illness. Be aware that your values and beliefs may distort your assessment of a client whose background differs from yours. To obtain the most accurate and useful general survey findings, remain as objective as possible and avoid imposing your values on the client.

During the general survey, attempt to assess the client's values and health beliefs accurately. Take care not to mistake cultural preferences in dress, manner, and physical appearance for abnormal behavior or signs of a physical or psychological disorder. For example, what you may consider poor hygiene might be considered normal in certain cultures. Likewise, behavior that may strike you as apathetic, seductive, or hostile might be a standard response to stress in clients from a particular family background.

Avoid stereotyping a client on the basis of ethnic or cultural background. Doing so tends to limit your appreciation of the client's uniqueness.

Documenting the general survey

The nurse documents general survey findings in a short, concise paragraph. Include only the information that you consider essential to communicating your overall impression of the client. Do not comment on everything you observe—only the most important points. For example, mention that the client has a facial rash, but do not describe the rash in detail until later, when documenting the complete physical assessment findings.

The following examples show how to document general assessment findings properly:

> Ms. Clemens is an alert, neatly dressed, slender, Black female, who looks her stated age of 30. She is relaxed, oriented to time, place, and person, and communicative. She speaks clearly and confidently. She shows no signs of distress.

> Mr. Gregorio is an elderly, obese, Caucasian male who is short of breath, gasps, and uses accessory respiratory muscles. He speaks sparingly and with effort; to aid in breathing, his arms are propped on an overbed table. He appears restless and anxious, but his speech is appropriate.

Vital signs

Assessment of vital signs—temperature, pulse, respirations, and blood pressure—is a basic nursing responsibility and an important method for measuring and monitoring vital body functions. Vital signs give insight into the function of specific organs—especially the heart and lungs—as well as entire body systems. The nurse obtains vital signs to establish baseline measurements, observe for trends, identify physiologic problems, and monitor a client's response to therapy.

During a complete physical assessment, the nurse will take all vital signs at once, or will integrate vital signs into different assessment steps. Because an abnormal finding can alert you to possible problems to investigate further as you proceed, you may prefer to take all vital signs at the beginning.

An ill client requires frequent vital sign assessment, with frequency depending on the nature and severity of the disorder. Expect to assess vital signs every 4 to 6 hours in a hospitalized client. In an acute situation, however, you may assess vital signs every 1 to 2 hours. After certain types of surgery and other procedures, a client may need extremely frequent monitoring—perhaps every 15 minutes. With any client, do not hesitate to obtain vital signs as often as you think appropriate.

When assessing vital signs, keep in mind that a single measurement usually proves far less clinically valuable than a series of measurements, which can substantiate a trend. In most cases, look for a change—from the normal range, from the client's normal measurement, or from previous measurements. Because vital signs reflect basic body functions, any significant change warrants further investigation.

General guidelines

To obtain accurate vital sign measurements, the nurse should keep the following guidelines in mind:

- Because physical and emotional stress can alter vital signs, have the client relax before you begin the assessment. Approach the client in a calm, unhurried manner and explain each step as you proceed.
- Develop and use a consistent system for obtaining vital signs; for example, check blood pressure, pulse, and respirations while taking the client's oral temperature. Also use a consistent method to assess each client's vital signs. For instance, if you or another nurse previously checked a client's temperature rectally, be sure to use the same route for subsequent measurements, as needed. (Be sure to document that the temperature was taken rectally.)
- If you obtain an unusual measurement or if you doubt a finding, repeat the measurement or, if possible, have another nurse repeat it. If you still feel uncertain, check your equipment and, if necessary, replace it and take another measurement.
- If you obtain an abnormal vital sign finding, maintain a calm, professional demeanor; an anxious expression or exclamation could upset the client. If the client expresses concern over repeated measurements, calmly explain that you obtained a slightly high or low measurement and just want to check it again.
- Consider how vital sign findings relate to each other and to other physical assessment findings. Some relationship will be significant. For example, a rapid pulse typically accompanies a high temperature; flushing com-

monly occurs with a temperature rise (from vasodilation, as the body attempts to eliminate heat); decreased level of consciousness frequently accompanies a blood pressure drop (from inadequate cerebral circulation).

• When assessing vital signs in an ill client, familiarize yourself with the client's medical diagnosis, treatment, and medication regimen, and consider how these factors can affect vital signs. In a client receiving propranolol, for instance, expect a slow pulse.

Temperature

Body temperature represents the difference between the amount of heat the body produces and the amount it loses. Normally, a negative feedback system controlled by the brain's hypothalamic thermoregulatory center maintains body temperature within fairly constant limits. This system balances the body's heat-producing mechanisms—metabolism, shivering, muscle contraction, disease, exercise, and increased thyroid activity—with its heat-losing mechanisms—radiation, conduction, convection, and evaporation.

When a heat-producing mechanism produces excessive heat, fever (hyperthermia) results. Conversely, overactivity of a heat-losing mechanism can lead to an abnormally low body temperature (hypothermia).

The nurse may measure and record temperature in degrees Fahrenheit (° F.) or degrees centigrade, or Celsius (° C.). To convert Fahrenheit to centigrade degrees, use this formula:

$$[°\text{ F.} - 32] \times \frac{5}{9} = °\text{ C.}$$

To convert centigrade to Fahrenheit degrees, use this formula:

$$[°\text{ C.} \times \frac{9}{5}] + 32 = °\text{ F.}$$

You can take a client's temperature by three routes: oral, rectal, or axillary. Unless the physician orders a specific route, choose the one that seems most appropriate for the client's age and physical condition. Whichever route you choose, document it on the client's chart.

The oral route offers maximum convenience for you and the client. Use this route for an alert adult, but make sure the client does not breathe through the mouth and has not drunk a hot or cold beverage or smoked a cigarette in the past 15 minutes; these factors could cause an inaccurate reading.

To obtain an oral temperature with a glass-mercury thermometer, place the thermometer tip under the front of the tongue. For the most accurate reading, leave it in place for about 7 minutes.

Avoid taking an oral temperature in a client who has an oral deformity or who has undergone recent oral surgery. Because it may break, a glass-mercury thermometer is contraindicated for oral temperature measurement in a young child, a confused client, and a client with a frequent cough, a seizure disorder, or chills that cause shaking.

You may take the temperature rectally when the oral route is inappropriate—for example, in an infant or a young child or in a weak, confused, or comatose client. To assess rectal temperature, place the client in a side-lying or prone position. Lubricate the thermometer bulb with a water-soluble lubricant and gently insert it into the anus—about 1″ to 1½″ (2.5 to 3 cm) in an adult and ½″ (1 cm) in a child or an infant. Hold the thermometer in place for about 3 minutes, and stay with the client during this time. Be aware that sometimes an alert adult client may prefer to insert the thermometer rather than have the nurse place it in position.

Avoid the rectal route in a client with an anal lesion, bleeding hemorrhoids, or a history of recent rectal surgery. This route also may be contraindicated in a client with a cardiac disorder because it may stimulate the vagus nerve, possibly leading to vasodilation and a decreased heart rate.

You may measure temperature by the axillary route in an alert client who has had oral surgery, who cannot close the lips around a thermometer because of a deformity, or who is wearing an oxygen mask. Many health care professionals prefer the axillary route for an infant or a small child because it eliminates the risks of thermometer breakage and rectal perforation.

To take an axillary reading, place the thermometer bulb in the client's axilla (armpit). Have the client hold the arm across the chest to keep the thermometer in place. (You may need to hold the thermometer in place if the client cannot.) Axillary temperature takes the longest to obtain: about 11 minutes.

When used by any route, an electronic thermometer provides the fastest temperature measurement, yielding highly accurate readings in about 30 seconds. Place this thermometer as you would any other, but remember to change the disposable cover on the probe for every client.

You may use other devices to measure body temperature—for example, an electronic rectal probe that provides continuous or instantaneous readouts, to allow close tracing of the course of a fever. Caring for a client on isolation precautions may require the use of a clinical dot disposable thermometer.

Normal and abnormal body temperatures. Normal body temperature ranges from about 96.8° F. to 99.5° F. (36° C. to 37.5° C.). When evaluating temperature, keep in mind that some persons have a high or low baseline temper-

The effect of age on vital signs

Normal vital sign ranges vary with age, as this chart shows.

AGE	TEMPERATURE ° Fahrenheit	° Celsius	PULSE RATE	RESPIRATORY RATE	BLOOD PRESSURE
Newborn	98.6 to 99.8	37 to 37.7	70 to 190	30 to 80	systolic: 50 to 52 diastolic: 25 to 30 mean: 35 to 40
3 years	98.5 to 99.5	36.9 to 37.5	80 to 125	20 to 30	systolic: 78 to 114 diastolic: 46 to 78
10 years	97.5 to 98.6	36.3 to 37	70 to 110	16 to 22	systolic: 90 to 132 diastolic: 56 to 86
16 years	97.6 to 98.8	36.4 to 37.1	55 to 100	15 to 20	systolic: 104 to 108 diastolic: 60 to 92
Adult	96.8 to 99.5	36 to 37.5	60 to 100	12 to 20	systolic: 95 to 140 diastolic: 60 to 90
Older adult	96.5 to 97.5	35.9 to 36.3	60 to 100	15 to 25	systolic: 140 to 160 diastolic: 70 to 90

ature. In a client with a baseline of 96.8° F. (36° C.), a temperature of 98.6° F. (37° C.) could indicate fever. Also, body temperature tends to vary throughout the day, dropping lowest in the early morning and peaking in late afternoon.

Other factors, such as age, sex, physical activity, and environmental conditions, can influence normal temperature ranges. Infants and children tend to have higher temperatures than adults, averaging more than 99° F. (37.2° C.) until age 3. (For details, see *The effect of age on vital signs*.) Relatively fast metabolism makes a child vulnerable to dramatically high fevers when ill; a child also is more likely to have temperature-related seizures. The older adult commonly has a lower body temperature, averaging about 97° F. (36.1° C.) and sometimes dropping to 95° F. (35° C.).

Women typically have higher temperatures than men. During the childbearing years, women experience a slight temperature rise for several days after ovulation; during the first several months of pregnancy, temperature remains elevated.

In any person, temperature may vary from normal levels during stress, such as from exercise, hard work, or exposure to extreme cold or heat. Temperature also depends upon organic body processes. Metabolic diseases, such as hyperthyroidism, and neurologic disorders, such as cerebral hemorrhage (which involves impairment of the hypothalamic regulatory center), can cause body temperature changes. Fever can develop as an inflammatory response to tissue destruction, such as after extensive surgery, during recovery from myocardial infarction, or when the body fights infection.

After obtaining the client's temperature, interpret your findings. Consider hyperthermia or hypothermia cause for concern; if persistent, an extremely high temperature (above 105° F. [40.6° C.]) or an extremely low temperature (below 93° F. [33.9° C.]) can cause death.

Pulse

When assessing a client's pulse, the nurse feels or hears the pressure wave of blood ejected from the heart as it surges through arteries. Each pulsation corresponds to a heartbeat. By assessing heartbeat characteristics, you can determine how well the heart handles its blood volume and, indirectly, how well it perfuses organs with oxygenated blood. Pulse assessment techniques include the following:

To assess a client's pulse, you can auscultate at the apex of the heart with a stethoscope or palpate a peripheral pulse with your fingers. Although either method can determine heart rate (beats per minute), auscultation proves superior for assessing heart rhythm (regularity).

You can palpate or auscultate the pulse in various locations. (For an illustration of these locations, see *Pulse sites*, page 96.) Usually, you assess the radial pulse be-

Pulse sites

This illustration shows the locations of the major peripheral arterial pulses and the apical pulse.

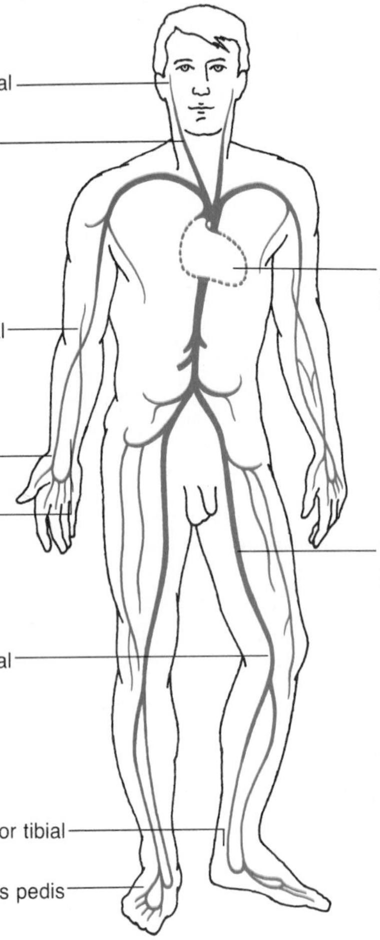

Temporal pulse
Carotid pulse
Brachial pulse
Radial pulse
Ulnar pulse
Popliteal pulse
Posterior tibial pulse
Dorsalis pedis pulse
Apical pulse
Femoral pulse

cause of its easy accessibility. To do this, palpate the radial artery with the pads of your index and middle fingers for 60 seconds while compressing the artery gently against the radial bone. Do not use your thumb because it has a pulse of its own that you could confuse with the client's pulse. Although some practitioners count the pulse for 15 seconds and multiply by 4, this practice is not desirable, especially if the client does not have a normal heart rate and rhythm). If you have trouble distinguishing a faint peripheral pulse from your own pulse, check another site.

If the client has a cast or splint, has a condition that impairs peripheral circulation (such as diabetes or vascular disease), or has undergone a recent invasive vascular procedure (such as angiography or surgery), you may need to check all peripheral pulses to ensure adequate circulation to an extremity. If you have difficulty finding a peripheral pulse, mark the pulse site with a wax marker for future reference. (When marking a pulse site this way, be sure to document it.)

In an emergency, you may palpate femoral and carotid pulses in a client with severe cardiovascular compromise. However, take care not to exert too much pressure against the carotid artery because this can stimulate the vagus nerve and cause reflex bradycardia. Also, do not press against both carotid pulses at once—this can interfere with cerebral circulation.

If the client has a cardiac dysrhythmia or is receiving a cardiac drug, such as digoxin, you may need to auscultate the apical pulse for 60 seconds. Before administering each scheduled drug dose, auscultate the apical rate by placing the diaphragm of the stethoscope over the apex of the heart (located at the lower border of the heart, at the fifth intercostal space $2\frac{3}{4}''$ to $3\frac{1}{2}''$ [7 to 9 cm] from the midsternal line). Listen closely and count the beats for 60 seconds.

To assess an infant's or a toddler's heart rate, auscultate the apical pulse or palpate the carotid or femoral pulse. Alternatively, you can observe and count pulsations of the anterior fontanelle.

The normal pulse rate varies with age, physical condition, and other factors. At birth, it averages about 125 beats per minute (BPM). Declining steadily to 100 BPM by age 4, the normal pulse rate should fall into the adult range of 60 to 100 BPM by adolescence. (To compare heart rates by age-groups, see *The effect of age on vital signs,* page 95.)

Usually, a pulse rate below 60 BPM (bradycardia) or above 100 BPM (tachycardia) is abnormal. However, even in a healthy person, various factors may cause the pulse rate to increase or decrease. An increase may result from sympathetic nervous system stimulation, such as from fear, anger, or pain; a decrease may stem from sleep, relaxation, or vagus nerve stimulation, such as from vomiting or suctioning.

A well-conditioned athlete may have a normal resting pulse rate below 60 BPM. During sustained exercise, the heart must pump harder and more rapidly to supply oxygen to other muscles. This extra work conditions the heart just as it conditions other muscles. Eventually, the heart does not require such rapid rates, causing a low pulse rate.

As you obtain the pulse rate, also assess pulse amplitude and rhythm. Document pulse amplitude (which reflects the strength of left ventricular contractions) by using a numerical scale or a descriptive term. (For more information, see *Documenting pulse amplitude.*)

Documenting pulse amplitude

To document pulse amplitude, the nurse may use a numerical scale or a descriptive term. Different health care facilities may use numerical scales that differ slightly. If you use a numerical scale, make sure it corresponds to the one used in your facility or by your colleagues. The scale shown here, along with the corresponding descriptions of pulse amplitude, is among the most commonly used. Remember, only +2 describes a normal pulse.

+3 = **bounding**—readily palpable, forceful, not easily obliterated by finger pressure

+2 = **normal**—easily palpable and obliterated only by strong finger pressure

+1 = **weak or thready**—hard to feel and easily obliterated by slight finger pressure

0 = **absent**—not discernible

When assessing pulse rhythm, you evaluate the regularity of the electrical conduction of the heart over time. Check the rhythm as you count the pulse rate over 60 seconds. Normally, rhythm should be regular, with approximately the same interval between pulsations. If you detect an irregular rhythm, describe its pattern. A predictably irregular rhythm sometimes occurs with respiration; this rarely signifies a pathologic disorder. A totally irregular rhythm (dysrhythmia) suggests a cardiovascular problem. With practice, you may be able to identify a specific dysrhythmia through palpation. However, you can best identify dysrhythmias by auscultating the heart or by obtaining an electrocardiogram (EKG). (For more information, see Chapter 11, Cardiovascular System.)

Occasionally, you may detect a pulse that fades on inspiration and strengthens on expiration. Known as a paradoxical pulse, this abnormailty can occur with deep breathing or such cardiac problems a as tamponade, in which the pericardium (the fibroserous sac covering the heart) fills with blood or fluid. A paradoxical pulse may indicate an emergency and always warrants further investigation.

If you detect an irregular pulse, auscultate the apical area and palpate the radial area simultaneously to identify a potential pulse deficit (difference between the two pulses). A pulse deficit occurs when a premature heartbeat cannot produce the wave of blood needed to fill the arteries; thus, peripheral radial artery pressure is too low to palpate every heartbeat. To calculate a pulse deficit, record apical and radial pulses separately for 60 seconds each or have another nurse record one pulse while you record the other for 60 seconds. Usually, you must obtain an EKG to confirm findings.

Respiration

During respiration, the lungs take in oxygen with each inspiration and expel carbon dioxide with each expiration. Respiration depends upon metabolism, the condition of respiratory muscles (mainly the diaphragm and intercostal muscles), and airway patency. Because the respiratory control center lies in the brain stem, respiratory rate and rhythm rely on normal neurologic function. (For more information about respiratory physiology and assessment, see Chapter 10, Respiratory System.)

When assessing respiration, focus on the rate, depth, and rhythm of each breath. Stay alert for other evidence of possible respiratory problems, such as cyanosis (bluish skin), chest pain, anxiety, restlessness, and confusion. A complaint of insufficient air intake or difficulty breathing always warrants further evaluation.

To determine the respiratory rate, count the number of respirations for 60 seconds. (One respiration consists of an inspiration and an expiration.) Do this as unobtrusively as possible—a client who knows that you are counting respirations may inadvertently alter the rate. In one unobtrusive method, you hold the client's wrist against the chest or abdomen as if checking the pulse rate. If respirations are too shallow to see a rise and fall of the chest wall, hold the back of your hand next to the client's nose and mouth to feel expirations.

As with other vital signs, the respiratory rate varies with age. In adults, it normally ranges from about 12 to 20 breaths per minute. In children, it tends to be faster. (For a comparision of age-related differences, see *The effect of age on vital signs,* page 95.)

The respiratory rate may increase with emotional stress, such as fear or anxiety; metabolic disorders, such as diabetes mellitus; lung tissue abnormalities, such as emphysema; and disorders that inhibit chest wall expansion, such as myasthenia gravis. The respiratory rate may decrease with nervous system depression, as from excessive sedation or anesthesia. Usually, an adult client with a respiratory rate above 30 or below 12 breaths per minute requires close observation and further evaluation.

Respiratory depth roughly reflects tidal volume—the amount of air taken in with each breath. In a healthy adult, tidal volume ranges from 300 to 500 ml. (The actual volume of inspired air can be measured only with special spirometry equipment.)

To estimate respiratory depth, observe the chest as it rises and falls and assess the effort required to breathe. Respirations should be quiet and easy. Note any abnormal breath sounds, such as wheezing. Describe respirations as shallow, moderate, or deep. Shallow

Respiratory patterns

When assessing a client's respirations, the nurse should determine their rate, rhythm, and depth. These schematic diagrams show different respiratory patterns.

Eupnea
Normal respiratory rate and rhythm

Tachypnea
Increased respiratory rate

Bradypnea
Slow but regular respirations

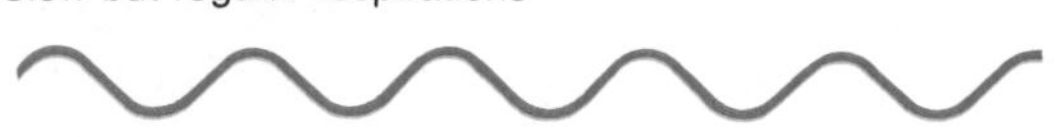

Apnea
Absence of breathing (may be periodic)

Hyperventilation
Deeper respirations; normal rate

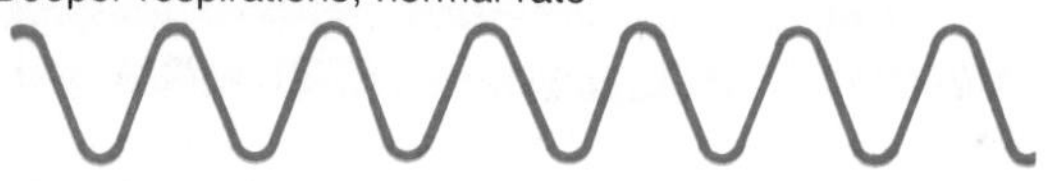

Cheyne-Stokes
Respirations that gradually become faster and deeper than normal, then slower; alternates with periods of apnea

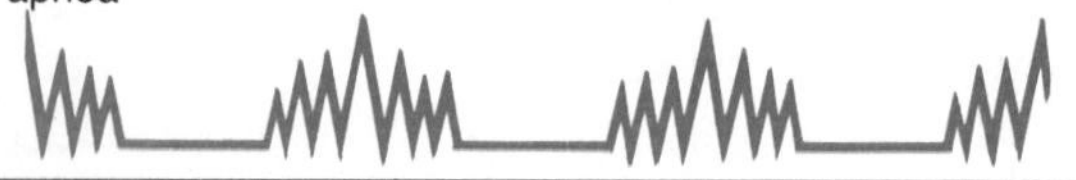

Biot's
Faster and deeper respirations than normal, with abrupt pauses between them; breaths have equal depth

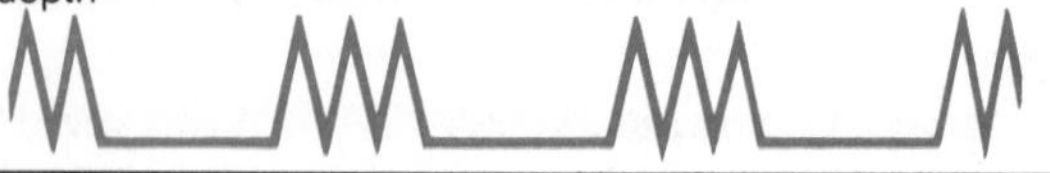

Kussmaul's
Faster and deeper respirations without pauses

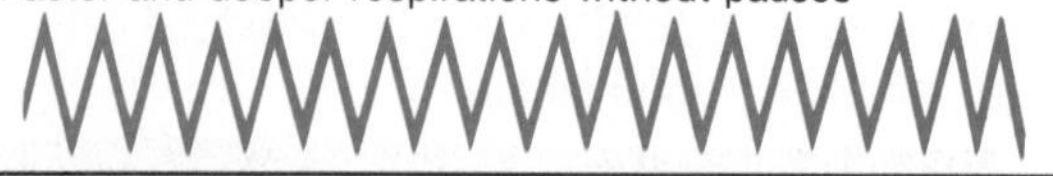

Apneustic
Prolonged, gasping inspiration followed by extremely short, inefficient expiration

breathing may indicate a chest injury, such as a broken rib; deep breathing, a neurologic disorder, such as a cerebrovascular accident.

Note the symmetry of chest wall expansion on inspiration. Skeletal deformity, broken ribs, and collapsed lung tissue can cause asymmetrical (unequal) expansion. Observe thoracic and abdominal muscle use. Women typically use thoracic muscles to breathe; men and children, abdominal muscles. You may see paradoxical breathing, a sign of respiratory distress characterized by movement of the chest and abdomen in opposition, producing a seesaw effect. This abnormal breathing tires the client quickly.

Also note any use of accessory respiratory muscles—scalenus, sternocleidomastoid, and abdominal muscles. Accessory muscle use sometimes occurs in labored breathing associated with chronic lung disease or respiratory distress. Labored breathing also may cause intercostal muscles to bulge or retract abnormally and may be accompanied by nasal flaring and lip pursing on expiration.

As you assess the respiratory rate and depth, note the respiratory rhythm, or pattern. Children and adults normally breathe with a regular rhythm, interspersing respirations with sighs (occasional deep, prolonged breaths that allow full lung expansion). Infants, on the other hand, typically have a variable respiratory pattern, interspersing rapid rates with short spells of apnea (absence of spontaneous respirations). Irregular rhythms in children or adults, such as Biot's or Cheyne-Stokes respirations, commonly result from neurologic disorders. (For a description of some abnormal rhythms, see *Respiratory patterns*.)

Blood pressure

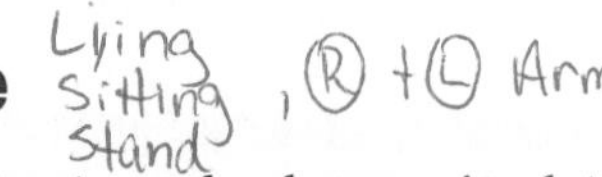

As the heart contracts and relaxes, circulating blood exerts pressure on inner arterial walls. Blood pressure measurement indirectly reflects this pressure and provides information about arterial resilience and resistance, cardiac output, circulatory status, and fluid balance—important indices of a client's overall health status.

Blood pressure measurement reflects two stages in the cardiac cycle. *Systolic pressure* refers to the maximum pressure exerted on the arterial wall at the peak of systole (left ventricular contraction). *Diastolic pressure* reflects minimum systemic arterial pressure, which occurs during diastole (left ventricular relaxation).

Diastolic pressure usually proves more diagnostically significant than systolic pressure; however, elevated systolic pressure signals an increased risk of

Measuring blood pressure

To assess a client's blood pressure accurately, the nurse should follow this procedure.

Preparing the client

Before beginning, make sure the client is relaxed and has not eaten or exercised in the past 30 minutes. The client can sit, stand, or lie down during blood pressure measurement.

Applying the cuff and stethoscope

To obtain a reading in an arm (the most common measurement site), wrap the sphygmomanometer cuff snugly around the arm 1″ (2.5 cm) above the antecubital area (the inner aspect of the elbow), with the cuff bladder centered over the brachial artery (see below). Most cuffs have arrows that should be placed over the brachial artery. Make sure to use the proper-sized cuff for the client.

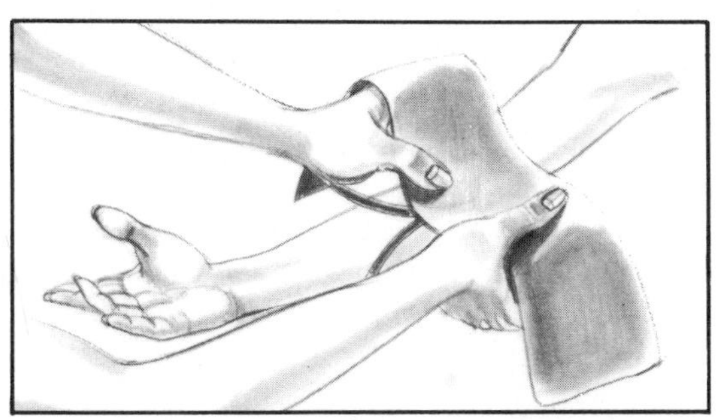

Keep the mercury manometer at eye level; if using an aneroid gauge, place it level with the client's arm. Keep the client's arm level with the heart. *Do not* use the client's muscle strength to hold up the arm; tension from muscle contraction can elevate systolic pressure. Have a recumbent client rest the arm at the side.

Then, palpate the brachial pulse just below and slightly medial to the antecubital area. Rapidly inflate the cuff to about 30 mm Hg above the level at which the pulsations disappear. Deflate the cuff slowly until you feel the pulse again. Then, deflate the cuff completely. Place the earpieces of the stethoscope in your ears and position the stethoscope head over the brachial artery, just distal to the cuff or slightly beneath it (see below). Generally, you will use the easy-to-handle, flat diaphragm to auscultate the pulse; however, you may need to use the bell if the client has a diminished or hard-to-locate pulse, because the bell detects the low-pitched sound of arterial blood flow more effectively.

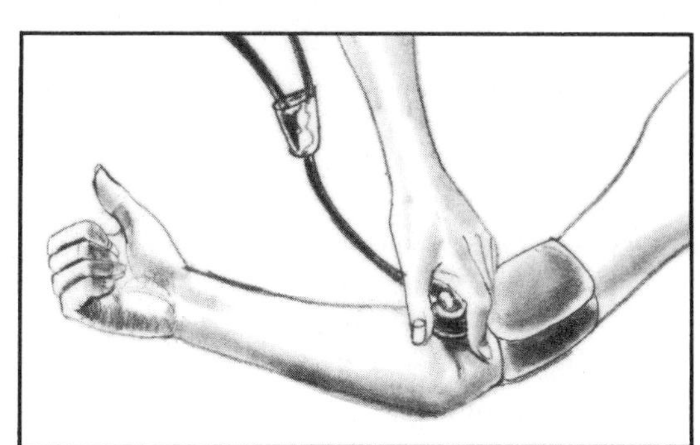

Obtaining the blood pressure reading

Watching the manometer, pump the bulb until the mercury column or aneroid gauge reaches about 30 mm Hg above the point at which the pulse disappeared. Then, slowly open the air valve and watch the mercury drop or the gauge needle descend. Release the pressure at a rate of about 3 mm Hg per second and listen for pulse sounds (Korotkoff sounds).

These sounds, which determine the blood pressure measurement, are classified as follows:

Phase I
Onset of clear, faint tapping, with intensity that increases to a thud or louder tap

Phase II
Tapping that changes to a soft, swishing sound

Phase III
Return of clear, crisp tapping sound

Phase IV (first diastolic sound)
Sound becomes muffled and takes on a blowing quality

Phase V (second diastolic sound)
Sound disappears.

As soon as you hear blood begin to pulse through the brachial artery, note the reading on the aneroid dial or mercury column. Reflecting phase I (the first Korotkoff sound), this sound coincides with the client's systolic pressure. Continue deflating the cuff, noting the point at which pulsations diminish or become muffled—phase IV (the fourth Korotkoff sound)—and then disappear—phase V (the fifth Korotkoff sound). For children and highly active adults, many authorities consider phase IV the most accurate reflection of blood pressure.

The American Heart Association and the World Health Organization recommend documenting phases I, IV, and V. However, phase IV is often not indicated in practice. To avoid confusion and make your measurements more useful, follow this format for recording blood pressure: systolic/muffling/disappearance (for example, 120/80/76).

cerebrovascular accident. The difference between systolic and diastolic readings, known as *pulse pressure,* has important diagnostic value in clients with such conditions as increased intracranial pressure, hypertension, cardiac malformations, and shock.

Many factors affect arterial blood pressure. Physical activity, emotional stress, and body position can cause wide fluctuations. Blood pressure also fluctuates in a 24-hour (circadian) pattern, dropping lowest in the late hours of sleep and peaking in the afternoon and evening.

Age also affects blood pressure. From infancy throughout childhood and adolescence, blood pressure increases gradually, then stabilizes as adulthood begins. In elderly persons, decreased vessel elasticity typically causes increased systolic pressure. (To compare age-related blood pressure variations, see *The effect of age on vital signs,* page 95.)

Assessing blood pressure

The nurse determines arterial blood pressure (measured in millimeters of mercury [mm Hg]) by using a sphygmomanometer and a stethoscope. Assess blood pressure in an arm or a leg by listening to brachial or popliteal artery pulsations. However, keep in mind that measurements taken over the popliteal artery in the leg produce higher systolic and lower diastolic readings than those obtained from the arm. (For information on how to measure, see *Measuring blood pressure,* page 99.)

If you cannot hear a pulse or have reason to doubt your blood pressure finding, recheck the pressure. To avoid venous engorgement from cuff pressure, wait 30 seconds between attempts.

In a client with venous congestion or hypertension, you may detect a silent period between systolic and diastolic sounds, when you cannot hear intervening pulse sounds. Known as the auscultatory gap, this phenomenon may cause you to underestimate the systolic or overestimate the diastolic reading significantly. To avoid either error, make sure to inflate the blood pressure cuff at least 30 mm Hg over the point at which the palpated pulse first disappeared.

When assessing a client's blood pressure for the first time, take measurements in both arms. Consider a slight pressure difference (5 to 10 mm Hg) between arms normal; a difference of 15 mm Hg or more may indicate cardiac disease, especially aortic coarctation (narrowing) or arterial obstruction.

In some cases, you may want to assess orthostatic (postural) blood pressure by taking readings with the client lying down, sitting, and standing, then checking for differences with each position change. Normally, blood pressure rises or falls slightly with a position change. A drop of 20 mm Hg or more, however, indicates orthostatic hypotension. Such a decrease, which usually causes dizziness, can result from hypovolemia, medication effects, or prolonged bed rest.

If you have difficulty auscultating a peripheral pulse when assessing an infant's blood pressure, use the flush method. First, pump the cuff around the infant's wrist or ankle to occlude the blood supply. As you release the pressure, the foot will flush as it reperfuses. The manometer reading coinciding with the flush approximates mean blood pressure (average of systolic and diastolic blood pressures).

If you cannot auscultate a pulse because the pressure is inaudible or because you do not have a stethoscope or Doppler probe, measure blood pressure by palpation. After applying the cuff and palpating the brachial pulse, inflate the cuff until the manometer reads 30 mm Hg above the point at which you can no longer palpate the pulse. Now, release the cuff pressure slowly, at a rate of approximately 2 to 3 mm Hg per heartbeat. While doing this, closely observe the manometer. The number that appears when you feel the first palpable pulsation is the systolic reading.

Because pulsations continue until the manometer reading falls to zero, you may have more difficulty determining the diastolic reading. Document a palpated blood pressure by writing, for example, "120/palpated."

Normal and abnormal blood pressure readings. Normal blood pressure varies greatly among individuals. In adults, normal systolic pressure ranges from 100 to 140 mm Hg; normal diastolic pressure, from 60 to 90 mm Hg. However, consider a series of blood pressure readings establishing a *trend* more important than an individual reading. A change of more than 20 mm Hg between readings, with no apparent reason for fluctuation (such as a position change or recent physical exertion) warrants further investigation.

Some clients normally have chronically low blood pressure. For most, however, consistent readings below 95 mm Hg systolic or 60 mm Hg diastolic indicate hypotension (low blood pressure). Hypotension may result from a condition that reduces total blood volume, such as severe hemorrhage, burns, or diarrhea, or from a condition that decreases cardiac output, such as myocardial infarction or congestive heart failure.

Consistently elevated readings—above 140 mm Hg systolic and 90 mm Hg diastolic—indicate hypertension (high blood pressure). Hypertension may be idiopathic (of unknown cause) or secondary to an underlying disorder, such as renal disease. (For more information, see Chapter 11, Cardiovascular System.)

Consider a pulse pressure difference greater than 40 mm Hg as abnormal. Such a difference can stem from increased systolic pressure caused by rigid, inflexible arteries, or it may be a classic sign of aortic insufficiency (backflow into the heart and consequent low diastolic readings, from aortic valve incompetence).

Documenting vital signs

The nurse records vital signs in an obvious place on the physical assessment documentation. If using a vital signs form, record vital signs in the space provided. Note any pertinent information as concisely as possible. In the following example, the client has a temperature of 98.8° F. (37.1° C.), measured orally; a pulse rate of 80 BPM, with regular rhythm and strong amplitude; a respiratory rate of 12 breaths per minute, with regular rhythm and unlabored quality; and blood pressure readings of 122/90/80 mm Hg measured with the client lying down, 122/88/80 mm Hg with the client sitting, and 120/90/82 mm Hg with the client standing:

T 98.8° F. (37.1° C.) orally
P 80, regular, +2
R 12, unlabored, regular, and deep
BP 122/90/80 lying; 122/88/80 sitting; 120/90/82 standing.

Height and weight measurements

With every client—in any setting—the nurse should record height and weight (anthropometric measurements) as part of the basic assessment profile. Although the general survey gives an overall impression of body size and type, height and weight measurements provide more specific information about a client's general health and nutritional status. In routine physical assessment, these measurements should be taken periodically throughout the client's life to help evaluate normal growth and development and to identify abnormal patterns of weight gain or loss—frequently an early sign of acute or chronic illness. (For information on determining optimal body weights as well as other anthropometric measurements such as midarm circumference and triceps skinfold, see Chapter 6, Nutritional Status.)

Accurate height and weight measurements also serve other important purposes. In children, they guide dosage calculations for various drugs; in adults, they help guide cancer chemotherapy and anesthesia administration, and they help evaluate the response to I.V. fluids, drugs, or nutritional therapy.

To weigh an adult or a child who can stand unassisted, use a standard platform scale with a balance beam. Before taking the measurement, balance the scale by moving the sliding weights to the *0* position and adjusting the movable knob on the back of the scale. Have the client remove shoes and wear only a gown or undergarments. Slide the weights down the bar until the indicator balances, and record weight to the nearest ½ lb (0.2 kg).

To weigh a client who cannot stand, use a bed scale—either a manual counterbalance scale or an electronic scale with a digital display. Make sure the scale has been calibrated and balanced before each use.

Weigh an infant in a small platform scale with a balance beam and curved sides to hold the infant in place. If possible, weigh the infant naked.

To measure height, use the sliding headpiece on the platform scale; this allows you to obtain weight and height measurements at the same time. To ensure accurate measurements, have the client remove shoes and stand straight, facing away from the scale with feet together and arms hanging relaxed at the sides. Lower the headpiece until it rests lightly on the crown of the head, and record the measurement to the nearest ¼" (0.6 cm). Instruct the client to remain standing straight, then remeasure; the two readings should be within ¼" of each other. Alternatively, you can measure an adult's height with a measuring tape attached to the wall.

To measure the height of a client who cannot stand, position the client supine on a bed. On the sheet, make a mark at the top of the client's head and another at the bottom of the foot. Then extend these marks to the side of the bed and measure the distance between the marks with a measuring tape.

To measure an infant's height, use a board with a sliding headpiece. Alternatively, place the infant on a large sheet of paper on the examining table, make a mark at the top of the head and at the heel of the extended leg, and measure the distance between the two marks with a measuring tape.

Chapter summary

This chapter discusses several aspects of the physical assessment and serves as a preface to the following chapters that address detailed assessment of various body systems. Chapter highlights include the following:

• The physical assessment begins with *subjective* findings, including the health history and review of systems. The *objective* portion follows. A dynamic, ongoing process, the physical assessment provides an opportunity to obtain extensive data about a client.
• The physical assessment parts discussed in this chapter are: general survey (initial observations of the client's appearance and behavior); vital sign measurements (assessment of temperature, pulse and respiration rates, and blood pressure); assessment of height and weight.
• Accurate physical assessment requires use of the nurse's senses and an intelligent, systematic approach. Special equipment is sometimes necessary. The four basic assessment techniques are inspection, palpation, percussion, and auscultation.
• The nurse may perform a complete assessment or a modified assessment in any setting. Either type of assessment can cause the client to become anxious, fearful, or uncomfortable. The nurse can take steps to minimize these feelings and to help ensure client comfort.
• The general survey provides vital information about the client's behavior and health status, and is usually documented in a one-paragraph summary. It includes observations of the client's sex, race, and approximate age as well as signs of distress; facial characteristics; body type, posture, and movements; speech; dress, grooming, and personal hygiene; and psychological state.
• Assessment of vital signs—temperature, pulse, respirations, and blood pressure—provides information about the function of specific organs, such as the heart and lungs, as well as entire body systems.
• Height and weight measurements provide more specific information than a general survey about a client's general health and nutritional status. These measurements help evaluate normal growth and development and detect abnormal patterns of weight gain or loss.

Study questions

1. What is the overall purpose of the physical assessment? What is the purpose of the general survey and what does it contribute to the physical assessment?

2. What equipment should you expect to gather for a basic assessment? How would you use this equipment?

3. A caring, supportive approach will enhance the assessment's effectiveness. What techniques can you use to put the client at ease and reduce stress during the assessment?

4. Several factors characterize a well-documented physical assessment. What are these factors and their importance?

5. Physical assessment of a pediatric client differs greatly from that of the adult. How would you describe these differences?

Selected references

Bolton, B. (1987). *Handbook of measurement and evaluation in rehabilitation* (2nd ed.). Baltimore: Brookes.
Cohen, S., Kenner, C., and Hollingsworth, A. (1991). *Maternal, neonatal, and women's health nursing.* Springhouse, PA: Springhouse Corp.
DeGowin, E., and DeGowin, R. (1987). *Bedside diagnostic examination* (5th ed.). New York: Macmillan.
Eliopoulos, C. (1987). *Gerontological nursing* (2nd ed.). Philadelphia: Lippincott.
Hoekelman, R., Blatman, S., Friedman, S., Nelson, M., and Seidel, H. (1987). *Primary pediatric care.* St. Louis: Mosby.
Sherman, J., and Fields, S. (1987). *Guide to patient evaluation* (5th ed.). New York: Elsevier.

Nursing research

Baker, N., Cerone, S., Gaze, N., and Knapp, T. (1984). The effect of type of thermometer and length of time inserted on oral temperature measurements of afebrile subjects. *Nursing Research,* 33(2), 109-111.
Garcia, C., and Gibner, J. (1990). A comparative study of temperatures in the elderly. *Nursing Homes,* 39(5/6), 21-23.
Hollerbach, A., and Sneed, N. (1990). Accuracy of radical pulse assessment by length of counting interval. *Heart & Lung,* 19(3), 258-264.
Nichols, G. (1966). Oral, axillary, and rectal temperature determinations and relationships. *Nursing Research,* 15(4), 307-310.*
Ruffolo, M. (1983). A comparison of oral and rectal temperature measurements on patients receiving oxygen by mask. *Nursing Research,* 32(6), 373-375.

*Landmark publication

UNIT THREE

Assessing Activity, Sleep, and Nutrition

Unit Three provides detailed information about assessing a client's activities of daily living, sleep and wake patterns, and nutritional status—three health promotion and protection patterns described briefly in Chapter 3, The Health History. These patterns require thorough assessment because they can provide important information about the client's health.

Activities of daily living, sleep patterns, and nutrition are interrelated and must be carefully balanced for physiologic and psychological health. For example, daily activity affects a client's ability to sleep; the quality of sleep affects a client's ability to carry out daily activities; proper nutrition provides the energy and nutrients the client needs for daily activities. Any alteration in these patterns can signal an actual or potential health problem.

Chapter 5
Activities of Daily Living and Sleep Patterns

Because daytime activities and sleep patterns affect each other significantly, Chapter 5 describes both and discusses the importance of a balance between them. First, the chapter describes how to assess the client's daytime activities, such as eating, attending to hygiene, dressing, working, playing, and going to school or work. Then, it explores sleep stages, normal sleep patterns, factors that promote or inhibit sleep, sleep disorders, and sleep pattern assessment.

Chapter 6
Nutritional Status

A nutritional status assessment evaluates the balance between nutrient intake and energy expenditure. Chapter 6 shows the nurse how to perform such an assessment. It begins by discussing the physiology of nutrition. Then it presents health history questions and physical assessment techniques that evaluate nutritional status, including inspection, palpation, and height, weight, and related body measurements. Finally, it describes how to document assessment findings.

Nursing diagnoses

Health history and observations or physical assessment findings serve as the basis for formulating nursing diagnoses related to activity, sleep, and nutrition. In turn, the nursing diagnoses form the basis for planning, implementing, and evaluating client care. Nursing diagnoses may include the following:

- Altered nutrition: less than body requirements, related to difficulty in chewing and swallowing
- Altered nutrition: more than body requirements, related to a calorie intake–energy expenditure imbalance
- Fluid volume deficit, related to nausea and vomiting
- Fluid volume excess, related to fluid retention
- Impaired physical mobility, related to flaccidity, atrophy, and weakness
- Impaired physical mobility, related to limitations imposed by hip spica cast
- Knowledge deficit, related to iron-rich foods
- Self-care deficit: feeding, related to loose dentures
- Sleep pattern disturbance: acute, related to anxiety
- Sleep pattern disturbance: chronic difficulty maintaining sleep, related to caffeine ingestion.

5

Activities of Daily Living and Sleep Patterns

Objectives

After reading and studying this chapter, you should be able to:

1. Discuss the importance of balance between activity and sleep in a client's life.
2. Describe the factors affecting activities of daily living.
3. Identify interview questions used to assess personal care, family responsibility, work, school, recreational, and socialization activities for an adult and for a child.
4. Describe rapid eye movement sleep and the four stages of non–rapid eye movement sleep.
5. Describe the factors affecting sleep.
6. Compare and contrast disorders of initiating and maintaining sleep, disorders of excessive daytime sleepiness, disorders of the sleep-wake cycle, and parasomnias.
7. Phrase representative interview questions that assess a client's sleep patterns.

Introduction

Maintaining a constant balance between daily activities and sleep is vital to the promotion and maintenance of physiologic and psychosocial health. Daily activity affects a person's ability to sleep soundly, and in turn, the quality of sleep affects a person's ability to carry out daily activities. Therefore, the nurse must carefully assess the client's ability to perform activities of daily living (ADLs), the client's ability to achieve and maintain restful sleep patterns, and the balance between the two. Alterations in ADLs or disturbances in sleep patterns can signal actual or potential health problems.

This chapter describes the importance of daily activities and sleep for children and adults, and provides guidelines for assessing these factors in different age-groups. It also offers specific assessment questions and rationales, and describes how to document assessment findings.

Activities of daily living

ADLs are the activities necessary to develop and maintain physiologic and psychosocial well-being. These include five components: personal care, family responsibility, work or school, recreation, and socialization. Being able to live independently hinges on a person's ability to perform necessary ADLs.

Participating in daily activities promotes physiologic health for children and adults. For example, in children, recreation promotes normal growth and development of the neuromuscular and musculoskeletal systems. In adults, physical activity encourages optimum functioning of each body system and frequently reduces risk factors associated with certain diseases. An active life-style helps preserve the normal structure and function of joints, bones, and muscles, and when combined with a controlled caloric intake, helps maintain ideal body weight.

Glossary

Activities of daily living (ADLs): activities necessary to develop and maintain physiologic and psychosocial well-being.
Biological rhythms: intrinsic, biological clocks that operate on cycles of hours, days, or months; they assist adjustment to the surrounding environment to maintain a person's internal balance.
Bruxism: teeth grinding during sleep.
Cognitive function: process of perceiving, organizing, and interpreting sensory stimuli to think and solve problems.
Disorders of excessive daytime sleepiness: sleep disorders characterized by difficulty remaining awake during the day.
Disorders of initiating and maintaining sleep: sleep disorders characterized by changes in sleep onset, or interrupted sleep. Commonly called insomnia.
Disorders of sleep-wake cycle: transient or chronic sleep disorders characterized by altered or disorganized circadian rhythms caused by shift rotation, jet lag, or other interruptions in the normal sleep cycle.
Dream: vivid, internally generated sensations and perceptions.
Enuresis: involuntary urination during sleep in an individual with normal bladder control; bedwetting.
Insomnia: disorder of initiating and maintaining sleep, which may be transient (if less than 3 weeks in duration) or chronic (if longer).
Narcolepsy: sleep disorder characterized by abnormal sleep tendencies and pathologic manifestations of REM sleep.
Nightmare: bad dream that does not cause arousal.
Night terrors: sudden, fearful partial arousal during Stage 3 or 4 sleep that the client cannot recall after awakening.
Non-rapid eye movement (NREM) sleep: phase of sleep consisting of four stages that progress from light to deep sleep.
Parasomnias: dysfunctions of sleep, sleep stages, or partial arousals. Examples include night terrors, somnambulism, or enuresis.
Psychosocial function: individual's ability to process past and present information to gain a realistic perspective of oneself, one's life, and others.
Rapid eye movement (REM) sleep: phase of sleep characterized by dreaming.
Sleep apnea, central: serious disorder of excessive daytime sleepiness characterized by an absence of airflow through the nose and mouth and by an absence of inspiratory effort during sleep.
Sleep apnea, obstructive: serious disorder of excessive daytime sleepiness characterized by a collapsed upper airway resulting in no airflow despite respiratory efforts during sleep.
Sleep apnea, mixed: serious disorder of excessive daytime sleepiness characterized by central and obstructive sleep apnea.
Somnambulism: sleepwalking.
Stress: nonspecific physical response to a demand, or stressor.

Performing ADLs also promotes psychosocial health. Recreation allows children to express emotions—such as joy, fear, and hostility—that encourage emotional growth and build self-concept. In adults, successfully completing ADLs provides a sense of accomplishment. Other activities, such as hobbies, help alleviate stress and tension or serve as a means of self-expression.

Factors affecting ADLs

A person's interest in and ability to perform necessary ADLs depend on several factors: age and developmental status, culture, physiologic health, cognitive function, psychosocial function, stress level, and biological rhythms. The nurse must be aware of these factors when performing the assessment.

Age and developmental status

A client's age and developmental status provide clues to the client's interests and abilities, as well as how the client might react to an inability to perform ADLs.

When progressing from infancy to adulthood, an individual gradually shifts from dependence to independence in performing the five ADL components. For example, an infant depends on parents to meet every need, but an older adolescent independently performs most of these necessary activities. An elderly adult, however, may find that normal physiologic changes threaten independent functioning unless adaptations are made. Acute and chronic illnesses, which frequently occur during the later years, also may disrupt a person's ability to perform ADLs. Therefore, consider the client's age and developmental level when assessing the level of independence and ability to assume responsibility for ADLs.

Culture

A person's culture—learned values, beliefs, customs, and behaviors—affects interests and roles, sometimes depending on sex. Traditionally in our culture, many teenage boys enjoy watching or participating in sports; many teenage girls enjoy talking about and experimenting with clothing, cosmetics, and hairstyles. As adults, men may assume the role of "bread-winner"; women may manage the household and care for the children.

However, a group's values and beliefs can change over time, allowing for altered roles and relationships. For example, in our society today, the dual-income family has become common, and the traditional male and female roles have evolved, making more choices available. Therefore, determine the influence of a person's cultural heritage as well as any changes in values and customs when assessing ADLs.

Physiologic health

Because a person's physiologic health affects the ability to participate in ADLs, consider the functional status of each body system when performing an assessment. For example, the nervous system gathers, translates, and organizes environmental information; the musculoskeletal system coordinates with the nervous system, allowing an individual to respond to sensory input by becoming mobile. A disruption of these systems by disease, such as a cerebrovascular accident (stroke), or traumatic injury, can alter or prevent certain ADLs. Also, the cardiopulmonary system furnishes the oxygen essential for body functioning. In turn, cardiovascular or pulmonary disease may force an individual to modify or restrict activity.

Cognitive function

The level of cognitive function also influences a person's ability to perform ADLs. Cognitive function refers to the process of perceiving, organizing, and interpreting sensory stimuli to think and solve problems.

Mental processes contributing to cognitive function include attention, memory, and intelligence. An alteration in any aspect of cognitive function may interfere with logical thinking or abstract reasoning and therefore prohibit independent performance of ADLs. For example, a disturbance in attention span and memory may prevent an individual from assuming many family or occupational responsibilities. However, that same individual may still be able to perform personal care activities independently.

During ADL assessment, analyze the client's level of cognitive function, and then use that information to formulate questions and to structure teaching in a manner appropriate to the client.

Psychosocial function

Psychosocial function refers to a person's ability to process past and present information in a manner that provides a realistic view of oneself, one's life, and others. This process involves a complex interaction between intrapersonal and interpersonal behaviors. Disturbances in intrapersonal behavior—for example, those caused by an altered self-concept or emotional instability—could interfere with an adult's performance of family or occupational responsibilities or with a child's school performance. Disturbances in interpersonal behavior—such as communication problems, impaired social interactions, or dysfunctions in role performance—also can affect a person's ability to perform ADLs. Use the assessment to discover any disturbances in a client's psychosocial health and to plan appropriate interventions with the client and the family.

Stress level

Stress is a nonspecific, physical response to any kind of demand. The factors that produce stress, called stressors, can originate from within the body or from the environment and can disrupt the body's equilibrium. Stressors can be physiologic, such as an injury, or psychological, such as the loss of a loved one.

Stress is necessary for normal growth and development. It can have a negative or a positive effect on a person's ability to participate in ADLs. For example, the stress of an upcoming test may motivate a student to study and learn; other types of stress can result in psychological discomfort, an inability to perform certain ADLs, or physical illness.

Whether a stressor produces positive or negative results depends on several factors, the first of which is the individual's perception. For example, a child usually views a best friend's move to another city differently than an adult would. In addition, the magnitude or intensity of the stressor affects the person's response. For example, a person who loses the use of a finger may view the situation as troubling but tolerable. However, a concert pianist or violinist would no doubt view losing the use of a finger as a severe stressor. The number of concurrent stressors as well as their frequency and duration also affects the type of response. Multiple, frequent, prolonged stressors often result in negative outcomes and can affect a person's ability to perform ADLs. Experiences with stress and past coping behaviors influence how a person will face new stressors.

Stress affects people of all ages and affects healthy functioning; therefore, assessing a client's stress level is essential. To perform an accurate assessment, evaluate the characteristics of the stressor, determine the client's perception of the stressor, and discover the client's method of coping. (For additional information on assessing stress, see Chapter 3, The Health History.)

Biological rhythms

Rhythmic biological clocks, known as biological rhythms, influence the functioning of humans. Understanding how biological rhythms affect daily activities is integral to assessing ADLs.

Biological rhythms help the organism adjust to the surrounding physical environment and maintain internal homeostasis (relative balance in the body's internal environment). Various biological rhythms, beginning by the third week of life and continuing thereafter, operate on cycles of hours, days, or months. One type of rhythm, the circadian rhythm, operates on a cycle of approximately 24 hours. Different circadian rhythms help regulate biological and behavioral activities, including sleep and wakefulness, body temperature, and hormone levels. For example, in a 24-hour period, the body temperature normally peaks between 4 p.m. and 8 p.m., and drops to its lowest level between 4 a.m. and 6 a.m.

Many factors contribute to an individual's circadian rhythms. Environmental factors such as the hours of daylight and darkness and the seasons of the year regulate many daily activities. These environmental cues establish the appropriate times to eat, work, and relax. Social factors such as work or school schedules, household routines, and social activities also influence circadian rhythms. Hospitalization, shift work, or stress can disrupt these circadian rhythms and can result in physical illness, psychological discomfort, or impaired cognition. For example, disrupted circadian rhythms can compromise the muscle strength and coordination required to perform a task or the attention, memory, and concentration needed to complete an activity. Once disrupted, a circadian rhythm may require up to several weeks to return to normal.

Assessing ADLs

A thorough assessment ascertains a client's functional status and identifies actual and potential health problems related to ADLs. In addition, such an assessment suggests interventions to help promote the client's independent function at home and in the community and provides a method for measuring progress.

Acute-care hospitals, rehabilitation centers, outpatient clinics, or long-term-care facilities are all potential locations for assessing ADLs. Ideally, however, the nurse will perform the assessment in the client's home. This allows a view of the client's ability to perform ADLs and reveals environmental resources and physical barriers.

The nurse uses the interview and observation to gather information on ADLs. During the interview, gather data from the client and the family. Focus on their perceptions of the client's ability to perform ADLs, and identify the client's and family's goals for functioning. Determine whether the client and the family have realistic views, have developed attainable goals, and have similar perspectives. Observe the client performing ADLs whenever possible. For the hospitalized client, this can occur subtly, while the client eats, bathes, or dresses, or, in certain instances, by directly asking the client to perform specific activities.

Use the assessment to ascertain the client's functional status in performing ADLs. Determine whether the client can function independently, if the client requires the assistance of a person or a device, or if the client depends totally on others. If the client needs assistance, determine the amount and type required. If the client depends on devices, inquire about the type of device and its adequacy in resolving the problem. Also evaluate the possible need for other devices.

Personal care activities

When determining a client's self-care status, first assess mobility. (For an in-depth discussion of assessing musculoskeletal functioning, see Chapter 18, Musculoskeletal System.) Then assess the client's ability to prepare and eat meals and to perform elimination, personal hygiene, and dressing and grooming activities. The following questions and rationales offer a guide to assessing the client's personal care activities:

Do you have any difficulty standing, walking, or climbing stairs? Can you get in and out of a chair? Can you get in and out of bed? What assistive devices do you use to aid in mobility? If the client uses a wheelchair, ask, *Can you propel the chair yourself?*

(RATIONALE: An alteration in mobility may hinder a client's ability to engage in other ADLs.)

Can you open packages and containers? Can you use utensils for eating? Can you cut your food? Do you have any other problems feeding yourself? What times do you usually eat? Who prepares your meals? Where do you eat your meals? With whom do you eat?

(RATIONALE: These questions help investigate the client's ability to prepare meals and to eat independently. The ability to feed oneself is an important personal care activity. Besides providing nourishment, meals may provide a time for socializing.)

Can you use the toilet alone, or do you require assistance? Do you have any problems with bowel or bladder control? If so, how do you manage these problems? Do you use any assistive devices for elimination, such as catheters or colostomy bags? If so, can you care for these devices? How have elimination problems affected your other activities?
(RATIONALE: An elimination problem can interfere with work, school, recreational, and socialization activities. These questions give the client an opportunity to discuss problems, fears, and anxieties regarding elimination, and give the nurse an opportunity to teach the client ways to manage these problems. Keep in mind that elimination activities are private matters to adults; the client or family may hesitate to discuss them because of embarrassment. Ask questions in a matter-of-fact way and try to put the client at ease.)

What are your usual bathing habits? Do you have any problems with personal hygiene and bathing? Can you get in and out of a tub or shower? Can you shave? Can you care for your teeth, hair, fingernails, and toenails? Can you care for your dentures, hearing aids, or any other prostheses?
(RATIONALE: For many clients, an inability to manage personal hygiene activities can reduce self-esteem and self-concept. These questions help investigate the client's ability to perform these activities. Remember that most clients consider personal hygiene activities to be private; they may hesitate to discuss problems. Also, some clients may have experienced a gradual, unnoticed decline in their ability to perform personal hygiene.)

Do you have any difficulties with dressing and grooming? If so, are these problems more pronounced on the left side, the right side, the upper part, or the lower part of your body? Can you fasten buttons, snaps, and zippers? Is dressing easier with certain types of clothing? If so, which kinds?
(RATIONALE: Musculoskeletal or neuromuscular abnormalities can disrupt fine or gross motor coordination, making dressing and grooming—activities that most adults perform independently—difficult for the client. To help prevent frustration with this normal ADL, suggest different types of clothing or assistive devices.)

Family responsibility activities

The family is the first and oldest social institution. It functions to nurture the young and to support its members. Interactions within the nuclear and the extended family depend on various evolving roles. For example, the young child depends totally on parents or others to perform the necessary ADLs. With time, the child gradually assumes responsibility for small chores. During the teenage years, the adolescent shifts focus away from the family and toward outside groups, triggering conflicts over role expectations and responsibilities. An adult, who may feel overwhelmed by responsibilities at home and at work, may feel a loss of control over life. Then, as old age approaches, a person may relinquish a home and the associated responsibilities. If the decision to do this is made by choice, the elderly client may view it as a freeing action that will result in more time for other activities. However, if financial difficulties or failing health force the decision, the client may grieve and feel a sense of loss.

The following questions and their rationales offer a guide to assessing family responsibilities associated with ADLs:

What are your living arrangements? Does your home need structural changes so that you can fulfill your family responsibilities and perform activities of daily living? Do you have any problems with food management, such as shopping or food preparation? Can you do your own laundry? What type of cleaning can you do? If you have a yard, can you care for it? Are you having any difficulties managing your money, such as getting to a bank? What arrangements have you made for child care? Does your family responsibility include caring for any sick or disabled persons in the home? If so, do you have any difficulties with this role? Do you care for a pet in your home?
(RATIONALE: These questions help investigate the structure and composition of the client's family, the client's developmental status, and the responsibilities the client has assumed in the family. A client who cannot perform usual family responsibility activities may develop role and relationship problems. Such a client may benefit from a referral to a social agency for help with such responsibilities as food management or child care.)

Work and school activities

Work is any formal activity that involves earning a living or preparing to earn a living. Work helps bind society together and ensures the survival of the individual in the social system. A person's work can provide individual identity, sense of worth, and fulfillment. However, work also can be a source of frustration, disappointment, and negative stress. If one loses the ability to work, income may decline, role relationships may change or may be sacrificed, and choices may diminish. Retirement can also be difficult; some people view it as the end of everything important. Others, however, await it eagerly as a new opportunity. Either way, retirement alters the individual's daily routine and power status.

For many people, particularly those who are young, school is their work. In our society, school educates individuals in tasks and interpersonal skills and prepares them for entry into the job market. School, like work, may offer intellectual stimulation, personal satisfaction, and interpersonal relationships. However, school also may create feelings of frustration and stress, and contribute to feelings of low self-esteem.

The following questions and their rationales offer a guide to assessing the client's work or school activities associated with ADLs:

What does your typical day involve? Do you work outside the home? Where and what type of work do you do? How many hours per week do you work? What is your work schedule like? Do you have any conflicts between your work schedule and other responsibilities or activities of daily living? What is your job like? Is work mainly a source of satisfaction or frustration? Do you participate in any volunteer work?
(RATIONALE: These questions help investigate the type of work the client participates in and the role of work in the client's life. A client with a heavy, stressful work schedule may feel that he or she is neglecting family and self, causing guilt feelings that add to the stress. Suggest stress reduction techniques for such a client.)

What do you see yourself doing in the future? How do you feel about retirement? What plans have you made for retirement?
(RATIONALE: These questions help investigate the client's view of retirement, including alterations in ADLs caused by retirement.)

Are you going to school? If so, where and for what purpose? What do you like most about school? What do you like least about school? Do you have any difficulties balancing school activities with other life responsibilities?
(RATIONALE: These questions help investigate the nature and demands of any schoolwork in which the client participates, and help assess the effects of school on other activities. A client whose school activities interfere with personal care activities, family responsibilities, or work activities may benefit from counseling.)

Recreational activities

People participate in play, recreation, and exercise—either alone or in groups—for amusement, entertainment, self-fulfillment, or self-improvement. These activities contribute to personal growth, offer an outlet for emotions, provide opportunities for friendships, and help bind communities.

For an adult, solitary or group recreation usually offers freedom from the constraints of work or school. Solitary recreational activities can provide relief from interpersonal interactions; group activities can offer a chance to socialize. Recreation can help adults escape from the concerns of work, or can offer an opportunity to review daily activities and make plans. Physical exercise has become a popular recreational activity for many adults. Although regular and reasonably strenuous physical exercise can improve health, irregular strenuous exercise can prove detrimental.

Ask the following questions to investigate the client's recreational activities:

What do you do when you're not working or in school? How do your days off differ from your work or school days? How much recreational time do you have in a day and in a week? Are you satisfied with the amount of your recreational time and what you can do during that time? With whom do you share your recreational time? How would you describe any physical exercise you perform? How often do you get physical exercise? Do you participate in any special exercise program? If so, what kind and for how long? How do you feel after you exercise? Has your physician ever restricted your activity or exercise? If so, why? What benefits have you gained from exercise?
(RATIONALE: These questions help investigate the type, amount, timing, purpose, and benefits of the client's recreational and physical exercise activities. A decrease in usual activity levels may result from a physical disorder, and may lead to an emotional problem, such as depression.)

Are you retired? If so, how would you describe your day? What recreational and exercise activities do you participate in now that you are retired?
(RATIONALE: These questions help discover the type of activities enjoyed by a retired client, who may have more time for recreation than a younger adult. For a retired client, recreation and exercise activities may take the place of work activities, providing stimulation, satisfaction, and interpersonal relationships.)

Socialization activities

Relationships with others significantly influence emotional, intellectual, and personality development. Each individual develops a social network depending on personal choice, occupation, place of residence, sex, age, developmental status, and family size. Ask the following questions to obtain information about the client's socialization activities:

What kinds of things do you do when you are alone? Can you use a phone, write clearly, and see well enough to enjoy reading or watching television? Do you have many close friends? Who would you confide in if you had a problem? Do you depend on your family for help? How often do you get together with family members? Can you travel outside the home? Which activities are you involved in outside your home? Do you belong to any social groups, such as clubs or church groups? If so, which ones? Do you drive your own car or use public transportation?
(RATIONALE: These questions help investigate the client's role in society, the structure of the client's social network, and any barriers to socialization the client may have. Illness, relocation, or the loss or change of a job can disrupt the client's usual social network, leading to social isolation, loneliness, and depression. Help such a client adjust by suggesting social activities that are available in the community.)

Developmental considerations

The nurse must devise special questions when assessing a child's ADLs. Try to include the child in the assessment; when this is not possible, direct the interview questions to the child's parent or guardian. Ask the following questions:

Does your child eat independently? Does your child use utensils or fingers to eat? Does your child eat with other members of the family?
(RATIONALE: The ability to feed oneself is an important personal care activity and, for a child, an important developmental step. A child who eats with other family members not only receives nourishment but also develops social skills.)

Is your child toilet trained? If so, when did this occur? Does your child have problems with incontinence during the day or bedwetting at night? How does your child communicate the need to eliminate? Does your child need any type of assistance with toileting?
(RATIONALE: These questions assess elimination activities, which are important milestones for children. They uncover any special needs the child may have so that these needs can be met during hospitalization, if necessary.)

Can your child get dressed alone? Does your child have any difficulties when dressing?
(RATIONALE: Children gradually assume responsibility for dressing and grooming—two important components of personal care activities. Slowness to assume these responsibilities may indicate a developmental lag.)

Where does your child go to school? In which grade is your child? What does your child enjoy most and least in school? Has your child's school performance changed recently? If so, in what way?
(RATIONALE: For most older children, school activities are their work activities. Questions such as these evaluate a child's involvement in, and feelings about, school.)

What is your child's daily schedule? Does your child prefer to play alone, with peers, or with adults? What are your child's favorite activities and toys? Which toys does your child use to feel more secure? Does your child participate in sports? If so, what types? How much time each day does your child have for play? What type of physical exercise does your child perform as a part of normal play?
(RATIONALE: These questions evaluate the type of play the child enjoys and the factors affecting it. Play provides the child with a sense of control, a means of self-expression, and a way to learn about the world. Play also encourages sensorimotor and intellectual development. Culture, sex, age, developmental level, and health status all may affect the type of play in which a child engages.)

Observations and documentation

During the assessment, observe the client for any signs of an inability to perform ADLs. For example, when the client enters the room and sits down, notice the degree of mobility. If the client moves stiffly or unsteadily or requires an assistive device, the client may have a mobility problem that affects other ADLs. Also evaluate gross and fine motor coordination. Alterations in gross motor coordination impair ambulation and the ability to move from one position to another; alterations in fine motor coordination hinder the performance of tasks such as buttoning clothes or writing.

Be sure to document all pertinent observations with other physical assessment findings in the objective portion of your notes. Then use this information and the subjective assessment data to develop nursing diagnoses for use in the nursing process.

Sleep patterns

Between 25% and 50% of all adults complain of sleeping difficulties. Although some of these difficulties last only a night or two, others are chronic and debilitating sleep disorders. Clients with altered sleep patterns can appear in various clinical settings. For example, hospitalized clients may have difficulty falling asleep because of anxiety and pain. College students may visit the student health clinic because they stay up late studying for many nights. Mothers of healthy toddlers may lack knowledge about appropriate bedtimes for their children and allow them to decide when they are ready for bed. Nurses and others who work shifts can experience recurrent sleep problems because of shift rotation.

The first steps in assessing a client's sleep patterns are identifying the factors affecting sleep, distinguishing between normal and abnormal sleep patterns, and knowing when to refer a client to a sleep disorder center for specialized diagnostic procedures and treatment. Then, after collecting appropriate data, the nurse can formulate a specific nursing diagnosis and plan interventions.

This section of the chapter discusses sleep stages, normal sleep patterns, factors that affect sleep patterns, and sleep disorders. It prepares the nurse to understand the sleep assessment, which is described at the end of this section.

Sleep stages

While awake, people move continuously and purposefully, think logically and progressively, and experience vivid, externally generated sensations and perceptions. During sleep, these processes change dramatically, varying during different stages as follows.

Most adults fall asleep in about 15 minutes, experience two to three brief arousals during the night, and then awake 6 to 10 hours later. During sleep, a person moves about every 15 to 30 minutes, remains immobile for 10 to 30 minutes, and then moves again. Movement and short arousals often occur with changes in sleep stages. Two types of sleep occur: rapid eye movement (REM) sleep and non–rapid eye movement (NREM) sleep. NREM sleep divides further into stages 1, 2, 3, and 4. (See *Stages of sleep*, page 112.)

Sleep stages occur in a repetitive cycle throughout the night. Most adults experience four to six complete sleep cycles per night, with the majority of delta sleep occurring early in the night and longer REM-sleep periods occurring in the early morning hours.

Normal sleep patterns

Sleep patterns (the amount of sleep and the routine time to go to sleep and to awaken) vary among individuals and across groups of people. Many factors, including work or school schedules, can affect the timing and duration of sleep. For example, approximately 27% of male employees and 16% of female employees work in rotating shifts. Older adolescents and college-age students often prefer to stay up late to study or participate in social activities. This may result in inadequate sleep and chronic daytime sleepiness.

Sleep patterns vary with each individual. Some people, called "larks," go to sleep early at night, arise early in the morning, and function well in the morning. In contrast, "owls" prefer to stay up late, have difficulty waking and functioning in the early morning, and function well at night. The sleep requirement, which varies from person to person, ranges from 4 to 10 hours. Some people have extremely short or extremely long sleep periods. For example, one healthy woman, age 70, regularly slept only 67 minutes per night. In contrast, Albert Einstein often slept 14 to 16 hours per day for several days in a row (Meddis, Pearson, and Langford, 1973).

On the average, healthy adults between ages 20 and 50 sleep approximately 7.5 hours each night and do not require regular daytime naps. Despite the admonitions of many that getting a "good night's sleep" every night is important, the loss of sleep for one or two nights is not harmful. In fact, the loss of one night's sleep produces a transient mood elevation in 40% to 75% of depressed clients (Gillin, 1983).

After reviewing the results of numerous studies on sleep deprivation, Parkes (1985) concluded that "the main effect of total sleep deprivation in man is not any striking alteration in mood, performance, or behaviour, but in sleepiness." Even after 112 hours of sleep deprivation, only 7 of 350 subjects studied by Tyler (1955) exhibited transient psychotic behaviors. Rather, advanced age, sensory deprivation, stress, history of psychiatric problems, severity of preoperative and postoperative illness, and length of stay in the intensive care unit all contribute to the possibility that a client will develop perceptual disturbances. However, chronic sleep deprivation alone, such as that experienced by clients suffering from prolonged sleep apnea (absence of spontaneous respirations during sleep), can cause memory difficulties and mood changes.

Stages of sleep

Normal sleep occurs in four stages. Stage 1 marks the transition between sleep and wakefulness. The eyes move in a slow, rolling fashion; thinking slows; reactions to external stimuli decrease; and movements become episodic and involuntary. However, many people state they feel awake during this stage of sleep. Stage 1 constitutes 5% to 10% of normal sleep.

Then, within 1 to 7 minutes of the onset of sleep, Stage 2 occurs. Thinking becomes fragmented. If awakened from Stage 2 sleep, people correctly report that they have been sleeping. Stage 2 sleep constitutes approximately 50% of nightly sleep.

Next, 30 to 45 minutes after the onset of sleep, stages 3 and 4 occur, lasting 15 to 30 minutes in young adults. During this period, people are difficult to arouse and, once awake, may need a few moments to become alert and oriented. Delta waves (as shown on an electroencephalogram, or EEG) occur during stages 3 and 4, so the two stages are often referred to as delta sleep. Stages 3 and 4 compose 10% to 20% of nightly sleep.

REM sleep, or dreaming sleep, occurs approximately 75 to 90 minutes after sleep onset in healthy adults. A person in REM sleep exhibits EEG activity resembling that of an awake person, has decreased or absent muscle tone, and displays rapid eye movements. During REM sleep, a person experiences dreams (vivid, internally generated sensations and perceptions), thinks illogical and bizarre thoughts, and cannot move voluntarily. The body temperature drops, and the respiratory rate, heart rate, and blood pressure change. Males of all ages experience erections during REM sleep. REM sleep occupies 20% to 25% of nightly sleep.

Factors affecting sleep patterns

A person's age, exercise level, personal habits, diet, environment, and mood all affect the quality and duration of sleep. Altering one or more of these factors, with the obvious exception of age, often can improve sleep.

Age

Sleeping patterns change over the life span. For example, few children experience difficulty falling asleep at night or remaining awake during the day. In contrast, many older adults complain of difficulties obtaining enough sleep, and frequently take hypnotic drugs to combat age-related changes in their sleep patterns. Individuals spend less time asleep as they grow older, with the most dramatic changes occurring during infancy and childhood. The type (stages) of sleep and the quality of sleep also change with maturation. (For more information, see *The effect of age on sleep patterns.*)

Infants, particularly newborns, sleep 16 to 20 hours each day. However, their sleep is not confined to one period (consolidated), but is fragmented with frequent nocturnal awakenings. EEG recordings reveal that infants shift into different sleep stages every 20 to 35 minutes and that sleep commences with a REM period. Infants do not have specific, identifiable sleep stages, but rather have an "active sleep" similar to REM sleep, and a "quiet sleep" similar to NREM sleep. During active sleep, infants exhibit rapid eye movements, increased pulse and respiratory rates, and various body movements. They experience an equal amount of REM and NREM sleep.

During the next few months of life, sleep stages become more distinct, and adult patterns begin to appear. In a child age 6 months, sleep begins with a NREM, rather than a REM, period. Total sleep time decreases to approximately 13 hours, and REM sleep decreases to 25% to 30% of total sleep. REM occurs 75 to 90 minutes after a 3-year-old begins to sleep, and sleep consolidates into one period at night and an afternoon nap. By age 5 or earlier, most children do not require afternoon naps.

Total sleep time decreases from age 4 (10 to 12 hours) to age 10 (9 to 10 hours). By this age, children experience deep, restorative sleep with few arousals. Younger children may experience nightmares (bad dreams during REM sleep), bedwetting (enuresis), sleepwalking (somnambulism), and night terrors (awakening in a fearful state); however, these problems usually disappear before puberty. During adolescence, total sleep time decreases to approximately 7½ hours. However, the need for sleep does not decrease, and may even increase. As a result, many adolescents are excessively drowsy throughout the day and may experience difficulties remaining alert in the classroom.

Most healthy adults experience few problems sleeping until after age 35. Then, sleep begins to lighten and the amount of Stages 3 and 4 sleep begins to decrease. Adults under age 60 may complain of problems falling asleep but, once asleep, do not have difficulty sustaining sleep.

The need for sleep does not decrease with aging. Because elderly people often have problems sustaining sleep, they may require a longer time in bed than younger adults to obtain an equal amount of sleep. Usually, older people require more time to fall asleep (sleep latency), experience more arousals and fragmented sleep, have less deep sleep, and are prone to waking early. After age 60, people have more Stages 1 and 2 sleep with little or no Stages 3 and 4 sleep. Interestingly enough, the percentage of REM sleep remains relatively constant. By age 70, an elderly client's sleep is no longer consolidated into one block, but often includes a daytime nap.

Exercise

Although many people advocate regular exercise as a method of improving sleep, little evidence suggests that exercise affects subsequent sleep in any way. Sporadic exercise probably has little effect on sleep, unless it is overly vigorous. Then it may cause pain or aching muscles, which can interfere with sleep. Vigorous exercise just before retiring at night may inhibit sleep.

Smoking

Tobacco smoking alters normal sleep patterns. On the average, cigarette smokers require almost twice the amount of time to fall asleep as nonsmokers. In addition, smokers have lighter sleep with more frequent arousals. Although smokers often complain of feeling tired and irritable when trying to quit smoking, their sleep improves immediately after successful nicotine withdrawal.

Caffeine

Caffeine ingestion often affects sleep. A single cup of coffee before bedtime is unlikely to disrupt sleep; however, two or more cups of coffee produce a significant increase in sleep latency and reduce total sleep time. Elderly clients are particularly sensitive to the arousal effects of caffeine. For instance, after consuming caffeinated beverages, elderly clients experience an average reduction in total sleep time by 2 hours, and a significant increase in sleep latency.

Alcohol

Although alcohol ingestion decreases arousals during the first half of the night, it increases the frequency of arousals during the second half. It also decreases REM sleep and makes it more fragmented. REM rebound (compensation for REM sleep deprivation by increasing total REM sleep by up to 60%) occurs with chronic alcoholism. Sleep patterns remain disturbed for several months after alcohol withdrawal.

Alcohol also exacerbates sleep apnea and sleep disturbances associated with aging. For example, healthy male snorers over age 40 suffered sleep apneas and other hypoxic events after ingesting alcohol during the evening.

Diet

Food intake also can affect sleep. For example, a person gaining weight may sleep longer and deeper than normal; a person losing weight may sleep for shorter periods and may have more fragmented sleep. Although many persons believe that tryptophan, an essential amino acid found in dairy products and other food, promotes sleep, little evidence substantiates this belief. In fact, research has shown that tryptophan ingestion has no effect on the onset or quality of sleep.

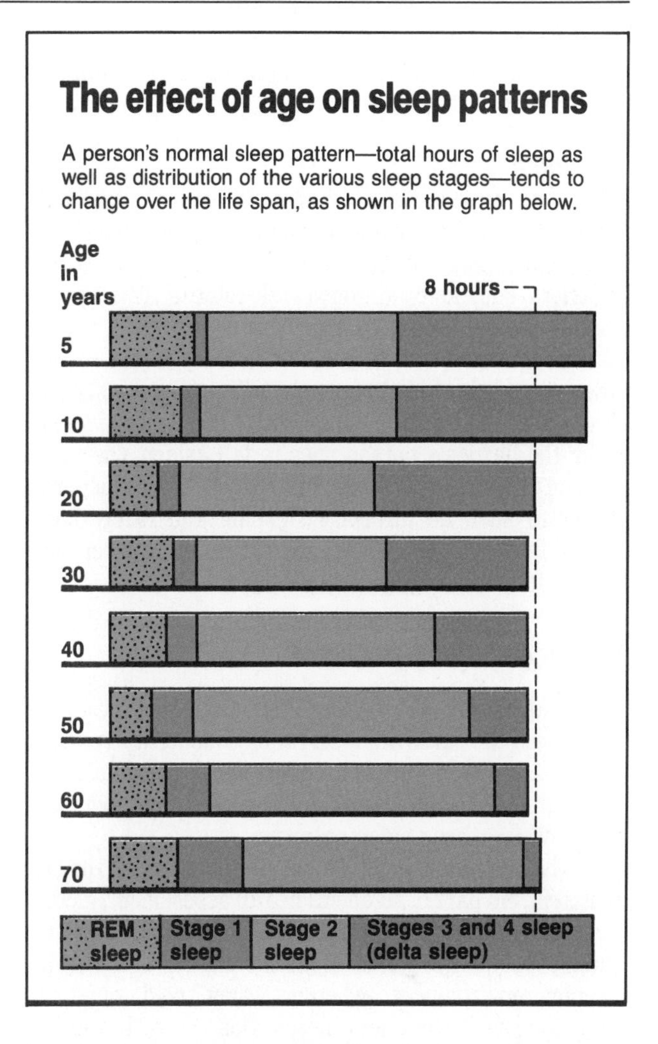

Environment

Of all the environmental conditions that can affect sleep, noise is particularly disruptive. Studies have demonstrated that an occasional loud noise is more bothersome than a constant noise, such as the sound of a fan or air conditioner. Episodic noise interrupts sleep and increases the amount of Stage 1 sleep. Moreover, arousals continue even after a person becomes accustomed to sleeping in a noisy environment.

Sleep also varies with environmental temperature. When the room temperature rises above 75°F. (23.9°C.), individuals have reduced REM and delta sleep, wake more often, move more frequently, and sometimes have a greater dream recall. Cool temperatures below 54° F. (12.2° C.) can produce unpleasant and emotional dreams.

Sleeping with a partner in the same bed also can

disrupt sleep. Sleep improves in quiet surroundings, in a comfortable bed, and without light and noise. Familiar surroundings also facilitate sleep.

Emotional factors

Mood and expectations strongly influence sleep patterns. Acute and chronic stress can increase arousal and inhibit sleep. In addition, stress may lead to maladaptive behaviors, such as conditioned wakefulness. This occurs when a person learns to associate wakefulness rather than sleep with being in bed, which leads to the expectation of not being able to fall asleep. The fear of insomnia becomes a self-fulfilling prophecy, triggering a vicious cycle: the harder a person tries to fall asleep, the more aroused the person becomes. In contrast, "good sleepers" expect to have no difficulty sleeping and rarely have trouble falling asleep. (For information about sleep disorders, see *Summary of sleep disorders*.)

Assessing sleep patterns

Asking questions about sleep during the health assessment gives the nurse an opportunity to teach and correct misconceptions as well as to collect subjective data about the client's sleep patterns. Use the following guidelines for assessing these sleep patterns.

The approach depends on the purpose of the assessment. As part of a general health assessment, gather basic data about the client's usual patterns of activity and sleep. Ask questions about the client's age, normal sleeping environment (whether warm, cold, quiet, or noisy), whether the client sleeps alone or with another person, and the usual time for retiring at night and rising in the morning. Ask open-ended questions about the quality of nighttime sleep and whether the client remains awake throughout the day. If the client feels satisfied with the quality and quantity of sleep, an extensive assessment is unnecessary. However, if the client complains about lack of sleep, excessive sleep, or a lack of daytime alertness—or if the client risks sleep disruption—perform a more detailed assessment. (For an overview of this type of assessment, see *Sleep pattern assessment*, page 116.)

In the case of a real or suspected problem, assess the nature and severity of the sleep problem, the daytime symptoms, and the client's normal sleep pattern. Gather more information about the client's health history and current physical status, current life events, and emotional and mental status. Also question the client's bed partner, and, in some cases, have the client prepare a sleep log.

Sleep-wake patterns

Ask the following questions to assess sleep-wake patterns for all clients:

How old are you?
(RATIONALE: Age and developmental status affect the amount, timing, and quality of sleep.)

What do you do for a living? What are your normal working hours?
(RATIONALE: Certain occupations require shift work, which can disrupt sleep.)

What time do you usually go to bed? What time do you usually wake up in the morning?
(RATIONALE: The usual times for retiring and arising provide accurate information about the duration of sleep.)

Do you fall asleep easily? Do you usually sleep all night without waking up? If awakened, do you fall asleep again quickly?
(RATIONALE: Difficulty falling asleep or staying asleep at night may indicate a sleep disorder. If so, this would indicate the need for a more detailed sleep assessment.)

Does anything help you sleep? Does anything make it more difficult to sleep?
(RATIONALE: The answers to these questions provide information about the use of sleeping aids, such as sedatives and hypnotics, and the client's bedtime rituals.)

Do you feel rested when you awaken in the morning?
(RATIONALE: A complaint of feeling tired upon awakening suggests insufficient sleep or a lack of restful sleep because of mood changes, medical problems, or a sleep disorder. In this instance, perform a more detailed assessment of the client's sleep patterns.)

Do you take naps during the day? Can you stay awake when driving, at work, and around the house?
(RATIONALE: Although daytime naps are common for children and elderly clients, most adults can remain awake and alert during the day. If the client has difficulty remaining awake when carrying out ADLs, perform a more detailed assessment.)

How is your health? Do you have any acute or chronic illnesses? What prescription and nonprescription medications do you take? Do you use alcohol or recreational drugs?
(RATIONALE: Certain medications, such as diet pills, and some illnesses, such as emphysema, can interfere with sleep.)

Summary of sleep disorders

Four major categories of sleep disorders exist: disorders of excessive daytime sleepiness, disorders of initiating and maintaining sleep, disorders of the sleep-wake cycle, and parasomnias (dysfunctions associated with sleep, sleep stages, or partial arousals). Each category includes several specific disorders, as described below.

Disorders of excessive daytime sleepiness

Narcolepsy
This disorder is characterized by abnormal sleep tendencies and pathologic manifestations of REM sleep. Brief attacks of sleep occur many times a day, during times of physical inactivity or when least expected, such as during a test, while at a traffic light, or while dancing. Some attacks occur without warning; others follow a period of drowsiness. Cataplexy, sleep paralysis, and hypnagogic hallucinations may also occur.

Sleep apnea
This disorder is characterized by transient failure to breathe during sleep. Three types of sleep apnea can occur: central, obstructive, and mixed. Clients with any type of untreated, severe sleep apnea are at risk for sudden cardiac arrest during sleep.

Central sleep apnea occurs when the client experiences inadequate airflow through the nose and mouth from an absence of inspiratory effort. During episodes of central apnea, ventilatory drive disappears, and nerve impulses to the respiratory muscles cease. Breathing recurs when nerve output resumes.

Obstructive sleep apnea occurs when the client's diaphragm and chest wall move with changes in intrathoracic pressure, but no air flows through the mouth or nose. The upper airway collapses, obstructing air movement, and blood oxygenation decreases, sometimes dramatically. The episode terminates when arousal restores muscle tone or when increasing respiratory efforts reopen the airway.

Mixed sleep apnea takes place when central and obstructive apneas occur in a single episode of airflow cessation.

Disorders of initiating and maintaining sleep

Insomnia
Up to 25% of all adults experience insomnia—inability to sleep—at some point. Insomnia may be transient or chronic. A subjective phenomenon, it most frequently affects female and elderly clients, as well as those who are neurotic, are thin, smoke cigarettes, or drink alcohol.

Transient insomnia refers to insomnia of less than 3 weeks in duration. It usually occurs with a brief illness, life crisis, new baby, bereavement, hypnotic withdrawal, travel, or temporary sleep deprivation. Rapid recovery usually occurs after a sleep disruption of 2 to 3 weeks.

Chronic insomnia may continue through life. Advanced age and medical, behavioral, and psychiatric problems frequently cause prolonged difficulties in obtaining restful sleep. Chronic insomnia may accompany another sleep disorder, such as sleep apnea.

Disorders of the sleep-wake cycle

Transient disorders
These include short-term problems with altered or disorganized circadian rhythms. Such problems may result from rapid time zone changes (jet lag) that require the client to be awake when normally asleep, and vice versa.

Chronic disorders
These include long-term problems with altered or disorganized circadian rhythms. These problems typically result from frequent shift rotation schedules that disrupt the internal body rhythms by requiring the client to be awake when normally asleep, and vice versa.

Parasomnias

Bruxism
Bruxism is teeth grinding during sleep. Like most parasomnias, it is not a serious disorder and rarely causes severe nocturnal sleep disturbances.

Enuresis
Commonly known as bedwetting, enuresis refers to involuntary urination during sleep in an individual with normal bladder control. Although most children gain bladder control by age 3 to 4, experts do not consider enuresis abnormal in children under age 5.

Night terrors
Night terrors cause a sudden fearful partial arousal from sleep during Stage 3 or 4. Upon awakening in the morning, the client has no memory of the episode. Although relatively uncommon, night terrors seem to recur in families and to afflict children more often than adults.

Somnambulism
Commonly known as sleepwalking, somnambulism occurs at least once in approximately 15% of all children between ages 5 and 12. Most children outgrow this behavior within 1 to 3 years. Adults rarely sleepwalk.

Sleep pattern assessment

When a client reports a sleep problem or is at risk for sleep disruption, assess the severity of the problem by following these basic steps. Obtain more detailed information, as needed, based on the client's responses to your questions.

1. Ask if the client has difficulty initiating and maintaining sleep. If so, carefully assess the duration of the problem as well as the client's habits, mood, stress level, snoring, and use of medications. Also, observe and document nighttime sleep.

2. Find out if the client is excessively sleepy during the day. If so, ask about the onset and duration of symptoms, type of problems encountered, presence of other symptoms, snoring, and character of nocturnal sleep. Also, observe and document the client's sleep patterns.

3. Determine if the client sleeps normally, but at an inappropriate time of day. Ask if the client must work evenings, nights, or rotating shifts. If so, assess how long difficulties have been present, and how the client has tried to resolve them.

4. Ask if the client sleepwalks, experiences night terrors or enuresis, or makes unexplained movements or noises at night. If so, check for a family history of these activities and a history of seizures. Also note the client's age and any stressors.

5. If no abnormal sleep patterns are present, no further assessment is needed. Provide preventive information, if appropriate. However, if abnormal sleep patterns are present, perform a detailed sleep assessment.

6. After the detailed sleep assessment, expect the physician to refer the client to a sleep disorder center if the client has symptoms of chronic insomnia, sleep apnea, narcolepsy, sleep-wake cycle disturbances, or nocturnal seizures. If no referral is needed, plan interventions with the client to normalize sleep patterns.

Are you satisfied with your sleep? If not, what bothers you about it?
(RATIONALE: The answer to this question uncovers the client's perception of sleep. If the client has concerns, perform a further assessment or, if indicated, educate the client about normal sleep patterns.)

Excessive daytime sleepiness

If the client's main complaint is excessive daytime sleepiness, thoroughly assess the client's sleep problem. Obtain information about the quality and duration of nighttime sleep. Also inquire about the circumstances that trigger sleepiness, and gather information about the onset and duration of these symptoms. Question the client about snoring or other symptoms, such as cataplexy (attacks of muscle weakness triggered by emotions), sleep paralysis, hypnagogic hallucinations (hallucinations during sleep), memory difficulties, morning headaches, and recent weight gain. Question the client's bed partner about the client's daytime drowsiness, snoring, breathing patterns at night, personality changes, and amount of restlessness during sleep. Document any complaints of sleepiness, irritability, difficulty concentrating, and loud snoring. Also discuss drug use, including alcohol and caffeine.

Ask the following questions to assess a client with excessive daytime sleepiness:

When did you first notice that you had difficulty staying awake during the day? Could you stay awake in high school or in college? Could you stay awake during your 20s or 30s?
(RATIONALE: The answers to these questions help pinpoint the onset of the symptoms. Also question the client's spouse, friends, or family members about the client's ability to stay awake during the day.)

Does your sleepiness cause you any difficulties? Can you stay awake while driving? Have you had any accidents because of sleepiness? Do you fall asleep at work, when talking, or while watching TV or reading? Do you fall asleep at unusual times and places?
(RATIONALE: Brief attacks of sleep during activity and rest may indicate narcolepsy or sleep apnea.)

Do you take naps? How long are the naps? Do you feel refreshed after a nap?
(RATIONALE: The responses to these questions provide information about whether the client can resist naps and about the duration of naps. Naps usually refresh clients with disorders of excessive daytime sleepiness, but only briefly.)

Does anything improve your alertness or make you especially sleepy?
(RATIONALE: The response to this question provides information about ways the client has tried to increase alertness and conditions that provoke sleepiness.)

Does anything unusual happen—such as a feeling of weakness or feeling that you will fall down—when you laugh, become angry, or feel startled or surprised?
(RATIONALE: Positive answers to these questions indicate cataplexy. If the symptoms exist, ask when they first

began and what circumstances trigger them. Refer a client with these symptoms to a sleep disorder center for definitive diagnosis and treatment.)

Have you ever felt momentarily paralyzed just before falling asleep or upon awakening?
(RATIONALE: If the client has experienced sleep paralysis, ask about onset and frequency. Sleep paralysis can be normal and does not by itself suggest a sleep disorder.)

Have you ever had dreams more frightening than nightmares, and so vivid that they seemed real? If so, when did these dreams occur? Did they occur while you were falling asleep, on awakening, or during the night?
(RATIONALE: These symptoms suggest hypnagogic hallucinations, which are vivid and realistic and usually occur while falling asleep or on awakening.)

Have you ever been told that you snore? If so, how loudly? Can people in the next room hear you? How about several rooms away? When did you start snoring? Has it recently become louder or more frequent?
(RATIONALE: Snoring often accompanies sleep apnea. The loudness of the snoring provides a rough index of the problem's severity. The client's bed partner is an excellent source for this information.)

Have you ever been told that you stop breathing at night, that you make grunting or snorting noises, or that you are a restless sleeper? If so, when did these things first happen? Have they recently increased in frequency?
(RATIONALE: Breathing difficulties and restless sleep commonly occur in a client with obstructive sleep apnea. The client's bed partner, and not the client, usually notices these signs and symptoms.)

Have you recently gained weight? Do you weigh more now than you did 5 years ago, 10 years ago, or 15 years ago? Has your clothing size increased in recent years?
(RATIONALE: Weight gain often triggers the onset of obstructive sleep apnea.)

Do you drink alcohol? If so, how much?
(RATIONALE: Alcohol exacerbates sleep apnea.)

Do you have headaches in the morning? How is your memory? Is it worse than it used to be? Have you been told that you are more irritable than you used to be?
(RATIONALE: Clients with sleep apnea frequently experience morning headaches, memory loss, and irritability. The client's spouse or family members are often the first to notice memory and personality changes.)

Does anyone else in your family have similar problems with sleep?
(RATIONALE: Approximately half of the clients with narcolepsy have family members who suffer from excessive sleepiness.)

Insomnia

For clients who report insomnia, design questions to elicit information about the client's mood, past and present stressors, current life events, sleeping habits, and beliefs about sleep. Also obtain information about sleep onset, duration, the age when difficulties first occurred, the stressors at that time, the timing of nocturnal sleep, snoring (especially in middle-aged, obese men), drug use, and related illnesses. Again, consider the client's perception of the problem, which may provide a basis for interventions that facilitate normal sleep. Ask the following questions to obtain this information:

When did you first notice that you had difficulty sleeping at night? What was going on in your life at that time? Were you ill, stressed, or having family problems?
(RATIONALE: These questions establish the approximate date of symptom onset and help identify the precipitating circumstances.)

Has the problem worsened, improved, or remained the same? Do you have problems every night or only once in a while?
(RATIONALE: Besides describing the severity of the complaint, the answers to these questions help assess for factors affecting the client's ability to sleep.)

What do you do when you can't sleep? Do you worry about not being able to sleep? Do you stare at the clock, get up and do something else, or take a sleeping pill?
(RATIONALE: Besides identifying the use of sleeping pills, these questions help identify behaviors that might increase sleeplessness.)

After a sleepless night, how do you feel the next day? Do you have difficulty staying awake? Do you take a nap?
(RATIONALE: Napping, particularly in the evening, may disrupt nocturnal sleep.)

Do you exercise regularly? If so, what time of day do you usually exercise?
(RATIONALE: Regular exercise, especially in the late afternoon, may facilitate sleep for some individuals. Irregular exercise or exercise just before retiring may inhibit sleep.)

(Text continues on page 120.)

Applying the nursing process

Assessment findings form the basis of the nursing process. Using them, the nurse formulates the nursing diagnoses and develops appropriate planning, implementation, and evaluation of the client's care.

The table below shows how the nurse can use data gained from assessment of a client's activities of daily living and sleep patterns in the nursing process for the client described in the case history (shown at right). In the first column, history and physical assessment data are followed by a paragraph of mental notes. These notes help the nurse make important mental connections among assessment findings, aiding in development of the nursing diagnoses and planning.

The second column presents several appropriate nursing diagnoses; however, the information in the remaining columns is based on the *first* nursing diagnosis. Although it is not part of the nursing process, documentation appears in the last column because of its importance. Documentation consists of an initial note using all components of the SOAPIE format and a follow-up note using the appropriate SOAPIE components.

ASSESSMENT	NURSING DIAGNOSES	PLANNING	IMPLEMENTATION
Subjective (history) data • Client reports having recent difficulty falling asleep and then awakening two or three times a night because of "strange noises in the building." • Client reports not feeling rested when she awakens and is having difficulty completing activities of daily living, especially home maintenance tasks, because of fatigue. • Client states that she has been napping for 1 to 2 hours in the afternoon, which is not her usual routine. • Client indicates that she has not changed her usual bedtime routine, which includes watching television and drinking one glass of wine. • Client sleeps with her husband in a double bed. **Objective (physical) data** • Vital signs: temperature 98.4° F. (36.9° C.), pulse 78 and regular, respirations 18 and regular, blood pressure 136/84. • Skin appears pale, with dark circles under both eyes and slightly puffy eyelids. • Client yawned several times during the interview and appeared lethargic. **Mental notes** *The change in environment may be contributing to the sleep disturbance. During the home visit, assess the environment for noise, lighting, and temperature. The client's feelings about her change in living arrangements may be contributing to her sleep problems.*	• Sleep pattern disturbance related to changes in home environment. • Potential for impaired home maintenance management related to sleep disturbance. • Potential for ineffective individual coping related to sleep disturbance.	**Goals** By the next home visit, the client will: • describe factors that inhibit sleep • return to her usual sleeping pattern • fall asleep within 15 to 30 minutes of going to bed • awaken feeling rested • perform activities of daily living without fatigue	• Help the client identify factors contributing to sleep disturbances, such as noise, room temperature, and light. • Help the client plan measures to eliminate or reduce environmental distractions, such as closing the bedroom door to reduce noise, closing the curtains to minimize light, and adjusting the thermostat to keep the room cool. • Obtain a list of the client's prescription and over-the-counter medications and evaluate them for any adverse effects on sleep. • Instruct the client to avoid caffeine-rich food or drinks, because caffeine is a stimulant that may interfere with sleep. • Instruct the client to avoid alcohol. • Encourage the client to engage in additional comfort measures at bedtime, including listening to relaxing music, reading, or taking a warm bath. • Encourage the client to minimize or eliminate daily naps to help promote the quality and quantity of nighttime sleep.

CASE HISTORY

Mrs. Jones, a 72-year-old female, has a history of hypertension. Three weeks ago, she moved with her husband of 44 years from their single-family home into a senior citizen apartment complex. While the visiting nurse checks her blood pressure, Mrs. Jones complains of having difficulty sleeping at night and of feeling tired and sluggish during the day.

EVALUATION

At the next follow-up visit, the client:
- identified at least two factors that interfere with sleep
- reported a return to her usual sleep pattern
- reported sufficient and restful sleep
- reported being able to perform usual home maintenance activities without fatigue.

DOCUMENTATION BASED ON NURSING PROCESS DATA

Initial

S Client states, "I am having trouble falling asleep and wake up several times during the night. My husband and I just moved to a new apartment, and I'm having trouble sleeping in a different place. I'm tired and have difficulty doing my usual activities during the day. I often have to take a nap, which is not my usual routine."

O Temperature 98.4° F. (36.9° C.), pulse 78 and regular, respirations 18 and regular, blood pressure 136/84. Skin pale, dark circles under the eyes. Eyelids appear puffy. Client yawned frequently during the interview.

A Sleep pattern disturbance related to changes in home environment.

P Identify factors interfering with client's sleep. Develop strategies to eliminate or reduce environmental disturbances. Discuss foods and medications that may interfere with restful sleep. Teach client additional measures to promote restful sleep.

I Discussed with client noise, temperature, light, and newness of surroundings as possible factors interfering with sleep. Taught strategies to reduce environmental disturbances, such as closing door and curtains. Discussed why reliance on sleeping medications is not advised and pointed out the effect of caffeine and alcohol consumption on sleep. Instructed client in relaxation techniques, such as a warm bath and reading at bedtime.

E Client identified factors that interfere with sleep and strategies to eliminate them. Client described the role of medications and food in the promotion of restful sleep. Client identified relaxation methods she will employ to promote sleep.

Follow-up

S Client states, "I only have trouble sleeping about one night per week. I have much more energy during the day to complete my chores."

O Temperature 98.4° F. (36.9° C.), pulse 74 and regular, respirations 20 and regular, blood pressure 160/92. No pallor, no circles under eyes or puffy eyelids noted. Client alert and talkative.

A Disturbance in sleep patterns has been markedly reduced. Client has returned to her baseline sleep and activity pattern.

P Encourage client to continue using the strategies that helped promote sleep.

Do you smoke cigarettes?
(RATIONALE: A smoker may have more difficulty falling asleep than a nonsmoker.)

Is your bedroom noisy or uncomfortably hot or cold? Does your bed partner snore or disrupt your sleep?
(RATIONALE: Noise [including snoring], a restless bed partner, or an uncomfortable room temperature can disrupt sleep.)

How would you describe your recent moods? Are you depressed or under stress?
(RATIONALE: Most insomnia results from anxiety or psychological problems.)

Do you have any other concerns about your sleep that you would like to discuss?
(RATIONALE: This open-ended question provides an opportunity to discuss concerns and reassure the client that the body obtains all the sleep it needs and that sleep loss rarely leads to illness or other problems.)

Developmental considerations

When assessing a child's sleep patterns, focus on normal changes in sleep, usual habits, and parental expectations rather than on abnormalities. Keep in mind, however, that sleep apnea and narcolepsy may occur during childhood. To assess a child's sleep patterns, ask the parents the following questions:

What is your child's usual bedtime and naptime? How long does your child sleep at night?
(RATIONALE: Evaluate the child's sleep patterns according to the child's age. Teach the parents about the normal changes that occur with age. For example, many 5 year olds stop taking naps.)

What is your child's usual bedtime routine? Does it include such activities as eating a snack, listening to a story, or brushing teeth?
(RATIONALE: Toddlers commonly have elaborate bedtime routines. Use this information to continue the child's usual bedtime routine during hospitalization. Also, if the child has difficulty falling asleep at night, assess the child's activities just before bedtime.)

Does your child have any particular security objects, such as a toy or a night-light? Does your child have any security behaviors, such as thumb sucking?
(RATIONALE: Use this information to continue the child's usual routine during hospitalization. Also, reassure parents that many children need security objects and behaviors, and will relinquish them with maturity.)

Does your child have any sleep difficulties? Does your child have difficulty falling asleep? Does your child awaken during the night (if not appropriate for the child's developmental age)? *Does your child have nightmares or night terrors? If so, please describe. Does your child wet the bed, snore, or breathe loudly?*
(RATIONALE: Many difficulties associated with bedtime and awakening at night occur because of inconsistent routines, a lack of parental limit-setting, and the parent's response to the child awakening at night. For example, feeding and holding the child whenever the child awakens at night positively reinforces nighttime awakenings. Reassure the parents that children commonly have night terrors and nightmares between ages 2 and 4. Provide information about enuresis, if appropriate. Also, loud, noisy breathing or snoring suggests sleep apnea, which requires referral to a sleep disorder center for evaluation and treatment.)

Do you have any other concerns about your child's sleep patterns that you would like to discuss?
(RATIONALE: This open-ended question gives the parents the opportunity to discuss any additional concerns.)

Observations and documentation

While assessing the client's sleep-wake patterns, observe for clues to a sleep disorder. If the client is hospitalized, note excessive daytime sleepiness or insomnia. Document this information along with vital signs and other objective (physical) assessment findings.

Then use this information along with subjective (history) data to formulate appropriate nursing diagnoses. Finally, use these diagnoses as the basis for the rest of the nursing process steps: planning, implementation, and evaluation of client care. (For a case study that shows how to apply the nursing process to a client with a variation in ADLs and sleep patterns, see *Applying the nursing process,* pages 118 and 119.)

Chapter summary

This chapter discusses the assessment of activities of daily living and sleep patterns. Here are chapter highlights:

- A balance between activities of daily living and sleep is vital for health maintenance.

• Factors affecting activities of daily living include age and developmental status, culture, physiologic health, cognitive function, psychosocial health, stress, and biological rhythms.
• Evaluating personal care activities, family responsibilities, work and school activities, recreation, and socialization are all aspects of assessing ADLs.
• Sleep patterns vary among individuals and groups of individuals.
• Two types of sleep exist: REM and NREM. NREM consists of four stages, ranging from light to deep sleep.
• Factors affecting sleep include age, exercise, smoking, caffeine and alcohol consumption, diet, environment, and emotional factors.
• The four major categories of sleep disorders are disorders of initiating and maintaining sleep, disorders of excessive daytime sleepiness, disorders of the sleep-wake cycle, and parasomnias.
• The nurse should perform a detailed sleep assessment on a client who complains of sleep problems, reports a lack of daytime alertness, or is at risk for sleep disruption.
• When planning nursing care for any client, the nurse should include strategies for helping the client maintain appropriate sleep patterns and document this information appropriately.

Study questions

1. Ralph Thompson, age 55, comes to the clinic for a follow-up evaluation of hypertension. During the visit, he mentions difficulty sleeping at night. What data should you obtain to assess Mr. Thompson's sleeping problem?

2. Ms. Jenkins brings her daughter Cindy, age 8, to the clinic for a routine checkup. During the interview, Ms. Jenkins expresses concern that, for the past several weeks, Cindy has "moped around the house" instead of engaging in normal play. When Cindy does play with her friends, the activity usually ends prematurely because of fighting. What factors should you explore to discover the reasons for Cindy's changed pattern of play? Why are these factors important? How would you document your findings?

3. How do sleep patterns change with age?

4. What factors are important when assessing a client with a sleep pattern disturbance?

5. Regina Johnson, age 68, was diagnosed with Parkinson's disease a year ago. She tells you she is having difficulty dressing herself. What questions would you ask to assess her ability to perform ADLs?

Selected references

Baker, T. (1985). Sleep apnea disorders: Introduction to sleep and sleep disorders. *Medical Clinics of North America*, 69(6), 1123-1152.

Balsmeyer, B. (1990). Sleep disturbances of the infant and toddler. *Pediatric Nursing*, 16(5), 447-452.

Bradley, T., and Philipson, E. (1985). Pathogenesis and pathophysiology of the obstructive sleep apnea syndrome. *Medical Clinics of North America*, 69(6), 1169-1185.

Browman, C., Sampson, M., and Yolles, S. (1984). Obstructive sleep apnea and body weight. *Chest*, 85(3), 435-438.

Buchanan, B. (1986). Functional assessment: Measurement with the Barthel Index and PULSES Profile. *Home Healthcare Nurse*, 4(6), 11-17.

Carnevali, D. (1985). A daily living functional health status perspective for nursing diagnosis and treatment in critical care nursing. *Heart & Lung*, 14(5), 437-443.

Carskadon, M., and Dement, W. (1987). Sleepiness in the normal adolescent. In C. Guilleminault (Ed.), *Sleep and its disorders in children*. New York: Raven Press.

Davies, A., et al. (1990). A method for assessing dressing skills in elderly patients. *British Journal of Occupational Therapy*, 53(7), 272-274.

Davis-Sharts, J. (1989). The elder and critical care: Sleep and mobility issues. *Nursing Clinics of North America*, 24(3), 755-767.

Dunlap, W., and Sands, D. (1987). Development of a set of instruments to assess independent living skills. *Journal of Rehabilitation*, 53(1), 58-62.

Emra, K., and Herrera, C. (1989). When your patient tells you he can't sleep. *RN*, 52(9), 79-80, 82, 84.

Gillin, J. (1983). The sleep therapies of depression. *Progress in Neuropsychopharmacology and Biological Psychiatry*, 2(7), 351-364.

Guilleminault, C. (1987). Disorders of arousal in children: Somnambulism and night terrors. In C. Guilleminault (Ed.), *Sleep and its disorders in children.* New York: Raven Press.

Hauri, P. (1985). Primary sleep disorders and insomnia. In T. Riley (Ed.), *Clinical aspects of sleep and sleep disturbances.* Stoneham, MA: Butterworth-Heinemann.

Lichtenstein, M., and Schaffner, W. (1985). Assessing activities of daily living. *Hospital Practice,* 20(5A), 8-9.

Malick, M., and Almasy, B. (1988). Assessment and evaluation—Life work tasks. In H. Hopkins and H. Smith (Eds.), *Willard and Spackman's occupational therapy* (7th ed.). Philadelphia: Lippincott.

Meddis, R., Pearson, A., and Langford, G. (1973). An extreme case of healthy insomnia. *Electroencephalography in Clinical Neurophysiology,* 35, 213-214.

Metzler, D., and Finesilver, C. (1990). When to worry if your patient can't sleep...Sleep apnea. *RN,* 53(3), 52-57.

Monjan, A. (1990). Sleep disorders of older people: Report of a consensus conference. *Health & Community Psychiatry,* 41(7), 743-744.

Mosey, A. (1986). *Psychosocial components of occupational therapy.* New York: Raven Press.

Parish, J., and Shepard, J. Jr. (1990). Cardiovascular effects of sleep disorders. *Chest,* 97(5), 1220-1226.

Parkes, J. (1985). *Sleep and its disorders.* Philadelphia: Saunders.

Rameizl, P. (1983). CADET: A self-care assessment tool. *Geriatric Nursing,* 4(6), 377-378.

Remmers, J. (1990). Sleeping and breathing. *Chest,* 97(3), 77-80S.

Selye, H. (1978). *The stress of life.* New York: McGraw-Hill.*

Shaver, J., and Giblin, E. (1989). Sleep. *Annual Review of Nursing Research,* 7, 71-93.

Smith, R., Morrow, M., Heitman, J., Rardin, W., Powelson, J., and Von, T. (1986). The effects of introducing the Klein-Bell ADL Scale in a rehabilitation service. *American Journal of Occupational Therapy,* 40(6), 420-424.

Tyler, D. (1955). Psychological change during experimental sleep deprivation. *Diseases of the Nervous System,* 16, 239-299.*

Nursing research

Ancoli-Israel, S., Klauber, M., and Kripke, D. (1989). Sleep apnea in female patients in a nursing home: Increased risk of mortality. *Chest,* 96(5), 1054-1058.

Aske, D. (1990). The correlation between mini-mental state examination scores and Katz ADL status among dementia patients. *Rehabilitation Nursing,* 15(3), 140-142, 146.

el Bayadi, S., Millman, R., Tishler, P., Rosenberg, C., Saliski, W., Boucher. M., and Redline, S. (1990). A family study of sleep apnea: Anatomic and physiologic interactions. *Chest,* 98(3), 554-559.

Biggs, A. (1990). Family caregiver versus nursing assessments of elderly self-care abilities...Biggs Elderly Self-Care Assessment Tool. *Journal of Gerontological Nursing,* 16(8), 11-16, 36-37.

Edwards, M. (1990). The reliability and validity of self-report activities of daily living scales. *Canadian Journal of Occupational Therapy,* 57(5), 273-278.

Frederiks, C., te Weirik, M., Visser, A.,and Sturmans, F. (1990). The functional status and utilization of care of elderly people living at home. *Journal of Community Health,* 15(5), 307-317.

Hanly, P., Millar, T., Steljes, D., Baert, R., Frais, M., and Kryger, M. (1989). Respiration and abnormal sleep in patients with congestive heart failure...Cheyne-Stokes respiration. *Chest,* 96(3), 480-488.

Johnson, S. (1989). Sleep pattern disturbance: Defining characteristics observable in practice. In R. Carroll-Baker (Ed.), *Classification of nursing diagnoses: Proceedings of the eighth NANDA conference.* Philadelphia: Lippincott.

*Landmark publication

6

Nutritional Status

Objectives

After reading and studying this chapter, you should be able to:

1. Discuss the relationship between nutrient intake and health.
2. Describe how pregnancy and lactation place the client at nutritional risk.
3. Give examples of appropriate health history questions to ask the client when assessing nutritional status.
4. Describe representative adverse effects of drugs on nutritional status.
5. Assess a client's dietary patterns using a dietary recall method.
6. Differentiate between normal and abnormal nutritional findings obtained by inspection, palpation, and anthropometric measurements.
7. Describe how to adapt assessment techniques for pediatric and elderly clients.
8. Describe the most important laboratory tests used to evaluate nutritional status.
9. Document nutrition assessment findings using the nursing process.

Introduction

From birth, the quality of a client's life is affected by the quality and quantity of nutrients consumed and used. The body's nutritional status—the balance between nutrient intake and energy expenditure or need—reflects the degree to which the physiologic need for nutrients is being met. Proper nutrition promotes growth, maintains health, and helps the body resist infection and recover from disease or surgery. Malnutrition impedes these natural processes.

Many people assume that malnutrition occurs only in underdeveloped countries. Unfortunately, this assumption is false. Malnutrition affects about two thirds of the world's population and occurs in people of every nationality, race, and age. In North America, certain groups—especially those with low incomes—run a particularly high risk of developing nutritional deficiencies. These groups include children, adolescents, pregnant or lactating women, and people over age 60. Malnutrition may be a primary disorder caused by insufficient nutrient intake, or a secondary disorder caused by a condition that impairs digestion, absorption, or use of nutrients or by a condition that increases nutrient requirements or excretion.

The nurse can encounter clients with nutritional disorders in settings that range from pediatric clinics to schools to hospitals, and the nurse's involvement in the client's nutritional status can vary. In some health care facilities, the nurse may have the primary responsibility for the client's nutritional assessment and care. In other settings, the nurse may refer the client to a specially trained dietitian who performs these functions. In still other facilities, the nurse may work with members of a nutritional support team to provide complete nutritional services.

Glossary

Amino acids: organic compounds that contain nitrogen and are the building blocks of protein.

Anabolism: one of two main phases of cell metabolism in which simple substances are combined to form complex substances.

Anorexia nervosa: eating disorder involving severe self-limitation of food intake; usually seen in teenage and young adult females.

Anthropometric measurements: measurements of the human body, including height, weight, body frame size, skinfold evaluation, and (in infants and young children) head and chest circumference.

Bulimia: eating disorder involving alternating periods of starvation and excessive food intake with self-induced vomiting and purging; usually seen in teenage and young adult females.

Calorie: standard unit of heat; the amount of energy it takes to raise the temperature of one gram of water one degree centigrade at atmospheric pressure.

Catabolism: one of two main phases in cell metabolism in which complex substances are broken down into simpler constituents.

Chylomicrons: lowest-density lipoproteins that carry fatty acids and cholesterol from the intestine to the blood and storage areas.

Chyme: nearly liquid mixture of partly digested food and digestive secretions found in the stomach and small intestine during digestion.

Complete protein food source: food source containing all essential amino acids.

Energy: capacity to do work, produce motion, or overcome resistance.

Glycogenesis: process by which glycogen is synthesized from glucose.

Glycogenolysis: process in which glycogen is reconverted to glucose.

High-density lipoproteins (HDLs): cholesterol carried by alpha-lipoproteins. HDLs are believed to serve as carriers that remove cholesterol from peripheral tissues and return it to the liver for catabolism and excretion; HDLs are also thought to inhibit cellular uptake of low-density lipoproteins. HDL values are inversely related to the risk of coronary atherosclerosis.

Incomplete protein food source: protein foods, such as vegetables and grains, that do not contain all essential amino acids.

Kilocalorie: standard unit of heat used in metabolic studies and used to express the energy value of food. One kilocalorie is the amount of heat it takes to raise the temperature of one kilogram of water one degree centigrade at atmospheric pressure. Also called a large calorie.

Kwashiorkor: disease related to protein deficiency; seen most often in severely malnourished children age 18 months to 3 years, but can occur in older children and adults in acute states of protein-poor intake and stress.

Lipogenesis: transformation of excess glucose into fatty acids.

Lipoprotein: protein bound to lipids containing various amounts of triglycerides, cholesterol, free fatty acids, and phospholipids.

Low-density lipoproteins (LDLs): beta-lipoproteins derived from very low-density lipoproteins (VLDL), approximately 50% cholesterol by weight. LDL values correlate closely with the risk of coronary atherosclerosis.

Marasmus: semistarvation caused by inadequate caloric intake or, more rarely, a metabolic defect.

Metabolic equivalent of a task (MET): measurement used to determine energy expenditure from activity; it refers to the amount of oxygen used per minute per kilogram of body weight.

Metabolism: complex process of chemical changes that determines the body's use of nutrients.

Mixed micelles: soluble complexes formed from bile salts coating fat globules of the small intestine.

Nitrogen balance: state of equilibrium in which nitrogen intake equals nitrogen excretion.

Pica: craving for and ingestion of substances not normally considered food, such as starch, dirt, clay, cornstarch, ashes, and plaster. Condition may be associated with pregnancy.

Saturated fatty acid: fatty acid chain that contains maximal hydrogen, but with no double bonds between the carbon atoms.

Unsaturated fatty acid: fatty acid chain that contains either one double bond (monounsaturated) or several double bonds (polyunsaturated) between the carbon atoms.

Very low-density lipoproteins (VLDLs): major carriers of triglycerides. Degradation of VLDLs is the major source of LDLs.

This chapter prepares the nurse for nutritional assessment in any setting. It begins with a discussion of the physiologic processes involved in nutrition. Then it presents health history questions that evaluate nutrition, highlighting specific questions for children and for pregnant, breast-feeding, and elderly clients. The chapter continues with a description of the physical assessment that evaluates nutritional status through inspection, palpation, and anthropometric measurements. Finally, it reviews the laboratory studies used for nutritional assessment and describes how to document assessment findings and use them in the nursing process.

Physiology review

An accurate nutritional assessment requires an understanding of the physiologic processes of ingestion, digestion, absorption, cell metabolism, and excretion. (For a detailed discussion of gastrointestinal anatomy and physiology, and of the digestive process, see Chapter 13, Gastrointestinal System.)

Ingestion, digestion, absorption, and excretion

Ingestion is the act of eating or taking food into the body; it is affected by age and cultural, psychological, socioeconomic, physiologic, and religious factors.

Digestion is a series of physical and chemical changes by which ingested food undergoes hydrolysis (addition of water) and is broken down in preparation for absorption.

Absorption of some nutrients occurs in the stomach. However, most nutrients are absorbed in the duodenal and jejunal segments of the small intestine, with the remainder absorbed in the ileum.

After absorption by any of these processes, water-soluble nutrient components from carbohydrates and proteins readily dissolve in plasma and enter the portal circulation en route to the liver. Fat and fat-soluble vitamins (A, D, E, and K) are absorbed as mixed micelles, soluble complexes formed from bile salts coating the fat globules in the small intestine. The bile salts, released after the micelles are absorbed into mucosal cells of the small intestine, reenter the intestinal lumen for reabsorption in the ileum and circulation to the liver for reuse.

The lipid components (diglycerides and monoglycerides) reform into triglycerides within the intestinal epithelial cells. They then circulate through the lymph vessels, through the systemic circulation, and into the liver.

Most of the water in the intestinal contents is absorbed in the intestines. The remaining water and related nutrients, such as minerals and vitamins, are absorbed in the colon, primarily in the proximal half. Electrolytes, principally sodium, are transported into the bloodstream from the colon. Bacteria in the colon synthesize vitamin K and some B complex vitamins, which are then absorbed from the colon.

Excretion is the process by which undigested food residue, including dietary fiber, inorganic matter such as minerals, metabolic waste products, and dietary excesses such as water-soluble vitamins (B complex and vitamin C), are eliminated through the large intestine, the kidneys, and to a lesser extent, the lungs and skin.

Metabolism

Cell metabolism is the complex process of chemical changes that determines the final use of nutrients by the body. The process is controlled by cellular enzymes and their coenzymes (many of which are vitamins), and by other cofactors and hormones.

The two main phases of cell metabolism are anabolism and catabolism. Anabolism includes the chemical changes by which simple substances combine to form more complex substances; this process produces new cellular materials and stores energy. Catabolism includes processes that break down complex substances into simpler constituents for energy production or excretion. The two processes occur continuously and simultaneously. When anabolism exceeds catabolism, the body gains weight; when catabolism exceeds anabolism, the body loses weight.

Energy

Energy is the capacity to do work. At the cellular level, metabolism provides energy in the form of adenosine triphosphate (ATP), a compound that cells need to function.

Three basic nutrients—proteins, carbohydrates, and fats—supply the energy needed for metabolism; vitamins and minerals also are necessary to the process.

Energy requirements include specific needs above and beyond the energy that the resting body needs to maintain life (basal metabolism). The basal metabolic rate (BMR) can be measured by direct and indirect calorimetry. (Direct calorimetry measures the amount of heat released by a client in an insulated chamber. Indirect calorimetry measures the amount of heat by determining the client's oxygen consumption and carbon dioxide excretion.) BMR is affected by lean body mass, gender, body growth, age, hormone levels, and health status.

Individual activity level also affects total energy needs. Activity levels may be expressed as kilocalories used per minute or in metabolic equivalents of a task (METs), which is the amount of oxygen used per minute per kilogram of body weight. One MET equals 3.5 ml oxygen per kilogram of body weight per minute. An individual at rest expends approximately 1 MET. One kilocalorie (1 Kcal) is the amount of heat required to raise 1 kg of water 1° C. at atmospheric pressure. It is the large calorie used in the study of metabolism and in the expression of the energy value of food.

4 Kcal

Carbohydrate metabolism

Carbohydrates, the primary source of energy, are composed of carbon, hydrogen, and oxygen, yielding 4 Kcal/g. Experts recommend that carbohydrates make up 50% to 60% of the daily dietary intake.

Carbohydrates, which are ingested as starches (complex carbohydrates) and sugars (simple carbohydrates), are the chief protein-sparing ingredients in a nutritionally sound diet. Carbohydrates are absorbed primarily as glucose; some are absorbed as fructose and galactose, but are converted to glucose by the liver. Once inside the cell, glucose is either metabolized to produce the energy needed to maintain cell life or stored as glycogen. Most of the energy produced by glucose metabolism is used to form the ATP found in the cytoplasm and nucleoplasm of all body cells. ATP is the principal storage form of immediately available energy for cell reactions. Complex carbohydrates, such as rice, pasta, or legumes, provide more energy than simple carbohydrates, such as sugar, ice cream, and candy.

Glucose storage occurs when the liver synthesizes glycogen (glycogenesis) from glucose. The liver subsequently reconverts glycogen to glucose (glycogenolysis) as needed. The liver can also transform excess glucose into fatty acids (lipogenesis) that may be stored as adipose (fat) tissue.

Excessive carbohydrate intake—especially of simple carbohydrates—can cause obesity, predisposing the client to many disorders, including cardiovascular disease and hypertension.

4 Kcal

Protein metabolism

Proteins are complex nitrogenous organic compounds composed of carbon, hydrogen, oxygen, and nitrogen atoms arranged as amino acids (organic compounds containing nitrogen). These basic structural units are joined by peptide bonds. One gram of protein yields 4 Kcal.

An adequate daily intake of protein is essential to health because proteins are necessary for growth, maintenance, and repair of all body tissue, as well as efficient performance of regulatory mechanisms.

Foods containing protein are made up of different numbers and kinds of amino acids. All protein food sources are not identical in quality: complete proteins, such as those found in poultry, fish, meat, eggs, milk, and cheese, can maintain body tissue and promote a normal growth rate; incomplete proteins, such as vegetables and grains, lack essential amino acids (organic compounds essential for nitrogen balance but not synthesized in the body).

To be absorbed, dietary protein must be broken down into amino acids and peptides. Amino acids are classified as essential and nonessential in terms of dietary requirements. Nonessential amino acids, which are as important as essential ones, can be produced by the body; therefore, they are not required in the diet.

Amino acids pass unchanged through the intestinal wall and are transported via the portal vein through the liver and into the general circulation; from there, each tissue type absorbs the specific amino acid it needs to make its protein.

The collected amino acids derived from protein digestion, absorption, and endogenous tissue breakdown form a reserve metabolic pool, which ensures the availability of a balanced mixture of amino acids to meet the energy needs of various organs and tissues.

Protein is not stored in the body. It has a limited life span and is constantly undergoing change (synthesis, degradation to amino acids, and resynthesis into new tissue proteins). The rate of protein turnover varies in different tissues. When energy demands of the body are unmet by the usual sources (available carbohydrate or fat), the body uses protein precursors to generate energy.

Nitrogen balance—when nitrogen intake equals nitrogen excretion—is a normal state for the healthy person, provided that caloric intake is adequate and protein intake exceeds the minimum requirement. Positive nitrogen balance occurs when nitrogen intake exceeds its output as, for example, during pregnancy or growth periods. Negative nitrogen balance occurs when nitrogen output exceeds intake. Negative balance may result from inadequate dietary protein intake, which causes tissue to break down to supply energy; inadequate quality of ingested dietary protein; or excessive tissue breakdown following stress, injury, immobilization, or disease.

9 Kcal

Fat metabolism

One gram of fat yields 9 Kcal. Fats should make up about 30% of the daily caloric intake—5% to 10% less than the amount ingested by the average American. Of that 30%, saturated fat consumption should account for only about 10%, and cholesterol should be limited to 300 mg per day. Fats are a major source of energy, and give taste and flavor to food. Because fats reduce gastric motility and remain in the stomach longer than other foods, they delay the onset of hunger sensations; thus they have high satiety value.

Like carbohydrates, fats are composed of carbon, hydrogen, and oxygen. However, fats have a smaller proportion of oxygen than carbohydrates and also differ in their structure and properties. The major fats are the glycerides (primarily triglycerides), phospholipids, and cholesterol.

Understanding lipoproteins

Synthesized chiefly in the liver, lipoproteins consist of lipids combined with plasma proteins. The four types of lipoprotein are chylomicrons, very low-density lipoproteins, low-density lipoproteins, and high-density lipoproteins.

Chylomicrons

The lowest-density lipoproteins, these consist mostly of triglycerides derived from dietary fat, with small amounts of protein and other lipids. In the form of chylomicrons, long-chain fatty acids and cholesterol move from the intestine to the blood and storage areas. An above-normal level of circulating chylomicrons (Type I hyperlipoproteinemia) has not been linked with coronary artery disease (CAD).

Chylomicrons

85% to 95% triglycerides

5% to 10% phospholipids

3% to 5% cholesterol

1% to 2% protein

Very low-density lipoproteins (VLDLs)

These contain mostly triglycerides with some phospholipids and cholesterol. Produced in the liver and small intestine, VLDLs transport glycerides. Obese and diabetic clients and, less commonly, young CAD clients may have above-normal VLDL levels (Type IV hyperlipoproteinemia).

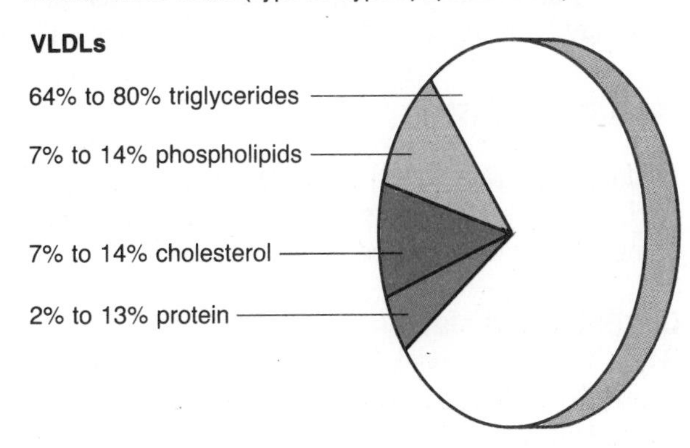

Low-density lipoproteins (LDLs)

These consist mainly of cholesterol, with comparatively few triglycerides. By-products of VLDL breakdown, LDLs have the highest atherogenic potential (conducive to forming plaques containing cholesterol and other lipid material in the arteries). An elevated LDL level (Type II hyperlipoproteinemia) commonly accompanies an elevated VLDL level.

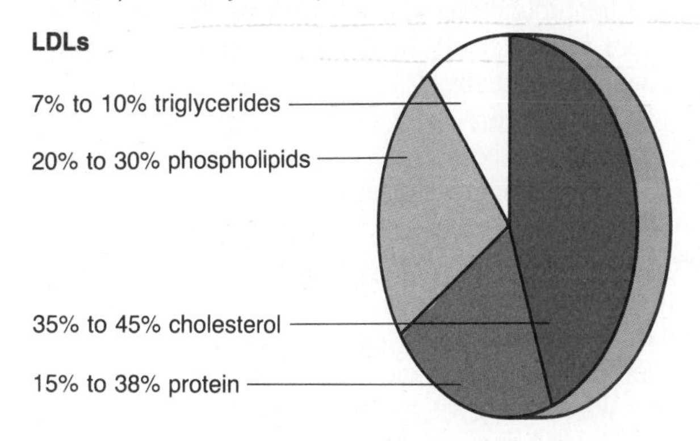

High-density lipoproteins (HDLs)

These substances—about half protein and half phospholipids, cholesterol, and triglycerides—may help remove excess cholesterol. Because persons with high HDL levels have a lower incidence of CAD, many researchers believe HDLs may help protect against CAD.

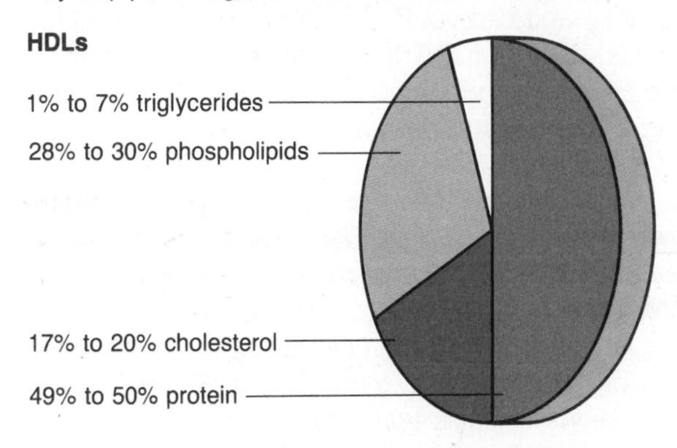

Adapted from Storz, N. "Metabolism and Nutrition: An Overview," p. 17, in *Metabolic Problems*. NurseReview Series. Springhouse, Pa.: Springhouse Corp., 1988.

Glycerides are the end product of fat digestion. They are used by the body cells for energy.

Phospholipids and cholesterol are formed by the liver. Phospholipids, which make up 95% of all blood lipids, serve several functions: they assist in the transport of fatty acids through the intestinal mucosa into the lymph; provide protective insulation of nerve fibers as myelin sheath; participate in phosphate tissue reactions; and form thromboplastin and some structural body elements. Cholesterol is used in the formation of cholic acid, which produces the bile salts necessary for fat digestion. It also is involved in the synthesis of provitamin D, helps form hormones (especially the adrenocortical steroids and the steroid sex hormones), and helps produce the water-resistant quality of the skin.

Together with phospholipids in the body cells, cholesterol helps form the insoluble cell membrane needed to maintain physical cellular integrity.

Fats are insoluble in water. However, when proteins combine with fats and phospholipids, the resulting lipoproteins can move through the aqueous medium of the blood. Lipoproteins contain proteins, triglycerides, cholesterol, phospholipids, and traces of related materials, including fat-soluble vitamins and steroid hormones. Lipoproteins are classified by density, which is determined by their percentage of protein. For example, a high-density lipoprotein contains a higher percentage of protein than a low-density lipoprotein. (For more information, see *Understanding lipoproteins*, page 127.)

Dietary fat carries fat-soluble vitamins A, D, E, and K. Some fat is necessary for the absorption of vitamin A and its precursor, carotene.

Fats not used for energy are synthesized into other lipids in the liver or stored as adipose tissue in subcutaneous tissue and in the abdominal cavity, where they insulate the body (reducing body heat loss in cold weather) and provide padding and protection for vital organs. When energy is needed, adipose tissue releases fatty acids and glycerol into the circulation.

Vitamins and minerals

Vitamins are biologically active organic compounds that are essential for normal metabolism; they contribute to enzyme reactions that facilitate the metabolism of amino acids, fats, and carbohydrates. They are also essential to normal growth and development. Although relatively small amounts of vitamins are needed, inadequate vitamin intake leads to deficiency states or disorders.

Vitamins are classified either as water-soluble (C and B complex) or fat-soluble (A, D, E, and K). Their activity in the body is affected by surgery, disease, medication, metabolic disorders, and trauma, especially multiple trauma. Because readily observable changes occur in the late stages of vitamin deficiency, the nurse must assess the client carefully for inadequate dietary intake and for subtle changes that may give early warning of vitamin depletion.

Minerals are also essential to good nutrition. They participate in the metabolism of many enzymes, in the membrane transfer of essential compounds, in the maintenance of acid-base balance (stable concentration of hydrogen ions in the body) and osmotic pressure (pressure on a semipermeable membrane separating a solution from a solvent), in the transmission of nerve impulses, and in muscle contractility. Minerals also contribute indirectly to the growth process; although requirements for individual minerals vary, the overall need is higher during growth periods—from birth to puberty—than in later life.

Minerals are constituents of skeletal structures and are present in hemoglobin, thyroxin, and vitamin B_{12}. Seven mineral elements—calcium, phosphorus, magnesium, sodium, chloride, potassium, and sulphur—are considered macronutrient or major minerals (greater than 0.005% of body weight). The others are considered micronutrient or trace minerals (less than 0.005% of body weight).

Trace minerals currently established as essential include zinc, iron, copper, iodine, cobalt, chromium, manganese, selenium, molybdenum, and fluorine.

Health history

The nutritional health history includes a dietary history, intake record, and psychosocial assessment. It can confirm good nutrition or detect an altered nutritional status and the need for more in-depth assessment and follow-up; it also identifies potential nutrition-related health problems, detects the need for education, and permits realistic planning for short- and long-term goals.

The questions in this section are designed to help the nurse evaluate the client's nutritional status. They include rationales that describe the significance of the answers and, where appropriate, nursing interventions that may be incorporated into the client's care plan.

Health and illness patterns

By following these guidelines, the nurse can use this part of the health history to help identify actual or potential nutrition-related health problems.

Current health status

Begin the assessment by inquiring about the client's current health status. Then explore factors related to nutritional status.

Have you had any recent change in diet? If so, can you describe the duration and specific changes? To what degree has your caloric intake increased or decreased?
(RATIONALE: A decreased intake contributes to weight loss and may lead to nutritional deficiency. An increased intake may lead to weight gain, but does not rule out nutritional deficiency.)

Have you experienced any unusual stress or trauma such as surgery, change in employment, or family illness?
(RATIONALE: Stress and trauma increase nutritional requirements of essential nutrients.)

Have you experienced any significant weight gain or loss, or a change in appetite, bowel habits, mobility, physical exercise, or life-style?
(RATIONALE: Significant changes may indicate an underlying disease. For example, weight gain may indicate an endocrine imbalance such as Cushing's syndrome or hypothyroidism; weight loss may be related to cancer, gastrointestinal disorders, diabetes mellitus, or hyperthyroidism.)

Do you take any prescription or over-the-counter medications, especially vitamin or mineral supplements or appetite suppressants? If so, what is the purpose, starting date, dose, and frequency of each? Do you use any "natural" or "health" foods? If so, which ones and how much of each do you use, and why?
(RATIONALE: The client's response to these questions may indicate a nutritional deficiency requiring supplementation, or that the client perceives a nutritional deficiency and self-prescribes. In other cases, the response may reveal routine drug use that can cause nutritional deficiencies or related problems. For more information, see *Adverse drug reactions*, page 130.)

Do you drink alcoholic beverages? If so, how much per day or week and what kind? How long have you been drinking alcohol?
(RATIONALE: Alcohol intake provides calories, but no essential nutrients. Chronic alcohol abuse may lead to malnutrition.)

Do you smoke or use chewing tobacco or snuff?
(RATIONALE: Use of tobacco products may affect taste, which in turn may affect appetite.)

How much per day do you consume of the following beverages: coffee, tea, cola, cocoa?
(RATIONALE: These beverages contain caffeine, a habit-forming stimulant that increases heart rate, respiration rate, blood pressure, and secretion of stress hormones. In moderate amounts of 50 to 200 mg/day, caffeine is relatively harmless. Intake of greater amounts can cause sensations of nervousness and intestinal discomfort. Clients who drink 8 or more cups of coffee may complain of insomnia, restlessness, agitation, palpitations, and recurring headaches. Sudden abstinence after long periods of even moderate daily intake can cause withdrawal symptoms, usually headache. For more information, see *Caffeine content of common beverages*, page 131.)

Past health status

During the next part of the health history, ask the following questions to explore the client's history for information related to nutritional health or disorders.

Have you had any major illnesses, trauma, extensive dental work, hospitalizations, or chronic medical conditions?
(RATIONALE: Any of these may affect the client's daily living patterns by interfering with the ability to walk, open food containers, shop for groceries, prepare food, or chew or swallow food, thereby altering nutritional intake.)

Do you have any food allergies? If so, please describe them.
(RATIONALE: Food allergies may have caused the client to eliminate certain foods, thus increasing the hazard of nutritional deficiencies. The nurse can use information about food allergies to help the client plan safe, balanced meals or to prevent the hospitalized client from being served food that can cause an allergic reaction.)

Have you ever had (or been told that you have) an eating disorder, such as anorexia nervosa or bulimia, or a problem with substance abuse?
(RATIONALE: These conditions compromise nutritional status.)

Have you followed a planned weight-loss or weight-gain program within the past 6 months? If so, please describe the program.
(RATIONALE: Because fad dieting can lead to altered nutritional status, explore the client's eating program to be sure that it is well balanced.)

Family health status

Next, explore possible genetic or familial disorders that may affect the client's nutritional status.

Do you have a family history of any of the following disorders: cardiovascular disease, Crohn's disease, diabetes mellitus, cancer, GI tract disorders, sickle-cell anemia, allergies, food intolerance (for example, lactose intolerance), or obesity?
(RATIONALE: These genetic or familial disorders may affect digestion or metabolism of food and can alter the client's nutritional status.)

Developmental considerations

Use the following questions as a guide in assessing individual developmental status.

Adverse drug reactions

When obtaining a nutritional health history, the nurse should ask about current drug use because many drugs can affect nutritional status. The chart below lists some commonly used drugs, along with possible nutrition-related adverse reactions associated with their use.

DRUG CLASS	DRUG	POSSIBLE ADVERSE REACTIONS
Antacids	calcium carbonate	Hypercalcemia, milk-alkali syndrome
	magnesium hydroxide	Fluid and electrolyte imbalances
	sodium bicarbonate	Metabolic alkalosis
Anti-infectives	amphotericin B	Hypokalemia, hypomagnesemia, reversible normochromic, normocytic anemia
	aminoglycosides	Sprue-like syndrome with steatorrhea, malabsorption, and electrolyte imbalance
	tetracyclines	Impaired absorption of calcium, magnesium, and iron
	sulfasalazine	Inhibition of folic acid absorption
Antilipemics	cholestyramine resin	Impaired folic acid or phosphorus absorption, steatorrhea, fat-soluble vitamin absorption with long-term use of high doses
	niacin	Hyperglycemia and abnormal glucose tolerance with long-term use of high doses
	cholestipol hydrochloride	Impaired absorption of vitamins A, D, E, and K
Antineoplastics	cisplatin	Severe electrolyte disturbances
	cyclophosphamide	Hyperkalemia, hyponatremia
Diuretics	thiazides	Hypokalemia, hypochloremic alkalosis, hypercalcemia, hypophosphatemia, hypomagnesemia
	bumetanide, furosemide	Hypokalemia, hypomagnesemia, hypochloremia, hyponatremia, hypocalcemia, metabolic alkalosis
	mannitol	Fluid and electrolyte imbalances
	amiloride hydrochloride, spironolactone, triamterene	Hyperkalemia
Steroids	prednisone, methylprednisolone, dexamethasone	Sodium retention, hypokalemic alkalosis, hypocalcemia
Miscellaneous agents	alcohol	Decreased vitamin B_{12} absorption; thiamine, magnesium, or folic acid deficiencies
	chlorpropamide, tolbutamide	Hyponatremia
	oral contraceptives	Decreased glucose tolerance, altered carbohydrate and lipid metabolism, folic acid or B_6 deficiency

Caffeine content of common beverages

Based on the chart below, the nurse can estimate the amount of caffeine the client consumes daily. Consumption of more than 200 mg per day can cause nervousness, intestinal discomfort, and other signs and symptoms.

BEVERAGE	CAFFEINE CONTENT
Coffee (brewed), 1 cup	85 mg
Coffee (instant), 1 cup	60 mg
Black tea (brewed), 1 cup	50 mg
Cola, 12 oz.	32 to 65 mg
Green tea (brewed), 1 cup	30 mg
Cocoa, 1 cup	8 mg
Decaffeinated coffee, 1 cup	3 mg

Pediatric client. Nutritional needs vary greatly as a child ages. The following questions help determine if those needs are being met. If the client is a very young child, direct questions to the parent or guardian. Be sure to conclude the pediatric health history by asking the parents if they have any questions or problems they would like to discuss.

Infant (newborn to age 1). Ask the following questions about a breast-fed or bottle-fed infant. For a bottle-fed infant, omit questions that relate specifically to breast-feeding.

If the infant is breast fed, how often and how long does he or she nurse at each breast? How much water does the infant drink, and how often? Do you use relief bottles? If so, what type of bottle or nipple do you use? What type of formula do you use, and how much and how often do you give it? Do you give the infant supplementary food or cereal? If so, how much?

(RATIONALE: During the 1st year of life, energy needs are high in relation to body size. The normal full-term neonate needs 110 to 120 calories per kg of body weight per 24 hours. Human milk and properly prepared formula supply adequate fluid intake under normal circumstances. A "rule-of-thumb" gauge for the fluid requirement for normal infants is approximately 100 ml of fluid per kilogram of body weight in a 24-hour period. Neither whole cow's milk nor skim milk is suitable for use in formula during the 1st year of life. Solid food is usually not introduced until the 4th to 6th month for formula-fed infants and the 6th month for breast-fed infants. Cereal is usually the first solid food added to the infant's diet. Strained fruits and vegetables may be introduced gradually at about the 6th month.)

Do you give supplementary vitamins? If so, what type do you use and how do you give them?

(RATIONALE: Information about vitamin supplementation helps provide an overall picture of an infant's nutrition.)

Toddler (age 1 to 3). Ask the following questions to evaluate a toddler's nutritional status.

How much fluid does your child drink in a typical 24-hour period? How much of it is milk (specify kind), juice, or carbonated drinks? Does the child drink from a cup? Does the child feed himself? How often and what kind of snacks are eaten? Is the child allergic to any foods? Does the child particularly like or dislike any food(s)?

(RATIONALE: Growth rate slows during this time, but muscle mass development and bone mineralization increase. [For a tool to evaluate the child's growth, see *Pediatric growth grids,* pages 134 and 135.] At the beginning of the toddler period (age 1), the child needs approximately 1,000 Kcal/day; the amount increases to 1,300 to 1,500 Kcal by the end of the toddler period (age 3). In developing autonomy, a toddler may refuse food at times.)

Preschooler (age 3 to 6). Ask the same questions as for a toddler as well as the following question.

Does the child attend a day-care center, nursery school, kindergarten, or other group?

(RATIONALE: The preschool period is one of continuing growth and of learning the family food patterns. A child who spends time at a day-care center, nursery school, or kindergarten will learn the food patterns of other groups as well, which may affect food habits.)

School-age child (age 6 to 12). Ask the same questions as for the toddler. Also pose these additional questions.

What does the child eat for breakfast? Does the child take lunch to school or eat the school lunch? Is the child involved in sports or other physical activities at school?

(RATIONALE: Body changes continue at a gradual rate during these years. Girls usually advance at a faster rate than boys. Breakfast is a particularly important meal during this time, preparing the child for learning and school activities. Food likes and dislikes continue in the established pattern, and may be affected by television viewing. Nutrition information usually is included in the curriculum. School-related activities may conflict with family meal times.)

Adolescent (age 12 to 18). To determine the nutritional intake of an adolescent client, ask the following questions about the type, amount, and frequency of foods eaten.

What do you eat in a typical day (24 hours)? What snacks and fluids do you consume? Do you use any alcohol, drugs, tobacco, caffeine (coffee, tea, cola, or cocoa), salt, or vitamin supplements? If so, what effects do they produce? Do you follow any special diets? Have you gained or lost weight recently?
(RATIONALE: Adolescence is a time of rapid growth, with the onset of puberty increasing nutritional requirements. The growth rate varies widely among individuals, and includes sex-related differences. The growth rate of boys is usually slower than that of girls; however, boys' total weight and height gains are usually greater than girls'.)

Pregnant client. Ask a pregnant client the following questions.

How have your eating patterns changed since you have become pregnant?
(RATIONALE: The nutritional status of the mother during pregnancy contributes to the future health of the child. An increase in protein and other nutrients—particularly calcium, iron, and folic acid—is needed during pregnancy. The daily requirement of folic acid is doubled during pregnancy, from 0.4 mg to 0.8 mg, because of increased fetal needs. Some pregnant women have pica [a craving for nonfood substances such as starch or clay].)

Are you taking any nutritional supplements such as vitamins?
(RATIONALE: Physicians usually prescribe supplements that contain all of the needed additional nutrients for pregnant clients. If the pregnant client is a teenager, the need for nutrients is greater from demands of the developing fetus added to the growth and development of the mother.)

How has your weight changed since you have become pregnant?
(RATIONALE: Caloric intake should be increased by about 300 kilocalories per day. Sometimes, however, a woman may overeat, believing she must eat for two. The weight gain should be at the rate of 0.5 to 1 pound per week, with approximately 4 pounds in the 1st trimester, 10 to 12 pounds in the 2nd trimester, and 8 to 10 pounds in the 3rd trimester.)

Are you currently breast-feeding another baby?
(RATIONALE: Breast-feeding is contraindicated during pregnancy because both processes increase nutritional requirements and compete for available nutrients.)

Breast-feeding client. The following questions help evaluate the nutritional status of a breast-feeding mother.

Do you have any questions regarding breast-feeding, or any personal concerns or problems? Have you noticed any changes or problems in your breasts? Is breast-feeding pleasurable?
(RATIONALE: A change in the mother's physical or emotional health can alter breast milk supply.)

Elderly client. Ask an elderly client the following questions.

Do you wear dentures? If so, do they interfere with your eating patterns in any way?
(RATIONALE: Poorly fitted dentures can decrease nutritional intake and limit variety in diet, predisposing the client to certain nutritional deficiencies.)

Do you have any disabilities or chronic conditions?
(RATIONALE: Some common conditions in elderly clients, such as degenerative joint disease, paralysis, and impaired vision from cataracts or glaucoma, can affect nutritional intake by limiting the client's mobility and therefore the ability to obtain, prepare, or eat food.)

Do you suffer from constipation or stool incontinence?
(RATIONALE: A decrease in intestinal motility characteristically accompanies aging; constipation also may be related to poor dietary intake, physical inactivity, or emotional stress, or may occur as an adverse reaction to drugs. Elderly clients often consume nutritionally inadequate diets of soft, refined foods that are low in residue and dietary fiber. Laxative abuse, another common problem in elderly clients, moves foods rapidly through the GI tract and subsequently decreases periods of digestion and absorption.)

Has your diet changed as you have grown older? If so, how?
(RATIONALE: Individual protein, vitamin, and mineral requirements usually remain the same during aging, while caloric needs decrease. Decreased activity may lower

energy requirements about 200 calories/day for men and women age 51 to 75, 400 calories/day for women over age 75, and 500 calories/day for men over age 75. Other physiologic changes can affect nutrition in an elderly client. For example, decreased renal function can cause greater susceptibility to dehydration and formation of renal calculi. A decreased salivary flow and diminished sense of taste may reduce the client's appetite and increase consumption of sweet and spicy foods. Other physiologic changes that can affect nutrition include loss of calcium and nitrogen [in nonambulatory clients], decreased enzyme activity and gastric secretions, and decreased intestinal motility.)

Do you participate in a community meal program for your main meals, or a "Meals on Wheels" program?
(RATIONALE: A change in economic status or the loss of a food program can alter meal planning and eliminate certain foods, thus placing the client at risk for a nutritional disorder.)

Health promotion and protection patterns

The nurse can ask the following questions to help determine what the client is doing to maintain an adequate nutritional intake and prevent deficiencies.

Health beliefs

These questions help in assessing the client's understanding of personal health.

Which particular foods do you believe you should eat at this time? Which particular foods do you believe you should not eat at this time? How would these foods affect your body?
(RATIONALE: Different cultural health beliefs exist concerning food intake and its relationship to health.)

Exercise and activity patterns

A client's level of activity may affect nutritional status. The following questions help assess this possibility.

How would you describe your usual activity patterns? Do you exercise? If so, what specific type of exercise do you do? How often do you exercise and for how many minutes? What time of day do you usually exercise?
(RATIONALE: The response will reveal if the client is active or sedentary and will help you determine the client's caloric requirements.)

What is the purpose of your exercise? Are you trying to achieve aerobic conditioning, control weight, or build muscle? Do you monitor the effect of the exercise through pulse, blood pressure, weight, or other measurement?
(RATIONALE: Answers to these questions may provide clues to the client's knowledge about the relationship of exercise to health, as well as the client's goals and sense of locus of control.)

Nutritional patterns

To assess the nutritional adequacy of the client's dietary intake and related factors, obtain a dietary history. Use any of the following methods: 24-hour diet recall, 3-day or 7- to 14-day dietary inventory or diary, food frequency form, or agency dietary history questionnaires. In a hospital or extended care facility, the 24-hour recall method is usually adequate. (For more information, see *Dietary recall methods*, page 136.) When compared with either the basic food groups or recommended dietary allowances, dietary intake data show where diet counseling is needed.

The basic food groups include the bread and cereal group (4 to 6 servings), the fruit group (2 to 4 servings), the vegetable group (3 to 5 servings), the meat group (2 to 3 servings), and the milk group (2 servings for adults and children, 3 for teenagers and pregnant or lactating women, and 4 for pregnant or lactating teenagers). Instruct the client to choose foods from these five food groups for an optimal diet, to include the minimum number of servings, and to limit totals as necessary to maintain desired body weight.

Stress and coping patterns

Understanding the degree of stress in the client's life, as well as the usual way of coping with stress, is helpful in the nurse's overall nutritional assessment. The client's responses to earlier questions on patterns of activity and nutrition, for example, provide clues to stressful situations. If the client did not give the reasons for any changes then, begin to explore the subject of stress with general questions.

Does the stress of your job, daily schedule, or other factors influence your eating patterns?
(RATIONALE: In many cases, employment, stress, and daily schedules interfere with mealtimes, predisposing the client to nutritional deficiencies.)

Do you use food or drink to help you get through stressful times?
(RATIONALE: Answers to this question will help identify whether the client uses food or drink as a coping mechanism. Individuals respond to stressful situations in different ways; they may increase or decrease food intake,

(Text continues on page 136.)

Pediatric growth grids

When assessing a child's nutritional status, the nurse uses a growth grid that correlates height and weight with age. To use a growth grid, follow these guidelines. First, select the appropriate grid for the child's sex. Find the child's height in the far left column and plot the point where it intersects the vertical line representing the child's age. Note where this point falls on the curved lines representing height percentiles. Repeat this procedure for the child's weight, using the information in the far right column and the bottom set of curved percentile lines.

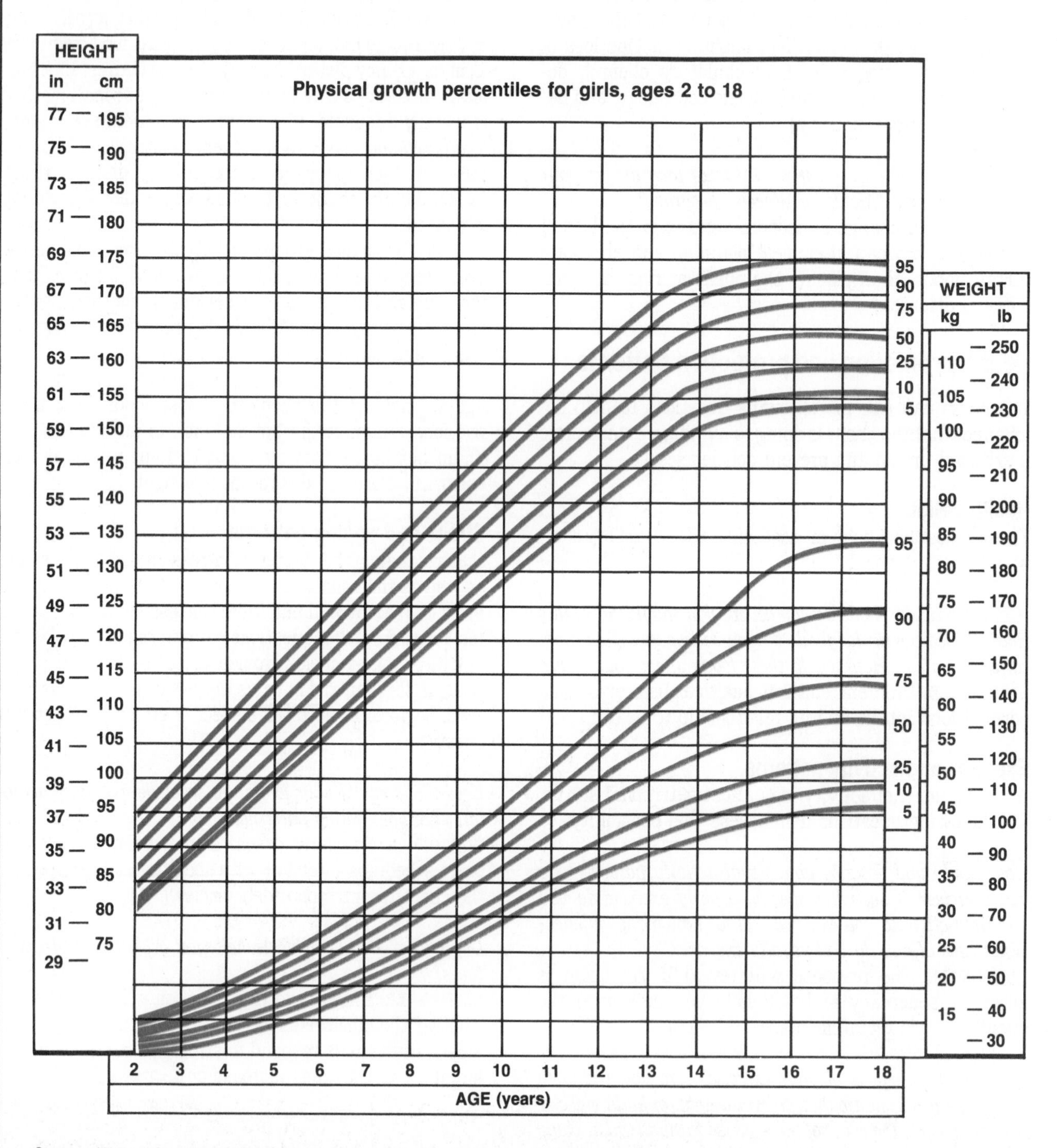

Courtesy of National Center for Health Statistics: Health Examination Survey Data. *Monthly Vital Statistics Report*, vol. 25, No. 3, June 1976.

Consider the child's growth normal if it falls between the 5th and 95th percentiles; abnormal if it falls below the 5th or above the 95th percentile, or if it sharply or suddenly deviates from the child's usual percentile.

Keep in mind that consistently abnormal measurements over time are more likely to indicate a problem than a single abnormal measurement, which can result from a normal growth spurt. Also, remember that children from different ethnic groups have different normal distributions on the growth grids.

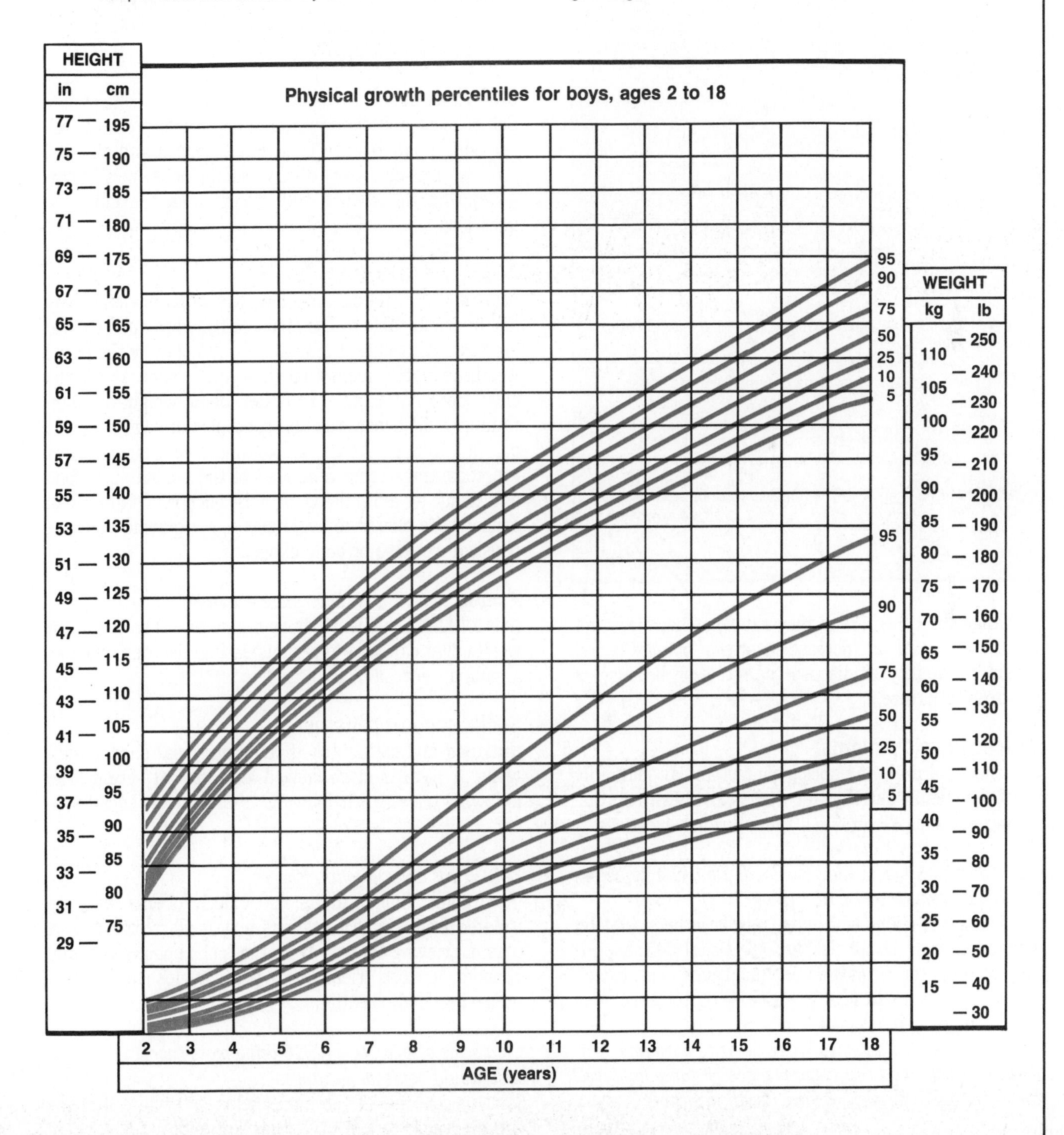

Dietary recall methods

The nurse can use one of several diet recall methods to assess a client's dietary patterns, as described below.

For the *24-hour dietary recall,* ask the client to recall everything taken as food or drink within the past 24 hours (or yesterday), the time it was taken, the amount, and how it was prepared. If the client is an infant or small child, determine the feeding schedule and the types and amounts of food and drink taken. (Determine if intake is adequate.) If the client is hospitalized, the 24-hour recall will not provide information regarding the usual dietary pattern; ask this client to write down 24-hour food intake on a "typical day."

When completing the *3-day* or *7- to 14-day dietary inventory* or *diary,* have the client record everything taken as food or fluid; the time it was taken; the amount; and if cooked, how prepared—that is, broiled, fried (in what), baked, boiled, stir-fried, microwaved. Also have the client record the place in which it was consumed, whether it was taken when alone or with others, and whether it was taken in response to a felt personal need, such as hunger or thirst, or for some other reason. This type of inventory is considered very reliable; however, a client may consciously or unconsciously modify the dietary intake during the recorded time.

The *food frequency form* provides an overview of the quality and variety of the foods eaten. Using the list of foods, the client indicates how often a particular food is eaten.

Agency *dietary history questionnaires* usually combine dietary intake inventory with questions about factors that affect food intake.

When completing any of the diet recall intake forms, be sure to ask the client to indicate the addition of any seasoning to the food.

or change the type of food they eat. The client may not be fully aware of an increase in stress, or may be reluctant to identify or discuss the situation because of its stressful nature.)

Socioeconomic patterns

Economic, cultural, and sociologic factors can markedly affect the client's nutritional patterns and health status. To uncover such factors, ask the following questions.

Where and how is your food prepared? Do you have access to adequate storage and refrigeration?

(RATIONALE: A client who must rely on others for food preparation may be at risk for nutritional deficiency if the food preparer is unavailable. Inadequate food storage and refrigeration can lead to nutritional problems.)

Do you receive food stamps, Social Security payments, supplemental Social Security payments, or assistance from welfare or the WIC (Women, Infant, Child) program?

(RATIONALE: A change in economic status or the loss of a food program can alter meal planning and eliminate certain foods, thus placing the client at risk for a nutritional disorder.)

Role and relationship patterns

This portion of the history is extremely important, because body image and relationships with others are frequently interrelated with food intake.

Self-concept

Self-concept and dietary intake are closely related. Advertising promotes the idea that thinness and physical prowess are necessary to achieve happiness and success. To explore the client's self-concept, ask the following questions.

Do you like yourself physically?

(RATIONALE: Children and adults who are overweight may feel uncomfortable by the focus on thinness and physical prowess. Self-concept may also be affected by the many weight-reduction plans that guarantee "success." If the client does not succeed in either losing weight or maintaining weight loss, the self-concept can easily become one of "failure." At the same time, overweight clients are constantly being reminded of the pleasures of food and drink by advertising. A self-concept of failure can cause these clients to avoid settings requiring vigorous physical exercise or body exposure.)

Are you content with your present weight?

(RATIONALE: The client's answer may reveal beliefs about weight that can lead to serious eating disorders such as anorexia nervosa or bulimia.)

Social support patterns

Nutrition and eating are affected by social support patterns. A meal is often viewed as a "social" event. The following questions help evaluate the client's social support.

Do you eat alone or with others?

(RATIONALE: Single adults and elderly clients who are isolated from support systems may neglect nutrition. A person grieving over the recent loss of a spouse, a family member, a close friend, or a pet may lose interest in preparing food or eating.)

On a scale of 1 to 10, with 10 being most important to you, how would you rate mealtimes?

(RATIONALE: Use of the scale helps determine if meals are enjoyed or endured. If they are endured, the client could develop an eating disorder such as bulimia.)

Physical assessment

The physical assessment may reveal clinical signs that the history and laboratory studies do not. Gross signs of malnutrition are readily apparent; however, many clients have hard-to-detect subclinical or marginal nutritional problems. The nurse should remember that overt clinical signs of altered nutritional status occur late in the course of the problem, and signs and symptoms suggesting nutritional problems can have nonnutritional causes. The following paragraphs describe steps for the nurse to follow during physical assessment.

The physical assessment includes inspection, palpation, and collection of anthropometric data (height and weight; body frame size; skinfold evaluation; and, in infants and children, head and chest size). In some instances, assessment also includes measurement of arm and arm muscle circumference. To prepare for the physical assessment, obtain a standing platform scale with height attachment; use an infant scale when appropriate and a stature measuring device if the client is a child. Also obtain skinfold calipers, a measuring tape, and a recumbent measuring board.

An adolescent or overweight client may be uncomfortable about having anthropometric measurements taken. Try to provide privacy and take a few minutes to establish rapport with the client before beginning this part of the assessment.

Inspection

Begin by inspecting the client's overall appearance, particularly the skin, hair, mouth (lips, teeth, gingivae, tongue, and mucus membrane), eyes, nails, posture, muscles, extremities, and thyroid gland. Generally, the skin should appear smooth, free of lesions, and appropriate for the client's age. The hair should be shiny. The mouth, mucous membranes, lips, tongue, and gingivae should be pink and free of lesions. The teeth should be intact, firmly attached to the gingivae, and contain few cavities. The eyes should be clear with pink conjunctiva. The nails should be smooth without cracks or fissures. The client's posture should be appropriate for age, and the movement of extremities and muscles should be symmetrical. The thyroid should not appear enlarged. (For more information about these structures and their normal assessment findings, see Chapter 7, Skin, Hair, and Nails; Chapter 8, Head and Neck; Chapter 9, Eyes and Ears; Chapter 18, Musculoskeletal System; and Chapter 20, Endocrine System.)

Abnormalities in these areas may suggest a nutritional deficiency. For example, inspection of the eyes may detect dry, rough conjunctiva accompanied by swelling and redness of the eyelids and a clouded cornea—signs of a vitamin A deficiency. A vitamin B_2 (riboflavin) deficiency could cause mild conjunctivitis; vitamin C (ascorbic acid) deficiency could cause hemorrhages in the ocular conjunctiva.

Inspection of the oral structures may reveal several abnormalities. Cheilosis (scales and fissure on the lips and mouth) may occur, indicating a vitamin B_2 deficiency. The mouth, tongue, and lips may appear reddened, suggesting a vitamin B_3 (niacin) deficiency. Cheilosis and a smooth tongue often accompany an iron deficiency. A client who exhibits swollen or bleeding gingivae may be suffering from a vitamin C deficiency. A client with a folic acid deficiency is more likely to demonstrate glossitis (tongue inflammation).

Many nutritional deficiencies can impair the musculoskeletal system. For example, marasmus (semistarvation caused by inadequate caloric intake or, more rarely, a metabolic defect) can cause growth retardation and muscle wasting; a severe thiamine deficiency can cause paralysis.

Palpation

Although less important than inspection for detecting nutritional deficiencies, palpation helps detect enlarged glands, including the thyroid, parotid, liver, spleen, and others that may indicate a nutrition-compromising disorder. Palpation may also reveal signs of deficiency when performed on the teeth and tongue. (For information about palpating the glands and the normal assessment findings, see Chapter 13, Gastrointestinal System, and Chapter 20, Endocrine System.)

Enlargement of a specific gland can indicate a particular nutritional deficiency. For example, thyroid enlargement is characteristic of iodine deficiency; liver or spleen enlargement may occur with an iron deficiency.

Loose teeth may suggest a vitamin C deficiency. Tongue palpation may reveal atrophy of the papillae, a common sign of a niacin deficiency.

Anthropometric measurements

Considering the client's height in relation to his weight may provide clues to undernutrition or to overnutrition.

(Text continues on page 142.)

Applying the nursing process

Assessment findings form the basis of the nursing process. Using them, the nurse formulates the nursing diagnoses and develops appropriate planning, implementation, and evaluation of the client's care.

The table below shows how the nurse can use nutritional assessment data in the nursing process for the client described in the case history (shown at right). In the first column, history and physical assessment data appear, followed by a paragraph of mental notes. These notes help the nurse make important mental connections among assessment findings, aiding in development of nursing diagnoses and planning.

The second column presents several appropriate nursing diagnoses; however, the information in the remaining columns is based on the *first* nursing diagnosis. Although it is not part of the nursing process, documentation appears in the last column because of its importance. Documentation consists of an initial note using all components of the SOAPIE format and a follow-up note using the appropriate SOAPIE components.

ASSESSMENT	NURSING DIAGNOSES	PLANNING	IMPLEMENTATION
Subjective (history) data • Client states, "I feel so tired and weak lately. I've had a poor appetite since my husband's death 3 months ago. I've been sleeping poorly since then, too." • Client reports, "I take a prescribed daily calcium supplement. Once or twice a week, I need a laxative. I take aspirin for occasional headaches and to calm my nerves when going to bed at night." • Client's 24-hour diet recall revealed intake of 2 cups of decaffeinated coffee and a slice of toast for breakfast, a small glass of juice at noon with "a roll and jelly" and "maybe a slice of cheese," and a glass of milk with a slice of bread and peanut butter in the evening. This had become a fairly regular diet pattern, although client occasionally opened a can of fruit for dessert or a snack. Before retiring, the client usually drank a glass of water after brushing her teeth. On the day a friend from church came to do the cleaning, client reported eating and drinking an increased amount with greater variety, because of the woman's encouragement. Use of the food diary for food intake before her spouse's death and the "flu episode" revealed a varied and complete diet. **Objective (physical) data** • Client appears tired and ready to cry. • Skin and mucous membranes dry and pale. Teeth intact; no evidence of gingivitis. Vision: myopia corrected with glasses, bifocals for reading. • Anthropometric measurements: Height 5′7″ (170.2 cm) without shoes. Weight 122 lb (55.5 kg). Body frame size: medium. Standard for this height and body frame is between 132 and 147 lb; client has lost 7.5% of body weight in 3 months. • Triceps skinfold, 16 mm; midarm circumference, 25 cm; midarm muscle circumference, 20 cm. **Mental notes** *The 24-hour diet recall reveals inadequate intake of fruits and vegetables, which can cause serious vitamin and mineral deficiencies. A diet low in fiber and roughage can lead to constipation.* *Decreased caloric intake and unbalanced diet can produce tired appearance. A 7.5% loss of body weight is a significant weight loss.*	• Altered nutrition: intake less than body requirements, related to decreased appetite after death of spouse. • Fluid volume deficit related to decreased fluid intake. • Sleep pattern disturbance related to grief over death of spouse. • Altered bowel elimination: constipation related to dietary intake. • Potential self-care deficit: hygiene, dressing, and grooming related to fatigue and weakness. • Impaired social interaction related to grief and fatigue.	**Goals** By the next visit, the client will: • report increase of daily fluid intake by 200 ml every 3 days until 1,800 ml per day has been reached. • document daily dietary intake from each of the five food groups, with emphasis on complex carbohydrates and protein foods. • report addition of 1 teaspoon of bran to cereal daily. • exhibit increase in body weight by 1 lb every 2 weeks for a total of 10 lb.	• Assess client's knowledge of food groups and nutrients. • Plan a conference between client and dietitian. • Explain the relationship of fiber and fluid intake to constipation. • Include client's preferences in scheduling daily fluid intake. • With client, develop a way for client to record fluid intake. • Discuss the relationship of exercise to appetite and sense of well-being. • Identify client's strengths: (1) interest in maintaining health; (2) healthy food intake before spouse's death; (3) health promotion activities, such as exercise classes, swimming, walking, and nonsmoking. • Weigh client every 3 days. Record, and work out a plan for client to take over this responsibility while in the hospital and after discharge. • Evaluate progress every 3 days.

CASE HISTORY

Mrs. Elsa Braun, age 72, was admitted to the hospital with a medical diagnosis of "unexplained weakness and weight loss."

EVALUATION	DOCUMENTATION BASED ON NURSING PROCESS DATA			
		Initial		**Follow-up**
At next visit, 3 days later, the client: • had increased fluid intake by 250 ml per day over the past 3 days. • was unaware of which foods belong to each of the five food groups. • reported taking 1 teaspoon of bran with cereal each morning, but still has constipation. • gained 2 lb over past 3 days.	**S**	Client states, "I feel so tired and weak lately. I've had a poor appetite since my husband's death 3 months ago. I've been sleeping poorly since then, too."	**S**	Client states, "I have to force myself to eat, but I know I need to."
	O	Client appears tired and close to tears. Vital signs: BP 120/82; pulse 76, regular; respirations irregular. Weight: 122 lb (55.5 kg). Height: 5′7″ (170.2 cm). Body frame: medium. Triceps skinfold: 16 mm; midarm circumference, 25 cm; midarm muscle circumference, 20 cm. Dry, pale skin. Teeth in good repair.	**O**	Weight has increased by 2 lb since admission 3 days ago. Intake record reveals an average of 1,250 ml of fluid daily, compared to 1,000 ml on admission.
	A	Altered nutrition: intake less than body requirements, related to decreased appetite after death of spouse. Client's measurements are at the 15th percentile, indicating mild depletion.	**A**	Client met with dietitian this a.m. to review five basic food groups. Client has not had a bowel movement in 2 days.
	P	Broaden dietary intake to include foods from the five basic food groups. Add bran to prevent constipation. Increase fluid intake. Increase body weight by 1 lb every 2 weeks for 5 weeks.	**P**	No bowel movement. Increase bran to 2 teaspoons.
	I	Teach client about five food groups. Teach client to keep a food diary. Weigh client every 3 days.	**I**	Bran increased to 2 teaspoons daily. Reinforced five basic food groups with client.
	E	Client wants to eat properly and take care of herself. She understands the importance of writing down what she eats every day.		

Evaluating body weight

Body frame size and height serve as the basis for evaluating the client's body weight. To make these basic anthropometric measurements, follow this procedure.

1. To determine the client's body frame size, first measure the wrist at its smallest circumference, just distal to the styloid process (wristbone) of the radius (the outer bone of the forearm on the thumb side) and ulna (the large inner bone of the forearm on the side opposite the thumb).

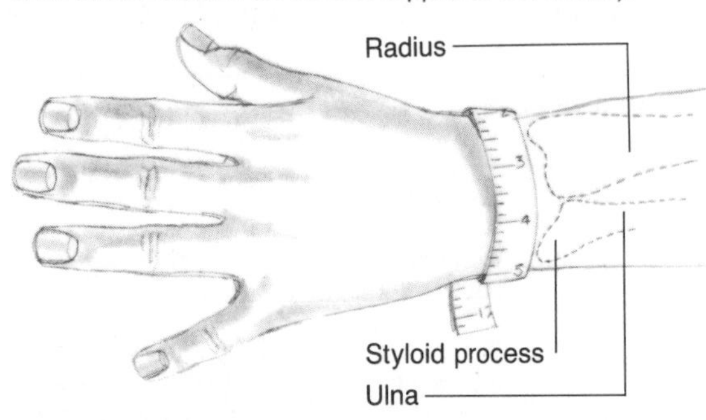

2. Next, obtain the client's height without shoes. Convert the height to centimeters. Then divide the client's wrist circumference into the height to obtain the r value:

$$r = \frac{\text{height (cm)}}{\text{wrist circumference (cm)}}$$

3. Find the client's r value on the chart below to determine body frame size.

	SMALL	MEDIUM	LARGE
Adult males	>10.4	9.6-10.4	<9.6
Adult females	>11.0	10.1-11.0	<10.1

Body frame size according to r value adapted with permission from Grant, J.P. *Handbook of Total Parenteral Nutrition.* Philadelphia: W.B. Saunders, 1980: p. 15.

4. Then obtain the client's weight and compare it to the tables below. The tables give standard weights, in pounds, for men and women from age 25 to 59 based on lowest mortality. They include the weight of indoor clothing (5 lb for men and 3 lb for women) and shoes (with 1″ heels).

Women

HEIGHT Ft	In	SMALL FRAME	MEDIUM FRAME	LARGE FRAME
4	10	102-111	109-121	118-131
4	11	103-113	111-123	120-134
5	0	104-115	113-126	122-137
5	1	106-118	115-129	125-140
5	2	108-121	118-132	128-143
5	3	111-124	121-135	131-147
5	4	114-127	124-138	134-151
5	5	117-130	127-141	137-155
5	6	120-133	130-144	140-159
5	7	123-136	133-147	143-163
5	8	126-139	136-150	146-167
5	9	129-142	139-153	149-170
5	10	132-145	142-156	152-173
5	11	135-148	145-159	155-176
6	0	138-151	148-162	158-179

Men

HEIGHT Ft	In	SMALL FRAME	MEDIUM FRAME	LARGE FRAME
5	2	128-134	131-141	138-150
5	3	130-136	133-143	140-153
5	4	132-138	135-145	142-156
5	5	134-140	137-148	144-160
5	6	136-142	139-151	146-164
5	7	138-145	142-154	149-168
5	8	140-148	145-157	152-172
5	9	142-151	148-160	155-176
5	10	144-154	151-163	158-180
5	11	146-157	154-166	161-184
6	0	149-160	157-170	164-188
6	1	152-164	160-174	168-192
6	2	155-168	164-178	172-197
6	3	158-172	167-182	176-202

Height and weight tables courtesy of Statistical Bulletin 1983, Metropolitan Life Insurance Company

Integrating assessment findings

Sometimes, a cluster of assessment findings will strongly suggest a particular nutritional disorder. In the chart below, column one shows groups of presenting signs and symptoms—the ones that make the client seek medical attention. Column two shows related assessment findings that the nurse may discover during the health history and physical assessment. The client may have one or more of these findings. Column three shows the possible disorder indicated by a cluster of these findings.

PRESENTING SIGNS AND SYMPTOMS	RELATED ASSESSMENT FINDINGS	POSSIBLE DISORDER
Weight loss, dry skin, weakness, frequent diarrhea, growth retardation in children, muscular wasting	Inadequate intake of proteins and calories Hospitalization for condition such as cancer, Crohn's disease, or cirrhosis Weight-height ratio 60% to 90% below standard Triceps skinfold thickness usually 60% below standard Midarm muscle circumference usually 60% to 90% below normal	Maramus (caloric deficiency)
Weight loss of more than 20% of body weight, emaciated appearance	Morbid fear of being fat and compulsion to be thin Inadequate intake of protein and calories coupled with avid exercising and refusal to eat Use of laxatives or diuretics to lose weight Dental caries Amenorrhea Susceptibility to infection Adolescent or young adult female Skeletal muscle atrophy, loss of fatty tissue Hypotension Blotchy or sallow skin, dryness or loss of scalp hair	Anorexia nervosa
Weakness, flaccid paralysis, lethargy, convulsions from electrolyte imbalances	Gorging followed by spontaneous or self-induced vomiting Ritualistic purging to maintain a desired weight level Use of laxatives and diuretics to lose weight Exaggerated dread of becoming fat Muscular weakness Adolescent or young adult female Erosion of dental enamel	Bulimia
Significant weight gain over time, skin thickening, pale striae, weakness, joint strain or pain possible	Pattern of overeating accompanied by decreased energy expenditure, or history of endocrine abnormality (less common) Weight-height ratio 20% or more above normal Triceps skinfold measurement indicating obesity	Obesity
Dry, scaly, rough skin with follicular hyperkeratosis, shrinking and hardening of mucous membranes, weakness, vague apathy possible, failure to thrive possible	Night blindness that may progress to permanent blindness Diet lacking in leafy green and yellow vegetables and fruits Fat malabsorption Dry, rough conjunctiva Swelling and redness of eyelids Clouded cornea, possibly with ulcerations	Vitamin A deficiency
Weight loss, emaciated appearance, pallor, especially in infants; subcutaneous edema in arms and legs possible; weakness; apathy; confusion; memory loss; anorexia; vomiting; constipation; abdominal pain; muscle cramps; paresthesias; polyneuritis; in severe cases, convulsions	Increased need for B_1 during fever or pregnancy Infants on low-protein diets Inadequate intake of whole or enriched breads or cereals, pork, beans, and nuts Malabsorption syndrome Chronic alcoholism Edema beginning in legs and moving upward Cardiomegaly with tachycardia Dyspnea possible Nystagmus possible	Thiamine (B_1) deficiency

Although an adult's self-report of height is usually correct, take a baseline measurement. (For a detailed explanation of this technique, see Chapter 4, Physical Assessment Skills.)

Body weight is the total weight of lean body mass (extracellular fluid, protoplasm, and bone) and fat. Comparison with standard measurments shows whether the client's weight, height, and body frame are above or below that standard, indicating whether the client is undernourished or overnourished. Measured daily, the client's weight reflects changes in hydration, which helps assess fluid retention and the effectiveness of diuretic therapy or dialysis.

Weigh the client yourself, if possible, to obtain an accurate baseline for comparison with ideal body weight, usual weight, and future weight. (For the correct way to weigh a client, see Chapter 4, Physical Assessment Skills.) Do not rely on client information; it may not include significant weight changes.

To determine ideal body weight for an adult client (age 18 and over), first determine body frame size. Then, based on body frame size, compare the client's height and weight with the values on a standard height-weight chart. (For an illustrated procedure, see *Evaluating body weight,* page 140.) After locating the client's ideal weight-for-height, use that value to calculate the percentage of ideal body weight that the client's present weight represents. Some authorities believe that any client who has had an unmonitored 10% weight loss over 6 months, or is either 20% above or 20% below the standard, is at risk for nutritional disorders and may need referral for medical evaluation and follow-up. (For more information about the abnormal findings associated with nutritional disorders, see *Integrating assessment findings,* page 141.)

Developmental considerations

Children and elderly clients require special techniques for physical assessment of nutritional status.

Pediatric clients

In a child under age 2, measure length with the child supine. Weigh an infant nude, because diapers vary greatly in weight. Use growth charts to compare the height and weight measurements; these charts reflect measurements of the population of American children taken as a whole. (For samples, see *Pediatric growth grids,* pages 134 and 135.) Plot the data on a growth chart. These charts show curved lines for specific per-

Measuring head and chest circumference

Head and chest circumference are anthropometric measurements taken as part of the physical assessment of infants and children. To obtain accurate results, the nurse follows these procedures.

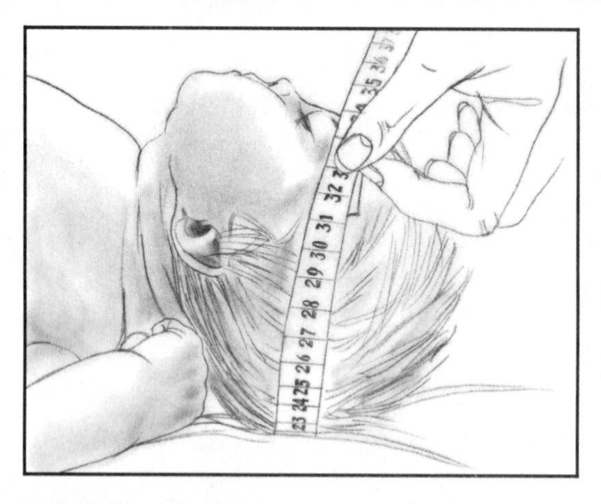

Head circumference
To measure an infant's head circumference, wrap a nonstretching measuring tape around the head just above the supraorbital ridges and over the most prominent part of the occiput.

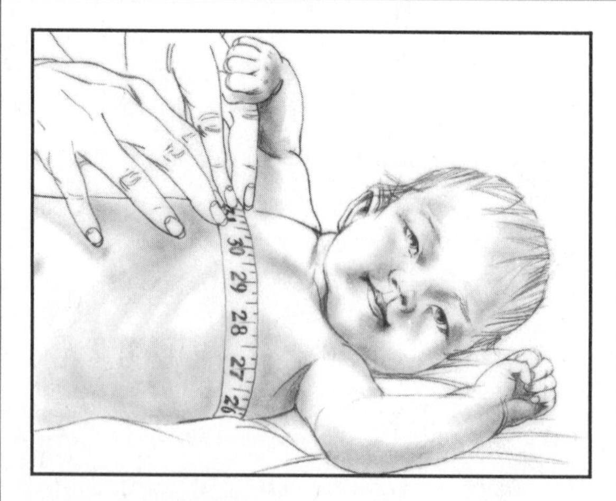

Chest circumference
To measure an infant's chest circumference, wrap the tape around the chest at the nipples. Take the measurement between inspiration and expiration.

ADVANCED ASSESSMENT SKILLS

Anthropometric arm measurements

Measurements of the midarm circumference, triceps skinfold thickness, and midarm muscle circumference provide information about skeletal muscle and adipose tissue, which helps indicate the client's protein and calorie reserves. The nurse follows this procedure.

1 Locate the midpoint on the client's upper arm using a nonstretching tape measure, and mark the midpoint with a felt-tip pen.

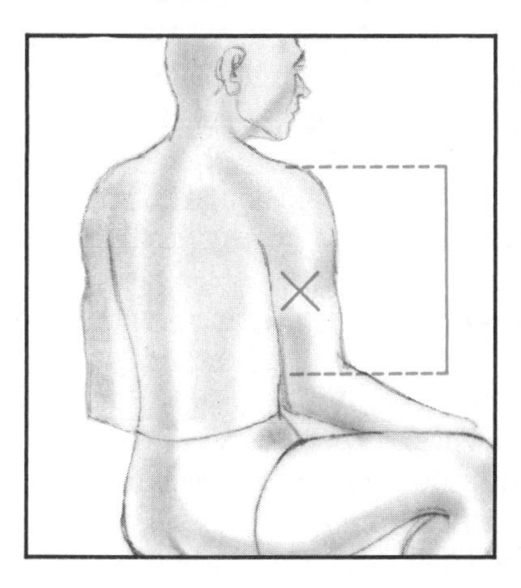

2 Determine the triceps skinfold thickness by grasping the client's skin between thumb and forefinger approximately 1 cm above the midpoint. Place the calipers at the midpoint and squeeze the calipers for about 3 seconds. Record the measurement registered on the handle gauge to the nearest 0.5 mm. Take two more readings, then average all three to compensate for possible error.

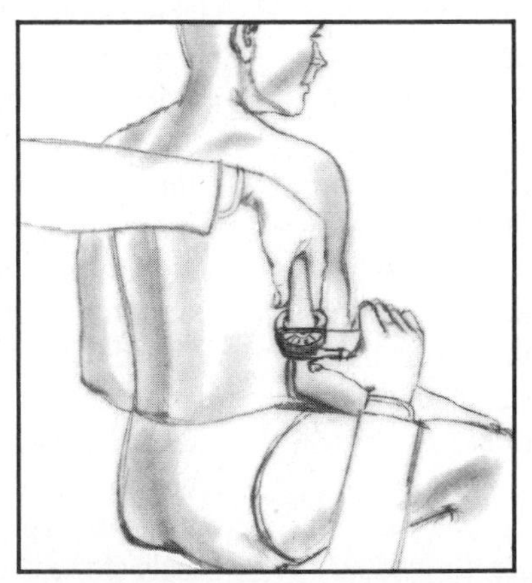

3 From the midpoint, measure the midarm circumference. Calculate midarm muscle circumference by multiplying the triceps skinfold thickness (in centimeters) by 3.143 and subtracting the result from the midarm circumference.

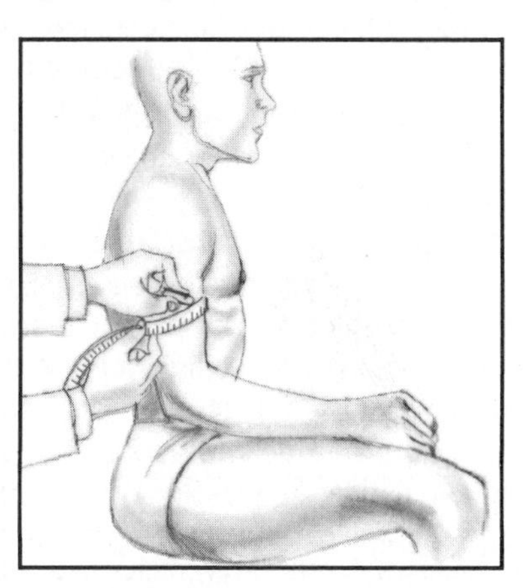

4 Record all three measurements as percentages of the standard measurements by using the following formula:

$$\frac{\text{actual measurement}}{\text{standard measurement}} \times 100$$

Compare the client's percentage measurement to the standard shown at right. A measurement less than 90% of the standard indicates caloric deprivation; a measurement over 90% indicates adequate or more than adequate energy reserves.

MEASUREMENT		STANDARD	90%
Triceps skinfold	Men	12.5 mm	11.3 mm
	Women	16.5 mm	14.9 mm
Midarm circumference	Men	29.3 cm	26.4 cm
	Women	28.5 cm	25.7 cm
Midarm muscle circumference	Men	25.3 cm	22.8 cm
	Women	23.2 cm	20.9 cm

Adapted with permission from Blackburn, G., Bistrian, B., Maini, B., Schlamm, H., and Smith, M., "Nutritional and Metabolic Assessment of the Hospital Patient." *The Journal of Parenteral and Enteral Nutrition* 1(1):11-22, 1977.

centiles (5th, 10th, 25th, 50th, 75th, 90th, and 95th), with curve values given for ages 2 to 18 for both males and females. Measurements that fall between the 5th and 95th percentiles represent normal growth for most clients.

When interpreting data, be aware that these charts are standardized according to growth rates of North American children; growth rates of other children may not conform to the charts.

A healthy growing child usually maintains the same relative position on the growth chart. For example, a child in the 20th percentile at age 3 will often remain in that percentile at age 5, 6, and so on. Moving up or down a percentile as the child grows older is not abnormal unless it reflects a progressively upward or downward trend. Check any values above the 90th or below the 10th percentiles for accuracy. Refer for evaluation any infant or child whose height-weight or height-age ratio falls below the 5th or above the 95th percentile.

Measure head and chest circumference in infants and children. (For an illustrated procedure, see *Measuring head and chest circumference*, page 142.) Because the brain grows rapidly in a child's first 2 years, head circumference can reflect abnormal rates of development, giving some indication of nutritional status. Chest circumference is routinely measured only in the newborn; measure it in older infants and young children with signs of a growth problem. As with height and weight, compare these measurements to standard growth charts.

Elderly clients

When assessing an elderly client, be sure to measure the height yourself. The client's self-report may be inaccurate because the client may be unaware of a height loss. Height decreases with age because of changes in intervertebral disks, vertebrae, and posture.

Advanced assessment skills

Midarm circumference, triceps skinfold thickness, and midarm muscle circumference provide a way to determine the amount of skeletal muscle and adipose tissue—which indicate protein and fat reserves. (For information about these procedures, see *Advanced assessment skills: Anthropometric arm measurements*, page 143.) Some health care facilities require that a dietitian perform these measurements.

If any of the above measurements fall between the 5th and 25th percentile, the client may be moderately nutritionally depleted; report this finding and conduct serial measurements. If the measurements fall at or below the 5th percentile, or at or above the 95th percentile, refer the client for medical evaluation.

Serial measurements reflect changes in nutritional status. Documenting the measurements on a graphic flow chart provides an excellent visual means of following trends, as well as the relationship between particular measurements over a particular time.

Documentation

To complete the nutritional assessment, the nurse must check the results of laboratory and diagnostic studies ordered for the client. (For a summary of common studies and their implications, see *Common laboratory studies.*)

Evaluation of history, physical, and laboratory data places the client in one of the four categories that describe nutritional status:

- Adequate nutrition. The client exhibits no deficits in body fat stores, lean body mass, visceral proteins, or immunocompetence.
- Marasmus. This deficiency state indicates depletion of body fat and lean body mass. Body weight is below the standard range, reflecting loss of muscle and fat. Decreased triceps skinfold thickness indicates loss of body fat; reduced arm muscle circumference reflects loss of skeletal muscle tissue. Serum albumin and transferrin levels are maintained by the breakdown of lean body mass, which provides the components necessary for synthesis of these proteins. Lean body mass breakdown can maintain normal albumin and transferrin levels until marasmus becomes severe.
- Depleted visceral protein (hypoalbuminemic malnutrition or kwashiorkor). This deficiency state indicates protein loss from the stress of trauma or infection. The development of anergy (decreased reaction to a specific antigen) and hypoalbuminemia reflects increasing impairment of visceral function. This type of malnutrition occurs in clients maintained for long periods on intravenous glucose infusions, which suppress the endogenous breakdown of lean body mass. Such suppression, with inadequate exogenous protein, limits the components available for the synthesis of the visceral proteins. Normal to excessive body fat and normal body weight are characteristic. Edema may occur.
- Marasmus combined with visceral protein depletion (marasmic kwashiorkor). This deficiency state results

Common laboratory studies

For a client with signs and symptoms of a nutritional disorder, various laboratory studies can provide valuable clues to the possible cause, as shown in the chart below. Keep in mind that abnormal findings may stem from a problem unrelated to nutrition. Remember also that values differ between laboratories; check the normal value range for the specific laboratory.

TEST AND SIGNIFICANCE	NORMAL VALUES OR FINDINGS	ABNORMAL FINDINGS	POSSIBLE NUTRITIONAL OR RELATED CAUSES OF ABNORMAL FINDINGS
Blood tests			
Hemoglobin This test measures hemoglobin, the blood component that provides oxygen-carrying capacity.	*Males:* 14 to 18 g/dl *Females:* 12 to 16 g/dl *Children:* 11 to 13 g/dl	Above-normal level	Polycythemia or dehydration
		Below-normal level	Anemia, massive or prolonged blood loss, hemolytic reactions to blood or blood products, increased red blood cell destruction, fluid retention causing hemodilution
Hematocrit A commonly performed test, hematocrit measures the percentage of red cells in total blood volume.	Concentration varies with the client's age and sex *Males:* 42% to 54% *Females:* 38% to 46% *Children:* 36% to 40%	Above-normal level	Polycythemia, dehydration, hemoconcentration from blood loss
		Below-normal level	Massive or prolonged blood loss, hemolysis, hemodilution
Red blood cell indices This blood test provides information about the size, hemoglobin concentration, and hemoglobin weight of an average red cell.	*Mean corpuscular volume (MCV):* 84 to 99/mu³/red cell	Above-normal level	Macrocytic anemia, sprue, alcoholism, vitamin B and folate deficiencies, malabsorption syndromes
		Below-normal level	Dehydration or chronic blood loss, microcytic or hypochromic anemia
	Mean corpuscular hemoglobin (MCH): 26 to 32 pg/red cell	Above-normal level	Macrocytic anemia
		Below-normal level	Microcytic anemia
	Mean corpuscular hemoglobin concentration (MCHC): 30% to 36%	Above-normal level	Dehydration
		Below-normal level	Microcytic or hypochromic anemia
Serum iron Commonly used to confirm iron deficiency, this test measures the amount of iron bound to transferrin.	*Males:* 70 to 150 μg/dl *Females:* 80 to 150 μg/dl Level normally peaks in the morning and drops at night	Below-normal level	Iron deficiency
Serum albumin This test measures serum levels of albumin, which maintains oncotic pressure and transports substances such as fatty acids, which are insoluble in water.	3.3 to 4.5 g/dl	Below-normal level	Possible visceral protein depletion, overhydration, pregnancy, decreased muscle mass
		Above-normal level	Underhydration; in all cases, results may mask nutritional implications.

continued

Common laboratory studies continued

TEST AND SIGNIFICANCE	NORMAL VALUES OR FINDINGS	ABNORMAL FINDINGS	POSSIBLE NUTRITIONAL OR RELATED CAUSES OF ABNORMAL FINDINGS
Serum transferrin (siderophilin) By determining the iron-transporting capacity of the blood, this test evaluates iron metabolism in iron-deficiency anemia.	250 to 390 μg/dl (65 to 170 μg usually bound to iron)	Above-normal level	Severe iron deficiency; elevations occur normally in children between ages 2½ and 10 and during the third trimester of pregnancy.
		Below-normal level	Visceral protein depletion
Total iron-binding capacity (TIBC) This test helps estimate total iron storage and evaluate nutritional status.	*Males:* 300 to 400 μg/dl *Females:* 300 to 450 μg/dl	Above-normal level	Iron deficiency
		Below-normal level	Protein-losing conditions (such as nephrotic syndrome, protein-losing enteropathy, and iron overload)
Total lymphocyte count (TLC) Besides helping to diagnose nutritional status, this test may suggest impaired immunocompetence.	1,500 to 3,000 mm^3 (TLC value stems from differential white blood cell [WBC] count)	Above-normal level	Viral infection (infection may mask malnutrition, which normally depresses TLC)
		Below-normal level	Protein-calorie malnutrition, possibly reflecting an impaired immune response; moderate malnutrition (900 to 1,400 mm^3), severe malnutrition (below 900 mm^3)
Total protein By measuring the protein content of the blood—a plasma nutrition source for body tissues—this test helps determine nutritional status and indicates hyperproteinemia or hypoproteinemia.	6 to 8 g/dl	Above-normal level	Dehydration
		Below-normal level	Malnutrition, protein-losing condition

from depleted fat reserves and lean body mass. Serum albumin and transferrin levels are below normal. Immunocompetence is impaired; edema may occur.

Based on the client's health history and physical assessment findings as well as the results of laboratory studies, the nurse can formulate appropriate nursing diagnoses that determine the planning, implementation, and evaluation of subsequent nursing care. (For a case study that shows how to apply the nursing process to a client with a nutritional disorder, see *Applying the nursing process,* pages 138 and 139.)

Recording the assessment findings is as important as the assessment itself. The nurse must document all data completely, including normal and abnormal findings.

The following example illustrates the documentation of some normal findings in a nutritional assessment:

> *Weight:* 150 lb
> *Height:* 5′10″
> *Vital signs:* within normal range (BP 126/82, T 98.4° F., P 82/minute, and R 18/minute). Body frame size, small. Triceps skinfold thickness, 12.4 mm; midarm circumference, 28.2 cm; midarm muscle circumference, 22.8 cm. No abnormalities noted on inspection. Skin without blemishes; nails short; hair shiny; mouth, tongue, and gingivae free of lesions. Extremities equal in size with normal range of motion. No glandular enlargement present.

The following example illustrates the documentation of some abnormal findings in a nutritional assessment:

> *Weight:* 138 lb
> *Height:* 5′11″
> *Vital signs:* within normal limits except for pulse (104/minute) and respiration (28/minute). Body frame size, large. Triceps skinfold thickness, 10 mm; midarm circumference, 22.8 cm; midarm muscle circumference, 20 cm. Eyes sunken and dry in appearance. Skin dry and scaly. Cheilosis present; glossitis present; nails split and spoon-shaped. Extremities thin. Client appears underweight. Splenic enlargement present.

Chapter summary

The nurse's comprehensive nutritional assessment of the client is essential. A complete nutritional assessment requires understanding the basic elements of adequate nutrition and the contribution of a thorough nutritional history. Besides developing the ability to recognize signs of nutritional deficiency or depletion from the history, physical assessment, and laboratory studies, the nurse must apply this information to planning goals for the client and overseeing their implementation, documentation, and evaluation. This chapter covers these important points:

- Maintenance of appropriate nutrition depends on the integrated physiologic processes of ingestion, digestion, absorption, metabolism, and excretion.
- Through a complex process of chemical changes, metabolism determines the body's use of carbohydrates, fats, and proteins.
- A comprehensive nutritional health history assists in identifying existing or potential nutrition-related problems. It should consider dietary habits.
- The health history also should assess the nutritional adequacy of the client's diet, through the use of such methods as the 24-hour diet recall, and the 3-day and 7- to 14-day diet inventories.
- Overt clinical signs of nutrition disorders found during physical assessment usually indicate an advanced deficiency state; subclinical or marginal nutritional problems are not easily detected.
- The techniques of physical assessment include inspection and palpation as well as anthropometric measurements that determine amounts of skeletal muscle and adipose tissue, providing information about protein and calorie reserves.
- Complete nutritional assessment includes reviewing laboratory studies to assess nutritional status. Common laboratory studies include hemoglobin and hematocrit levels, red blood cell indices, serum iron level, serum albumin level, serum transferrin level, total iron-binding capacity, total lymphocyte count, and total protein level.
- The nursing process helps identify actual or potential nutritional problems and establish measures to resolve them.

Study questions

1. A client asks for information on dietary requirements, including the best sources of carbohydrates. What facts do you provide?

2. Mrs. Adams brings her daughter Kirsten, age 4 months, to the clinic. Kirsten is listless, refuses food and fluid, and appears pale. After weighing Kirsten, you find that she is 8 lb, 5 oz. You notice that she sucks weakly on a pacifier. How would you record the following information related to your nursing assesesment of Kirsten?

- history (subjective) assessment
- physical (objective) assessment
- assessment techniques and equipment
- two appropriate nursing diagnoses
- documentation of findings.

3. Karen McNulty, age 18, is pregnant and comes to the prenatal clinic for a checkup. Because of her age and condition, Mrs. McNulty is at nutritional risk. What health history questions would you ask Mrs. McNulty to assess her nutritional status?

4. What four factors contribute to malnutrition in elderly clients?

5. What assessment techniques are used to determine a client's nutritional status? Correlate the assessment techniques with the body systems involved.

Selected references

Balkam, J. (1986). Guidelines for drug therapy during lactation. *JOGNN,* 15(1), 65-70.

Behm, R. (1985). A special recipe to banish constipation. *Geriatric Nursing,* 6(4), 216-217.

Bishop, C., and Petchey, S. (1987). Estimation of the mid-upper arm circumference measurement error. *Journal of the American Dietetic Association,* 87(4), 469-473.

Blackburn, G., Bistrian, B., Maini, B., Schlamm, H., and Smith, M. (1977). Nutritional and metabolic assessment of the hospital patient. *Journal of Parenteral and Enteral Nutrition,* 1(1), 11-22.

Collinsworth, R., and Boyle, K. (1989). Nutritional assessment of the elderly. *Journal of Gerontological Nursing,* 15(12), 17-21, 38-39.

Drugay, M. (1986). Nutrition evaluation: Who needs it? *Journal of Gerontological Nursing,* 12(4), 14-18.

Fanelli, M., and Abernathy, M. (1986). A nutritional questionnaire for older adults. *The Gerontologist,* 26(2), 192-197.

Fiatarone, M. (1990). Nutrition in the geriatric patient. *Hospital Practice,* 25(9A), 38, 40, 45+.

Franz, M., Bar, P., Holler, H., Powers, M., Wheeler, M., and Wylie, R. (1987). Exchange lists: Revised 1986. *Journal of the American Dietetic Association,* 87(1), 28-34.

Grant, J. (1980). *Handbook of parenteral nutrition.* Philadelphia: Saunders.

Hamaqui, E., Krasnopolsky-Levine, E., and Lefkowitz, R. (1990). Nutritional support in an AIDS patient. *Nutrition in Clinical Practice,* 5(2), 63-67.

Hytten, F. (1990). Nutritional requirements in pregnancy: What should the pregnant woman be eating? *Midwifery,* 6(2), 93-98.

Jensen, M., and Bobak, I. (1989). *Maternity and gynecologic care: The nurse and the family* (4th ed.). St. Louis: Mosby.

Keithley, J. (1985). Nutritional assessment of the patient undergoing surgery. *Heart & Lung,* 14(5), 449-455.

Krause, M., and Mahan, L. (1984). *Food, nutrition, and diet therapy* (7th ed.). Philadelphia: Saunders.

Leonard, L. (1984). Pregnancy and the underweight woman. *MCN,* 9(5), 331-335.

Lerman, R. (1986). Malnutrition in hospitalized patients. *Hospital Practice,* 21(3A), 22-31.

National Center for Health Statistics: Health Examination Survey Data. (1976). *Monthly Vital Statistics Report,* 25(3).

Ream, S., Murray, S., Nath C., and Ponte, C. (1985). Infant nutrition and supplements. *JOGNN,* 14(5), 371-376.

Roe, D. (1992). *Geriatric nutrition* (3rd ed.). Englewood Cliffs, NJ: Prentice-Hall.

Schlenker, E. (1984). *Nutrition in aging.* St. Louis: Mosby.

Shuran, M., and Nelson, R. (1986). Updated nutritional assessment and support of the elderly. *Geriatrics,* 41(7), 48-70.

Storz, N. (1988). Metabolism and nutrition: An overview. In NurseReview Series, *Metabolic Problems.* Springhouse, PA: Springhouse Corp.

Stotts, N., and Washington, D. (1990). Nutrition: A critical component of wound healing. *AACN Clinical Issues in Critical Care Nursing,* 1(3), 585-594.

Whitney, E., and Hamilton, E. (1990). *Understanding nutrition* (5th ed.). St. Paul, MN: West Publishing.

Wink, D. (1985). Getting through the maze of infant formulas. *AJN,* 85(4), 388-392.

Nursing research

Bunston, T., and Breton, M. (1990). The eating patterns and problems of homeless women. *Women and Health,* 16(1), 43-62.

Ifft, D., Engstrom, J., Meier, P., Kavanaugh, K., and Yousef, C. (1989). Reliability of head circumference measurements for preterm infants. *Neonatal Network,* 8(3), 41-46.

Lakin, J., Steen, S., and Oppliger, R. (1990). Eating behaviors, weight loss methods, and nutrition practices among high school wrestlers. *Journal of Community Health Nursing,* 7(4), 223-234.

Mohs, M., Watson, R., and Leonard-Greene, T. (1990). Nutritional effects of marijuana, heroin, cocaine, and nicotine. *Journal of the American Dietetic Association,* 90(9), 1261-1267.

Myers, S., et al. (1990). Consistent wound care and nutritional support in treatment. *Decubitus,* 3(3), 16-19, 22-24, 28.

Pete, J. (1989). Newborn infants' preference for sterile water versus five-percent glucose and water. *Journal of Pediatric Nursing,* 4(4), 263-267.

Prendergast, J., Coe, R., Chavez, M., Romeis, J., Miller, D., and Wolinsky, F. (1989). Clinical validation of a nutritional risk index. *Journal of Community Health,* 14(3), 125-135.

Schols, A., Mostert, R., Soeters, P., Greve, L., and Wouters, E. (1989). Inventory of nutritional status in patients with COPD. *Chest,* 96(2), 247-249.

Suitor, C., Gardner, J., and Feldstein, M. (1990). Characteristics of diet among a culturally diverse group of low-income pregnant women. *Journal of the American Dietetic Association,* 90(4), 543-549.

Vetter, N., Lewis, P., Charny, M., and Farrow, S. (1990). Dietary habits and beliefs of elderly people. *Health Visitor,* 63(8), 263-265.

Wood, A. (1991). Factors affecting reciprocity between nurses and preterm infants during feeding. *Journal of Perinatal and Neonatal Nursing,* 4(4), 62-70.

UNIT FOUR

Assessing Body Structures and Systems

Unit Four applies the general information from Units One, Two, and Three to assessments of specific body structures and systems. Throughout its 14 chapters, this unit focuses on health, describing normal assessment findings for healthy clients.

The nurse who recognizes normal findings can recognize health—with all its normal variations—during client assessment in any health care setting. This skill enables the nurse to identify abnormal assessment findings accurately, providing the basis for developing nursing diagnoses and plans for client care. Perhaps most important, the ability to recognize normal findings builds the nurse's self-confidence in promoting, maintaining, and restoring client health—the nurse's primary responsibility.

During assessment, the nurse has a dual role: concentrating on one body structure, system, or concern; and assessing and caring for a client whose health is compromised. The nurse also must be able to integrate assessment findings and view the client's health holistically—mind, body, and spirit. Assessment findings provide the basis for nursing actions.

To prepare the nurse to perform assessments, all 14 chapters in Unit Four follow a similar format. In each chapter, the first section reviews anatomy and physiology of the body structure or system being assessed, explaining the structures and physiologic processes that affect assessment findings. The second section explains how to gather health history data for the body structure or system under discussion. It groups health history questions into three categories: health and illness patterns, health promotion and protection patterns, and role and relationship patterns. To help the nurse establish a trusting relationship with the client, this section begins with the least sensitive questions, then advances to more personal ones. A rationale follows each question or group of questions to explain its significance. When appropriate, the rationale includes nursing interventions that are important to client care. To help the nurse evaluate the client's medication history, this section includes a chart of commonly used drugs that may cause adverse reactions in the body structure or system under discussion.

The next section discusses physical assessment by describing how to prepare the client for asssessment of a specific body structure or system, and explaining how to inspect, palpate, percuss, and auscultate the structures of that part or system. It also illustrates more advanced assessment techniques, as needed. This section discusses normal findings and common abnormal findings and their significance, and includes a chart that helps the nurse associate clusters of abnormal assessment findings with common disorders of the body structure or system under discussion. As appropriate, this section explores developmental and cultural differences that the nurse needs to be aware of during physical assessment.

The last major section in each chapter addresses integration and documentation of assessment findings. To help the nurse gather further assessment information and integrate it properly, this section contains a chart of common laboratory studies that evaluate the body structure or system under discussion. This chart describes the tests, normal and abnormal test results, and possible causes of abnormal results.

As an example of integration and documentation of assessment findings, each chapter includes a chart that applies the nursing process to a case study. The chart works through each step of the nursing process: assessment (history and physical data), nursing diagnoses, planning, implementation, and evaluation. Then it provides sample documentation using the SOAPIE method.

Chapter 7
Skin, Hair, and Nails

The largest body system, the skin serves as a protector, temperature regulator, and sense organ. In fact, the skin is so extensive and performs such different functions that it affects—and is affected by—all other body systems. The nurse must assess the skin carefully, because skin changes may result from minor skin disorders or major dysfunctions in other body systems.

When assessing a client with a skin disorder, the nurse must keep in mind that skin appearance is closely linked to self-image. Therefore, skin changes can have a profound psychological impact on a client. To help the nurse reduce this impact and assess the client effectively, Chapter 7 addresses psychological, developmental, and cultural considerations. It also details the nomenclature and descriptors for skin lesions, such as macules and papules.

Chapter 7 describes the anatomy and physiology of the hair and nails and helps the nurse identify and assess for abnormalities in these structures.

Chapter 8
Head and Neck

Chapter 8 discusses general assessment of the head and neck structures. (Separate chapters explore the specific organs, such as the eyes and ears.) For example, it describes how to inspect and palpate the skull for size and shape and inspect the face for symmetry, shape, and expression. It also explains how to assess the nose, sinuses, oral mucosa, teeth, tongue, oropharynx, tonsils, and other visible nasal and oral structures.

Chapter 8 details inspection and palpation of the neck muscles and bones. It touches on assessment of neck structures related to other body systems, such as the trachea, thyroid gland, cervical lymph nodes, carotid arteries, and jugular veins. It also describes two advanced assessment skills: direct inspection of the nostrils using a nasal speculum and transillumination of the sinuses.

Chapter 9
Eyes and Ears

Because vision and hearing help the client communicate and understand, a client with an eye or ear disorder may need a nursing assessment that evaluates social isolation, coping, self-concept, safety, and health care maintenance. The health history section describes these assessments.

The physical assessment section highlights vision and hearing tests. Then it describes two advanced assessment skills: the ophthalmoscopic examination, which assesses inner eye structures, and the otoscopic examination, which assesses the external ear, tympanic membranes, and other middle ear structures.

Chapter 10
Respiratory System

Respiratory assessment represents an essential part of all assessments, including routine health evaluations and screenings. It assumes even greater importance in acute care settings where rapid changes in respiratory status demand immediate intervention to prevent severe consequences—possibly even death.

Chapter 10 includes health history questions and physical assessment techniques that enable the nurse to detect early changes in respiratory function, thus allowing timely interventions. They also provide information that the nurse can use to formulate nursing diagnoses that help improve the quality of life, especially for a client with a chronic respiratory problem. The chapter describes two advanced assessment skills: palpating tactile fremitus and measuring diaphragmatic excursion.

Chapter 11
Cardiovascular System

Chapter 11 reviews the structures and functions of the cardiovascular system, highlighting the mechanical and electrical events of the cardiac cycle. Its health history questions help the nurse identify risk factors of cardiovascular disease, evaluate major signs and symptoms, and investigate client behaviors that promote or detract from cardiovascular health.

The chapter covers these physical assessment techniques: precordial inspection, palpation, percussion, and auscultation; and assessment of the neck veins, major arteries, and peripheral pulses. Its advanced assessment skills section explains how to interpret the jugular venous pulse waves and how to recognize abnormal heart sounds.

Chapter 12
Female and Male Breasts

Because breast assessment can detect breast cancer at an early stage, Chapter 12 stresses the nurse's role in promoting breast self-examination and regular professional examination. After describing the anatomy and physiology of the male and female breasts and axillae, the chapter discusses the changes associated with breast maturation.

Its health history section focuses on detecting risk factors of breast cancer, such as family history. Its physical assessment section emphasizes a sensitive nursing approach to inspection and palpation of the breasts and axillae.

Chapter 13 Gastrointestinal System

Chapter 13 describes how to assess the client's gastrointestinal (GI) function. It points out that a trusting nurse-client relationship is a prerequisite for most GI assessments, because many clients consider bowel function a private matter and have difficulty discussing it.

The health history questions examine the relationship of GI signs and symptoms to food intake, especially hot or cold fluids, alcohol, spicy foods, and foods that are high in fat or carbohydrates. They also explore physical or emotional stressors. The physical assessment section describes techniques for assessing the abdomen and includes the advanced assessment skills of percussing and palpating the liver.

Chapter 14 Urinary System

A client with a urinary disorder may exhibit signs and symptoms that range from subtle and mild to obvious and severe. Through urinary system assessment, the nurse can detect disorders in other body systems, such as the cardiovascular or endocrine system. If the urinary system is not thoroughly assessed, the nurse may overlook valuable clues to a more severe disorder.

The chapter explains the connections between the urinary system and other body systems. It provides health history questions and describes how to inspect, palpate, percuss, and auscultate the urinary system. It also includes one advanced palpation technique: capturing the kidney.

Chapter 15 Female Reproductive System

Disorders of the female reproductive system not only cause physical problems, but may raise psychological concerns about such factors as sexual maturity and childbearing. To assess either type of problem, the nurse must be especially sensitive to the client's fears or anxieties about reproductive and sexual problems. To that end, the chapter provides information about physiologic problems and psychological implications.

Basic assessment includes inspection and palpation of the external genitalia. Advanced assessment techniques include using a vaginal speculum and bimanual palpation of the internal pelvic organs.

Chapter 16 Male Reproductive System

Because assessment of the male reproductive system can be uncomfortable for the client and the nurse, Chapter 16 shows how the nurse can use the health history to gain insights into the client's needs and develop a trusting relationship. It guides the nurse in understanding the client's beliefs and values and in presenting facts without bias. The chapter provides information about the structures and functions of the male reproductive organs and clearly explains how to assess them.

Chapter 16 describes two basic assessment techniques: inspection and palpation of the external male genitalia. It also explains one advanced technique: palpation of the prostate and rectum.

Chapter 17 Nervous System

The neurologic assessment particularly challenges the nurse because of the system's complexities. Accordingly, Chapter 17 begins by reviewing the anatomy and physiology of the central and peripheral nervous systems as well as reflex responses. Then it describes how to obtain useful health history information and explains how to perform both the basic neurologic screening and the complete neurologic assessment, including basic tests for cerebral, motor, sensory, cranial nerve, and reflex functioning. Its advanced assessment section describes evaluating brain stem function and performing more detailed assessments of the sensory system, cerebellar function, and reflexes.

Chapter 18 Musculoskeletal System

When a general assessment reveals musculoskeletal signs or symptoms, the nurse must be able to evaluate the client's musculoskeletal system in greater detail. Chapter 18 describes all the components of a comprehensive musculoskeletal assessment.

The physical assessment section of this chapter emphasizes systematic evaluation of body symmetry, posture, gait, and muscle and joint function. It explains how to perform musculoskeletal tests and identifies normal findings. Its advanced assessment section describes how to identify musculoskeletal abnormalities.

Chapter 19 Immune System and Blood

Most body systems are composed of organ groups. Unlike other systems, the immune system is made up of billions of circulating cells and widely distributed lymph nodes; the blood-forming system is composed of bone marrow and blood cells that circulate throughout the body. As a result, the immune system and blood can directly affect—and be affected by—every organ system.

Although some immune and blood disorders cause obvious, identifiable signs and symptoms, others produce subtle effects that may be easily overlooked. For this reason, Chapter 19 provides detailed information about the history and physical assessment of the immune system and blood. It alerts the nurse to obvious signs and symptoms of disorders in these systems as well as the nonspecific effects of these disorders, which can appear in any body system. Its advanced assessment techniques include percussing and palpating the spleen.

Chapter 20
Endocrine System

Because the endocrine system regulates homeostasis and many body functions, it profoundly affects the client's overall health. This explains why an endocrine disorder can cause a wide range of signs and symptoms, such as fatigue, weakness, weight changes, abnormal sexual maturity, sexual dysfunction, mental status changes, or extreme thirst and frequent urination.

Chapter 20 helps the nurse identify and assess endocrine signs and symptoms, including seemingly unrelated or vague endocrine effects that may appear as changes in multiple body systems.

Nursing diagnoses

Health history and physical assessment findings serve the nurse as a basis for formulating nursing diagnoses. In turn, the nursing diagnoses help the nurse plan, implement, and evaluate client care. In each chapter of Unit Four, a case study illustrates this process. Depending on a client's needs, appropriate nursing diagnoses may include the following:

- Activity intolerance, related to increasing calf pain
- Activity intolerance, related to insufficient oxygenation
- Altered comfort: chronic pain, related to muscle spasm and tension in the neck
- Altered nutrition: less than body requirements, related to difficulty in chewing and swallowing
- Altered thought processes, related to sensory loss with age
- Altered sexuality patterns related to feelings of undesirability
- Anxiety, related to cardiac palpitations
- Disturbance in self-concept: body image, related to flaky, scaling skin
- Fear, related to outcome of breast surgery
- Fluid volume deficit, related to nausea and vomiting
- Fluid volume excess, related to fluid retention
- Impaired communication: verbal, related to aphasia
- Impaired physical mobility, related to flaccidity, atrophy, and weakness
- Impaired skin integrity, related to friction and pressure from bed rest
- Ineffective airway clearance, related to retained secretions
- Ineffective breathing pattern, related to stress
- Ineffective family coping: compromised, related to diagnosis of breast cancer in wife (mother)
- Ineffective individual coping, related to ototoxic hearing loss
- Ineffective thermoregulation, related to hypermetabolism
- Potential for infection, related to immunodeficiency
- Potential for infection, related to unsanitary living conditions
- Potential for injury, related to decreased vision
- Potential for injury, related to scratching of pruritic skin lesions
- Potential for injury: skin breakdown, related to irritation and moisture
- Self-care deficit: bathing, dressing, and toileting, related to dyspnea
- Self-care deficit: feeding, related to poor-fitting dentures
- Self-care deficit: toileting, related to management of new colostomy
- Sexual dysfunction, related to adverse effects of antihypertensive therapy
- Sexual dysfunction, related to chest pain and dyspnea
- Sexual dysfunction, related to vaginal dryness
- Social isolation, related to changes in saliva production
- Spiritual distress, related to conflict between religious beliefs and health regimen that requires the use of birth control methods
- Urinary retention, related to inability to stand during voiding.

7

Skin, Hair, and Nails

Objectives

After reading and studying this chapter, you should be able to:

1. Compare the composition and function of the epidermis with those of the dermis.
2. Describe how the skin protects, assists with sensory perception, assists thermoregulation, affects vitamin synthesis, and aids in excretion.
3. Describe normal hair, nails, sebaceous glands, and sweat glands and their primary functions.
4. Give examples of appropriate health history questions for assessment of the skin, hair, and nails.
5. Identify representative adverse reactions from drugs that may affect the skin.
6. Identify behavior patterns harmful to the skin.
7. Describe how to assess the client's skin by inspection and palpation.
8. Differentiate between normal and abnormal skin conditions.
9. Describe the characteristics of common skin lesions, using appropriate terminology.
10. Use the nursing process to document nursing care for a client with a specific skin disorder.

Introduction

The largest body system, the skin and its appendages (the hair, nails, and certain glands) protect underlying structures, help regulate body temperature, and serve as a sensory organ. Because changes in the skin can indicate health changes, assessment of this system is an essential part of the total physical assessment.

Skin disorders affect clients of all ages: infants develop diaper rash; children may acquire diseases such as chicken pox (varicella) and measles (rubella) that cause skin eruptions; and adults may readily contract a wide variety of skin lesions (discontinuities in the skin), such as the vesicular eruption from poison ivy *(Rhus radicans)*. A client with a skin disorder is treated in a physician's office or other outpatient health care facility. However, the nurse also may encounter a client with skin lesions, such as a rash from an adverse drug reaction, in an inpatient facility.

In some cultures, the appearance of the skin has great importance and any alteration is viewed negatively. In Western societies, efforts to enhance skin appearance have resulted in the expenditure of money and time, not always with beneficial results. Makeup and other skin or hair care products can cause skin disturbances, and suntanning can cause skin cancer. Because many cultures view skin disease as shameful, a client may be embarrassed by the disorder as well as by its location—for example, in the genital area. In such instances, the client may avoid seeking prompt treatment.

This chapter on the skin, hair, and nails (the integumentary system) reviews the anatomy and physiology of the skin and its appendages (hair, nails, and certain glands). It provides a framework for performing a health history and physical assessment of the skin, using the techniques of inspection and palpation. It also includes developmental, racial, and psychosocial considerations, and documentation samples.

Glossary

Alopecia: partial or complete hair loss caused by normal aging, endocrine disorders, drug reactions, chemotherapeutic agents, or skin disorders.
Anhidrosis: abnormally decreased perspiration, which may be caused by neurologic and skin disorders; congenital, atrophic, or traumatic changes to sweat glands; and use of certain drugs.
Annular: ring-shaped; characteristic of a skin lesion surrounding a clear, normal skin area.
Arciform: arc-shaped; characteristic of a lesion forming an arc or curve.
Confluent: fused or blended; characteristic of merging skin lesions.
Demarcation: clear border or end point, as a skin lesion with a clearly marked border.
Dermatome: skin area supplied with sensory nerve fibers from a single spinal nerve root.
Diffuse: generalized or widespread, in contrast to localized or regionalized.
Discrete: separate and distinct; characteristic of individual, well-demarcated lesions.
Ecchymosis: bruise; large, irregularly shaped hemorrhagic area, ranging from purple or purplish blue to green, yellow, and brown.
Eczema: superficial dermatitis characterized by oozing vesicles and crust formation.
Endogenous: caused by internal factors. For example, itching (pruritus) can result from an endogenous cause, such as uremia (failure of the kidneys to excrete urea).
Exanthem: lesion that characterizes an eruptive disease, such as rubeola or varicella.
Exogenous: caused by external factors. For example, pruritus and vesicles can result from an exogenous cause, such as skin contact with poison ivy.
Focal: in a limited area; as in focal skin lesions.
Herpetiform: patterned along the course of cutaneous nerves; characteristic of clusters of vesicles that appear with some herpesviruses.
Hirsutism: excessive body hair, especially a masculine distribution in women caused by heredity, hormonal dysfunction, porphyria, or medication.
Hyperhidrosis: abnormally increased perspiration, often caused by heat, hyperthyroidism, strong emotion, menopause, or infection.
Intertrigo: erythematous irritation involving the skin folds, such as the axillae, the folds underneath the breasts, or the inner thighs.
Iris (target lesions): bull's-eye pattern; characteristic of some round, raised bullae.
Lichenification: skin thickening and hardening, often caused by repeated scratching of a pruritic lesion.
Linear: in a straight line, as in linear skin lesions.
Localized: in one area only, as in localized skin lesions.
Macule: skin eruption with thickened or discolored areas that are flush with the skin surface.
Nevus: pigmented, congenital skin blemish, usually benign, but may become malignant. Also called a mole or birthmark.
Nummular: coin-shaped; characteristic of vesicular or scaling lesions associated with dermatitis.
Papule: small, solid, raised skin lesion.
Paronychia: infection of skin fold at a nail margin.
Pedunculated: on a stalk or stem, as in the cutaneous skin tags found in elderly clients.
Petechiae: small, 1- to 3-mm, red or purple hemorrhagic spots, possibly from vascular leaks or decreased platelet count.
Photosensitivity reaction: reaction occurring in areas commonly exposed to sun. This type of reaction may be direct, such as that caused by sunburn, or indirect, such as that caused by systemic or topical drugs.
Pruritus: itching that usually leads to scratching, which often results in secondary infection; can be caused by skin irritation.
Serpiginous: having a wavy, wandering, snakelike margin, such as a lesion in some skin disorders.
Telangiectasis: spot on the skin, usually formed by superficial vasodilation.
Verruca: rough, warty skin lesion.
Vesicle: small, thin-walled, raised skin lesion filled with clear fluid; a blister.

Anatomy and physiology review

The skin (integument) is the largest body system. Its two distinct layers, the epidermis and dermis, lie above a third layer of subcutaneous fat (sometimes called the hypodermis). Numerous epidermal appendages occur throughout the skin: hair, nails, sebaceous glands, and two types of sweat glands—apocrine glands found in the axilla and groin near hair follicles, and eccrine glands located over most of the body (except the lips). As a whole, this organ system covers an area of $10\frac{3}{4}$ to $21\frac{1}{2}$ ft^2 (1 to 2 m^2) and accounts for about 15% of body weight. (For an illustration and description of the layers of the skin, see *Anatomy of the skin,* pages 156 and 157; for a description of the hair, nails, and glands, see *Appendages of the skin,* page 158.)

Functions of the skin

The skin protects underlying tissues and provides sensory perception. It also plays an important role in body temperature and blood pressure regulation, as well as vitamin synthesis and excretion.

Protection. The epidermis protects against trauma, noxious chemicals, and invasion by microorganisms. Langerhans' cells enhance the immune response by helping lymphocytes process antigens entering the epidermis. Melanocytes protect the skin by producing melanin to help filter ultraviolet light (irradiation). The intact skin also protects the body by limiting water and electrolyte excretion.

Sensory perception. This function is performed by sensory nerve fibers that carry impulses to the central nervous system and by autonomic nerve fibers that carry impulses to smooth muscles in the walls of the dermal blood vessels, to the muscles around the hair roots, and to the sweat glands. Sensory nerve fibers originate in dorsal nerve roots and supply specific areas of the skin known as dermatomes. Through these fibers, the skin can transmit various sensations, including temperature, touch, pressure, pain, and itching. Itching is unique to the skin and mucous membranes, and the mechanism by which it occurs is not completely understood. The skin also indicates emotion through color change, as in the blush of embarrassment, the pallor of fear, or the redness of anger.

Temperature and blood pressure regulation. Abundant nerves, blood vessels, and eccrine glands within the dermis assist thermoregulation. When the skin is exposed to cold or internal body temperature falls, the blood vessels constrict in response to stimuli from the autonomic nervous system. This decreases blood flow through the skin and conserves body heat. When the skin is too hot or internal body temperature rises, the small arteries in the dermis dilate. Increased blood flow through these vessels reduces body heat. If this does not adequately decrease body temperature, the eccrine glands act to increase sweat production; subsequent evaporation cools the skin. Dermal blood vessels also assist the regulation of systemic blood pressure by vasoconstriction.

Vitamin synthesis. The skin affects vitamin synthesis by forming vitamin D_3 (cholecalciferol) in response to ultraviolet light. Vitamin D_3 plays a role in preventing rickets, a condition caused by vitamin D, calcium, and phosphorus deficiency. Characterized by abnormal bone formation and osteomalacia (bone softening), rickets particularly affects persons with inadequate dietary intake of vitamin D_3.

Excretion. The skin is also an excretory organ; the sweat glands excrete sweat, which contains water, electrolytes, urea, and lactic acid. The skin maintains body surface integrity by migration and shedding. It can repair surface wounds by intensifying normal cell replacement mechanisms. However, regeneration will not occur if the dermal layer is destroyed. The sebaceous glands produce sebum—a mixture of keratin, fat, and cellulose debris. Combined with sweat, sebum forms a moist, oily, acidic film that is mildly antibacterial and antifungal and that protects the skin surface.

Developmental considerations

The skin, hair, and nails undergo changes as a client grows and develops.

Pediatric clients

Premature neonates have lighter skin than full-term neonates because of undeveloped melanin. Subcutaneous fat stores increase during the last trimester of gestation and throughout the first year of life. After age 1, these fat stores decrease gradually until adolescence; the process then reverses and fat stores increase 1 year before an adolescent's height spurt.

The neonate usually sheds much of the stratum corneum by desquamation (skin sloughing) beginning in the first few days of life. At birth, the neonate's body is covered with vernix caseosa, a mixture of sebum and keratinized epidermal cells that protected the skin in the fluid environment of the uterus. This covering is gradually washed, wiped, or worn away shortly after birth. Vernix is more prominent in premature than full-term neonates and may be less apparent in post-term neonates in whom desquamation has already begun.

Pregnant clients

Pregnancy increases fat stores, which may separate as the demands of the enlarging abdomen exceed the elastic limit of increasingly fragile connective tissue in the dermis. Pregnancy also increases peripheral vasodilation and capillary development, increasing skin blood flow and sweat and sebaceous gland activity. Facial hyperpigmentation (mask of pregnancy) and linea nigra (a line of pigmentation down the center of the abdomen to the pubis) result from hormonal influences. Hair growth may increase, nails may become brittle, and spider angiomas and varicose veins may appear.

Anatomy of the skin

As this illustration shows, the skin is a complex structure containing cells, blood vessels, hair follicles, glands, and other networks.

Epidermis

The epidermis, the outermost layer of skin, varies in thickness from less than 0.1 mm on the eyelids to more than 1 mm on the palms of the hands and soles of the feet. The epidermis is composed of avascular, stratified squamous (scaly or platelike) epithelial tissue, which contains two layers: a superficial keratinized, horny layer of cells (stratum corneum) and a deeper germinal (basal cell) layer. The germinal layer produces new cells to replace the superficial keratinized cells that are continuously shed or worn away.

The deepest part of the germinal layer contains specialized cells known as melanocytes, which produce the brown pigment, melanin, and disperse it to the surrounding epithe-

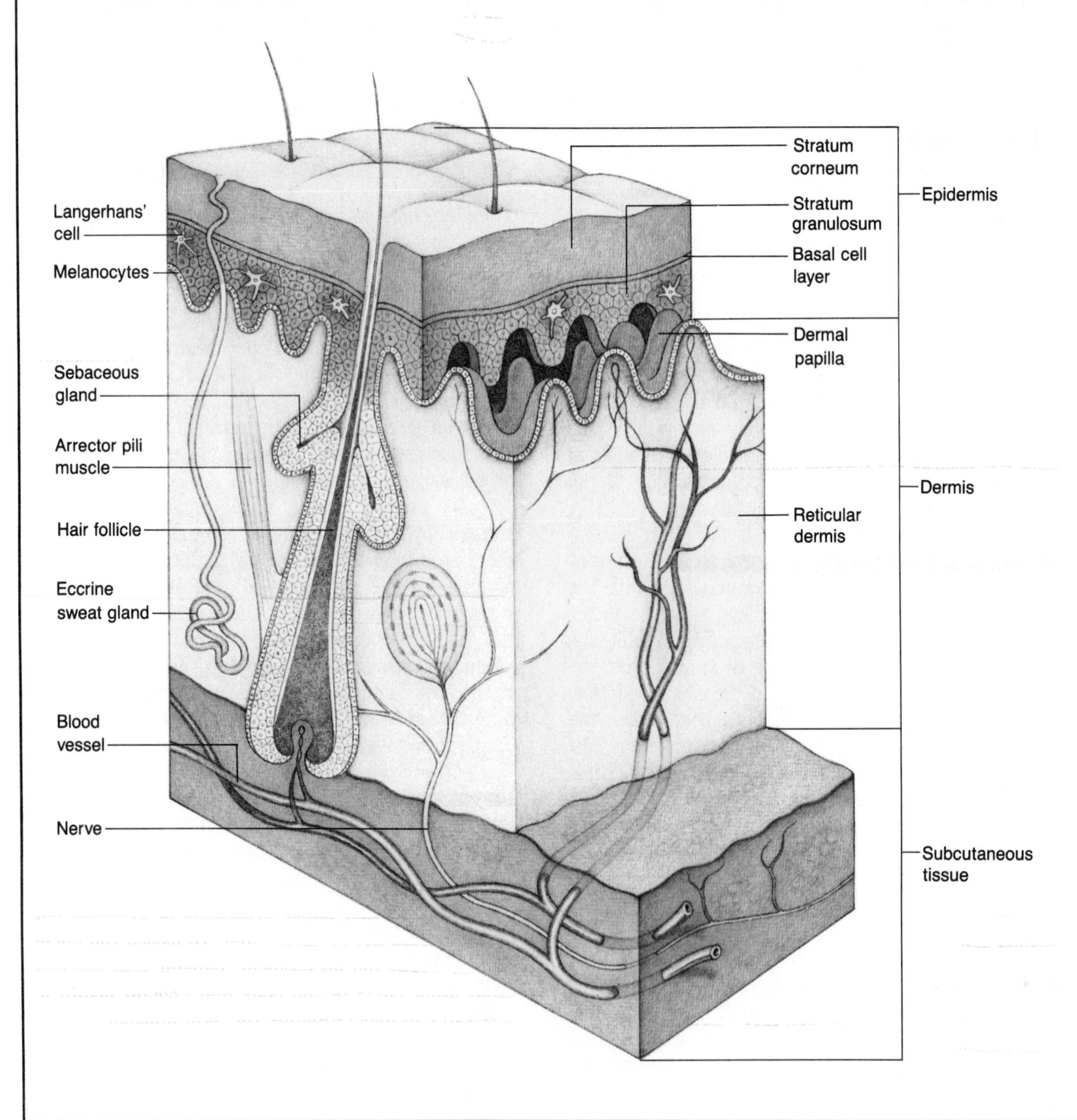

lial cells where it accumulates in the cytoplasm (the major substance composing the cell). Melanin is the most significant determinant of skin color and is normally produced at a steady, continuous rate. All people have approximately the same number of melanocytes; however, dark-skinned individuals produce more melanin. Melanin primarily serves to filter ultraviolet irradiation (light). Exposure to ultraviolet light can stimulate melanin production.

After mitosis (cell division) occurs in the germinal layer, epithelial cells undergo a series of physical and metabolic changes as they migrate to the outermost part of the stratum corneum, a journey that takes approximately 14 days. As these cells migrate, they flatten and lose water as their intracellular substances move into the intercellular space. Enzymes released from within these cells destroy the nucleus and convert the remaining intracellular contents to a tough, insoluble substance known as keratin. The residual cellular membranes and keratin of these tightly arranged cells form the stratum corneum.

Langerhans' cells are specialized cells interspersed among the keratinized cells below the stratum corneum. Langerhans' cells have an immunologic function and assist in the initial processing of antigens (substances that cause antibody formation) that enter the epidermis. Epidermal cells are usually shed from the surface as epidermal dust in 14 days.

Dermis

The dermis (corium), the second layer of skin, is an elastic system that contains and supports blood vessels, lymphatic vessels, nerves, and epidermal appendages (hair and eccrine, apocrine, and sebaceous glands).

Extracellular material called matrix makes up most of the dermis; matrix contains various connective tissue fibers (collagen, elastin, and reticular fibers). Collagen, a protein, gives strength to the dermis; elastin makes the skin pliable; and reticular fibers bind the collagen and elastin fibers together. The matrix and connective tissue fibers are produced by spindle-shaped connective tissue cells (dermal fibroblasts), which become part of the matrix as it forms. Fibers are loosely arranged in the papillary dermis, but more tightly packed in the deeper reticular dermis. Two layers compose the dermis: the superficial papillary dermis and the reticular dermis.

Papillary dermis

This dermal layer is studded with fingerlike projections (papillae) that nourish the epidermal cells. The epidermis lies over these papillae and bulges downward to fill the spaces. A collagenous membrane known as the basement membrane lies between the epidermis and dermis, holding them together.

Reticular dermis

This dermal layer covers a layer of subcutaneous tissue (adipose layer or panniculus adiposus), a specialized layer primarily composed of fat cells. It insulates the body to conserve heat, acts as a mechanical shock absorber, and provides energy.

Elderly clients

The following skin functions normally decline with aging: injury response, barrier function, cell replacement, chemical clearance, immune response, mechanical protection, sensory response, thermoregulation, sweat production, sebum production, and vitamin D production. These changes can affect the health of an elderly client. For example, a decline in immune response increases the client's susceptibility to disease. A decline in cell replacement increases the incidence of atrophy and other conditions, such as poor wound healing, and increases the risk of injury, infection, and morbidity from surgical procedures.

With age, a decline in protective function reduces the skin's ability to react to irritants. However, the incidence of allergic contact dermatitis (skin inflammation) also declines, because cell-mediated immune responses diminish simultaneously. Unfortunately, the combination of decreased immune response and impaired healing is thought to increase the risk of skin carcinoma.

Aging thins the subcutaneous fat layer, especially in the extremities. When elastin and collagen fibers shrink in size and number, creases form in the epidermis. Decreasing sebum production causes dry skin. Additional skin changes occur throughout life in response to nutrition.

Decreasing peripheral circulation slows nail growth. All nails develop longitudinal ridges, become brittle, and split readily; the toenails, especially, become thick, hard, and yellow. Fungal (mycotic) infections and peripheral vascular disease may also cause nail changes.

Health history

Skin assessment begins with a complete health history, which includes information that can tell the nurse a considerable amount about the client's skin, hair, and nails.

When assessing the skin, remember that skin disorders may involve or stem from other organ system problems, and that minor symptoms or systemic complaints should not be discounted. To lessen the client's anxiety about the assessment, explain that questions about other parts of the body and general health are necessary to understanding the skin problem.

Appendages of the skin

The skin appendages—hair, nails, and sebaceous, eccrine, and apocrine glands—derive from the epidermis and may extend into the dermal layers.

Hair

Hair and hair follicles, epithelial structures, cover the body except for the palms, soles, and mucocutaneous junctions (areas where skin and mucous membranes meet.)

A hair consists of a long, slender shaft composed of keratin, with an expanded lower end (bulb or root) indented on its undersurface by a cluster of connective tissue and blood vessels called a hair papilla. Matrix cells in the bulb produce hair and have a rapid mitosis rate that can be affected by nutrition, disease, or medications. Each hair lies within an epithelial-lined sheath called a hair follicle. Melanocytes are located in the hair matrix. Hair color depends on the amount of melanin incorporated into the hair as it grows. Sebaceous glands secrete sebum into the hair follicle. A bundle of smooth muscle fibers (arrector pili) extends through the dermis to attach to the base of the hair follicle. Contraction of these muscles causes hair to stand on end. Hair follicles also have a rich blood and nerve supply.

Hair has a repetitive and constant growth pattern with a growing phase (anagen), a transitional phase (catagen), and a resting phase (telogen).

Sebaceous glands

These glands occur in all parts of the skin, except on the palms and soles. They vary in size and number and are most prominent on the scalp, face, and upper torso and in the anogenital region.

Sebaceous glands derive from the epidermis and consist of a group of lobules that open into a single duct. Sebum, a lipid substance, is produced within the lobule and secreted into the hair follicle or directly onto the skin via the sebaceous duct. Sebum may help waterproof the hair and skin and promote the absorption of fat-soluble substances into the dermis. Sebum may be involved in the production of vitamin D_3 and may have some antibacterial function.

Eccrine glands

These widely distributed coiled glands produce an odorless, watery fluid with a sodium concentration equal to that of plasma. Derived from the epidermis, the eccrine glands are located in the dermal layer. A duct from the secretory coils passes through the dermis and epidermis and opens onto the skin surface. Eccrine glands in the palms and soles secrete fluid primarily in response to emotional stress, such as taking a test. The remaining 3 million eccrine glands respond primarily to thermal stress, effectively regulating temperature. As external or body temperature increases, eccrine glands increase sweat production. As the sweat evaporates, heat dissipates.

Apocrine glands

Located primarily in the axillary and anogenital areas, the apocrine glands have a coiled secretory portion that lies deeper in the dermis than the eccrine glands. A duct connects the apocrine glands to the upper portion of the hair follicle. Apocrine glands, which begin to function at puberty, have no known biologic function. Bacterial decomposition of the fluid produced by these glands causes body odor.

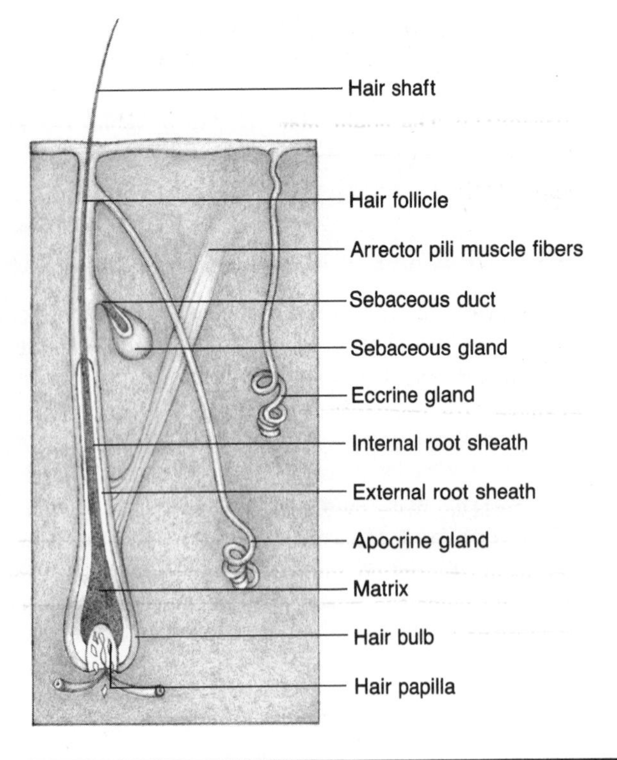

Nails

Like hair, nails are specialized types of keratin situated over the distal surface of the end of each digit (finger or toe). The nail plate, surrounded on three sides by the nail folds (cuticles), lies on the nail bed; the germinative nail matrix, which extends proximally for about 5 mm beneath the nail fold, forms the nail plate. The distal portion of the matrix shows through the nail as a pale semilunar area, the lunula. The translucent nail plate distal to the lunula exposes the nail bed. The vascular bed imparts the characteristic pink appearance under the nails.

Fingernails grow at a fairly continuous rate of about 0.1 mm per day; toenails grow at a slightly slower rate.

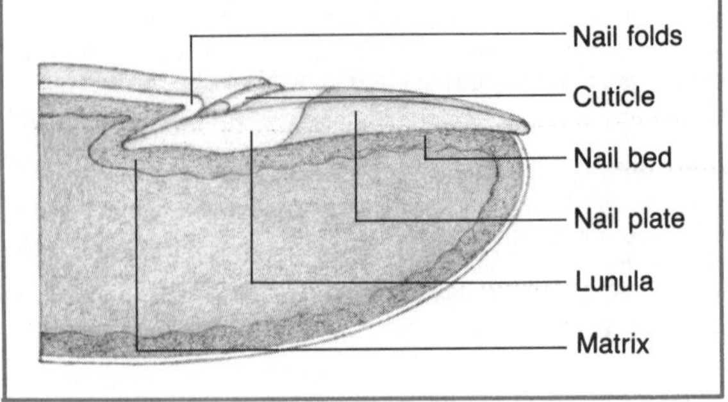

Begin with questions about present problems, followed by a full investigation of the client's health and illness patterns, health promotion and protection patterns, and role and relationship patterns. Start with the least sensitive or threatening questions in each section, and end with questions that may cause embarrassment or anxiety, such as those related to sexual matters. Be sure to use terms that are familiar to the client.

During the skin assessment, obtain as much information as possible about the client's general health, and begin to make pertinent observations. These observations may provide additional insight into the problem and serve as a guide for further data collection. Also observe the degree and appropriateness of the client's concern for the skin problem, noting whether the concern seems overstated or understated. Many skin disorders are exacerbated by emotional stress. (*Note: Skin change* refers to variation from normal; *skin disorder* refers to problems affecting function.)

Health and illness patterns

To assess important health and illness patterns, explore the client's current, past, and family health status as well as developmental status.

Current health status

Because current health status will be the client's predominant interest, begin the interview with this subject. Carefully document presenting signs and symptoms in the client's words. Then use the *PQRST* method to obtain a complete description of these complaints. (For a detailed explanation of this method, see *Symptom analysis* in Chapter 3, The Health History.) To assess the client's current health status further, ask the following questions:

What aspect of your skin problem bothers you the most?
(RATIONALE: This question allows the client to identify the most important personal aspect of the problem, even though other concerns are apparent. For example, the client may be more concerned with itching than with change in appearance.)

Where on your body did the skin problem begin?
(RATIONALE: Explain the importance of identifying the original site of the problem. Otherwise, a client who is too embarrassed to indicate an area considered private, such as the genitalia, may name another area as the origin of the problem instead.)

When did you first notice these changes?
(RATIONALE: Knowing the progression of the skin changes can provide important information.)

Please describe the initial problem in as much detail as possible, even if that problem has already disappeared. Can you also describe how the problem spread and in what order other areas were affected?
(RATIONALE: The shape, size, color, location, and distribution of the problem give clues to the cause of the disorder. So do the sensations associated with it and any pattern of migration. For example, chicken pox [varicella] spreads from the trunk to the limbs; shingles [herpes zoster] spreads in a distinct pattern along cutaneous nerve endings.)

Do you have other symptoms?
(RATIONALE: Symptoms in other body systems may be associated with certain skin disorders. For example, systemic prodromal symptoms such as malaise and anorexia are associated with chicken pox.)

How does your skin feel?
(RATIONALE: Try to obtain the client's description before asking about specific sensations, such as itching, burning, stinging, tingling, numbness, pain, tenderness, malaise, or achiness.)

Have you noticed skin changes in other areas?
(RATIONALE: The client may feel too embarrassed to discuss certain body areas and may select others to discuss and exhibit instead. This question will help pinpoint the original site if it has not already been identified.)

Can you relate the skin problem to a cause or event, such as stress, contact with a particular substance, or a change in activities?
(RATIONALE: The client may be able to relate the skin problem to a clearly defined cause or event, which may help establish its etiology.)

Does anything make the problem worse?
(RATIONALE: Aggravating factors are part of the diagnostic pattern for many skin disorders. Ask specifically about changes related to food, heat, cold, exercise, sunlight, stress, pregnancy, and menstruation. Shingles, for example, are frequently aggravated by sunlight, menstruation, or stress.)

Does anything make the problem better?
(RATIONALE: A positive answer, with specific drug or treatment description, may help the physician plan treatment and helps the nurse plan appropriate nursing interventions.)

Does the problem seem to be resolving or improving?
(RATIONALE: If the problem is resolving without treatment, the physician may want to watch and wait rather than treat it.)

Have you used any home remedies to try to resolve your problem, such as medications, compresses, lotions, creams, or ointments? Have you used any prescription or over-the-counter drugs?
(RATIONALE: If a home remedy is not harmful and the client believes it helps, try to incorporate it into the care plan. Especially note the client's use of antibiotics or other drugs that may exacerbate the disorder. For additional information, see *Adverse drug reactions,* pages 162 and 163.)

Have you recently had any other illnesses, such as heart problems, muscle aches, or infections?
(RATIONALE: A review of body systems effectively elicits information on health problems that may affect the skin.)

Have you noticed any unusual overall or patchy hair loss?
(RATIONALE: Overall hair loss may result from systemic illness or any treatment that affects the hair growth cycle, such as chemotherapy for cancer. Patchy hair loss may stem from hair care products, hairstyles, scalp infections, or infestations, such as lice [pediculosis].)

Have you noticed any changes in your nails?
(RATIONALE: Nail changes from aging are exacerbated by peripheral vascular disease; other systemic illnesses also may cause negative changes.)

Past health status

During this part of the health history, explore the client's medical history for additional related information.

Have you recently experienced any fever, malaise, or upper respiratory or gastrointestinal problems?
(RATIONALE: Many common skin eruptions are related to viral infections. Recent infections and illnesses as well as treatment regimens may contribute to skin disorders.)

Have you ever experienced anything similar?
(RATIONALE: Some skin disorders, such as psoriasis, can recur.)

Have you had any allergic reactions to medications, foods, or other substances such as cosmetics?
(RATIONALE: Past and present allergies, including those caused by cutaneous, ingested, or inhaled allergens, may predispose the client to other skin disorders.)

Family health status

When inquiring about family health status, try to elicit information suggesting a familial tendency to skin disease and allergies.

Has anyone in your family had a skin problem? If so, what was it and when did it occur?
(RATIONALE: Some skin disorders, such as allergic dermatitis, acne, or psoriasis, have familial tendencies; contagious skin problems, such as chicken pox and scabies, may be transmitted to the client from a family member.)

Has anyone in your family had an allergy? If so, what was it and how was it treated?
(RATIONALE: The client's problem may stem from an allergy that may be identified through knowledge of allergies in other family members.)

Developmental considerations

If the client is young, pregnant, or elderly, investigate developmental status by exploring areas related to developmental skin changes and age-related skin disorders.

Pediatric client. Encourage a child to participate in the interview as fully as age permits, relying on the parent or guardian for information the child cannot provide. Be sure to include the following questions:

Is the infant breast-fed or formula-fed?
(RATIONALE: Breast-fed infants have fewer allergies because they are not exposed to foreign proteins as early as formula-fed infants.)

Has the child had any skin problems related to a particular formula or food added to the diet?
(RATIONALE: Food allergies often manifest as skin problems in infants and young children.)

Has your infant had any diaper rashes that did not clear up readily with over-the-counter skin preparations?
(RATIONALE: Severe, unremitting diaper rashes may be caused by infection.)

What kind of diapers do you use? If cloth diapers, how do you wash them?
(RATIONALE: Severe, unremitting diaper rash may result from diapers that are not changed frequently enough or diapers that are not washed properly.)

How often do you bathe your infant?
(RATIONALE: Too-frequent bathing can lead to skin problems, including dry skin with excessive desquamation. Conversely, infrequent bathing can lead to intertrigo [a superficial dermatitis in the skin folds] or cradle cap [a sebaceous hair and skin cell collection on the scalp].)

What products do you use on the infant's skin?
(RATIONALE: The infant may be allergic to soaps or other skin preparations, especially if they contain perfumes.)

How do you dress the infant in hot weather and in cold weather?
(RATIONALE: Rashes may develop in intertriginous areas [areas where skin surfaces oppose, for example, in the skin folds of the groin] when an infant is dressed too warmly.)

Is your child attending nursery school? Do you have an older child in kindergarten or elementary school?
(RATIONALE: Contact with other children increases early exposure to communicable diseases with exanthems [skin eruptions accompanied by inflammation], such as measles or scarlet fever.)

Do you have pets in your home? Does the child sleep with stuffed animals?
(RATIONALE: Contact with pets and stuffed animals exposes the child to animal dander and collected dust, which may cause an allergic reaction.)

Has the child been scratching the scalp? Does the skin or scalp scale in circular patterns? Has the child lost an unusual amount of hair? Has the child been pulling his or her own hair?
(RATIONALE: The child may have pediculosis or ringworm [tinea capitis]. Both conditions injure the hair roots, weaken hair follicles, and may damage hair. A hair-pulling habit [trichotillomania] may cause patchy hair loss.)

Has the child ever had warts? If so, on which body surfaces? How were they treated?
(RATIONALE: Warts are a viral condition. Warts on the soles of the feet may be painful. Warts on the genitalia may be a sign of sexual abuse by a person with venereal warts.)

For a school-age child or an adolescent, ask the following questions to assess additional developmental considerations:

Do you play where you might come in contact with bugs, weeds, or bushes?
(RATIONALE: A child may develop transient or permanent hypersensitivity to insect bites or contact dermatitis from plant oils. The resulting itching can lead to scratching, excoriation, and possibly infection.)

What do you usually eat each day, including junk food?
(RATIONALE: Allergies to food containing milk, wheat, or corn commonly cause skin rashes.)

Have you had any bad cuts or scrapes from falls or other accidents? If so, how long did it take for them to heal?
(RATIONALE: Knowing about previous healing patterns is important to determine wound-healing capacity.)

Do you bite your nails? Do you twirl or otherwise play with your hair?
(RATIONALE: The client may develop nail infections from nail-biting and pattern baldness [alopecia] from playing with the hair.)

Does your face, upper back, or chest ever break out? If so, how do you feel about your skin appearance?
(RATIONALE: The adolescent may be self-conscious about acne and reluctant to talk about it until you establish a rapport. Knowing what exacerbates the problem, how the client feels about it, and what skin preparations are used can help establish an effective therapeutic regimen.)

Pregnant client. Keep in mind that pregnancy alters the thickness of the subcutaneous fat layer, stretches and increases the vascularity of the dermal layer, and increases the activity of sweat and sebaceous glands. It also can cause other changes in the skin, hair, and nails. Itching (pruritus) may require only symptomatic treatment; however, any rash has the potential for infection and requires serious attention. To assess a pregnant client, ask the following question:

Have you noticed any changes in your skin during your pregnancy?
(RATIONALE: The answer provides an opportunity to discuss normal changes with the client and to explore abnormal changes more fully.)

Elderly client. When assessing an elderly client, ask the following questions:

Adverse drug reactions

When obtaining a health history to assess a client's skin, the nurse should ask about current drug use. Many drugs affect the skin; some can cause permanent damage. For example, penicillins can cause urticaria (hives) and maculopapular rashes. The chart below presents some commonly used drugs that may cause adverse skin reactions.

DRUG CLASS	DRUG	POSSIBLE ADVERSE REACTIONS
Adrenocorticosteroids	methylprednisolone, prednisone	Urticaria, skin atrophy and thinning, acne, facial erythema, striae, allergic dermatitis, petechiae, ecchymoses
Anticonvulsants	phenytoin sodium	Morbilliform (measleslike) rash, excessive hair growth
	ethosuximide	Urticaria, pruritic (itchy) and erythematous (reddened) rashes
Antimalarial	chloroquine phosphate	Pruritus; pigmentary skin changes, eruptions resembling lichen planus (with prolonged therapy)
Antineoplastic agents	bleomycin sulfate	Skin toxicity may be accompanied by hypoesthesia that may progress to hyperesthesia, urticaria, erythematous swelling, hyperpigmentation, patchy hyperkeratosis, alopecia
	busulfan	Cheilosis, melanoderma (increased melanin in the skin), urticaria, dry skin, alopecia, anhidrosis (absent or deficient sweating)
	cyclophosphamide	Skin and fingernail pigmentation, alopecia
Barbiturates	pentobarbital sodium, phenobarbital	Urticaria; maculopapular, morbilliform, or scarlatiniform rash
Cephalosporins	cefazolin sodium, cefoxitin sodium, cefuroxime sodium, ceftriaxone sodium, cefotaxime sodium	Rash, pruritus, urticaria, erythema multiforme
Gold salts	auranofin, gold sodium thiomalate	Rash, pruritus, photosensitivity, urticaria
Nonsteroidal anti-inflammatory agents	diflunisal	Rash, pruritus, erythema multiforme, Stevens-Johnson syndrome
	ibuprofen	Rash, erythema multiforme, Stevens-Johnson syndrome
	sulindac	Rash, pruritus, photosensitivity, erythema multiforme, Stevens-Johnson syndrome
Oral antidiabetic agents	all types	Photosensitivity, various skin eruptions
Penicillins	amoxicillin trihydrate, ampicillin, penicillin G potassium, penicillin V potassium, nafcillin, mezlocillin	Urticaria, erythema, maculopapular rash, pruritus
Phenothiazines	chlorpromazine hydrochloride, thioridazine hydrochloride, trifluoperazine hydrochloride	Dermatoses, pruritus, marked photosensitivity, urticaria, erythema, eczema, exfoliative dermatitis

Adverse drug reactions continued

DRUG CLASS	DRUG	POSSIBLE ADVERSE REACTIONS
Sulfonamides	co-trimoxazole, sulfamethoxazole, sulfasalazine, sulfisoxazole	Rash, pruritus, erythema nodosum, erythema multiforme, Stevens-Johnson syndrome, exfoliative dermatitis, photosensitivity
	griseofulvin	Rash, urticaria, photosensitivity, lupus erythematosus or lupuslike syndrome
Tetracyclines	demeclocycline hydrochloride, doxycycline hyclate, tetracycline hydrochloride	Photosensitivity
Miscellaneous agents	allopurinol	Pruritic maculopapular rash, exfoliative dermatitis, urticaria, erythematous dermatitis
	captopril	Maculopapular rash, pruritus, erythema
	corticotropin (ACTH)	Urticaria, pruritus, scarlatiniform exanthema, skin atrophy and thinning, acne, facial erythema, hyperpigmentation
	oral contraceptives (estrogen with progesterone)	Chloasma or melasma, rash, urticaria, erythema multiforme, erythema nodosum, pruritus, acne
	furosemide	Purpura, photosensitivity, rash, urticaria, exfoliative dermatitis, erythema multiforme
	isotretinoin	Cheilitis, dry skin, pruritus, palmoplantar desquamation, skin fragility, skin infections, photosensitivity

How has your skin changed as you have aged?
(RATIONALE: The answer allows you to assess the client's perception of changes and provides an opportunity to discuss and clarify normal changes and explore abnormal ones.)

How do you feel about the skin changes you have noticed?
(RATIONALE: The changing body image may lower the client's self-image and self-esteem.)

Have you had any recent falls or other accidents?
(RATIONALE: Answers may explain later physical findings such as bruising, scrapes, burns, or other skin injuries.)

Have you noticed any difference in healing of wounds or sores?
(RATIONALE: Healing capacity decreases with age; diseases, such as diabetes mellitus and peripheral vascular disease, also affect healing.)

Do external temperature changes, touch, pressure, or pain affect your skin?
(RATIONALE: With normal aging, these sensations decrease as the number of skin receptors transmitting sensations to the central nervous system decreases.)

Have you developed more moles recently? If so, where? Have any of your moles changed in appearance, become painful, developed a discharge, or bled?
(RATIONALE: The number of moles normally increases with age. Warts that rub against clothing may become painful. However, changes in their appearance—including changes in color—,drainage, or bleeding may indicate cancer.)

B. Health promotion and protection patterns

To continue the health history, determine the client's personal habits, sleep and wake patterns, and typical daily activities. Ask the following questions to identify factors in the client's environment that may cause or aggravate skin disorders and to determine how the client's life-style relates to the skin problem:

What do you think makes a person's skin healthy?
(RATIONALE: This explores the client's ideas and knowledge about what constitutes healthy skin.)

What do you do to try to keep your skin healthy? What things would you like to do for your skin but feel unable to do?
(RATIONALE: The answer to this question helps reveal the client's skin care routine and beliefs.)

What type of soap and skin creams or lotions do you use? Do you use ointment, oil, or styling spray on your hair? How often do you shampoo and what product do you use? Do you use makeup or scents? If so, what type? Do you shave with a blade or an electric razor? Do you use a depilatory? Do you color your hair?
(RATIONALE: Skin changes, contact dermatitis, or allergy may result from cosmetics and grooming practices. Information on personal habits such as grooming are pertinent for some skin disturbances, particularly those localized to a body area. For example, dying the hair may have preceded scalp or hair changes.)

How would you describe your usual skin exposure to the sun? Do you wear a sun block or cover your skin with clothing before going out in the sun?
(RATIONALE: This question investigates the client's sun protection practices and the potential for exacerbating age-related changes and skin cancers.)

How do you cut your nails?
(RATIONALE: Improper nail cutting can cause infections or ingrown nails. This question provides an opportunity to teach correct nail-cutting technique.)

Has your sleep pattern changed recently? Are you sleeping more or less? Is your sleep interrupted? If so, by what?
(RATIONALE: Recent changes in sleep patterns may reflect increased stress or disruption by some symptom. Itching, for example, may seem more intense at night. Itching and night sweats may indicate an underlying systemic disease, such as renal or hepatic disease.)

What type of work do you do or have you done?
(RATIONALE: Skin disorders may be caused by exposure to occupational substances, such as paint, aerosol sprays, petroleum products, weed killers, and cleaning solvents.)

What are your recreational activities? Do these activities expose you to sun or other light, chemicals or other toxins, animals, the outdoors, or foreign travel?
(RATIONALE: Recreational activities such as craft work, gardening, camping, outdoor sports, and tanning may expose the client to sources of skin problems. Foreign travel may expose the client to skin diseases that are uncommon in North America.)

Have you recently experienced any stress or emotional problems, such as an unplanned work change or a broken relationship? How have you handled these problems?
(RATIONALE: Stress may contribute to some skin diseases, and some skin diseases may cause stress because of changes in the client's self-image.)

What concerns do you have about your skin problem and its treatment?
(RATIONALE: Many treatments for skin disorders are expensive and time consuming, limiting the client's ability to carry out the regimen. The client may express concern about the cost of medications.)

c. Role and relationship patterns

Once client trust has been established, explore sensitive areas of physical appearance and social or sexual practices related to the skin disorder. Such questions might include:

How has your skin problem affected your daily activities?
(RATIONALE: This line of questioning may provide information on limitations related to physical or emotional discomfort or distress. For example, gloves may be required when washing dishes because pain occurs when water contacts the affected area.)

How does the affected area look to you?
(RATIONALE: Skin appearance is important to the client because it provides an initial impression to others. The client's perception of this appearance can affect self-image, self-esteem, and participation in activities.)

How does this rash or skin lesion make you feel? How have these skin changes affected your relationships with others? How do you feel about going out socially?
(RATIONALE: A client with noticeable skin lesions may report that others make unkind remarks or move away, making the person feel unclean, embarrassed, and isolated. Such a client may choose to limit social contact to avoid emotional discomfort.)

Has your skin problem interfered with your role as a spouse (or student, parent, or other) or with your sexuality?
(RATIONALE: The client's self-esteem and sexual feelings and expression may be severely diminished. Do not un-

derestimate the psychological ramifications of skin disease or the need to provide the client with an opportunity to discuss such feelings.)

Physical assessment

When performing the physical assessment, the nurse must keep in mind that cultural and ethnic influences can predispose the client to some illnesses and may affect skin and mucous membrane coloring as well as hair texture and distribution. Ethnic background may influence customs and social relationships, whereas specific dietary influences, rituals, and folk practices may affect the incidence, morbidity, and treatment of skin disorders. The social and sexual practices of some subgroups place them at risk for acquired immunodeficiency syndrome (AIDS) and skin lesions, such as herpesvirus and fungal infections.

To assess the client's skin, hair, and nails thoroughly, the nurse must evaluate features that reflect skin composition and function, such as body weight, fluid balance, general appearance, and related body systems. The following provides guidelines.

Preparing for skin, hair, and nail assessment

Physical assessment of the skin, hair, and nails requires inspection and palpation. Before beginning, wash your hands. Implementation of these techniques demands good observation skills, but requires only simple equipment, including:

- bright, even light source (preferably natural light or overhead fluorescent lights) for a clear view of the skin
- penlight and tongue depressor to evaluate the oral mucosa
- centimeter rule (preferably clear lucite) to measure skin lesions and evaluate color change in response to pressure
- magnifying glass and a flashlight with a transilluminator (the flashlight permits close inspection of color and elevation of the lesion borders, and the transilluminator helps identify fluid-filled cysts or masses)
- Wood's lamp (an ultraviolet light) to assess fluorescent lesions, such as those in fungal infections
- gloves for palpating moist lesions or mucous membranes.

Be sure to warm the room. This will make the client comfortable and will prevent cold-induced vasoconstriction, which may affect skin color.

When assessing the skin, protect the client's modesty as much as possible by appropriate draping. Expose areas for inspection and palpation sequentially; for example, first the left arm and then the right arm. Assess the entire skin surface during other parts of the nursing assessment or procedures. For example, at the beginning of the examination, observe the scalp and hair, then assess facial skin closely while assessing the pupils. Assess neck skin and jugular vein distention together, and combine the chest and back assessment with heart and lung auscultation.

Also assess the skin while the client is changing into bedclothes during admission or bathing. In some instances, assessment procedures and client teaching can be combined; for example, by teaching the client how to prevent wound infection while assessing a leg ulcer during a dressing change.

A systematic approach to assessment includes inspection and palpation of all of the skin, hair, nails, and mucous membranes, even if the client reports only a local lesion. The client may not recognize subtle skin changes or asymptomatic skin disturbances, such as an early melanoma located on the back. Also, the client may be too embarrassed to mention a lesion in the genital area.

Failure to assess the entire skin surface can lead to incorrect diagnosis and care planning. For example, consider a male client with a pruritic (itchy), papular (raised) rash and excoriations (injury caused by scratching or abrasion) between the fingers. Inspection limited to the local lesions may suggest something the client has handled as a probable cause, leading to a review of potential environmental causes. However, inspection of the rest of the skin may uncover similar lesions on the flexor surfaces of the wrists, or on the forearms, areolae, penis, and buttocks, indicating infestation with scabies (a contagious parasitic disorder).

During the assessment, be alert for any variations in lesion color, vascular supply, and pattern compared to other lesions. Also check for their distribution over the whole body.

Body weight, fluid balance, general appearance, and related body systems

To assess fluid status, weigh the client at the same time on the same scale every day, and make sure that the client wears the same amount of clothing. If this is not possible, record and document the differences. Recent weight changes (over the previous 48 hours) reflect changes in fluid status rather than body mass and may affect skin turgor (resiliency). As needed, record and measure daily fluid intake and output. (For details on assessing fluid balance and weight, see Chapter 14, Urinary System.)

Compare the client's stated age with the general appearance. Long-term excessive sun exposure, acute or chronic illness, and long-term smoking can cause a client to look older than his or her actual age.

Skin diseases associated with systemic disorders may also affect the mucous membranes, which normally appear smooth and moist with a consistent pink color and an intact surface. Blood vessels usually do not predominate. The most readily examined mucous membranes include the conjunctiva and the oral mucosa. (For a description of assessing the conjunctiva, see Chapter 9, Eyes and Ears; for a description of assessing the oral mucosa, see Chapter 8, Head and Neck.) Pale mucous membranes may indicate anemia; a blue tinge (cyanosis) may indicate excess carbon dioxide in the blood. Mucous membrane cyanosis indicates central cyanosis; that is, cyanosis produced because arterial blood lacks oxygen saturation as a result of either a cardiac or pulmonary problem.

Dry mucous membranes suggest dehydration. Other mucous membrane conditions and lesions may be caused by pressure; burns; actinic (sun) damage; contact with tobacco, chemicals, and allergens; drug reactions; infections with viruses, bacteria, spirochetes, fungi, or animal parasites; or systemic causes, including leukemia, thrombocytopenia, pernicious anemia, metabolic disorders, collagen vascular disease, autoimmune disease, and underlying cancers. Because skin disorders may result from metabolic, endocrine, gastrointestinal, hepatic, cardiovascular, blood, pulmonary, renal, or psychological disorders, always correlate skin findings with findings from other body system assessments.

Inspection

During this part of the assessment, inspect the skin, hair, and nails.

Skin

Begin the physical assessment of the skin by observing the client's overall appearance from a distance of 3′ to 6′, noting complexion, general color, color variations, and general appearance (such as neat and clean versus dirty and unkempt). Note any body odor, especially unusual odors such as mustiness or sourness. (Be aware that a short time in contact with an odor may lessen your sensitivity.) Particular odors are associated with some skin problems; for example, a distinct, sickly sweet odor is a sign of a *Pseudomonas* infection.

Because abnormal skin variations require identification and description, note disturbances in pigmentation (light or dark areas compared to the rest of the skin), freckles, moles (nevi), and tanning (usually considered normal variations). Usually benign, nevi that occur in large numbers (up to 40) or change in size and appearance may indicate cancer. Freckles and nevi are examples of focal or localized hyperpigmentation (increased pigmentation).

Color. Skin color varies from person to person, depending on race and ethnic origin. These variations usually range from whitish pink to ruddy with olive or yellow tones, or to warm yellow, brown, or black. Oxyhemoglobin (oxygen combined with hemoglobin) in the red blood cells imparts a warm, lively color to healthy skin. Skin color also varies normally in different parts of the body, although overall coloring should remain fairly even—especially within a body region. For example, the face, neck, hands, and arms frequently darken from sun exposure; the areola of the nipple is darker than the surrounding breast; and the genitalia also may have a darker color. Some alterations in the normal pattern of pigmentation may result from changes in melanocyte distribution or function, which may cause either increased pigmentation (hyperpigmentation)—such as in birthmarks and freckles—or decreased pigmentation (hypopigmentation)—which can lead to vitiligo (a complete lack of pigment).

Vascular changes. Inspection detects vascular changes; however, palpate to differentiate these from nonvascular changes. Because the epidermis has no vasculature, all vascular lesions (even those visible in the epidermis) originate in the dermis. Some skin areas readily reflect vascular changes; for example, the flush areas across the cheeks, nose, neck, upper chest, and genitalia often demonstrate an increased pinkness in response to the vasodilation of blushing, excitement, sexual stimulation, or fever.

Alterations in skin vasculature usually appear as red pigmented lesions. Some vascular lesions occur in persons in good health. For example, blood vessel hypertrophy (enlargement) may result in hemangiomas, which vary from bright red to purple. Usually soft and easily compressed, hemangiomas range from 1 to 3 mm in diameter. These lesions blanch (lose color or fade) slightly when palpated and compressed. To demonstrate blanching, press on the lesion with the lucite rule, and observe and note the color change. Permanently dilated superficial blood vessels (telangiectasia or spider veins) can indicate disease, but frequently are normal.

Skin lesions. Throughout the assessment, carefully observe and document any lesion according to the following considerations:

- Morphology (clinical description) of the lesion. Note size (measure and record its dimensions), shape or configuration, color, elevation or depression, pedunculation (connection to the skin by a stem or stalk), and texture. Note odor, color, consistency, and amount of exudate. Use a flashlight to assess the color of the lesion and elevation of its borders. Use a transilluminator to assess fluid in a lesion by darkening the room and placing the tip of the transilluminator against the side of the lesion; a fluid-filled lesion glows red, whereas a solid lesion does not. Use a Wood's lamp to assess fungal lesions and a magnifying glass to inspect tiny lesions.

Identifying lesion morphology is the most crucial part of the physical assessment because morphology often is closely related to histology (microscopic anatomy). To aid the physician's diagnosis, describe lesions accurately, keeping in mind that two or more types can coexist. In some cases, lesions change during the natural course of a disease. For example, the rash of chicken pox begins with macules that progress rapidly to papules, then to vesicles, and finally to pustules and crusts. Scratching, rubbing, and applying medication also may alter the original, or primary, lesion. These modified lesions are described as secondary lesions.

- Distribution. Lesion distribution may vary with the disease progression or external factors. Note the pattern on first inspection; many skin disorders involve specific skin areas. Assessment of distribution includes the extent of involvement; the pattern of involvement (such as symmetry or distribution in areas that are exposed to sunlight); and characteristic locations, such as dermatomes (along cutaneous nerve endings), flexor or extensor surfaces, intertriginous areas, or palms or soles.
- Location (related to total skin area). Note whether the pattern of lesions is local (in one small area), regional (in one large area), or general (over the entire body). Also note which areas they affect, such as flexor or extensor surfaces, along cutaneous nerve endings, along clothing or jewelry lines, or if they appear randomly.
- Configuration or pattern (arrangement of lesions in relation to each other). Configuration may help determine the cause. Note whether lesions are discrete (separate and distinct), coalesced or confluent (fused or blended), grouped (positioned close together), diffuse (scattered), linear (arranged in a line), annular (distributed in a ring), or arciform (arranged in a curve or arc). Also note gyrate or polycyclic (concentric), herpetiform (along the course of cutaneous nerves), and iris configurations. (For illustrations, see *Assessing lesion distribution and configuration,* pages 168 and 169.)

Document lesion configurations carefully because some diseases have definite, readily identifiable configurations. Herpes zoster vesicles, for example, characteristically appear in a linear pattern; those of herpes simplex usually appear in groups.

- Individual characteristics. Assessment involves descriptive terms, such as annular, iris, linear, round, oval, and arciform, as well as a description of color and consistency or "feel" of the lesion. For example, a lesion may be pink or red, or red in the center and pink at the edges, and soft or firm in consistency.

Besides lesions, document the characteristics of any breaks or other skin changes, including abrasions, scratches, cuts, bruises, and scars from previous injuries.

Hair and scalp

When assessing the hair, note its quantity, texture, color, and distribution. Hair distribution varies greatly among individuals and is affected by race and ethnic origin. For example, a client of Mediterranean origin may have more profuse body hair than an Asian client. Cultural differences in hygiene, grooming, and hair arrangement may affect the appearance of scalp hair. For example, traction from repeated braiding may cause scalp hair loss.

Assessment of the scalp should reveal a clean surface, free of debris, with equal distribution of hair follicles. Variations in hair growth and distribution, including hereditary baldness and excessive facial hair, occur naturally and are not preventable.

Nails

Careful nail assessment provides information that reflects not only health status but also life-style, self-esteem, and level of self-care. Inspect the nails for color, consistency, smoothness, symmetry, and freedom from ridges and cracks as well as for length, jagged or bitten edges, and cleanliness.

Assess the angle between the fingernail and the nail base (usually about 160 degrees) by placing the lucite ruler across the dorsal surface of the finger and the nail, and observing the angle formed where the proximal nail fold meets the nail plate. In clubbing (abnormal enlargement of the distal phalanges from decreased oxygen supply to peripheral tissues), this angle reaches 180 degrees or more. (For additional information on clubbing, see *Finger clubbing* in Chapter 10, Respiratory System.) Caucasians normally have pink nail beds (easily visible through the translucent nail), whereas those of dark-skinned persons may appear brown, with occasional longitudinal lines.

Assessing lesion distribution and configuration

When a client has skin lesions, the nurse must assess their distribution and configuration. This information may help pinpoint the cause of the lesions.

Distribution

To assess distribution, note the location of all lesions. Then characterize this distribution pattern as localized (over a small area), regionalized (over a larger area), or generalized (over the whole body). Further characterize lesion distribution, if possible, by one of the distribution patterns shown in the illustration below.

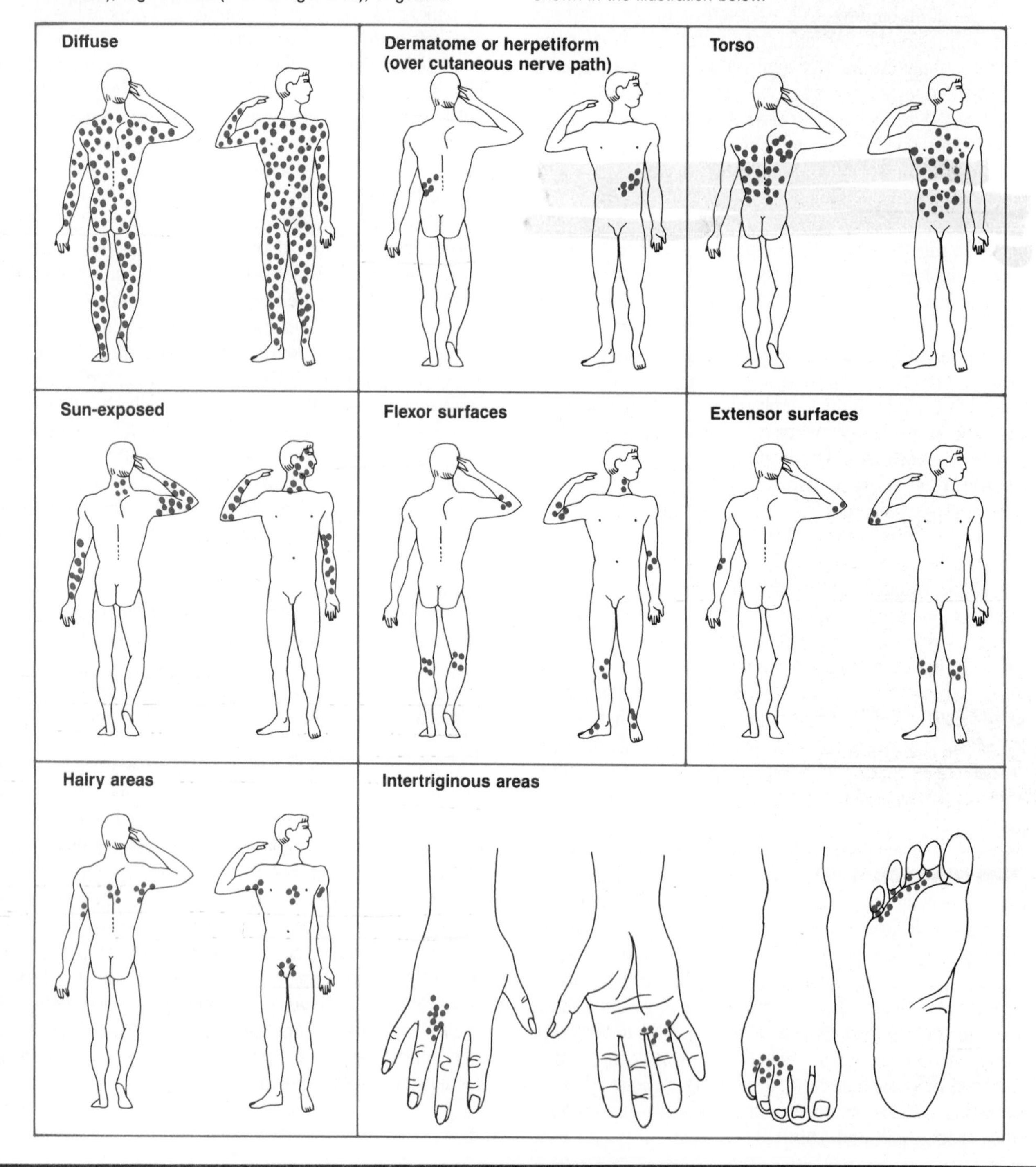

Configuration

To assess configuration, observe the relationship of the lesions to each other. Then characterize the configuration by one of the patterns illustrated in the chart below.

Discrete Individual lesions are separate and distinct.	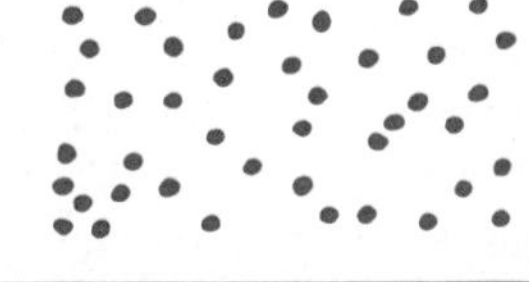
Grouped Lesions are clustered together.	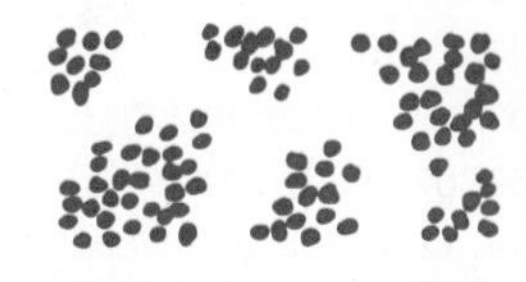
Confluent Lesions merge so that discrete lesions are not visible or palpable.	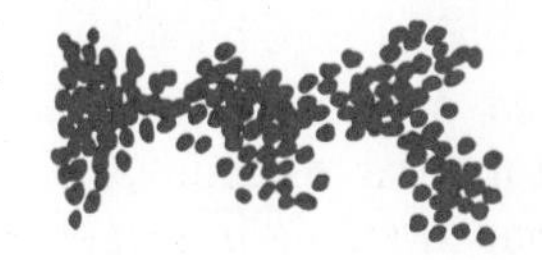
Linear Lesions form a line.	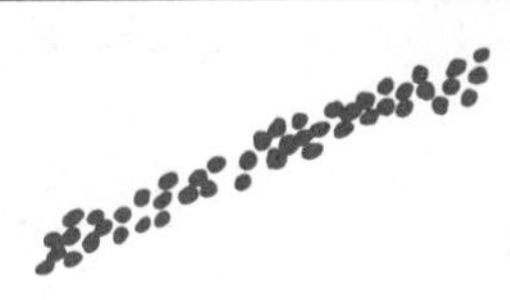
Annular (circular) Lesions are arranged in a single ring or circle.	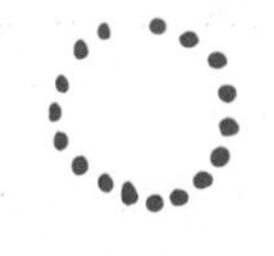
Polycyclic Lesions are arranged in concentric circles.	
Arciform Lesions form arcs or curves.	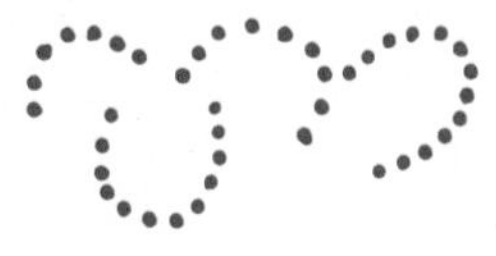
Reticular Lesions form a meshlike network.	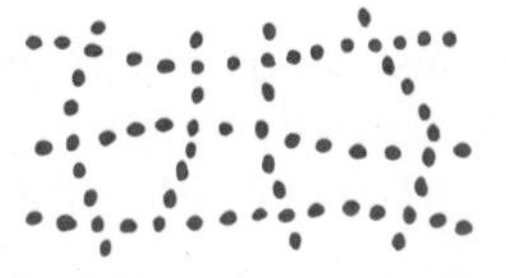

Abnormal findings

Some of the most common disorders of the skin, hair, and nails are discussed below.

Skin

Generalized or diffuse hyperpigmentation usually accompanies a systemic disorder, such as Addison's disease, nutritional deficiencies, or drug reactions. Focal, macular hypopigmented lesions occur in vitiligo (characterized by the complete absence of melanocytes) and postinflammatory hypopigmentation. (For a summary of abnormal skin color variations, see *Skin color variations,* page 170.)

Other abnormal skin variations include hypertrophic changes from increased numbers of cells. Such changes usually involve the epidermis and include scales, papules, plaques, and lichenification (skin thickening and hardening from continuous irritation, such as rubbing). Dermal layer changes frequently involve the connective tissue and may cause nodules. Skin thickening or induration may follow collagen buildup, a change associated with epidermal hypertrophy. Hypertrophy of subcutaneous fat is visible only if tissue mass significantly increases, as in obesity. Small local accumulations of fat are called lipomas.

Thinning or atrophy of the skin accompanies aging and may follow long-term use of topical steroids, giving the skin a smooth or finely wrinkled appearance. Atrophy of the dermis usually follows destruction of dermal tissue by an inflammatory condition. Such atrophy appears as a skin depression.

Erosions (ulcerations) may accompany atrophy. Erosions result from superficial damage, such as maceration and excoriation. Dried exudate from erosions forms crusts. Erosions may involve the entire thickness of the epidermis and subcutaneous layers. (For illustrations of common abnormal skin lesions, see *Primary and secondary skin lesions,* pages 172 and 173.)

Inspection may reveal a wide variety of vascular lesions. It may detect flushing, hemangiomas (small, usually benign tumors consisting of blood vessels) and telangiectasia (permanent dilation of groups of superficial capillaries, common in pregnancy and hepatic cirrhosis). Erythema (a blanchable redness caused by vasodilation) may be localized or generalized and may accompany wheals (a condition in which intravascular fluid leaves the capillaries, causing local edema). Purpura occurs when blood seeps into the dermis after blood vessel disruption. With palpable (papular) purpura, purple raised lesions may represent an inflammatory process disrupting the blood vessel walls, such as sepsis or collagen vascular disease; an adverse reaction to some

Skin color variations

During the physical assessment, the nurse should inspect the client's skin, particularly noting any variation from its normal color. Skin color variations in certain areas of the body may indicate a particular condition, as shown below.

COLOR	DISTRIBUTION	POSSIBLE CAUSE
Absent	Small circumscribed areas	Vitiligo
	Generalized	Albinism
Blue	Around lips (circumoral pallor)	Cyanosis
	Generalized	Cyanosis
Deep red	Generalized	Polycythemia vera (increased red blood cell count)
Pink	Local or generalized	Erythema (superficial capillary dilation and congestion)
Tan to brown	Face patches	Chloasma of pregnancy; "butterfly" rash of lupus erythematosus
Tan to brown-bronze	Generalized	Addison's disease (not related to sun exposure)
Yellow	Sclera	Jaundice from liver dysfunction
	Generalized	Jaundice from liver dysfunction
Yellow-orange	Palms, soles, and face; not sclera	Carotenemia (carotene in the blood)

drugs; or edematous disseminated intravascular coagulation. Such lesions herald the progress of a potentially fatal condition. Nonpalpable (macular) purpura produces macular purple lesions and occurs secondary to clotting disorders or capillary fragility. Immediately report either type of purpura to the physician for further evaluation.

Additional vascular lesions may occur, such as a cherry angioma (round, raised, bright red, 1- to 3-mm lesion that usually appears on the trunk, partially blanches, and is more frequent with age), a spider angioma (round central lesion of up to 2 mm, surrounded by fine vascular "legs," that appears on upper half of body, blanches with pressure, and may accompany liver disease, vitamin B deficiency, or pregnancy), ecchymosis or bruise (large, irregularly shaped hemorrhagic area, ranging from purple or purplish blue to green, yellow, and brown), or petechiae (small, 1- to 3-mm, red or purple hemorrhagic spots, possibly from vascular leaks or decreased platelet count).

Changes in the sebaceous glands also may cause skin changes. Increased sebum production, for example, causes the skin to look and feel oily, but does not necessarily cause skin lesions. Blockage or impaction of a sebaceous gland outlet causes formation of a comedo (blackhead); surface exposure of the blocking material to air causes the characteristic darkening. Milia (whiteheads), also caused by blockage, remain light in color because air does not reach the blocking material. Inflammation around the follicles may cause formation of pustules, papules, nodules, and cysts, resulting in acne.

Sweat gland changes also may cause observable differences. Anhidrosis (absence of sweat) results from atrophic changes in sweat glands. Atrophy of all sweat glands (an extremely rare and serious disorder) prevents regulation of core body temperature. Hyperhidrosis (increased sweating) often causes embarrassment; the client may have continually wet skin or may experience extreme sweating in response to such stimuli as highly seasoned or excessively hot foods, or emotional stress. Blockage of eccrine sweat glands may cause milaria (commonly called prickly heat or heat rash), which is characterized by pruritus, erythema, small papules, and vesicles.

Hair

Hair loss (alopecia), whether normal or pathologic, may be diffuse or patchy. Diffuse hair loss may be caused by hormonal and genetic changes (male or female pattern hair loss), systemic infections, hypothyroidism, or a reaction to chemicals or medications. Anticancer drugs commonly cause hair loss because of their effects on rapidly dividing cells. Patchy hair loss may accompany scalp infections such as ringworm, which typically produces reddened bald patches with broken-off hair stumps; bacterial infections of the scalp (folliculitis, furuncles, and carbuncles); secondary syphilis; and chicken pox. Traumatic alopecia (hair loss caused by plucking or breaking the hair) may be caused by permanent waving, hot combs or pony tails, or trichotillomania.

Nails

Exogenous causes of nail color changes include contact with such agents as silver nitrate or gentian violet, cosmetics, occupational chemicals, and trauma. Endogenous causes include poisons, drugs, lymphatic disease, endocrine disorders, cardiovascular disorders, metabolic and congenital disorders, and infection. White spots or streaks on the nails (leukonychia) may result from trauma, cardiovascular or liver disease, or renal failure. Yellow nails may accompany lymphatic abnormalities or thyrotoxicosis, but also come from nicotine staining in heavy cigarette smokers. Green nails usually suggest *Pseudomonas* infection; blue nails may be caused by drugs (distal discoloration only) or vascular disease. Gastrointestinal disease or nutritional disorders may cause bright pink nails. Renal disease causes a pigmentary change: a vertical brown line at the free edge of the nail.

Additional nail abnormalities may be present. Beau's lines (transverse depressions in all nails) may signal severe, acute illness; malnutrition; or anemia. Fingernail clubbing, which causes fingertip enlargement and a spongy, swollen nail base, often indicates a cardiopulmonary disorder. Koilonychia (spoon-shaped nails with a concave curve) is associated with chronic eczema, nail bed tumor, systemic diseases, and anemia. Onycholysis (partial separation of distal nail edge) may occur in heart disease and other chronic disorders. Paronychia (erythema, swelling, and thickening of the skin around the nail edges) usually results from monilia but may also occur with diabetes, bacterial infections, third-stage syphilis, and leprosy. Pterygium (nail matrix inflammation accompanied by fusion of the proximal nail fold to the nail bed) may indicate peripheral vascular disease, trauma, or lichen planus.

Palpation

Use the following guidelines for palpation of the skin. Wear gloves when palpating moist skin lesions, and explain to the client that gloves protect the client, the nurse, and other clients. (Few skin lesions are infectious. Routine use of gloves during palpation reduces the ability to detect minor tactile variations.) Also, wash your hands before touching the client, after touching any mucous membranes or lesions, and before touching another client, even when using gloves.

Skin

Palpation allows assessment of skin texture, consistency, temperature, moisture, and turgor. It also permits evaluation of changes or tenderness of particular lesions. Touching the skin reassures the client that you are not afraid of making physical contact.

Texture and consistency. Skin texture refers to smoothness or coarseness; consistency refers to changes in skin thickness or firmness and relates more to changes associated with lesions. Always note the general texture of the skin and the location of any changes, such as roughness. Skin texture may vary with age and nutrition, as in the thin, fragile skin of an elderly or emaciated client. Skin thickness also varies with age and body area. For example, thin skin covers the eyelids, whereas thick skin covers the soles, palms, elbows, and other areas that are subjected to local pressure or rubbing.

Temperature. Assess temperature by using the dorsal surfaces of your fingers or hands, which are most sensitive to temperature perception. The skin should feel warm to cool, and areas should feel the same bilaterally. Assess for bilateral symmetry by palpating similar areas simultaneously, placing your right hand on the client's left side and your left hand on the client's right, then crossing hands so that each assesses the opposite side. A temperature change felt over one area by both hands indicates a change in the client's temperature; a change noted in similar areas by one hand indicates that your hands have different temperatures; such a finding requires a second assessment by another nurse with even hand temperatures.

Moisture. Assess for moisture with the relatively dry dorsal surface of your hands and fingers to prevent confusing the client's moisture with yours. Moisture normally varies in different parts of the body. The greatest amounts are found on the palms, soles, and skin folds (intertriginous areas). Remember that the skin has a thermoregulatory function involving the production and evaporation of sweat, which varies with body and environmental temperature and exercise.

Turgor. Assess skin turgor (elasticity) by gently grasping and pulling up a fold of skin, releasing it, and observing how quickly it returns to normal shape. Normal skin usually resumes its flat shape immediately. This technique also assesses skin mobility, which may be diminished in connective tissue disorders.

Lesions. Palpating skin lesions provides details about their morphology, distribution, location, and configuration, as described earlier. When documenting assessed lesions, remember that a complete description is usually more helpful than specific nomenclature.

Hair

To palpate the client's hair, rub a few strands between the index finger and thumb. Feel for dryness, brittleness, oiliness, and thickness.

Primary and secondary skin lesions

Primary skin lesions appear on previously healthy skin in response to disease or external irritation. Secondary lesions result from changes in the primary lesion, usually related to the disease process. Arranged alphabetically, the chart below illustrates the most common primary and secondary lesions.

PRIMARY LESIONS

Bulla
Fluid-filled lesion greater than 2 cm (¾″) in diameter (also called a blister); for example, severe poison oak or ivy dermatitis, bullous pemphigoid, second-degree burn

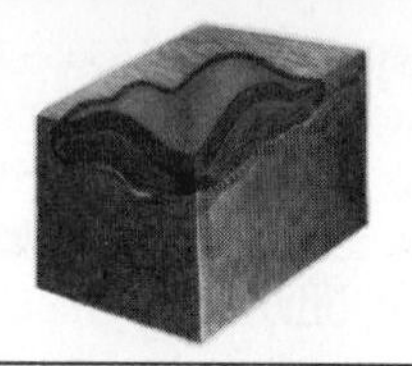

Comedo
Plugged pilosebaceous duct, exfoliative, formed from sebum and keratin; for example, blackhead (open comedo), whitehead (closed comedo)

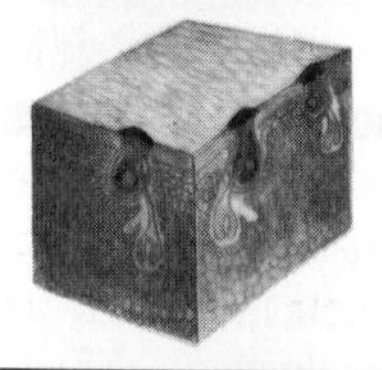

Cyst
Semisolid or fluid-filled encapsulated mass extending deep into dermis; for example, acne

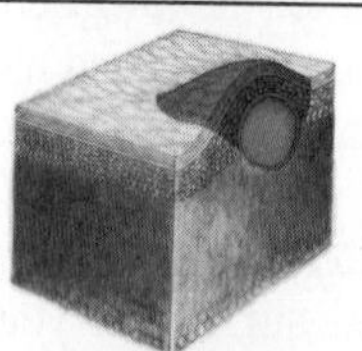

Macule
Flat, pigmented, circumscribed area less than 1 cm (⅜″) in diameter; for example, freckle, rubella

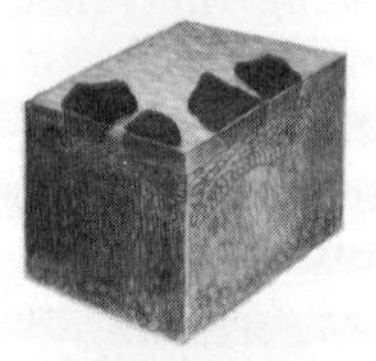

Nodule
Firm, raised lesion; deeper than a papule, extending into dermal layer; 0.5 to 2 cm (¼″ to ¾″) in diameter; for example, intradermal nevus

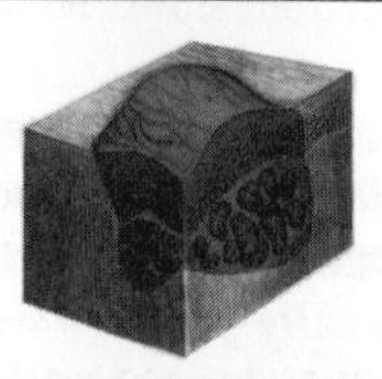

Papule
Firm, inflammatory, raised lesion up to 0.5 cm (¼″) in diameter; may be same color as skin or pigmented; for example, acne papule, lichen planus

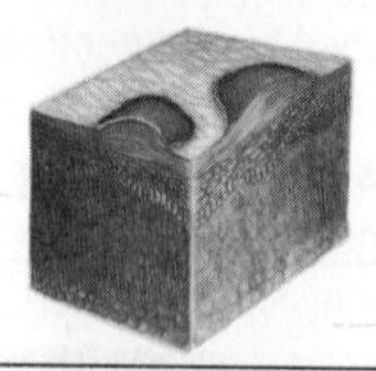

Patch
Flat, pigmented, circumscribed area greater than 1 cm (⅜″) in diameter; for example, herald patch (pityriasis rosea)

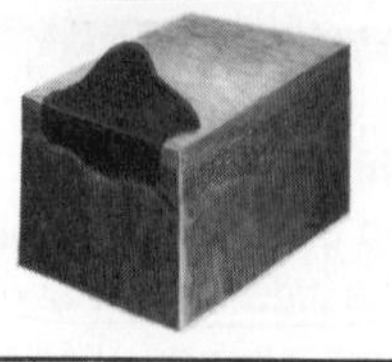

Plaque
Circumscribed, solid, elevated lesion greater than 1 cm (⅜″) in diameter. Elevation above skin surface occupies larger surface area in comparison with height; for example, psoriasis

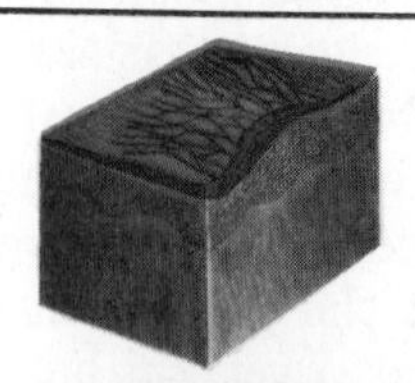

Pustule
Raised, circumscribed lesion usually less than 1 cm (⅜″) in diameter; contains purulent material, making it a yellow-white color; for example, acne pustule, impetigo, furuncle

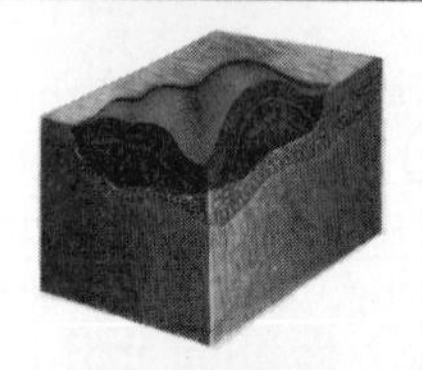

Tumor
Elevated solid lesion larger than 2 cm (¾″) in diameter, extending into dermal and subcutaneous layers; for example, dermatofibroma

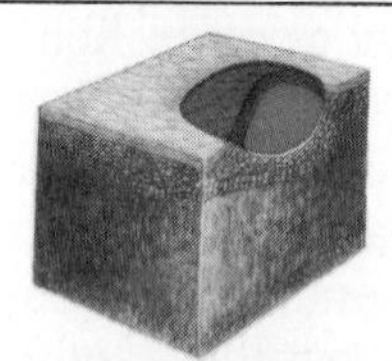

Vesicle
Raised, circumscribed, fluid-filled lesion less than 0.5 cm (¼″) in diameter; for example, chicken pox, herpes simplex

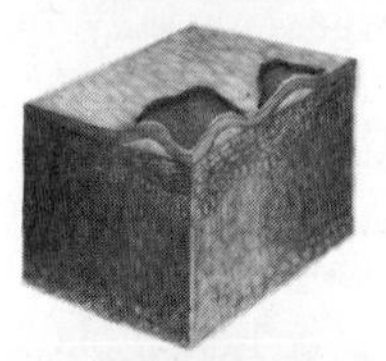

Wheal
Raised, firm lesion with intense localized skin edema, varying in size and shape; color varies from pale pink to red; disappears in hours; for example, hive (urticaria), insect bite

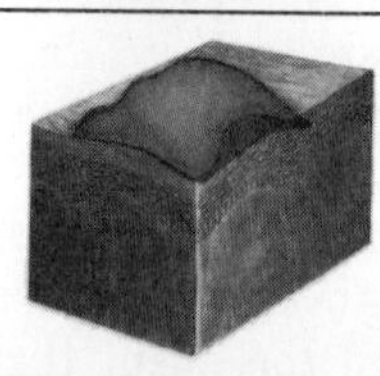

SECONDARY LESIONS

Atrophy
Thinning of skin surface at site of disorder; for example, striae, aging skin

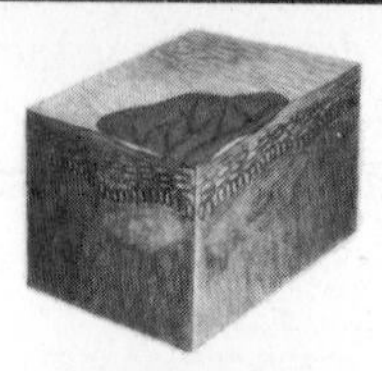

Crust
Dried sebum, serous, sanguineous, or purulent exudate, overlaying an erosion or weeping vesicle, bulla, or pustule; for example, impetigo

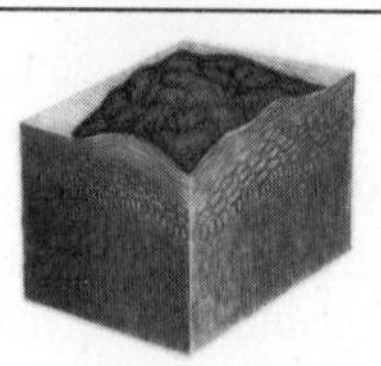

Erosion
Circumscribed lesion involving loss of superficial epidermis; for example, rug burn, abrasion

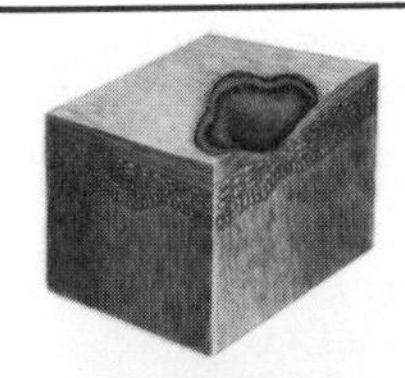

Excoriation
Linear scratched or abraded areas, often self-induced; for example, abraded acne lesions, eczema

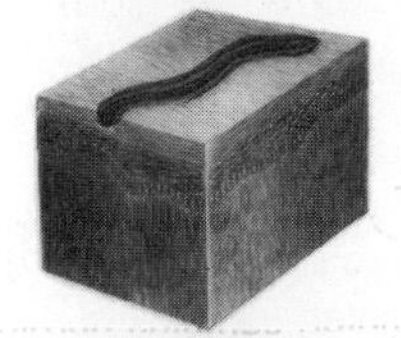

Fissure
Linear cracking of the skin extending into the dermal layer; for example, hand dermatitis (chapped skin)

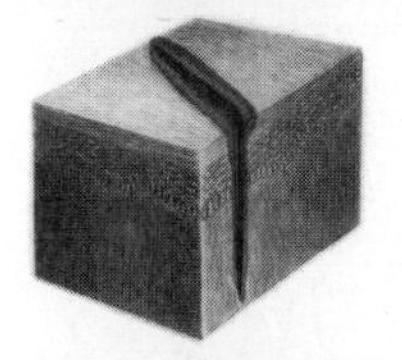

Keloid
Thick, red, or dark firm scar formed by hyperplasia of fibrous tissue; more frequent in Blacks and Asians; for example, surgical incision

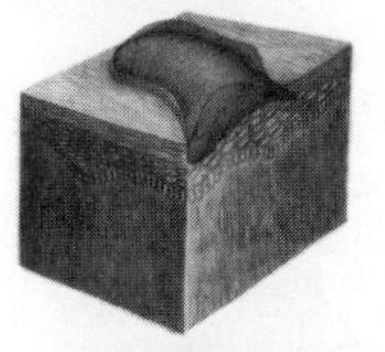

Lichenification
Thickened, prominent skin markings caused by constant rubbing; for example, chronic atopic dermatitis

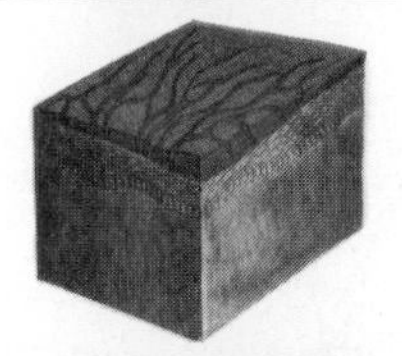

Scale
Thin, dry flakes of shedding skin; for example, psoriasis, dry skin, newborn desquamation

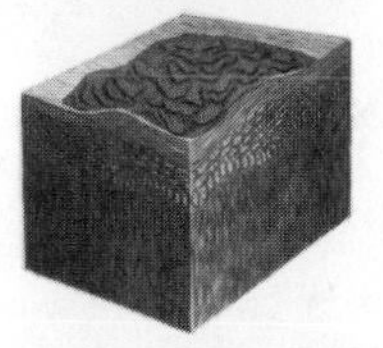

Scar
Fibrous tissue caused by trauma, deep inflammation, or surgical incision; red and raised (recent), pink and flat (6 weeks), or pale and depressed (old); for example, a healed surgical incision

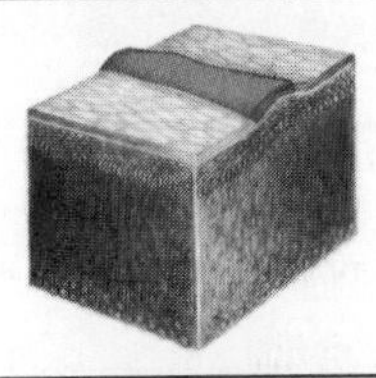

Ulcer
Epidermal and dermal destruction, may extend into subcutaneous tissue; usually heals with scarring; for example, decubitus or stasis ulcer

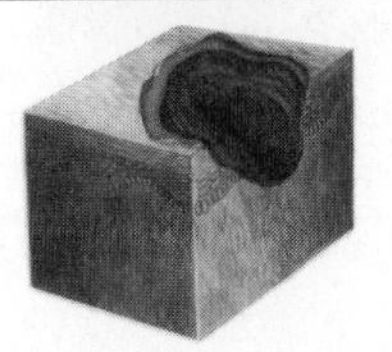

Nails

When palpating the nails, assess the nail base for firmness and the nail for firm adherence to the nail bed; sponginess and swelling accompany clubbing. To simulate clubbing, gently squeeze the lateral nail folds of one finger between the thumb and middle finger for a few seconds, then press on the lunula with your index finger.

Abnormal findings

Skin texture may vary with disease, as in the smooth, soft skin of hyperthyroidism or the coarse, dry skin of hypothyroidism. Dermal flow may affect skin temperature; for example, the entire skin surface may feel warm in a client with vasodilation from a fever, whereas it may feel cold in a client in shock because of local constriction of peripheral blood vessels. Localized temperature changes may also reflect underlying conditions. For example, localized warmth may indicate inflammation or infection, whereas coolness of the legs may indicate decreased peripheral circulation related to arteriosclerosis. Although skin feels drier in the winter months, severe dryness can indicate dehydration. Increased perspiration may result from abnormally increased sweat gland function.

When assessing skin turgor, abnormal findings are described as *tenting* because of the shape the pinched skin assumes. Decreased turgor may occur in the elderly client because of decreased elastin content, but it more commonly results from dehydration; increased turgor may occur with edema.

Essential hypertrichosis (hirsutism, or the excessive growth of hair) occurs in women on the face and legs; the amount ranges from a few hairs to extreme overgrowth. Suspect an underlying endocrine disorder in recent hypertrichosis.

Gentle pressure on the nail causes blanching of the nail bed as blood is forced out of the capillaries; color should return rapidly on release of pressure as blood returns to the capillaries. Known as capillary refill, this maneuver evaluates both central cyanosis (when accompanied by mucosal cyanosis) and peripheral cyanosis (independent of mucosal cyanosis) related to reduced peripheral blood supply. (For some common abnormal assessment findings associated with the skin, hair, and nails, see *Integrating assessment findings,* page 174.)

Cultural considerations

Normal skin variations in a dark-skinned client require careful assessment. A pigmented line of demarcation (Futcher's line) that extends diagonally from the shoul-

Integrating assessment findings

Sometimes, a cluster of assessment findings will strongly suggest a particular skin, hair, or nail disorder. In the chart below, column one shows groups of presenting signs and symptoms—the ones that make the client seek medical attention. Column two shows related assessment findings that the nurse may discover during the health history and physical assessment. The client may exhibit one or more of these findings. Column three shows the possible disorder indicated by a cluster of these findings.

PRESENTING SIGNS AND SYMPTOMS	RELATED ASSESSMENT FINDINGS	POSSIBLE DISORDER
Itching; small, very fragile vesicles that, when broken, exude liquid that dries and forms honey-colored crusts; usually occurs on face but may occur anywhere	Young age (most common in children) Hot weather Overcrowded living quarters Poor skin hygiene Anemia Malnutrition Minor skin trauma	Impetigo
Macular or maculopapular eruption on trunk that rarely spreads to the arms, neck, face, and legs and that fades within 24 hours	Exposure to infected person 7 to 17 days previously Sudden high fever 3 or 4 days before rash Age 6 months to 3 years Inflamed pharynx	Exanthema subitum (roseola infantum)
Small grouped vesicles around genitals and mouth	Infant delivered vaginally by infected mother Adolescent or adult who has had sexual contact with infected person	Herpes simplex
Mild to severe itching; inflamed papules caused by scratching	Visible lice Exposure to infected persons Overcrowded living quarters	Pediculosis (lice)
Mild itching; rash that begins with faint macules on hairline, neck, and cheeks; increases to maculopapular rash on entire face, neck, and upper arms; spreads to back, abdomen, arms, thighs, and lower legs	Exposure to infected person 10 to 14 days previously Koplick's spots (white patches on oral mucosa) Generalized lymphadenopathy Conjunctivitis Cold, conjunctivitis, fever, and cough before rash appears	Rubeola (measles)
Maculopapular rash on face that spreads to trunk	Exposure to infected person 14 to 21 days previously No symptoms before rash in children Headache, malaise, anorexia before rash in adolescents Conjunctivitis Low-grade fever Posterior cervical and postauricular lymphadenopathy Joint pain	Rubella (German measles)
Itching, especially at night; excoriated and sometimes erythematous papules, 1 cm (3/8") long; lesion about 1 cm long in straight or zigzag line, with a black dot at end	Exposure to infected person Lesions on interdigital webs on hands, creases of wrists, elbows, breasts, buttocks, and penis Microscopic mites and nits in scraping from intact lesion	Scabies
Very mild itching on scalp; small spreading papules that may become inflamed, pus-filled lesions; patchy hair loss with scaling	Exposure to infected person Patchy hair loss Infected areas that appear green under Wood's lamp Microscopic hyphae	Tinea capitis (scalp ringworm)
Itching; urticaria around vesicle; initially, crops of small red papules and clear vesicles on red base; vesicles break and then dry, causing crust formation; begins on trunk and spreads to face and scalp; may leave scars	Exposure to infected person 13 to 21 days previously Malaise and anorexia before rash Temperate area Late fall, winter, and spring Slight fever	Varicella (chicken pox)

der to the elbow, and deep pigmentation of ridges in the palm, occur normally in some individuals with dark skin.

Yellow-brown pigmentation of the sclera in a Black client is normal and does not indicate jaundice. The Black client may normally have a freckled or patchy-appearing oral mucosa, with dark brown or even blue gingivae; do not confuse such coloring with cyanosis.

Common skin disorders also appear differently on dark skin. Lesions that are deep red in Caucasians may be deep purple in Blacks. Many inflammatory conditions may lead to chronic pigmentary changes. Blacks, for example, are more likely to develop keloids (hypertrophic scarring) and pomade acne, a condition affecting predominantly the forehead and temples in adults as well as children. Pomade acne, which is caused by pomades (greasy creams and oils) used on the hair and scalp, may leave a hyperpigmented area when it clears. Pomade application may have cultural significance for a Black client, who may be reluctant to stop the practice. Some skin inflammations, such as pityriasis rosea, may leave hypopigmentation in dark-skinned clients.

Developmental considerations

Many normal age-related changes affect the skin, hair, and nails. For example, the skin of infants, children, and adolescents differs markedly from adult skin. Keep these normal variations in mind to help allay client concerns during the assessment.

Pediatric client

The thin, delicate skin of an infant may appear mottled from the development of the cutaneous capillary network. An infant with less subcutaneous tissue may appear redder than one with thicker subcutaneous tissue. A dark-skinned infant may appear lighter at birth than at age 2 to 3 months, when melanocytes are fully functional. A normal physiologic jaundice (related to the destruction of excess red blood cells) may occur 2 to 3 days after birth but should resolve in about a week.

Although the full-term infant has all necessary skin structures at birth, most of these structures are functionally immature. For example, nails remain quite thin for the first 18 months. The premature infant has soft nails and light-appearing skin because of incomplete melanization and less prominent accumulation of sebum (vernix caseosa). The immature sweat glands of the premature infant may also interfere with thermoregulation. Desquamation (shedding of the epidermis) normally begins a few days after birth, especially on the infant's wrist and ankle creases. Neonates may have profuse hair or no hair at all; hair present at birth is usually shed within the first 3 months. Most abundant on the scalp, face, and genitals, sebaceous glands secrete sebum, which may contribute to cradle cap (sebum accumulation manifested as a yellow, greasy crusting with matted hair). The skin of a dehydrated or malnourished infant or young child readily demonstrates tenting in response to skin turgor tests.

Other normal skin variations in an infant may distress the parents. Provide information and reassure the parents that the changes are normal. (For a description of these variations, see *Normal neonatal skin lesions*, page 176.)

Diaper dermatitis (rash), also common in infants, may result from numerous causes, such as infrequent diaper changes, poor hygiene, psoriasis, seborrhea, and candidiasis. The condition, which first appears as a smooth erythematous eruption, with or without scales and vesicles, tends to spare the skin creases. Establish the underlying cause before initiating therapy. For example, candidiasis, a superficial fungal infection, commonly occurs in the diaper area as a scaly, red, papular rash, and on the oral mucosa as a widespread creamy or bluish white film; both manifestations require antifungal treatment.

Viral and bacterial infections that commonly occur in children also cause many skin lesions. Between infancy and puberty, the skin changes very little, although the texture may coarsen. Changes in hair texture and distribution and sebaceous and sweat gland activity increase at puberty.

The adolescent client may be particularly modest, so take special care to preserve privacy while conducting skin, hair, and nail assessment. During inspection, look for increased skin oiliness and perspiration, as well as increased hair oiliness that often leads to excessive hair washing, which can dry the scalp. Assess for characteristic adult body odor from functional maturation of apocrine glands, as well as pubic and axillary hair, and male or female body hair patterns. Darkening and coarsening of body hair often alarms a female client, who may begin to shave the legs or axillae or use a depilatory; this sometimes causes skin irritation or eruptions. The adolescent male client develops facial hair and may be concerned if growth does not match that of peers in coarseness or heaviness. Acne, which commonly affects the prepubertal and adolescent client, also causes much concern. Lesions typically occur as comedones, papules, pustules, nodules, and cysts on the face, back, and upper chest. Try to present these findings in a matter-of-fact, yet concerned, manner while conveying understanding of acne as a problem. Establishing a trusting, caring relationship while assessing the adolescent client in-

Normal neonatal skin lesions

When assessing a neonate, the nurse should inspect the skin carefully for normal skin lesions, as shown below. If such lesions are present, document them and reassure the parents that these lesions are normal.

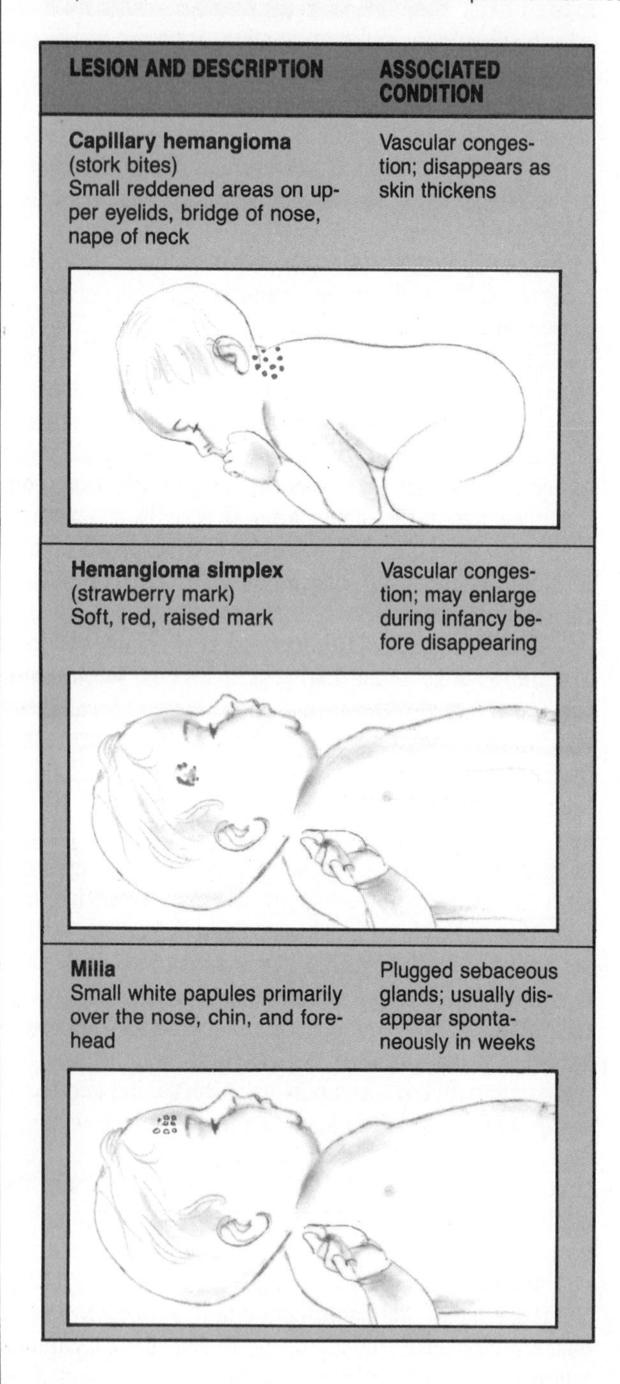

LESION AND DESCRIPTION	ASSOCIATED CONDITION
Capillary hemangioma (stork bites) Small reddened areas on upper eyelids, bridge of nose, nape of neck	Vascular congestion; disappears as skin thickens
Hemangioma simplex (strawberry mark) Soft, red, raised mark	Vascular congestion; may enlarge during infancy before disappearing
Milia Small white papules primarily over the nose, chin, and forehead	Plugged sebaceous glands; usually disappear spontaneously in weeks

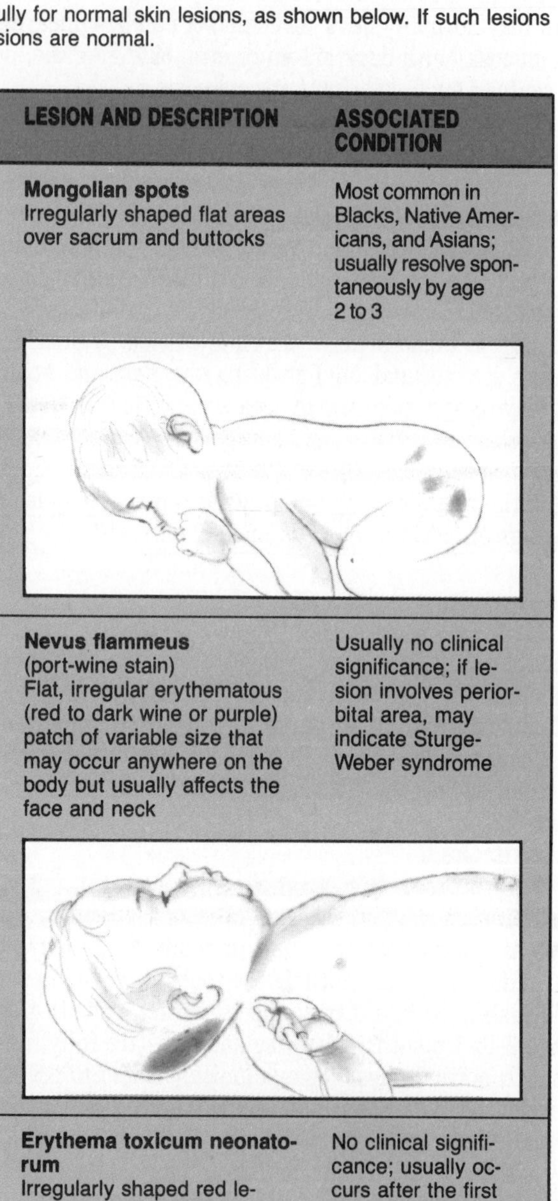

LESION AND DESCRIPTION	ASSOCIATED CONDITION
Mongolian spots Irregularly shaped flat areas over sacrum and buttocks	Most common in Blacks, Native Americans, and Asians; usually resolve spontaneously by age 2 to 3
Nevus flammeus (port-wine stain) Flat, irregular erythematous (red to dark wine or purple) patch of variable size that may occur anywhere on the body but usually affects the face and neck	Usually no clinical significance; if lesion involves periorbital area, may indicate Sturge-Weber syndrome
Erythema toxicum neonatorum Irregularly shaped red lesions, some with white central papules	No clinical significance; usually occurs after the first day of life and resolves within a week

creases cooperation during planning and implementation of skin care and treatment regimens.

Pregnant client

The skin, hair, and nails may also be affected by pregnancy. Melanocyte activity increases and may cause generalized hyperpigmentation. Scars, moles, and the areola of the nipple tend to darken, and a brownish black streak (linea nigra) may appear on the midline of the abdomen in a pregnant client. The client may also experience a darkening of facial skin, known as chloasma or the mask of pregnancy. Other common manifestations of pregnancy include striae (stretch marks), spider angiomas, varicose veins, brittle nails, and increased sweating. A pregnant client also may experience hair changes, such as straightening, increased oiliness, or partial hair loss.

Elderly client

In the elderly client, the epidermis may thin and flatten so that it looks like parchment, and blood vessels may become more visible. Skin permeability also makes the skin more susceptible to absorption. The dermis becomes less elastic from loss of collagen and elastin fibers, and wrinkles develop. The subcutaneous tissue layer may decrease, resulting in increased bony prominence and less protection from pressure. Decreased numbers of functioning sebaceous and sweat glands cause skin dryness and impair thermoregulation. Although usually age-related, the same changes may be caused by photo-aging (actinic damage from sun exposure) at a younger age.

Gray or white hair commonly occurs in the elderly client because of decreased numbers of functioning melanocytes. Changes in hair-growth stages within the hair follicles, decreased androgen production in the elderly male client, and decreased ratio of estrogen to androgen in the elderly female client may cause changes in hair distribution, including baldness; the growth of coarse hair in men's ears and on women's faces; and the loss of axillary and pubic hair.

Decreased peripheral circulation, particularly in the toes, typically increases the thickness and fragility of the toenails and turns them yellow.

Documentation

To determine what the assessment findings may indicate, the nurse reviews and integrates the data collected from the health history and physical assessment of the skin, hair, and nails. The nurse also reviews data about related body structures as well as vital signs and other statistics.

Assessment constitutes the first step in the nursing process. The nurse uses the assessment findings to formulate appropriate nursing diagnoses, which allow planning, implementation, and evaluation of client care. (For a case study that shows how to apply the nursing process to a client with a skin disorder, see *Applying the nursing process,* pages 178 and 179.)

Upon completing the assessment, document the data fully, including normal and abnormal findings. The following example shows correct documentation of normal physical assessment findings:

Weight: 134 lb
Vital signs: Temperature 98.6° F., pulse 72 and regular, respirations 18 and regular, blood pressure 130/70.
Black female client, age 60. Skin warm to touch; color medium brown; smooth and pliable, with minimal wrinkling and good turgor. Skin somewhat thickened and rough on extensor surfaces of knees and elbows; calluses noted on soles of feet, with corn on great left toe. Two vitiliginous patches on left anterior calf, approximately 1½" and 2" (3.81 and 5.08 cm) in diameter. About 15 to 20 dark-brown to black, rough, dry, flat nevi 0.5 to 1 cm in diameter, scattered on thorax, more posterior than anterior.

Mucous membranes moist, slight bluish brown cast throughout oral mucosa. Palpebral conjunctiva also brownish, and bulbar conjunctiva yellowish.

Scalp hair is coarse, tightly curled terminal hair with even distribution, showing some graying on crown, worn short (1½") all over head. Skin is moist in intertriginous areas of small dependent breasts.

Nails well-groomed, with good capillary refill, normal 160-degree angle on fingernails, some thickening and longitudinal ridges on toenails.

The following example shows correct documentation of abnormal physical assessment findings:

Weight: 100 lb
Vital signs: Temperature 99° F., pulse 100 and irregular, respirations 20 and regular, blood pressure 90/60.
Female client, Caucasian, age 27. Takes Motrin prescribed by gynecologist t.i.d. x 3d before menses,

(Text continues on page 180.)

Applying the nursing process

Assessment findings form the basis of the nursing process. Using them, the nurse formulates the nursing diagnoses and develops appropriate planning, implementation, and evaluation of the client's care.

The table below shows how the nurse can use skin, hair, and nail assessment data in the nursing process for the client described in the case history (shown at right). In the first column, history and physical assessment data appear, followed by a paragraph of mental notes. These notes help the nurse make important mental connections among assessment findings, aiding in development of the nursing diagnoses and planning.

The second column contains several appropriate nursing diagnoses; however, the information in the remaining columns is based on the *first* nursing diagnosis. Although it is not part of the nursing process, documentation appears in the last column because of its importance. Documentation consists of an initial note using all components of the SOAPIE format and a follow-up note using the appropriate SOAPIE components.

ASSESSMENT	NURSING DIAGNOSES	PLANNING	IMPLEMENTATION
Subjective (history) data • Client states, "I have been under a lot of stress since starting law school 6 months ago. Then, 4 months ago, I noticed some faint redness and inflammation over my elbows and knees, with itchiness." • Client says redness progressed to large raised patches with silver scales that now involve the skin over the buttocks. • Client reports that on a scale of 1 to 10 (least to most severe), itchiness is an 8 and worsens on hot, humid days. • Client states, "I tried moisturizers, calamine lotion, and aloe, but they didn't help. This condition is embarrassing because I look dirty." **Objective (physical) data** • Oral mucosa clear. Skin dry; no scalp lesions, no hair loss. • Large (12 x 5 cm) erythematous plaques with silver scales noted over knees and elbows with multiple plaques (4 x 5 cm) over buttocks and on right thigh; multiple scratch marks around lesions. • Nails pitted. Onycholysis noted on right index and ring fingers and left index and middle fingers. **Mental notes** *Considered along with assessment findings, the client's complaints suggest psoriasis. Emotional stress may play a role in the development of the psoriasis, and a poor body image caused by a chronic skin disorder is apt to increase the stress. Besides obtaining treatment for the condition, client needs to learn how to deal with stress.*	• Ineffective individual coping related to change in body image. • Potential for injury related to pruritus. • Alteration in skin integrity related to scaly lesions.	**Goals** Before leaving the clinic today, the client will: • identify effective coping strategies to deal with changes in appearance • identify stressful life situations and devise ways to lessen stress, including relaxation-response classes • discuss her medical diagnosis, treatment, and prognosis. At the next follow-up visit, the client will: • state the coping strategies used to deal with changes in appearance • discuss the measures taken to lessen stress.	• Allow time for the client to discuss feelings about the skin disorder. • Discuss with the client past methods of dealing with stress and how those methods can be used again. • Make referral to appropriate support groups. • Teach client about the causes and treatment of psoriasis. Give client a booklet about psoriasis to read at home.

CASE HISTORY

Ms. Julie Roman, age 21, is a single Caucasian female law student. She has noted changes in her skin over the past 4 months.

EVALUATION	DOCUMENTATION BASED ON NURSING PROCESS DATA			
		Initial		**Follow-up**
At the next follow-up visit, the client: • reported joining a class to learn relaxation response to alleviate stress and hiring a typist to type school papers, to allow more free time with friends • reported less distress related to appearance of skin, after joining a support group run by the American Psoriasis Foundation, and no longer feeling alone in distress over the disease.	**S**	Client states, "The doctor told me I have psoriasis and I'll have it forever! It started with redness, and now I have these ugly silver patches on my elbows, knees, and buttocks." Client reports severe itchiness (8 on a severity scale of 1 to 10). Says she started law school 6 months ago and finds it harder than she expected. She feels depressed about her appearance.	**S**	Client says, "I came for a refill of the medication Dr. Simmons prescribed for me. I read the booklet you gave me and I understand the disease better. I'm continuing to attend the relaxation-response class and the support group. I'm still worried about school, which is harder than I expected, and the competition is fierce!"
	O	Skin: Large (12 x 5 cm) erythematous plaques with silver scales over knees and elbows, with multiple plaques (4 x 5 cm) over buttocks and on right thigh. Multiple scratch marks around lesions. Nails pitted, onycholysis in four nails (right index and ring, left index and middle fingers). Tearful at present. Earlier in visit, mentioned interest in learning relaxation response.	**O**	Skin of knees and elbows shows less erythema. Scratch marks fading around plaque areas. Client calm but serious, and still expresses worry over school.
	A	Ineffective individual coping related to change in body image. Client is depressed about changes in appearance and stressed about school.	**A**	Anxiety reduced, coping improved as evidenced by attendance at relaxation-response class and support group.
	P	Allow time for client to discuss feelings about skin appearance. Provide emotional support. Assist client with stress-reduction measures. Reinforce that psoriasis is a disease characterized by remissions and exacerbations. Make referral to psoriasis support group.	**P**	Plan monthly follow-up visits for next 3 months, then every other month. Refer client to school counselor to discuss strategies for balancing an academic work load with other life demands.
	I	Gave client information about relaxation-response class and psoriasis support group being held at the hospital. Explained signs and symptoms, causes, and treatment of psoriasis.		
	E	Client enjoyed relaxation response, reported having used a variation of it in past. Will encourage continued use.		

sometimes q.i.d. during days 1 and 2. Skin color golden tan from recent beach vacation, pale white in areas covered by bikini. No scars, no exanthems over body surface except facial lesion; skin has good turgor. Skin scent flowery perfume. Skin thickened and somewhat lichenified at flexor surfaces of both arms and popliteal areas (client was allergic to wool as a child, used to scratch these areas constantly, still avoids wool against skin). Lesion on upper lip at border: small group of ruptured vesicles coated with yellow crust. Center of largest vesicle ulcerated and painful to manipulation or touch with gloved hand. (Client says constant annoyance #3 on 1 to 10 scale, increases to #5 or #6 when touched; tried coating lesions with camphor ice.)

Mucous membranes moist, oral mucosa pink, with thick, rough, erythematous area inside lower lip on right side. Palpebral conjunctiva pale.

Terminal scalp hair bleached pale blond, worn long and permed; many broken hair ends noted, dark roots in some areas, some scalp irritation with scaling at nape of neck and above ears.

Nails clean and well-groomed, toenails short and polished, fingernails long, tapered, and polished.

Chapter summary

This chapter focuses on anatomic, physiologic, and assessment norms of the skin, hair, and nails. It includes the following points:

- The skin has two distinct layers, the epidermis and the dermis, overlying a layer of subcutaneous fat. Epidermal appendages include the hair, nails, and sebaceous, apocrine, and eccrine glands.
- The surface skin layer, the epidermis, is further divided into two layers: a superficial keratinized layer of cells that can be shed or worn away and a deeper germinal layer, in contact with the dermis. The dermis also contains two layers: papillary and reticular. A collagenous membrane (the basement membrane) anchors the epidermis to the papillary dermis along its fingerlike projections. The subcutaneous fat layer beneath the dermis acts as a mechanical and thermal insulator.
- Skin appendages include hair, nails, and glands. Adult hair consists of two types: coarse terminal scalp and pubic hair, and finer vellus hair that covers all other body surfaces except the palms, soles, and mucocutaneous junctions. Nails, which derive from a special keratin, are situated over the dorsal surface at the distal end of each digit. The underlying vascular nail bed gives the nail plate its pink color. Nails protect the digits. The skin contains the sebaceous glands and the sweat glands; the latter include apocrine and eccrine glands.
- The skin affects or is affected by every body system. Problems seen in the skin may arise from disorders elsewhere in the body. Thus, skin assessment makes an important contribution to the assessment and management of any illness, as well as primary skin disorders.
- Skin assessment includes a thorough health history followed by careful inspection and palpation.
- When conducting a skin health history, the nurse can establish trust by providing a comfortable environment and using terms that are familiar to the client. Without such rapport, the client may be embarrassed to discuss or reveal lesions on private parts of the body.
- When physically assessing the skin, the nurse first evaluates the client's body weight, fluid status, general appearance, and vital signs, then uses inspection and palpation to assess all skin areas and appendages, including mucous membranes of the mouth and eyes.
- The nurse assesses the skin for color, consistency, temperature, turgor, and lesions, comparing similar body areas.
- When assessing primary skin lesions, the nurse notes their morphology, distribution, location, and configuration as well as secondary changes that may have occurred.
- During physical assessment, the nurse can recognize common skin lesions and document them by their descriptive characteristics as well as by their nomenclature.
- The nurse documents all assessment findings and uses them in the nursing process to plan, implement, and evaluate the client's nursing care.

Study questions

1. How would you compare the location, secretions, and function of the apocrine, eccrine, and sebaceous glands of the skin?

2. You have been assigned to the newborn nursery. What are three normal skin variations of the newborn about which parents may express concern?

3. What effects do each of the following conditions have on the skin?
- anemia
- decreased oxygenation
- fever
- liver disease
- pregnancy

4. What harmful effects on the skin, hair, and nails can the following behaviors produce?
- taking excessively hot showers and baths
- long-term braiding or corn-rowing of hair
- exposing unprotected skin to cleaning solvents
- sunbathing or using a tanning booth

5. John Peterson, age 44, has been admitted with a fever of 102° F. (38.9° C.); red, puffy eyes; and a generalized red, raised rash with a few small blisters of 2 days' duration. He also reports discomfort from superficial, eroded lesions in his mouth.

During the interview, Mr. Peterson asks you to dim the lights because they bother his eyes. He says he has had a seizure disorder for the past 5 years, which until recently was well controlled. He began taking phenytoin sodium (Dilantin) a few days ago.

How would you relate the following information in an assessment of Mr. Peterson?
- history (subjective) assessment data
- physical (objective) assessment data
- assessment techniques and equipment
- two nursing diagnoses
- documentation of your findings.

Selected references

Assessment. (1986). Nurse's Reference Library. Springhouse, PA: Springhouse Corp.

Baran, R., and Dawber, R. (Eds.). (1984). *Diseases of the nails and their management.* St. Louis: Mosby-Year Book.

Beavan, D., and Brooks, S. (1984). *Color atlas of the nail in clinical diagnosis.* Chicago: Year Book.

Blaylock, B. (1990). Pressure ulcers: A review. *Dermatology Nursing,* 2(5), 278-282.

Burton, J. (1985). *Essentials of dermatology* (2nd ed.). New York: Churchill Livingstone.

Cooper, D. (1990). Human wound assessment: Status report and implications for clinicians. *AACN Clinical Issues in Critical Care Nursing,* 1(3), 553-565.

Delauney, W., and Land, W. (1984). *Principles and practice of dermatology* (2nd ed.). Stoneham, MA: Butterworth-Heinemann.

DeWitt, S. (1990). Nursing assessment of the skin and dermatologic lesions. *Nursing Clinics of North America,* 25(1), 235-245.

Dobson, R., and Abele, D. (1985). *The practice of dermatology.* Philadelphia: Harper & Row.

Fitzpatrick, T., Eisen, A., Wolff, K., Freedberg, I., and Austen, K. (Eds.). *Dermatology in general medicine* (3rd ed.). New York: McGraw-Hill.

Grove, G. (1986). Physiologic changes in older skin. *Dermatologic Clinics,* 4(3), 425-432.

Harris, M., and Peters, D. (1990). Impaired skin integrity: A nursing diagnosis—A nursing challenge. *Home Healthcare Nurse,* 8(5), 33-38.

Jones, P., and Millman, A. (1990). Wound healing and the aged patient. *Nursing Clinics of North America,* 25(1), 263-277.

Kleinsmith, D., and Perricone, N. (1986). Common skin problems in the elderly. *Dermatologic Clinics,* 4(3), 485-499.

Lookingbill, D., and Marks, J. (1986). *Principles of dermatology.* Philadelphia: Saunders.

Malloy, M., and Perez-Woods, R. (1991). Neonatal skin care: Prevention of skin breakdown. *Pediatric Nursing,* 17(1), 41-48.

Moschella, S., and Hurley, H. (1985). *Dermatology* (2nd ed.). Philadelphia: Saunders.

Rook, A., Parish, L., and Beare, J. (Eds.). (1986). *Practical management of the dermatologic patient.* Philadelphia: Lippincott.

Rook, A., Savin, J., and Wilkinson, D. (1986). *Textbook of dermatology* (4th ed.). London: Blackwell Scientific.

Zviak, C. (1986). *The science of hair care.* New York: Marcel Dekker.

Nursing research

Choudhuri, M., et al. (1990). Efficiency of skin sterilization for a venipuncture with the use of commercially available alcohol or iodine pads. *American Journal of Infection Control,* 18(2), 82-85.

Olson, B. (1989). Effects of massage for prevention of pressure ulcers. *Decubitus,* 2(4) 32-37.

8

Head and Neck

Objectives

After reading and studying this chapter, you should be able to:

1. Discuss the normal anatomy and physiology of the head and neck.
2. Give examples of appropriate health history questions to ask the client when assessing the head and neck.
3. Identify representative adverse drug reactions that affect the head and neck.
4. Describe how to inspect, palpate, percuss, and auscultate the structures of the head and neck.
5. Describe the normal findings of a head and neck assessment for clients of all ages.
6. Describe common abnormalities that may be found in head and neck assessment.
7. Demonstrate how to use a nasal speculum.
8. Document head and neck assessment findings.

Introduction

This chapter covers the skills needed to assess the head, neck, and associated structures, including the face, nose, paranasal sinuses, mouth, and oropharynx. Each major structure is discussed separately, providing detailed information on the various organs in this body region. Chapter 21, Complete and Partial Assessments, discusses how to use this information in a typical head-to-toe assessment.

The head and neck support and protect the brain, sensory organs, and other structures. Because of these functions, they are among the first structures to evaluate in the assessment process.

The health history has particular importance in a head and neck assessment because of the wide range of disorders that can affect these structures. For example, a client with chronic neck stiffness may have a history of trauma from an automobile accident, or may disclose—through the health history—a long-term, stressful work environment. Although either condition can cause chronic neck stiffness, each requires different nursing interventions and treatment.

The nurse must consider history-taking especially important when a client complains of a common symptom, such as a headache. Because headaches occur frequently, many people ignore them and do not seek medical attention. About 90% of headaches result from benign causes, but the remaining 10% may produce serious consequences if not evaluated further.

Normal head and face appearance varies greatly between individuals and between age-groups. Differences require careful evaluation to distinguish between actual abnormalities and normal variations.

Anatomy and physiology review

This section discusses the normal structures and functions of the head, face, nose, sinuses, mouth, and neck. (For an illustration of important head and neck structures, see *Anatomy of the head and neck*, pages 184 and 185.)

Glossary

Bruxism: grinding of the teeth, especially during sleep.
Cheilitis: abnormal lip condition characterized by inflammation and cracking. The various forms of cheilitis include those caused by excessive exposure to sunlight and chemical irritants.
Cheilosis: lip and mouth disorder marked by scales and fissures, characteristic of riboflavin deficiency.
Choanae: funnel-shaped openings between the nasopharynx and the nasal cavity.
Fontanels: membrane-covered spaces between the bones of an infant's cranium.
Frenulum: restraining band of tissue, such as that attaching the posterior tongue to the floor of the mouth.
Gingivae: gums.
Gingivitis: acute or chronic inflammation of the gums.
Hydrocephalus or **hydrocephaly:** pathologic condition characterized by an abnormal accumulation of cerebrospinal fluid, causing head enlargement.
Malocclusion: abnormal positioning of the upper and lower teeth that prevents correct jaw alignment and chewing.
Mastication: chewing.
Microcephaly or **micrencephaly:** congenital anomaly characterized by an abnormally small head and an underdeveloped brain, resulting in mental retardation.
Nares: openings of the nasal cavities; nostrils.
Nasolabial folds: creases extending from the angle of the nose to the corner of the mouth.
Palpebral fissures: openings between the eyelids.
Papillae: small, nipple-shaped projections, as on the tongue.
Pharynx: tubular structure that extends from the base of the skull to the esophagus. A muscular structure lined with mucous membranes, the pharynx is divided into the nasopharynx, the oropharynx, and the laryngopharynx.
Sutures: immovable joints between the bones of the cranium.
Temporomandibular joint: connecting point between the mandible and the temporal bone. Usually abbreviated as TMJ.
Turbinates: bony internal nasal walls.
Uvula: small, cone-shaped mass that hangs from the soft palate and is composed of muscle and mucous membranes.

Head and face

Within the head, the skull is composed of eight cranial bones: the frontal bone, the right and left temporal bones, the right and left parietal bones, and the ethmoid, sphenoid, and occipital bones. (For an illustration of the major cranial and facial bones of an adult and the cranial bones, sutures, and fontanels in an infant, see *Comparison of the adult and infant skull,* page 186.)

The scalp and hair form the major integumentary structures of the head. (For anatomic and physiologic details about these structures, see Chapter 7, Skin, Hair, and Nails.)

The face is composed of 14 bones: the vomer and mandible; the right and left maxillae and inferior nasal conchae; and the right and left nasal, zygomatic, lacrimal, and palatine bones. Together with the other cranial bones, the facial bones protect and support the underlying structures, including the brain, eyes, and mucous membranes of the nose and mouth. The maxilla and mandible also support the teeth, which have their roots imbedded in these bones. The mandible, the only movable bone of the head and face, plays a major role in chewing (mastication) and a minor role in forming speech sounds. The area where the mandible and the temporal bone join is known as the temporomandibular joint.

The complex facial muscles provide the structure needed for expression and chewing. Cranial nerve VII (the facial nerve) innervates the facial muscles. Facial sensations are mediated by cranial nerve V (the trigeminal nerve).

The major facial artery, known as the temporal artery, is located bilaterally, extending from the front of the ear to the inner canthus of the eye—that part closest to the nose.

External landmarks of the face include the nasolabial folds—the creases extending from the angle of the nose to the corner of the mouth—and the palpebral fissures—the openings between the eyelids.

Nose, sinuses, mouth, and neck

The nose is the sensory organ for smell. It is also responsible for warming, filtering, and humidifying inhaled air.

The sinuses, which are hollow, air-filled cavities, lie within the facial bones. They include the frontal, sphenoidal, ethmoidal, and maxillary sinuses. The mucous membrane lining the sinuses is the same as that in the nasal cavity, which makes the sinuses prone to infections from the same viruses and bacteria that cause upper respiratory tract infections. The sinuses aid voice

(Text continues on page 187.)

Anatomy of the head and neck

Before assessing the head and neck, the nurse should be familiar with their structures.

Nose

The nose consists of bone and cartilage; the upper third is bone and the lower two thirds, cartilage. Innervated by cranial nerve I (the olfactory nerve), the nose is the sensory organ for smell. The vestibule, which is the area just inside the nostrils (nares), is lined with cilia—tiny hairs that filter inhaled air. The nostrils are separated by the nasal septum. The three turbinates—the superior, middle, and inferior—are curved, bony structures separated by grooves called meatuses. The turbinates and their mucosal covering aid breathing by warming, filtering, and humidifying inhaled air. Posterior air passages known as choanae lead to the oropharynx.

Mouth

The mouth contains the tongue, gingivae, teeth, and salivary glands. The tongue is covered with papillae (small, nipple-shaped projections), giving it a rough surface. It is attached to the floor of the mouth by a frenulum (a restrain-

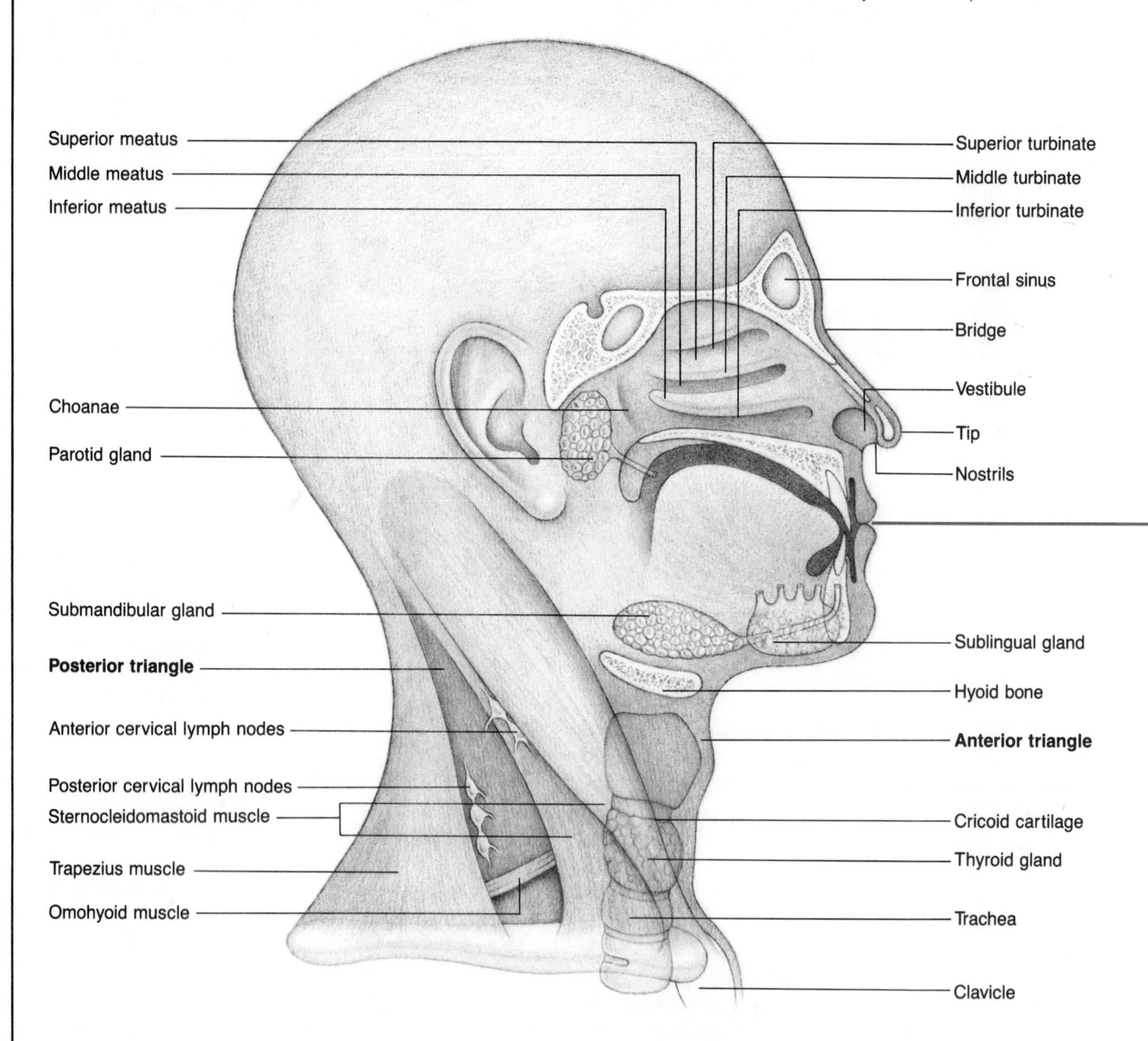

ing band of tissue). The gingivae cover the necks and roots of the teeth.

In the mouth, the anterior and posterior pillars form a cavity that houses the tonsils. The three pairs of salivary glands—parotid, sublingual, and submandibular—secrete into the mouth. The parotid glands are located just in front of and below the external ear; their openings, known as Stensen's ducts, lie in the buccal membrane near the second upper molar. The sublingual glands lie in the mouth under the tongue and open into the floor of the mouth posterior to the openings of Wharton's ducts. The mucosa is raised to cover them. The submandibular glands lie below and in front of the parotid glands. Wharton's ducts, the openings for the submandibular glands, open on the floor of the mouth on either side of the frenulum of the lower lip.

Neck

The cervical vertebrae, ligaments, and the major neck and shoulder muscles – the trapezius and sternocleidomastoid muscles – support the neck and allow it to move. These muscles and adjoining bones create two anatomic landmarks, the anterior and posterior triangles.

The anterior triangle of the neck lies between the sternocleidomastoid muscles and the mandible; it contains the hyoid bone, cricoid cartilage (the uppermost ring of tracheal cartilage), trachea, thyroid gland, and anterior cervical lymph nodes. The posterior triangle of the neck is bordered by the trapezius and sternocleidomastoid muscles and the clavicle; it contains the posterior cervical lymph nodes. The omohyoid muscle runs below the base of the posterior triangle.

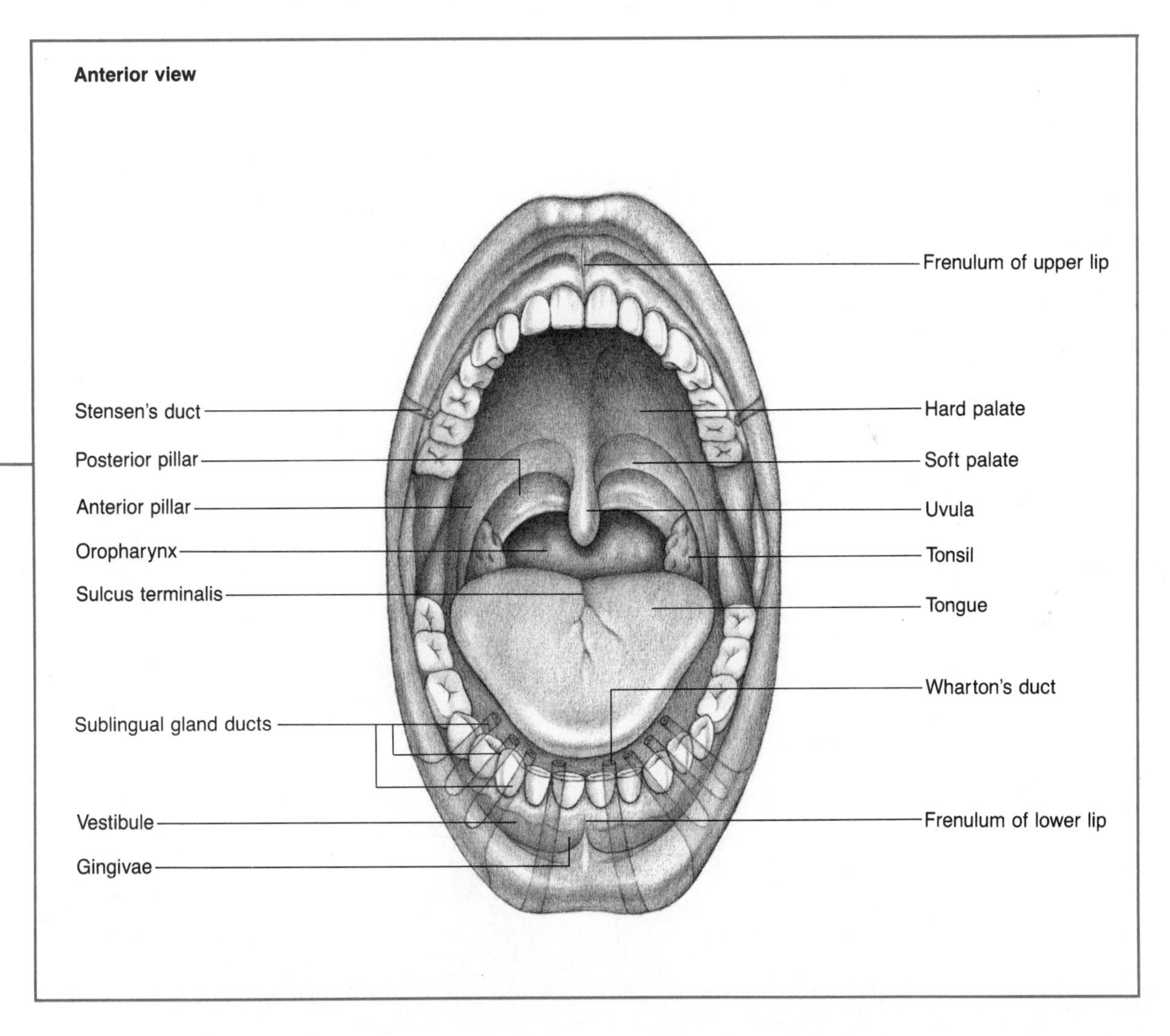

Comparison of the adult and infant skull

In an adult skull, the cranial bones are joined by fixed joints called sutures. In an infant skull, the cranial bones are joined by membranous spaces known as fontanels, located at the junctions of major sutures.

For several days after birth, a neonate's skull may be molded or elongated from the pressure that was exerted as it passed through the vaginal canal. Within a week after birth, a neonate's skull is usually round, with an anterior and posterior prominence. The fontanels, which allow such flexibility, also allow the cranium to accommodate brain growth in children under age 2. Normally, the anterior fontanel measures between 1⅝" and 2⅜" (4 and 6 cm) at birth and closes between age 7 and 18 months; the posterior fontanel measures between ⅜" and ¾" (1 and 2 cm) at birth and closes by age 2 months.

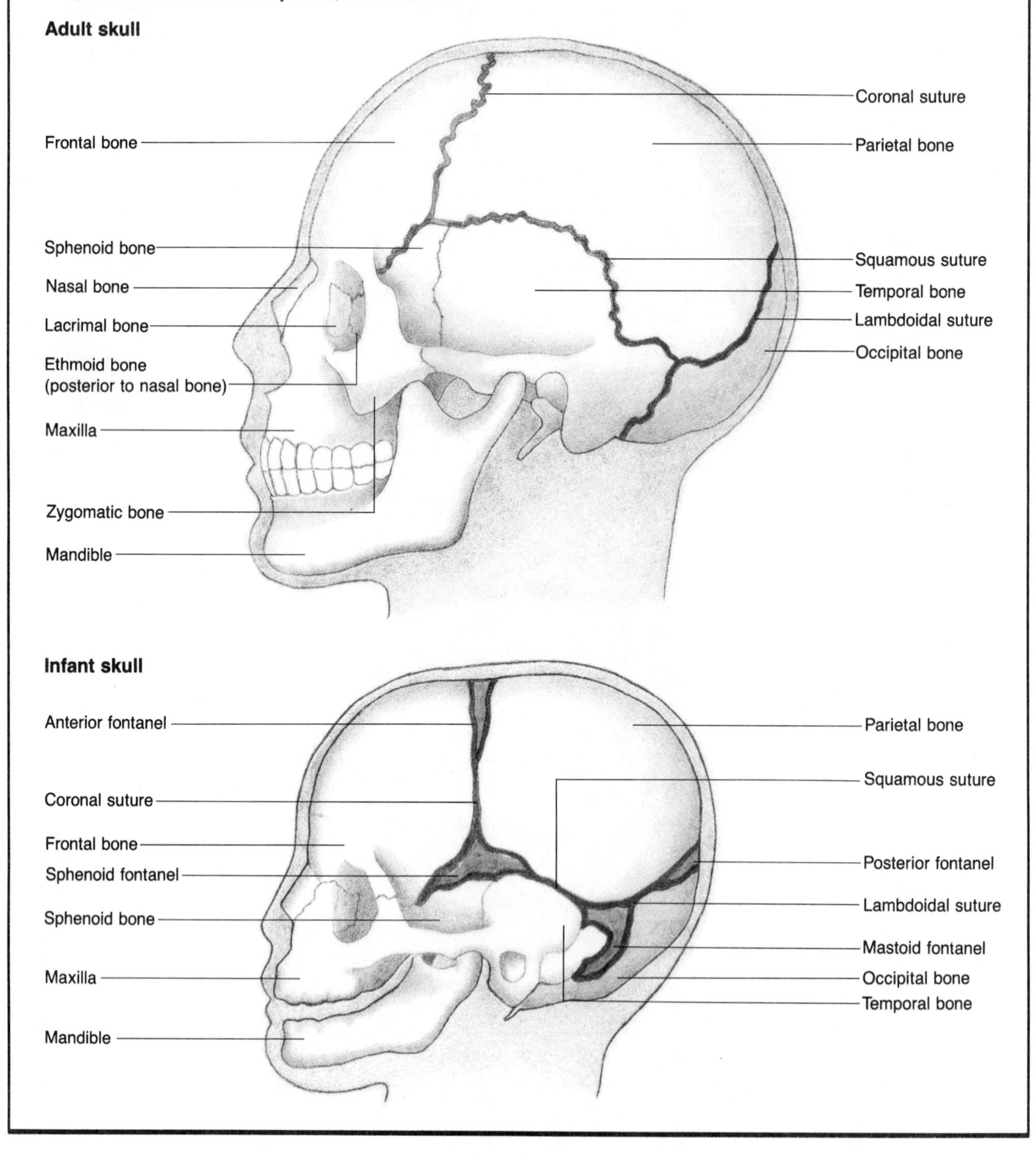

resonance and also may warm, humidify, and filter inhaled air (although this latter function has not been clearly established).

The mouth is surrounded by the lips anteriorly and the soft palate and uvula (a small, cone-shaped muscle that hangs from the soft palate and is lined with mucous membrane) posteriorly. The mandibular bone, covered with loose, mobile tissue, forms the floor of the mouth; the hard and soft palates form the roof of the mouth.

The neck includes the cervical vertebrae, ligaments, and neck and shoulder muscles. (For an illustration of important structures in the nose, mouth, and neck, see *Anatomy of the head and neck*, pages 184 and 185.) The posterior neck houses the cervical vertebrae, the cervical spinal nerves, and some fibers of cranial nerve XI (spinal accessory nerve). Cervical spinal nerves I through IV form the cervical plexus, which supplies sensory ability to the back of the head, front of the neck, and upper part of the shoulders and provides motor control of the neck muscles. Cervical spinal nerves III and IV also innervate the diaphragm, the primary muscle of respiration. Cervical spinal nerves V through VIII form the brachial plexus, innervating the scapular, pectoral, and deltoid muscles. Cranial nerve XI controls the trapezius and sternocleidomastoid muscles.

The neck also houses several other structures, including the trachea, neck vessels, lymph nodes, and thyroid gland. (For information about these structures, see Chapter 10, Respiratory System; Chapter 11, Cardiovascular System; Chapter 19, Immune System and Blood; and Chapter 20, Endocrine System, respectively.)

Health history

Because of the many structures involved in the head and neck, the nurse should construct health history questions that elicit information on topics as diverse as headaches and oral hygiene.

When assessing a client with recent head or neck trauma, the nurse should gather information about the chief complaint and current status but postpone taking the complete health history until X-rays have been taken, to prevent further injury from head or neck movement.

The questions in this section are designed to help evaluate the client's head, neck, and related structures. They include rationales that describe the significance of the answers and, where appropriate, nursing interventions to incorporate into the client's care plan.

Health and illness patterns

The nurse begins compiling the health history by investigating the client's current, past, and family health status, and then applies the PQRST method to obtain a complete description of any symptoms the client reports. (For a detailed explanation of the PQRST method, see *Symptom analysis* in Chapter 3.) The following questions will help elicit the most valuable information.

Have you ever had head trauma, skull surgery, or jaw or facial fractures? If so, when? What events came before and what happened afterward?
(RATIONALE: Head trauma, skull surgery, or jaw or facial fractures can change the configuration of the skull or face, producing abnormalities that should be fully evaluated during physical assessment. Events before and after the trauma or surgery—for instance, common sequelae such as frequent headaches or blurred vision—provide clues for further questioning.)

Do you have frequent headaches? If so, how often do they occur? What precedes them and what relieves them? Do they occur at a particular time of day? What part of your head do they affect? How would you describe the pain?
(RATIONALE: Answers to these questions can help differentiate one type of headache from another. For example, muscle contraction headaches usually produce a tight sensation in the occipital or temporal areas and are relieved by mild analgesics. Vascular headaches produce a throbbing, typically unilateral pain that is not relieved by analgesics. Headaches from brain tumors are typically intermittent, deep-seated, and dull at the tumor site. They may be especially intense in the morning.)

Have you ever had any swelling over your face, jaws, or mastoid process? (Point out the mastoid area, located just behind the client's ear.) *If so, when did it occur?*
(RATIONALE: Jaw swelling suggests an abscessed tooth or other dental problem. Facial swelling may be caused by a local problem, such as an abscessed tooth, sinusitis, or salivary gland cancer; or by a systemic problem, such as an allergic reaction or nephrotic syndrome. Mastoid swelling may arise from lymph node infection.)

Do you have a history of sinus infections or tenderness?
(RATIONALE: Sinus infections tend to recur in those persons susceptible to such infections. Tenderness usually accompanies sinus infections.)

Do you have any nasal discharge or postnasal drip? If so, describe it. When does it occur?
(RATIONALE: Nasal discharge and postnasal drip typically result from infections, allergies, or environmental irritants. Thick, tenacious, purulent discharge suggests infection; a watery discharge suggests an allergy or irritant. Certain types of allergies, such as hay fever, occur only at specific times of the year.)

Do you have frequent or prolonged nosebleeds?
(RATIONALE: Epistaxis [nosebleed] can occur with overuse of nasal sprays, from elevated blood pressure, and from other problems such as hematopoietic disorders, including leukemia and thrombocytopenia. Analyzing the symptoms can help identify the probable cause.)

What over-the-counter and prescription medications do you currently use?
(RATIONALE: Over-the-counter and prescription medications can produce numerous adverse reactions that can affect the nose, gingivae, teeth, and other head and neck structures. For further information, see *Adverse drug reactions.*)

Have you had any mouth lesions, ulcers, or cold sores? If so, how would you describe them? How long have you had them? Do they recur?
(RATIONALE: Among the various disorders causing mouth lesions are: the fungal infection candidiasis, which produces soft, white, elevated plaques; herpes simplex, which produces vesicles [cold sores] that rupture and leave a painful, crusting ulcer that often recurs; and gonorrhea, which causes painful lip ulcerations and rough, red, bleeding gingivae.)

Do you have any difficulty swallowing or chewing? If so, how would you describe this difficulty? Does it occur all the time, or only when you eat or drink?
(RATIONALE: Calculi in the parotid gland interfere with normal salivation and cause difficult swallowing [dysphagia]. Painful swallowing accompanied by hoarseness may indicate cancer of the larynx or esophagus. Difficult chewing and swallowing may result from dental problems, such as malocclusion, or from neuromuscular disorders, such as myasthenia gravis.)

Have you experienced any hoarseness or noticed any changes in the sound of your voice?
(RATIONALE: A positive response warrants further investigation; these signs can occur with numerous disorders, ranging from a sinus or tonsil infection to a tumor.)

Do you have any allergies that cause breathing difficulty and a sensation that your throat is closing? If so, when do these symptoms typically occur and how do you deal with them?
(RATIONALE: Documenting any known allergies and effective treatment measures will be valuable if the client is subsequently exposed to the offending allergen.)

Have you ever had a neck injury or experienced difficulty moving your neck in any direction? If so, how would you describe the problem? When did it occur and what, if anything, helped relieve it?
(RATIONALE: Disorders as diverse as neck sprain and cervical lymphadenitis [inflamed lymph nodes in the neck] can cause pain and tenderness and restrict the range of motion in the neck.)

Have you ever had neck surgery? If so, when and why?
(RATIONALE: In a client who has had unilateral carotid endarterectomy, expect to hear bruits [low-pitched sounds caused by turbulent blood flow] when auscultating the opposite side.)

Developmental considerations

These additional questions help in assessing a pediatric or an elderly client.

Pediatric client. The child's parent or guardian should answer the following questions during the health history:

Is your drinking water treated with fluoride?
(RATIONALE: Fluoride helps prevent dental caries, especially in children. If the water is unfluoridated, ask what other measures the family takes to prevent caries.)

Does the child use a pacifier or suck his thumb?
(RATIONALE: These habits misalign the upper teeth as they erupt.)

When did the child begin teething?
(RATIONALE: If the child's dentition is progressing slowly, check for other developmental lags.)

Does the child have tonsils? If not, when were they removed?
(RATIONALE: A child with intact tonsils is at greater risk for frequent streptococcal throat infections, which could lead to chronic tonsillitis.)

Elderly client. The elderly client should answer the following questions during the health history:

Adverse drug reactions

When obtaining a health history to assess a client's head and neck, the nurse must ask about current drug use. Many of the commonly used drugs listed below can produce adverse reactions in the head and neck, including gingivitis (gum inflammation), alopecia (hair loss), and epistaxis (nosebleed).

DRUG CLASS	DRUG	POSSIBLE ADVERSE REACTIONS
Anticholinergics	atropine, scopolamine, glycopyrrolate, propantheline, belladonna alkaloids, dicyclomine, hyoscyamine	Decreased salivation, dry mouth
Anticonvulsants	phenytoin sodium	Gingival hyperplasia
Antidepressants	All agents, including amitriptyline and nortriptyline	Dry mouth
Antihypertensives	guanabenz, clonidine, methyldopa	Dry mouth
Antilipemics	clofibrate	Dry brittle hair, alopecia
Antineoplastics	bleomycin sulfate	Ulcerated tongue and lips, alopecia
	dactinomycin	Mouth lesions, alopecia
	melphalan	Mouth lesions
	mitomycin	Mouth lesions, alopecia
	methotrexate	Gingivitis, mouth lesions, alopecia
	cyclophosphamide	Mouth lesions, alopecia
	vincristine sulfate	Mouth lesions, alopecia
	chlorambucil	Mouth lesions
	uracil mustard	Mouth lesions
	cisplatin	Gingival platinum line, alopecia
	hydroxyurea	Mouth lesions
	fluorouracil	Alopecia, epistaxis
	doxorubicin	Mouth lesions, alopecia
	cytarabine	Mouth lesions, alopecia
	daunorubicin	Mouth lesions, alopecia
	etoposide	Alopecia
Cardiac agents	disopyramide phosphate	dry mouth
Genitourinary smooth-muscle relaxants	flavoxate, oxybutynin	Dry mouth

continued

Adverse drug reactions continued

DRUG CLASS	DRUG	POSSIBLE ADVERSE REACTIONS
Gold salts	gold sodium thiomalate	Gingivitis, mouth lesions
	auranofin	Mouth lesions
Nonsteroidal anti-inflammatory agents	indomethacin	Gingival lesions
	ibuprofen	Dry mouth, gingival lesions
Miscellaneous agents	lithium salts	Dry mouth, dry hair, alopecia
	metoclopramide	Dry mouth, glossal or periorbital edema
	penicillamine	Mouth lesions
	isotretinoin	Inflamed lips, epistaxis, dry mouth
	allopurinol	Alopecia
	propranolol	Hyperkeratosis and psoriasis of the scalp, alopecia
	guanethidine sulfate	Nasal stuffiness, dry mouth
	edrophonium	Increased salivation
	pyridostigmine	Increased salivation, increased tracheobronchial secretions
	fluorides	Staining or mottling of teeth
	warfarin sodium	Epistaxis with excessive dosage
	amphetamines	Dry mouth, continuous chewing or bruxism (tooth grinding) with prolonged use
	tetracycline	Enamel hypoplasia and permanent yellow-gray to brown tooth discoloration in children under age 8 and in offspring of pregnant clients

Do you wear dentures? If so, how well do they fit?
(RATIONALE: Ill-fitting dentures can cause reluctance to speak, difficulty with eating, or gingival lesions in an elderly client.)

Health promotion and protection patterns

The following questions will help the nurse assess any behavioral patterns that may affect the client's health status.

Do you smoke a pipe?
(RATIONALE: Pipe smoking increases the risk of lip and mouth cancer.)

Do you chew tobacco or use snuff?
(RATIONALE: These practices greatly increase the risk of mouth cancer.)

If you suffer from headaches or tightness in the neck or jaw, what do you do for relief? Does relaxation, exercise, or massage help you? Does headache or neck or jaw tightness correlate with lack of sleep, missed meals, or stress?
(RATIONALE: Inadequate sleep, nutrition, or relaxation can produce stress, which can cause headaches or tight-

ness in the neck or jaw. Health protection behaviors that relieve the pain or tightness may benefit the client. Examples include meditation and massage.)

Does your job require long hours of sitting, such as at a computer terminal?
(RATIONALE: Sitting in a particular position for long hours can cause headaches and tightness in the neck or jaw.)

Do you grind your teeth?
(RATIONALE: Bruxism [grinding of teeth, especially while asleep] can be a sign of stress. The client may benefit from learning stress-reduction techniques, which may eliminate bruxism.)

Does your job put you at risk for head injury? If so, do you wear a hard hat? Do you participate in any sports that require a helmet? Do you wear a seat belt when you are in an automobile?
(RATIONALE: The answers to these questions will show how highly the client regards personal safety. They may also point out a need for safety teaching.)

What are your mouth-care habits? How often do you brush and floss your teeth? When was your last dental examination?
(RATIONALE: These questions elicit information about the client's dental health habits. If several years have passed since the last dental examination, the client needs counseling to pay more attention to proper dental hygiene and to visit a dentist.)

Role and relationship patterns

A head or neck problem can affect the way a client feels about roles and relationships with others. The following questions can reveal such difficulties.

Does your head or neck problem affect the way you feel about yourself or the way you relate to your family?
(RATIONALE: Chronic headaches or neck or jaw tightness may result from family stress. The chronic discomfort can then trigger further stress by lowering the client's self-esteem and interfering with family and social activities. More symptoms then follow. Stress-reduction techniques may help relieve the problem, breaking the cycle of stress-symptoms-stress.)

Has your head or neck problem interfered with your activities of daily living or normal sexual activity?
(RATIONALE: If activities of daily living or sexual activity are affected, exercises that strengthen the head and neck may help the client. Alternative sexual positions may help relieve strain or pressure on the head or neck.)

Physical assessment

This section discusses examining the client's head and face, nose and sinuses, mouth and oropharynx, and neck. It notes normal and abnormal findings for each of these areas, and provides assessment modifications that accommodate the special needs of children, pregnant women, and elderly clients.

On first meeting the client, the nurse should observe the overall appearance and body movements; look for head or neck tilting, facial grimacing, or other signs of discomfort; and note if the client is holding or rubbing any part of the head or neck. This quick survey can reveal stiff or painful areas that require further assessment.

Next, the nurse evaluates the client's respirations. Because cervical spinal nerves III and IV innervate the diaphragm, labored respirations and incomplete diaphragmatic excursion may point to a problem affecting these nerves. (For more information, see *Advanced assessment skills: Measurement of diaphragmatic excursion* in Chapter 10, Respiratory System.) A client with these signs should be watched closely for signs of respiratory distress.

For a complete head and neck assessment, the nurse employs the four major examination techniques—inspection, palpation, percussion, and auscultation—and the following equipment: stethoscope, tape measure, glass of water, tongue depressor, gloves, 4″ × 4″ gauze pad, small flashlight, and nasal speculum or ophthalmoscope handle with nasal attachment.

To begin the hands-on assessment, the nurse washes his or her hands and asks the client to be seated and to remove any wig or hairpiece.

Examining the head and face

To perform this part of the physical assessment, the nurse should follow these steps:

First, note the client's spontaneous facial expression. Inspect the head and face for any abnormalities in size, shape, contour, or symmetry. Observe the client's head; it should be erect and midline, and the client should be able to hold it still. Inspect the face for symmetry, paying particular attention to the palpebral fissures and nasolabial folds. Check that the eyes are equidistant both midline and laterally and that they align horizontally with the helix, the prominent outer rim of the ear. Also look for facial lesions, rash, swelling, or redness. Note any tics, twitching, or other abnormal movements. Keep in mind that certain facial features are characteristic of race; for example, the prominent epicanthal folds (vertical folds of skin over the inner canthus of the eye) in Asians.

Examine the scalp and hair, observing how the hair is distributed on the scalp and, in men, on the bearded region of the face. (For more information about this part of the assessment, see Chapter 7, Skin, Hair, and Nails.)

Note the client's facial expression; it can be a clue to the client's psychological state, or it can reveal physical distress or pain.

Note facial color. Pallor or cyanosis (bluish skin tone) usually appears first in the oral mucous membranes. Either may also appear around the lips or other areas of the face. Yellow skin and sclera may indicate jaundice.

Palpate

After inspecting, palpate the head and face to learn more about their condition. Use your fingertips to discriminate skin surface textures and the pads of your fingers to determine the configuration and consistency of bony structures or skin lesions.

First, palpate the head for symmetry and contour; then palpate the scalp, using a gentle rotary movement of the fingertips. The head should feel symmetrical and free of lumps or other lesions. It should not be tender to the touch. The scalp also should be free from dryness, lesions, or scars and should move freely over the skull. The hair should not feel excessively dry, oily, or brittle.

Next, gently palpate the face to assess skin tone and facial contours. Palpate bilaterally, using both hands simultaneously. The face should feel smooth, and the client should not feel any tenderness or pain. (*Note:* In children and premenopausal women, facial skin is usually softer and smoother; in adult men and postmenopausal women, it is rougher and less elastic.) Facial contours should feel symmetrical, with no swelling, edema, or masses.

Evaluate facial skin turgor by palpating the skin of the cheeks for recoil. To do so, gently grasp the cheek between your thumb and index finger, lift it slightly, then release. The skin should return quickly to its normal position; failure to do so may indicate muscle weakness or inadequate hydration. Simultaneously palpate the muscles on both sides of the face while the client smiles, frowns, grits the teeth, and puffs out the cheeks. This maneuver evaluates facial muscle tone. Check for symmetrical muscle movement with each of these maneuvers.

Palpating the temporomandibular joints

The nurse palpates the temporomandibular joints (located anterior to and slightly below the auricle) to assess jaw function. To palpate this area, the nurse places the middle three fingers of each hand bilaterally over each joint, then gently presses on the joints as the client opens and closes the mouth. The nurse evaluates the joints for movability, approximation (drawing of bones together), and discomfort. Normally, this process should be smooth and painless for the client.

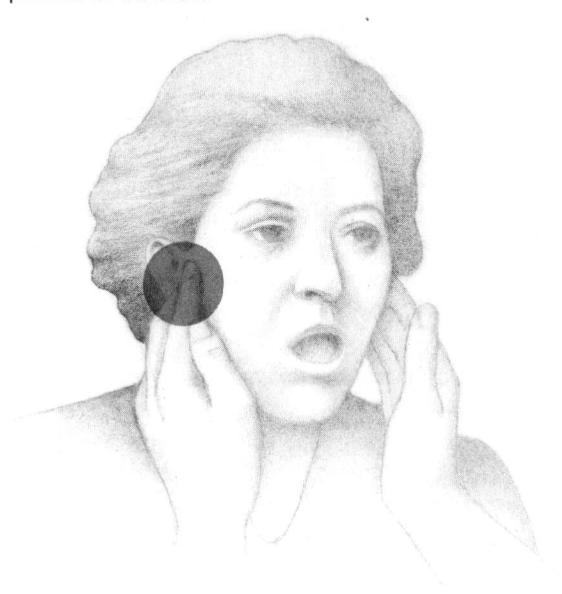

Temporomandibular joint structures

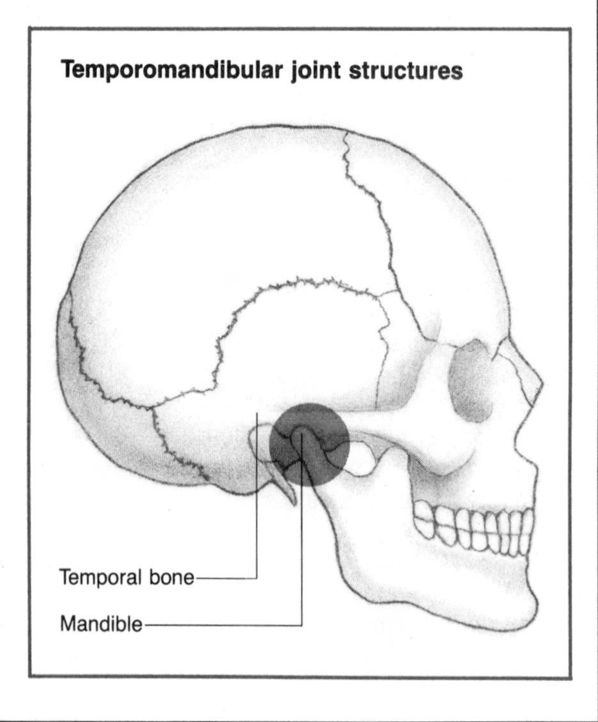

When palpating the face, be sure to check the temporal artery pulses; they should be of equal strength and rhythm.

Palpate the temporomandibular joints (located anterior to and slightly below the auricle) to evaluate how easily they move, whether they are properly aligned (approximation), and whether they cause any discomfort. (For more information, see *Palpating the temporomandibular joints.*) The temporomandibular joints should move smoothly and without pain.

Finally, auscultate over the major vessels of the head—the periorbital, temporal, and occipital arteries—using the bell of the stethoscope. Be particularly careful over any arteries that feel hard, ropelike, or tender on palpation. Auscultation should not reveal any sounds in these arteries. If you detect any bruits, notify the physician for further evaluation.

Abnormal findings

Skull deformities may result from various causes, including head trauma and surgical removal of part of the skull. In an adult, an abnormally large head may indicate acromegaly, a disorder of excessive growth hormone characterized by enlarged and thickened skull bones, increased length of the mandible, and increased prominence of the nose and forehead.

Abnormalities in facial color, shape, or symmetry may stem from a systemic disorder. For example, periorbital and facial edema and cyanosis of the lips, nose, and cheeks may occur in congestive heart failure and other serious cardiovascular disorders. Periorbital edema may also be seen in renal disease. A blank or mask-like facial expression may indicate Parkinson's disease. Facial pallor can be caused by shock or anemia. Yellow skin and sclera suggest jaundice, usually from liver disease.

Certain hormonal imbalances produce characteristic facial abnormalities. Hyperthyroidism (Graves' disease), which causes exophthalmos (eyeball protrusion) and elevation of the upper eyelids, can make a client stare or look startled. In many cases, hypothyroidism progresses to myxedema, creating puffy, dry skin; coarse features; and a dull expression.

In Cushing's syndrome, a rare disorder of increased adrenal hormone production, the face assumes a characteristic rounded "moon" shape, with red cheeks, increased facial hair, and possibly edema. These characteristics may also result from prolonged use or high doses of steroid medications, such as cortisone.

(Second)

Examining the nose and sinuses

For this part of the physical assessment, the nurse should follow these steps:

Inspect the nose for symmetry and contour, noting any areas of deformity, swelling, or discoloration. To assess nasal symmetry, ask the client to tilt the head back, then observe the position of the nasal septum. The septum should be aligned with the bridge of the nose. With the head in the same position, evaluate flaring of the nostrils (nares). Some flaring during quiet breathing is normal, but marked flaring may indicate respiratory distress. Although the external appearance of the nose may vary slightly between individuals and according to developmental age, the nose should be intact and symmetrical, with no edema or deformity. Note the character and amount of any drainage from the nostrils.

Next, palpate the nose, checking for any painful or tender areas, swelling, or deformities. Evaluate nostril patency by gently occluding one nostril with your finger and having the client exhale through the other.

To assess the paranasal sinuses, inspect, palpate, and percuss the frontal and maxillary sinuses. (The ethmoidal and sphenoidal sinuses lie above the middle and superior turbinates of the lateral nasal walls and cannot be assessed.) To assess the frontal and maxillary sinuses, first inspect the external skin surfaces above and lateral to the nose for inflammation or edema. Then palpate and percuss these sinuses. (For illustrated procedures, see *Palpating and percussing the sinuses,* page 194.)

If the nose and sinuses require more extensive assessment, use the advanced techniques of direct inspection and transillumination. (For illustrated procedures, see *Advanced assessment skills: Direct inspection,* page 195, and *Advanced assessment skills: Transillumination,* page 196.)

Abnormal findings

Inspection of the nose may reveal asymmetrical bones or cartilages, causing a deviation to one side. Marked flaring of the nostrils may indicate respiratory distress, especially in a child. The character of drainage from the nostrils provides clues to its origin. Bloody drainage may be minor from frequent blowing, or major from a spontaneous or traumatic epistaxis. Thick white, yellow, or green drainage usually occurs with infection. Clear, thin drainage may be associated with rhinitis (runny nose) or, more seriously, with cerebrospinal fluid leakage from a basilar skull fracture. Nonpatent nostrils may indicate simple nasal congestion, a nasal fracture, or a deviated septum.

Pain or discomfort elicited by sinus palpation may indicate sinus congestion or infection. Swelling over sinus areas may also indicate congestion or infection.

Palpating and percussing the sinuses

Although the head contains four paranasal sinuses, only two—the frontal and maxillary sinuses—can be assessed. (In children under age 8, the frontal sinuses are usually too small to examine.) The other two—the ethmoidal and sphenoidal sinuses—are inaccessible. The nurse should be familiar with their locations, however, to ensure accurate assessment. After inspecting the paranasal sinuses, the nurse palpates and percusses them using the following techniques:

Sinus locations

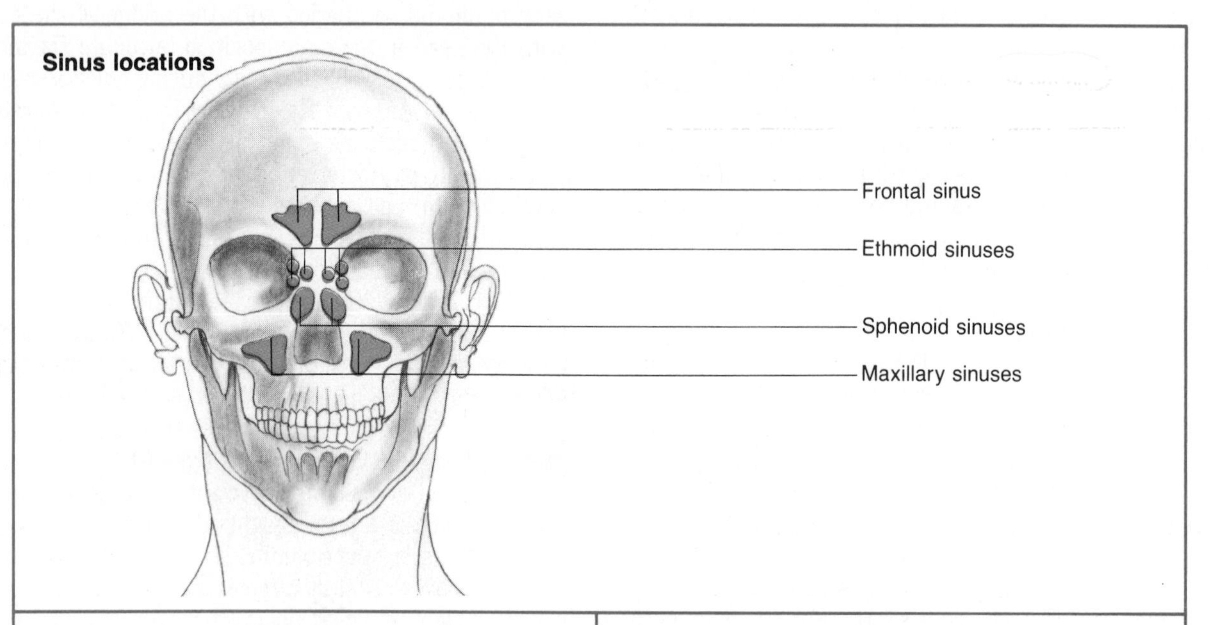

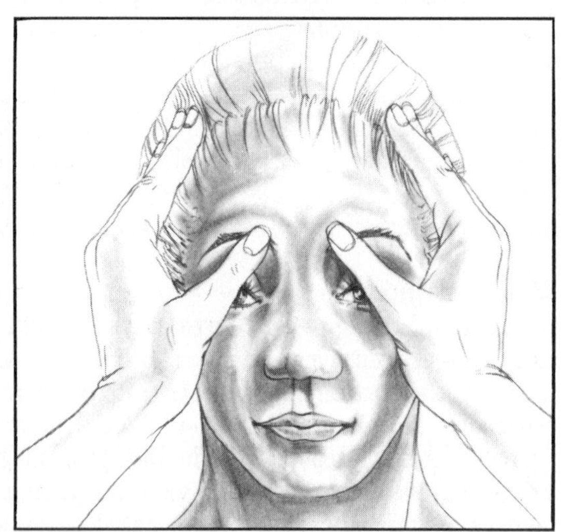

Palpation
To palpate the frontal sinuses, place the thumbs above the eye just under the bony ridge of the upper orbit. Place the fingertips on the forehead and apply gentle pressure as shown here. Then palpate the maxillary sinuses by applying gentle pressure with the index and middle fingers (or thumbs) on each side of the nose in the area immediately below the zygomatic bone (cheekbone).

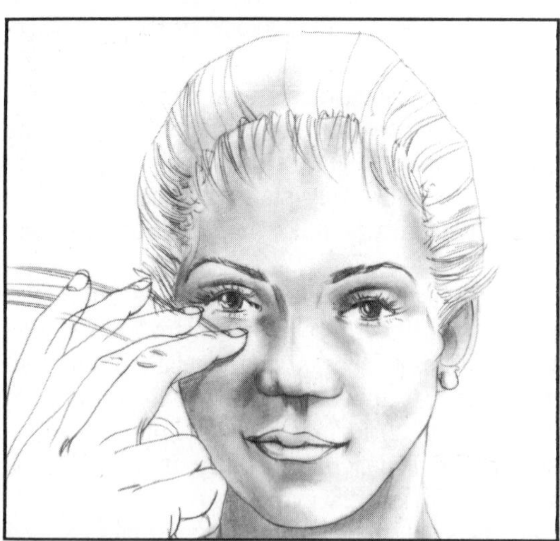

Percussion
Percuss the frontal sinuses by gently tapping the index or middle finger just above the eyebrows. Then percuss the maxillary sinuses by tapping the index or middle finger on both sides of the nose beneath the eye in line with the pupils as shown here.

ADVANCED ASSESSMENT SKILLS

Direct inspection

To assess the nostrils more thoroughly, the nurse uses direct inspection. Direct inspection is performed with a nasal speculum and a small flashlight, or an ophthalmoscope handle with a nasal tip. A nasal speculum is not used to assess infants or toddlers, because their nostrils are too small for the sharp speculum blades. A flashlight will do. To inspect the internal nostrils, the nurse follows these steps:

1 Facing the seated client, insert the tip of the closed speculum into the nostril up to the point at which the blade widens. Then slowly open the speculum as wide as possible (without causing the client discomfort) to allow visibility. If necessary, ask the client to tilt the head back. Move as necessary to examine the structures. Shine a small flashlight into the nostril to illuminate the area.

2 Examine one nostril at a time. The mucosa should be moist, pink to red, and free of lesions and polyps. Observe the choana (posterior air passage), variable amounts of cilia, the middle and inferior turbinates, and below each turbinate, the meatus. Direct inspection should disclose no excessive drainage, edema, or inflammation of the nasal mucosa. The nasolacrimal duct drains into the inferior meatus, and most of the paranasal sinuses drain into the middle meatus. Note the color, patency, and presence of any exudate in each nostril. When direct inspection is completed, close the speculum before removing it.

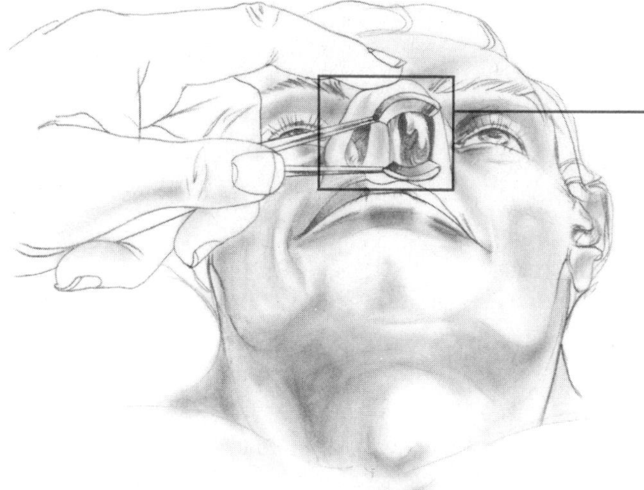

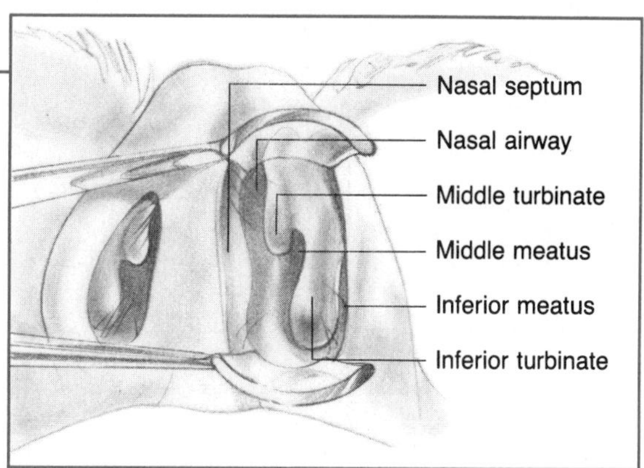

Examining the mouth and oropharynx

For this part of the physical assessment, the nurse should follow these steps:

Put on examination gloves, and ask the client to remove any partial or complete dentures to see the inside of the mouth and throat more clearly. Note how the dentures fit and how easily the client can remove them.

Next, note any unusual breath odors. Inspect the oral mucosa by inserting a tongue depressor between the teeth and the cheek to examine the membranous tissue. It should be moist, smooth, and free of lesions. Small, yellowish-white raised lesions, known as Fordyce's spots, are the normal sebaceous glands of the buccal mucosa. Assess Stensen's duct openings—small, white-rimmed openings located at the level of the second molar in each cheek—for tenderness and inflammation. Note the color of the mucosa; it is usually pink, although dark-skinned clients may have bluish-tinted or patchily pigmented mucosa.

When examining the oral mucosa, observe the gingivae and teeth. Gingival surfaces should appear pink, moist, and slightly irregular, with no spongy or edematous areas. The edges of the teeth should be clearly defined, with a shallow crevice visible between the gingivae and teeth.

Note any missing, broken, loose, or repaired teeth. An adult normally has up to 32 teeth. (For more information, see *Dentition of temporary and permanent teeth,* page 197.) Check tooth color, which normally varies from bright white to ivory. Tooth edges should be smooth, with no areas of unusual wear. To assess for occlusion

ADVANCED ASSESSMENT SKILLS

Transillumination

If sinus palpation and percussion cause tenderness, transillumination of the frontal and maxillary sinuses will help the nurse fully evaluate these structures. This technique, which may be performed on clients over age 8, requires a small flashlight or an ophthalmoscope handle with a transilluminator head. It is performed in these two steps:

1 Darken the room and place the flashlight against the orbital bone immediately below the eyebrow. Hold one hand over the end of the transilluminator and the skin surface being assessed. Usually, a reddish glow (illumination) will be visible above the sinus area. Lack of illumination may indicate frontal sinus congestion. Extreme illumination may occur in an elderly client because of reduced subcutaneous facial fat. Repeat this procedure to assess the other frontal sinus.

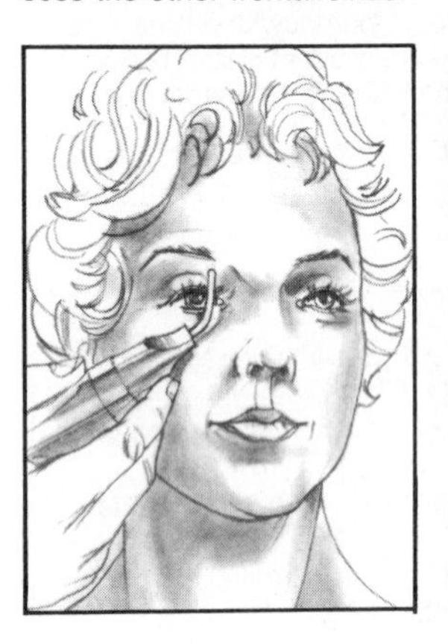

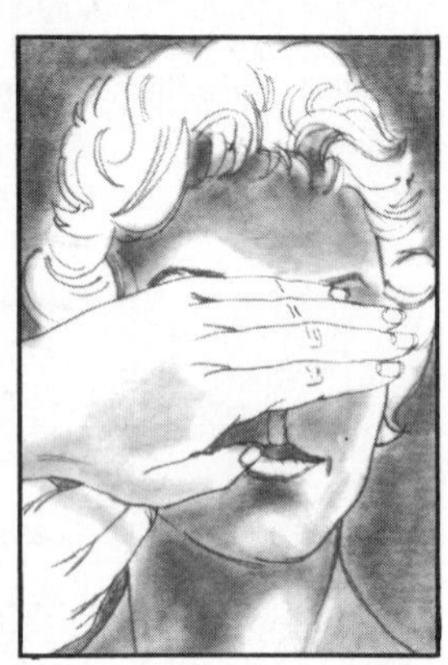

2 To transilluminate the maxillary sinuses, place the transilluminator beneath the center of the eye, lateral to the nose. Ask the client to open the mouth. A soft glow should illuminate the hard palate and allow you to see the sinuses above.

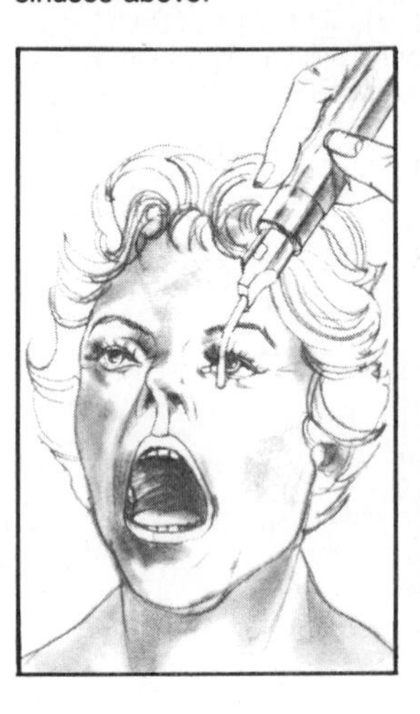

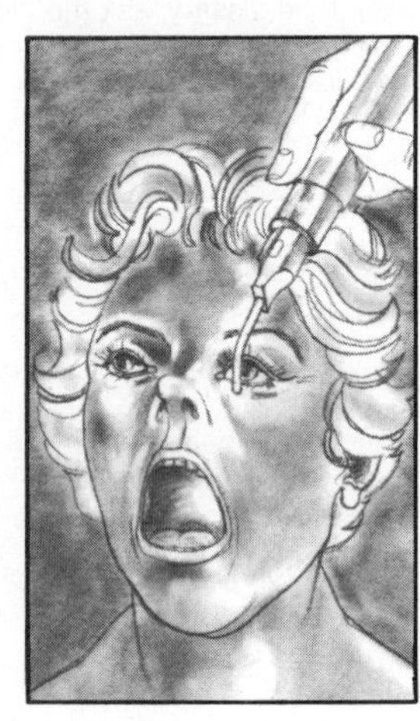

of the upper and lower jaw, ask the client to close the mouth gently. The upper teeth should extend slightly beyond and over the lower teeth.

Inspecting the tongue will provide valuable information about the client's hydration status and the function of cranial nerve XII (the hypoglossal nerve), which controls the motor function of the tongue. The tongue should appear pink and slightly rough with a midline depression and a V-shaped division (sulcus terminalis) separating the anterior two thirds from the posterior third. The tongue should fit comfortably into the floor of the mouth. It may be covered with a thin white film that can be scraped off easily with a tongue depressor. Note any lesions that are not removed easily or that cause bleeding when removed. Geographic tongue (superficial, irregular areas of the tongue that have exposed tips of the papillae) is normal.

The position of the tongue in the mouth helps evaluate the functioning of cranial nerve XII, which controls tongue movement. To perform this assessment, ask the client to stick out the tongue, and observe for midline positioning, voluntary movement, and tremors.

Next, ask the client to touch the tip of the tongue to the roof of the mouth, and observe the underside for any lesions or other abnormalities. The bottom surface of the tongue should be smoother and pinker than the top surface.

As the client keeps the tongue against the roof of the mouth, inspect the lingual frenulum (the membrane that anchors the tongue to the floor) and the submandibular (Wharton's) ducts. The sublingual fold under the tongue contains salivary glands that provide oral lubrication and assist with digestion. The fold should appear pink and moist.

Also inspect the hard and soft palates. They should appear pink to light red in color, with symmetrical lines. Normally, the hard palate is rougher and a lighter pink than the soft palate. Note and describe any deformities, lesions, or areas of tenderness or inflammation.

Observe the tonsils for unilateral or bilateral enlargement. Grade tonsil size on a scale of 0 to +4. A grade of 0 (normal) indicates that both tonsils are behind

Dentition of temporary and permanent teeth

Temporary teeth

Normal dentition changes with age. A child may have up to 20 temporary teeth, also called deciduous or baby teeth. The first tooth usually erupts by age 6 months; all temporary teeth usually are shed between age 6 and 13.

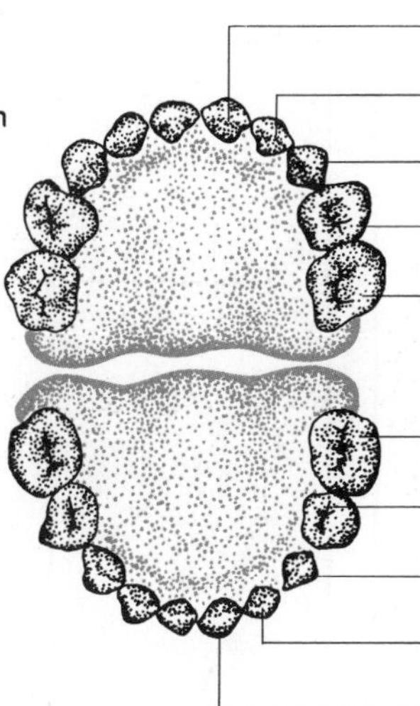

MAXILLARY

Central incisor: 6 to 8 months

Lateral incisor: 7 to 12 months

Canine: 16 to 20 months

First molar: 12 to 16 months

Second molar: 20 to 30 months

MANDIBULAR

Second molar: 18 to 22 months

First molar: 16 to 24 months

Canine: 14 to 18 months

Lateral incisor: 7 to 9 months

Central incisor: 6 to 8 months

Permanent teeth

An adult normally has 32 permanent teeth. The lower permanent teeth usually erupt earlier than the upper ones. The third molars (wisdom teeth) erupt last, usually appearing after age 17.

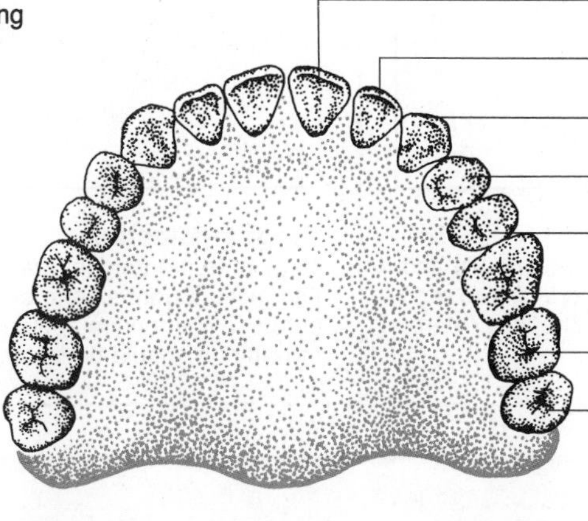

MAXILLARY

Central incisor: 7 to 8 years

Lateral incisor: 7 to 10 years

Canine: 9 to 14 years

First premolar: 9 to 13 years

Second premolar: 10 to 14 years

First molar: 5 to 8 years

Second molar: 10 to 14 years

Third molar: 17 to 24 years

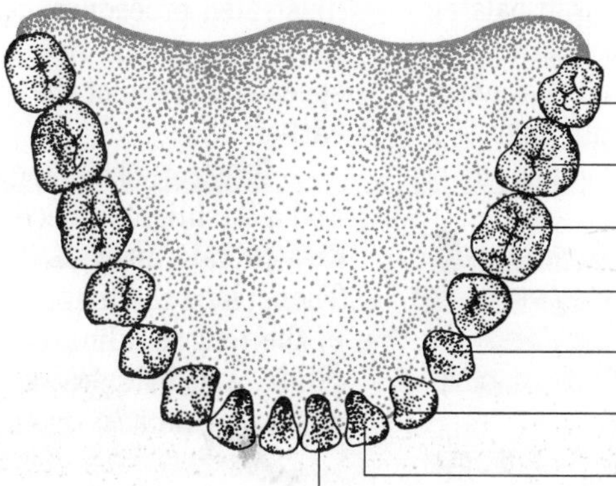

MANDIBULAR

Third molar: 17 to 24 years

Second molar: 10 to 14 years

First molar: 5 to 8 years

Second premolar: 10 to 14 years

First premolar: 9 to 13 years

Canine: 9 to 14 years

Lateral incisor: 7 to 10 years

Central incisor: 7 to 8 years

Palpating the lips and tongue

To assess the mouth, the nurse palpates the lips and tongue.

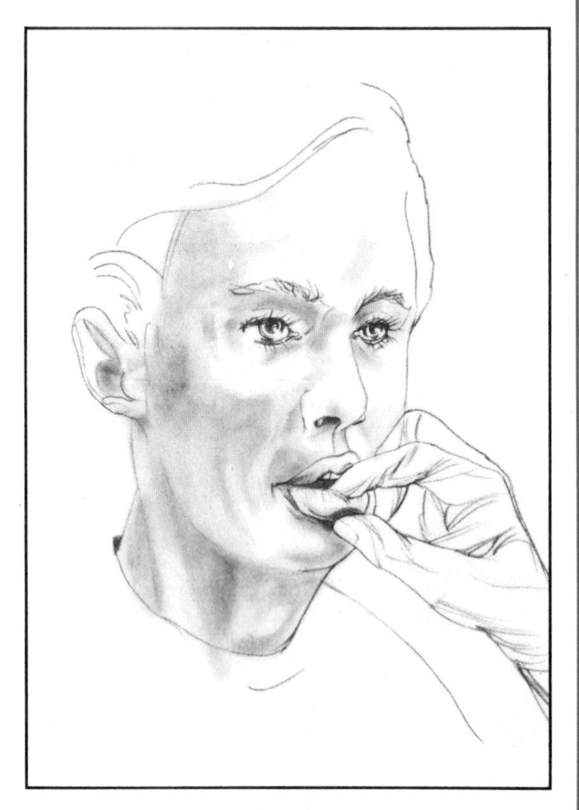

Lip palpation
To palpate the lips, gently pull down on the lower lip and up on the upper lip. The lips should be soft, pink to red in color, symmetrical with good muscle tone, and free of lesions, lumps, ulcers, and edema.

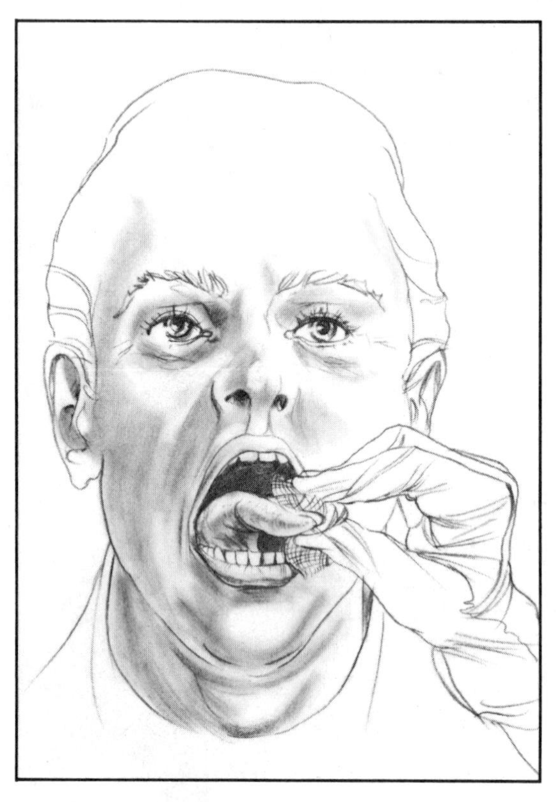

Tongue palpation
To palpate the tongue, grasp it with a 4″ x 4″ gauze pad and move it from side to side while examining the lateral borders. The tongue should be slightly rough and freely movable. It should be intact.

the pillars (the supporting structures of the soft palate); +1, that the tonsils are peaking from the pillars; +2, that the tonsils are between the pillars and the uvula; +3, that the tonsils are touching the uvula; and +4, that one or both tonsils are extending to the midline of the oropharynx.

Inspect the maxillary mucobuccal fold (the membrane that attaches the upper lip to the gingivae) and the labial frenulum (the membrane that attaches the lower lip to the gingivae) for irritation or signs of inflammation.

Palpate the upper and lower lips and the tongue to evaluate muscle tone and surface structure. (For an illustrated procedure, see *Palpating the lips and tongue.*) As you move the lips and tongue during palpation, inspect any areas of the gingivae that were not examined earlier.

Examine the oropharynx, using a tongue depressor and a flashlight, if necessary. Observe the position, size, and overall appearance of the uvula and the tonsils. Then, place the tongue depressor firmly on the midpoint of the tongue, almost far enough back to elicit the gag reflex, and ask the client to say "ah." The soft palate and uvula should rise symmetrically.

The last step of the basic mouth and oropharynx assessment involves evaluating the gag reflex. With the tongue depressor, gently touch the posterior aspect of the tongue. (*Note:* Use this technique cautiously in a client with nausea; it may induce vomiting.) Gagging during this maneuver indicates that cranial nerves IX and X (the glossopharyngeal and vagus nerves) are intact.

Abnormal findings

An unusual breath odor may indicate a serious systemic disorder. For example, an ammonia breath odor may be caused by chronic renal failure; a fecal breath odor, by a GI obstruction or disorder; and a fruity breath odor, by diabetic or starvation ketoacidosis.

Abnormalities of the oral mucosa may point to various disorders. Reddened mucosa often results from infection; cyanotic mucosa may indicate hypoxia (oxygen deficiency). Pale mucous membranes may indicate anemia. Mucous membrane ulcers may be related to inadequate nutrition or infection. Small areas of white scar tissue may indicate chronic irritation from friction of irregular tooth surfaces or from biting the mucous membrane while chewing. Leukoplakia, a thickened white patch on the buccal membrane, may be precancerous. Inflammation of the mucobuccal fold or labial frenulum can be caused by ill-fitting dentures. Inflamed or painful Stensen's duct openings may indicate parotid gland infection.

Marginal redness, retraction, swelling, or bleeding of the gingivae may be signs of gingivitis. Absent or broken teeth, cavities, or malocclusion (improper alignment of the upper and lower teeth) can cause chewing difficulties, tooth discoloration, or bruxism. Worn and flattened tooth edges may indicate bruxism.

Lips that are asymmetrical, cracked, fissured, or bleeding may suggest cheilitis. Abnormally pale lips may indicate that the client is cold; cyanotic lips may indicate coldness or hypoxia. Lip dryness and cracking may accompany a febrile illness, although cracking, especially at the corners of the lips, may also occur from vitamin B_6 deficiency or improper hygiene. Inflammation and lumps in the submaxillary glands may indicate stones or cysts.

On the tongue, a smooth dorsal surface, beefy red color, white coating, or patches on the anterior surface suggest an infection. Deviation of the tongue to one side may indicate a problem with cranial nerve XII. Nodules or ulcers, especially on the base of the tongue, may be cancerous.

Note decreased or absent gag reflex, which suggests possible neurologic dysfunction and increases the client's risk of aspiration. Deviation of the uvula to one side when the client says "ah" could indicate pathology of cranial nerve IX or X. Record the direction and extent of any deviation.

Examining the neck

For this part of the physical assessment, the nurse should follow these steps:

Begin by inspecting the skin for lesions and by palpating for masses along the chains of lymph nodes. (For further information, see Chapter 19, Immune System and Blood, and Chapter 20, Endocrine System.) Also observe the major neck vessel area, looking for jugular vein distention and visible pulsations in the carotid and jugular veins. (For more information, see Chapter 11, Cardiovascular System.) The neck should be free of masses, lymph node enlargement, or venous distention.

Next, check the neck muscles for strength and symmetry. Have the client move the neck through its entire range of motion, including extension, flexion, and lateral bending; it should be supple, moving easily and without discomfort. (For more information about the major neck muscles, see Chapter 18, Musculoskeletal System.)

Assessment of the underlying structures of the posterior neck, which houses the cervical vertebrae and the cervical spinal nerves, is especially important. To evaluate innervation of the neck, shoulder, and upper arm muscles, have the client slowly and carefully rotate the neck through the entire range of motion, then shrug the shoulders and lift the arms.

Inspect the midline of the neck for thyroid gland swelling. Then, carefully palpate the trachea. The cricoid cartilage (the uppermost ring of the trachea) will be palpable in the midline, just below the thyroid cartilage. To determine the position of the trachea, place your index finger or thumb along each side of the trachea and assess the space between the trachea and the sternocleidomastoid muscle. The space should be equal on each side; narrowing on either side indicates tracheal deviation to that side. A client with a short, thick, muscular neck is more difficult to examine; apply slightly more pressure during palpation.

To assess the ability to swallow, have the client sip from a glass of water with the head tipped back slightly. Normally, the larynx, trachea, and thyroid will rise with swallowing.

Palpate down the posterior neck over the bony prominences of the cervical vertebrae, checking for any tenderness. Then, palpate on either side of the bony prominences to assess alignment.

Using the bell of the stethoscope, auscultate over the major vessels in the neck, particularly the carotid arteries. Pay particular attention to any arteries that feel hard, ropelike, or tender on palpation. Normally, auscultation of these vessels detects no sounds.

Integrating assessment findings

Sometimes, a cluster of assessment findings will strongly suggest a particular head or neck disorder. In the chart below, column one shows groups of presenting signs and symptoms—the ones that make the client seek medical attention. Column two shows related assessment findings that the nurse may discover during the health history and physical assessment. The client may exhibit one or more of these findings. Column three shows the possible disorder indicated by a cluster of these findings.

PRESENTING SIGNS AND SYMPTOMS	RELATED ASSESSMENT FINDINGS	POSSIBLE DISORDER
In an infant, an enlarged head that the infant has difficulty holding upright; enlarged, tense fontanels and sunset eyes (downward eye position with the sclera visible above the irises); suture separation	Anterior fontanel above 6 cm in diameter Bulging fontanel Head circumference above 95th percentile and increasing weekly Sunset eyes Dilated scalp veins Glow throughout cranium on transillumination Ventricular enlargement on computed tomography scan	Hydrocephaly
Limited range of motion in neck, pain with movement, complaints of stress and tension	Limited range of motion in neck Pain on movement or palpation Palpable muscle tenseness and spasm Cervical spine changes on X-ray	Osteoporosis, arthritis, or ankylosing spondylitis
Inflamed, painful gingivae; usually no difficulty swallowing	Reddened or bleeding gingivae Change in normal gingival contours	Gingivitis
Tongue pain, dysphagia, difficulty speaking and chewing	Reddened, ulcerated, swollen tongue Swelling that may obstruct airway Tongue irritation, ill-fitting dentures, recent ingestion of spicy foods, or allergy to toothpaste or mouthwash	Glossitis

Abnormal findings

Neck pain and stiffness can result from many disorders, including trauma, cervical arthritis, and osteoporosis. If you detect tracheal deviation, consider the possibility of a neck or mediastinal tumor. Muscle spasm and tenderness result from simple tension in many cases, but may be caused by a neck injury that does not involve the vertebrae. Nuchal rigidity (severe muscle stiffness at the nape of the neck) is a characteristic symptom of meningitis. Bruits heard on auscultation of neck vessels may indicate atherosclerosis in an elderly client and cerebrovascular anomalies in a child. (For more information about selected common disorders and their associated findings, see *Integrating assessment findings.*)

Developmental considerations

To assess the head and neck of a child, pregnant woman, or elderly client, the nurse will need to modify some assessment techniques used to evaluate structures and will need to take into account certain developmental considerations. The following paragraphs provide guidelines for modified assessments.

Pediatric clients

To assess the head of a child under age 2, measure the head circumference and assess the fontanels. Head circumference measurements provide information about nutritional and growth disturbances. To measure circumference, wrap a nonstretchable tape measure around the widest part of the head and record the measurement in centimeters. Compare the measurement to the normal range for the child's age-group. (For information on this procedure, see *Measuring head circumference* in Chapter 6, Nutritional Status.) Note any abnormally large or small measurements, which may require further evaluation by a physician.

Assess the fontanels—particularly the large anterior fontanel—by inspecting and then gently palpating with the pads of the index and middle fingers. The fontanels should feel soft, yet firm, and appear almost flush with the scalp surface with slight visible pulsations. For the most accurate findings, examine the fontanels when the infant is quiet and seated upright. Pressure from postural changes or intense crying can cause the fontanels to bulge or seem abnormally tense. Also palpate the sutures; they should feel smooth and not override one another or feel separated.

When examining a neonate's head and face, remember that the shape may be altered by the molding that occurs during vaginal delivery or by premature closing of the sutures (craniosynostosis). Slight asymmetry of the head can occur when an infant always sleeps in one position. Instruct the parents or guardian to change the infant's position regularly to help prevent or correct this mild deformity.

Also be aware that congenital syndromes can alter a child's facial appearance. For example, a child with congenital hypothyroidism (cretinism) will have coarse facial features, a low hairline, and sparse eyebrows. Down's syndrome may be manifested by a small rounded head; prominent epicanthal folds; small, low-set ears; and oblique palpebral fissues.

Usually, the bridge of an infant's nose is slightly flattened. Because most infants under age 6 months breathe only through the nose, not through the mouth, assess airway patency by occluding one nostril at a time and evaluating airflow through the other nostril.

Count the teeth and compare the number to the normal range for the child's age-group.

In an infant, an unusually large or small tongue may indicate a congenital abnormality. Macroglossia (grossly enlarged tongue) may occur in cretinism, Down's syndrome, and other disorders. An enlarged, protruding tongue is frequently seen in mental retardation or cleft palate (a congenital defect characterized by a fissure in the middle of the palate). A tight frenulum is a congenital abnormality that prevents the child from touching the tip of the tongue to the upper lip.

Assess the oropharynx while the infant is crying. Evaluate the tonsils according to the child's developmental stage. Normal tonsils are small in the neonate, then increase in size until the child reaches adolescence, then shrink afterward. In an infant, raised white spots known as Epstein's pearls may normally occur along the gum line or on the hard palate. These spots usually disappear a few weeks after birth. Sucking lesions (small, papillae-like projections) are also normal on the buccal membranes of infants.

Light palpation of an infant's lips should elicit the sucking reflex. Very thin lips accompany some mental retardation syndromes. One or more fissures in the upper lip may indicate cleft lip, a congenital defect.

An infant's neck should move easily in all directions. However, the muscles are not sufficiently developed to enable an infant to turn the head from side to side until about age 2 weeks; to lift the head 90 degrees when prone until about age 2 months; or to hold the head upright when seated until about age 3 months. Both infants and young children normally have very short necks.

Pregnant clients

Many women past 16 weeks of gestation develop a blotchy, brownish hyperpigmentation of the face, especially on the forehead and cheeks. This pigmentation characterizes melasma, the "mask of pregnancy," a cosmetically bothersome but otherwise benign skin disorder. Slight gingival swelling may also be normal during pregnancy.

Elderly clients

Typically, an elderly client's face is wrinkled because of an overall reduction in subcutaneous fat. This fat loss may also make the nose seem more prominent or the bony ridges over the brow more noticeable. Sometimes in a thin elderly client, the temporal artery may be visible under the forehead skin. The technique for auscultating it, however, can remain the same.

An elderly client usually exhibits some gingival recession and may have loose teeth and gingival inflammation. With aging, salivary output decreases. This may cause dryness of the mucous membranes, which may interfere with chewing and make the membranes more susceptible to breakdown. Longitudinal or latitudinal fissures in the tongue can also occur with aging.

Many elderly clients experience decreased range of motion or neck pain from osteoporosis, arthritis, or other disorders. When assessing range of motion in such a client, instruct the client to move slowly and carefully to avoid pain.

Documentation

To understand the significance of the assessment findings and form a clear picture of a client's health status, the nurse should carefully review the physical assessment information about the client's head, face, nose, sinuses, mouth, oropharynx, and neck, as well as the health history findings.

Based on this information, the nurse can formulate appropriate nursing diagnoses, which determine how to plan, implement, and evaluate subsequent nursing care. (For a case study that shows how to apply the nursing

Applying the nursing process

Assessment findings form the basis of the nursing process. Using them, the nurse formulates nursing diagnoses and develops appropriate planning, implementation, and evaluation of the client's care.

The table below shows how the nurse can use head and neck assessment data in the nursing process for the client described in the case history (shown at right). In the first column, history and physical data appear, followed by a paragraph of mental notes. These notes help the nurse make important mental connections among assessment findings, aiding in development of the nursing diagnoses and planning.

The second column presents several appropriate nursing diagnoses; however, the information in the remaining columns is based on the *first* nursing diagnosis. Because of its importance, documentation of the nursing process appears in the last column. Documentation consists of an initial note using all components of the SOAPIE format and a follow-up note using the appropriate SOAPIE components.

ASSESSMENT	NURSING DIAGNOSES	PLANNING	IMPLEMENTATION
Subjective (history) data • Client states, "My neck hurts whenever I nod or turn my head." • Pain wakes her at night. • Client has no history of fever or upper respiratory infection. • Client has no history of thyroid problems. • Client experiences no other discomfort or pain. • Client has not noticed any swelling in neck. • Client was passenger in car that was hit from behind 2 days ago when stopped at a stoplight. • Client did not strike dashboard or windshield. • Two aspirins t.i.d. do not relieve pain. **Objective (physical) data** • Client unable to perform range of motion due to pain. • Neck palpation reveals muscle spasm and pain with passive range of motion. • Remainder of head and neck examination normal. • Temperature 98.6° F. (37° C.). **Mental notes** *Severe muscle spasm will respond to warm compresses as well as medications. Need to provide instructions. Need to determine if Ms. Wilson is open to relaxation techniques to relax muscles and relieve spasm. If so, teach her.*	• Knowledge deficit related to cause and self-care of neck symptoms. • Alteration in comfort related to muscle spasm. • Impaired physical mobility related to neck pain and muscle spasm.	**Goals** Before leaving the clinic today, the client will: • Obtain pain relief. • Be able to achieve self-care. • Learn when to see the physician. • Understand the physiologic reasons for pain. • Verbalize potential adverse reactions to over-the-counter analgesics.	• Teach Ms. Wilson why whiplash causes muscle spasm and neck pain. • Explain proper application of warm compresses to the neck t.i.d. • Instruct her to increase aspirin doses to 600 mg every 4 hours as prescribed. Discuss potential adverse reactions. • Instruct her to see the physician if her symptoms have not improved in 48 hours. • Advise her to use a cervical collar to support the neck and reduce pain. • Call her in 2 days to check her progress.

process to a client with a neck complaint, see *Applying the nursing process.*)

Proper documentation is an essential element in organizing assessment data and making it available to other members of the health care team. The nurse needs to document all data completely, including normal and abnormal findings.

The following illustrates the documentation of some normal physical findings in a head and neck assessment:

> Client observed with head held upright. Facial features are symmetrical. Facial skin appears pink and free of lesions. Palpation of head and face detects no lumps, lesions, or tenderness. Temporal artery pulses are equal bilaterally. Temporomandibular joint approximates. Auscultation of the vessels of the head reveals no bruits. The nose is

CASE HISTORY

Janet Wilson, age 26, comes to the outpatient clinic complaining of neck pain with any movement. Ms. Wilson grimaces in pain and holds her neck.

EVALUATION		DOCUMENTATION BASED ON NURSING PROCESS DATA		
By the end of the clinic visit, the client: • Verbalized self-care instructions. • Had no questions about the instructions. • Explained potential adverse reactions to aspirin therapy. During the follow-up phone call, the client: • Reported minimal pain and full range of motion.		**Initial**		**Follow-up**
	S	Client came to walk-in nursing clinic complaining of neck pain of 36-hour duration. Has not had fever or noticed "lumps" in neck. Was passenger in stopped car that was rear-ended by another car going 10 miles an hour. Client denies hitting dashboard or windshield.	**S**	Phone call—client states, "I still have a lot of pain. I can hardly turn my neck to the left. I've been taking the aspirin but now my stomach's upset and burning. I can't wear that collar."
	O	Range of motion severely limited because of pain. Unable to flex and rotate neck. Palpation reveals tenderness and muscle spasm with passive range of motion. Cervical vertebrae nonmovable with palpation. Temperature 98.6° F. (37° C.).	**O**	Neck pain increased and range of motion decreased. Gastric irritation from aspirin.
	A	Knowledge deficit related to cause and self-care of neck symptoms.	**P**	Client to return to clinic to see physician. Will continue warm compresses. Client to try buffered aspirin. Encourage again to wear cervical collar.
	P	Teach client about physiologic causes and proper self-care of neck symptoms.		
	I	Instructed client to apply warm compresses t.i.d. and to take 600 mg of aspirin every 4 hours. Recommended cervical collar. Will call in 48 hours for follow-up.		
	E	Client repeated aspirin dosage instructions and potential adverse reactions without difficulty. Understands need for physician evaluation if symptoms not reduced in 48 hours.		

symmetrical with no drainage from the nostrils; palpation shows no tenderness. Frontal and maxillary sinuses are not tender when palpated and percussed. Mucosa of the mouth and oropharynx are pink and moist; teeth are intact. Inspection and palpation of lips, gingivae, and tongue reveal no lesions or ulcerations. Neck is taut and firm; no tenderness elicited on palpation; range of motion normal.

The following illustrates the documentation of some abnormal physical findings in a head and neck assessment:

> Client observed with head bending slightly to the right with a droop of the right eye and right corner of the mouth. Palpation of the head and face reveals a tender, 1-cm lump under the left eye over the orbital bone. Temporal pulses are +1 on the right

and +2 on the left. Temporomandibular joint on the right side does not approximate. Auscultation of head vessels uncovers a bruit in the right temporal artery. The nose is symmetrical, but a cloudy discharge is noted from the nostrils. Palpation of the frontal and maxillary sinuses elicits tenderness. The tongue shifts slightly to the right on examination, but appears pink and moist. The gingivae are erythematous and edematous, and bleed slightly when palpated. Palpation of neck muscles detects tightness on the left side. Range of motion is severely limited because of pain; client cannot flex and rotate the neck. Palpation reveals tenderness and muscle spasm with passive range of motion.

Chapter summary

This chapter discusses anatomic, physiologic, and assessment norms of the head and neck structures, including the nose, sinuses, mouth, and oropharynx. Here are the highlights of this chapter:

- The eight bones of the cranium are joined by immobile joints called sutures. These bones, together with the 14 bones of the face, protect and support the brain, eyes, and other structures. The sinuses are hollow structures within the facial bones. The nose is composed of bone and cartilage. The mouth includes the lips, tongue, mucosa, gingivae, teeth, and salivary glands.
- The neck is held erect by the sternocleidomastoid muscle, trapezius muscle, ligaments, and the cervical vertebrae. These structures form the anterior and posterior triangles, which are assessment landmarks.
- During a nursing assessment of the head and neck, the nurse uses health history questions that evaluate the client's health and illness patterns. These questions focus on head and neck injuries, fractures, surgery, swelling, infections, range of motion, nasal discharge, mouth lesions, swallowing, chewing, voice changes, nosebleeds, and allergies.
- To assess health promotion and protection patterns, the nurse asks questions that uncover information about smoking, headache relief, neck tightness relief, occupational stresses, risk of head injury, and mouth care patterns.
- To assess role and relationship patterns, the nurse asks questions that uncover the effects of a head or neck problem on the client's self-concept, family relationships, and activities of daily living.
- The nurse begins the basic assessment with inspection and palpation of the head and face, followed by auscultation of the vessels in the head; inspection and palpation of the nose; inspection, palpation, and percussion of the frontal and maxillary sinuses; inspection of the mouth (including the lips, tongue, mucosa, gingivae, teeth, and salivary glands) and oropharynx; palpation of the lips and tongue; inspection and palpation of the neck; and auscultation of the carotid arteries.
- To perform a basic head and neck assessment in a child, the nurse includes two additional steps: palpation of the fontanels and measurement of head circumference. Normal findings can vary greatly between adults and children, especially in dentition, tonsil size, and breathing patterns. Pregnant and elderly clients may also exhibit differences in normal findings.
- The nurse applies advanced assessment skills as needed. These include direct inspection of the nostrils by flashlight and nasal speculum or by ophthalmoscope handle with nasal attachment, illumination of the septum, and transillumination of the sinuses with a flashlight or an ophthalmoscope handle with transillumination head.
- The nurse documents all assessment findings and uses them in the nursing process to plan and evaluate the client's care.

Study questions

1. The head and neck contain various anatomic structures. What are these structures and which techniques can you use to assess them?

2. For a client with a head or neck problem, which health history questions are the most important to ask? Why?

3. A child's head and neck differ greatly from those of an elderly client. What differences in physical assessment findings can you expect to see?

4. Janet Gray, age 68, comes to the outpatient clinic complaining of chronic neck pain that she has had for 2 months. She has no history of fever or recent injury. How would you report the following information related to your nursing assessment of Ms. Gray?
- history (subjective) assessment data
- physical (objective) assessment data
- assessment techniques and equipment
- two nursing diagnoses
- documentation of findings.

5. Lisa Nelson, age 5, is brought to the emergency department by her mother. Lisa complains of a sore throat, and her mother says she has had a fever of 102° to 103° F. for the past 24 hours. Lisa has been reluctant to eat or drink because of her sore throat. How would you report the following information related to your nursing assessment of Lisa?
- history (subjective) assessment data
- physical (objective) assessment data
- assessment techniques and equipment
- two nursing diagnoses
- documentation of findings.

Selected references

Bowers, A., and Thompson, J. (1992). *Clinical manual of health assessment* (4th ed.). St. Louis: Mosby-Year Book.

DiIorio, C., and Price, M. (1990). Swallowing: An assessment guide. *AJN,* 90(7), 38-41.

Dornbrand, L., Hoole, A., Fletcher, R., and Picard, C. (Eds.). (1985). *Manual of clinical problems in adult ambulatory care.* Boston: Little, Brown.

Dychtwald, K. (1986). *Wellness and health promotion for the elderly.* Rockville, MD: Aspen Systems.

Isaacs, J. (1988). Differentiating neck masses. *Emergency Medicine,* 20(18), 59-61, 64, 67, 69.

Jones, D., Lepley, M., and Baker, B. (Eds.) (1984). *Health assessment across the lifespan.* St. Louis: Mosby-Year Book.

McEvoy, G. (Ed.). (1992). *American Hospital Formulary Service drug information.* Bethesda, MD: American Society of Hospital Pharmacists.

Murray, R., and Zentner, J. (1985). *Nursing concepts for health promotion* (3rd ed.). Englewood Cliffs, NJ: Prentice-Hall.

Pinnell, N., and Meneses, M. (1986). *The nursing process theory: Application and related processes.* East Norwalk, CT: Appleton & Lange.

Wong, D., and Whaley, L. (1990). *Clinical handbook of pediatric nursing* (3rd ed.). St. Louis: Mosby.

Nursing research

Braun, B., and Amundson, L. (1989). Quantitative assessment of head and shoulder posture. *Archives of Physical Medicine and Rehabilitation,* 70(4), 322-329.

Budreau, G. (1989). The perceived attractiveness of preterm infants with cranial molding. *JOGNN,* 18(1), 38-44.

Dewan, N., et al. (1990). Smell and taste function in subjects with chronic obstructive pulmonary disease: Effect of long-term oxygen via nasal cannulas. *Chest,* 97(3), 595-599.

Niehaus, C., Meiller, T., and Peterson, D. (1987). Oral complications in children during cancer therapy. *Cancer Nursing,* 10(1), 15-20.

Pople, J., and Oliver, D. (1986). Oral thrush in hospice patients. *Nursing Times,* 82(45), 34-35.

Winn, D., and Pickle, L. (1986). Smoking tobacco and cancer in women: Implications for cancer research. *Women's Health,* 11(3/4), 253-266.

9

Eyes and Ears

Objectives

After reading and studying this chapter, you should be able to:

1. Describe the components of the internal and external eye.
2. Describe the physiology of vision.
3. Demonstrate the five acuity tests performed for vision testing.
4. Explain how vision testing for children under age 7 differs from that for adults.
5. Compare common eye assessment findings for an elderly client with those for a young adult.
6. Demonstrate how to assess the external and internal eye of an adult and a child.
7. Discuss possible adverse effects of drugs on vision.
8. Explain the function of the structures of the external, middle, and inner ear.
9. Describe the physiology of hearing.
10. Demonstrate how to assess the external and internal ear of an adult and a child.
11. Discuss possible adverse effects of drugs on hearing.
12. Use the nursing process to document assessment findings for a client with a common eye or ear ailment.

Introduction

Although the eyes and ears differ in structure and function, they share several important features. For example, they are two of the main sources of perception, responsible for the senses of sight and hearing. They usually are assessed sequentially. Because of their proximity, the ears usually are examined immediately after the eyes in the complete physical assessment. However, in a child under age 5, the eyes and ears are usually examined last. In addition, the eyes and ears may be evaluated with similar techniques: screening tests (for vision or hearing), inspection, palpation, and advanced assessment skills (using an ophthalmoscope or an otoscope).

Clients with an inflamed or injured eye, a foreign body in the eye, or an earache can be any age and usually are not acutely ill. However, eye and ear disorders can signal a serious neurologic problem, such as a brain tumor or an acoustic nerve (cranial nerve VIII) damaged by an adverse drug reaction. Regardless of the cause, the nurse should keep in mind that, because vision and hearing are vital, a client may be especially anxious about an eye or ear disorder.

This chapter reviews the anatomy and physiology of the eye and discusses how to obtain a pertinent health history of the client's problem and past health. The chapter describes how to perform a systematic physical assessment of the eye, beginning with screenings of vision, color perception, and extraocular muscle function and proceeding to inspection and palpation. It discusses differences in assessment procedures for children, adults, and elderly clients and allows for ethnic considerations. The chapter presents normal and abnormal findings and discusses the use of the ophthalmoscope.

This chapter presents similar information about the anatomy and physiology of the ear and includes pertinent health history questions for a client with an ear disorder. The physical assessment of the ear highlights inspection, palpation, hearing screening, and otoscopic examination.

Glossary

Accommodation reflex: adjustment of the eyes for near vision, consisting of pupillary constriction, convergence of the eyes, and increased convexity of the lens.

Amblyopia: reduced vision in an eye that appears structurally normal during ophthalmoscopic examination.

Aqueous humor: watery, clear fluid circulating in the anterior and posterior chambers of the eye.

Astigmatism: abnormal eye condition in which a light ray does not focus clearly on the retina, but rather spreads over a diffuse area. Astigmatism occurs when the curve of the cornea or lens is not even in all parts. It causes blurred vision and discomfort during close eye work.

Cataract: abnormal, progressive loss of lens transparency in the eye. Most cataracts result from degenerative changes that occur after age 50.

Conductive hearing loss: hearing loss caused by blockage of sound waves from the external to the middle or inner ear. It may result from a cerumen obstruction, middle ear inflammation, or sclerosis of the ear bones.

Consensual reaction: reflex stimulation of one body side or part resulting from the stimulation of the opposite side or another body part. For example, a consensual reaction to light occurs when the client's right pupil constricts when the nurse illuminates the left pupil.

Diplopia: double vision caused by defective functioning of the extraocular muscles or by a disorder of the nerves that innervate the muscles.

Esotropia: form of strabismus (misalignment of the axis of the eye) characterized by an inward deviation of one eye relative to the other eye. Also called convergent strabismus.

Exophthalmos: abnormal protrusion of one or both eyeballs caused by trauma, intracranial lesions, intraorbital disorders, or systemic disease such as hyperthyroidism.

Exotropia: form of strabismus (misalignment of the axis of the eye) characterized by the outward deviation of one eye relative to the other eye. Also called divergent strabismus.

Glaucoma: abnormal condition of elevated intraocular pressure caused by obstruction of the outflow of aqueous humor. In acute (closed-angle) glaucoma, the angle narrows between the iris and cornea, and the pupil dilates markedly. The iris folds and blocks the exit of aqueous humor from the anterior chamber. In chronic (open-angle) glaucoma, the pressure builds slowly, with the obstruction probably in Schlemm's canal.

Hordeolum: purulent infection of the meibomian (sebaceous) glands of the eyelid, often caused by a staphylococcal infection. Also called a stye.

Hyperopia: refractive error causing the light rays entering the eye to focus behind the retina. Also called farsightedness.

Miosis: contraction of the sphincter muscle of the iris, causing the pupil to constrict. Stimulation of the pupillary light reflex, or certain drugs such as morphine sulfate, cause miosis.

Mixed hearing loss: hearing loss caused by a combination of conductive and sensorineural hearing disorders.

Mydriasis: pupil dilation caused by contraction of the dilator muscle of the iris. Certain drugs, such as atropine sulfate, cause mydriasis.

Myopia: refractive error resulting from eyeball elongation, which causes light rays entering the eye parallel to the optic axis to focus in front of the retina. Also called nearsightedness.

Papilledema: optic disk swelling visible during ophthalmoscopic examination. Increased intracranial pressure, malignant hypertension, or thrombosis of the central retinal vein all cause papilledema.

Presbyopia: vision defect caused by a loss of elasticity in the lens of the eye. Also called farsightedness, presbyopia commonly develops with aging.

Sensorineural hearing loss: hearing loss caused by damage to inner ear structures, such as the organ of Corti, or by damage to cranial nerve VIII (the acoustic nerve). Also called nerve deafness.

Tinnitus: ringing or tinkling sound in one or both ears. Tinnitus may be caused by trauma, inner ear disease, ossification of the bones of the inner ear, aging, or cerumen pressing on the tympanic membrane or occluding the external auditory canal.

Vertigo: sensation of movement of self or surroundings, caused by disease of the inner ear or the vestibular branch of the acoustic nerve.

Anatomy and physiology review: The eye

The eye is the sensory organ of sight that transmits visual images to the brain for interpretation. The eyeball is about 1″ (2.5 cm) in diameter and occupies the bony orbit, a skull cavity formed anteriorly by the frontal, maxillary, zygomatic, acromial, sphenoid, ethmoid, and palatine bones. Nerves, adipose tissue, and blood vessels cushion and nourish the eye posteriorly.

Extraocular (external) and intraocular (internal) structures form the eye, and extraocular muscles and nerves control it.

Extraocular muscles and structures

The extraocular muscles and structures work together to support and protect the eyes.

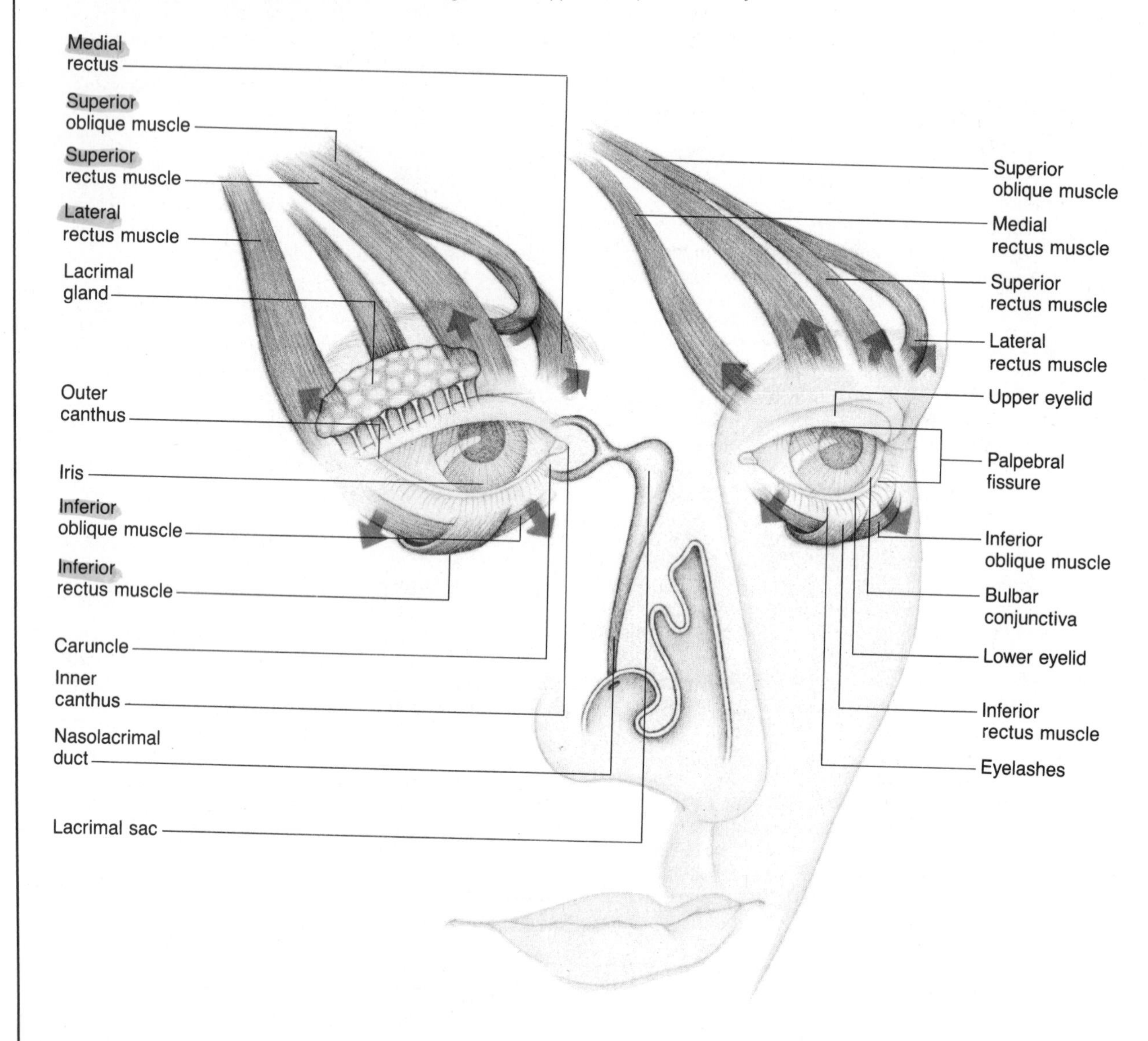

Extraocular muscles

By functioning together, the extraocular muscles hold both eyes parallel and create binocular vision (both eyes directed at the same object at the same time). The superior and inferior rectus muscles move the eye up and down on a transverse axis; the medial and lateral rectus muscles move the eye toward the nose and toward the temple on an anteroposterior axis; and the superior and inferior oblique muscles move the eye to the right and left on a vertical axis.

Extraocular structures

The eyelids, conjunctivae, and lacrimal apparatus form the extraocular structures of the eye.

Eyelids

Also called palpebrae, the eyelids are loose folds of skin covering the anterior eye. The eyelids protect the eye from foreign bodies, regulate the entrance of light, and distribute tears over the eye by blinking. The lid margins contain hair follicles, which in turn contain eyelashes and sebaceous glands. When closed, the upper and lower eyelids cover the eye completely. When open, the upper eyelid extends beyond the limbus (the junction of the cornea and the sclera) and covers a small portion of the iris. The lower lid margin lies even with, or just below, the limbus. The palpebral fissure, which is the distance between the lid margins, should be equal in both eyes.

Conjunctivae

Serving to protect the eye from foreign bodies, the conjunctivae are clear, transparent membranes, continuous with the skin. The palpebral conjunctiva lines the highly vascular eyelids and therefore appears shiny pink or red. The bulbar conjunctiva, which contains many small blood vessels, joins the palpebral portion and loosely covers the sclera. At the limbus, the bulbar conjunctiva merges with the corneal epithelium.

A small, fleshy elevation called the caruncle sits at the nasal corner of the conjunctivae. Along the border of thick connective tissue at the free edge of the eyelid is the tarsal plate, containing meibomian glands in vertical columns, which create the appearance of light yellow streaks. These glands secrete sebum (composed of keratin, fat, and cellular debris) onto the posterior lid margins to retain tears and keep the eye lubricated.

Lacrimal apparatus

Composed of lacrimal glands, the punctum, the lacrimal sac, and the nasolacrimal duct, the lacrimal apparatus lubricates and protects the cornea and the conjunctivae by producing and absorbing tears.

Located anterior and lateral to the eye, the lacrimal glands secrete tears to cleanse and moisten the eye's surface. After washing across the eyeball, the tears drain through the punctum. The punctum, which is the only visible portion of the lacrimal apparatus, is a tiny opening at the medial junction of the upper and lower eyelids. From there, the tears flow through the lacrimal canals into the lacrimal sac, which sits in a groove in the lacrimal bone in the medial part of the orbit. They then drain through the nasolacrimal duct and into the nose.

Extraocular nerves, muscles, and structures

Six cranial nerves—the optic (II), oculomotor (III), trochlear (IV), trigeminal (V), abducens (VI), and facial (VII)—innervate the eye, the ocular muscles, and the lacrimal apparatus. (For a discussion of cranial nerves, see Chapter 17, Nervous System.)

The coordinated action of six eye muscles—the superior, inferior, medial, and lateral rectus muscles, and the superior and inferior oblique muscles—controls eye movement. Extraocular structures—the eyelids, conjunctivae, and lacrimal apparatus—protect and lubricate the eye. (For more information and an illustration, see *Extraocular muscles and structures.*)

Intraocular structures

The nurse can easily view several anterior intraocular structures, including the sclera, cornea, anterior chamber, iris, and pupil. Some intraocular structures are visible only with the use of an ophthalmoscope or other instrument. These include the lens, the posterior chamber, the ciliary body, the vitreous humor, and the three layers of the eyeball: the posterior sclera, the choroid, and the retina.

The retina is the innermost layer of the eyeball and contains neural tissue to receive visual images. The reddish-orange color of the retina results from its deep pigment layers and extensive vascular supply. The color varies with the client's complexion.

Ophthalmoscopic (funduscopic) examination of the posterior portion of the eye (the fundus) allows the nurse to view the retinal blood vessels, the optic disk, the physiologic cup of the optic disk, the macula, and the fovea centralis. (For an illustration, see *Intraocular structures,* pages 210 and 211.)

Physiology of vision

Every object reflects light. For an individual to perceive an object clearly, the reflected light must pass through the intraocular structures, including the cornea, anterior chamber, pupil, lens, and vitreous humor. The retina focuses the light into an upside-down and reversed image. This stimulates nerve impulses to travel from the retina through the optic nerve and optic tract to the visual cortex of the occipital lobe, which then interprets the image. (For an illustration, see *The vision pathway,* page 212.)

Intraocular structures

The nurse can view some intraocular structures, such as the sclera, cornea, iris, pupil, and anterior chamber, through inspection. However, others, such as the retina, must be seen through an ophthalmoscope.

Sclera and cornea

The white sclera coats the outside of the eyeball, maintaining its size and form. The cornea replaces the sclera over the pupil and the iris. The cornea is a smooth, avascular, transparent tissue merging with the bulbar conjunctiva at the limbus. Kept moist by tears, the cornea is very sensitive to touch (mediated by the ophthalmic branch of cranial nerve V, the trigeminal nerve).

Iris, pupil, and anterior chamber

The iris is a circular contractile disk containing smooth and radial muscles and perforated in the center by the pupil. Numerous smooth muscle fibers varying in color compose the surface of the iris, giving the eye its color.

Pupils should be equal and round and, depending on the client's age, from 3 to 7 mm in diameter. Infants have small pupils that become larger during childhood and then progressively decrease throughout adulthood and into old age. The posterior portion of the iris contains involuntary dilator and sphincter muscles that regulate light entry by controlling pupil size.

The anterior chamber is filled with a clear, watery fluid called aqueous humor. This fluid drains away from the anterior chamber through the canal of Schlemm.

Lens and ciliary body

Located directly behind the iris at the pupillary opening, the lens of the eye acts like a camera lens, refracting and focusing light onto the retina. The lens, composed of transparent fibers in an elastic membrane called the lens capsule, contains no blood vessels, nerves, or connective tissue. The ciliary body (the thickened part of the vascular coat of the eye that joins the iris and choroid) controls the lens thickness and, together with the coordinated action of the muscles in the iris, regulates the light focused through the lens onto the retina.

Posterior chamber

This small space directly posterior to the iris but anterior to the lens is filled with aqueous humor.

Vitreous humor

Consisting of a thick, gelatinous material, the vitreous humor fills the space behind the lens. There, it maintains the placement of the retina and the spherical shape of the eyeball.

Posterior sclera and choroid

A white, opaque, fibrous layer, the posterior sclera covers the posterior five sixths of the eyeball, continues back to the dural sheath, and covers the optic nerve. The choroid, which lines the recessed portion of the eyeball beneath the sclera, contains many small arteries and veins.

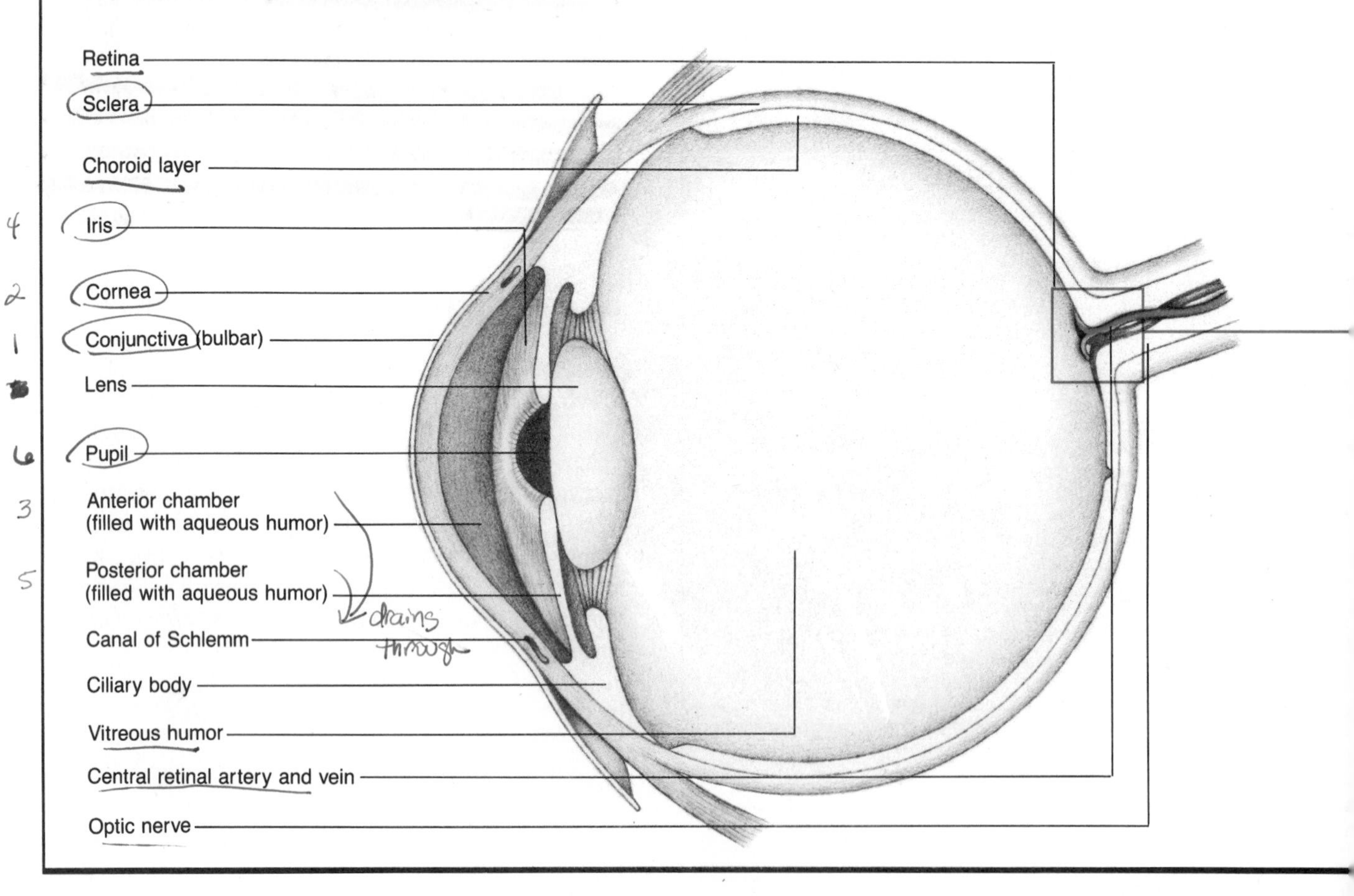

Retina

The innermost coat of the eyeball, the retina's main function is to receive visual stimuli and send them to the brain. Each of the four sets of retinal vessels, visible through an ophthalmoscope, contains a transparent arteriole and vein. The arterioles are 25% smaller than the veins and brighter in color. Arterioles and veins become progressively thinner as they leave the optic disk, intertwining as they extend to the periphery of the retina. Each set of vessels supplies a particular quadrant of the retina: superonasal, inferonasal, inferotemporal, and superotemporal.

The optic disk is a well-defined, 1.5-mm round or oval area within the nasal portion of the retina. The yellow to creamy pink disk allows the optic nerve to enter the retina at a point called the nerve head. A whitish to grayish crescent of scleral tissue may be present on the lateral side of the disk.

The physiologic cup is a light-colored depression within the optic disk on the temporal side. The cup covers one quarter to one third of the disk but does not extend completely to the margin.

Photoreceptor neurons called rods and cones compose the visual receptors of the retina. These receptors, which are not visible through an ophthalmoscope, allow for color vision. The rods, concentrated toward the periphery of the retina, respond to low-intensity light and shades of gray, and the cones, concentrated in the fovea centralis, respond to bright light and color.

Located laterally to the optic disk is the macula, which is slightly darker than the rest of the retina and without visible retinal vessels. Because its borders are poorly defined, the macula is difficult to see.

The fovea centralis, a slight depression in the center of the macula, appears as a bright reflection in ophthalmoscopic examination. Because the fovea contains the heaviest concentration of cones, it is a main receiver of vision and color.

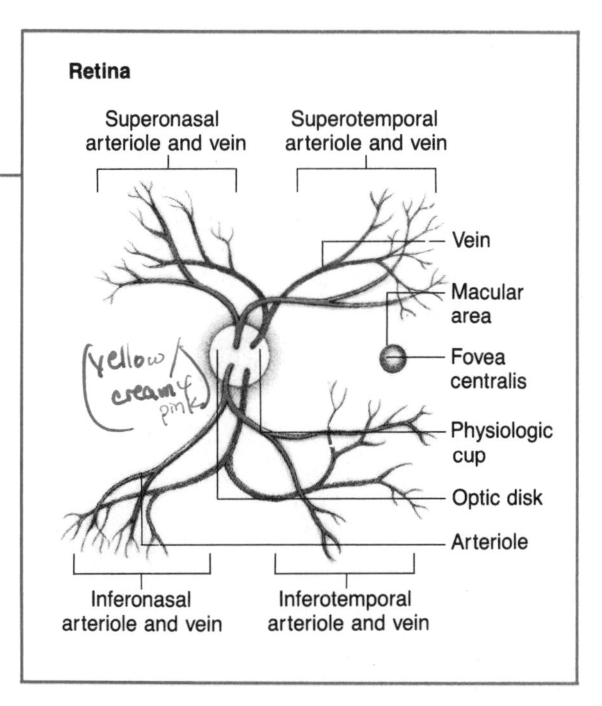

Health history: The eye

To obtain an accurate and complete health history, adjust questions to the client's specific complaint and compare the answers with the results of the physical assessment. In the case of a well client, ask more general history questions about the eye.

Further modify questions according to the client's age—for example, by asking a child if the writing on the school chalkboard is readable or by asking an elderly client about peripheral vision, visual acuity, problems with glare, glaucoma testing, and the functioning of the lacrimal glands.

The questions in this section are designed to help you evaluate the client's eyes fully. They include rationales that describe the significance of the answers and, where appropriate, nursing interventions that may be incorporated into the client's care plan.

Health and illness patterns

To assess important health and illness patterns, use the following guidelines to explore the client's current, past, and family health status, as well as the developmental status.

Current health status

Begin the interview by asking about the client's current eye health status. Carefully document the chief complaint in the client's own words. Using the PQRST method, question the client for a complete description of this problem and any others. (For a detailed explanation of this method, see *Symptom analysis* in Chapter 3, The Health History.)

During the interview, observe the client's eye movements and focusing ability for clues to visual acuity and eye muscle coordination. To investigate further, ask the following questions about eye function.

Do you have any problems with your eyes?

(RATIONALE: Besides indicating visual disturbances, problems with the eyes can indicate other conditions, such as diabetes, hypertension, or neurologic disorders.)

Do you wear or have you ever worn corrective lenses? If so, for how long?

(RATIONALE: This establishes how long the client has had a vision disorder and informs the nurse of the client's need to wear corrective lenses during the visual acuity check.)

The vision pathway

Intraocular structures perceive and form images and send them along the vision pathway to the brain for interpretation. To interpret these images properly, the brain relies on vision pathway structures to create the proper visual fields.

Image perception and formation

Normally, the cornea, aqueous humor, lens, and vitreous humor refract light rays from an object, focusing them on the fovea of the retina, where an inverted and reversed image clearly forms. Within the retina, rods and cones turn the projected image into an impulse and transmit it to the optic nerve. The impulse travels to the optic chiasm where the two optic nerves unite, split again into two optic tracts, and then continue into the optic section of the cerebral cortex. There, the inverted and reversed image on the retina changes back to its original form.

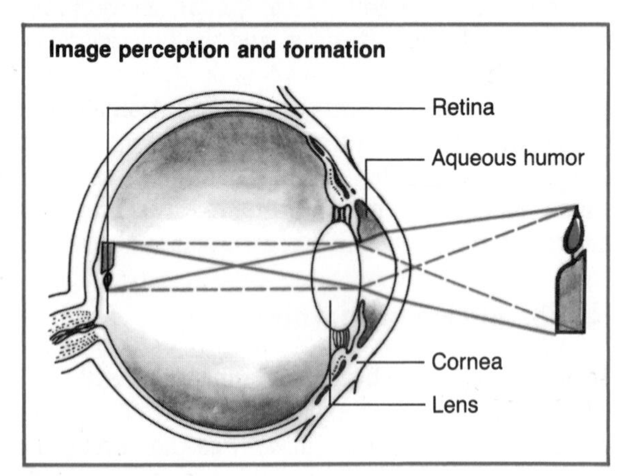

Visual fields

In the optic chiasm, fibers from the nasal aspects of both retinas cross to opposite sides, and fibers from the temporal portions remain uncrossed. Both crossed and uncrossed fibers form the optic tracts. Injury to one of the optic nerves can cause blindness in the corresponding eye; an injury or lesion in the optic chiasm can cause partial vision loss (for example, loss of the two temporal visual fields).

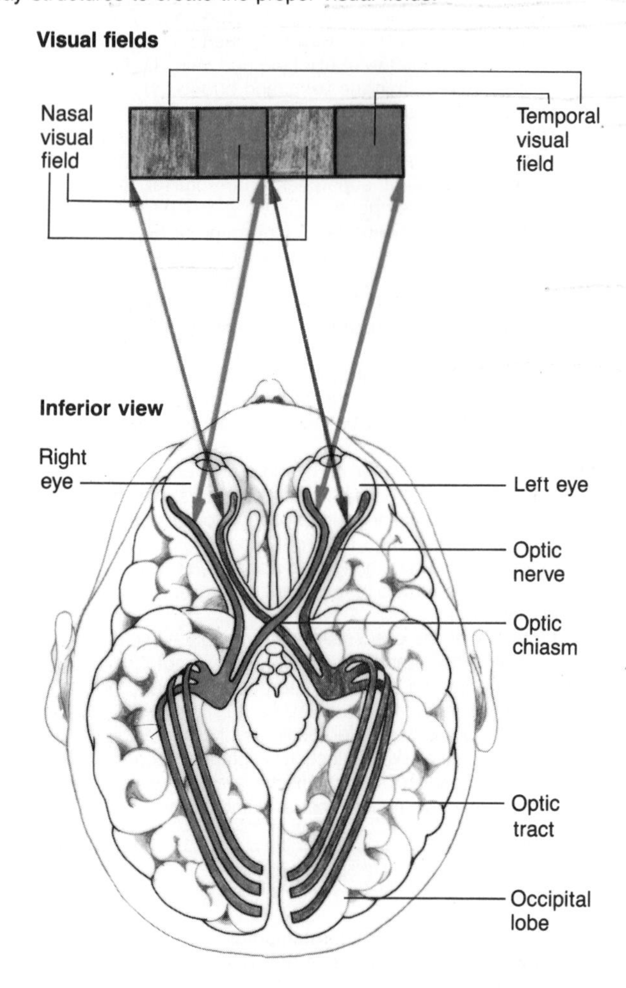

If you wear corrective lenses, are they glasses or hard or soft contact lenses?
(RATIONALE: Improperly fitted contact lenses or prolonged wearing of contact lenses can cause eye inflammation and corneal abrasions. Wearers of soft lenses are especially vulnerable to conjunctival inflammation and infection because the lenses, worn for long periods of time, can irritate the eye.)

For what eye condition do you wear corrective lenses?
(RATIONALE: Besides providing information about any existing eye condition, the answer allows the nurse to adjust the diopters for ophthalmoscopic examination of nearsightedness or farsightedness.)

If you wear corrective lenses, do you wear them all the time or just for certain activities, such as reading or driving?
(RATIONALE: The answer provides information about the severity and type of visual disturbance.)

If you once wore corrective lenses and have stopped wearing them, why and when did you stop?
(RATIONALE: Eyestrain or excessive tearing may occur if the client is not wearing necessary lenses.)

Past health status

During the next part of the health history, ask the following questions to gather additional information about the client's eyes.

When did you last have your lenses changed?
(RATIONALE: A recent lens change with continued visual disturbances could indicate an underlying health problem, such as a brain tumor.)

Have you ever had blurred vision?
(RATIONALE: Blurred vision can indicate a need for corrective lenses or suggest a neurologic disorder, such as a brain tumor, or an endocrine disorder, such as diabetic retinopathy.)

Have you ever seen spots or floaters, or halos around lights? If yes, is this a sudden change or has it occurred for a while?
(RATIONALE: The sudden appearance of spots, floaters, or halos may indicate a retinal detachment or glaucoma. Chronic appearance of spots or floaters is a common normal occurrence in elderly and myopic clients.)

Do you suffer from frequent eye infections or inflammation?
(RATIONALE: Frequent infections or inflammation can indicate low resistance to infection, eyestrain, allergies, or occupational or environmental exposure to an irritant.)

Have you ever had eye surgery?
(RATIONALE: A history of eye surgery may indicate glaucoma, cataracts, or injuries—such as detached retina—that may appear as abnormalities on ophthalmoscopic examination.)

Have you ever had an eye injury?
(RATIONALE: Injuries, such as from a penetrating foreign body, can distort the ophthalmoscopic examination.)

Do you often have styes?
(RATIONALE: Styes [hordeolums], infected meibomian or zeisian glands, tend to recur.)

Do you have a history of high blood pressure?
(RATIONALE: High blood pressure can cause arteriosclerosis of the retinal blood vessels and visual disturbances.)

Do you have a history of diabetes?
(RATIONALE: Diabetes causes noninflammatory changes in the retina [retinopathy] that can lead to blindness.)

Are you currently taking any prescription medications for your eyes? If so, which medications and how often?
(RATIONALE: Prescription eye medications should alert the nurse to an eye disorder. For example, a client who is taking pilocarpine probably has glaucoma.)

What other medications are you taking, including prescription drugs, over-the-counter (OTC) *medications, and home remedies?*
(RATIONALE: Certain medications can cause visual disturbances. For more information, see *Adverse drug reactions,* pages 214 and 215.)

Family health status

Next, investigate the eye health of the client's family by asking the following question.

Has anyone in your family ever been treated for cataracts, glaucoma, or blindness?
(RATIONALE: These conditions have a familial tendency.)

Developmental considerations

For pediatric and elderly clients, be sure to investigate developmental status by exploring additional areas of the health history.

Pediatric client. When assessing a child who is old enough to participate, include the child along with the parent or guardian in the interview by using age-appropriate words. For an infant, gather information about visual acuity and eye muscle coordination by observing the steadiness of the infant's gaze at the parent's face or nearby objects.

For additional information about the child's developmental status, ask the following questions:

Does your infant gaze at you or other objects and blink at bright lights or quick, nearby movements?
(RATIONALE: Failure to gaze and blink appropriately could indicate impaired vision.)

Are the child's eyes ever crossed or do both eyes ever move in different directions?
(RATIONALE: These abnormal movements suggest impaired eye muscle coordination.)

Does the child often rub his eyes?
(RATIONALE: Frequent rubbing could indicate visual disturbances or eye inflammation.)

Does the child squint frequently?
(RATIONALE: Squinting implies visual disturbances, such as farsightedness or light sensitivity.)

Does the child often bump into, or have difficulty picking up, objects?
(RATIONALE: A positive response indicates astigmatism. Astigmatism distorts or blurs vision because of an irregularly shaped lens.)

Adverse drug reactions

When assessing a client's eye, the nurse should ask the client about current drug use. Many drugs can cause adverse effects that can mimic signs or symptoms of various diseases or damage the eye, resulting in optic neuritis or other ocular problems.

DRUG CLASS	DRUG	POSSIBLE ADVERSE REACTIONS
Aminoglycosides	All aminoglycosides	Optic neuritis with blurred vision, scotomas (areas of depressed vision surrounded by an area of less depressed vision), enlargement of the blind spot
Antiarrhythmics	quinidine sulfate	Blurred vision, color perception disturbances, night blindness, mydriasis, photophobia, diplopia, reduced visual fields, scotomas, optic neuritis
	flecainide acetate	Blurred vision, difficulty focusing, spots before eyes, diplopia (double vision), photophobia (light sensitivity), nystagmus (abnormal lateral movements of the eyes)
Anticholinergic agents	All types	Blurred vision, cycloplegia (paralysis of visual muscles responsible for accommodation), mydriasis (pupil dilation), photophobia
Anti-infectives	chloramphenicol	Optic neuritis, decreased visual acuity
	norfloxacin	Visual disturbances
	sulfisoxazole	Periorbital edema, conjunctival and scleral injection
Anti-inflammatory agents	All nonsteroidal anti-inflammatory agents	Blurred vision, color vision changes, decreased visual acuity, corneal opacity, optic neuritis
Antineoplastics	cisplatin	Optic neuritis, papilledema, cerebral blindness
	tamoxifen	Retinopathy, corneal opacities, decreased visual acuity
Antitubercular agents	isoniazid, pyrazinamide, ethambutol	Optic neuritis, decreased visual acuity, loss of red-green color perception, central and peripheral scotomas (ethambutol only)
Cardiotonic glycosides	digitalis leaf, digoxin, and digitalis	Altered color vision, photophobia, diplopia, halos or borders on objects
Diuretics	amiloride	Visual disturbances
	hydrochlorothiazide	Altered color vision, transient blurred vision
Genitourinary smooth muscle relaxants	flavoxate	Blurred vision, disturbed accommodation
	oxybutynin	Transient blurred vision, cycloplegia, mydriasis
Glucocorticoids	prednisone and others	Exophthalmos (abnormal protrusion of the eyeball), increased intraocular pressure, cataracts, increased susceptibility to secondary fungal and viral eye infections

Adverse drug reactions continued

DRUG CLASS	DRUG	POSSIBLE ADVERSE REACTIONS
Phenothiazines	All phenothiazines	Abnormal corneal lens pigmentation
	chlorpromazine	Cataracts, retinopathy, visual impairment
Miscellaneous agents	carbamazepine	Blurred vision, transient diplopia, visual hallucinations
	oral contraceptives (estrogen with progesterone)	Worsening of myopia or astigmatism, intolerance to contact lenses, neuro-ocular lesions
	isotretinoin	Conjunctivitis, dry eyes, corneal opacities, eye irritation
	loxapine	Blurred vision, pigmentary changes
	metrizamide	Diplopia, amblyopia, photophobia, eye flickering, blurred vision
	pentazocine hydrochloride	Blurred vision, focusing difficulty, nystagmus, diplopia, miosis (pupil constriction)
	vitamin D	Photophobia, calcific conjunctivitis (with vitamin D intoxication)

If school-age, does the child have to sit at the front of the room to see the chalkboard? Does the child sit close to the television at home?
(RATIONALE: If so, the child could be nearsighted.)

If school-age, how is the child's progress in school?
(RATIONALE: Poor progress in school could indicate a visual disturbance.)

Elderly client. For an elderly client, the nurse should ask the following questions about eye disorders common to aging:

Do your eyes feel dry?
(RATIONALE: Dry eyes or a feeling of sand or grittiness is common in elderly clients because of decreased lacrimal gland secretion.)

Do you have difficulty seeing in front of you but not to the sides?
(RATIONALE: In macular degeneration, which is common in elderly clients, central vision deteriorates, but peripheral vision remains intact.)

Do you have problems with glare?
(RATIONALE: As the lens thickens and yellows with age, excessive light becomes an irritant.)

Do you have any problems discerning colors?
(RATIONALE: The thickening and yellowing of the lens also makes blues and purples look green.)

Do you have difficulty seeing at night?
(RATIONALE: Lens opacity that occurs with cataracts causes night blindness.)

Health promotion and protection patterns

Questions related to health promotion and protection patterns indicate the client's involvement in personal health care. The nurse should ask the following questions to elicit this information.

When was your last eye examination? What were the results?
(RATIONALE: Besides suggesting the importance of eye examinations to the client, the question may reveal changes that caused the client to have an examination. If that examination was more than 2 years ago, suggest another one.)

Does your health insurance cover eye examinations and lenses?
(RATIONALE: If not, the client may forgo eye examinations or buying lenses for economic reasons.)

Does your occupation require close use of your eyes, such as long-term reading or prolonged use of a video display terminal?)
(RATIONALE: These activities can cause severe eyestrain and dryness. Instruct the client to take periodic breaks to rest the eyes.)

Does the air where you work or live contain anything that causes you eye problems?
(RATIONALE: Cigarette smoke, formaldehyde insulation, or occupational materials such as glues or chemicals can cause eye irritation.)

Do you wear goggles when working with power tools, chain saws, or table saws, or when engaging in sports that might irritate or endanger the eye, such as swimming, fencing, or playing racquetball?
(RATIONALE: Serious eye irritation or injury can occur with these activities. If the client does not wear goggles, provide instruction about eye safety.)

Role and relationship patterns

Vision disturbances can influence many roles and relationships. To discover the extent of this influence, the nurse should ask the client the following questions.

If you wear glasses, are they a problem for you?
(RATIONALE: Some clients, especially children and adolescents, may feel less attractive with glasses and may not wear them as prescribed. If this is so, provide instruction about eye health.)

If you are visually impaired, do you have difficulty fulfilling home or work obligations?
(RATIONALE: Visual impairment can seriously affect the client's ability to carry out a role. For example, a homemaker may have to depend on another person to help with housework. If this is the case, refer the client to an occupational health therapist, who can help the client make necessary adjustments in the environment.)

If you are visually impaired, are your social activities curtailed? If so, to what extent?
(RATIONALE: Some clients may avoid social activities because of poor vision. If so, refer the client to special activities or support groups for those who are visually impaired.)

Physical assessment: The eye

Assessment of the eye includes testing the client's vision and extraocular muscles, inspecting and palpating external ocular structures, and inspecting internal structures with an ophthalmoscope. Because inspection and palpation can cause eye irritation and tearing, the nurse should test the client's vision before inspecting and palpating. The client usually remains seated for the eye assessment.

For a basic eye assessment, obtain a Snellen eye chart, a piece of newsprint, an eye occluder or a 3 x 5 card, a penlight, a wisp of cotton, a pencil or other narrow cylindrical article, and, for the advanced assessment, an ophthalmoscope. Wash your hands before beginning the assessment.

Vision

Prepare for the assessment by washing your hands. Then test visual functions, including near and distant visual acuity, color perception, and peripheral vision. Perform the vision tests in a room that is well-lit, but where you can control the amount of light.

Distance vision

To test the distance vision of a client who can read English, use the Snellen alphabet chart containing various-sized letters. For clients who are illiterate or who cannot speak English, use the Snellen E chart, which displays the letter in varying sizes and positions. The client indicates the position of the E by duplicating the position with his or her fingers. (For an illustration of the Snellen eye charts, see *Basic assessment equipment* in Chapter 4, Physical Assessment Skills.)

The Snellen chart contains lines of letters that decrease in size with each succeeding line, with each line labeled with a number containing a numerator and a denominator. The numerator, which is always 20, is the distance in feet between the chart and the client. (Be certain to position the client 20′ from the chart.) The denominator, which ranges from 10 to 200, indicates from what distance a normal eye can read the chart. For example, if the client reads a line identified by the numbers 20/20, this means that the client can read from

20′ what a person with normal vision can also read from 20′. However, if the client can only read a line identified by the numbers 20/100, this means that the client must read from 20′ what a person with normal vision can read from 100′. On the other hand, if the client can read a line labeled 20/10, this means that the client can read at 20′ what a person with normal vision must read from 10′.

Test each eye separately by covering first one eye and then the other with an opaque 3 x 5 card or an eye occluder. Afterward, test the client's binocular vision by having the client read the chart with both eyes uncovered. The client who normally wears corrective lenses for distance vision should wear them for the test. Start with the line marked 20/20. If the client reads more than two letters incorrectly, go up to the next line (20/25). Continue until the client can read a line correctly with no more than two errors. That line indicates the client's distance visual acuity. If the client reads the 20/20 line correctly, move down until the client makes more than two mistakes. The last line read with fewer than two mistakes indicates the client's distance visual acuity. Retest any client with a score of 20/30 or greater in 1 week; if the results remain the same, refer the client to a specialist for a complete examination.

Near vision

Test the client's near vision by holding either a Snellen chart or a card with newsprint 12″ to 14″ (30.5 to 35.5 cm) in front of the client's eyes. The client who normally wears reading glasses should wear them for the test. As with distance vision, test each eye separately and then together. Any client who complains of blurring with the card at 12″ to 14″, or is unable to read it accurately, needs to be retested and then referred to an ophthalmologist if necessary. Keep in mind that a client who is illiterate may be too embarrassed to say so. If a client seems to be struggling to read the type, or stares at it without attempting to read, change to the Snellen E chart.

Color perception

Color blindness is usually an inherited, sex-linked recessive trait passed from mothers to male offspring. People with color blindness cannot distinguish among red, green, and blue.

Among the many tests to detect color blindness, the most common involves asking a client to identify patterns of colored dots on colored plates. The client who cannot discern colors will miss the patterns. Early detection of color blindness allows the child to learn to compensate for the deficit and also alerts teachers to the student's special needs. Color perception testing is also important during adolescence, before the young adult makes an occupational choice.

Record the results of visual acuity testing for each eye separately and for both eyes together, noting whether or not the client wears corrective lenses. Also record the results of the color perception test.

Abnormal findings

Poor near vision, especially in clients over age 45, can indicate presbyopia, a condition in which the lens loses elasticity and the ciliary muscles begin to weaken. Poor near vision also can result from cataracts.

Extraocular muscle function

To assess extraocular muscle function, the nurse must use the following techniques. First, inspect the eyes for position and alignment, making sure they are parallel. Next, perform the following tests: the six cardinal positions of gaze test, the cover-uncover test, and the corneal light reflex test. (For illustrated procedures, see *Testing extraocular muscle function,* pages 218 and 219.)

The six cardinal positions of gaze test evaluates the function of each of the six extraocular muscles and tests the cranial nerves responsible for their movement (cranial nerves III, IV, and VI). The normal eye muscles work together so that when the right eye moves upward and inward, the left eye moves upward and outward.

The cover-uncover test assesses the fusion reflex, which makes binocular vision possible. The fusion reflex results from adequate extraocular muscle balance, which keeps the eyes parallel and on the same axis as the working muscles.

The corneal light reflex test assesses the ability of the extraocular muscles to hold the eyes steady, or parallel, when fixed on an object.

If an adult client fails one of these tests, schedule that client for a retest within a month. However, if a child fails one test, or if an adult fails more than one test, retesting should be done in 2 weeks. Refer any client who fails the second screening to an ophthalmologist. The referral is especially important for a child, because an extraocular muscle imbalance can cause the eyes to cross (strabismus).

Abnormal findings

Disturbances in ocular muscle balance prevent parallel eye movement. Such disturbances are caused by an abnormally long or short muscle or by a weakness or paralysis of the extraocular muscles resulting from a defect or a lesion in the nerve supplying those muscles.

Testing extraocular muscle function

To assess a client's extraocular muscle function, the nurse should perform three tests—the six cardinal positions of gaze test, the cover-uncover test, and the corneal light reflex test.

Six cardinal positions of gaze test

Sit directly in front of the client, and ask the client to remain still while you hold a cylindrical object, such as a pencil, directly in front of, and about 18″ (46 cm) away from, the client's nose.

Ask the client to watch the object as you move it clockwise through each of the six cardinal positions, returning the object to midpoint after each movement.

Throughout the test, the client's eyes should remain parallel as they move. Note any abnormal findings, such as nystagmus or the deviation of one eye away from the object.

Lateral | **Superior** | **Inferior**

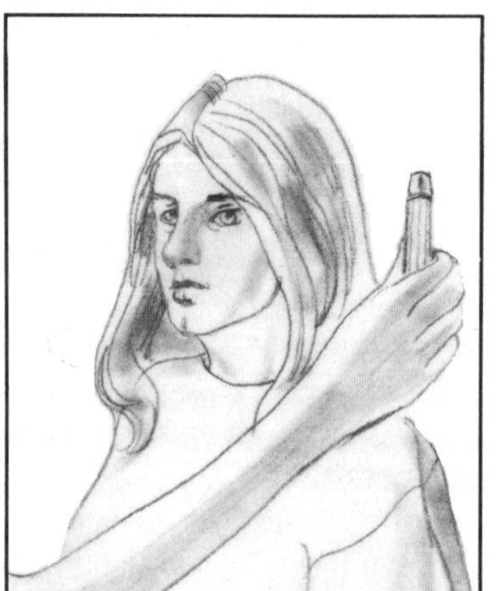

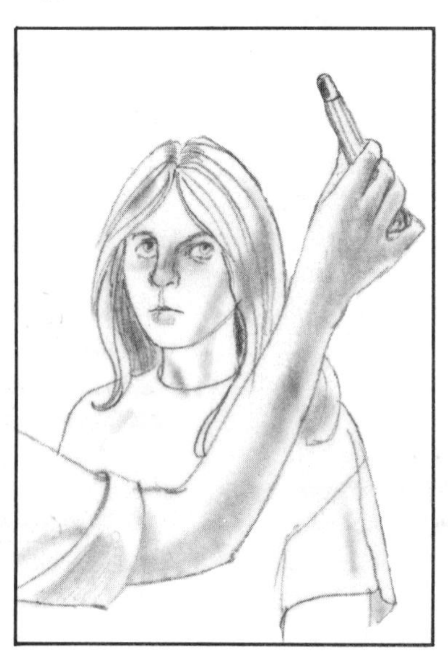

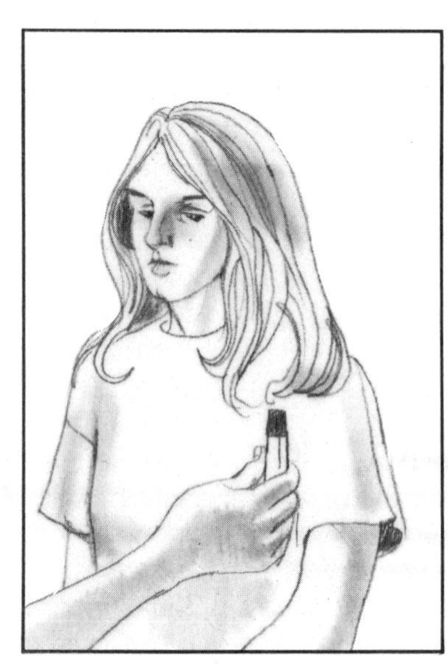

1. | **2.** | **3.**

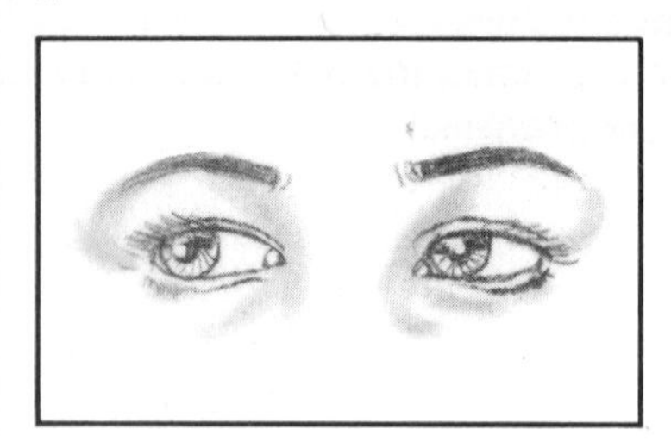

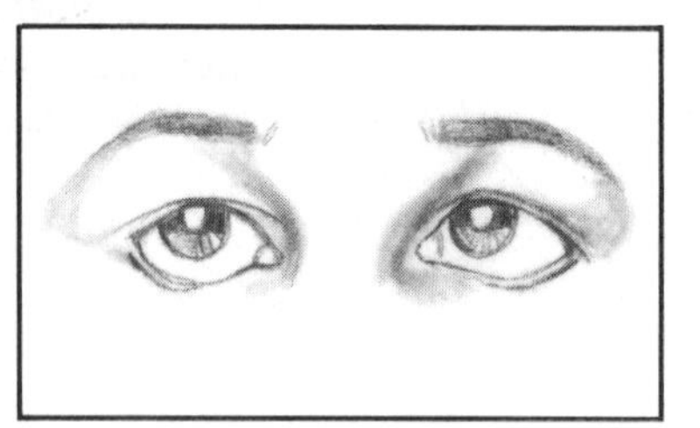

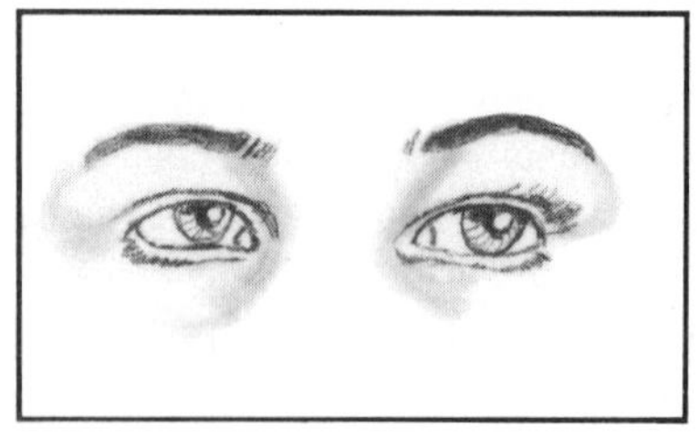

4. | **5.** | **6.**

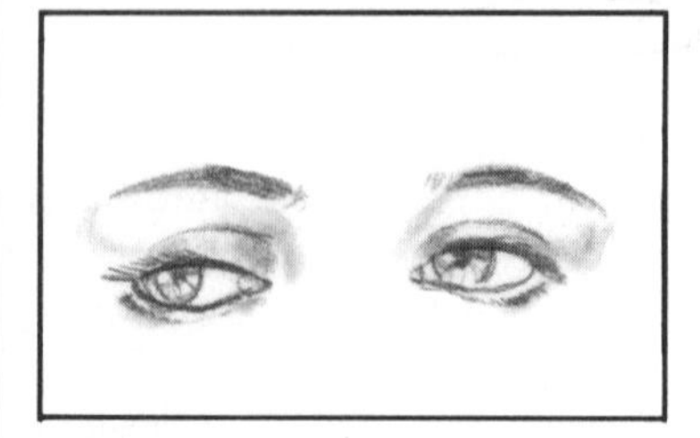

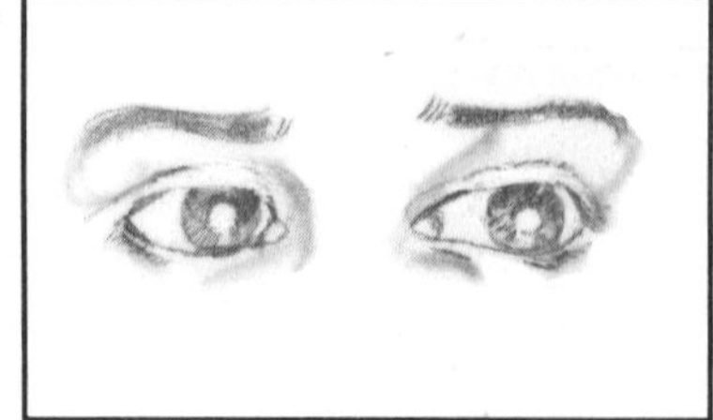

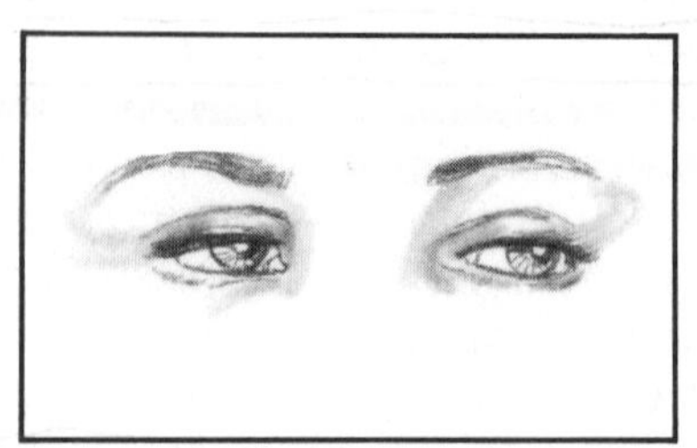

Cover-uncover test
Have the client stare at an object on a distant wall directly opposite. Cover the client's left eye with an opaque card and observe the uncovered right eye for movement or wandering.

Next, remove the card from the left eye. The left eye should remain steady, without moving or wandering. Repeat the procedure on the right eye.

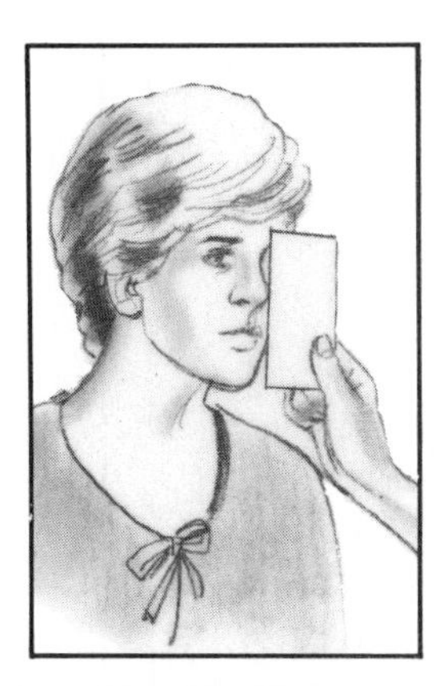

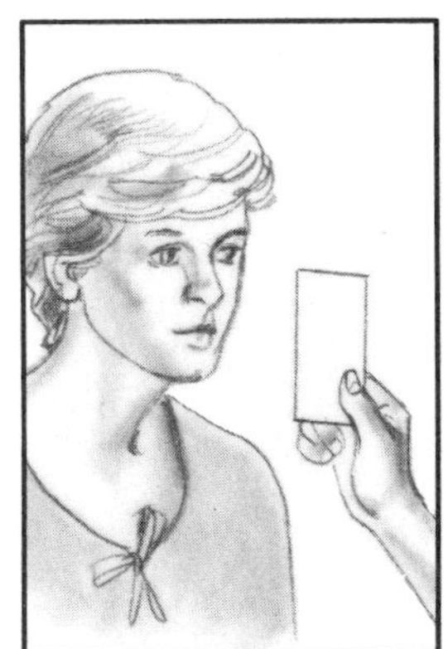

Corneal light reflex test
Ask the client to stare straight ahead while you shine a penlight on the bridge of the client's nose from a distance of 12″ to 15″ (30.5 to 38 cm). Check to make sure that the cornea relects the light in exactly the same place in both eyes. An asymmetrical reflex indicates a muscle imbalance causing the eye to deviate from the fixed point.

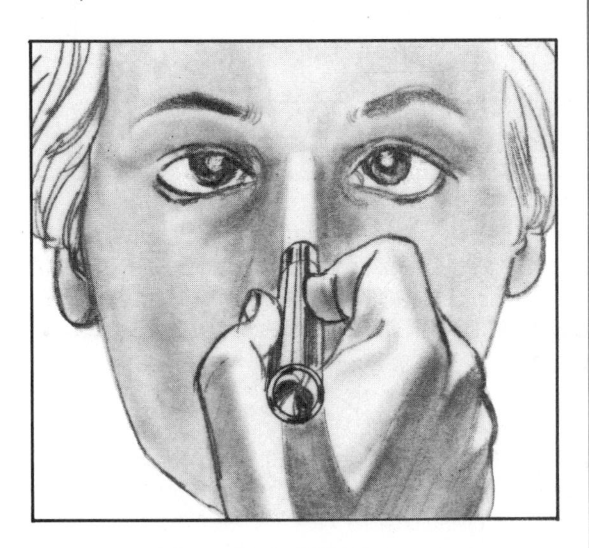

Testing the six cardinal positions of gaze can reveal exophoria, a mild outward deviation of the eye, or esophoria, an inward deviation; both are caused by muscle weakness. Tropia is a more severe ocular muscle weakness that produces a permanent misalignment of the optic axes of the eyes (strabismus) in which the eyes turn outward (exotropia) or inward (esotropia).

Testing muscle balance can uncover strabismus, which is an important first step in preserving the client's vision. If strabismus remains untreated, the affected eye will weaken from disuse (amblyopia). This results because the optic cortex receives two images instead of one, suppresses one of the images to avoid diplopia, and causes a "lazy," or nonfunctioning, eye. Phoria is a mild weakness of these muscles.

Peripheral vision

Assessment of peripheral vision tests the optic nerve (cranial nerve II) and measures the ability of the retina to receive stimuli from the periphery of its field. The nurse can grossly evaluate peripheral vision by assessing visual fields, which compares the client's peripheral vision with the nurse's. However, because this assumes that the nurse has normal vision, this test can be subjective and inaccurate. (For an illustrated procedure, see *Testing peripheral vision,* page 220.)

Abnormal findings

A client's decreased peripheral vision, along with a history of seeing rainbows or halos around lights, can indicate glaucoma. The nurse should refer a client with these symptoms for further studies.

Visual field defects, indicated by decreased peripheral vision, can result from lesions on the retina, in the occipital lobe, or at any point along the optic nerve. Because nerves from both eyes cross at the optic chiasm and both optic tracts terminate in the occipital lobe, lesions in either of these locations affect the visual fields of both eyes. However, damage or lesions on one optic nerve affect the visual field in that eye only.

Inspection

After performing vision testing, perform the following assessment techniques. Inspect the eyelids, eyelashes, eyeball, and lacrimal apparatus. Also inspect the conjunctiva, sclera, cornea, anterior chamber, iris, and pupil. Use an ophthalmoscope to assess the vitreous humor and retina.

Testing peripheral vision

To test peripheral visual fields, the nurse should follow this procedure. Sit facing the client, about 2′ (60 cm) away, with your eyes at the same level as the client's. Have the client stare straight ahead. Cover one of your eyes with an opaque cover or your hand and ask the client to cover the eye directly opposite your covered eye. Next, bring an object, such as a pencil, from the periphery of the superior field toward the center of the field of vision, as shown in the illustration below. The object should be equidistant between you and the client. Ask the client to tell you the moment the object appears. If your peripheral vision is intact, you and the client should see the object at the same time.

Repeat the procedure clockwise at 45-degree angles, checking the superior, inferior, temporal, and nasal visual fields, as shown in the diagram at right. When testing the temporal field, you will have difficulty moving the pencil far enough out so that neither person can see it. So test the temporal field by placing the pencil somewhat behind the client and out of the client's visual field.

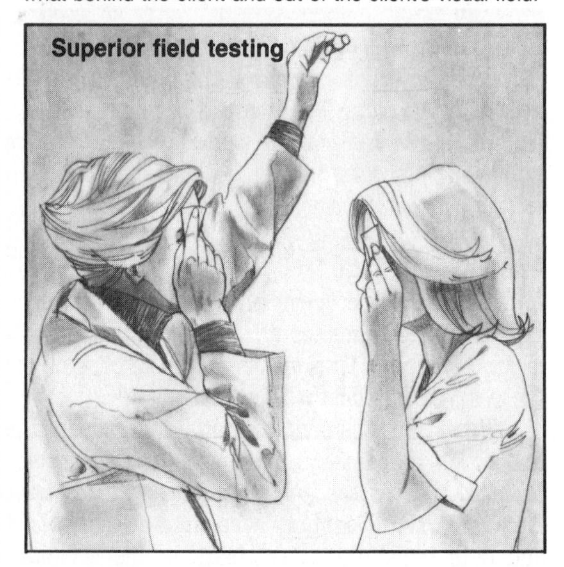

Slowly bring the pencil around until the client can see it.

The normal field of vision is about 50 degrees upward, 60 degrees medially, 70 degrees downward, and 110 degrees laterally. Remember that this test discovers only large peripheral vision defects, such as blindness in one quarter to one half of the visual field.

Positions for peripheral vision testing

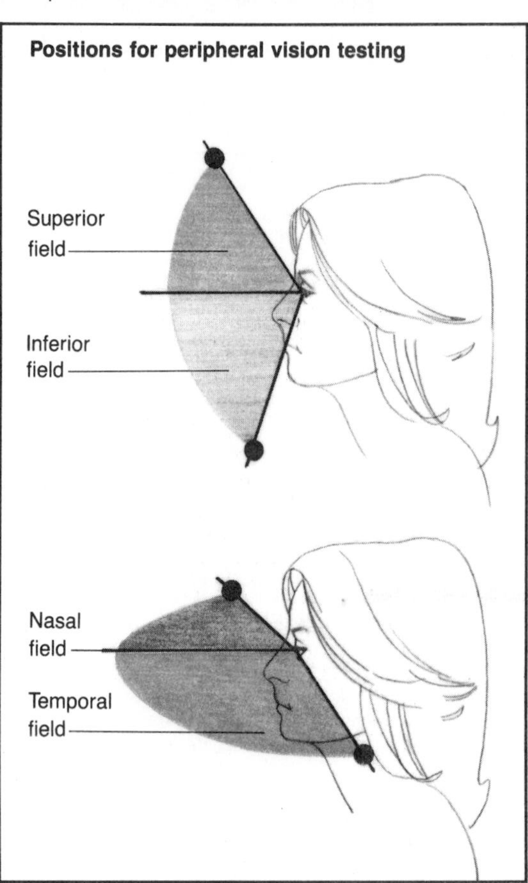

Eyelids, eyelashes, eyeball, and lacrimal apparatus

Inspect these structures for general appearance. The eyes are normally bright and clear. The eyelids should close completely over the sclera, and when opened, the margins of the upper eyelids should fall between the superior pupil margin and the superior limbus, covering a small portion of the iris. The eyelids should be free from edema, scaling, or lesions, and the eyelashes should curve outward and be equally distributed along the upper and lower eyelid margins. The color of the eyelids should be consistent with the client's complexion. Inspect the palpebral folds for symmetry and the eyes for nystagmus (involuntary oscillations of the eyes) and lid lag (unequal eyelid movement). Further inspect the eyes for excessive tearing or dryness and the puncta for inflammation and swelling.

Conjunctiva and sclera

Next, inspect the bulbar and palpebral portions of the conjunctiva for clarity. (For an illustrated procedure, see *Inspecting the conjunctivae*.)

View the white sclera through the bulbar portion of the conjunctiva. The conjunctiva should be free from hyperemic (engorged) blood vessels and drainage.

Inspecting the conjunctivae

While assessing the external eye structures, follow these steps to inspect the bulbar conjunctiva over the sclera (white portion of the eye visible anteriorly) and the palpebral conjunctiva on the inner portion of the upper eyelid.

Bulbar conjunctiva
To inspect the bulbar conjunctiva, gently separate the eyelids with your thumb or index finger. Ask the client to look up, down, left, and right as you examine the eye.

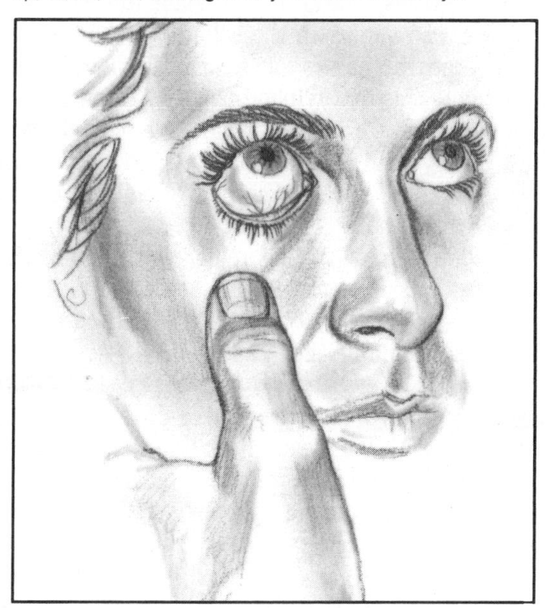

Palpebral conjunctiva
1. Check the palpebral conjunctiva only if you suspect a foreign body or if the client complains of eyelid pain. To examine the upper conjunctiva, hold the upper eyelashes and press on the tarsal border with a cotton-tipped applicator to evert the eyelid. Ask the client to look down. This technique requires skill to avoid client discomfort. Hold the lashes to the brow and examine the conjunctiva, which should be pink and free from swelling.

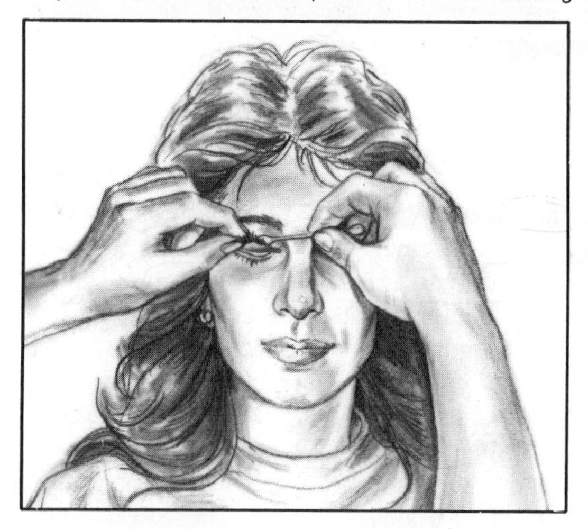

2. To return the eyelid to its normal position, release the eyelashes and ask the client to look upward. If this does not invert the eyelid, grasp the eyelashes and gently pull them forward.

Inspect the color of the sclera. Although it is normally white, clients with dark complexions, such as Blacks and those from the Middle East, may have small, dark-pigmented spots on the sclera.

Cornea, anterior chamber, and iris

To inspect the cornea and anterior chamber, shine a penlight into the client's eye from several side angles (tangentially). Normally, the cornea and anterior chamber are clear and transparent. Calculate the depth of the anterior chamber from the side by figuring the distance between the cornea and the iris. The iris should illuminate with the side lighting. The surface of the cornea normally appears shiny and bright without any scars or irregularities.

Test for corneal sensitivity, which indicates intact functioning of the sensory fibers of cranial nerve V (trigeminal nerve) and motor nerve fibers of cranial nerve VII (facial nerve), by lightly stroking a wisp of cotton across the corneal surface. The lids of both eyes should close when you touch either cornea. Use a separate piece of cotton for each eye to avoid cross-contamination.

Inspect the iris for shape, which should appear flat when viewed from the side, and color.

Pupil

Consentual

Examine the pupil of each eye for equality of size, shape, reaction to light, and accommodation. To test pupillary reaction to light, darken the room, and, with the client staring straight ahead at a fixed point, sweep a beam from a penlight from the side of the left eye to the center of its pupil. Both pupils should respond; the pupil receiving the direct light constricts directly, while the other pupil constricts simultaneously and consensually. Now test the pupil of the right eye. The pupils should react immediately, equally, and briskly (within 1 to 2 seconds). If the results are inconclusive, wait 15 to 30 seconds and try again. The pupils should be round and equal before and after the light flash.

To test for accommodation, ask the client to stare at an object across the room. Normally, the pupils should dilate. Then ask the client to stare at your index finger or at a pencil held about 2′ (60 cm) away. The pupils should constrict and converge equally on the object. To document a normal pupil assessment, use the abbreviation PERRLA (which stands for: pupils equal, round, reactive to light, and accommodation) and the terms direct and consensual.

Abnormal findings

Common problems related to the external eye structures include ptosis, ectropion, and entropion.

In ptosis, the upper eyelid falls below the middle of the iris. An oculomotor nerve lesion or a congenital condition in children can cause the eyelid to fall at or below the pupil (called lid lag). When the eyelid margin falls above the limbus and some sclera is visible (as in exophthalmos), hyperthyroidism may be the cause.

In some clients, especially elderly clients, the eyelids lose their elasticity and turn outward (ectropion). In many cases, the everted eyelid obstructs the punctum, thus blocking tear drainage and resulting in excessive tearing. Inward turning of the eyelid (entropion) results from eyelid spasms or scar tissue on the lids from frequent styes. If left untreated, the inward-turned eyelashes can irritate the cornea and cause a corneal abrasion.

Also observe the lid for any lumps that could be styes. Search the anterior chamber for any visible material, such as blood spots, which would be abnormal.

Other common eye abnormalities that can indicate a minor or serious disorder include allergic, viral, or bacterial conjunctivitis; scleral color changes; corneal abrasions; lens changes; abnormalities in pupil size; or an inability to move the eyes in a parallel fashion.

Conjunctivitis is usually self-limiting and does not cause permanent damage. On occasion, conjunctivitis may become chronic, causing degenerative changes and damage from repeated attacks. However, bacterial conjunctivitis is a contagious disease (pinkeye) and usually requires antibiotic therapy to prevent its spread. Conjunctivitis is characterized by yellow or green purulent drainage accompanied by conjunctival vessel engorgement. The eyes may be matted closed upon awakening. Occasionally, upper respiratory tract infections may produce purulent eye drainage in children because of the proximity of the lacrimal duct to the nose. Purulent material in the lacrimal apparatus also can cause conjunctivitis. Elderly clients are more likely to experience viral conjunctivitis, which is also contagious and can cause corneal scarring. Viral conjunctivitis does not produce purulent exudate and does not require antibiotic therapy.

Scleral color change usually indicates a potentially severe systemic problem. Jaundice from liver disease manifests itself first in the sclera, which becomes yellow (scleral icterus). Pallor from anemia and cyanosis from hypoxia also appear in the sclera.

Corneal abrasions cause corneal inflammation, pain, and light sensitivity (photophobia). Corneal abrasions can occur after prolonged wearing of contact lenses or after injury from a foreign object, such as a fragment of metal or glass. Suspected corneal abrasions need referral to an ophthalmologist.

If a portion of the iris remains unilluminated when lit from the side, a change in the depth of the anterior chamber—such as that caused by increased intracranial pressure—could be the cause.

A cataract is an opacity in the lens that can assume various shapes and colors. For example, some look like pieces of coral and others look like crystals. Cataracts can be congenital or, in a young adult or a child, can result from a metabolic disorder such as diabetes mellitus. However, most cataracts result when the lens degenerates from aging.

About 5% of the population has a difference in pupil size (anisocoria). Usually, however, pupil inequality results from central nervous system disorders or trauma. Any irregularity in the contour of the pupil may result from trauma or iritis. Pupillary constriction (miosis) occurs after using narcotics or the medication prescribed for glaucoma (pilocarpine). Occasionally, the acute swelling of sinusitis can constrict nerves and cause pupillary constriction. Also, pupillary enlargement (mydriasis) can result from trauma or a systemic reaction to sympathomimetic and parasympathetic drugs. A client age 45 or over may suffer from reduced accommodation to near vision (presbyopia).

Palpation

After inspection, the nurse should follow these steps to palpate the eye and related structures. Gently palpate the eyelids for swelling and tenderness. Next, palpate ① the eyeball by placing the tips of both index fingers on the eyelids over the sclera while the client looks down. The eyeballs should feel equally firm.

Next, palpate the lacrimal sac by pressing the index ② finger against the client's lower orbital rim on the side

Integrating assessment findings

Sometimes, a cluster of assessment findings will strongly suggest a particular eye disorder. In the chart below, column one shows groups of presenting signs and symptoms—the ones that make the client seek medical attention. Column two shows related assessment findings that the nurse may discover during the health history and physical assessment. The client may exhibit one or more of these findings. Column three shows the possible disorder indicated by a cluster of these findings.

PRESENTING SIGNS AND SYMPTOMS	RELATED ASSESSMENT FINDINGS	POSSIBLE DISORDER
Acute eye pain and tenderness with purulent green or yellow discharge	Gradual onset of pain, tenderness, and swelling Red and swollen eyelid sebaceous gland Outward pointing eyelash Swollen eyelid sebaceous gland pointing into conjunctival side of eyelid Positive culture and sensitivity tests for bacterial infection	Hordeolum (stye)
Itching and foreign body sensation in eye with redness and discharge	Enlarged regional nodes; reddened conjunctiva; sticky, crusty eyelids; and purulent drainage Photophobia Increased tearing Reddened cornea and conjunctiva; pseudoptosis, especially apparent in early morning	Conjunctivitis, infections
Pain in eye, blinking, increased tearing, and blurred vision	History of trauma to eye Contact lens use Injected cornea Irregular corneal surface apparent with light Visible ulcer outline upon instillation of fluorescein dye Decreased visual acuity on visual acuity testing	Corneal abrasion
Gradual bilateral loss of peripheral vision; halos around lights; decreased visual acuity, especially at night	Familial, genetically determined lens changes from systemic disorders Cupping and atrophy of optic disk on ophthalmoscopic examination Loss of peripheral vision on visual field testing Increased intraocular pressure on tonometer examination	Chronic open-angle glaucoma
Photophobia; gradual blurring and loss of vision; changes in color perception; halos around lights	Advanced age History of lens trauma from foreign body or intraocular disease History of diabetes Visible white area behind pupil on inspection with penlight Lens opacification on ophthalmoscopic examination Decreased visual acuity on visual acuity testing Absence of red reflex	Cataract

closest to the client's nose. While pressing, observe the punctum for any abnormal regurgitation of purulent material or excessive tears, which could indicate blockage of the nasolacrimal duct.

Abnormal findings

Excessive hardness of the eyeball could indicate increased intraocular pressure.

Eyelid edema without inflammation can indicate potentially serious systemic conditions such as glomerulonephritis, heart disease, nephrotic syndrome, and thyroid deficiency. Periorbital edema is seen in frontal sinusitis and nephrosis. A potentially serious condition, called periorbital cellulitis, produces both edema and inflammation, which, unless treated immediately, can cause brain abscess because of the proximity of the orbit to the brain. Less serious causes of eyelid edema and inflammation include severe sinusitis, allergies, and an allergic response to medication. (For some common abnormalities associated with the eye, see *Integrating assessment findings*.)

Developmental and ethnic considerations

The nurse should consider the following differences in methods and procedures when assessing the eyes of pediatric, elderly, Asian, or Black clients.

Pediatric client

To perform a successful and accurate eye assessment on a preschooler, consider the child's age and behavioral development. Also consider appropriate methods of allaying the child's anxiety before the examination and diverting the child's attention during the examination. For example, use a brightly colored toy, piece of yarn, or puppet to divert a toddler's or preschooler's attention while you inspect external ocular structures, perform the cover-uncover test, test pupillary functions, assess the corneal light reflex, and check the six cardinal positions of gaze. The parent can assist with the examination by soothing, distracting, or holding the infant or child.

Generally speaking, infants and children under school age will not be able to cooperate long enough for you to perform an ophthalmoscopic examination (funduscopy) or an assessment of visual fields. However, checking for the presence of a red reflex (bright orange glow in the pupil) is essential. (See *Advanced assessment skills: Ophthalmoscopic examination.*) Visual acuity varies with age. For example, 20/200 is normal for an infant and 20/30 is normal for a child age 2 to 3. Although visual acuity assessment is not possible in children under age 30 months, assess an infant's vision by quickly passing a light or an object toward the infant's eyes while checking for a blink reflex. For children age 30 to 42 months, use the Denver Eye Screening Examination (DESE) to assess visual acuity and ocular mobility. In children age 7 and under, use either the DESE or the Snellen E chart to test visual acuity.

In addition, some researchers have found the Stycar test from England to be accurate in children age 2 and older. It contains easily recognized letters, such as "X," "0," "C," and "V"; the child points out matching letters. Charts also exist picturing cows, horses, and boats; however, since the child may not be familiar with the objects pictured, these charts are less accurate than the Stycar.

Researchers (Brown and Collar, 1982) have had greater success assessing children who have been prescreened, or prepared, for the eye examination. The preparation involves playing a matching game using Stycar letters with the child for 2 weeks before the examination. During the first week, the parents and child simply play the matching game. During the second week, parents introduce an eye patch similar to that used for tests like the cover-uncover test. Then, in the third week, the nurse screens the child. Researchers discovered that, after following this routine, the amount of time required to perform a visual acuity screening on children age 2½ to 3 decreased.

Common visual acuity problems in children include myopia (nearsightedness), hyperopia (farsightedness), and astigmatism (irregular lens or cornea).

Careful testing of the infant's and young child's extraocular muscle function can uncover different types of strabismus. Noncomitant or paralytic strabismus occurs from a paralyzed ocular muscle, usually as a result of eye trauma. This type of strabismus often is not apparent when a child stares straight ahead but will appear during a test of the six cardinal positions of gaze. Paralytic strabismus should resolve 1 to 2 months after the trauma. Concomitant strabismus (which occurs regardless of the direction in which the eyes are gazing) is common in infants but should resolve by age 6 months. Until then, the infant merits close watching. Some children exhibit a tendency toward strabismus only when ill or tired (phoria). Ask the parents whether they have noticed this type of strabismus.

Brief periods of involuntary, rapid, jerking eye movements (nystagmus) are normal in an infant who is not yet focusing. However, if the nystagmus is continuous, the infant requires further examination by a specialist. All children may normally demonstrate a slight nystagmus when gazing to either side.

The results of a normal eye assessment are the same for a child as for an adult, except for acuity and muscle balance. Children under age 7 or 8 do not have normal 20/20 vision, and no infants under age 6 months have parallel muscle balance. Children over age 6 months who fail muscle balance assessments twice within a 2-week period need further evaluation by an ophthalmologist. Check color perception in children age 3 or over if the parent indicates that the child has learned to identify colors.

Elderly client

Although assessment procedures for the elderly client are the same as those for a younger adult, the findings vary because of normal changes from aging. Checking peripheral vision and the red reflex is especially important in the elderly client.

With aging, the eyebrows and eyelashes thin as the number of hair follicles decreases. The eyes may appear sunken because of decreased fatty tissue around them;

they also may appear dry and lackluster because the lacrimal glands lessen tear production. Common complaints in elderly clients are dry eyes and a gritty feeling upon blinking. The gritty feeling is an irritation and can occasionally cause increased tearing.

Other external eye changes include possible laxness of the eyelids, which predisposes the client to eversion or inversion of the lower lid, and pseudoptosis (drooping of the upper lid caused by aging, not by a neurologic problem). A thickening of the bulbar conjunctiva on the nasal side (pinguecula) and an accumulation of yellow lipid substances on the eyelid (xanthelasmas) also may occur. Other noticeable changes include clouding of the cornea and small, somewhat fixed pupils, both of which are caused by sclerotic changes in the iris.

An elderly client's cornea may exhibit a thin, gray-white surrounding ring resulting from lipid deposits. This finding, called arcus senilis, is normal in elderly clients. Most clients over age 85 will show almost no pupil reaction to accommodation, and only one third will react to light. Also, as the lens thickens and yellows, the client's perception of light diminishes and colors become distorted, with blues and purples appearing green. The yellow lens also causes problems with glare and decreases visual acuity in dim light. Therefore, elderly clients require more light to read, embroider, or perform other fine work. Also, because of a loss of elasticity and transparency of the lens, the elderly client has decreased ability to discriminate clear objects, such as windows, and also may have difficulty with distance perception.

Peripheral vision may also normally decrease in elderly clients. Because intraocular fluid reabsorption decreases, glaucoma may occur. A client experiencing a sudden decrease in peripheral vision and complaining of eye pain requires an immediate evaluation by an ophthalmologist. These are symptoms of acute glaucoma, a medical emergency.

Ethnic considerations

An ethnic variation that may be noted when assessing the eyes occurs in Asian persons, who have skin folds covering the inner canthus. These folds, called epicanthal folds, also occur in persons with Down's syndrome.

Black people, and others with dark skin, may have small, darkly pigmented spots on the sclera (muddy sclera). A Black person's corneas may have a gray-blue hue, and the optic disk and retina are darker orange or darker red than those of a fair-skinned client.

Advanced assessment skills

After becoming proficient at basic eye assessment techniques, the nurse is ready to learn the more advanced techniques of ophthalmoscopic examination and tonometry. (For information on the ophthalmoscope, see Chapter 4, Physical Assessment Skills.)

Ophthalmoscopic examination

The nurse should follow these steps to perform an advanced eye examination. (For an illustrated procedure, see *Advanced assessment skills: Ophthalmoscopic examination,* pages 226 and 227.) Before beginning an ophthalmoscopic examination, practice holding and using the instrument until you feel comfortable with it. Turn on the ophthalmoscope by depressing the button of the rheostat on the handle and then turning the rheostat clockwise to increase light intensity. To learn how the apertures look and work, project the light onto a white piece of paper while moving the aperture selection lever through its various settings.

Each lens on the ophthalmoscope has a magnification value, called a diopter. The lens value, which appears in an illuminated opening on the front of the ophthalmoscope, ranges from +40 to −20. The positive diopters are black; the negative diopters are red. The lens system compensates for the examiner's vision and can correct for client myopia or hyperopia, but not for astigmatism. The "0" lens is glass without any refraction. The nurse with normal vision should set the lens at 0 and then slowly move toward a positive number, such as 6 or 8, or until the client's optic disk becomes sharply focused.

An ophthalmoscopic examination can detect many disorders of the optic disk and retina, but the technique, and the interpretation of abnormalities, requires skill, experience, and knowledge. Three of the major optic disk pathologies detected by ophthalmoscopic examination are papilledema, optic atrophy, and glaucoma.

Papilledema usually occurs with increased intracranial pressure, such as that resulting from severe hypertension, eclampsia, brain tumor, or subdural hematoma. The increased pressure in the brain inhibits normal venous return from the eye. Therefore, blood backs up and fluid starts to leak around the optic disk, causing the disk and the optic nerve to swell. To the examiner, the borders of the optic disk look hazy and blurred. These blurred borders are the major diagnostic sign of papilledema.

Optic atrophy occurs when optic nerve fibers die; the disk vessels also disappear. Because the vessels

ADVANCED ASSESSMENT SKILLS

Ophthalmoscopic examination

An ophthalmoscope can help the nurse identify inner eye abnormalities. To perform an ophthalmoscopic examination, place the client in a darkened or semidarkened room, with neither you nor the client wearing glasses unless you are very myopic or astigmatic. Contact lenses may be worn by you or the client.

1 Sit or stand in front of the client with your head about 1½′ (45 cm) in front of and about 15 degrees to the right of the client's line of vision in the right eye. Hold the ophthalmoscope in your right hand with the viewing aperture as close to your right eye as possible. Place your left thumb on the client's right eyebrow to prevent hitting the client with the ophthalmoscope as you move in close. Keep your right index finger on the lens selector to adjust the lens as necessary, as shown here. To examine the left eye, perform these steps on the client's left side.

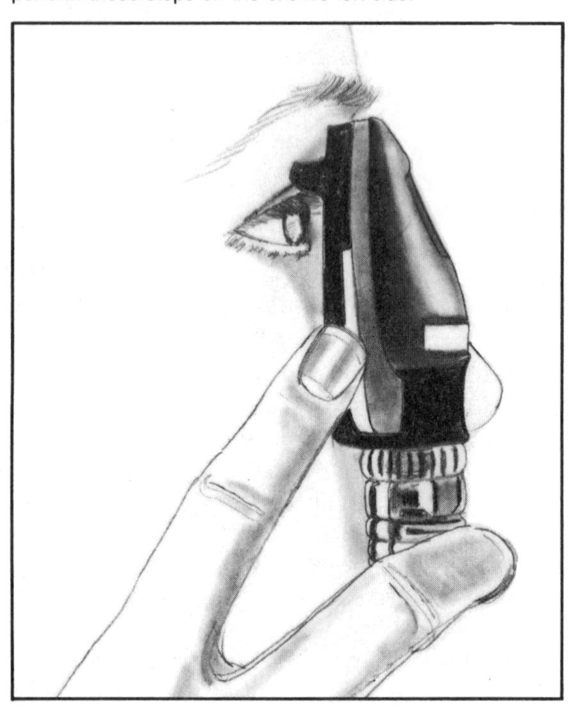

2 Instruct the client to look straight ahead at a fixed point on the wall at eye level. Also instruct the client that, although blinking during the examination is acceptable, the eyes must remain still. Next, approaching from an oblique angle about 15″ (38 cm) out and with the diopter at 0, focus a small circle of light on the pupil, as shown here. Look for the orange-red glow of the red reflex, which should be sharp and distinct through the pupil. The red reflex indicates that the lens is free from opacity and clouding.

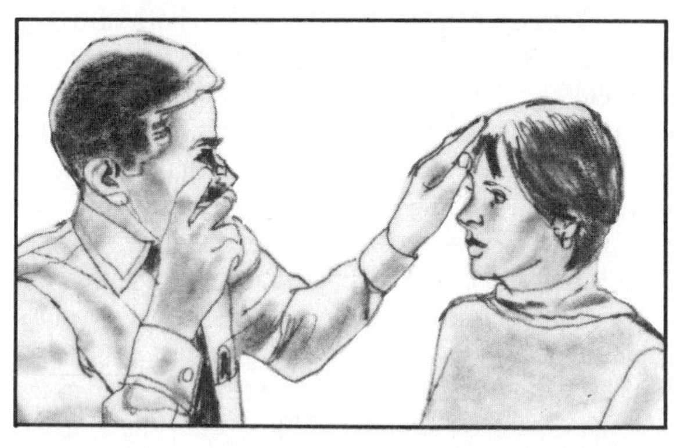

3 Move closer to the client, changing the lens with your forefinger to keep the retinal structures in focus, as shown here.

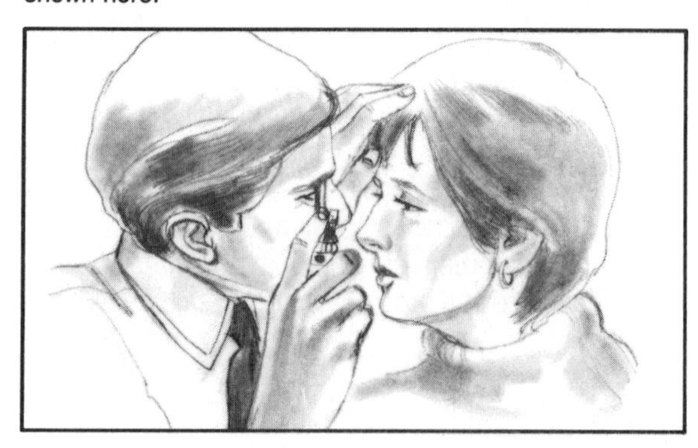

provide the optic disk with its normal pinkish color, an optic disk that has atrophied appears white or pale on ophthalmoscopic examination.

Glaucoma occurs when the outflow of aqueous humor becomes blocked, causing pressure to build within the eye. The increased pressure changes the optic disk shape from round to cupped. Check for cupping by inspecting the retinal vessels as they emerge from the center and exit over the disk margin. With glaucomatous cupping, the vessels seem to disappear at the disk rim and then reappear at a slightly different position just past the rim.

Examining the retinal vessels and retinal background for abnormalities is also an important component of the ophthalmoscopic examination. Hypertension and other systemic diseases can cause changes at the arteriovenous (AV) crossings, such as an apparent nar-

4 Change to a positive diopter to view the vitreous humor, observing for any opacity.

5 Next, view the retina, using a strong negative lens. Look for a retinal blood vessel, and follow that vessel toward the client's nose, rotating the lens selector to keep the vessel in focus. Because focusing depends on both your and the client's refractive status, the lens diopters may differ for almost every client. Carefully examine all the retinal structures, including the retinal vessels, the optic disk, the retinal background, the macula, and the fovea.

6 Examine the vessels for their color, the size ratio of arterioles to veins, the arteriole light reflex, and the arteriovenous (AV) crossing. The crossing points should be smooth, without nicks or narrowings, and the vessels should be free of exudate, bleeding, and narrowing. Retinal vessels normally have an AV ratio of 2:3 or 4:5.

7 Evaluate the color of the retinal structures. The retina should be light yellow to orange and the background free from hemorrhages, aneurysms, and exudates. The optic disk, located on the nasal side of the retina, should be orange-red with distinct margins. The physiologic cup is normally yellow-white and readily visible.

8 Examine the macula last because it is very light-sensitive. The macula, which is darker than the rest of the retinal background, is free of vessels and located temporally to the optic disk. The fovea centralis is a slight depression in the center of the macula. You may find locating the macula difficult, so ask the client to look directly at the light. Be careful to limit the time the light shines on the fovea and macula, because they are points for central vision. The client will become uncomfortable if the light shines too long on these structures.

rowing or blocking of the vein where an arteriole crosses over (called AV nicking). Nicking occurs when an abnormally opaque arteriole with sclerotic edges conceals the underlying vein to varying degrees. Tortuous and engorged veins occur with atherosclerosis, diabetes, multiple myeloma (malignant neoplasm of the bone marrow), polycythemia (abnormal increase of erythrocytes in the blood), and leukemia.

Hemorrhages and exudates (cellular debris) in the retinal background are always pathologic. Superficial hemorrhages are flame-shaped; deeper ones are round and blotchy. Tiny, discrete red spots with smooth edges in the macula are usually the microaneurysms seen in diabetes.

Two types of retinal exudates also occur: hard and soft. Hard exudates are creamy or yellow with well-defined borders. Soft exudates (cottonwool patches) are small areas of necrosis in the arteriole (microinfarctions). They appear as dense, grayish retinal infiltrates with irregular borders. Cottonwool patches occur with hypertension, subacute bacterial endocarditis, lupus, and papilledema.

Many disease-related changes in the eye are painless and do not interfere with vision; therefore, a client may provide no subjective findings. These eye changes may be the first sign of a problem elsewhere in the body. For example, the retinal changes associated with hypertension may be the first indicator of this often silent systemic disease.

Macular degeneration, which is common in elderly clients, is confirmed by ophthalmoscopic examination as the absence of the centrally located fovea centralis. The client will complain of poor central vision, but peripheral vision remains intact.

During the ophthalmoscopic examination, identify exudates and hemorrhages in the retina in relation to the disk diameter (DD), or the size of the optic disk. For example, an exudate may be said to be 1 DD in size and located at 2 o'clock in the right eye.

Although the ophthalmoscopic examination is not commonly performed on children under age 6, at least assess for the presence of a red reflex. To accomplish this, set the ophthalmoscope at 0 diopters and focus the light on the pupil. The red reflex should flash, easily visible, indicating that the lens is clear and free of opacity. Refer any infant or child without a visible red reflex to an ophthalmologist to rule out congenital cataracts or other serious disorders. Children age 6 and over can cooperate for a full ophthalmoscopic examination and for the remainder of the eye assessment.

On an elderly client, an ophthalmoscopic examination will reveal a pale fundus, mildly narrowed retinal vessels, and a decrease in the brightness of the macular and foveal reflexes. Granular pigmentation may also occur in the macula. Occasionally, benign degenerative hyaline deposits, called drusen, appear in the fundi as haphazard gray or yellow spots.

Tonometry

Tonometry measures intraocular pressure by indenting the anesthetized cornea. When using Schiotz' tonometer,

(Text continues on page 230.)

Applying the nursing process

Assessment findings form the basis of the nursing process. Using them, the nurse formulates the nursing diagnoses and develops appropriate planning, implementation, and evaluation of the client's care.

The table below shows how the nurse can use eye assessment data in the nursing process for the client described in the case history (shown at right). In the first column, history and physical assessment data appear, followed by a paragraph of mental notes. These notes help the nurse make important mental connections among assessment findings, aiding in development of the nursing diagnoses and planning.

The second column presents several appropriate nursing diagnoses. However, the information in the remaining columns is based on the *first* nursing diagnosis. Although it is not a part of the nursing process, documentation appears in the last column because of its importance. Documentation consists of an initial note using all components of the SOAPIE format and a follow-up note using the appropriate SOAPIE components.

ASSESSMENT	NURSING DIAGNOSES	PLANNING	IMPLEMENTATION
Subjective (history) data • Client states, "I can't see things from the side as well as I used to." • Client reports that he has been diabetic for 22 years and is to take insulin, 80 U Semilente, daily. Client states, "I don't take insulin every day, just when I eat a lot of sugar." • Client says he does not test blood for glucose level with glucometer. • Client has family history of diabetes and glaucoma. • Last eye examination, 12 years ago. **Objective (physical) data** • Temperature 99° F., pulse 92 and regular, respirations 24 and regular, blood pressure 170/100. • Peripheral pulses nonpalpable in dorsalis pedis and in popliteals. • Dry skin on legs and feet. • Carotid arteries have bruits bilaterally. • Visual acuity 20/30 each eye and both eyes. • Visual field testing reveals lowered peripheral vision bilaterally. • Inspection of eyes shows white sclera and conjunctiva free of drainage. No eyelid edema is present. • Ophthalmoscopic examination reveals 2:4 AV ratio with AV nicking. Optic disk reveals early glaucomatous cupping. Retinal background reveals several whitish yellow exudates, 3 DD from disk at 1 and 4 o'clock bilaterally. Several small exudates on macula bilaterally. • Blood glucose 300 mg/dl nonfasting with glucometer. **Mental notes** *Client needs thorough diabetes education because he does not take insulin daily and demonstrates a poor understanding of diabetes.* *He also needs education on glaucoma and, even more important, on how diabetic retinopathy may be causing his vision problems.* *He needs to reach an understanding of his responsibility for his health.*	• Knowledge deficit related to relationship between vision changes and diabetes. • Alteration in visual sensation related to increased ocular pressure, decreased peripheral vision, and funduscopic abnormalities. • Alteration in tissue perfusion related to decreased peripheral pulses.	**Goals** Before leaving the clinic today, the client will: • verbalize the importance of seeing a physician. At the next follow-up visit, the client will: • discuss the effects of diabetes on vision. • discuss how keeping diabetes in control will prevent added retinopathy. • describe how he plans to follow his diabetic regimen and discuss why it is important. • be able to verbalize his anger and frustration over having a chronic illness. • demonstrate how to use a glucometer to test blood glucose levels.	• Instruct the client to call a physician to schedule an appointment. • Instruct the client on the various aspects of the diabetic regimen and the importance of complying with the regimen. • Explain the effects of diabetes on his vision, and also explain the other potential complications resulting from noncompliance with the diabetic regimen. • Instruct client to expect a follow-up phone call in 1 week and a home visit later in the month. • Suggest that the client join a diabetes education group that also provides emotional support. • Teach client how to use a blood glucometer to test blood glucose levels.

CASE HISTORY

James Curran, age 52, is a married Caucasian male who works as a middle manager for a computer manufacturing firm. A known diabetic, Mr. Curran comes to the clinic complaining of difficulty seeing objects to the side.

EVALUATION

At the next follow-up visit, the client:
- verbalized fear, anger, and frustration with the health care system and over having a chronic illness.
- related the effects of diabetes on vision.
- stated that he visited his family physician and ophthalmologist and that he is trying to take his insulin daily after first checking his blood glucose level.
- demonstrated the use of a glucometer.
- declined a home visit, but said he would call again in 2 weeks to follow up.

DOCUMENTION BASED ON NURSING PROCESS DATA

Initial

	Initial
S	Client states, "I can't see things from the side as well as I used to." Client states he has had diabetes for 22 years and that, "I only take insulin when I've eaten too much sugar." Family history of diabetes and glaucoma. Last eye examination 12 years ago. No complaints of eye pain, discharge, infection, or injury. Wears glasses to read.
O	Temperature 99° F.; pulse 92 and regular; respirations 24 and regular; blood pressure 170/100. PERRLA direct and consensual. Cover-uncover test, six cardinal positions of gaze, corneal light reflex revealed no abnormalities. Peripheral vision revealed visual field deficits laterally in each eye. Visual acuity 20/30 O.D., O.S., and together. Ophthalmoscopic examination demonstrated 2:4 AV ratio with nicking. Exudates of 3 DD from disk at 1 and 4 o'clock bilaterally. Maculas have several white exudates bilaterally.
A	Knowledge deficit related to relationship between vision changes and diabetes.
P	Teach client about the need to see a physician and about the eye complications that can result from diabetes. Instruct the client in the use of a glucometer. Instruct client that nurse will follow up with a phone call and a visit.
I	Called client's physician and scheduled appointments. Taught client how to use glucometer to test blood glucose levels. Instructed client on the potential complications of noncompliance. Will follow up with phone call in 1 week.
E	Client verbalized fear, anger, and frustration with health care system and at having a chronic illness. Able to relate the effects of diabetes on vision.

	Follow-up
S	Follow-up phone call. Client stated he is being treated for glaucoma by an ophthalmologist recommended by his family physician. "I'm trying to remember to take insulin every day and to test my blood for sugar with this machine."
O	"I still can't see what's going on to the side of me, and the doctor can't tell me when I will get better."
A	Client needs continued follow-up to be taught about glaucoma.
P	Client needs continued follow-up and support to increase compliance with diabetic regimen.
I	Provide client with home visit and follow-up phone calls.
E	Call family physician and ophthalmologist to discuss case and to gain their support for client teaching efforts.

a normal pressure reading is below 20 mm Hg. Other tonometers have different normal values. All adults over age 40 should have an annual tonometric examination, which only experienced examiners should perform.

Documentation: The eye

To understand the significance of eye assessment findings, first review the health history findings and compare those findings to the physical assessment findings, including the results of the vision testing. A thorough history, including a complete review of systems, will help link subjective symptoms with objective findings. Carefully complete this process to avoid missing a potentially serious problem in the presence of a seemingly minor objective finding.

Because the eyes are such complex and vital structures, almost all of the eye disorders detected will require physician referral.

If the analysis of eye assessment data reveals no problems, simply educate the client about proper eye care. For example, instruct the client about the necessary frequency of eye assessments and how to avoid injuries. Discuss the importance of special eye care for clients with a chronic illness, such as diabetes, or the medications required for clients with an eye disorder, such as glaucoma.

Gathering the assessment data is the first step in the nursing process. Based on this data, you should be able to assign appropriate nursing diagnoses, allowing you to plan, implement, and evaluate the client's nursing care. (For a case study that shows how to apply the nursing process to a client with an eye disorder, see *Applying the nursing process,* pages 228 and 229.)

After completing the assessment, be sure to document the data completely, including normal and abnormal findings.

The following example illustrates how to document some normal physical assessment findings for the eye:

> Palpebral fissures symmetrical. No periorbital edema. Snellen alphabet chart demonstrates 20/20 vision in both eyes without corrective lenses. Cover-uncover test demonstrates no wandering or abnormal movements of eye. Six cardinal extraocular positions are equal in all planes with no abnormal movements. Corneal light reflex normal bilaterally. PERRLA direct and consensual. Sclera, conjunctiva, and cornea clear bilaterally. Red reflex present bilaterally.

The following example illustrates how to document some abnormal physical assessment findings for the eye:

> Snellen alphabet chart demonstrates visual acuity of 20/50 in right eye; 20/30 in left eye with corrective lenses. Cover-uncover test: right eye deviates outward when cover removed; left eye, no deviation. Corneal light reflex at 8 o'clock in right eye, center of pupil in left eye. Six cardinal positions are not equilateral on all axes. Right eye does not have full range of motion laterally as does left eye. Scleral conjunctiva has red area to right of right pupil. Corneas opaque bilaterally. Arcus senilis with lipid deposits on corners. Right pupil smaller than left; responds sluggishly to light. Red reflex not present on right.

Be sure to document the other steps of the nursing process—nursing diagnosis, planning, implementation, and evaluation—as they are applied to the client with an eye disorder.

Anatomy and physiology review: The ear

The ear, a sensory organ with the functions of hearing and maintaining equilibrium, contains three anatomic parts—the external ear, the middle ear, and the inner ear. The external flap, called the auricle or pinna, and the external auditory canal compose the external ear. The eardrum (tympanic membrane) separates the external from the middle ear at the proximal portion of the auditory canal. The middle ear is a small, air-filled cavity in the temporal bone that contains three small bones—the malleus, incus, and stapes. It leads to the inner ear, a bony and membranous labyrinth.

The auricle picks up sound waves and channels them into the auditory canal where they strike the tympanic membrane, which vibrates and, in turn, vibrates the handle of the malleus. The vibrations travel from the malleus to the incus, to the stapes, through the oval window, and through the fluid in the cochlea to the round window. The membrane covering the round window shakes the delicate hair cells in the organ of Corti, which stimulates the sensory endings of the cochlear branch of the acoustic nerve (cranial nerve VIII). The nerve sends the impulses to the auditory area of the temporal lobe in the brain, which then interprets the sound. (For an illustration, see *Structures and functions of the ear,* pages 232 and 233.)

Health history: The ear

Before beginning the interview, ascertain if the client hears well. If a hearing problem exists, look directly at the client and speak clearly when interviewing. Keep in mind that hearing problems can seriously affect the client's ability to carry out activities of daily living and can adversely affect every aspect of the client's life.

The questions in this section are designed to help you evaluate the client's ears fully. They include rationales that describe the significance of the answers and, where appropriate, nursing interventions that may be incorporated into the client's care plan.

Health and illness patterns

To assess current health and illness patterns related to the ear, use the following guidelines to explore the client's current, past, and family health status, as well as the developmental status.

Current health status

Because current health status is foremost in the client's mind, begin the interview by exploring this topic. Carefully document the chief complaint in the client's own words. Using the PQRST method, ask for a complete description of the problem. (For a detailed explanation of this method, see *Symptom analysis* in Chapter 3, The Health History.)

Have you recently noticed any difference in your hearing in one or both ears?
(RATIONALE: The pattern of hearing loss gives clues about its cause. For example, unilateral hearing loss could be caused by a polyp on the affected side. Sudden hearing loss may be caused by a rupture of the tympanic membrane. Unilateral, intermittent hearing loss could be caused by Meniere's disease.)

Do you have ear pain?
(RATIONALE: Ear pain can indicate a middle or inner ear infection, an ear canal obstruction by earwax [cerumen] or a foreign body, or temporomandibular joint infection.)

Do you ever have trouble with earwax? If so, what do you do for it?
(RATIONALE: Using cotton-tipped swabs to clear the ear canal can cause injury. Also, the overuse of home remedies or OTC products can cause skin abrasion in the external ear canal and lead to infection.)

Past health status

During the next part of the health history, ask the following questions to gather additional information about the client's ears.

Have you had an ear injury? If so, describe the injury and treatment.
(RATIONALE: Some injuries can cause permanent hearing impairment.)

Have you ever experienced ringing or crackling in your ears?
(RATIONALE: Tinnitus can result from hypertension, ossicle dislocation, or a blockage by cerumen, whereas crackling occurs because of fluid in the middle ear.)

Have you recently had a foreign body in your ear?
(RATIONALE: A recent history of a foreign body in the ear may explain an infection. Also, if the foreign body caused trauma to the external canal, an otoscopic assessment can be very painful, so proceed carefully.)

Do you suffer from frequent ear infections?
(RATIONALE: Chronic otitis media can cause a gradual hearing loss.)

Have you had drainage from your ears? If so, when and how was it treated?
(RATIONALE: Cloudy otorrhea [drainage from the ear] could be caused by serous fluid pressure buildup from an allergy, which ruptures the tympanic membrane. Clear, watery otorrhea could be cerebrospinal fluid [CSF] from a basilar skull fracture. Bloody, purulent otorrhea could be caused by otitis media.)

Have you had problems with balance, dizziness, or vertigo?
(RATIONALE: Vertigo can indicate a neurologic or otologic disorder. Dizziness is not caused by an ear disorder but may be caused by inadequate blood flow and blood supply to the brain.)

Structures and functions of the ear

These illustrations show how hearing occurs through the anatomic structures of the external, middle, and inner ear.

External ear

The cartilaginous antihelix, crux of the helix, lobule, antitragus, and concha together form the auricle (pinna). The tragus, which is not visible in the cutaway below, is anterior to the external opening. Although not part of the external ear, the mastoid process is an important bony landmark posterior to the lower part of the auricle.

The outer third of the external auditory canal is cartilage covered by thin, sensitive skin, and the inner two thirds is bone covered by thin skin. The adult client's external canal leads inward, downward, and forward to the middle ear.

Middle ear

The tympanic membrane separates the middle from the external ear at the proximal portion of the auditory canal. Composed of layers of skin, fibrous tissue, and mucous membrane, the tympanic membrane appears pearly gray, shiny, and translucent. The auditory canal stretches most of the membrane, called the pars tensa, tightly inward; however, a superior portion of the membrane, called the pars flaccida, hangs loosely and covers the short process of the malleus. The center of the membrane (the umbo) covers the long process of the malleus. Around the outer border of the membrane is a pale, white, fibrous ring (the annulus).

The external canal leads into the middle ear—a small, air-filled cavity in the temporal bone. Within this cavity, three small bones (auditory ossicles) link together to transmit sound. These bones are the malleus (hammer), the incus (anvil), and the stapes (stirrup).

During an otoscopic examination, the nurse should be able to see these tympanic membrane landmarks: the handle of the malleus, the short process of the malleus, the umbo, and the cone of light (the light reflex) that fans down from the umbo.

The stapes sits in an opening called the oval window (fenestra ovalis), through which sound vibrations travel to the

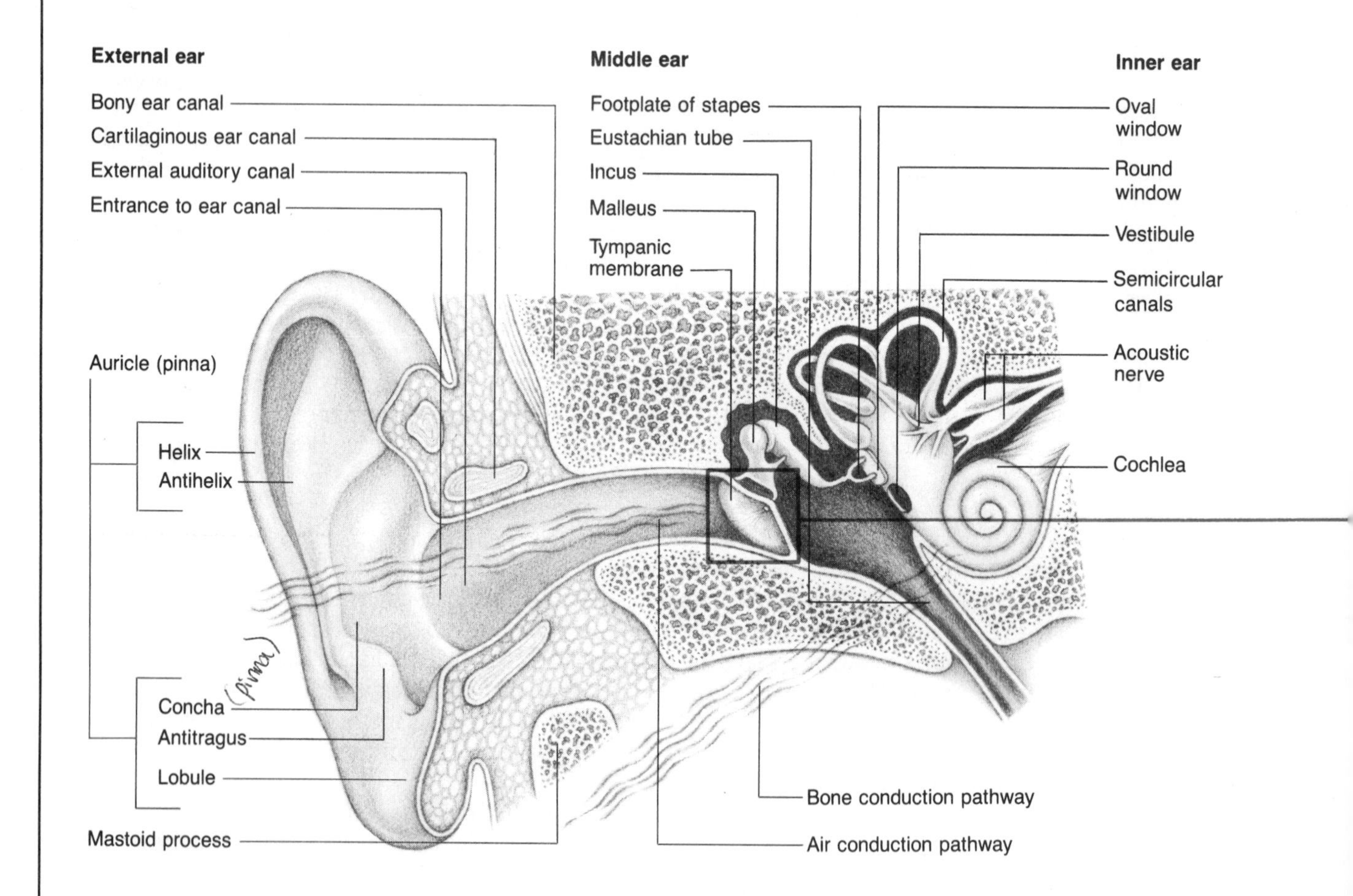

inner ear. Covered by a membrane, the round window (fenestra rotunda) opens the middle ear to the inner ear. The eustachian tube, which connects the middle ear with the nasopharynx, equalizes pressure between the inner and outer surfaces of the tympanic membrane.

Inner ear
A bony and a membranous labyrinth combine to form the inner ear. The bony labyrinth consists of the vestibule, the cochlea, and the semicircular canals. The latter contain sensory epithelium for maintaining a sense of position and equilibrium, and the cochlea contains the organ of Corti for transmitting sound to the cochlear branch of the acoustic nerve (cranial nerve VIII). The vestibular branch of the acoustic nerve contains peripheral nerve fibers that terminate in the epithelium of the semicircular canals, and the central branch terminates in the medulla at the vestibular nucleus.

The hearing pathways
For hearing to occur, sound waves travel through the ear by two pathways: air conduction and bone conduction, as indicated by the wavy red lines in the illustration on the left. Air conduction occurs when sound waves travel in the air through the external and middle ear to the inner ear. Bone conduction occurs when sound waves travel through bone to the inner ear.

The vibrations transmitted through air and bone stimulate nerve impulses in the inner ear. The cochlear branch of the acoustic nerve transmits these vibrations to the auditory area of the cerebral cortex, where the temporal lobe of the brain interprets the sound.

Otoscopic view of the tympanic membrane

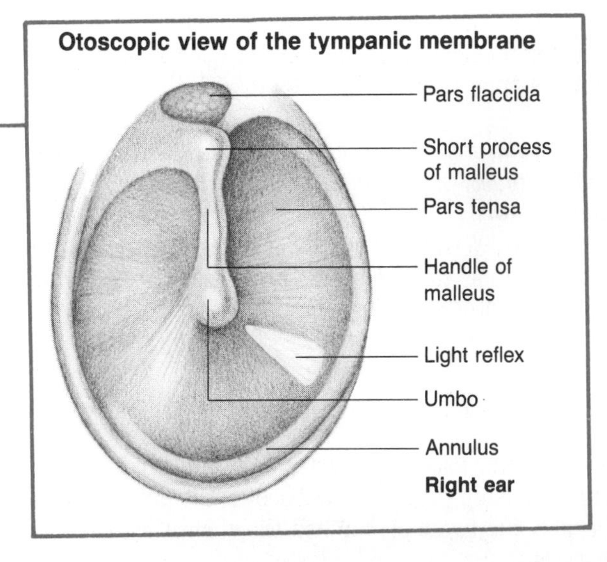

ototoxic

Have you been taking any prescription or over-the-counter medications or home remedies for your ears or for any other conditions? If so, which medications and how often?
(RATIONALE: Certain medications, such as aspirin, taken for other conditions can affect hearing. For more information, see *Adverse drug reactions,* page 234.)

Has anyone in your family had hearing problems?
(RATIONALE: Otosclerosis is a hereditary disorder that begins between age 20 and 30 as unilateral conductive hearing loss and progresses to bilateral mixed hearing loss.)

Developmental considerations

Young children frequently have ear disorders, and many elderly clients suffer from hearing impairment. The nurse must pose additional questions if the client is young or elderly.

Pediatric client. When assessing a child, try to involve the parent or guardian and the child in the interview. However, keep in mind that a child with an ear infection may be irritable from a high fever and severe pain. To assess the child, ask the following questions:

Does the infant respond to loud or unusual noises?
(RATIONALE: A negative response could indicate a hearing loss. In this case, refer the infant to a specialist for further evaluation.)

If over age 6 months, does the infant babble?
(RATIONALE: Failure to babble after 6 months could indicate a hearing impairment. Refer the infant to a specialist for further evaluation.)

If over age 15 months, does the toddler rely on gestures and make no attempt at sound?
(RATIONALE: Making no attempt to speak beyond the appropriate developmental age could indicate a hearing loss. Refer such a toddler to a specialist for further evaluation.)

Is the toddler speaking appropriately for his or her age?
(RATIONALE: Problems with speech development can indicate a hearing impairment.)

Have you noticed the child tugging at either ear?
(RATIONALE: This is often a sign of an ear infection.)

Have you noticed any coordination problems?
(RATIONALE: Inner ear infections can affect equilibrium.)

Adverse drug reactions

When assessing a client's ear, the nurse should ask the client about current drug use. Many drugs can cause adverse effects that can mimic signs or symptoms of various diseases or damage the cochlea or vestibule of the ear, resulting in tinnitus, vertigo, or hearing loss.

DRUG CLASS	DRUG	POSSIBLE ADVERSE REACTIONS
Aminoglycosides	All aminoglycosides	Tinnitus, vertigo, hearing loss
Anti-inflammatory agents	All nonsteroidal anti-inflammatory agents (such as diflunisal, ibuprofen, and indomethacin)	Tinnitus, vertigo, hearing loss
Antimalarials	quinine	Tinnitus, vertigo, hearing loss
Diuretics	furosemide and bumetanide	Tinnitus, vertigo, hearing loss (with too-rapid I.V. administration)
Nonnarcotic analgesics and antipyretics	All salicylates and all combination products containing salicylates	Tinnitus, dizziness, hearing loss (with high dose or long-term therapy)
Miscellaneous agents	capreomycin, cisplatin, ethacrynic acid, quinidine sulfate, and vancomycin	Tinnitus, vertigo, hearing loss

Has the child had meningitis, recurrent otitis media, mumps, or encephalitis?
(RATIONALE: Any of these conditions can cause hearing loss.)

Elderly client. When assessing an elderly client, ask these additional questions:

Have you noticed any change in your hearing recently?
(RATIONALE: Elderly clients commonly develop presbycusis—a physiologic hearing loss that usually affects those over age 50.)

Do you wear a hearing aid? If so, for how long? How do you care for it?
(RATIONALE: If the client wears a hearing aid, be especially careful to speak clearly and directly. Also, some clients who hear poorly refuse to wear a hearing aid because they do not want to accept that they have a hearing problem.)

Health promotion and protection patterns

To continue the health history, the nurse should use the following guidelines to ask about the client's personal health habits and occupational health patterns related to the ear.

When was your last ear examination or hearing test? What were the results?
(RATIONALE: The answer to this question could suggest the importance of preventive health care to the client. The last examination date also can serve for assessing recent changes.)

Do you have any other concerns about your ears or other symptoms that I haven't asked you about?
(RATIONALE: The client may have a different perception of the ear problem. This open-ended question gives the client the opportunity to discuss it with the nurse.)

Do you work around loud equipment, such as heavy machinery, airguns, or airplanes? If so, do you wear ear protectors?
(RATIONALE: Working around loud machinery for long periods of time can cause hearing loss. However, the client can prevent this type of loss by using earguards. Teach the client the importance of wearing them.)

Role and relationship patterns

Ear disorders, especially hearing loss, can affect role and relationship patterns. To discover the extent of this influence, the nurse should ask the client the following questions.

Does your hearing difficulty interfere with your activities of daily living?

(RATIONALE: A client who has a hearing problem may not want to work or perform regular chores such as shopping. If so, refer the client to an occupational therapist.)

Does your hearing difficulty affect your relationships with other people? If so, how?
(RATIONALE: The spouse or friends of a client with a hearing loss may become impatient with the hearing-impaired person. Many times, the client will feel left out of conversations, especially if background noise makes hearing even more difficult. The client may withdraw rather than try to understand the conversation.)

Physical assessment: The ear

Physical assessment of the ear includes inspection, palpation, hearing screening, and otoscopic examination. The nurse cannot inspect structures of the middle and inner ear but can assess their functioning through hearing screening.

Equipment required for a basic ear assessment includes an otoscope, a tuning fork, a watch, and for the advanced assessment, an otoscope.

Inspection

Inspection and palpation are usually performed simultaneously, but this section describes each separately to clarify the techniques used in each procedure. Prepare for the assessment by washing your hands. Then seat the adult client and begin inspecting the external ear structures. The auricle should cross a line approximated from the outer canthus of the eye to the protuberance of the occiput. The ear position should be almost vertical, with no more than a 10-degree lateral-posterior slant.

Next, inspect the ear for color and size. The ears should be similarly shaped, colored the same as the face, and sized in proportion to the head. However, ear shape and size vary greatly within the population, so obtain information about what other family members' ears look like before concluding that an abnormality exists.

Inspect the ear for drainage, nodules, or lesions. Some ears normally drain large amounts of cerumen. Also check behind the ear for inflammation, masses, or lesions.

Abnormal findings

A deviation in the alignment of the auricle, such as ears below the lateral angle of the eye (low-set ears), suggests renal abnormalities or chromosomal abnormalities such as Down's syndrome. For this reason, carefully observe ear position and alignment in newborns and infants.

Underlying vasomotor disorders can cause pale or excessively red ears. Fevers can also cause red ears. Abnormally large, small, or unusually shaped ears can be a familial trait, an abnormality, or the result of an injury.

Purulent drainage usually indicates an infection, whereas drainage that is clear or bloody could be CSF leaking after head trauma.

Palpation

After the inspection, palpate the external ear and the mastoid process to discover any areas of tenderness, swelling, nodules, or lesions and then gently pull the helix of the ear backward to determine the presence of pain or tenderness.

Abnormal findings

An edematous or sensitive tragus can indicate an inflammation or infection of the external or middle ear. Pain or tenderness in the external canal on palpation of the helix, along with a noticeable yellow or serous purulent discharge, can also result from an external or middle ear infection that could be either viral or bacterial. Many times, the client reports a history of frequent swimming.

Auditory function screening

The most common causes of hearing loss result from conduction problems, neural problems, or problems with the auditory center from injury or damage.

Conduction deafness occurs from interference with the functioning of external and middle ear structures. For example, a cerumen plug in the canal, otitis media, a membrane rupture, or sclerosis of the ossicles can all cause the tympanic membrane to fail to vibrate, resulting in a conduction deafness.

Sensorineural deafness results from damage to inner ear structures, such as the organ of Corti, or from damage to cranial nerve VIII. Central deafness, also a sensorineural deafness, occurs after damage to the auditory area of the temporal lobe in the brain, such as from a cerebrovascular accident or a central nervous system lesion.

Gross hearing screening

Perform two gross screenings of hearing: the whispered or spoken voice test and the watch tick test. For the voice test, have the client occlude one ear with a finger. Test the other ear by standing behind the client at a distance of 1′ to 2′ (30 to 60 cm) and whispering a word or phrase. A client with normal acuity should be able to repeat what was whispered.

The watch tick test evaluates the client's ability to hear high-frequency sounds. Gradually move a watch until the client can no longer hear the ticking, which should occur when the watch is about 5″ (13 cm) away. These are crude methods, so use these tests with other forms of auditory screening.

Use the remaining auditory screening tests—Weber's and the Rinne tests—to evaluate the client for the presence of conduction or sensorineural hearing loss. The Schwabach test is another auditory screening test but is very subjective and not included. Conduct the tests with a tuning fork with frequencies of 500 to 1,000 cycles per second. The tuning fork tests air conduction (sound transmission by air through the canal, the tympanic membrane, the ossicles, and the cochlea to the acoustic nerve) and bone conduction (transmission of sound through the bones of the skull to the cochlea and acoustic nerve).

Weber's test

This test evaluates bone conduction. Perform the test by placing a vibrating tuning fork on the top of the client's head at midline or in the middle of the client's forehead. The client should perceive the sound equally in both ears. If the client has a conductive hearing loss, the sound will be heard in (lateralize to) the ear that has the conductive loss because the sound is being conducted directly through the bone to the ear. If the client has a sensorineural hearing loss in one ear, the sound will lateralize to the unimpaired ear because nerve damage in the impaired ear prevents hearing. Document a normal Weber's test by recording a negative lateralization of sound.

Rinne test

This test compares bone conduction to air conduction in both ears. Assess bone conduction by placing the base of a vibrating tuning fork on the mastoid process, noting how many seconds pass before the client can no longer hear it. Then, quickly place the still-vibrating tuning fork with the tines parallel to the client's auricle near the ear canal (to test air conduction). Hold the tuning fork in this position until the client no longer hears the tone. Note how many seconds the client can hear the tone. Repeat the test on the other ear. Because sound traveling through air remains audible twice as long (a 2:1 ratio) as sound traveling through bone, a sound heard for 10 seconds by bone conduction should be heard for 20 seconds by air conduction. If the client reports hearing the sound longer through bone conduction, the client has a conductive loss. In a sensorineural loss, the client will report hearing the sound longer through air conduction, but the ratio will not be a normal 2:1. (For some common abnormalities associated with the ear, see *Integrating assessment findings.*)

Developmental and ethnic considerations

Techniques and findings of ear assessments vary according to a client's age. An ear assessment of an infant, toddler, or preschooler can be very challenging; for that reason, you may want to perform it last. A father or mother can hold the infant in his or her lap, then immobilize the infant's head with one hand and the arms with the other.

Testing auditory function with a tuning fork is not possible with young children because of their lack of understanding of the procedure and their inability to verbalize well. However, you should evaluate an infant's or young child's responses to voices and a rattle to rule out a congenital hearing problem.

In elderly clients, the external structure of the ear, such as the auricle, may have lost adipose tissue and the cartilage may be harder. The skin and cerumen in the external auditory canal may be dry and flaky.

Elderly clients lose hair cells in the organ of Corti, which impairs the client's hearing of high-pitched tones. Sclerosis of the ossicles in the middle ear impairs the transmission of sound, and a loss of ganglion cells in the cochlea and neurons in the auditory cortex affects sound perception. All of these changes result in both sensorineural and conductive hearing loss, which may become apparent upon performance of Weber's, the Rinne, and the Schwabach tests.

Presbycusis, a sensorineural hearing loss of high-frequency tones that eventually leads to a loss of all frequencies, also occurs with advancing age. Consonants become difficult to hear, and, as a result, many words become hard to understand. Minimize this handicap by standing in front of the elderly client when you speak. This allows the client to watch your lips for clues to the inaudible consonants.

The only ethnic consideration related to assessing the ear is the difference in the color of cerumen in Blacks and other dark-skinned clients when compared to lighter-

Integrating assessment findings

Sometimes, a cluster of assessment findings will strongly suggest a particular ear disorder. In the chart below, column one shows groups of presenting signs and symptoms—the ones that make the client seek medical attention. Column two shows related assessment findings that the nurse may discover during the health history and physical assessment. The client may exhibit one or more of these findings. Column three shows the possible disorder indicated by a cluster of these findings.

PRESENTING SIGNS AND SYMPTOMS	RELATED ASSESSMENT FINDINGS	POSSIBLE DISORDER
Mild to severe ear pain aggravated by palpation of the auricle or tragus	History of swimming Moist, hot climate Cleaning ears with sharp object Allergy to hair spray Lymphadenopathy Low-pitched tinnitus Yellow discharge (may also be bloody, serous, or cheesy) Foul-smelling, tenacious discharge	Acute otitis externa
Severe, deep, throbbing head pain accompanied by a hearing loss	Purulent discharge if tympanic membrane is pierced Vertigo or dizziness accompanied by nausea Tinnitus Recent upper respiratory tract infection or measles, allergies, adenoid hypertrophy, fever, or chills Sudden cessation of pain when tympanic membrane ruptures Hyperemic tympanic membrane, minimal retraction with dull red landmarks obscured Normal or pus-filled canals	Acute otitis media
Sudden vertigo lasting from minutes to hours; low buzz tinnitus in one ear	Fluctuating low-frequency sensorineural hearing loss, usually in one ear Vertigo that can last from minutes to hours with occurrences weeks to months apart Abnormal audiography Recurrent episodes; asymptomatic between attacks Altered activities of daily living	Meniere's disease
Hearing loss; sudden or gradual vertigo; tinnitus in both ears, usually high-pitched	Use of ototoxic medication Ataxia (impaired coordination of movement) Normal otoscopic examination Permanent deafness possible	Ototoxicity
Severe itching of entire ear; discharge; mild vertigo or dizziness; mild, low-pitched tinnitus	History of recurrent psoriasis or other dermatosis Allergy to hair spray, hair dye, or nail polish Lymphadenopathy Red, thick, excoriated auricle and canal, possibly with crusting Insensitive canal and tympanic membrane	Chronic otitis externa
Progressive hearing loss, tinnitus	Family history of otosclerosis Conductive hearing loss, worsening with pregnancy Slight dizziness or vertigo Faint, pink blush behind tympanic membrane Soft speech despite hearing loss	Otosclerosis
Intermittent ear pain, sensation of ear canal blockage, occasional dizziness, tinnitus	History of exposure to pressure change, such as during air travel Retracted, reddened tympanic membrane Air bubbles in middle ear space	Eustachian tube blockage

ADVANCED ASSESSMENT SKILLS

Otoscopic examination

The nurse can perform an otoscopic examination to assess the tympanic membrane and other internal ear structures. To do so, follow these steps.

Before inserting the speculum into the ear, inspect the canal opening for a foreign body or discharge. Palpate the tragus and pull up the auricle to assess for tenderness. If tenderness is present, the client may have external otitis media; therefore, do not insert the speculum because pain is likely to result. Also inspect the external auditory canal before proceeding.

1 After determining that inserting the otoscope is safe, tip the adult client's head to the side opposite from the ear being assessed. Straighten the canal by grasping the superior posterior auricle between your thumb and index finger and pulling it up and back as shown here.

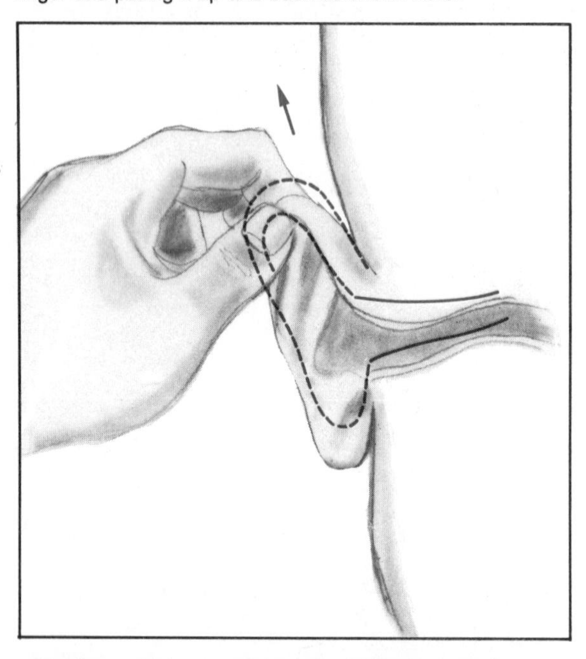

2 Then grasp the otoscope in your dominant hand with the handle parallel to the client's head and the speculum at the client's ear. Hold the otoscope firmly against the client's head, as shown here, to prevent jerking the speculum against the external canal. Examination of the external canal normally reveals varying amounts of hair and cerumen because the distal third of the canal contains hair follicles and sebaceous and ceruminous glands. Note the color of the cerumen—old cerumen is usually dry and grayish brown in color. Excessive cerumen can conceal the tympanic membrane and can also be a factor in reduced hearing ability or in a conductive hearing loss. Occasionally, hard, black cerumen plugs may require removal to allow you to see the tympanic membrane. The external canal should be free from inflammation and scaling.

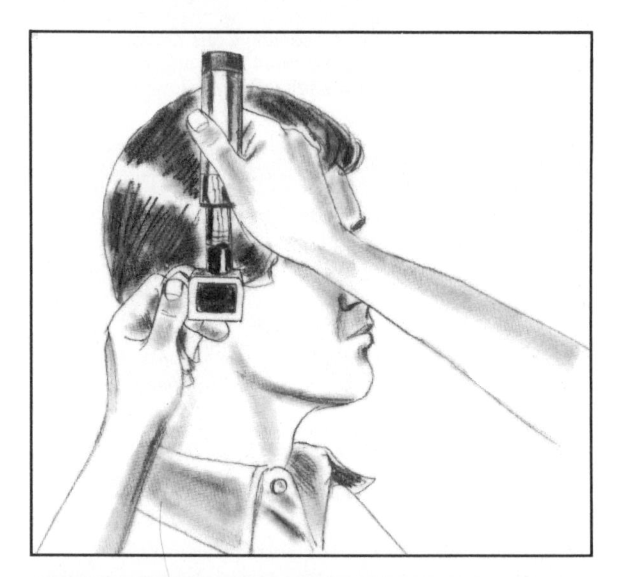

3 The inner two thirds of the canal is sensitive to pressure, so insert the speculum gently to avoid causing the client pain. Gently rotate the angle of the speculum as needed to gain a complete view of the tympanic membrane.

4 Inspect the tympanic membrane at the end of the canal, which should glisten and be translucent and pearly gray, with the annulus appearing white and denser than the rest of the membrane. The inferior edge of the tympanic membrane is posterior to the outside, and the superior edge is anterior. Look for bulging, retraction, or perforations at the periphery of the tympanic membrane.

Next, check the light reflex, which is in the anterior inferior quadrant in the 5 o'clock position in the right tympanic membrane and in the 7 o'clock position in the left. The light reflex usually appears as a bright cone of light with its point directed at the umbo and its base at the periphery of the tympanic membrane.

Also examine the malleus. The handle of the malleus originates in the superior hemisphere of the tympanic membrane and, when viewed through the membrane, looks like a dense whitish streak. The malleus attaches to the center of the tympanic membrane at the umbo.

At the top portion of the handle are the malleolar folds, where you can normally see the small white projection of the short process of the malleus.

Adjusting the technique for a pediatric client

Prepare a toddler or preschooler for an otoscopic examination by allowing the child to hold the equipment and "blow out" the light. Stroking the child's arm with the speculum can also reduce the fear of pain and facilitate the otoscopy. However, for some children, the examination will be difficult despite the preparation and distraction. In these instances, perform the examination as quickly as you can while the parent restrains the child.

1 To perform an otoscopic examination on an infant or toddler, pull the auricle down and back to straighten the canal, as shown here.

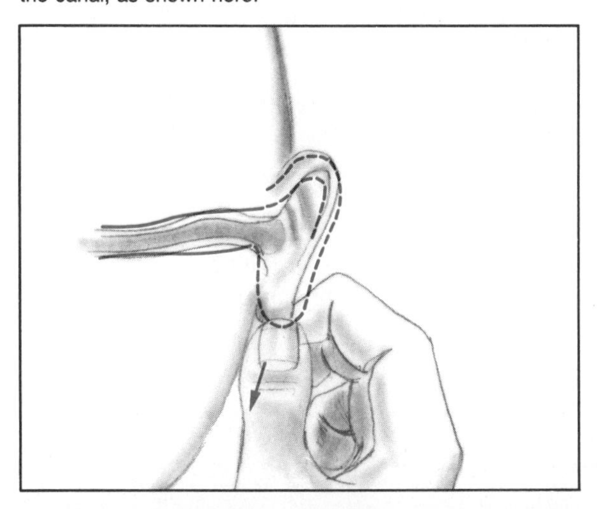

2 Brace your hand against the child's head, as shown here, to avoid traumatizing the canal with the speculum in case the child moves.

The tympanic membrane and its landmarks will have the same norms as in an adult, except for the light reflex, which is diffuse in an infant. If an infant is crying, the increased intracranial pressure will cause the membrane to turn pink or even red. Only experienced examiners can rule out tympanic membrane disease under those conditions. Talking softly and distracting the infant may reduce the likelihood of crying.

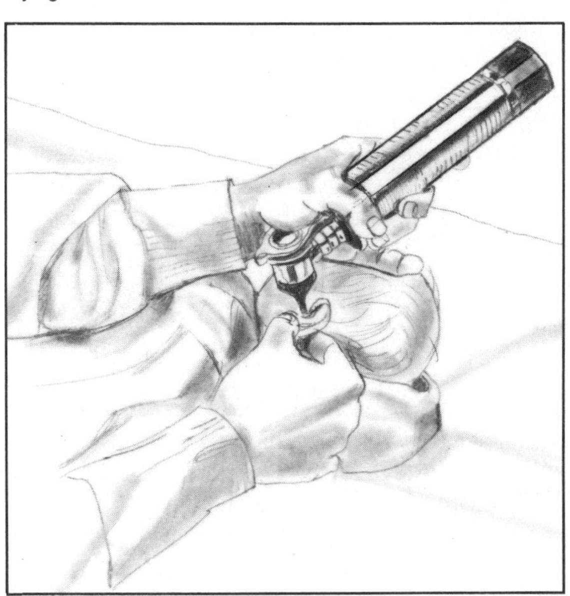

skinned ones. Dark-skinned persons normally have darker orange or brown cerumen, whereas fair-skinned persons have yellow cerumen.

Advanced assessment skills

Advanced assessment skills include the otoscopic examination.

Otoscopic examination

Before beginning the inspection of the canal and the tympanic membrane, become familiar with the function of the otoscope. (For a description of the otoscope and its use, see Chapter 4, Physical Assessment Skills.) The handles used for the otoscope and the ophthalmoscope are interchangeable. Use the following procedure. First, turn on the light for the otoscope by turning the rheostat. The light should be bright; if the light has a dull orange glow, the batteries are low. Also, use a speculum that fits comfortably in the client's external ear canal. Speculums range in diameter from 2 to 9 mm. Use the largest speculum possible for a comfortable examination. The light should reflect from the end of the speculum and not off to the side. When you feel comfortable with this piece of equipment, perform the otoscopic examination. (For an illustrated procedure, see *Advanced assessment skills: Otoscopic examination*.)

While performing this procedure, keep in mind that tympanic membranes vary slightly in size, shape, color, and clarity of landmarks. You may need to inspect numerous healthy tympanic membranes to be able to recognize an abnormal one.

If the client has otitis media, the tympanic membrane will be inflamed (hyperemic) in the initial stages. The light reflex (cone of light seen on the tympanic membrane during otoscopic examination) decreases and then disappears as the membrane swells. You will not be able to see the other landmarks, such as the umbo and the long process. Immediately refer a client with these symptoms to a physician for medication to prevent tympanic membrane perforation.

A retracted membrane can indicate serous otitis media, which often occurs during an upper respiratory infection. When the eustachian tube swells, negative pressure increases in the middle ear. This pulls the tympanic membrane back against the ossicles, accentuating the bony landmarks of the tympanic membrane. The light reflex is diffused rather than cone-shaped. Air fluid levels may appear behind the tympanic membrane, with the fluid color being amber. This change in fluid color changes the tympanic membrane from dull gray to orange-red.

Children are at risk for middle ear infections because of the transmission of viruses and bacteria from the upper respiratory tract to the middle ear via the nasopharynx and the eustachian tube. Children need careful, frequent otoscopic examinations to rule out hearing impairment caused by chronic infections.

In some elderly clients, the tympanic membrane appears thickened with a diminished light reflex.

Documentation: The ear

To understand the significance of ear assessment findings, review the health history findings and compare them to the physical assessment findings, including the results of the auditory testing. A thorough history, including a complete review of systems, will help link subjective symptoms with objective findings and prevent you from missing a potentially serious problem.

Almost all ear disorders detected will require physician referral. However, if the ear assessment data reveal no problems, simply educate the client about proper ear care. For example, instruct the client about the necessary frequency of ear assessments and how to avoid injuries.

Assessment data represent the first step in the nursing process. Based on this data, develop appropriate nursing diagnoses, which serve as the basis for planning, implementing, and evaluating the client's nursing care.

After completing the assessment, be sure to document the data completely, including normal and abnormal findings.

The following example illustrates how to document some normal physical assessment findings for the ear:

> Ears equal in size and symmetrical in position. Color same as skin. No masses palpated on either auricle. No tenderness. Tympanic membrane pearly gray bilaterally; contour slightly conical with a concavity at the umbo. Light reflex at 5 o'clock on the right and 7 o'clock on the left. Weber's and Rinne tests normal bilaterally; no lateralization on Weber's test. Rinne shows air and bone conduction at normal 2:1 ratio (30 seconds: 15 seconds) bilaterally.

The following example illustrates how to document some abnormal physical assessment findings for the ear:

> Right ear larger than left. Reddened raised mass, warm to touch, about 1 cm in diameter on lobe of right ear. Left tympanic membrane white with cone of light at 3 o'clock. Several small white scars on distal portion of membrane. Right tympanic membrane gray-white with long, jagged scar across midsection. Light reflex at 5 o'clock. Weber's test lateralized to right ear with bone conduction longer than air conduction on Rinne test. Rinne test on left shows air conduction 3 times longer than that of bone conduction (30 seconds: 10 seconds).

Be sure to document the other steps of the nursing process—nursing diagnosis, planning, implementation, and evaluation—as they are applied to the client with an ear disorder.

Chapter summary

To assess the client's eyes and ears effectively, the nurse should rely on pertinent health history data and physical assessment findings. Chapter 9 describes how to gather and integrate this information. Here are the chapter highlights:

- The eyelids, conjunctivae, and lacrimal apparatus form the extraocular structures of the eye.
- Six muscles—four rectus and two oblique—control eye movement. To assess the functioning of these extraocular muscles, use the six cardinal points of gaze test, the cover-uncover test, and the corneal light reflex test.
- Retinal structures include the optic disk, four sets of retinal blood vessels, the macula, and the fovea centralis. To view these structures, use an ophthalmoscope.
- When obtaining a health history, be sure to ask the client the date of the last eye examination. The answer provides information about how well the client takes care of health needs and serves as a basis for health teaching.
- When obtaining the health history, also ask what medications the client is taking. The answer might reveal if the client is self-treating an eye condition. Also, many medications can cause vision disorders.
- To assess the client's vision, perform visual acuity tests for near and distance vision, and assess extraocular muscle function.

• When performing an eye assessment on a child, use different tools, as appropriate—for example, the Snellen E chart or Stycar cards instead of the Snellen alphabet chart when testing visual acuity.
• Document all eye assessment findings and use them in the nursing process to plan, implement, and evaluate the client's care.
• The auricle and the external auditory canal compose the external ear. The tympanic membrane separates the external ear from the middle ear, which contains the three ossicles—the malleus, incus, and stapes. The inner ear contains the bony labyrinth, which houses the vestibule, the cochlea, and the semicircular canals.
• When obtaining a health history for a client with an ear disorder, the nurse should be sure to ask the client the date of the last ear examination. The answer provides information about how well the client takes care of health needs and serves as a basis for health teaching.
• During the health history, also discuss the client's medication use, particularly noting any drugs that may be used to self-treat an ear condition or that can cause hearing disorders.
• The basic assessment techniques for the ear include inspection, palpation, and auditory screening. The advanced assessment technique is the otoscopic examination.
• To view the tympanic membrane and the bulge of the handle of the malleus, use an otoscope. The other middle and inner ear structures are not visible with an otoscope.
• When conducting a hearing screening, use the voice, a watch, and a tuning fork. The voice and watch tick test are gross screenings. Weber's and the Rinne tests—both performed with a tuning fork—evaluate air and bone conduction.
• Document normal and abnormal assessment findings for the ear, and use them in the nursing process to plan, implement, and evaluate the client's care.

Study questions

1. When your eyes see an object, such as a red rose, how do they transmit its image to the brain? (Describe this process in terms of the anatomy and physiology of the eye.)

2. When a client reports an eye problem, such as blurred vision, what techniques should you use to collect physical assessment data about the eye?

3. When your ears hear a sound, such as a musical note, how do they transmit its perception to the brain? (Describe this process in terms of the anatomy and physiology of the ear.)

4. When inspecting the right ear canal and tympanic membrane, what normal findings should you expect to see? What three common abnormal findings might you see? What could cause these abnormal findings?

5. Mrs. Traynor brings her son Tim, age 6 months, to the outpatient clinic because he has had a fever of 101° to 102° F. (38.3° to 38.9° C.) for the past 24 hours. She reports that he was fussy yesterday, awoke three times last night, and has been fussy today. He is drinking well but has a decreased appetite. Mrs. Traynor noticed him pulling on his ears. How would you document the following information related to your nursing assessment of Tim?
• history (subjective) assessment data
• physical (objective) assessment data
• assessment techniques and equipment
• nursing diagnoses
• documentation of your findings.

Selected references

Alexander, M., and Brown, M. (1979). *Pediatric history taking and physical diagnosis for nurses* (2nd ed.). New York: McGraw-Hill.

Beauchamp, G., and Sanet, R. (1989). Recommendations for conducting screening of children with learning disability. *School Nurse*, 5(4), 29-30.

Boyd-Monk, H. (1990). Assessing acquired ocular disease. *Nursing Clinics of North America*, 25(4), 811-822.

Carotenuto, R., and Bullock, J. (1981). *Physical assessment of the gerontologic client.* Philadelphia: Davis.

Cohen, K., and Bryne, S. (1989). The role of the nurse in assisting with eye examinations on premature infants. *Neonatal Network*, 8(2), 31-35.

Dornbrand, L., Hoole, R., Fletcher, R., and Pickard, C. (Eds.). (1985). *Manual of clinical problems in adult ambulatory care.* Boston: Little, Brown.

Dychtwald, K. (1986). *Wellness and health promotion for the elderly.* Rockville, MD: Aspen Systems.

Mulrow, C. (1991). Screening for hearing impairment in the elderly. *Hospital Practice (Office),* 26(2A), 79, 83-86.

Pinnell, N., and Meneses, M. (1986). *The nursing process: Theory, application and related processes.* East Norwalk, CT: Appleton & Lange.

Sanet, R., and Ellis, G. (1990). What is the most effective vision screening tool to use with pre-school-age children in early childhood programs? *School Nurse,* 6(1), 27-30.

Sapira, J., and Scheiderman, H. (1990). The funduscopic examination: How to make the most of it. *Consultant,* 30(6), 22-27.

Wong, D., and Whaley, L. (1990). *Clinical handbook of pediatric nursing* (3rd ed.). St. Louis: Mosby.

Nursing research

Barber, N., and Kilmon, C. (1989). Reactions to tympanic temperature measurement in an ambulatory setting. *Pediatric Nursing,* 15(5), 477-481.

Brown, M. (1975). Vision screening of preschool children. How to check on visual acuity and heterophobia as part of a routine physical examination. *Clinical Pediatrics,* 14(10), 968-973.*

Brown, M., and Collar, M. (1982). Effects of prior preparation on the preschooler's vision and hearing screening...prior preparation by parents in the home. *MCN,* 7(5), 323-329.

Lewis-Cullinan, C., and Janken, J. (1990). Effect of cerumen removal on the hearing ability of geriatric patients. *Journal of Advanced Nursing,* 15(5), 594-600.

Lingua, R., Levin, L., and Azen, S. (1987). Comparison of the succinylcholine-induced ocular position and the postoperative alignment in strabismus. *Journal of Ophthalmic Nursing Technology,* 6(1), 7-13.

Newman, D. (1990). Assessment of hearing loss in elderly people: The feasibility of a nurse-administered screening test. *Journal of Advanced Nursing,* 15(4), 400-409.

*Landmark publication.

10

Respiratory System

Objectives

After reading and studying this chapter, you should be able to:

1. Identify the anatomic structures of the respiratory system.
2. Explain external and internal respiration.
3. Describe the mechanics of respiration.
4. Gather appropriate health history information for a client with a respiratory disorder.
5. Demonstrate how to inspect, palpate, percuss, and auscultate respiratory system structures.
6. Describe the normal assessment findings detected by inspection, palpation, percussion, and auscultation of the respiratory system.
7. Describe the most common abnormal assessment findings detected by inspection, palpation, percussion, and auscultation of the respiratory system.
8. Describe three advanced skills for respiratory assessment: tactile fremitus palpation, diaphragmatic excursion measurement, and voice resonance auscultation.
9. Describe the laboratory tests that help assess respiratory function.
10. Document respiratory assessment findings using nursing process data.

Introduction

After a brief discussion of respiratory system anatomy and physiology, the chapter emphasizes important questions to ask and areas to discuss during the health history. It considers the application of pertinent health history data to the physical assessment of the upper and lower airways and explains how to inspect, palpate, percuss, and auscultate respiratory structures correctly. (For details about assessing the nose, sinuses, and mouth, see Chapter 8, Head and Neck.) The chapter presents the respiratory diseases most frequently encountered during a respiratory assessment and discusses how to incorporate the assessment findings and laboratory results into proper documentation for a client with a specific respiratory disorder.

Because the body depends on the respiratory system to survive, respiratory assessment constitutes a critical aspect of a client's health evaluation. The respiratory system functions primarily to maintain the exchange of oxygen and carbon dioxide in the lungs and tissues and to regulate the acid-base balance (stable concentration of hydrogen ions in body fluids). Any change in this system affects every other body system. In chronic respiratory disease, changes in pulmonary status occur slowly, allowing the client's body time to adapt to the gradual hypoxia. However, acute respiratory changes, such as a pneumothorax or aspiration pneumonia, create a sudden hypoxia. Because this does not allow the body time to adapt, death may result.

Environmental factors, such as air pollution and cigarette smoke, may also cause or exacerbate respiratory changes. Even second-hand cigarette smoke can cause respiratory problems, especially in very young or very old clients.

Changes in other body systems may also reduce the ability of the lungs to provide oxygen. For example, a client with poor cardiac function may suffer from decreased tissue oxygenation, causing the lungs to work harder to provide oxygen. Any acute disease state in-

Glossary

Accessory muscles: muscles used for forced inspiration and active expiration, including the internal intercostal, pectoral, scalenus, sternocleidomastoid, trapezius, and abdominal rectus muscles.

Acid-base balance: condition existing when the net rate at which the body produces acids or bases equals the net rate at which acids or bases are excreted. The result of acid-base balance is a stable concentration of hydrogen ions in body fluids.

Angle of Louis: angle located between the manubrium and the body of the sternum.

Bradypnea: respiratory rate less than the normal range for age-group, which may indicate a physiologic or pathologic process such as a central nervous system disturbance or metabolic alkalosis.

Bronchophony: increased referred voice sounds auscultated in the periphery of the lungs. When auscultating a client who exhibits bronchophony, the word "ninety-nine" reverberates clearly over areas of consolidation and sounds muffled over other areas.

Chronic obstructive pulmonary disease (COPD): disease involving airway obstruction, such as asthma, chronic bronchitis, or emphysema.

Clubbing: abnormal enlargement of the distal phalanges associated with peripheral tissue hypoxia, characterized by the loss of the angle between the skin and nail base.

Consolidation: solidification of part of the lung into a dense mass from fluid or infection. In a client with consolidation, percussion over the lung produces dull sounds.

Costal angle: area between the two lower borders of the rib cage near the xiphoid process.

Crackles: short, moist, explosive sounds produced by air passing through liquid in the airways. Also called rales.

Cyanosis: bluish or purplish color of the skin and mucous membranes caused by reduced oxygen levels in the arterial blood.

Diaphragmatic excursion: percussion technique used to determine the depth of diaphragm movement between inspiration and expiration.

Diffusion: movement of molecules across a semipermeable membrane from an area of greater to lesser concentration.

Dyspnea: subjective feeling of shortness of breath.

Egophony: increased referred voice sounds auscultated in the periphery of the lung. When auscultating a client who exhibits egophony, the sound "e" will sound like "a" and have a nasal, bleating quality.

Elastance: tendency of lung tissue and the chest wall to recoil and return to their original sizes.

Eupnea: respiratory rate within normal range for an age-group.

External respiration: gas movement from pulmonary airways into alveoli and capillaries, which occurs via ventilation, perfusion, and diffusion.

Hilum: hollow depression on mediastinal surface of each lung where the bronchus, blood vessels, nerves, and lymphatics enter.

Hypercapnia: elevated carbon dioxide levels in arterial blood, which may appear in a client with chronic obstructive pulmonary disease.

Hyperpnea: deep or labored respirations that occur normally with exercise and abnormally with pain, fever, or metabolic acidosis.

Hyperventilation: ventilation rate that exceeds the rate metabolically necessary for respiratory gas exchange. It results from an increased frequency of breathing, an increase in the amount of air inhaled and exhaled, or both, and causes an excessive oxygen intake along with a loss of carbon dioxide. It may occur with anxiety and metabolic acidosis.

Hypopnea: Shallow respirations occurring normally in well-conditioned athletes and abnormally in those with brain stem damage.

Hypoventilation: abnormally reduced rate and depth of respiration resulting in an inadequate volume of air in the alveoli for gas exchange along with excess carbon dioxide retention.

Hypoxemia: abnormal oxygen deficiency in arterial blood caused by decreased alveolar oxygen tension or hypoventilation.

Hypoxia: oxygen deficiency caused by a reduced oxygen-carrying capacity of the blood (as seen in anemia), insufficient oxygen in inspired air (as at high altitudes or in heavily polluted areas), impaired tissue use of oxygen (as in edema in an arm or leg), or a blood flow inadequate to transport oxygen (as in shock).

Internal respiration: gas exchange between red blood cells and tissue cells.

Intrapleural pressure: constant negative pressure in the intrapleural spaces, which occurs with normal breathing.

Metabolic acidosis: condition resulting from excess absorption or retention of acid or from excess excretion of bicarbonate.

Metabolic alkalosis: condition resulting from excess excretion of acid or from retention of bicarbonate.

Pulmonary perfusion: blood supply primarily of the pulmonary circulation, which allows for gas diffusion at the alveolar and capillary levels.

Respiratory acidosis: condition resulting from decreased excretion of carbon dioxide by the lungs. This condition increases hydrogen ion concentrations.

Respiratory alkalosis: condition resulting from excess excretion of carbon dioxide by the lungs. This condition decreases hydrogen ion concentrations.

Glossary continued

Respiratory excursion: palpation technique that evaluates symmetry of chest expansion. A finding of asymmetry could indicate pneumothorax or pleural effusion on the side with reduced excursion.

Rhonchi: bubbling sounds produced by air passing through fluid-filled airways. Also called gurgles.

Tachypnea: persistent, rapid, shallow breathing, such as occurs as a protective splinting measure against the pain of pleurisy or a fractured rib.

Tactile fremitus: voice sounds palpated on the chest wall surface. Normally, the palpation of vibrations made by voice sounds decreases as the examiner's hands move from the center to the periphery of the lungs. Equal or increased tactile fremitus indicates consolidation in the palpated area.

Transairway pressure: pressure gradient between the mouth and the alveolar spaces.

Ventilation: gas movement and distribution into and out of the pulmonary airways.

Wheezes: musical sounds of lower pitch than crackles, produced by air passing through narrowed airways.

Whispered pectoriloquy: increased voice resonance auscultated in the periphery of the lung. In a client with whispered pectoriloquy, the words "one-two-three" sound clear over areas of consolidation but muffled over normal areas.

creases the oxygen demand of the body and therefore increases the work load of the lungs. Also, a debilitating, acute disease makes a client more susceptible to secondary infections, which may also affect the lungs.

Even a mild illness can promote respiratory complications. For instance, common postanesthesia hypoventilation can develop into lung collapse (atelectasis) that may, if left untreated, result in pneumonia. Even antibiotic therapy for a minor infection may alter the client's normal lung flora, allowing pneumonia to develop. Regardless of the cause, changes in lung function can create acid-base disturbances, tissue hypoxia, and even sudden death.

Correct assessment techniques help the nurse detect respiratory problems early. In turn, this allows quick intervention, which may prevent serious complications.

Anatomy and physiology review

The respiratory system consists of the upper and lower airways, and the thoracic cage. Besides exchanging oxygen and carbon dioxide in the lungs and tissues, the respiratory system helps regulate the acid-base balance in the body. (For more information, see *Respiratory system structures,* pages 246 and 247.)

Respiratory tract

glottis

The nose, mouth, nasopharynx, oropharynx, laryngopharynx, and larynx (voice box) compose the upper airways of the respiratory tract. These structures allow air passage; warm and humidify inspired air; provide for taste, smell, and mastication; and operate involuntary protective responses, or defense mechanisms. These mechanisms, which include sneezing, coughing, gagging, and spasm, protect the respiratory system against infection and foreign body inhalation.

Composed of the bronchi and the lungs, the lower airways of the respiratory tract also employ cough and spasm as defense mechanisms. Beginning at the bottom of the trachea, the bronchi split into right and left branches. Growing progressively smaller, the right and left mainstem bronchi further divide into secondary and tertiary bronchi, then into bronchioles, and finally into alveoli.

The lungs hang suspended in the right and left pleural cavities at the hilum, which is a pleural cavity depression where the bronchi, blood vessels, nerves, and lymphatics enter the lungs. Formed by the pleural membrane, the pleural cavities contain a lining of thin tissue, called the parietal pleural membrane. This membrane doubles back onto itself to form the outer covering of the lungs, called the visceral pleural membrane. To decrease irritation caused by lung expansion and contraction, a lubricant coats both membranes. A minute space, called the pleural space, exists between the membranes. This space exerts a slight negative pressure, which facilitates lung expansion and contraction.

The mainstem bronchi enter the pleural cavities at the hilum. The right mainstem bronchus, which is

(Text continues on page 248.)

Respiratory system structures

The respiratory system consists of the upper and lower airways and the thoracic cage. These structures work together to effect the vital exchange of oxygen and carbon dioxide in the lungs.

Upper and lower airways

The upper airways include the nose, mouth, nasopharynx, oropharynx, laryngopharynx, and larynx. In normal respiration, air enters the upper airways from the nasal cavity through two oval-shaped openings, called the choanae, and flows into the nasopharynx and oropharynx. Situated posterior to the nasal cavity and the choanae, the nasopharynx contains the pharyngeal tonsils (adenoids) and eustachian tubes; the oropharynx, which lies behind the oral cavity, contains the palatine tonsils and the uvula. From the oropharynx, air flows through the laryngopharynx and into the larynx.

The larynx incorporates several structures: the epiglottis, which is a movable flap of cartilage that covers the entrance to the lower airways during swallowing; vocal cords, which are mucous membrane folds that vibrate to produce voice sounds; and the glottis, which is an opening that allows air to pass into the lower airways.

The lower airways include the trachea, bronchi, lungs, bronchioles, and alveoli. Sixteen to twenty C-shaped cartilage rings—which are rigid in the front and covered with a thick, slightly expandable membrane in the back—form the trachea. The trachea extends from the cricoid cartilage in the neck to the carina, a ridge projecting from the lowest tracheal cartilage at the level of the second rib at the midsternal line.

The trachea then bifurcates into the right and left mainstem bronchi at the manubrial-sternal junction (angle of Louis) anteriorly, or at the level of the fourth thoracic vertebra posteriorly. These bronchi divide into five secondary bronchi and enter the lungs at the hilum. Each secondary bronchus enters a lung lobe. Within each lobe, the secondary bronchi branch into tertiary bronchi, bronchioles, and finally into alveoli.

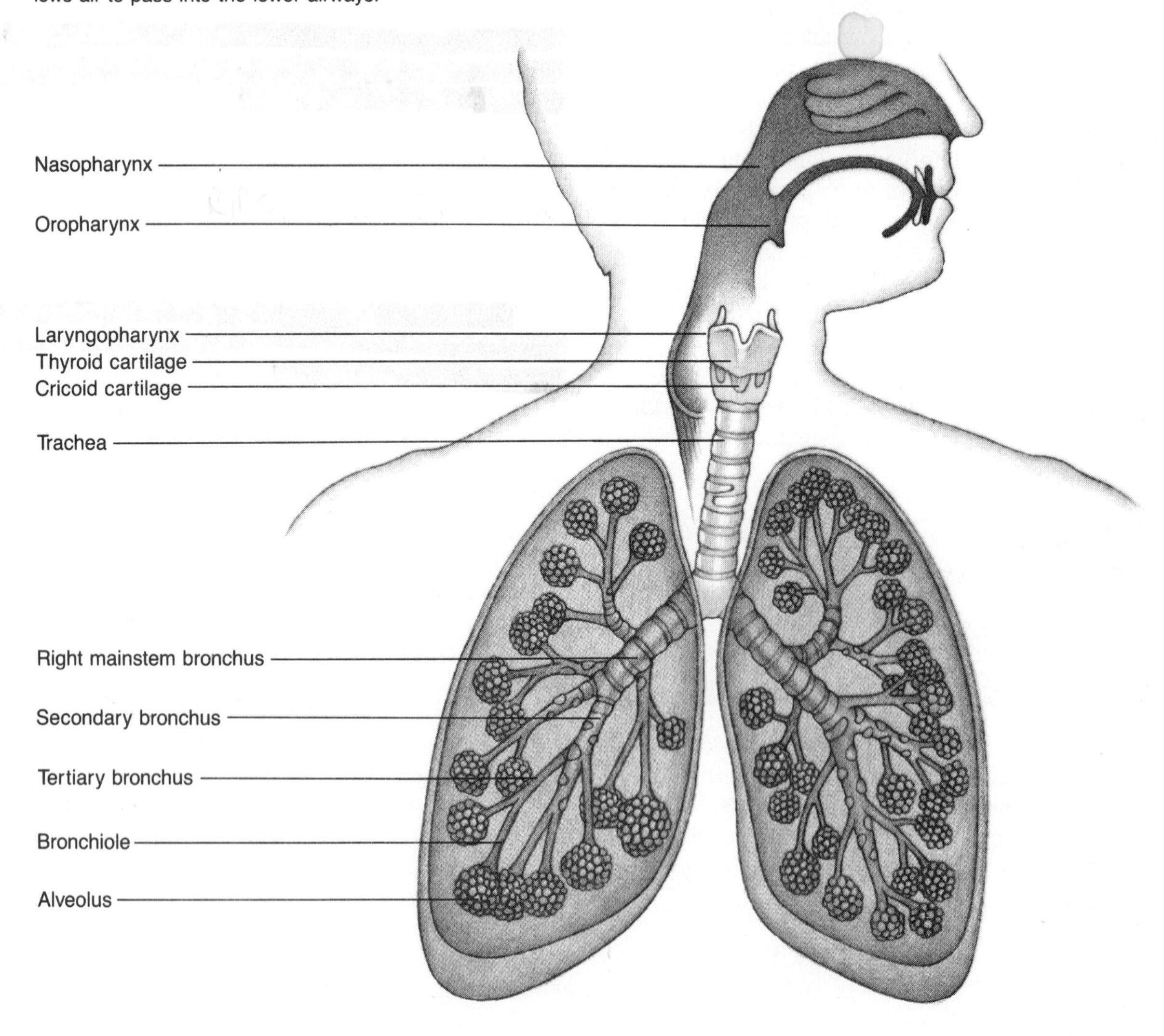

Thoracic cage and location of lung lobes

The thoracic cage includes the ribs, sternum, and vertebrae. These structures—along with the imaginary lines—act as landmarks that help identify underlying structures.

For example, the base or bottom of each lung rests anteriorly at the level of the sixth rib at the midclavicular line and the eighth rib at the midaxillary line. The apices (the pointed upper parts of the lungs) extend about 3/4" to 1 1/2" (2 to 4 cm) above the inner aspects of the clavicles. Posteriorly, the lungs extend from the cervical area to the level of the tenth thoracic spinous process (T10). On deep inspiration, the lungs may descend to the twelfth thoracic spinous process (T12).

Beneath the thoracic cage, the right lung divides into three lobes; the left lung, into two lobes. In the anterior thorax, the right upper lobe ends level with the fourth rib in the midclavicular line and with the fifth rib in the midaxillary line. Because of this sloping angle, the right middle lobe extends triangularly from the fourth to the sixth rib in the midclavicular line and to the fifth rib in the midaxillary line. Because the left lung does not have a middle lobe, the upper lobe ends level with the sixth rib in the midclavicular line and level with the fifth rib in the midaxillary line.

In the posterior thorax, an imaginary line stretching from the level of the T3 spinous process along the inferior border of the scapulae and to the fifth rib at the midaxillary line separates the upper lobes of both lungs. The upper lobes exist above the T3 spinous process; the lower lobes exist below the T3 spinous process and extend to the level of the T10 spinous process.

The right and left lateral rib cages cover the lobes of the right and left lungs respectively. Beneath these structures, the lungs extend from just above the clavicles to the level of the eighth rib. The left lateral thorax allows access to two lobes; the right lateral thorax, to three lobes.

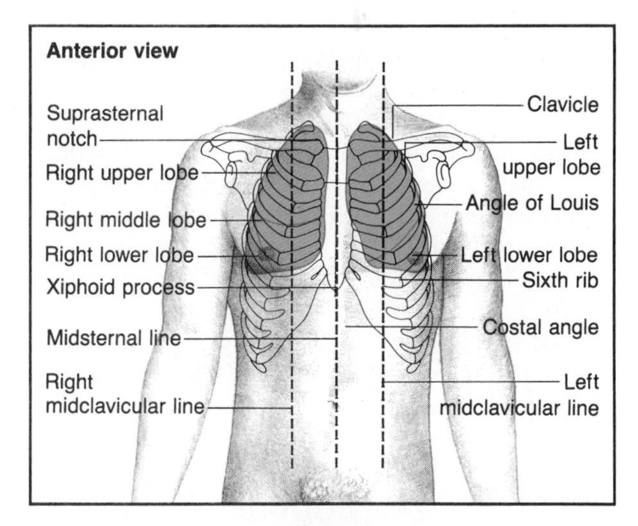

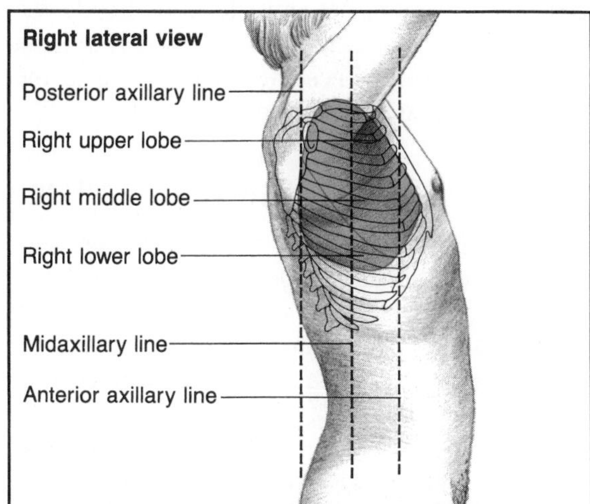

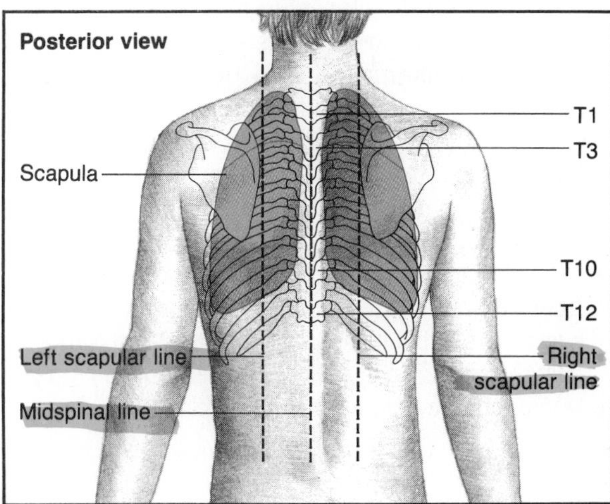

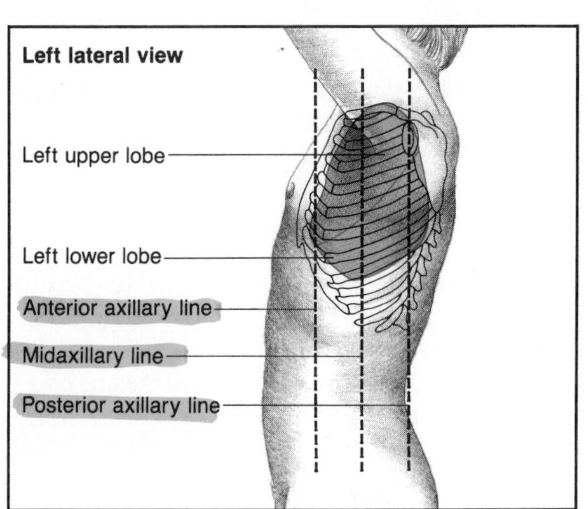

shorter, wider, and more vertical than the left mainstem bronchus, supplies air to the right lung, and the left mainstem bronchus supplies air to the left lung. The right lung, which is larger, consists of three lobes and handles 55% of the gas exchange. The smaller left lung consists of only two lobes and extends slightly lower in the thorax; it is crowded by the heart, which also lies in the left side of the chest.

At the hilum, the mainstem bronchi divide into five secondary (lobar) bronchi, each leading to a separate lobe of the lung. The right bronchus divides to supply the upper, middle, and lower lobes of the right lung, and the left bronchus divides to supply the upper and lower lobes of the left lung. The lobar bronchi further divide into tertiary (segmental) bronchi, which carry air to smaller bronchopleural segments. Within these segments, the bronchi continue to divide into progressively smaller bronchi and bronchioles. The larger bronchi consist of cartilage, smooth muscle, and epithelium; however, as the bronchi become smaller, they lose first the cartilage and then the smooth muscle, until, finally, the smallest (respiratory) bronchioles consist of only a single layer of epithelial cells. These bronchioles lead to the alveoli, where gas exchange begins.

Thoracic cage

Composed of bone and cartilage, the thoracic cage supports and protects the lungs. The vertebral column and twelve pairs of ribs form the posterior portion of the thoracic cage, support and protect the thorax, and allow for lung expansion and contraction. Posteriorly, certain landmarks aid identification of specific vertebrae. In 90% of the population, the most prominent vertebra on a flexed neck is cervical vertebra seven (C7); for the remaining 10%, it is thoracic vertebra one (T1). So, to locate a specific vertebra, the nurse can count down along the vertebrae from T1. The ribs, which form the major portion of the thoracic cage, extend from the thoracic vertebrae toward the anterior thorax. They are numbered from top to bottom, like the vertebrae.

The anterior thoracic cage—the manubrium, sternum, xiphoid process, and ribs—also protects the mediastinal organs (heart, aorta, and great vessels, such as the left pulmonary artery and superior vena cava) that lie between the right and left pleural cavities. Ribs one through seven attach directly to the sternum; ribs eight through ten attach to the cartilage of the preceding rib. The other two pairs of ribs are "free-floating"; they do not attach to any part of the anterior thoracic cage. Rib eleven ends anterolaterally, and rib twelve ends laterally. The lower parts of the rib cage (the costal margins) near the xiphoid process form the borders of the costal angle—an angle of approximately 90 degrees in a normal client.

Just above the anterior thorax is a depression called the suprasternal notch. Because the suprasternal notch is not covered by the rib cage like the rest of the thorax, it allows access to the trachea and aortic pulsation for palpation.

Inspiration and expiration

Breathing involves two actions: inspiration, an active process, and expiration, a relatively passive one. Both actions rely on the functioning of the muscles of respiration and the effects of pressure differences in the lungs. (For an illustration, see *The mechanics of respiration,* pages 250 and 251.)

Pulmonary blood flow

Pulmonary circulation perfuses the lungs, allowing gas exchange to occur. It begins at the pulmonary artery of the right ventricle. From there, blood flows through the main pulmonary arteries into the pleural cavities and the main bronchi. Then it flows through progressively smaller vessels until it reaches the single-celled endothelial capillaries that intertwine around the alveoli. Here, oxygen and carbon dioxide diffusion takes place. After passing through the pulmonary capillaries, the blood flows through progressively larger vessels, enters the main pulmonary veins, and flows back into the left atrium. (For a detailed illustration of this process, see *The pulmonary blood supply.*)

External and internal respiration

Effective respiration requires gas exchange in the lungs (external respiration) and in the tissues (internal respiration).

External respiration occurs through ventilation (gas distribution into and out of the pulmonary airways), pulmonary perfusion (blood flow from the right side of the heart, through the pulmonary circulation, and into the left side of the heart), and diffusion (gas movement from an area of greater to lesser concentration through a semipermeable membrane). Internal respiration occurs only through diffusion. These processes are vital to maintain adequate oxygenation and acid-base balance.

Ventilation

The nervous, musculoskeletal, and pulmonary systems all contribute to the lung pressure changes required for

(Text continues on page 252.)

The pulmonary blood supply

The respiratory and circulatory systems work closely to transport gases to and from the lungs. This relationship is indicated by the arrows in the illustration.

The right and left pulmonary arteries carry deoxygenated blood (blood with low oxygen levels) from the right side of the heart to the lungs. These arteries divide into distal branches, called arterioles, which eventually terminate as a concentrated capillary network in the alveoli and alveolar sacs where gas exchange occurs. The end branches of the pulmonary veins, called venules, collect the oxygenated blood from the capillaries and transport it to larger vessels, which lead to the pulmonary veins. The pulmonary veins enter the left side of the heart and deliver the oxygenated blood for distribution throughout the body.

During the gas exchange process, oxygen and carbon dioxide continuously diffuse across a very thin pulmonary membrane. To understand the direction of movement, remember that gases travel from areas of greater to lesser pressure. Carbon dioxide diffuses from the venous end of the capillary into the alveolus, and oxygen diffuses from the alveolus into the capillary.

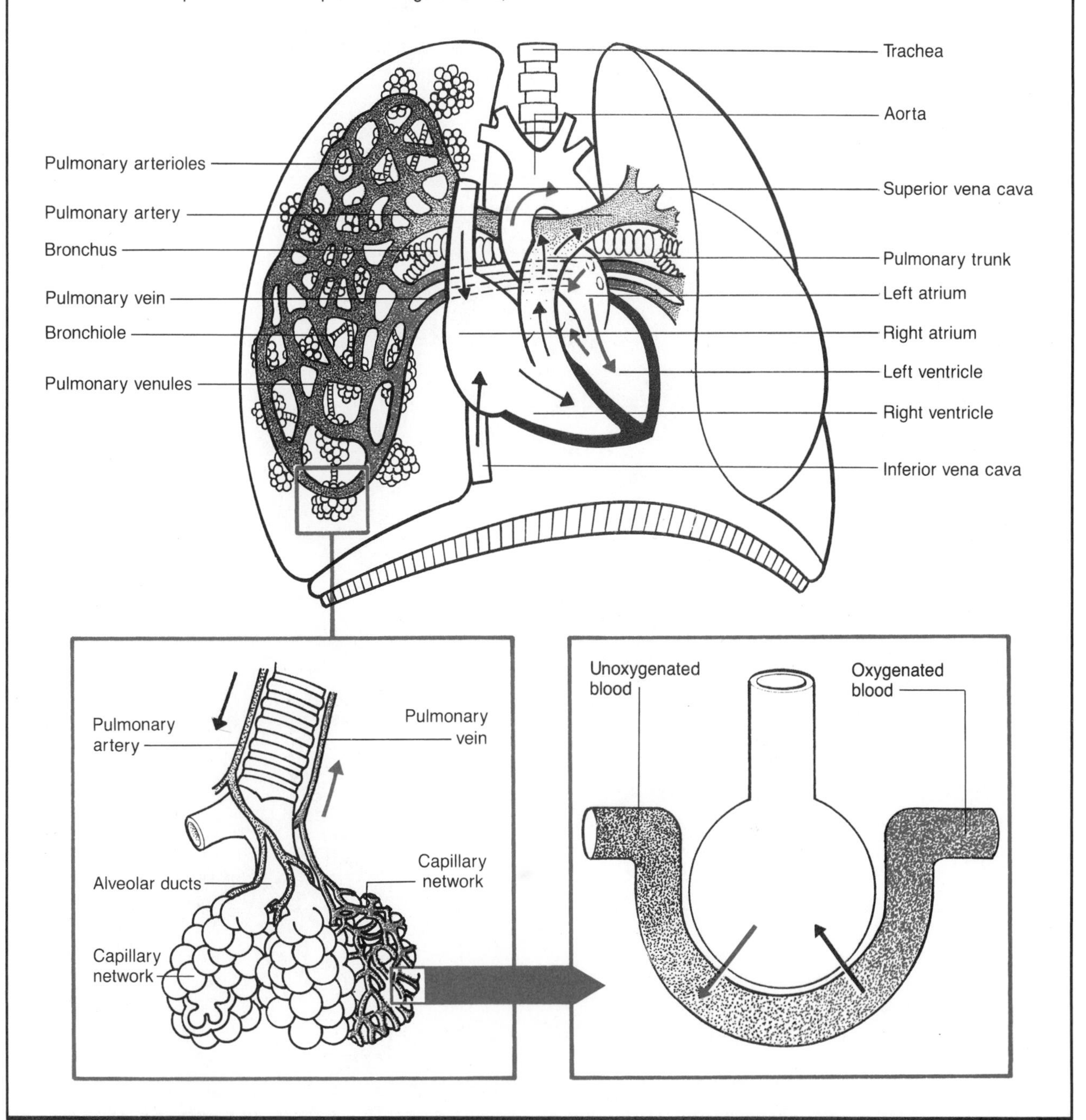

The mechanics of respiration

The muscles of respiration help the chest cavity expand and contract. The air pressure differences between the outside air and the lungs help produce air movement. Together, these actions allow inspiration and expiration.

Muscles of respiration

During normal respiration, the external intercostal muscles assist the diaphragm—the major muscle of respiration. The diaphragm descends to lengthen the chest cavity, while the external intercostal muscles—located between and along the lower borders of the ribs—contract to expand the anteroposterior diameter. This coordinated action causes inspiration. Rising of the diaphragm and relaxation of the intercostal muscles causes expiration.

During exercise, when the body requires increased oxygenation, or in certain disease states that require forced inspiration and active expiration, the accessory muscles of respiration also participate. These include the internal intercostals on the inner surface of the ribs, the sternocleidomastoids on the sides of the neck, the scalenus in the neck, and the abdominal rectus muscles.

During forced inspiration, the sternocleidomastoid muscles raise the sternum, and the scalenus muscles elevate, fix, and expand the upper chest. During active expiration, the internal intercostals contract to decrease the transverse diameter of the chest and the abdominal muscles pull down the lower chest, thus depressing the lower ribs.

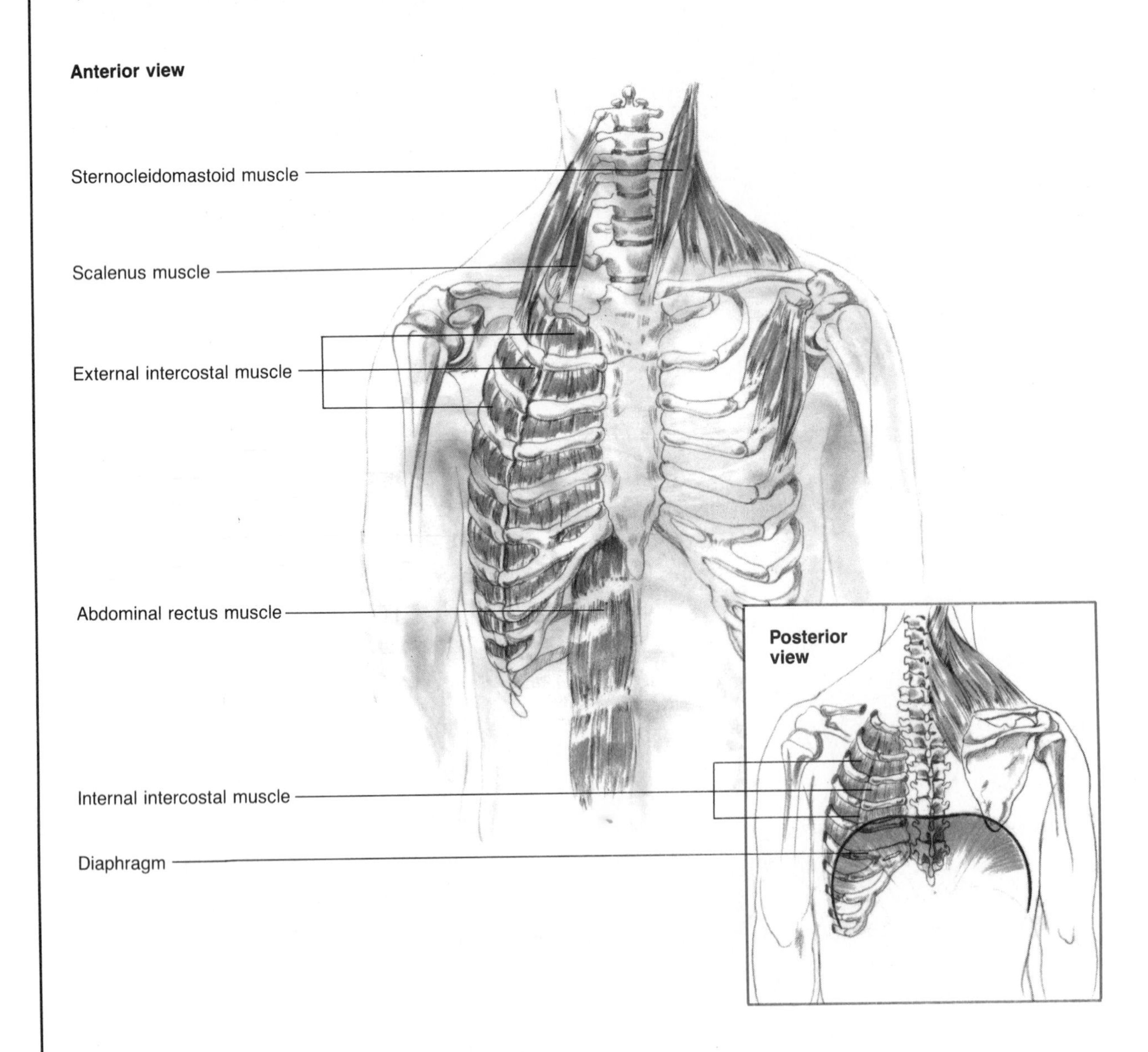

Air pressure differences
During inspiration and expiration, pressure differences allow the bellows-like movement of air in and out of the lungs. All gases move from an area of greater pressure to one of lesser pressure.

Resting phase
During the resting phase (occurring at the end of inspiration and expiration), no pressure difference exists between the atmosphere and the alveoli, and, thus, no airflow occurs. The negative intrapleural pressure prevents the lungs from collapsing.

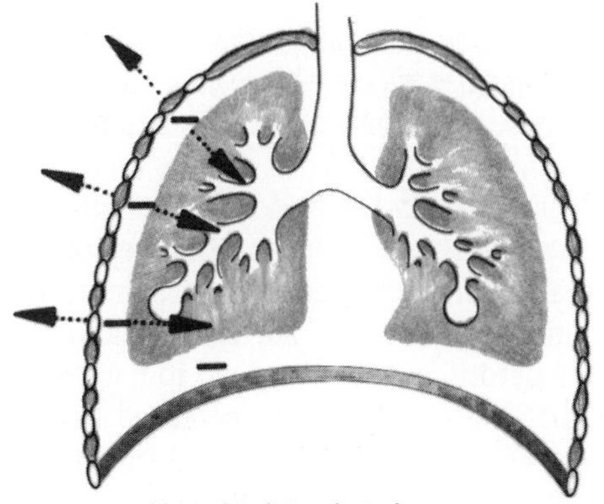

Negative intrapleural pressure

Inspiration
On inspiration, as the diaphragm descends and the chest cavity expands, intrapulmonary negative pressure builds. Then, as the lungs expand, the negative pressure transfers to the alveolar spaces, creating a pressure difference between the atmosphere and the alveoli. Because gas moves from an area of greater to lesser concentration, this pressure difference—called the transairway pressure gradient—moves gas through the upper airways and into the top of the lower airways, creating the first step in ventilation.

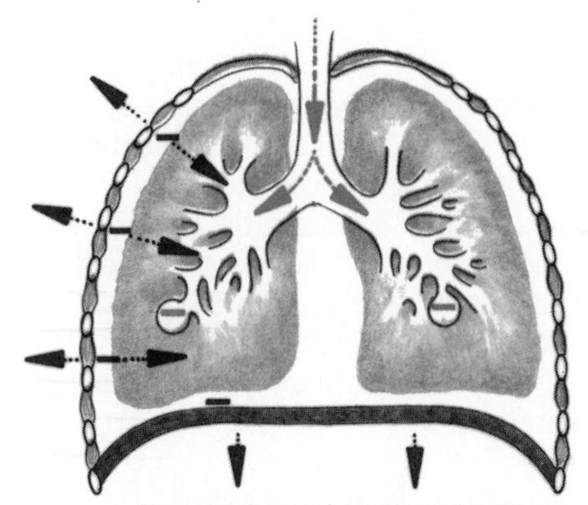

Negative intrapulmonary pressure

Expiration
On expiration, the diaphragm rises and the chest cavity contracts. Intrapleural pressure rises, but remains negative. As the chest cavity further compresses the lungs, lung pressure rises above atmospheric pressure. This creates a positive intrapulmonary pressure, forcing air out of the lungs, into the trachea, and into the atmosphere.

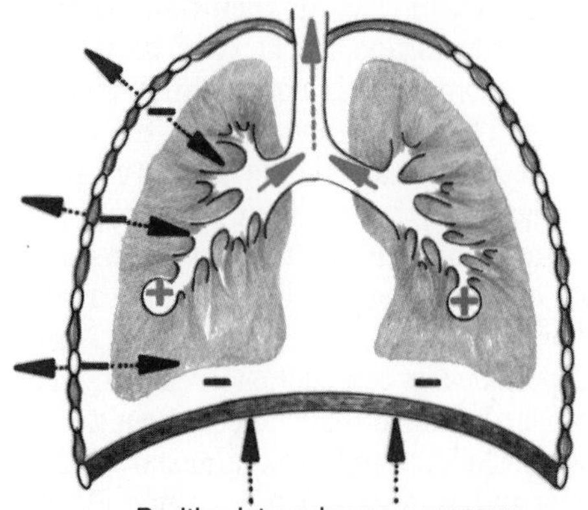

Positive intrapulmonary pressure

EXTERNAL RESPIRATION

A. Ventilation (cont).

adequate ventilation. Dysfunction in any of these systems increases breathing effort and decreases breathing effectiveness.

1. **Nervous system effect.** Although ventilation is largely involuntary, individuals can control the rate and depth of ventilation, such as by performing breathing exercises to reduce stress. Involuntary breathing results from neurogenic stimulation of the respiratory center in the medulla and the pons. The medulla controls the rate and depth of respiration; the pons moderates the rhythm or smoothness of the switch from inspiration to expiration. Specialized neurovascular tissue alters these phases of the breathing process automatically and instantaneously.

When carbon dioxide in the blood diffuses into the cerebrospinal fluid, specialized tissue in the respiratory center of the brain stem responds. At the same time, peripheral chemoreceptors in the aortic arch and the bifurcation of the carotid arteries respond to decreased oxygen levels in the blood. When an increased carbon dioxide level or a decreased oxygen level is noted, the respiratory center of the medulla responds by initiating respiration.

2. **Musculoskeletal system effect.** The adult thorax is a movable structure whose shape can be altered by chest muscle contraction. The medulla controls respiration primarily through stimulating the contraction of the diaphragm and the external intercostals, the major muscles of breathing. The diaphragm descends to expand the length of the chest cavity while the external intercostals contract to expand the anteroposterior diameter. These actions produce the intrapulmonary pressure changes that cause inspiration.

3. **Pulmonary system effect.** During inspiration, air flows through the right and left mainstem bronchi into increasingly smaller bronchi. The air then flows through bronchioles, alveolar ducts, and aveolar sacs, until reaching the alveolar membrane. This normal airflow distribution can be altered by the airflow pattern, the volume and location of the functional reserve capacity (air remaining in the alveoli to prevent their collapse during respiration), the amount of intrapulmonary resistance, and the presence of lung disease. If disrupted, the airflow distribution follows the path of least resistance. For example, an intrapulmonary obstruction or forced inspiration would cause the air to distribute unevenly.

Other musculoskeletal and intrapulmonary factors can affect airflow and, in turn, affect breathing. Normal breathing requires active inspiration and passive expiration; forced breathing demands active inspiration and expiration. Forced breathing, such as with emphysema, calls the accessory muscles of respiration into action, which require additional oxygen to work. This results in less efficient respiration with a possibly increased workload.

Other alterations in airflow, which also may demand additional energy, increase oxygen consumption, and cause respiratory muscle fatigue, include changes in compliance (distensibility of the lungs and thorax), elastance (the tendency of the lungs and chest wall to return to their resting states), and resistance (interference with airflow in the tracheobronchial tree).

B. Pulmonary perfusion

Another mechanism that aids external respiration is perfusion. Pulmonary blood flow allows gas exchange at the alveolar levels; however, many factors can negatively affect gas transport to the alveoli. For example, a cardiac output less than the average of 5 liters/minute reduces blood flow, which can lead to a reduced gas exchange. Also, elevated pulmonary and systemic resistance reduces blood flow, and abnormal or insufficient hemoglobin will pick up less oxygen for exchange. Gravity can affect oxygen and carbon dioxide transport positively by influencing pulmonary circulation. Gravity pulls unoxygenated blood to the lower and middle lung lobes, where most of the tidal volume also flows. This results in an ideal ventilation-perfusion match, which maximizes pulmonary gas exchange and promotes maintenance of acid-base balance by allowing excretion of carbon dioxide.

C. Diffusion

Diffusion aids external and internal respiration. It occurs when oxygen and carbon dioxide move between the alveoli and the capillaries. Partial pressure—the pressure exerted by one gas in a mixture of gases—dictates the direction of movement, which is always from an area of greater concentration to one of lesser concentration. In the process, oxygen moves across the alveolar and capillary membranes, dissolves in the plasma, and then passes through the red blood cell (RBC) membrane, while carbon dioxide moves in the opposite direction.

Successful diffusion requires an intact alveolocapillary membrane. Both the alveolar epithelium and the capillary endothelium are composed of a single layer of cells. Between these layers are minute interstitial spaces filled with elastin and collagen. Normally, oxygen and carbon dioxide move easily through all of these layers. Oxygen moves from the alveoli into the bloodstream, and carbon dioxide (the by-product of metabolism) diffuses from the blood into the alveoli. Most transported

Chest contours of different age-groups

The following illustrations compare the chest contours of an infant, toddler, adult, and elderly adult. An infant has a rounded thorax, with an anteroposterior diameter equal to or slightly greater than the lateral diameter. By the time the infant has grown into a toddler, the lateral diameter of the chest has grown broader than the anteroposterior diameter. By adulthood, the lateral diameter of the chest is broader by up to twice the anteroposterior diameter. Then, in the elderly adult, the chest again exhibits an increased anteroposterior diameter as the result of changes in the spine from aging.

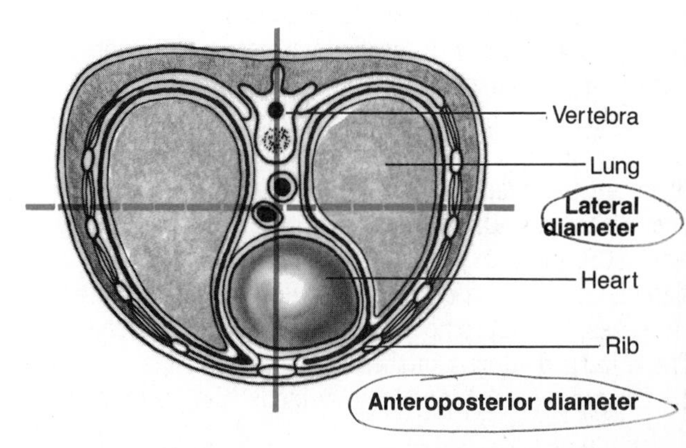

Infant

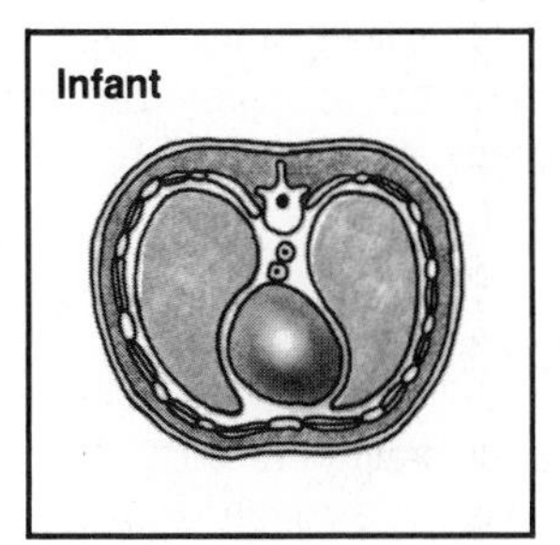

Toddler

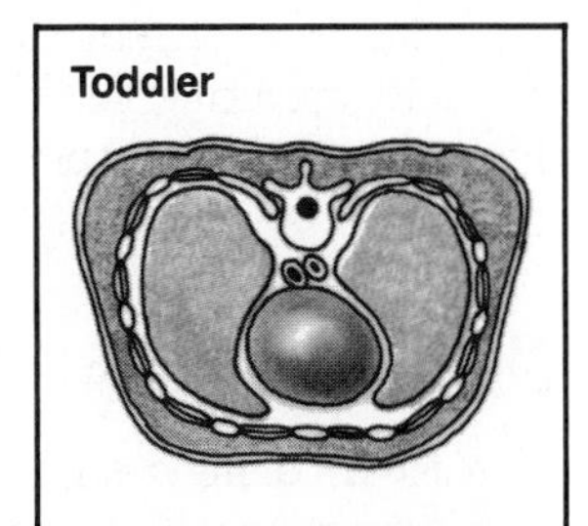

Adult

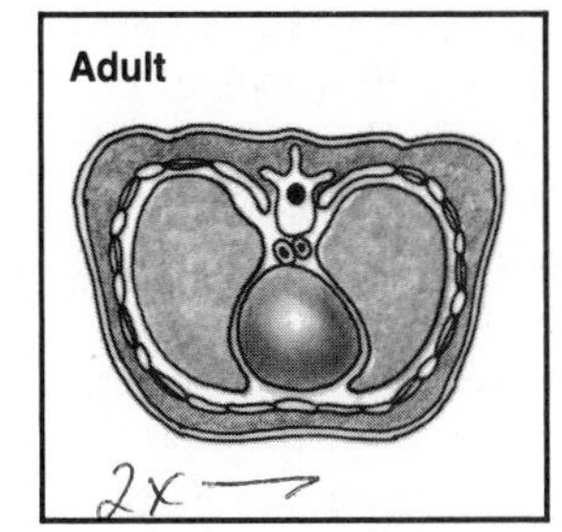

Elderly adult

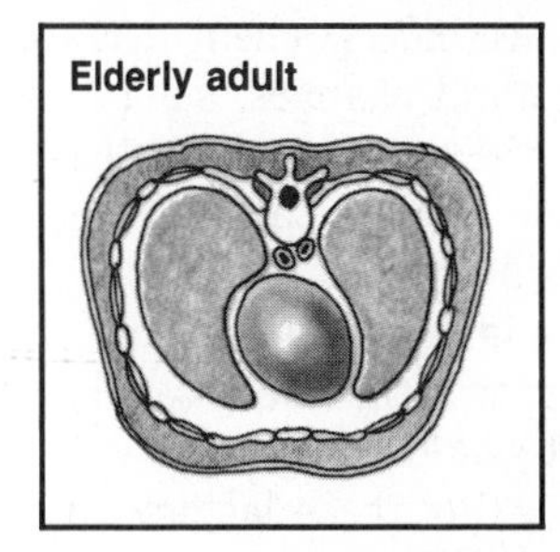

oxygen binds with hemoglobin to form oxyhemoglobin, while a small portion dissolves in the plasma (measurable as the partial pressure of oxygen—PaO_2). Hemoglobin has an affinity for oxygen, which causes RBCs to release carbon dioxide and take up oxygen.

After oxygen binds to hemoglobin, the RBCs travel to the tissues. At this point, the blood cells contain more oxygen and the tissue cells contain more carbon dioxide. Internal respiration occurs when, through cellular diffusion, the RBCs release oxygen and absorb carbon dioxide. The RBCs then transport the carbon dioxide back to the lungs for removal during expiration.

Acid-base balance

Through external and internal respiration, the lungs help maintain acid-base balance in the body. Oxygen taken up in the lungs is transported to the tissues by the circulatory system, which exchanges it for the carbon dioxide produced by cellular metabolism. Because carbon dioxide is more soluble than oxygen, it dissolves in the blood, the majority forming bicarbonate (base) and smaller amounts forming carbonic acid (acid).

The lungs control bicarbonate levels by converting it to carbon dioxide and water for excretion. In response to signals from the medulla, the lungs can change the rate and depth of respiration. This change allows for adjustment of the amount of carbon dioxide lost to help maintain acid-base balance. For example, in metabolic alkalosis (a condition resulting from excess bicarbonate retention), the rate and depth of respiration decrease so that carbon dioxide can be retained, which increases carbonic acid levels. In metabolic acidosis (a condition resulting from excess acid retention) the lungs increase the rate and depth of respiration to exhale excess carbon dioxide, which reduces carbonic acid levels.

When the lungs function inadequately, they can actually produce an acid-base imbalance. For example, they can cause respiratory acidosis by hypoventilation (reduced rate and depth of respiration), which causes carbon dioxide retention. The lungs can also cause respiratory alkalosis by hyperventilation (increased rate of respiration), which causes exhalation of increased amounts of carbon dioxide.

Developmental considerations

The respiratory system changes anatomically and physiologically with age. (For illustrations, see *Chest contours of different age-groups.*) For example, an infant or young child may have weak respiratory muscles and small airways, which increase the risk of respiratory problems. A child may also have an immature immune system, which could hinder recovery from a respiratory infection. Therefore, a child will require an especially thorough respiratory assessment.

Other developmental factors also affect the respiratory system. For example, a pregnant client experiences an increase in tidal volume and respiratory rate. These changes allow a pregnant client to consume almost 20% more oxygen than normal, and decrease her plasma carbon dioxide levels. Alveolar ventilation also increases, which promotes a more efficient gas exchange. The enlarged uterus pushes the thoracic cage and the diaphragm upward and also widens the base of the thorax.

An elderly client may exhibit some characteristic structural changes, such as a barrel chest, spinal deformities, or costal cartilage calcification, which increase thoracic cage stiffness. This stiffness, combined with decreased respiratory muscle strength, often results in high residual air volumes during expiration. Changes in the alveolocapillary membrane structure may limit gas exchange.

All of these factors can affect oxygen and carbon dioxide diffusion and can make an elderly client more susceptible to severe respiratory diseases. However, an elderly client may adjust to the limited gas exchange and may be asymptomatic until illness, surgery, or reduced mobility stresses the breathing process. Therefore, the nurse should be alert for early signs of pneumonia, atelectasis, aspiration, and other respiratory disorders when assessing an elderly client. Another abnormality common in elderly clients is tracheal deviation from kyphosis, a pronounced dorsal curvature of the thoracic spine.

Kyphosis

Health history

To obtain an accurate and meaningful client health history, the nurse should employ good assessment techniques, using these guidelines.

Before beginning, quickly assess the client for signs of acute respiratory distress, such as restlessness, anxiety, inability to follow conversation, or noisy or labored respirations. If the client displays these signs, obtain help, and, if possible, question the client's family about the current problem. Then, when the client is breathing comfortably, proceed with the full health history.

Begin the health history by reviewing the general factors affecting lung function, such as the client's age, sex, and type of living environment. Next, ask specific questions related to respiratory problems. Keep in mind that the client suffering from hypoxemia (low blood oxygen level), hypoxia (oxygen deficiency caused by reduced oxygen-carrying capacity, insufficient oxygen in inspired air, impaired tissue use of oxygen, or inadequate blood flow for transporting oxygen), or hypercapnia (high carbon dioxide levels in the blood) may have periods of confusion, inattentiveness, or sleepiness. If so, assess the client's ability to answer questions appropriately. If necessary, postpone the health history until after the client has rested or until family members are available to clarify and verify answers. Also, ask questions that can be easily understood and easily answered. A client suffering from shortness of breath (dyspnea) may have difficulty speaking. In this instance, complete the health history in several short interviews to avoid tiring the client.

Health and illness patterns

The most common signs and symptoms related to the respiratory system include dyspnea, cough, sputum production, and chest pain or discomfort. Using the PQRST method, thoroughly investigate all of these complaints. (For an explanation of this method, see *Symptom analysis* in Chapter 3, The Health History.)

Current health status

During this part of the health history, find out as much as possible about the client's chief complaint by posing the following questions.

Signs + symptoms

Do you have shortness of breath? If so, is it constant or intermittent? Does position, medication, or relaxation relieve it? Do your lips or nail beds ever turn blue? Does body position, time of day, or a particular activity affect your breathing? How many stairs can you climb, or blocks can you walk, before you feel short of breath?

(RATIONALE: A distressing symptom, dyspnea can result from various respiratory disorders. Although dyspnea may begin suddenly in relation to a specific activity, it usually develops gradually and insidiously. The client may have unconsciously made life-style changes to compensate for dyspnea, making the exact time of onset difficult to determine. Intermittent attacks may result from asthma, whereas dyspnea during sleep [paroxysmal nocturnal dyspnea] or dyspnea that requires the client to sit or stand to breathe normally [orthopnea] may indicate chronic lung disease or cardiac dysfunction. Dyspnea aggravated by activity suggests poor ventilation and perfusion or inefficient breathing mechanisms.)

Do you have a cough? If so, does it sound dry, hacking, barking, or congested? Does it usually occur at a certain time of day?
(RATIONALE: Cough, whether productive or nonproductive, usually indicates a respiratory disorder. Severe cough may disrupt activities of daily living, cause chest pain, or result in acute respiratory distress. Early-morning cough may result from a chronic airway inflammation caused by smoking; late-afternoon cough may indicate exposure to irritants at work; evening cough may suggest chronic postnasal drip, sinusitis, or gastric reflux with nocturnal aspiration. Dry cough may signal a cardiac condition; barking cough, croup or influenza; hacking cough, pneumonia; and congested cough, a cold, pneumonia, or bronchitis.)

Do you cough up sputum? If so, how much do you cough up each day? What color is it? How does it smell? Is it thick or thin? What time of day do you cough up the most sputum?
(RATIONALE: Sputum production accompanies a cough when the hairlike processes of the mucous membranes [cilia] attempt to clear debris from the airway by a wavelike, upward motion. In small amounts and with sufficient fluidity, sputum production serves to maintain airway hygiene and patency. Normal mucus is thin, clear to white, tasteless, odorless, and scant. Mucoid sputum may suggest tracheobronchitis or asthma; yellow or green sputum, bacterial infection; rust-colored sputum, pneumonia, pulmonary infarction, or tuberculosis [TB]; pink and frothy sputum, pulmonary edema.)

Do you have chest pain? If so, is it constant or intermittent? Is it localized? Does any activity produce pain? Does pain occur when you breathe normally or when you breathe deeply?
(RATIONALE: Chest pain may have a cardiac, pulmonary, or musculoskeletal origin. The characteristics of the pain help determine the probable origin. For example, pain that increases with deep breathing may be pulmonary [pleuritic] in origin. Musculoskeletal chest pain may mimic lung dysfunction. The lungs themselves have no pain-sensitive nerve endings, but the thoracic muscles, parietal pleura, and tracheobronchial tree do. Therefore, pulmonary chest pain may be a late sign of lung disease. For additional information on differentiating types of chest pain, see *Evaluating chest pain* in Chapter 11, Cardiovascular System.)

Past health status

Questions related to previous illnesses, injuries, and surgeries provide clues to assessment findings.

Have you had any lung problems such as asthma or tuberculosis? If so, what type? How long did they last and what treatment did you receive?
(RATIONALE: Frequent upper respiratory infections may indicate an underlying respiratory problem.)

Have you been exposed to anyone who has a respiratory disease?
(RATIONALE: Certain respiratory disorders, such as influenza, pneumonia, and other infections, are highly contagious.)

Have you had chest surgery or any diagnostic study of the pulmonary system? If so, what type, and why did you have it?
(RATIONALE: Previous diagnostic studies—such as bronchoscopy, arterial blood gas analysis, and sputum cultures—or a thoracotomy or other chest surgery can reveal a history of, or predisposition to, respiratory disorders.)

How many pillows do you sleep on? Does this number represent a change in your previous number?
(RATIONALE: The need for more than one pillow could indicate nocturnal dyspnea that has developed over time. The client may not realize that using more than one pillow relates to a breathing problem.)

Do you have allergies that flare up in different seasons? If so, what causes them? Do they cause runny nose, itching eyes, congestion, or other symptoms? What do you do to relieve these symptoms?
(RATIONALE: A client with allergies may use over-the-counter [OTC] drugs and inhalers, which could interact with medications ordered by the physician. Answers to these questions also reveal the use of common household remedies, and whether they are successful.)

Do you smoke tobacco? If so, for how long have you been smoking, and how much do you smoke?
(RATIONALE: Cigarette, cigar, or pipe smoking can predispose a smoker to various respiratory disorders. Information about pack years [the number of packs smoked per day multiplied by the number of years of smoking] can indicate the severity of the problem.)

Do you ever use over-the-counter nasal sprays or inhalers? If so, how frequently?
(RATIONALE: A client who uses OTC nasal sprays and inhalers too frequently may develop a tolerance and may have to use the spray more often for relief. Overuse of nasal inhalers may also cause rebound nasal congestion, characterized by red, swollen nasal mucosa.)

Do you take any over-the-counter or prescription medications for your respiratory difficulties? If so, which medications? How often do you take them? When did you last take these medications?

(RATIONALE: Medications taken by the client provide important clues to specific respiratory disorders. Breathing problems are often self-treated, so inquire about prescription and nonprescription drugs. Also ask about drugs that may be used as part of respiratory therapy, because the client may not identify these as medications.)

What other medications do you take? How frequently do you take them?
(RATIONALE: Many drugs can cause respiratory depression and other adverse respiratory reactions. For further information, see *Adverse drug reactions.*)

Do you use a nebulizer or other breathing treatment? If so, what is it used to treat, what dose of medication do you use, and how often do you take a treatment? Do you ever have any side effects from the treatment? Do you follow special instructions for using therapy? When did you last have a treatment?
(RATIONALE: Use of a nebulizer or other breathing treatment at home may indicate a chronic respiratory disorder. If hospitalized, the client would probably require continuation of the same home breathing treatments.)

Do you use oxygen at home? If so, do you use a cannula or mask? Do you use it continuously or intermittently? What is the liter flow rate at rest and with activity? Must you follow any special instructions for use?
(RATIONALE: Use of oxygen therapy at home may indicate a chronic respiratory disorder. Learn the client's maintenance amount as a baseline for future adjustments, and determine the client's awareness of necessary precautions.)

How long have you been on home oxygen? Who is your supplier? Does your insurance cover the cost of oxygen therapy?
(RATIONALE: Sometimes economics prevents clients from complying with ordered treatments. If financial considerations prevent proper oxygen supply, refer the client to a social worker.)

Have you ever been vaccinated against flu or pneumonia?
(RATIONALE: Expect the very young, very old, and those with chronic respiratory disease to have been vaccinated. If such a client has not been vaccinated, plan to educate the client about the protection that vaccinations provide.)
Pneumo-vax (1x life)

Family health status

Obtain a family history of respiratory illness as well as an overview of the family structure and support systems. A client with a chronic respiratory disease may eventually need a good deal of family assistance.

Has any member of your family had emphysema, asthma, respiratory allergies, or tuberculosis?
(RATIONALE: A family predisposition to emphysema and allergies may exist. If a family member has had TB, find out when the client may have been exposed to determine the need for a tuberculin skin test.)

Status of physiologic systems

When gathering information about a client with a respiratory problem, look at other body systems that may show symptoms related to the primary problem.

In the last 1 to 2 months, have you had fever, chills, fatigue, or night sweats?
(RATIONALE: These symptoms are associated with TB.)

Have you ever had a blood test that showed you had anemia? If so, when?
(RATIONALE: Anemia decreases the ability of the blood to carry oxygen because of reduced RBCs and hemoglobin. This, in turn, leads to fatigue, dyspnea, and orthopnea.)

Do you periodically suffer from sinus pain, nasal discharge, or postnasal drip?
(RATIONALE: These signs and symptoms may suggest allergies or sinus infection.)

Do you suffer from a bad taste in your mouth or bad breath?
(RATIONALE: These signs and symptoms could indicate a sinus or pulmonary infection, such as an abscess or bronchiectasis.)

Do you suffer from ankle edema or shortness of breath at night?
(RATIONALE: These effects may be related to right-sided congestive heart failure.)

Have you noticed any weight change recently?
(RATIONALE: A weight gain could indicate fluid accumulation from right-sided congestive heart failure, whereas weight loss could indicate generalized body wasting associated with a disease such as lung cancer.)

Do you ever feel confused, restless, or faint?
(RATIONALE: Any of these symptoms could result from lack of oxygen to the brain, as seen in the chronic obstructive pulmonary disease [COPD] client who has elevated carbon dioxide levels and decreased oxygen levels.)

Developmental considerations

During the health history, ask these questions of a pediatric or elderly client.

Adverse drug reactions

Many drugs can cause adverse respiratory reactions, such as dyspnea and respiratory depression. To help determine the cause of a client's respiratory problem, the nurse must obtain information about the use of over-the-counter and prescription medications.

DRUG CLASS	DRUG	POSSIBLE ADVERSE REACTIONS
Adrenergic agents (sympathomimetics)	epinephrine hydrochloride	Dyspnea, paradoxical bronchospasms
Adrenergic blockers (sympatholytics)	methysergide maleate	Nasal congestion; pulmonary fibrosis, resulting in dyspnea, tightness, chest pain, pleural friction rubs, effusion
Alkylating agents	busulfan	Irreversible pulmonary fibrosis (busulfan lung)
	carmustine	Pulmonary infiltrates, fibrosis
	cyclophosphamide	Pulmonary fibrosis (with high doses)
	melphalan	Pneumonitis
Antiarrhythmics	amiodarone hydrochloride	Interstitial pneumonitis, pulmonary fibrosis
Antibiotic antineoplastic agents	bleomycin sulfate	Fine crackles, dyspnea (early signs of pulmonary toxicity); interstitial pneumonitis
	mitomycin	Dyspnea, cough, hemoptysis, pulmonary infiltrates
Antihypertensives	enalapril maleate	Cough
	guanethidine sulfate	Nasal congestion
	guanabenz acetate	Nasal congestion
	reserpine	Nasal congestion
Anti-infectives	polymyxin B sulfate	Respiratory paralysis
Antimetabolites	methotrexate sodium	Pneumonitis
Beta-blockers	propranolol hydrochloride	Bronchospasm, particularly in clients with a history of asthma
	metoprolol tartrate	Bronchospasm, dyspnea, wheezing
	atenolol	Bronchospasm (with high doses)
Cholinergic agents	bethanecol chloride	Bronchoconstriction (with subcutaneous administration)
	neostigmine bromide	Increased bronchial secretions, bronchospasm
Gold salts	aurothioglucose, gold sodium thiomalate	Pulmonary infiltrates, interstitial pneumonitis, interstitial fibrosis, "gold" bronchitis
Narcotic analgesics	All types	Respiratory depression

continued

Adverse drug reactions continued

DRUG CLASS	DRUG	POSSIBLE ADVERSE REACTIONS
Nonsteroidal anti-inflammatory agents	aspirin	Bronchospasm
	ibuprofen	Bronchospasm, dyspnea
	indomethacin	Bronchospasm, dyspnea
Penicillins	All types	Anaphylaxis
Sedatives and hypnotics	All types	Respiratory depression, apnea
Urinary tract antiseptics	nitrofurantoin, nitrofurantoin macrocrystals	Pulmonary sensitivity reactions, such as cough, chest pain, dyspnea, pulmonary infiltrates; interstitial pneumonitis (with prolonged use)
Miscellaneous agents	cromolyn sodium	Cough, wheezing
	levodopa	Excessive nasal discharge, hoarseness, episodic hyperventilation, bizarre breathing patterns
	thiamine hydrochloride	Tightness of throat, respiratory distress, cyanosis, pulmonary edema (with I.V. administration)

Pediatric client. Ask the parent or guardian the following questions:

Did the mother have any pregnancy-related problems? Was the pregnancy carried to full term? If not, what care did the infant require?
(RATIONALE: A premature infant may have an underdeveloped respiratory system at birth.)

Did the infant have respiratory problems at birth? If so, how were they treated?
(RATIONALE: The nurse should know if problems were temporary, which the parent may forget about unless asked, or if residual respiratory difficulty continues and how it is treated.)

Does the infant suffer from frequent congestion, runny nose, or colds?
(RATIONALE: If yes, ask about the parents' smoking habits. Second-hand smoke can cause frequent congestion and other respiratory problems in infants.)

Does shortness of breath interfere with the infant's ability to suck a bottle?
(RATIONALE: If yes, the infant will require referral to a physician.)

Does the child cough at night? If so, does the cough awaken the child?
(RATIONALE: A hacking cough could mean tracheobronchitis with epiglottitis, which could lead to airway obstruction.)

Does coughing or shortness of breath interfere with the child's play or school activities?
(RATIONALE: Asthma and dyspnea may interfere with the child's usual activities.)

Elderly client. When assessing an elderly client, ask these questions:

Are you aware of any changes in your breathing patterns? Do you become easily fatigued when climbing stairs? Do you have trouble breathing when lying flat? Do you seem to have more colds that last longer?
(RATIONALE: Elderly clients are susceptible to breathing problems from limited chest wall and respiratory muscle strength. Their altered immune systems may increase their susceptibility to colds and respiratory infections.)

Health promotion and protection patterns

To assess health promotion and protection patterns, ask these questions about the client's occupation, home remedies, sleep and activity patterns, and stress. Also ask about home and work environments, which often contain irritants that may trigger or aggravate breathing problems.

When was your last chest X-ray? Tuberculosis test?
(RATIONALE: Preventive and screening behaviors provide information about the client's self-care patterns and possible teaching opportunities.)

Which home remedies do you use for respiratory problems?
(RATIONALE: Using the client's belief system aids compliance and healing. For example, a client's care plan could include a simple, traditional home remedy, such as herbal tea with honey.)

Have your sleep patterns changed because of breathing problems?
(RATIONALE: Changes in sleep patterns could lead to fatigue. In a client with COPD, such changes could make breathing even more tiring.)

Does your breathing problem affect your daily activities? Which activities can you manage without assistance? Which activities can you manage with assistance? Which activities are you unable to manage? What or who provides assistance when you need it? How do your current activities compare with those before your breathing problems?
(RATIONALE: These questions uncover the client's perceived need for help and also provide information that might suggest the need for follow-up care and services.)

Do you have any hobbies that expose you to respiratory irritants, such as glues, paints, and sprays?
(RATIONALE: The client who engages in such hobbies may need to increase the ventilation in the room when working with these agents. Also instruct the client to wear a protective mask.)

Do you have any breathing difficulty when eating? Do you eat three large meals or several small meals?
(RATIONALE: Clients with chronic respiratory disorders often eat small, frequent meals to reduce dyspnea and effortful breathing.)

Does stress at home or work affect your breathing?
(RATIONALE: Asthmatics and others may be able to identify an action-reaction cycle that includes stress and dyspnea.)

Do you have any special measures for stress management? If so, what are they?
(RATIONALE: Established stress-reduction measures should be incorporated into the care plan. If the client has none, explore the topic further, and teach the client an appropriate stress-reducing exercise.)

Can you afford the medication, equipment, and oxygen required for your health?
(RATIONALE: Often, noncompliance occurs because of economic reasons, not a lack of interest or understanding. If finances are a problem, refer the client to a social worker.)

How many people live with you? Do you have pets? Does the fur, or do the feathers, bother you? What type of home heating do you have? Is anything in your home a respiratory irritant, such as fresh paint, cleaning sprays, or heavy cigarette smoke?
(RATIONALE: The home environment is of special importance to a client with a respiratory problem. Data gathered from these questions can help the nurse and client plan for positive changes in the environment.)

What is your current occupation? What were your previous occupations? Are you exposed to any known respiratory irritants at work? Do you use safety measures during exposure?
(RATIONALE: Certain occupations, such as mining, chemical manufacturing, and working in a smoke-filled office, can expose a client to respiratory irritants. If the client does not have adequate protection, plan to provide information about job safety and regulations.)

Role and relationship patterns

Besides physical status, many factors can affect a client's health. The type of illness, its severity and duration, and its prognosis are important considerations. Other factors, such as emotional, psychological, cultural, and religious constraints, may be just as important, or perhaps even more important, than physical stressors in enhancing or reducing the client's ability to deal with the pulmonary disease.

What impact has your disease had on you and on your family? Are you able to meet family responsibilities? If not, is this a problem?
(RATIONALE: If the client cannot meet expected role responsibilities, additional stress and family conflict may result.)

How have family members reacted to your respiratory illness? Whom among family and friends can you count on in time of need?

(RATIONALE: Many clients with chronic respiratory illness need a great deal of assistance. Learn whether the client will require outside help, and, if so, help the client make the necessary plans. Many clients with chronic breathing problems often feel depressed and isolated from their family. Explore these concerns with the client during the health history.)

How has your breathing problem affected your sexual activity? Have you found ways to decrease the effect of breathing problems on sexual activity? Would you care to discuss them?

(RATIONALE: A client with a breathing problem may be overwhelmed during sexual activity. To help the client overcome this problem, discuss alternate ways to obtain sexual satisfaction, such as using less tiring positions and touching.)

Physical assessment

Before assessing the respiratory system, the nurse must inspect the client's skin as well as upper and lower extremities (arms and legs). This allows an overview of the client's clinical status and also permits an assessment of the degree of peripheral oxygenation. A dusky or bluish skin tint (cyanosis) may indicate a decreased oxygen content in the arterial blood.

Differentiating between central cyanosis and peripheral cyanosis is important. Central cyanosis results from prolonged hypoxia and affects all body organs. It may appear in clients with right-to-left cardiac shunting or a pulmonary disease that causes hypoxemia, such as chronic bronchitis. The cyanosis appears on the buccal mucosa, tongue, and lips, or in other highly vascular areas, such as the nail beds.

On the other hand, peripheral cyanosis results from vasoconstriction, vascular occlusion, or a reduced cardiac output. Often seen in clients after exposure to the cold, peripheral cyanosis appears in the nail beds and sometimes in the lips. Peripheral cyanosis does not affect the mucous membranes.

Dark-skinned clients may be more difficult to assess for central cyanosis. In these clients, the most accurate areas to inspect for cyanosis are the oral mucous membranes and lips. If a dark-skinned client has central cyanosis, these areas will appear ashen gray rather than the bluish tint found in light-skinned clients. Facial skin may appear pale gray or ashen in a cyanotic black-skinned client, and yellowish-brown in a cyanotic brown-skinned client.

For all clients, the nurse then assesses the client's fingertips and toes for abnormal enlargement. This condition, called clubbing, results from chronic tissue hypoxia. Nail thinning accompanied by an abnormal alteration of the angle of the finger and toe bases distinguishes clubbing. (For details, see *Finger clubbing*.)

Preparation for respiratory assessment

After gaining an overall picture of the client's oxygenation, the nurse should proceed with assessment of the respiratory system, using the following guidelines. (For information about assessment of the upper airways, see Chapter 8, Head and Neck.) Physical assessment of the respiratory system requires a quiet, well-lit environment and specific equipment, such as a stethoscope with a diaphragm (or pediatric diaphragm), a felt-tipped marking pen, a ruler, and a tape measure.

For basic assessment of the chest and lungs, use inspection, palpation, percussion, and auscultation. Be familiar with all of the equipment and techniques before using them on a client. (For a description of these techniques, see Chapter 4, Physical Assessment Skills.) More advanced assessment skills include palpation of tactile fremitus, measurement of diaphragmatic excursion, and auscultation of voice resonance.

Positioning the client properly is essential for an effective respiratory assessment. If possible, have the client sit in a position that allows access to the anterior and posterior thorax. Provide the client with a gown that offers easy access to the chest and back without requiring unnecessary exposure. Make sure the client is not cold, because shivering may alter breathing patterns. If the client cannot sit up, use the supine semi-Fowler's position to assess the anterior chest wall and the side-lying position to assess the posterior thorax. However, be aware that these positions may cause some distortion of findings. If the client is an infant or small child, seat the child on the parent's lap.

When performing the assessment, you may find it easiest to inspect, palpate, percuss, and auscultate the anterior chest first and then the posterior. However, this section covers inspection of the whole chest, then palpation, percussion, and auscultation of the whole chest.

Finger clubbing

To assess for chronic tissue hypoxia, the nurse must check the client's fingers for clubbing. Normally, the angle between the fingernail and the point where the nail enters the skin is about 160 degrees, as shown at the left below. Clubbing occurs when that angle increases to 180 degrees or more, as shown at the right. With uncertain findings, double-check by asking the client to place the first phalanges of each forefinger together, as shown. Normal, concave nail bases create a small, diamond-shaped space when the forefingers are placed together. Clubbing fingers are convex at the nail bases, and touch without leaving a space when placed together.

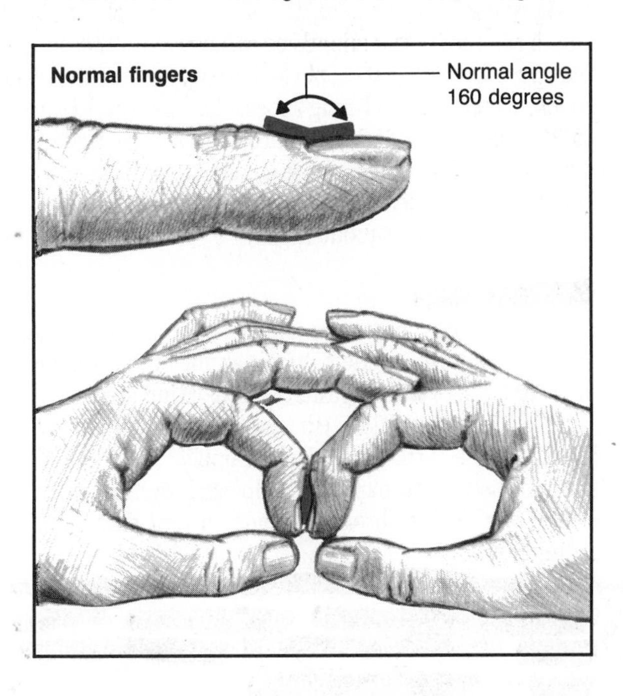

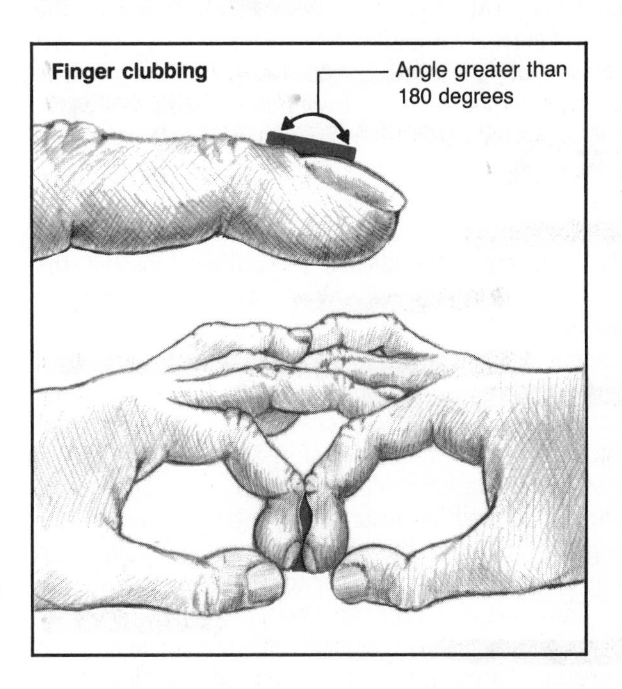

Inspection

Basic assessment of respiratory function requires inspection of the rate, rhythm, and quality of respirations as well as inspection of chest configuration, chest symmetry, skin condition, and accessory muscle use. It should also include assessment for nasal flaring. Accomplish these steps by inspecting the client's breathing and the anterior and posterior thorax, and noting any abnormal findings.

Respiration

Because respiratory rates vary with age, be aware of the normal rate range for the client being assessed. If a client is eupneic, the respiratory rate is within the normal range for the client's age group. (For specific ranges, see *How age affects vital signs* in Chapter 4, Physical Assessment Skills.)

When assessing respiratory rate, count the number of respirations, each composed of an inspiration and an expiration, for 1 full minute. For an infant or a client with periodic or irregular breathing, monitor the respirations for more than 1 minute to determine the rate accurately. Assess the duration of any periods lacking spontaneous respiration (apnea), and alert the physician to any actual or suspected alteration in the breathing pattern. Also note any abnormal respiratory patterns, such as tachypnea (persistent, rapid, shallow breathing) and bradypnea (abnormally decreased respiratory rate). (For more information, see *Respiratory patterns* in Chapter 4, Physical Assessment Skills.)

Assess the quality of respiration by observing the type and depth of breathing. Also assess the method of ventilation by having the client lie in a supine position to expose the chest and abdominal walls. Adult female clients often exhibit thoracic breathing, which involves an upward and outward motion of the chest; infants, males, and sleeping clients most often exhibit abdominal breathing, using the abdominal muscles. Clients with COPD may exhibit pursed-lip breathing, which prevents small airway collapse during exhalation. Forced inspiration or expiration may alter assessment findings; therefore, ask the client to breathe quietly.

Note the depth of quiet breathing, assessing for shallow chest wall expansion (hypopnea) or unusually deep chest wall expansion (hyperpnea). Assessing the depth of quiet breathing is based on the nurse's judgment; therefore, be sure to use the terms *hypopnea* or *hyperpnea,* not *hypoventilation* or *hyperventilation.* Detecting hypoventilation or hyperventilation requires a measurement of $Paco_2$ levels.

Anterior thorax

After assessing the client's respirations, inspect the thorax for structural deformities, such as a concave or convex curvature of the anterior chest wall over the sternum. Inspect between and around the ribs for visible sinking of soft tissues (retractions). Also assess the client's respiratory pattern, checking for symmetry, and look for any abnormalities in skin color or alterations in muscle tone. For future documentation, note the location of any abnormalities according to regions delineated by imaginary lines in the thorax. (For illustrations, see *Respiratory system structures,* pages 246 and 247.)

Initially inspect the chest wall to identify the shape of the thoracic cage. In an adult, the thorax should have a greater diameter laterally (from side to side) than anteroposteriorly (from front to back).

Note the angle between the ribs and the sternum at the point immediately above the xiphoid process. This angle, called the costal angle, should be less than 90 degrees in an adult; it widens if the chest wall is chronically expanded, caused by hypertrophy (enlargement) of the intercostal muscles.

To inspect the anterior chest for symmetry of movement, have the client lie in a supine position. Stand at the foot of the bed and carefully observe the client's quiet and deep breathing for equal expansion of the chest wall. At the same time, be alert for the abnormal collapse of part of the chest wall during inspiration along with an abnormal expansion of the same area during expiration (paradoxical movement). Paradoxical movement indicates a loss of normal chest wall function.

Next, check for the use of the accessory muscles of respiration by observing the sternocleidomastoid, scalenus, and trapezius muscles in the shoulders and neck. During normal inhalation and exhalation, the diaphragm and external intercostal muscles alone should easily maintain the breathing process. Hypertrophy of any of the accessory muscles may indicate frequent use, especially if found in an elderly client, but may be normal in a well-conditioned athlete. Also observe the position the client assumes to breathe. A client depending on accessory muscles may assume a "tripod position," which involves resting the arms on the knees or on the sides of a chair.

Observe the client's skin on the anterior chest for any unusual color, lumps, or lesions, and note the location of any abnormality. Unless the client has been exposed to significant sun or heat, the skin on the chest should match the rest of the client's complexion. Further inspect the chest for the location of the underlying ribs and other bones, cartilage, and lung lobes. An abnormality noted on the skin may reflect a problem in the underlying structure. Also check for any chest wall scars from surgery. If the client did not mention surgery during the health history, ask about it now.

Posterior thorax

To inspect the posterior chest, observe the client's breathing again. A client who cannot sit in a backless chair or lean forward against a supporting structure can lie in a lateral position. However, this may distort findings in some situations. For example, an obese client may not be able to expand the lower lung fully from the lateral position, so breath sounds on that side would be diminished.

Assess the posterior chest wall for the same characteristics as the anterior: chest structure, respiratory pattern, symmetry of expansion, skin color and muscle tone, and accessory muscle use.

Abnormal findings

During inspection, note all abnormal findings. For example, a unilateral absence of chest movement may indicate previous surgical removal of that lung, a bronchial obstruction, or a collapsed lung caused by air or fluid in the pleural space; delayed chest movement may indicate congestion or consolidation of the underlying lung; paradoxical movement often occurs after trauma or incorrectly performed chest compression during cardiopulmonary resuscitation.

Inspection also may reveal structural deformities of the chest wall resulting from defects of the sternum, rib cage, or vertebral column. These deformities have many variations and may be congenital, acute, or progressive. A concave sternal depression—called a funnel chest (pectus excavatum)—or a convex deformity—called a pigeon chest (pectus carinatum)—are two sternal defects that can hinder breathing by preventing full chest expansion. Also, COPD may cause a rounded chest wall (barrel chest). (For illustrations, see *Common chest deformities.*)

Common chest deformities

Inspecting the client's anterior chest for deviations in size or shape is important. Normally, the anteroposterior diameter is less than the lateral diameter. The illustrations below demonstrate three common deformities and show signs, associated conditions, and physical characteristics typical of each. For each deformity, a cross-sectional view compares the anteroposterior and lateral diameters of the normal chest to that of the deformed chest (as indicated by the dotted line).

Funnel chest (Pectus excavatum)

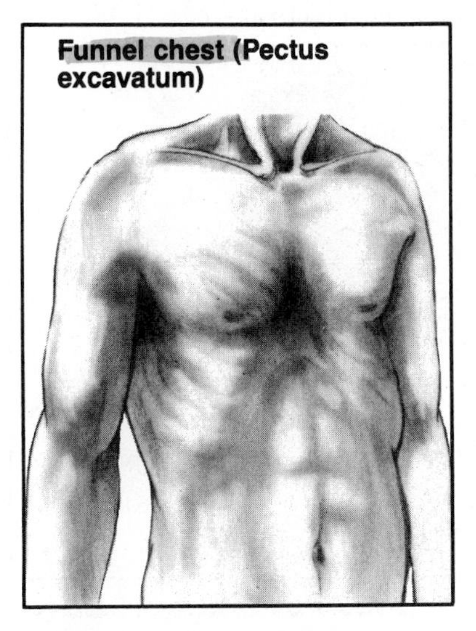

Signs and associated conditions
- Postural disorders, such as forward displacement of neck and shoulders
- Upper thoracic kyphosis
- Protuberant abdomen
- Functional heart murmur

Physical characteristics
- Sinking or funnel-shaped depression of lower sternum
- Diminished anteroposterior chest diameter
- Slightly increases the lateral diameter

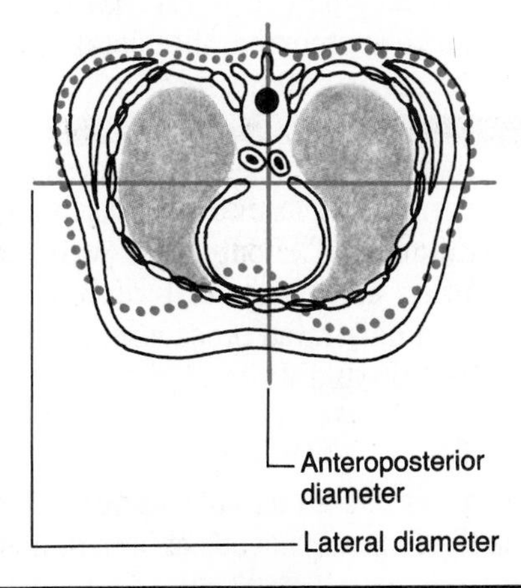

Pigeon chest (Pectus carinatum)

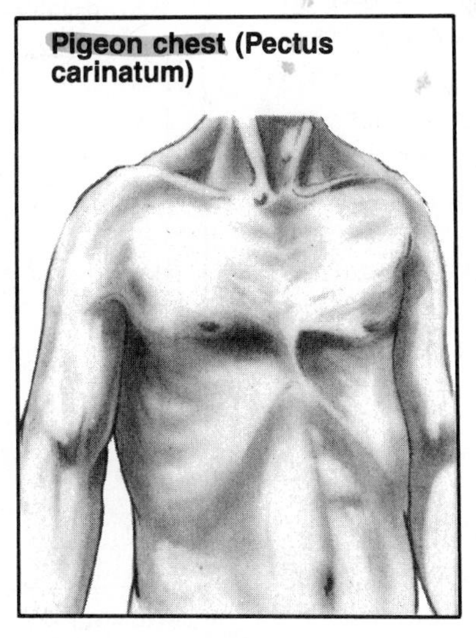

Signs and associated conditions
- Functional cardiovascular or respiratory disorders

Physical characteristics
- Projection of sternum beyond frontal plane of abdomen. Evident in two variations: projection greatest at xiphoid process; projection greatest at or near center of sternum
- Increased anteroposterior diameter
- Greatly decreased lateral diameter at the front of the chest

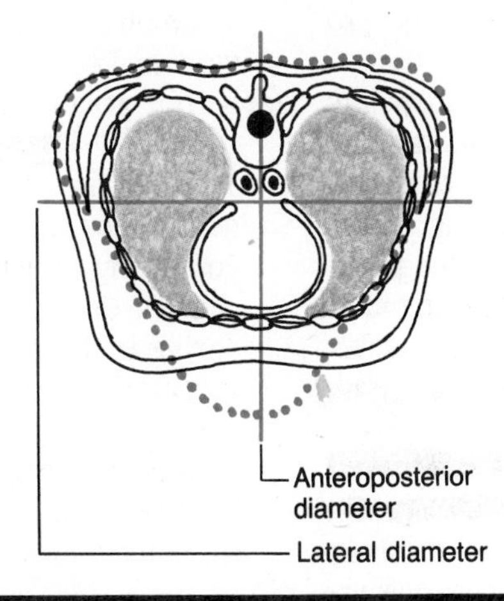

Barrel chest

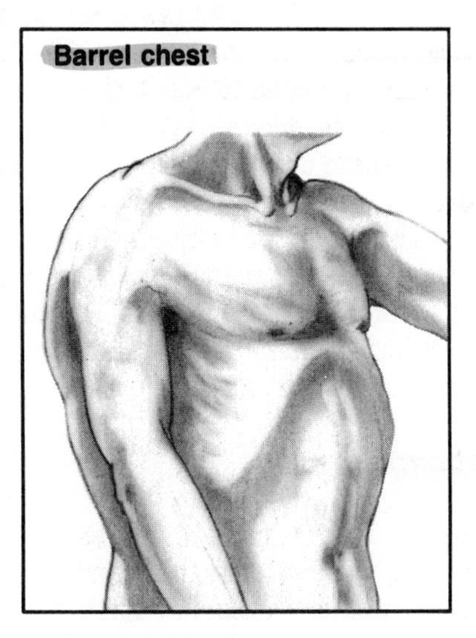

Signs and associated conditions
- Chronic respiratory disorders
- Increasing dyspnea
- Chronic cough
- Wheezing

Physical characteristics
- Enlarged anteroposterior and lateral chest dimensions; chest appears barrel-shaped
- Prominent accessory muscles
- Prominent sternal angle
- Thoracic kyphosis

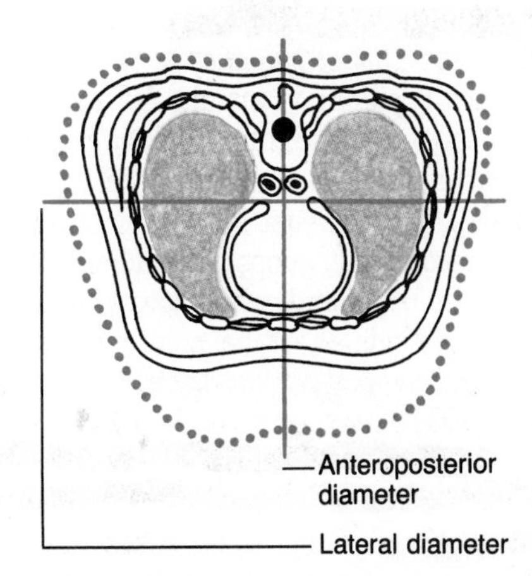

Other structural deformities of the posterior thorax that may alter ventilation include an anterior curvature of the lumbar spine (lordosis), a lateral curvature of the spine (scoliosis), an exaggeration of the anteroposterior spine (kyphosis), and a lateral and anteroposterior curvature of the spine (kyphoscoliosis). These deformities can compress one lung while allowing an overexpansion of the opposite lung, eventually leading to respiratory dysfunction. Acute changes in the thoracic wall from trauma, such as fractured ribs or a flail chest (fractures of two or more ribs in two or more places), also alter the ventilatory process by allowing uneven chest expansion. These deformities also cause pain, which leads to shallow breathing, increasing the respiratory distress.

Nonstructural abnormalities found on inspection include visible vein paths (superficial venous patterns), which could indicate underlying vascular or heart disease. Rib prominence suggests malnutrition, and a layer of fat over the ribs indicates obesity.

Palpation

Palpation of the trachea and the anterior and posterior thorax can detect structural and skin abnormalities, areas of pain, and chest asymmetry.

Trachea and anterior thorax

First, palpate the trachea for position. (For an illustrated procedure, see *Trachea palpation.*) Observe the client to determine whether the client uses accessory neck muscles to breathe.

Next, palpate the suprasternal notch. In most clients, the arch of the aorta lies close to the surface just behind the suprasternal notch. Use your fingertips to gently evaluate the strength and regularity of the client's aortic pulsations there.

Then palpate the thorax to assess the skin and underlying tissues for density. (For an illustrated procedure, see *Thorax palpation.*)

Gentle palpation should not cause the client any pain; therefore, assess any complaints of pain for localization, radiation, and severity. Be especially careful to palpate any areas that looked abnormal during inspection. If necessary, support the client during the procedure with one hand while using your other hand to palpate one side at a time, continuing to compare sides. Note any unusual findings, such as masses, crepitus, skin irregularities, or painful areas.

If a client complains of chest pain, attempt to differentiate the cause of the pain through palpation of the anterior chest. Certain disorders—such as musculoskeletal pain, an irritation of the nerves covering the xiphoid process, or an inflammation of the cartilage connecting the bony ribs to the sternum (costochondritis)—cause increased pain during palpation. These disorders may also produce pain during inspiration, causing the client to breathe shallowly to decrease discomfort. On the other hand, palpation does not increase pain caused by cardiac or pulmonary disorders, such as angina or pleurisy.

Next, palpate the costal angle. The area around the xiphoid process contains many nerve endings, so be gentle to avoid causing the client pain. If a client frequently uses the internal intercostal muscles to breathe, these muscles will eventually pull the chest cavity upward and outward. If this has occurred, the costal angle will be greater than the normal 90 degrees.

Also, use a technique called respiratory excursion to assess the anterior thorax for symmetrical chest movement. Respiratory excursion, performed anteriorly and posteriorly, provides information about chest wall expansion during inspiration and chest wall contraction during expiration. (For an illustrated procedure, see *Respiratory excursion* pages 266 and 267.)

Posterior thorax

Palpate the posterior thorax in a similar manner, using the palmar surface of the fingertips of one or both hands.

Trachea palpation

To palpate the trachea, the nurse proceeds as follows: Stand in front of the client and place one thumb on either side of the trachea above the suprasternal notch. Gently slide both thumbs, at equal speed, out along the upper edge of the client's clavicle until you reach the sternocleidomastoid muscle. Each thumb should have covered an equal distance, indicating a midline trachea.

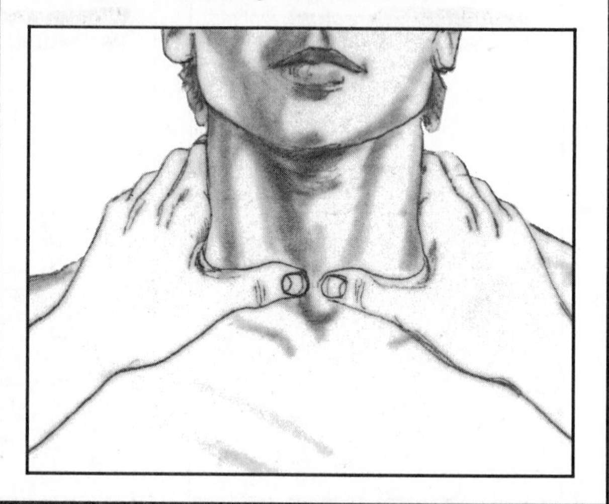

Sound travels more easily thru solid structure

Thorax palpation

Using the fingertips and palmar surfaces of one or both hands, the nurse should palpate the thorax systematically and in a circular motion, alternating palpation from one side of the thorax to the other.

Palpation

To palpate the anterior thorax, begin in the supraclavicular area, as shown. Then follow the sequence, as illustrated, progressing to the infraclavicular, sternal, xiphoid, rib, and axillary areas. Begin posterior palpation in the supraclavicular area, move to the area between the scapulae (interscapular), then below the scapulae (infrascapular), and down to the lateral walls of the thorax.

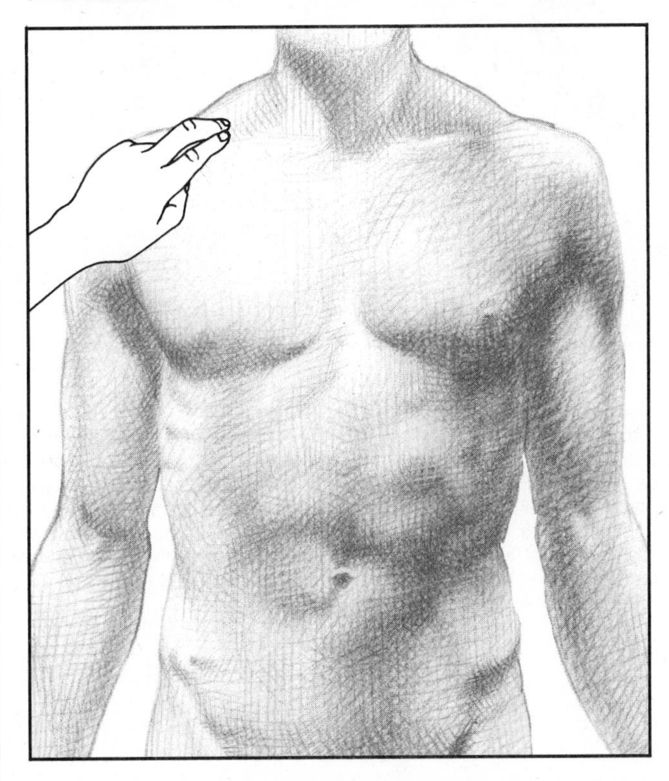

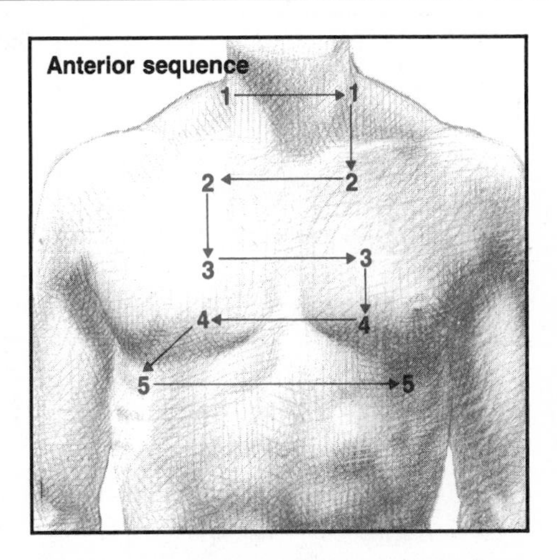

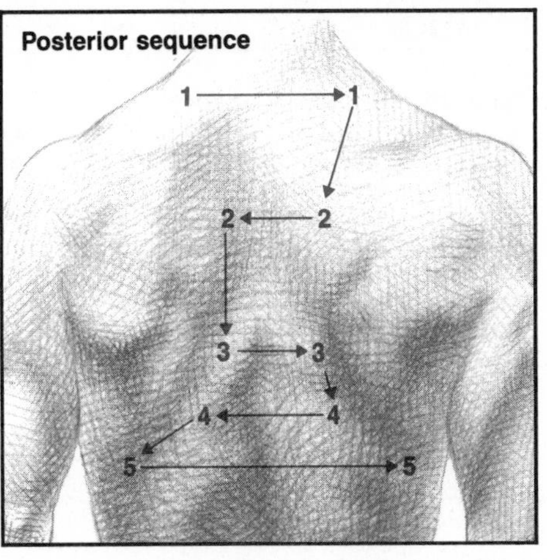

(For an illustration, see *Thorax palpation.*) During the process, identify bony structures, such as the vertebrae and the scapulae.

To determine the location of any abnormalities, identify the first thoracic vertebra (with the client's head tipped forward) and count the number of spinous processes from this landmark to the abnormal finding. Use this reference point for documentation. Also identify the inferior scapular tips and medial borders of both bones to define the margins of the upper and lower lung lobes posteriorly. Locate and describe all abnormalities in relation to these landmarks. Once again, assessment includes an evaluation of abnormalities, such as use of accessory muscles or complaints of pain.

Next, assess posterior respiratory excursion in a manner similar to the anterior assessment. (For an illustrated procedure, see *Respiratory excursion*, pages 266 and 267.)

Abnormal findings

Palpation may show that the trachea is not midline. This could result from a collapse of lung tissue (atelectasis), thyroid enlargement, or fluid accumulation in the air

Respiratory excursion

To assess anterior and posterior respiratory excursion, the nurse should follow these steps.

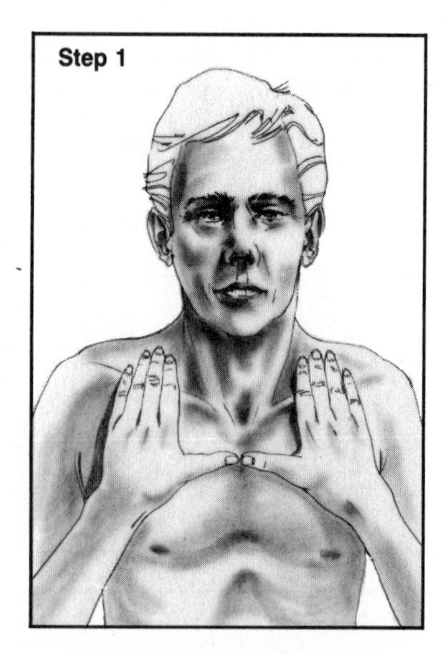

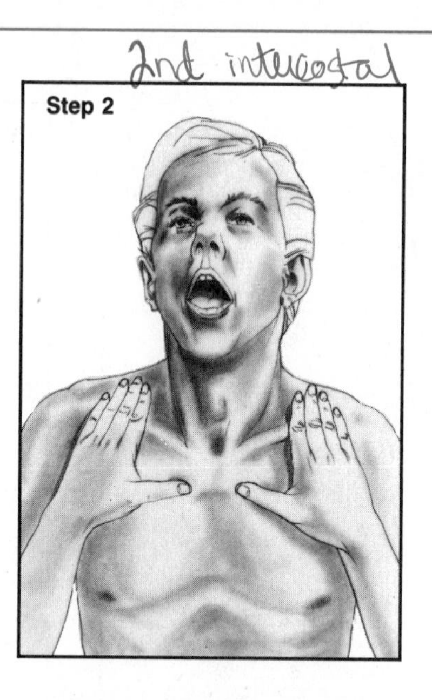

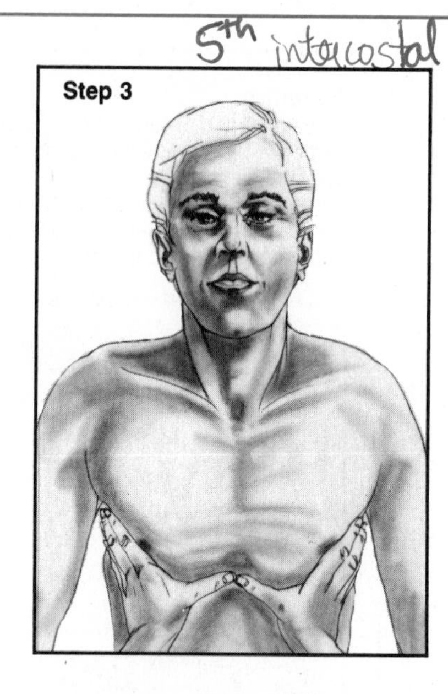

Anterior respiratory excursion

Assess respiratory excursion in three areas on the client's anterior thorax. For all three areas, stand in front of the client, who may either sit or stand.

To assess the first area, place your hands on the anterior chest wall, thumbs equidistant from the sternum, with the rest of your fingers spread over the lateral thorax. To identify equal thumb placement, locate the second rib on either side of the client's sternum, and place your thumbs on the tissue directly below those ribs in the second intercostal space (Step 1). Do not apply pressure, as this may alter the client's inspiration effort.

Instruct the client to take a deep breath. During the inspiration, observe the separation of your thumbs; they should separate simultaneously and equally to a distance several centimeters from the sternum (Step 2).

To assess respiratory excursion in the second area, place your thumbs at the fifth intercostal space and repeat the procedure (Steps 3 and 4).

spaces of the lungs (pleural effusion). A tumor, a collapsed lung (pneumothorax), or nodal enlargement may also displace the trachea to one side.

Tenderness on palpation of the anterior chest could indicate musculoskeletal inflammation, especially if the client complains of chest pain of unknown origin.

Palpation producing a crackly sound similar to the noise of crumpling cellophane paper suggests crepitus. Report this sign to the physician immediately, because 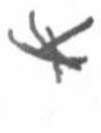 crepitus indicates air leakage into the subcutaneous tissue from a rupture somewhere in the respiratory system.

An absence or delay of chest movement during respiratory excursion may indicate a previous surgical removal of the lung, complete or partial obstruction of the airway or underlying lung, or diaphragmatic dysfunction on the affected side.

Percussion

Percussion helps determine the boundaries of the lungs and how much gas, liquid, or solid exists in the lungs. Percussion can effectively assess structures as deep as 1¾″ to 3″ (4.5 to 8 cm). To percuss the thorax, practice to become competent with the procedure. Also become familiar with the sounds elicited. (For general infor-

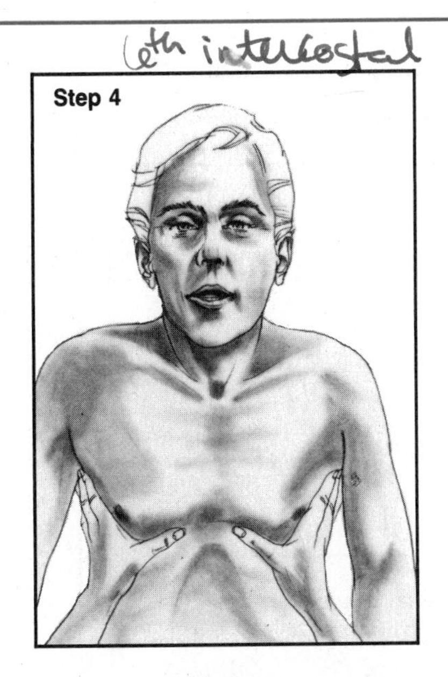

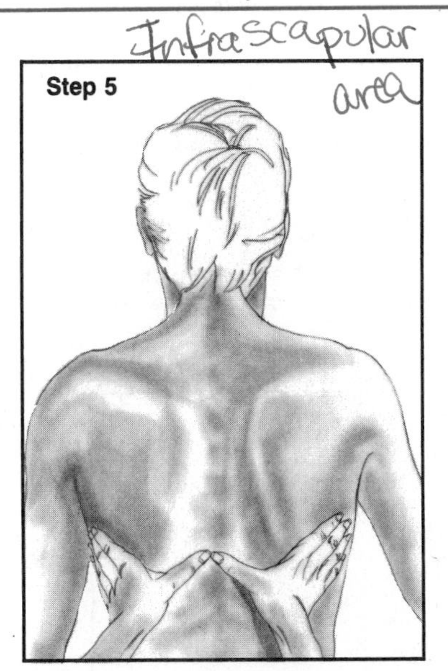

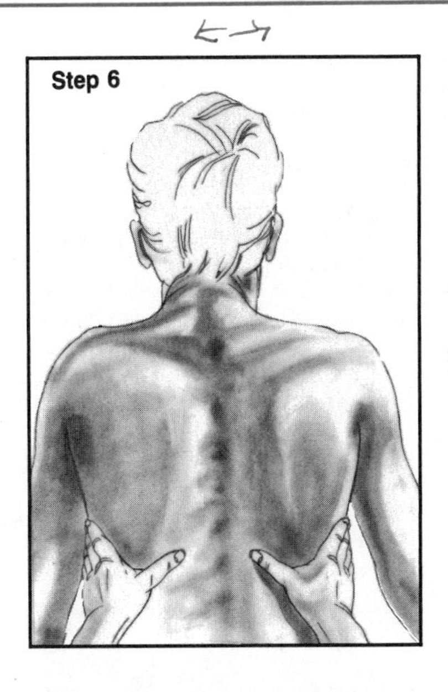

To assess respiratory excursion in the third area, place your thumbs at the sixth intercostal space and repeat the procedure. In a female client with pendulous breasts, thumb placement may be difficult to evaluate, and the technique may cause embarrassment; therefore, perform posterior respiratory excursion in this instance.

Posterior respiratory excursion
Assess respiratory excursion in two locations on the client's posterior thorax.

Stand behind the client and place your thumbs in the infrascapular area on either side of the spine at the level of the tenth rib. Grasp the lateral rib cage and rest your palms gently over the lateroposterior surface (Step 5). Avoid applying excessive pressure to prevent restricting the client's breath-

As the client inhales, the posterior chest should move upward and outward and your thumbs should move apart (Step 6). When the client exhales, your thumbs should return to midline and again touch.

Repeat the procedure after placing your thumbs equally lateral to the vertebral column in the interscapular area, with your fingers extending into the axillary area. Instruct the client to take a deep breath while you watch for simultaneous, equal separation of your thumbs.

mation about percussion techniques, see Chapter 4, Physical Assessment Skills.)

The most frequently used technique is mediate percussion, which involves striking one finger with another. Immediate percussion, which requires direct tapping on the chest to elicit sound, produces vibrations that are somewhat more difficult to identify.

To percuss correctly, follow these guidelines. Perform percussion in a quiet environment, and proceed systematically, percussing the anterior, lateral, and posterior chest over the intercostal spaces. (For an illustrated procedure, see *Thorax percussion,* page 268.) Avoid percussing over bones, such as over the manubrium, sternum, xiphoid, clavicles, ribs, vertebrae, or scapulae. Because of their denseness, bones produce a dull sound on percussion, and therefore yield no useful information. Percussion over a healthy lung elicits a resonant sound—hollow and loud, with a low pitch and long duration.

To percuss the anterior chest, have the client sit facing forward, hands resting at the side of the body. Following the anterior percussion sequence, percuss and compare sound variations from one side to the other. Anterior chest percussion should produce resonance from below the clavicle to the fifth intercostal space on the right (where dullness occurs close to the liver) and to the third intercostal space on the left (where dullness occurs near the heart).

Thorax percussion

When percussing a client's thorax, the nurse should always use mediate percussion and follow the same sequence, comparing sound variations from one side to the other. This helps ensure consistency and prevents the nurse from overlooking any important findings. Auscultation follows the same sequence as percussion.

Percussion

To percuss the anterior thorax, place your hands over the lung apices in the supraclavicular area. Then proceed downward, moving from side to side at 1½" to 2" (3- to 5-cm) intervals.

To percuss the lateral thorax, start at the axilla and move down the side of the rib cage, percussing between the ribs as shown.

To percuss the posterior thorax, progress in a zigzag fashion from the suprascapular to the interscapular to infrascapular areas, avoiding the vertebral column and the scapulae as shown.

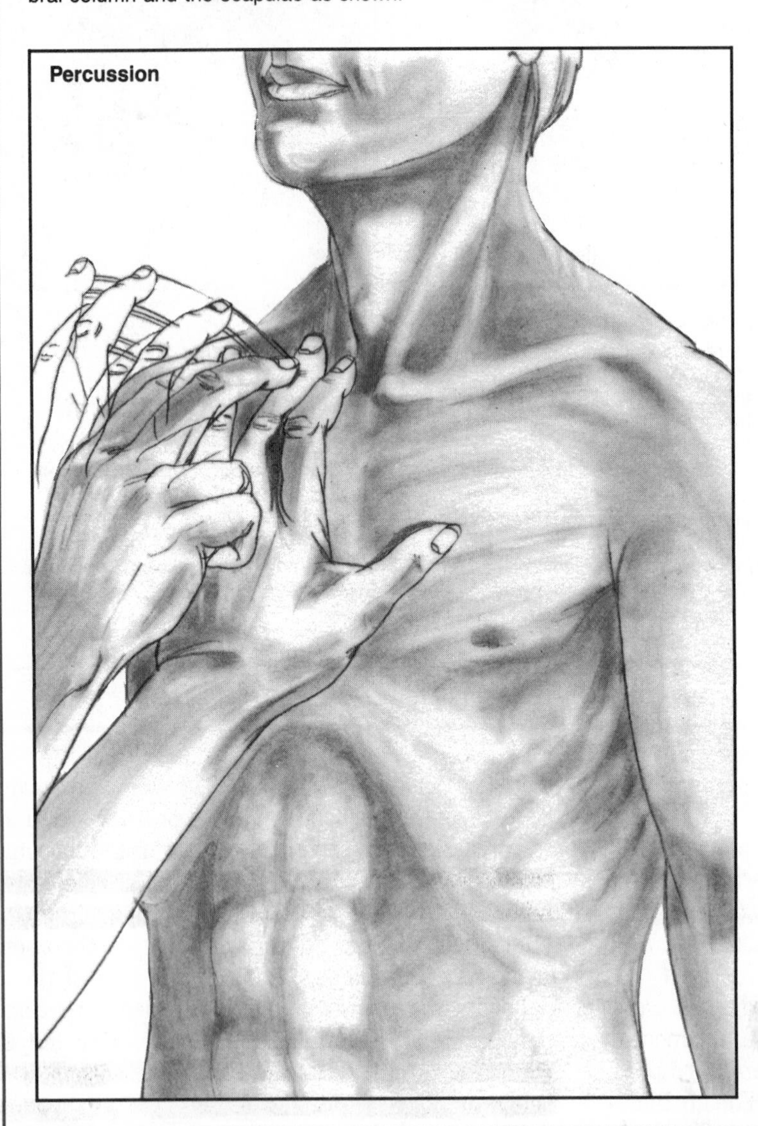

Anterior sequence

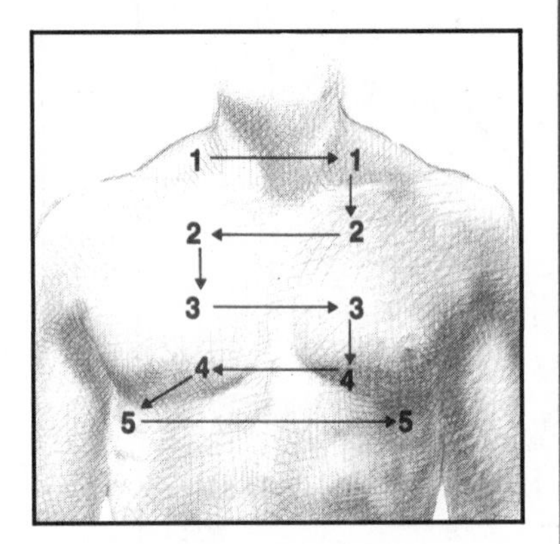

Left lateral sequence

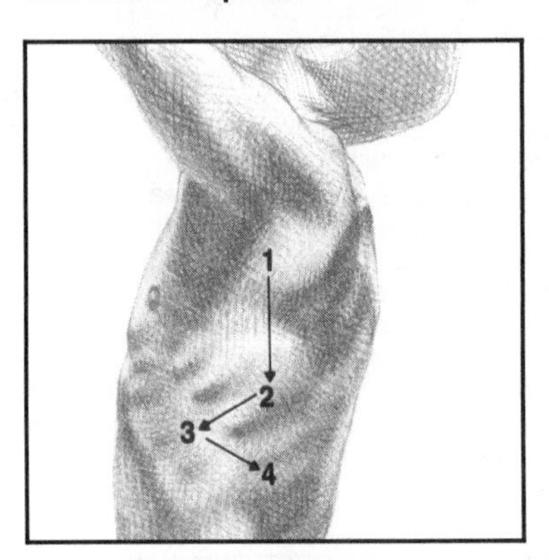

Posterior sequence

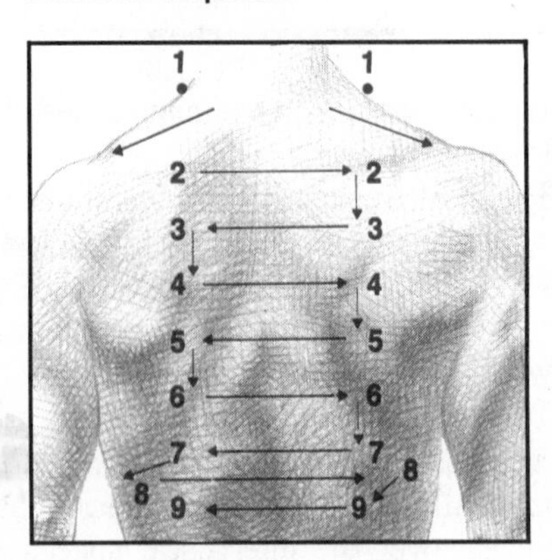

Next, percuss the lateral chest to obtain information about the left upper and lower lobes, and about the right upper, middle, and lower lobes. The client's left arm should be positioned on the client's head. Repeat the same sequence on the right side. Lateral chest percussion should produce resonance to the sixth or eighth intercostal space.

Finally, percuss the posterior thorax according to the percussion sequence. Posterior percussion should sound resonant to the level of T10.

Abnormal findings

Hyperresonance and dullness are the most frequent abnormal percussion findings. Hyperresonance may result from air in the pleural space, which may be caused by a pneumothorax or overinflation of the lung, such as occurs with COPD. Dullness may result from a consolidation of fluid or tissue, which may occur with pneumonia or atelectasis.

Auscultation

Auscultate the anterior, lateral, and posterior thorax to detect normal as well as abnormal breath sounds. To auscultate the thorax of an adult, first warm the stethoscope between your hands and then place the diaphragm of the stethoscope directly on the client's skin. Clothing or linen interferes with accurate auscultation.

If the client has significant hair growth over the areas to be auscultated, wet the hair to decrease sound blurring. Instruct the client to take deep breaths through the mouth (nose breathing may alter the findings), and caution the client against breathing too deeply or too rapidly to prevent light-headedness or dizziness.

Anterior and lateral thorax

Systematically assess the anterior and lateral thorax for normal as well as abnormal breath sounds, following the same sequence as that used for percussion. (For an illustration of this sequence, see *Thorax percussion*.) Begin at the upper lobes, and move from side to side and down.

Auscultate a point first on one side of the chest and then auscultate the same point on the other side of the chest, comparing findings. Always assess one full breath (inspiration and expiration) at each point.

To assess the right middle lung lobe, auscultate breath sounds laterally at the level of the fourth to the sixth intercostal spaces, following the lateral auscultation sequence, which is the same as the lateral percussion sequence. Although difficult to assess, especially in a female client with large breasts, the right middle lobe is a frequent site of aspiration pneumonia, so it requires special attention.

Normal breath sounds include bronchial (tracheal), bronchovesicular, and vesicular sounds. Bronchial sounds, which are harsh and discontinuous, occur over the trachea; they are prolonged during expiration. Bronchovesicular sounds, medium-pitched and continuous, occur over the upper third of the sternum anteriorly and in the interscapular area posteriorly. Bronchovesicular sounds are equally audible during inspiration and expiration. Vesicular sounds, low-pitched and continuous, occur in the periphery of the lungs, and are prolonged during inspiration. (For more information, see *Normal breath sounds,* page 270.)

Classify normal and abnormal breath sounds according to location, intensity (amplitude), characteristic sound, pitch (tone), and duration during the inspiratory and expiratory phases. When assessing duration, time the inspiratory and expiratory phases to determine the ratio. Also, when classifying sounds, keep in mind that higher-pitched breath sounds have a higher tone than lower-pitched ones, and that louder breath sounds have more intensity than softer ones. When describing specific sounds, identify the quality using specific terms such as *high-pitched* or *harsh*.

For the last step in auscultation, identify the inspiratory and expiratory phase of normal and abnormal breath sounds and then determine whether the sound occurs during inspiration, expiration, or both. Do this by placing one hand on the client's chest wall during auscultation: If the sound occurs as the thorax expands, it is part of inspiration; if the sound occurs as the thorax contracts, it is part of expiration.

During auscultation, first identify normal breath sounds and then assess and identify abnormal sounds. Practice auscultation on a normal chest to gain confidence. Specific breath sounds occur normally only in certain locations; therefore, the same sound heard anywhere else in the lung field constitutes an important abnormality requiring appropriate documentation.

Posterior thorax

The auscultation sequence for the posterior thorax follows the same pattern as the percussion sequence. During auscultation, remain aware of the client's breathing pattern. Breathing too rapidly or deeply causes an excessive loss of carbon dioxide that may result in vertigo or syncope.

In a normal adult, adolescent, or older child, bronchovesicular breath sounds (the sound of air moving through the bronchial airways) should occur over the interscapular area; vesicular breath sounds (the sound

Normal breath sounds

The illustrations below show the location of the various breath sounds. Bronchial (tracheal) sounds result from air passing over the walls of the trachea. They are heard best over the trachea as loud, high-pitched sounds. Their ratio of inspiration to expiration is 1:2. Bronchovesicular sounds result from transitional airflow moving through the branches and convergences of the smaller bronchi and bronchioles. These soft, breezy sounds are pitched about two notes lower than bronchial sounds. Anteriorly, they are heard near the mainstem bronchi in the first and second intercostal spaces; posteriorly, between the scapulae. Their inspiration-expiration ratio is 1:1. Vesicular sounds result from laminar airflow moving through the alveolar ducts and alveoli at low flow rates. They are heard best in the periphery of the lungs, but are inaudible over the scapulae. These soft, swishy, breezy sounds are about two notes lower than bronchovesicular sounds. Their inspiration-expiration ratio is 3:1.

Anterior chest

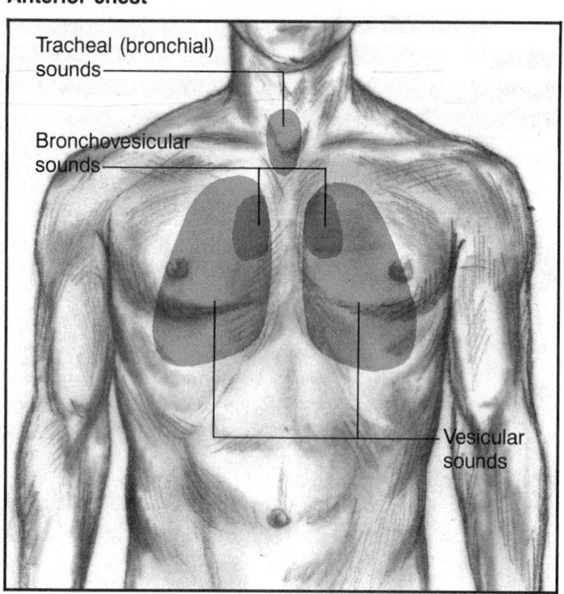

Posterior chest

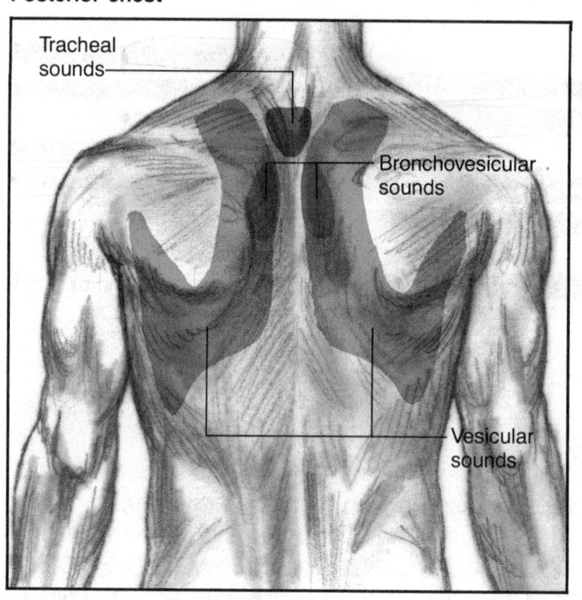

of air moving through the alveoli) should occur in the suprascapular and infrascapular areas. Note any absent, decreased, or adventitious breath sounds. For example, bronchovesicular sounds auscultated in the periphery of the lungs are adventitious. Crackles and rhonchi (gurgles) are also adventitious; if you hear them, instruct the client to cough, and then listen again.

Abnormal findings

Document adventitious breath sounds by labeling the sound or describing its characteristics. Although either method is correct, most nurses currently use a description of the sound with or without a label. Adventitious breath sounds may indicate fluid within alveoli, opening of compressed alveoli, secretions in small or large airways, narrowed airways, or pleural membrane inflammation.

Certain adventitious breath sounds, including crackles, wheezes, rhonchi, and pleural friction rubs, may appear in any lung lobe. (For further information, see *Abnormal breath sounds*.)

When assessing the client, note all abnormal findings; by the end of the assessment, a cluster of signs and symptoms may point to a particular disorder. (For signs and symptoms of some common respiratory problems, see *Integrating assessment findings*, pages 272 and 273.)

Developmental considerations

When assessing a pediatric, pregnant, or elderly client, modify assessment techniques to accommodate the client's developmental differences. Follow these guidelines.

Pediatric clients

For the most effective assessment, have a parent hold the child, either on the examination table or in the parent's arms. Auscultate the child's lungs first, before per-

Abnormal breath sounds

Air moving through the tracheo-broncho-alveolar system normally produces tracheal, bronchial, bronchovesicular, and vesicular breath sounds. Abnormal (adventitious) breath sounds occur when air passes through narrowed airways or moisture, or when the membranes lining the chest cavity and the lungs become inflamed. These sounds include crackles, wheezes, rhonchi, and pleural friction rubs.

The nurse can use this chart as a guide to assess abnormal breath sounds and to document findings.

TYPE	LOCATION	CAUSE	DESCRIPTION
Abnormal breath sounds in adult and pediatric clients			
Crackles (rales)	Anywhere; in lung bases initially, usually heard during inspiration. Also in dependent lung portions of bedridden clients. If crackles clear with coughing, they are not pathologic.	Air passing through moisture, especially in the small airways and alveoli, with pulmonary edema	Light crackling, popping, nonmusical sound, like hairs being rubbed together. Further classified by pitch: high, medium, or low
Wheezes	Anywhere; heard during inspiration or expiration. If wheezes clear with coughing, they may be coming from the trachea or larger upper airways	Fluid or secretions in the large airways or airways narrowed by mucus or bronchospasm	Whistling sound; can be described as sonorous, bubbling, moaning, musical, sibilant and rumbling, crackling, groaning
Rhonchi (gurgles)	Central airways; heard during inspiration and expiration	Air passing through fluid-filled airways, as in upper respiratory tract infection	Bubbling sound
Pleural friction rub	Lateral lung field; heard during inspiration and expiration (with client in upright position)	Inflamed parietal and visceral pleural linings rubbing together	Superficial squeaking or grating sound, like pieces of sandpaper being rubbed together
Additional abnormal breath sounds in pediatric clients			
Grunting	Central airways; heard during expiration	Physiologic retention of air in lungs to prevent alveolar collapse	Grunting noise
Stridor	Trachea; heard during inspiration	Forced movement of air through edematous upper airway	Crowing noise

forming any other assessment procedure, to avoid having the child cry. Crying increases the respiratory rate and creates noise that interferes with clear auscultation. Demonstrate any equipment on a parent or doll first, to help increase the child's cooperativeness.

Before inspecting an infant's respiratory system, first inspect the skin. Infants have a thin layer of subcutaneous tissue, making cyanosis a more reliable sign of respiratory distress in them than in adults. Inspect the chest wall to gain further information about respiratory status. More cartilage than bone composes a child's thoracic cage and, because less subcutaneous tissue is present to mask findings, chest wall movement should be more visible during breathing. Infants and children often exhibit abdominal breathing or paradoxical breathing. Paradoxical breathing, which occurs when the chest and abdomen do not work together to expand and contract during inspiration and expiration, results because of the child's immature respiratory center and weak chest muscles.

Next, observe for changes in thoracic structures, which are also easier to evaluate in an infant or child than in an adult. Assess an infant's chest circumference by snugly wrapping a tape measure around the chest at the nipple line. Rather than drawing a conclusion based on a single measurement, consider several measurements taken during the child's first 2 years to detect a trend.

Integrating assessment findings

Sometimes, a cluster of assessment findings will strongly suggest a particular respiratory system disorder. In the chart below, column one shows groups of presenting signs and symptoms—the ones that make the client seek medical attention. Column two shows related assessment findings that the nurse may discover during the health history and physical assessment. The client may exhibit one or more of these findings. Column three shows the possible disorder indicated by a cluster of these findings.

PRESENTING SIGNS AND SYMPTOMS	RELATED ASSESSMENT FINDINGS	POSSIBLE DISORDER
Dry cough progressing to productive cough, severe dyspnea with audible wheezing	Allergic response to exposure to known agents, such as animal dander or pollen Recent stress, exercise, or occupational exposure to respiratory irritant Tachycardia Pale, slightly cyanotic skin Sitting forward Nasal flaring Use of accessory respiratory muscles	Asthma
Chronic, productive cough in the mornings, for at least 3 months of the year for 2 consecutive years; hemoptysis (bloody sputum) possible; dyspnea with chest infection	Exposure to air pollution, inorganic or organic dusts, or noxious gases Cigarette smoking Genetic predisposition Frequent respiratory infections Bluish complexion Overweight Barrel chest Dullness on percussion Prolonged expiratory phase Sibilant and sonorous wheezes and crackles Labored respirations Tachypnea Orthopnea Neck vein distention on expiration	Chronic bronchitis
Moderate dyspnea; pleuritic (sudden, sharp) chest pain	History of dizziness, emphysema, or tuberculosis Spontaneous, sudden onset of dyspnea Crepitus Tracheal deviation Limited respiratory excursion on one side No tactile fremitus Resonance or hyperresonance on percussion Decreased or absent breath or voice sounds No adventitious sounds Slender body build	Closed pneumothorax
Cough with scant mucus production; dyspnea that progresses slowly to severe dyspnea on exertion	Genetic predisposition Cigarette smoking Acute, recurring respiratory illness Exposure to environmental hazards Under age 60 Reddish complexion Increased anteroposterior diameter of thorax Use of accessory respiratory muscles Decreased respiratory and diaphragmatic excursion bilaterally Decreased tactile fremitus Hyperresonance on percussion Breath sounds distant with prolonged expiration, occasionally wheezing Pursed lips when breathing Abnormal chest X-ray, pulmonary function test, arterial blood gas analysis, and hematocrit	Emphysema

Integrating assessment findings continued

PRESENTING SIGNS AND SYMPTOMS	RELATED ASSESSMENT FINDINGS	POSSIBLE DISORDER
Harsh cough; severe, increasing dyspnea	Sudden onset of sore throat, drooling, fever, and stridor Age 3 to 7 Wheezing Decreased breath sounds Hoarseness Cyanosis Retractions Restlessness Anxiety	Epiglottitis
Productive cough with mucoid, purulent sputum; dyspnea on exertion; pleuritic chest pain	Occurs in very young and very old Possible aspiration of vomitus Impaired mucus transport, as in neuromuscular or chronic obstructive diseases Fever Tachycardia Tachypnea Inspiratory crackles Percussion dull or flat over consolidated area	Pneumonia

The mean chest circumference at birth is about 13″ (33 cm), usually ¾″ to 1⅛″ (2 to 3 cm) smaller than the head circumference, and about 18½″ (47 cm) at 1 year. Normally, infants demonstrate a basically round thoracic structure; however, the ratio of chest width to chest depth varies with age from 1:2 to 5:7.

Infants and children seldom exhibit hypertrophy of the accessory muscles of respiration. However, they may exhibit bulging or retractions during inspiration and expiration—a sign of breathing difficulty. The intercostals often bulge during infant respiratory distress, while the suprasternal, substernal, and abdominal muscles retract. These findings also may appear in adults, especially small or thin clients. Infants commonly use only the abdominal muscles to breathe until age 6 or 7, when the thoracic intercostal muscles take over.

Infants and toddlers have small chest surfaces; therefore, limit palpation to an assessment of the suprasternal notch. Chest palpation becomes appropriate around age 4 or 5.

Percussion is usually unreliable because of the disproportionate size between an infant's chest and an adult's fingers.

Use a stethoscope with an appropriately sized diaphragm to auscultate a child. Because of a child's small chest size, fewer auscultation sites exist. (For illustrations, see *Auscultation sequence for children,* page 274.) An infant's breath sounds are louder and harsher than an adult's because an infant's chest is thinner and more resonant. Otherwise, normal breath sounds for this age-group are identical to those for adults. Grunting (deep, low-pitched sounds at the end of each breath) and stridor (loud, harsh, musical sounds resulting from tracheal or laryngeal obstruction) also may be heard, sometimes even without equipment.

Pregnant clients

These clients normally exhibit an increased costal angle, up to 103 degrees by the third trimester. As a result, the lower rib cage appears to flare out. As the uterus enlarges, the woman's breathing becomes more thoracic than abdominal. Also, the internal organs become crowded, which causes deeper respirations, increased sighing, and increased dyspnea. The respiratory rate and depth may increase during the second and third trimesters to meet the growing oxygenation and ventilation needs of the mother and fetus.

Elderly clients

These clients' thoracic structure typically becomes rounder, and the anteroposterior chest increases in relation to the lateral diameter. This is caused by changes in the

Auscultation sequence for children

Infants and young children have fewer auscultation sites and exhibit fewer types of breath sounds. These clients have audible tracheal and bronchial sounds, the same as in an adult. However, an infant's or young child's lungs exhibit bronchovesicular sounds throughout the chest, and also exhibit undifferentiated vesicular sounds.

Auscultation

To auscultate a child's anterior chest, begin just below the right clavicle, as shown. Continue to auscultate the anterior chest, following the illustrated auscultation sequence. Then auscultate the posterior chest, following the illustrated auscultation sequence.

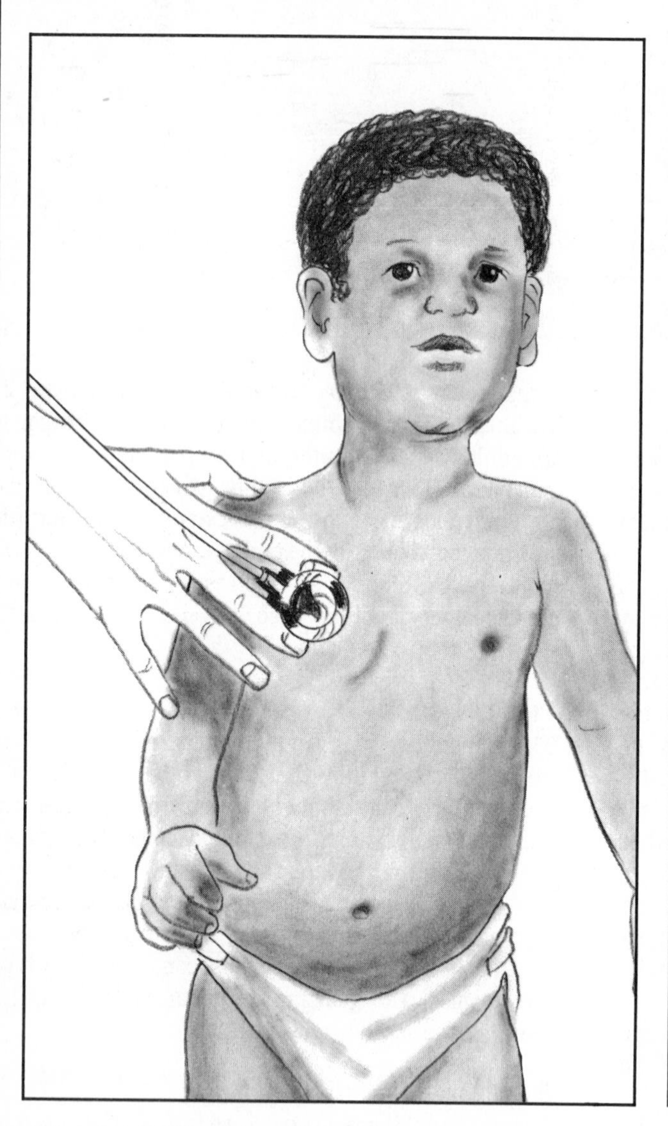

Anterior sequence

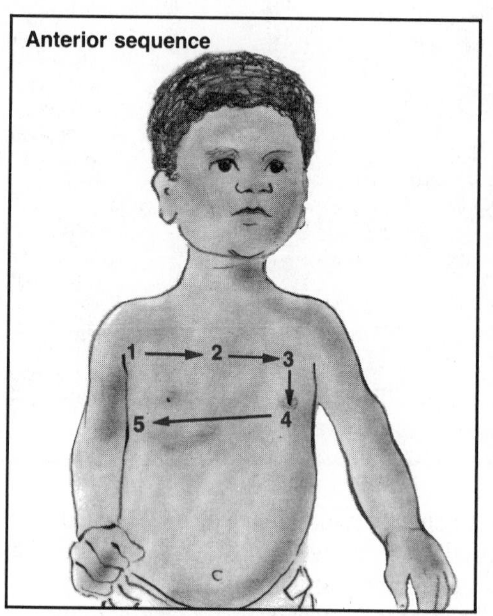

Posterior sequence

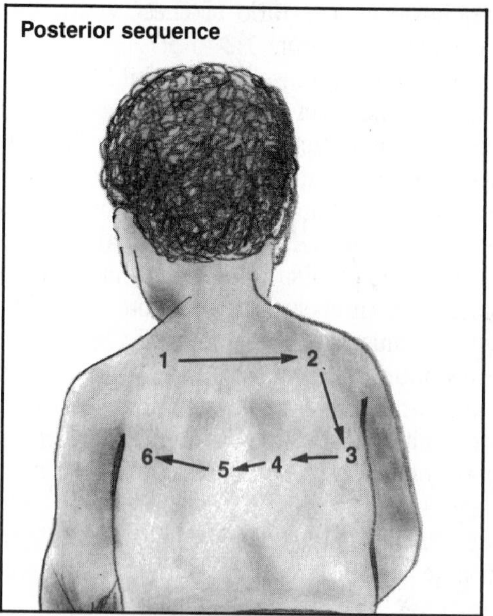

thoracic and lumbar spine. Also, because of calcification of the rib articulations, elderly clients may use accessory muscles to breathe. Percussion may produce hyperresonant sounds because of the decreased distensibility of the lung tissue. Also, for clients with suspected atelectasis, begin auscultation at the base of the lungs rather than at the apices; atelectic crackles may disappear as the client repeatedly takes deep breaths. Keep in mind that a decreased cough reflex also increases the risk of aspiration for this age-group.

Advanced assessment skills

Advanced pulmonary assessment skills include palpation of tactile fremitus, measurement of diaphragmatic excursion, and auscultation of voice resonance.

Tactile fremitus

Because sound travels more easily through solid structures than through air, assessing tactile fremitus—which is the palpation of voice vibrations—provides valuable information about the contents of the lungs. (For an illustrated procedure, see *Advanced assessment skills: Palpation for tactile fremitus*.)

The vocalizations should produce vibrations of equal intensity on both sides of the chest. Normally, vibrations should occur in the upper chest, close to the bronchi, and then decrease and finally disappear toward the periphery of the lungs.

Conditions that cause more air than normal to be blocked or trapped in the lungs, such as emphysema or pneumothorax, result in decreased tactile fremitus. Conditions causing a consolidation of tissue or fluid in a portion of the pleural area, such as lung tumor or some types of pneumonia, result in increased tactile fremitus. A grating feeling may signify a pleural friction rub.

Diaphragmatic excursion

This advanced assessment technique allows the nurse to evaluate the movement of the diaphragm—the primary muscle of respiration. (For an illustrated procedure, see *Advanced assessment skills: Measurement of diaphragmatic excursion*, page 278.)

Normal diaphragmatic excursion is 1¼" to 2¼" (3 to 6 cm). Failure of the diaphragm to contract down may indicate paralysis or muscle flattening, a condition that may be caused by COPD.

(Text continues on page 278.)

ADVANCED ASSESSMENT SKILLS

Palpation for tactile fremitus

The nurse should follow this procedure to assess tactile fremitus.

1 Place your open palm flat against the client's chest without touching the chest with your fingers.

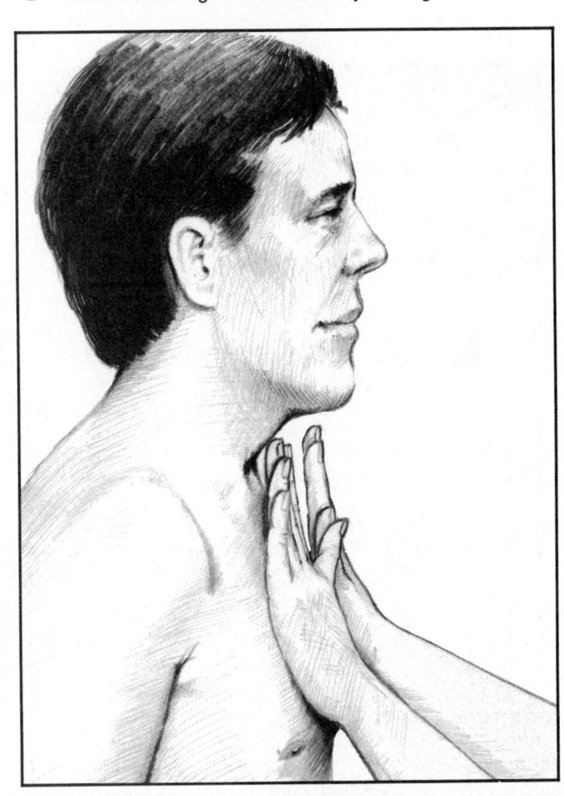

2 Ask the client to repeat a resonant phrase like "ninety-nine" as you systematically move your hands over the client's chest from the central airways to the lung periphery and back. You should feel vibrations of equal intensity on either side of the chest. The fremitus normally occurs in the upper chest, close to the bronchi, and feels strongest at the second intercostal space on either side of the sternum. Little or no fremitus should occur in the lower chest. The intensity of the vibrations varies according to the thickness and structure of the client's chest wall as well as the client's voice intensity and pitch.

3 Repeat this procedure on the posterior thorax. Always proceed in a systematic manner from the top of the suprascapular, interscapular, infrascapular, and hypochondriac areas (areas found at the level of the fifth and tenth intercostal spaces to the right and left of midline).

Applying the nursing process

Assessment findings form the basis of the nursing process. Using them, the nurse formulates the nursing diagnoses and develops appropriate planning, implementation, and evaluation of the client's care.

The table below shows how the nurse can use respiratory system assessment data in the nursing process for the client described in the case history (shown at right). In the first column, history and physical assessment data appear, followed by a paragraph of mental notes. These notes help the nurse make important mental connections among assessment findings, aiding in development of the nursing diagnoses and planning.

The second column presents several appropriate nursing diagnoses; however, the information in the remaining three columns is based on the *first* nursing diagnosis. Although it is not part of the nursing process, documentation appears in the last column because of its importance. Documentation consists of an initial note using all components of the SOAPIE format and a follow-up note using the appropriate SOAPIE components.

ASSESSMENT	NURSING DIAGNOSES	PLANNING	IMPLEMENTATION
Subjective (history) data • Client's chief complaint is dyspnea, which has worsened, especially with activity. • Client reports that the dyspnea interrupts his sleep and prevents him from walking more than one-half block without resting. • He reports a poor appetite and a 15-pound weight loss over the past 3 months. • Morning cough produces about 2 ounces of thin, white, nonodorous mucus. • Client reports smoking history of 40 pack years (two packs per day for 20 years). • Currently smoking one pack per day. Denies any exposure to respiratory irritants. **Objective (physical) data** • Male appearing to be of stated age, slightly dyspneic at rest but in no acute respiratory distress. Alert and cooperative. • Assumed "tripod" positioning—sat forward in chair with arms resting on sides of chair. • Respiratory rate 26 per minute with prolonged expiratory phase. Temperature 98.6° F. orally, pulse slightly irregular at 96, blood pressure 128/80. • Chest expansion equal. Barrel chest noted. Hypertrophy of sternocleidomastoid muscles. No retractions noted. Shallow chest movement during breathing. Costal angle increased. • Skin pink, warm, and dry. • Slight clubbing and decreased capillary refill in the fingernail beds. • No lesions, crepitus, or painful areas palpated. • Decreased tactile fremitus and hyperresonance to percussion throughout both lungs. • Auscultation reveals decreased vesicular breath sounds in both lung bases. Prolonged expiration and scattered expiratory wheezes in both bases. • Arterial blood gas analysis reveals Pa_{CO_2} 60 mm Hg and Pa_{CO_2} 55 mm Hg. **Mental notes** *Client has a long smoking history. Smoking has decreased with retirement, which is surprising because it often increases when a person has free time. His smoking may have been a response to his management job. Use of tripod position and accessory muscles of respiration could mean a chronic, rather than acute, problem. The client may have chronic obstructive pulmonary disease (COPD), which would require considerable teaching and further evaluation.*	• Ineffective breathing pattern related to decreased lung compliance and air trapping. • Knowledge deficit related to disease process and its treatment. • Impaired gas exchange related to inadequate air flow in and out of the lungs. • Activity intolerance related to dyspnea. • Sleep pattern disturbance related to respiratory distress. • Potential for alteration in nutrition: less than body requirements, related to dyspnea. • Potential for alteration in body image related to chronic illness.	**Goals** By the next follow-up visit, the client will: • verbalize his understanding of the disease process, including its causes and risk factors and the importance of patterned breathing. • take all medication as prescribed. • participate in all facets of prescribed therapy.	• Explain normal lung anatomy and physiology, using audiovisual aids if possible. • Define COPD and explain the gradual progression and irreversibility of the disease process. • Explain the purpose of patterned breathing for clients with COPD; demonstrate the correct techniques and have the client demonstrate them. • Review the most common signs and symptoms associated with the disease: dyspnea, especially with exertion; fatigue; cough; occasional mucus production; weight loss; rapid heart rate; irregular pulse; and use of accessory muscles to help with breathing from limited diaphragm function. • Provide information about smoking cessation groups in the community. • Explain the importance of avoiding fumes, respiratory irritants, temperature extremes, exposure to upper respiratory infections. • Explain the purpose of any equipment to be used at home.

CASE STUDY

Joseph Jones, age 66, a retired store manager, comes to the clinic with a major complaint of dyspnea (shortness of breath). Mr. Jones states that the dyspnea has become progressively worse over the past month.

EVALUATION

At the next follow-up visit, the client:
- verbalized an understanding of his disease.
- expressed the need for further practice of patterned breathing.
- reported enrolling in a smoking cessation group.
- has avoided risk factors.
- has complied with his medication therapy.
- has complied with his oxygen therapy.

DOCUMENTATION BASED ON NURSING PROCESS DATA

Initial

S Client states, "I get short of breath when I try to do anything. Why is this happening to me?"

O Respiratory rate 26 per minute with prolonged expiratory phase. Facial grimacing, foot shuffling, chain smoking, and speaking in short sentences. Hypertrophy of accessory muscles of ventilation. Barrel chest. Assumes "tripod" position in chair. Decreased tactile fremitus and hyperresonance to percussion throughout both lungs. Decreased vesicular breath sounds and scattered wheezes bilaterally. Expiratory phase prolonged with expiratory wheezes in both bases. Arterial blood gas analysis: PaO_2 60 mm Hg, $PaCO_2$ 55 mm Hg.

A Ineffective breathing pattern related to decreased lung compliance and air trapping. Client compensating with position and pursed lip breathing.

P Client showing interest in learning patterned breathing and understanding COPD. Initial history indicated that client can see well enough to read pamphlets and view audiovisuals. Client expresses the desire to have his family participate in learning about respiratory problems and therapy.

I Begin teaching about medications, activity, and breathing patterns. Review physiology of respiratory system. Discuss causes and risk factors of respiratory disorders.

E Reviewed current medications with client and family to maximize effectiveness. Suggested scheduling all daily activities to maximize oxygen conservation and allow for rest periods. Reviewed patterns of breathing and encouraged using the patterns, especially during activity, such as walking up stairs.

Follow-up

S Client states he is experiencing less shortness of breath and is able to manage increased activity.

O Respiratory rate 22 and not labored. Wheezes no longer audible on auscultation. Arterial blood gas analysis: PaO_2 65 mm Hg, $PaCO_2$ 50 mm Hg. Client demonstrates proper breathing patterns when climbing stairs to entrance. Otherwise unchanged since initial note.

A Client returned to clinic showing improved activity tolerance and verbalizing compliance with medical therapy.

P Provided information from Lung Association on "Freedom from Smoking" program. Client to review and be prepared to discuss it at the next visit.

E Client verbalized his motivation to stop smoking and his interest in continuing with the stop-smoking group.

ADVANCED ASSESSMENT SKILLS

Measurement of diaphragmatic excursion

The nurse should follow this procedure to assess diaphragmatic excursion.

1 Instruct the client to take a deep breath and hold it while you percuss down the right side of the posterior thorax. Begin at the lower border of the scapula and continue until the percussion note changes from resonance to dullness, which identifies the location of the diaphragm. Using a washable, felt-tipped pen, mark this point with a small line.

2 Instruct the client to take a few normal breaths. Then ask the client to exhale completely and hold it while you percuss again to locate the point where the resonant sounds become dull. Mark this point with a small line.

3 Repeat this entire procedure on the left side of the posterior thorax. Keep in mind that the diaphragm usually sits slightly higher on the right side than on the left because of the position of the liver.

4 Next, using a tape measure or ruler, measure the distance between the two marks on each side of the chest, as shown here. The distance between these two marks reflects diaphragmatic excursion—the distance that the diaphragm travels between inhalation and exhalation.

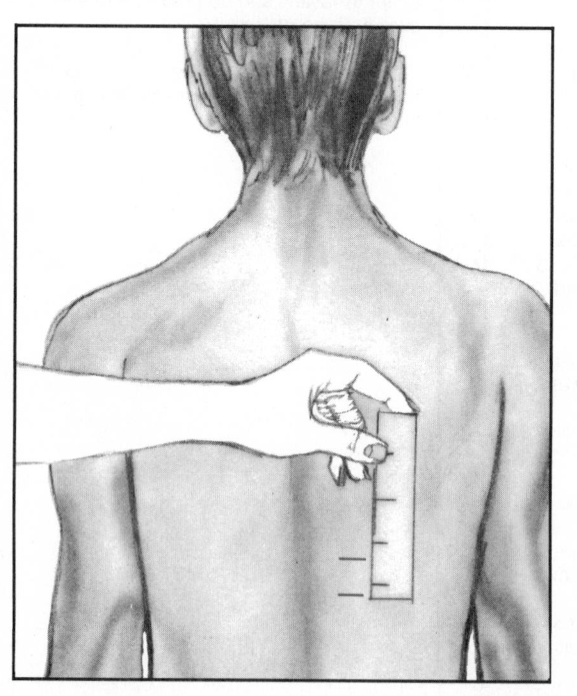

Voice resonance

To assess voice resonance, instruct the client to say "ninety-nine." As the client speaks, auscultate in the usual sequence. The voice normally sounds muffled and indistinct during auscultation. The sound appears loudest medially and softest in the lung periphery. However, conditions causing lung tissue consolidation cause bronchophony and the increased resonance that allows you to hear "ninety-nine" clearly during auscultation.

To test any increased resonance further, ask the client to repeat the letter "e," which should sound muffled and indistinct on auscultation. If the letter sounds like "a" and the voice sounds nasal or bleating, you have heard egophony.

To perform another test for increased resonance, ask the client to whisper the words "one-two-three." On auscultation, these words should be barely audible. If the words sound distinct and understandable, you have heard whispered pectoriloquy, which suggests lung tissue consolidation resulting from conditions such as a lung tumor, pneumonia, or pulmonary fibrosis. It occurs because sound vibrations travel with greater intensity through a solid structure than through a normal, air-filled lung.

Documentation

To understand the significance of assessment findings and form a clear picture of the client's health status, the nurse must carefully review the physical assessment information about the client's respiratory system as well as the health history findings and laboratory study results. (For more information, see *Common laboratory studies*.) Based on these data, the nurse can formulate appropriate nursing diagnoses, which determine how to plan, implement, and evaluate nursing care. (For a case study that shows how to apply the nursing process to a client with a respiratory disorder, see *Applying the nursing process*, pages 276 and 277.)

Proper documentation is an essential element in organizing assessment findings and making them available to other members of the health care team. Be sure to document all data completely, including normal and abnormal findings.

Remember to be specific when documenting the nursing process data. For example, document the type of breathing observed by including a description along

Common laboratory studies

For a client with respiratory signs and symptoms, various laboratory studies can provide valuable clues to possible causes, as shown in the chart below. (*Note:* Keep in mind that abnormal findings may stem from a problem unrelated to the respiratory system.) Remember that values differ between laboratories, and check the normal value range for the specific laboratory.

TEST AND SIGNIFICANCE	NORMAL VALUES OR FINDINGS	ABNORMAL FINDINGS	POSSIBLE RESPIRATORY OR RELATED CAUSES OF ABNORMAL FINDINGS
Blood tests			
Arterial blood gas (ABG) analysis This test evaluates gas exchange in the lungs by measuring the partial pressures of oxygen (PaO_2) and carbon dioxide ($PaCO_2$) and the pH of arterial blood. PaO_2 indicates how much oxygen the lungs deliver to the blood, and the $PaCO_2$ indicates how efficiently the lungs eliminate carbon dioxide. The pH indicates the acid-base level of the blood by measuring the hydrogen ion concentration. Blood gas measurements also show the amount of bicarbonate ions (HCO_3^-) and the oxygen (O_2) saturation of the blood.	*PaO_2:* 75 to 100 mm Hg *$PaCO_2$:* 35 to 45 mm Hg *pH:* 7.35 to 7.42 *HCO_3^-:* 22 to 26 mEq/liter *O_2 saturation:* 94% to 100%	pH less than 7.35; $PaCO_2$ greater than 45 mm Hg (Respiratory acidosis)	CNS depression from drugs, injury, or disease; asphyxia; hypoventilation caused by pulmonary, cardiac, musculoskeletal, or neuromuscular disease
		pH greater than 7.42; $PaCO_2$ less than 35 mm Hg (Respiratory alkalosis)	Hyperventilation from anxiety or pain; respiratory stimulation by drugs, disease, hypoxia, fever, or high room temperature
		pH less than 7.35; HCO_3^- less than 22 mEq/liter (Metabolic acidosis)	HCO_3^- depletion caused by renal disease, diarrhea, or small-bowel fistulas; excess production of organic acids related to hepatic disease, endocrine disorders, hypoxia, shock, or drug intoxication
		pH greater than 7.42; HCO_3^- greater than 26 mEq/liter (Metabolic alkalosis)	Loss of hydrochloric acid from prolonged gastric suctioning, loss of potassium from increased renal excretion as in diuretic therapy or steroid overdose, excessive alkali ingestion
Red blood cell (RBC) count This test reports the number of RBCs found in a microliter of whole blood. The main function of the RBC is to maintain a high concentration of circulating hemoglobin.	*Males:* 4.5 to 6.2 million/μl venous blood *Females:* 4.2 to 5.4 million/μl venous blood *Children:* 4.6 to 4.8 million/μl venous blood *Newborns:* 4.4 to 5.8 million/μl capillary blood	Increased RBCs	Polycythemia, severe diarrhea, dehydration
		Decreased RBCs	Anemia, hemorrhage
Total hemoglobin This test measures the grams of hemoglobin found in a deciliter of whole blood. Hemoglobin enables the RBC to carry oxygen from the lungs and carbon dioxide from the tissues.	*Males:* 14 to 18 g/dl *Females:* 12 to 16 g/dl *Children:* 11 to 13 g/dl *Newborns:* 17 to 22 g/dl	Increased hemoglobin	Polycythemia, chronic obstructive pulmonary disease, living in high altitudes
		Decreased hemoglobin	Anemia, hemorrhage, overhydration with intravenous fluids
Sputum tests			
Sputum culture and sensitivity This test is used to assess the presence of pathogens in expectorated or evacuated sputum. Also used to plan treatment for pathogens detected.	Normal throat flora, such as alphahemolytic streptococci or diphtheroids	Pathogenic organisms, such as *Streptococcus pneumoniae, Mycobacterium tuberculosis,* and *Legionella pneumophila*	Pneumonia, Legionnaires' disease, tuberculosis

with the label. If a client exhibits Cheyne-Stokes respirations, with 30-second periods of apnea followed by rapid, deep respirations for 75 seconds, include all of those details in the documentation. Be sure to document any retractions, chest wall asymmetry, or bulging of the intercostal muscles. Also document the location of any abnormal finding, noting any differences between the right and left side.

The following sample illustrates proper documentation of normal respiratory findings during physical assessment:

> *Weight:* 165 lb
> *Height:* 5′10″
> *Vital signs:* Temperature 98.6° F., pulse 70 and regular, respirations 18 and unlabored, blood pressure 120/80.
> Well-developed male, who looks to be his stated age of 42, in no acute distress. Sitting quietly during interview. Alert and cooperative. Ruddy complexion. Skin warm and dry. Chest symmetrical with equal expansion. Abdominal breather without accessory muscle use. No retractions noted. Palpation of anterior, posterior, and lateral chest walls reveals no areas of pain, swelling, lesions, or crepitus. Costal angle 90 degrees; not painful during palpation. Percussion resonant throughout peripheral lung lobes. Diaphragmatic excursion of 3 cm from level of T10 to T12. Auscultation reveals vesicular breath sounds in the peripheral lung lobes and bronchovesicular breath sounds anteriorly and posteriorly over the central airways.

The following sample illustrates proper documentation of abnormal respiratory findings during physical assessment:

> *Height:* 5′6″
> *Weight:* 124 lb
> *Vital signs:* Temperature 99.2° F., pulse 104 and regular, respirations 36 and labored with use of accessory muscles and pursed-lip breathing, blood pressure 168/96.
> Thin, barrel-chested male appearing older than his stated age of 56. Complexion has a bluish cast. Chest expansion symmetrical, but minimal movement. Palpation of anterior, posterior, and lateral chest walls reveals crepitus over left lower lobe. Percussion over all chest walls reveals hyperresonance. Breath sounds decreased over the left lower lobe with prolonged expiration.

Chapter summary

Gathering pertinent history data, performing respiratory assessment techniques, and evaluating appropriate laboratory studies are all important aspects of assessing the client's respiratory system effectively. Chapter 10 describes how to gather and integrate this information. Here are the chapter highlights:

- The respiratory system includes the upper airways, the lower airways, and the thoracic cage, which protects the lungs. The nose, mouth, nasopharynx, oropharynx, laryngopharynx, and larynx compose the upper airways. The trachea, bronchi, and lungs compose the lower airways.
- The respiratory system basically functions to exchange oxygen and carbon dioxide in the lungs and tissues, and to maintain the acid-base balance in the body.
- Comprehensive respiratory assessment begins with an in-depth health history, which should investigate the chief complaint in detail. The most common respiratory complaints include dyspnea, cough, sputum production, and chest pain. Investigate the severity of any of these symptoms to help evaluate their effect on the client's life-style.
- The health history should include questions about the client's past health status, family health status, physiologic system status, and developmental status. Also include questions about the client's health promotion and protection behaviors and role and relationship patterns. Be especially alert for a history of pulmonary risk factors or exposure to respiratory irritants.
- To assess the client's oxygenation, inspect for cyanosis of the skin and clubbing of the fingers and toes.
- The physical assessment of the respiratory system should include inspection, palpation, percussion, and auscultation. Begin the inspection by assessing the client's respiratory rate, depth, and pattern. Continue the assessment with inspection of the thoracic shape, chest wall symmetry, chest expansion, and use of accessory muscles of respiration.
- Assessment of the thorax should include palpation of the trachea and suprasternal notch as well as assessment of respiratory excursion for chest symmetry.
- Mediate percussion of the thorax helps determine the presence of gas, liquids, or solids in the lungs. Dullness to percussion may indicate a solid structure, mass, or consolidation at the location of the sound.
- Use the diaphragm of the stethoscope to auscultate for abnormal breath sounds. Perform auscultation in a

side-to-side pattern, moving from top to bottom and comparing audible sounds on one side of the chest to sounds in the same location on the opposite side of the chest.
- Advanced respiratory assessment skills include assessment of tactile fremitus, diaphragmatic excursion, and voice resonance.
- Pertinent laboratory studies, such as arterial blood gas analysis, red blood cell count, and sputum culture and sensitivity, provide valuable clues to the causes of abnormal findings.
- Incorporating respiratory assessment findings into the nursing process enables the nurse to plan, implement, and evaluate the client's care.

Study questions

1. What are the four most common signs and symptoms of respiratory dysfunction and why must they be thoroughly explored during assessment?

2. You may need to assess for respiratory excursion, diaphragmatic excursion, tactile fremitus, and egophony in a client with a respiratory disorder. How would you describe the step-by-step procedure to perform each assessment?

3. Mr. Egars, age 72, comes to the clinic complaining of shortness of breath, an inability to catch his breath after climbing a flight of stairs, and the need to sleep on more pillows than usual. What health history questions would you ask Mr. Egars to assess his respiratory problem?

4. Mrs. Miner, age 26, brings her son Timmy, age 4, to the office for a well-family visit. As you assess their respiratory systems, how would you modify your auscultation technique, and what differences in normal breath sounds would you expect to find?

5. Mrs. Lund, age 62, is admitted to the hospital from the emergency department. She reports having shortness of breath, a productive cough, fever, and chest pain that worsens with deep breathing and coughing. When you assess Mrs. Lund's vital signs, you find that her temperature is 102.4° F. (rectally), her blood pressure is 160/92 mm Hg, her pulse is 120 and regular, and her respiratory rate is 32 with deep, regular respirations. How would you report the following information related to your nursing assessment of Mrs. Lund?
- history (subjective) assessment data
- physical (objective) assessment data
- two appropriate nursing diagnoses
- assessment techniques and equipment
- documentation of findings.

Selected references

Carlson, K. (1989). Assessing a child's chest. *RN,* 52(11), 26-32.

Gift, A. (1989). A dyspnea assessment guide. *Critical Care Nurse,* 9(8), 79, 82-84, 86-88.

Hazinski, M. (1991). *Nursing care of the critically ill child* (2nd ed.). St. Louis: Mosby.

Henry, J. (1991). *Clinical diagnosis and management by laboratory methods* (18th ed.). Philadelphia: Saunders.

LeBlanc, K., and Forestell, F. (1990). Assessment of the neonatal respiratory system. *AACN Clinical Issues in Critical Care Nursing,* 1(2), 401-408.

Loudon, R., and Murphy, R. (1984). State of the art: Lung sounds. *American Review of Respiratory Disease,* 130(4), 663-673.

McEvoy, G. (Ed.). (1992). *American Hospital Formulary Service drug information.* Bethesda, MD: American Society of Hospital Pharmacists.

Pasterkamp, H., Montgomery, M., and Wiebicke, W. (1987). Nomenclature used by health care professionals to describe breath sounds in asthma. *Chest,* 92(2), 346-352.

Merenstein, G., Kaplan, D., and Rosenberg, A. (1990). *Silver, Kempe, Bruyn, and Fulginiti's handbook of pediatrics* (16th ed.). East Norwalk, CT: Appleton & Lange.

Whaley, L., and Wong, D. (1991). *Nursing care of infants and children* (4th ed.). St. Louis: Mosby.

Nursing research

Gift, A., and Cahill, C. (1990). Psychophysiologic aspects of dyspnea in chronic obstructive pulmonary disease: A pilot study. *Heart and Lung,* 19(3), 252-257.

Neuspiel, D., et al. (1989). Parental smoking and postinfancy wheezing in children: A prospective cohort study. *American Journal of Public Health,* 79(2), 168-171.

11

Cardiovascular System

Objectives

After reading and studying this chapter, you should be able to:

1. Identify the chambers and valves of the heart.
2. Trace the blood flow through the pulmonary, systemic, and coronary circulations.
3. Explain the events of the cardiac cycle.
4. Write interview questions that help evaluate cardiovascular health.
5. Describe the significance of these risk factors on cardiac disease: heredity, sex, race, age; hypertension, smoking, hyperlipidemia, diabetes mellitus; obesity, inactivity, stress, diet; left ventricular hypertrophy, oral contraceptives, gout, environment.
6. Explain the adverse effects of certain drugs on the cardiovascular system.
7. Differentiate between normal and abnormal findings during inspection and palpation of the cardiovascular system.
8. Demonstrate auscultation of the aortic, pulmonic, tricuspid, and mitral (or apical) areas, and describe the heart sounds normally heard at each one.
9. Describe accentuated, diminished, persistent, and paradoxical heart sounds and their significance.
10. Explain the purpose of the creatinine phosphokinase, lactic dehydrogenase, triglyceride, and lipoprotein cholesterol fractionation tests used to evaluate the cardiovascular system.
11. Document cardiovascular assessment findings using the nursing process.

Introduction

The cardiovascular system consists of the heart and blood vessels. The heart, a strong pump, and the blood vessels, long conduits, deliver blood—and the oxygen, nutrients, metabolites, and hormones that it carries—to the body's cells. In the cells, the blood picks up waste products and delivers them to target organs for detoxification and excretion.

The nurse's assessment of the cardiovascular system is important because cardiovascular disease is the most prevalent health care problem—and the most common cause of death—in the United States. Every year, more than 25,000 children are born with congenital heart disease, and more than 1.5 million adults experience myocardial infarctions (heart attacks). About 35 million Americans have hypertension (elevated blood pressure that consistently exceeds 140/90 mm Hg).

Because of the prevalence of congenital and acquired cardiovascular disorders, the nurse must be able to assess cardiac health and evaluate a sick client's response to therapy and ability to resume activities of daily living. Chapter 11 prepares the reader for these responsibilities. Because an understanding of cardiovascular structures and functions is essential to assessment, the chapter begins with a review of normal anatomy and physiology. Next, it describes how to obtain a cardiovascular health history and how to inspect, palpate, percuss, and auscultate the cardiovascular system. The advanced assessment section explains how to detect abnormal heart sounds, such as murmurs, clicks, and snaps.

Glossary

Afterload: pressure in the arteries leading from the ventricle that must be overcome for ejection to occur.

Angina: chest pain characterized as a squeezing or crushing sensation or a feeling of heaviness or tightness; caused by an inadequate oxygen supply to the myocardium when the work load of the heart is increased.

Atherosclerosis: disorder characterized by accumulation of lipids, calcium, and blood clotting products in the inner layer of arterial walls. As the debris accumulates, the vessel lumen narrows, causing ischemia in the organs supplied by the vessel. In the coronary arteries, ischemia occurs when the vessels are narrowed by 70% or more.

Bradycardia: circulatory condition characterized by a slow heart rate below 60 beats/minute in an adult.

Bruit: abnormal, murmurlike heart sound auscultated over a major vessel with turbulent blood flow.

Cardiac cycle: period from the beginning of one heartbeat to the beginning of the next.

Cardiac output: amount of blood ejected from the heart in 1 minute.

Click: high-pitched abnormal heart sound auscultated at the apex during mid- to late systole; it usually precedes a late systolic murmur.

Contractility: capacity for shortening or contracting in response to a stimulus, as in the ventricle, which contracts after electrical stimulation.

Corrigan's pulse: bounding pulse in which a great surge precedes a sudden absence of force or fullness; also called a water-hammer pulse.

Cyanosis: bluish discoloration of the skin and mucous membranes; a common sign of cardiovascular disease.

Diastole: period of ventricular relaxation when blood crosses the open mitral and tricuspid valves and fills the ventricular chambers.

Dyspnea: shortness of breath; a common symptom of cardiovascular disease.

Edema: fluid accumulation in interstitial tissues that causes swelling; a common sign of cardiovascular disease.

Gallop: abnormal heart rhythm characterized by a low-pitched extra sound during diastole; a general term for the extra heart sounds, S_3 and S_4.

Heave: strong outward thrust palpated over the chest during systole; also called a lift.

Hyperlipidemia: excess lipids in the plasma.

Hypertension: elevated blood pressure that consistently exceeds 140/90 mm Hg in an adult.

Ischemia: decreased blood supply to a body organ or tissue, which interferes with normal organ or tissue function.

Murmur: vibrating, blowing, or rumbling noise that is longer than a heart sound and may be heard over any cardiac auscultatory site. It results from turbulent blood flow through the heart and may be pathologic or nonpathologic.

Myocardial infarction (MI): interruption of the local blood supply to part of the heart muscle that causes necrosis (death) of muscle tissue.

Palpitations: sensation of pounding, racing, or skipped heartbeats; a common symptom of cardiovascular disease.

Pericardial friction rub: a harsh, scratching, scraping, or creaking sound auscultated at the third left intercostal space that may occur throughout systole or diastole or both.

Preload: blood volume in the ventricle at the end of diastole.

Pulse: regular expansion and contraction of arteries produced by pressure waves that occur as the left ventricle ejects blood.

Pulse pressure: difference between the systolic and diastolic blood pressures, normally 30 to 50 mm Hg.

Pulsus alternans: abnormal pulse rhythm with regular alternation of weak and strong beats.

Pulsus bigeminus: abnormal pulse rhythm in which premature beats alternate with sinus beats.

Pulsus bisferiens: abnormal pulse rhythm with a strong upstroke, downstroke, and second upstroke during systole.

Pulsus paradoxus or **paradoxical pulse:** abnormal pulse rhythm with markedly decreased amplitude during inspiration.

Regurgitation: backward flow of blood through the heart across a valve that does not close completely.

S_1 or **first heart sound:** normal heart sound that signals the beginning of systole; the *lub* of *lub-dub*.

S_2 or **second heart sound:** normal heart sound that signals the beginning of diastole; the *dub* of *lub-dub*.

S_3 or **ventricular gallop:** low-pitched extra heart sound auscultated in the tricuspid or mitral area during early to mid-diastole; caused by left ventricular failure associated with such disorders as myocardial infarction or mitral insufficiency.

S_4 or **atrial gallop:** low-pitched extra heart sound auscultated in the tricuspid or mitral area late in diastole just before S_1; caused by such disorders as hypertension or aortic stenosis.

Septal defect: defect or opening in the wall separating two heart chambers.

Snap: high-pitched abnormal heart sound auscultated medial to the apex along the lower left sternal border just after S_2.

continued

Glossary continued

Splitting: auscultation of a single heart sound as two separate sounds. Splitting can occur with S_1 or S_2 and may be normal or abnormal.
Stroke volume: output of each ventricle at every contraction.
Summation gallop: abnormal heart sound that combines S_3 and S_4 into a single loud sound auscultated in mid-diastole.
Syncope: faintness, especially after changing positions; a common symptom of cardiovascular disease.
Systole: period of ventricular contraction when the ventricles eject blood through the open aortic and pulmonic valves into the aorta and pulmonary artery.
Tachycardia: circulatory condition characterized by a fast heart rate exceeding 100 beats/minute in an adult.
Thrill: fine vibration, caused by turbulent blood flow, that may be palpated over the precordium.
Valvular insufficiency: inability of the heart valves to close properly, resulting in regurgitation (backward flow) of blood.
Valvular stenosis: narrowing or constriction of the heart valves that prevents them from opening properly.

Although the chapter emphasizes health, it also describes some common cardiovascular disorders as a nurse's aid to interpreting abnormal findings. It explains how to integrate and document assessment findings and how to use them as the first step in the nursing process.

Anatomy and physiology review

The heart and blood vessels deliver oxygenated blood to the body tissues and remove waste substances.

The heart

A four-chambered muscle, the heart weighs approximately 10½ to 12½ oz (300 to 350 g) in an adult male and 9 to 10½ oz (250 to 300 g) in an adult female—about 0.5% of total body weight. Roughly cone-shaped, it measures approximately 3½" (9 cm) wide and 4¾" (12 cm) long—about the size of a closed fist. It lies substernally in the mediastinum, between the second and sixth ribs. About one third of the heart lies to the right of the midsternal line; the remainder, to the left.

In most people, the heart rests obliquely in the chest, with the right side almost in front of the left, the broad part at the top, and the pointed end (apex) at the bottom. However, heart position varies with body build. For example, in a tall, thin person, the heart lies more vertically; in a short, stocky person, it lies more horizontally. Because the heart is hollow, blood can flow through its chambers. When the heart muscle contracts, it pumps the blood through the arteries. (For more information about heart structures, see *Anatomy of the heart,* pages 286 and 287.)

Chambers and valves

The heart contains four chambers and four valves. The two superior chambers are the right and left atria and the two inferior chambers are the right and left ventricles. The atria are small, thin-walled, holding chambers for blood that returns to the heart from the veins of the body. The ventricles are large, thick-walled chambers. The left ventricle is larger than the right because it must contract with enough force to eject blood into the aorta and the rest of the body.

Four valves keep the blood flowing in one direction through the heart: two atrioventricular (AV) valves and two semilunar (SL) valves. The AV valves separate the atria from the ventricles. The right AV valve lies between the right atrium and the right ventricle. It is known as the tricuspid valve because it has three triangular cusps, or leaflets. The left AV valve lies between the left atrium and the left ventricle. It is called the mitral, or bicuspid, valve because it has two cusps.

The SL valves are the pulmonic and aortic valves. The pulmonic valve lies between the right ventricle and the pulmonary artery. The aortic valve lies between the left ventricle and the aorta. Each SL valve has three cusps that are shaped like half-moons. Both SL valves open and close passively in response to pressure changes caused by ventricular contraction and blood ejection.

A coordinated sequence of events controls blood flow through the chambers and valves of the heart. The AV valves open and close in response to ventricular contraction and papillary muscle relaxation. When the ventricles relax during diastole, the AV valves open, allowing blood to flow from the atria into the ventricles. The atria contract late in diastole and force the remaining blood into the ventricles. The AV valves shut as the ventricles contract during systole, preventing regurgitation (backflow) of blood into the atria.

When the ventricles contract during systole, the resulting pressure forces the SL valves to open, which allows blood to flow into the pulmonary artery and the aorta. When the ventricles relax, the SL valves close, preventing regurgitation into the ventricles.

Blood circulation

A vast network of vessels—about 60,000 miles (96,558 km) of arteries, arterioles, capillaries, venules, and veins—keeps the blood circulating to and from every functioning cell in the body. This network has two basic branches: the pulmonary circulation and the systemic circulation. (For an illustration, see *Circulatory system,* pages 288 and 289.)

Through the pulmonary circulation, blood travels to the lungs to pick up oxygen and liberate carbon dioxide. Through the systemic circulation, blood carries oxygen and other nutrients to body cells and transports waste products for excretion. A specialized part of the systemic circulation, known as the coronary circulation, supplies blood to the heart itself.

Pulmonary circulation

Unoxygenated blood travels from the right ventricle through the pulmonic SL valve into the pulmonary arteries. Then it passes through progressively smaller arteries and arterioles into the capillaries of the lungs. Eventually, the blood reaches the alveoli, where it exchanges carbon dioxide for oxygen. (For more information, see Chapter 10, Respiratory System.) The oxygenated blood then returns via venules and veins to the pulmonary veins, which carry it back to the left atrium of the heart.

Systemic circulation

The major artery—the aorta—branches into vessels that supply specific organs or areas of the body. Three major branches arise from the arch of the aorta: the left common carotid, the left subclavian, and the innominate arteries. These vessels supply the brain, upper extremities (arms), and upper chest. As the aorta descends through the thorax and abdomen, its branches supply gastrointestinal and genitourinary organs as well as the spinal column and the lower chest and abdominal muscles. Then the aorta divides into the iliac arteries, which further divide into femoral arteries.

The pumping action of the heart that forces blood through the arteries is palpable at specific sites as the pulse (regular arterial expansion and contraction). (For more information, see *Pulse sites* in Chapter 4, Physical Assessment Skills.) Pulse assessment can therefore provide information about peripheral arterial circulation.

As the arteries divide into smaller units, the number of vessels increases dramatically, which increases the area that can be perfused (supplied with blood). At the end of the arterioles and the beginning of the capillaries lie strong sphincters that control blood flow into the tissues. They dilate to permit more flow when needed, close to shunt blood to areas with a greater need, or constrict to increase the blood pressure. Pressure drops slowly from 100 mm Hg in the aorta to 10 to 30 mm Hg in the capillaries.

Although the capillary bed contains the smallest vessels, it supplies blood to the largest area. Capillary pressure is very low, and the slow-flowing blood allows for the exchange of nutrients, oxygen, and carbon dioxide between body cells and the capillaries. From the capillaries, blood flows into venules and, eventually, into veins. Venous pressure continues to decrease from 10 mm Hg in the venules to 0 to 6 mm Hg in the right atrium. Valves in the veins prevent blood backflow, and the pumping action of skeletal muscles assists venous return to the right side of the heart. The veins merge until they form two main branches—the superior and inferior vena cava—that return blood to the right atrium.

Coronary circulation

The blood flowing through the heart chambers does not exchange oxygen and other nutrients with the myocardial cells. Instead, blood circulating through the coronary arteries supplies the myocardium. (For more information, see *Coronary blood supply,* page 291.)

Cardiac conduction system

An electrical conduction system regulates myocardial contraction. This system has two subdivisions: the extrinsic conduction system, which includes the nerve fibers of the autonomic nervous system (ANS); and the intrinsic conduction system, which includes specialized nerves and fibers in the heart.

(Text continues on page 290.)

Anatomy of the heart

The bony structures of the chest protect the heart, which lies obliquely in the chest, with two thirds of it located to the left of the sternum. The base of the heart (the superior portion, where the ascending aorta and pulmonary trunk emerge and the superior vena cava enters) corresponds to the level of the third costal cartilage. The apex of the heart (the inferior portion that points down and to the left) is normally located at the fifth left intercostal space, at the midclavicular line. The right end of the inferior surface lies under the sixth or seventh chondrosternal junction.

Within the chest, the lungs surround the heart laterally and superiorly. The esophagus lies posterior to the heart; the diaphragm, inferior to it. Because membranes attach the heart to the diaphragm, the heart changes position with each respiration. It moves down and to the right during inspiration, up and to the left during expiration.

Cardiac structures

The structures of the heart include the pericardium, three layers of the heart wall, four chambers, and four valves.

The pericardium (a closed, serous sac) surrounds the heart and roots of the great vessels. It has two layers: an inner (visceral) layer that forms the epicardium and an outer (parietal) layer that is continuous with the covering of the great vessels. The pericardial space between the visceral and parietal layers normally contains 10 to 20 ml of serous fluid. This fluid allows the epicardium and parietal pericardium to glide smoothly without friction during heart muscle contraction and relaxation.

The heart wall consists of three layers: endocardium, myocardium, and epicardium. The endocardium forms the inner layer, which provides a smooth surface for the internal structures of the heart. The myocardium, the thick middle

Heart position

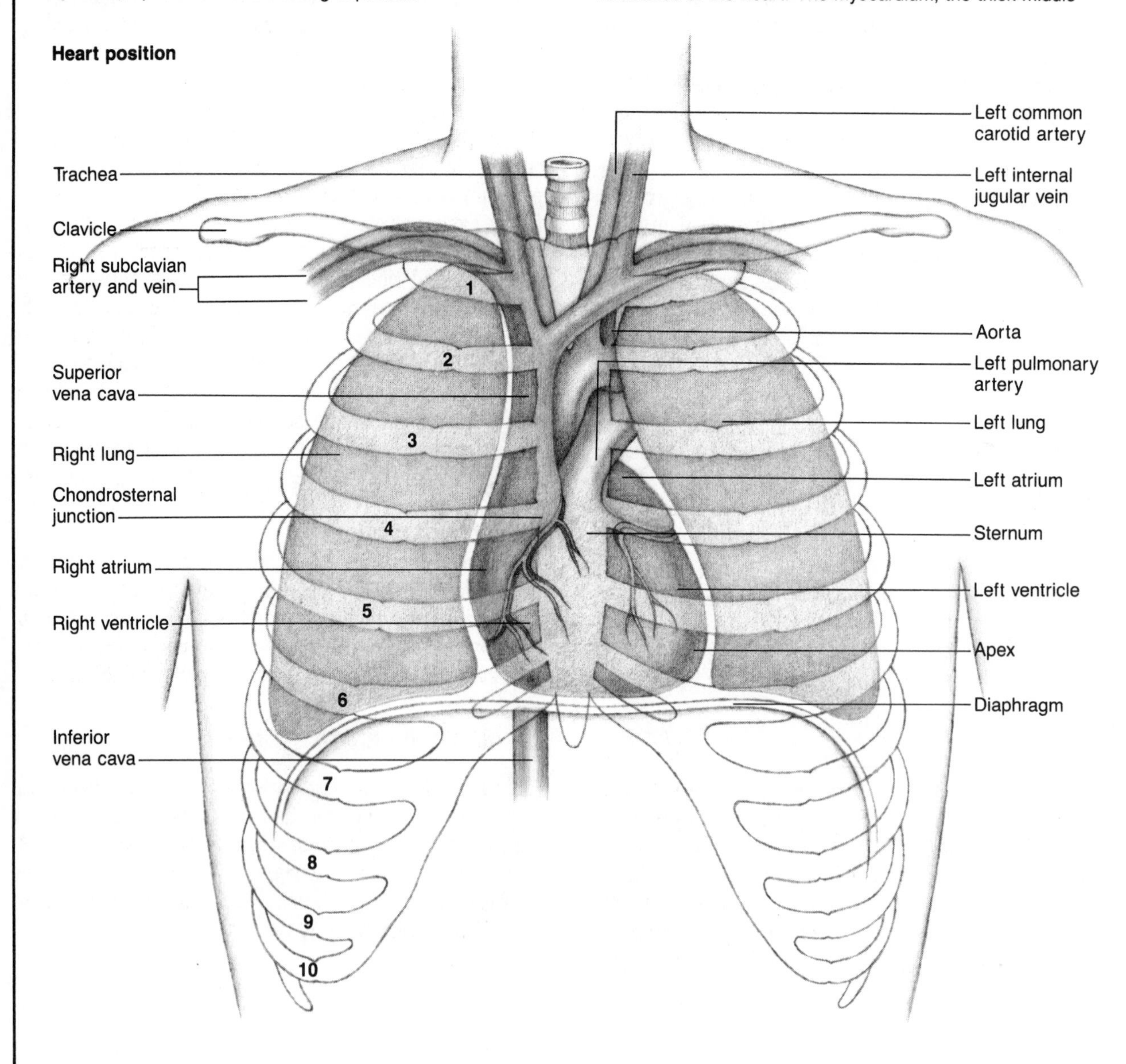

layer, is composed of muscle fibers that are responsible for contraction. The epicardium, which is continuous with the pericardial lining, forms the thin outermost layer.

The heart chambers include the right and left atria and the right and left ventricles. The right atrium lies in front and to the right of the left atrium, from which it is separated by the interatrial septum. It receives blood from the superior and inferior venae cavae. The right ventricle lies behind the sternum and forms the largest part of the sternocostal surface and inferior border of the heart. Its posterior wall is formed by the interventricular septum. The left atrium forms the upper part of the left border of the heart, extending to the left of and behind the right atrium. Its posterior aspect forms most of the base of the heart. The left ventricle forms the apex and most of the left border of the heart.

Heart valves include the atrioventricular (tricuspid and mitral) and the semilunar (pulmonic and aortic). The tricuspid valve is located at the right atrioventricular orifice and consists of three triangular cusps. The strong chordae tendineae attach the cusps of this valve to the papillary muscles in the right ventricle. The mitral valve is located at the left atrioventricular opening. Its two cusps attach to papillary muscles by chordae tendineae in the left ventricle. The two semilunar valves have three cusps each and are located at the orifices of the pulmonary artery and the aorta.

The chambers and valves work together to guide the blood flow through the heart. (The arrows in the illustration show how the blood flows.) The right heart, which includes the right atrium and right ventricle separated by the tricuspid valve, receives the venous blood from the body and pumps it to the lungs for oxygenation. The left heart, which consists of the left atrium and left ventricle separated by the mitral valve, receives oxygenated blood from the lungs and pumps it to all body tissues.

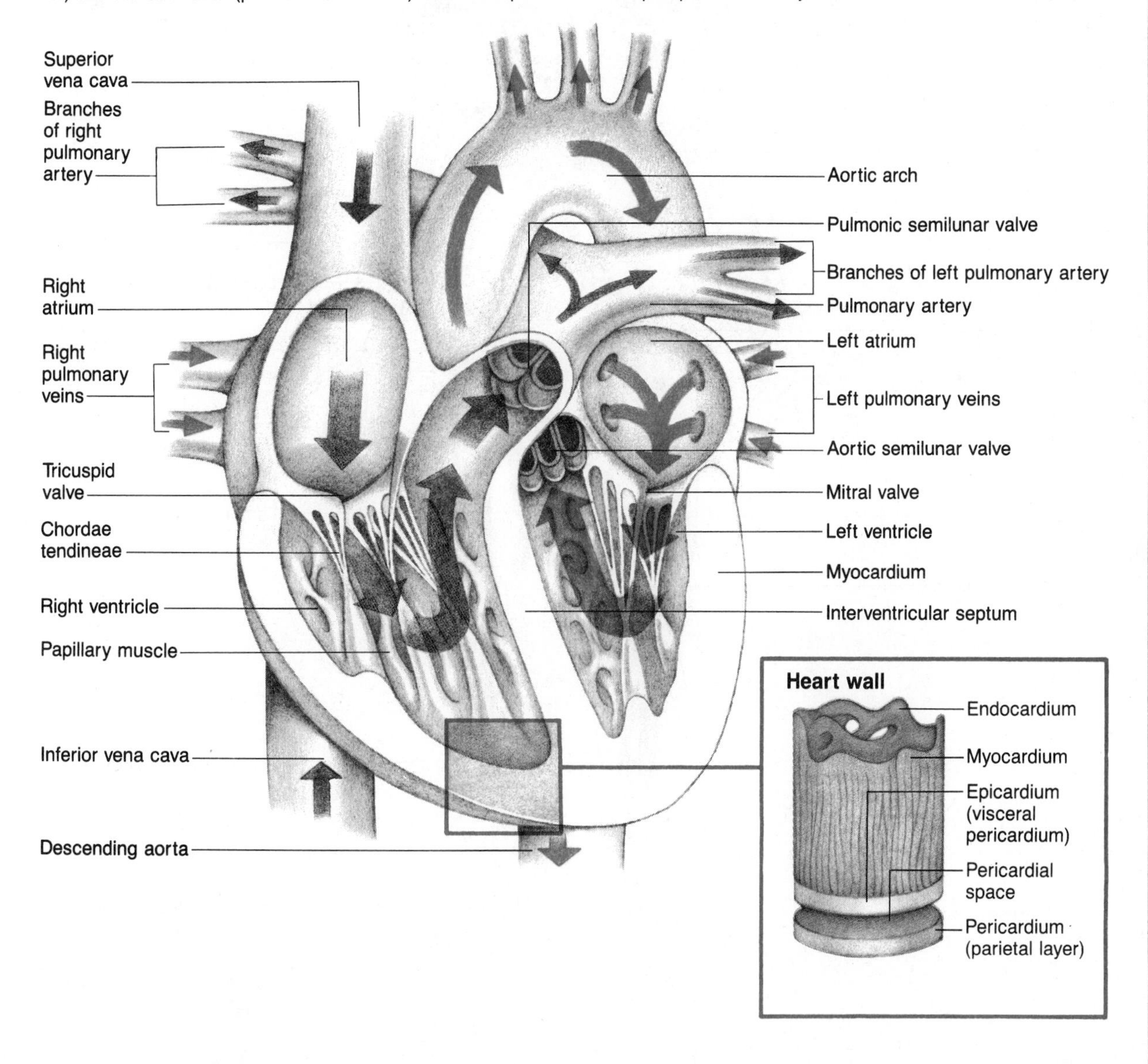

Circulatory system

The heart is the center of the circulatory system, keeping about 10 pints (4¾ liters) of blood in constant circulation in an adult. It pumps this blood through a vast network of vessels, which deliver blood to and from every functioning cell in the body. The illustration below shows the anatomic placement of some vessels of the circulatory system.

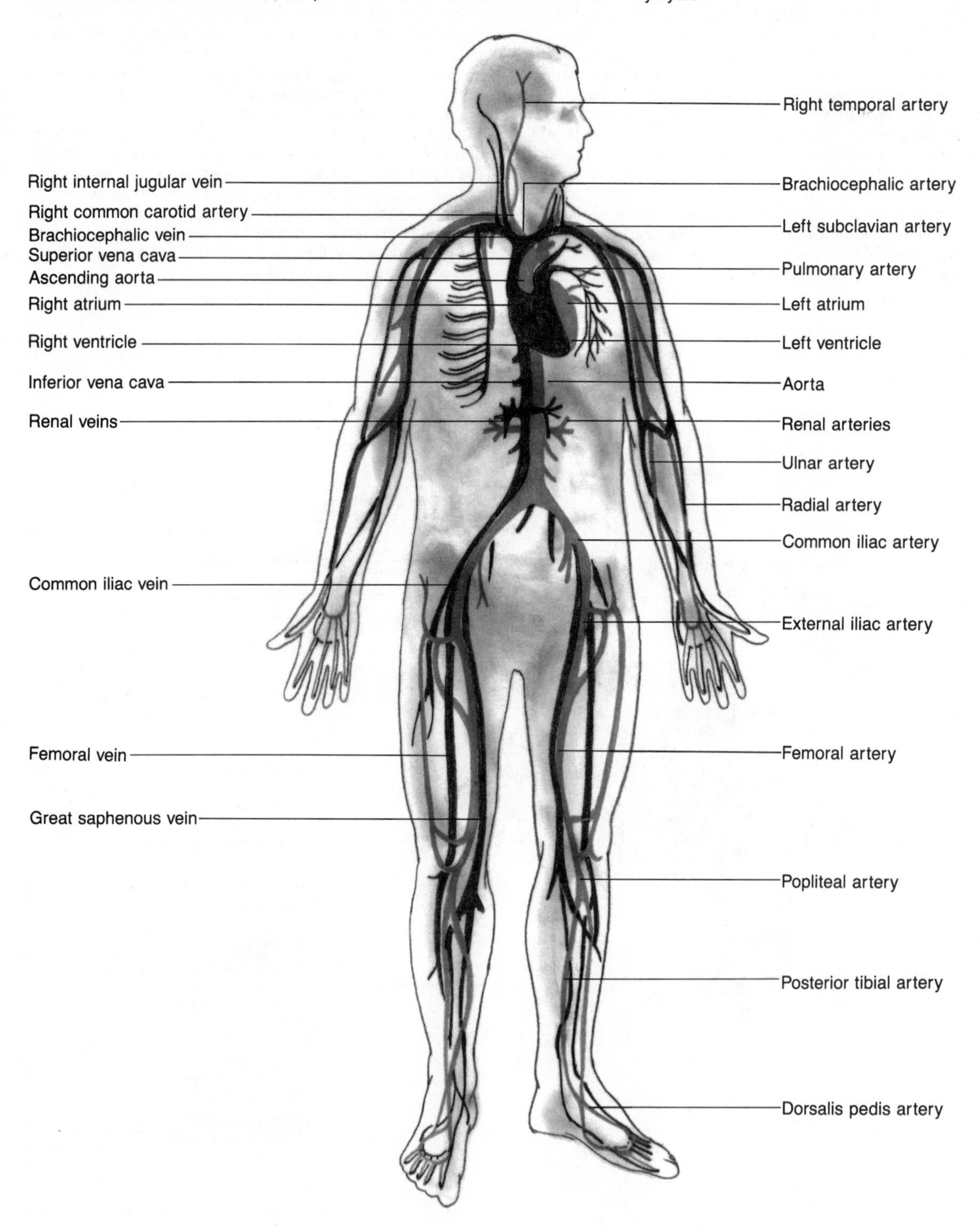

Schematic of blood circulation and vessels

The illustration at right provides a schematic of the blood circulation, showing how the blood leaves the heart, reaches a body structure, exchanges nutrients and gases at the capillary level, and returns to the heart.

As blood moves through the circulatory system, it travels through five distinct types of blood vessels: arteries, arterioles, capillaries, venules, and veins. (See illustrations below.) The structure of these vessels reflects differences in blood pressure. All vessels other than capillaries have an outer layer known as the tunica adventitia. Arteries have thick, muscular walls (tunica media) to accommodate blood flow at high speeds and pressures. Arterioles have thinner walls than arteries, and they can constrict or dilate as needed to control blood flow to the capillaries. The capillaries are microscopic vessels with walls composed of a single layer of endothelial cells. Venules gather blood from the capillaries but have thinner walls than arterioles. Similarly, veins have thinner walls than arteries but have larger diameters because of the low blood pressures required for return of venous blood to the heart. Veins of the arms, legs, and neck have valves that open in the direction of blood flow to prevent venous backflow.

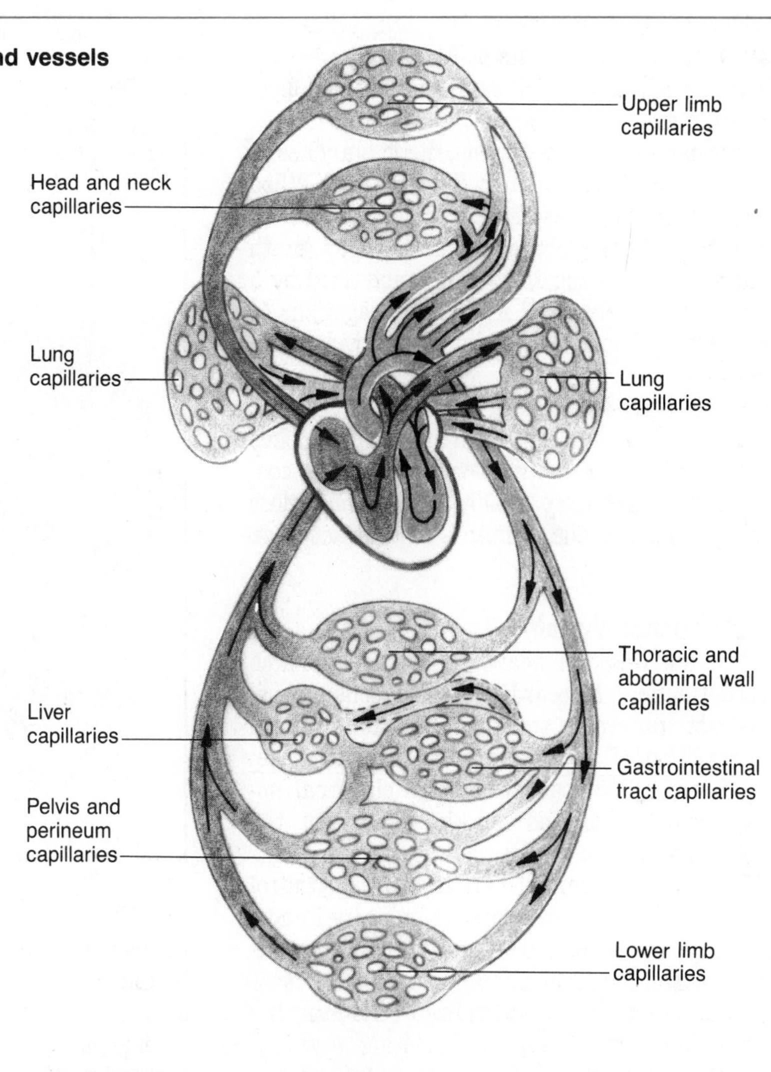

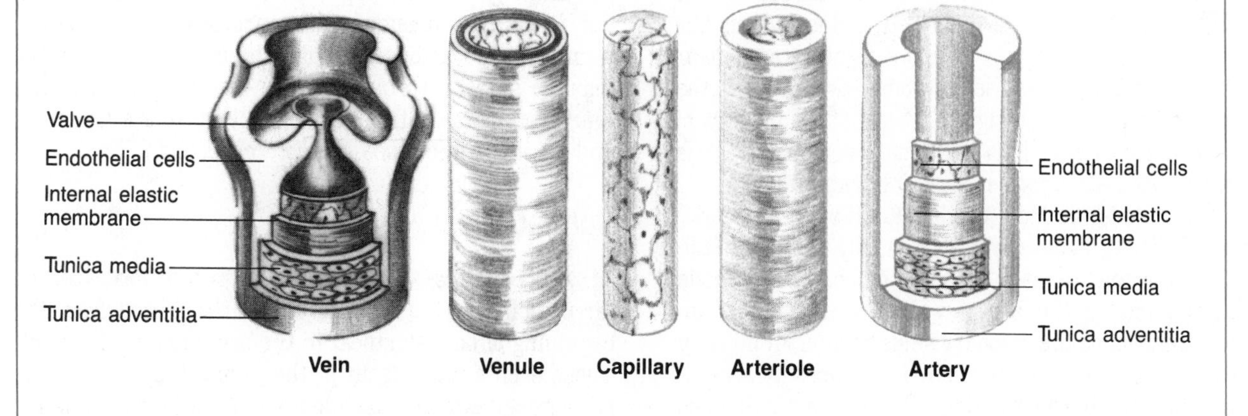

Extrinsic conduction system

This system controls cardiac contractility primarily through the action of the ANS, which regulates heart action by involuntarily increasing or decreasing it to meet the individual's metabolic needs. The ANS influences electrical conduction through its sympathetic and parasympathetic branches. It also alters the strength of myocardial contraction.

The sympathetic and parasympathetic branches of the ANS control cardiac function in different ways. When the body is at rest, the parasympathetic nervous system controls the heart through branches of the vagus (tenth cranial) nerve. The resting state is characterized by a slow heart rate and electrical impulse propagation. At rest, the energy-efficient body requires relatively little cardiac effort.

When the body becomes active, the sympathetic nervous system takes control through the nerve branches of the sympathetic chain. It stimulates the intrinsic conduction system to fire more rapidly and conduct more quickly, and stimulates the ventricles to contract more forcibly.

Intrinsic conduction system

This system initiates the heartbeat and coordinates chamber contraction. Myocardial muscle cells, which have indistinct transverse striations, provide strength during contraction. They also have specialized pacemaker cells that allow conduction of an electrical impulse. This impulse spreads quickly throughout the muscle cell network, causing a generalized contraction.

Although any myocardial muscle cell can control the rate and rhythm of contractions (a property known as automaticity) under certain circumstances, the pacemaker cells normally initiate and conduct impulses more rapidly and uniformly. These specialized cells form the conduction system and control heart rate and rhythm.

Normally, the sinoatrial (SA) node serves as the driving pacemaker of the heart. It is located on the endocardial surface of the anterior right atrium, near the superior vena cava. The SA node firing spreads the impulse throughout the right and left atria, by way of intranodal pathways. This electrical event normally is followed by a mechanical one: atrial contraction.

The impulse is then conducted through the atrioventricular (AV) node, normally the only electrical connection between the atria and ventricles. The AV node is located low in the septal wall of the right atrium immediately above the coronary sinus opening. It initially slows the impulse, delaying ventricular activity and allowing blood to fill from the atria. Then conduction speeds through the AV node and the bundle of His, a network of fibers.

Cardiac conduction

In the intrinsic conduction system of the heart, each electrical impulse travels from the sinoatrial (SA) node via intranodal pathways to the myocardial muscle cells of the atria, producing atrial contraction. The impulse slows momentarily as it passes through the atrioventricular (AV) node to the bundle of His. Then it travels down the left and right bundle branches to Purkinje fibers, which stimulate ventricular contraction.

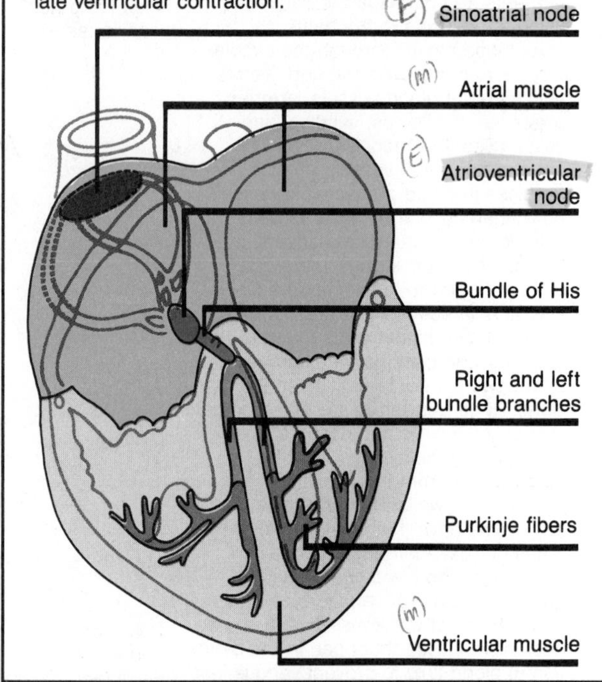

The bundle of His arises in the AV node and continues along the right intraventricular septum. It divides in the ventricular septum to form the right and left bundle branches. Its fibers rapidly spread the impulse throughout both ventricles. The distal portions of the left and right bundle branches are Purkinje fibers that fan across the subendocardial surface of the ventricles, from the endocardium through the myocardium. As the impulse spreads throughout the distal conduction system, it prompts ventricular contraction. (For a summary and an illustration, see *Cardiac conduction*.)

Cardiac cycle

All the electrical and mechanical events described so far combine in the cardiac cycle (the period from the beginning of one heartbeat to the beginning of the next). These events must occur in the proper order and to the proper degree to provide adequate blood flow to all parts of the body. The amount of blood that the heart pumps in 1 minute (the cardiac output) is determined by the stroke volume (the amount of blood ejected with each

Coronary blood supply

Two coronary arteries and their branches supply the heart with oxygenated blood; seven cardiac veins remove oxygen-depleted blood from it. During left ventricular contraction, blood is ejected into the aorta. Next, the ventricular muscle relaxes, allowing the coronary arteries to fill passively and nourish the heart muscle.

The right coronary artery supplies blood to the right atrium, part of the left atrium, most of the right ventricle, and the inferior part of the left ventricle.

The left coronary artery, which divides into the left anterior descending and circumflex arteries, supplies blood to the left atrium, most of the left ventricle, and most of the interventricular septum. Many collateral arteries connect the branches of the right and left coronary arteries.

The largest cardiac vein, the coronary sinus, lies in the posterior part of the coronary sulcus (groove) and opens into the right atrium. Most of the major cardiac veins empty into the coronary sinus, except for the anterior cardiac veins, which empty directly into the chambers of the heart in most people.

Anterior view

Left coronary artery
Right coronary artery
Left anterior descending artery
Great cardiac vein
Anterior cardiac veins
Small cardiac vein

Posterior view

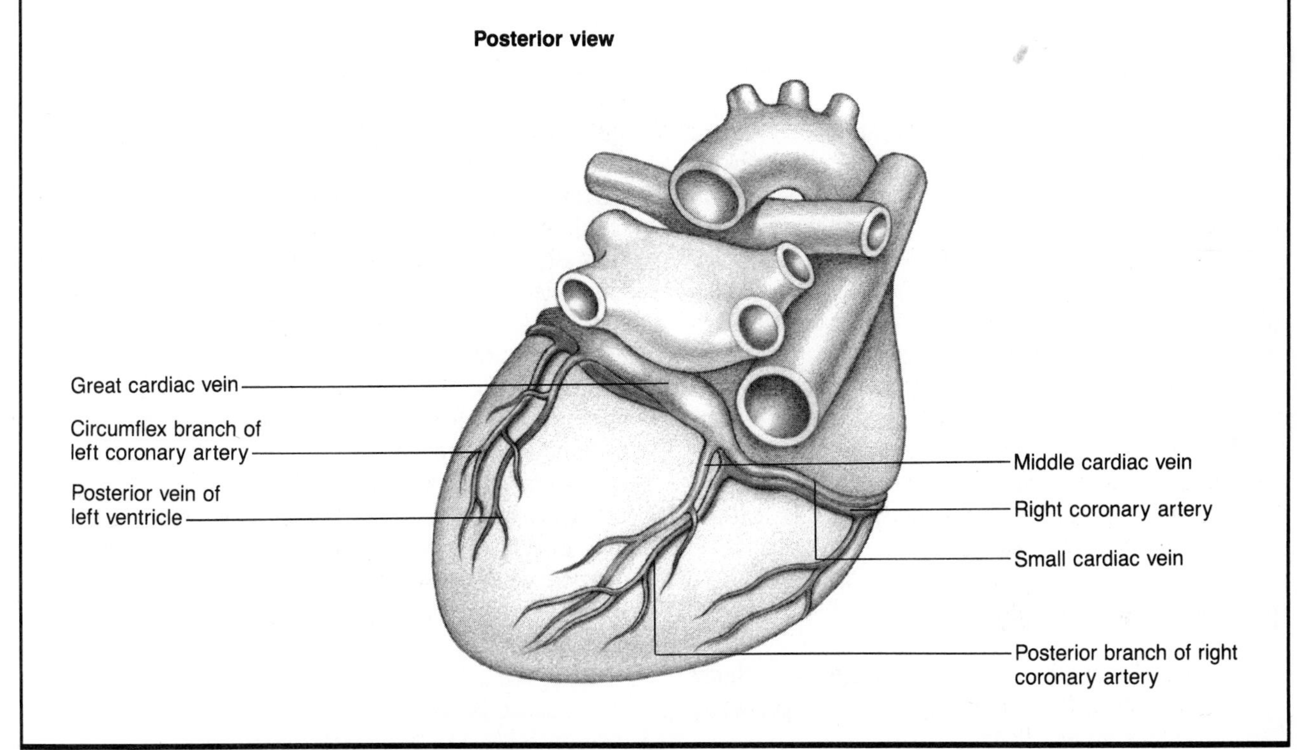

Events in the cardiac cycle

Basically, the cardiac cycle has two phases: systole, when the ventricles contract, ejecting blood into the aorta and the pulmonary artery; and diastole, when the ventricles relax and the atria contract.

At the beginning of systole, increasing ventricular pressure forces the mitral and tricuspid valves to shut. The closing of these atrioventricular (AV) valves produces the first heart sound, known as S_1 or the *lub* of *lub-dub*. The ventricular pressure builds until it exceeds that in the pulmonary artery and aorta. Then the aortic and pulmonic semilunar (SL) valves open and the ventricles eject blood into the arteries.

As the ventricles empty and relax, ventricular pressure falls below that in the pulmonary artery and the aorta. The SL valves close, producing the second heart sound, S_2 or the *dub* of *lub-dub,* and marking the end of systole. As the ventricles relax during diastole, the pressure in the ventricles is less than that in the atria. The AV valves open and blood begins to flow into the ventricles from the atria. When the ventricles become full near the end of diastole, the atria contract to send the rest of the blood to the ventricles. Ventricular pressure is now greater than atrial pressure. The AV valves close, marking the beginning of systole and repetition of the cardiac cycle.

Events on the right side of the heart occur a fraction of a second after events on the left side because the pressure is lower on the right side of the heart.

Systole

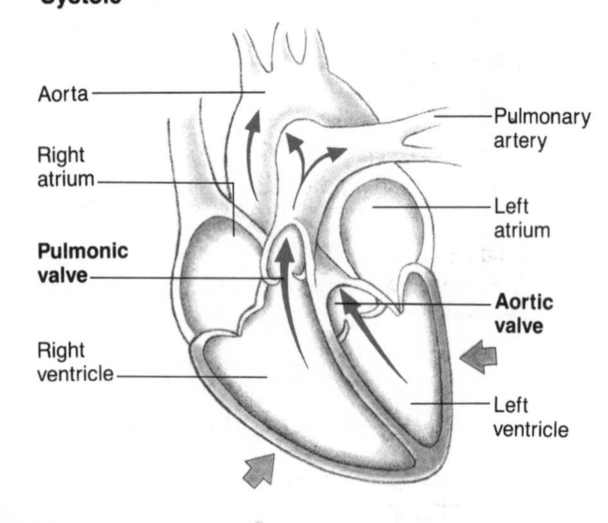

Diastole

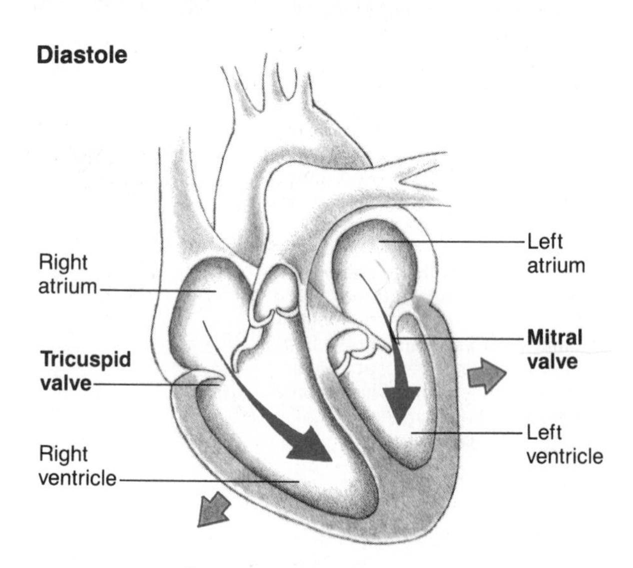

beat multiplied by the number of beats per minute). Stroke volume depends on three major factors: preload (the blood volume in the ventricles at the end of diastole), afterload (the pressure in the arteries leading from the ventricles that must be overcome for ejection to occur), and contractility (the inherent ability of the myocardium to contract normally). Although these factors can be measured only by sophisticated monitoring equipment, the nurse must be aware of them during physical assessment. A knowledge of these events promotes the nurse's understanding of cardiovascular assessment findings because many cardiac dysfunctions cause abnormal findings that correlate with the cardiac cycle. (For more information, see *Events in the cardiac cycle.*)

Developmental considerations

The heart and major blood vessels change as the body develops and ages. Notable changes occur in pediatric, pregnant, and elderly clients.

Pediatric clients

In relation to body size, a child's heart is roughly proportional in size to an adult's heart. In infants and children under age 7, however, the heart lies more horizontally. As a result, its apex lies higher—below the fourth left intercostal space.

Pregnant clients

Pregnancy normally increases the maternal blood volume by 30% to 40%. Because the heart must work harder to handle this added volume, its rate and strength of contraction increase. As the uterus enlarges, it displaces the heart forward, upward, and to the left.

During pregnancy, hormonal changes cause vasodilation, which increases venous capacity. The enlarging uterus exerts pressure on the inferior vena cava and iliac veins, increasing venous pressure. This, in turn, causes edema in the lower extremities (legs and feet) and varicose veins in the legs and genitals.

Elderly clients

With age, the heart rate slows and the strength of contraction decreases, reducing the amount of blood ejected by the ventricles. The conduction system also changes. The number of pacemaker cells in the SA and AV nodes decreases, as does the number of Purkinje fibers. Fibrous changes in conduction tissues can interfere with electrical function.

A decrease in myocardial elasticity and contractility along with fibrous changes in the heart valves can interfere with the mechanical function of the heart. Because of these changes, the heart takes longer to return to its resting rate after stress or exercise.

Calcification of the aorta and other arterial walls can occur with age, leading to vessel dilation, tortuosity, and loss of elasticity. These changes increase peripheral vascular resistance, requiring the heart to work harder to circulate the blood.

Health history

The cardiovascular health history that the nurse obtains should focus on client risk factors and any signs and symptoms of heart disease. The history should also assess client behaviors that promote cardiovascular health as well as those that jeopardize it. This part of the health history can uncover the need for teaching clients about behaviors that should be changed and can provide an opportunity to encourage the client to continue healthful behaviors.

Risk factors are characteristics that increase a client's chance of developing a specific disease. For cardiac disease, major risk factors include heredity, sex, race, age, hypertension, cigarette smoking, hyperlipidemia, and diabetes mellitus. Obesity, inactivity, stress, and diet contribute to the risk of cardiac disease. Other risk factors include left ventricular hypertrophy, oral contraceptive use, gout, and environmental factors. (For more information, see *Risk factors of cardiac disease,* pages 294 and 295.)

The major signs and symptoms of cardiac disease include chest pain, dyspnea (shortness of breath) with or without coughing, syncope (dizziness), edema (swelling), palpitations (sensation of pounding, racing, or skipped heartbeats), fatigue, and cyanosis (bluish discoloration of the skin and mucous membranes).

When obtaining a cardiovascular health history, the nurse should adapt the terminology to the client's chronologic and mental age, educational level, and emotional state. Also watch for verbal and nonverbal clues that indicate the client's understanding of the questions.

The questions in this section will help the nurse evaluate the client's cardiovascular system. Their rationales describe the significance of the client's answers and, where appropriate, nursing interventions that may be incorporated into the client's care plan.

Health and illness patterns

The cardiovascular health history should begin with questions that assess the client's health and illness patterns. Questions should thoroughly cover the client's current and past health status as well as the family health and developmental status.

Current health status

Because current health is foremost in the client's mind, begin the interview by exploring this topic with the following questions. Carefully document the chief complaint in the client's own words. Using the PQRST method, ask the client to describe completely this complaint and any others. (For a detailed explanation of this method, see *Symptom analysis* in Chapter 3, The Health History.) To investigate the client's current health status, ask the following questions:

Do you ever have chest pain or discomfort? If so, how would you characterize the pain? Where in your chest do you feel the pain? Does it radiate to any other area? How would you describe the pain? How long have you been having this chest pain? How long does an attack last?
(RATIONALE: Chest pain can result from many cardiac disorders, such as angina, myocardial infarction, and pericarditis [pericardial inflammation]. It can also result from pulmonary and gastroesophageal disorders. The client's answers to these questions should aid in determining the source of the chest pain. For more information, see *Evaluating chest pain,* pages 296 and 297.)

Do you ever experience shortness of breath? If so, is it accompanied by coughing?
(RATIONALE: Dyspnea commonly results from congestive heart failure. As the degree of heart failure increases, lung congestion occurs, leading to dyspnea and coughing.

Risk factors of cardiac disease

Because a client can have coronary atherosclerosis for years without signs or symptoms, the nurse should carefully evaluate risk factors when obtaining a cardiovascular health history. Some risk factors can be altered to reduce the probability of a client's developing cardiac disease, but when two or more risk factors—whether unalterable or alterable—are present, the risk of disease is greater than the sum of the factors.

Unalterable risk factors

Heredity
The occurrence of cardiac disease or hyperlipidemia in a blood relative before age 55 increases a client's risk of cardiac disease.

Sex
More men develop cardiac disease than women, and at a younger age. Before menopause, women have only one sixth the rate of cardiac disease as men in the same age-group. The difference narrows dramatically after a woman's menopause. By age 75, women become as likely as men to develop cardiac disease.

Race
Black women of all ages and Black men under age 45 have a higher incidence of hypertension than Causasian men and women of comparable ages, which increases the risk of cardiac disease in Blacks.

Age
The death rate from cardiac disease increases with age. Clients age 60 have three times the rate of disease found in clients age 45.

Alterable risk factors

Hypertension
Hypertension (consistently high blood pressure exceeding 140/90 mm Hg) poses a major risk of cardiac disease. It is more prevalent in Black, elderly, and obese clients and in those who use oral contraceptives. It usually can be controlled with exercise, a low-sodium diet, stress reduction techniques, and antihypertensive agents.

Cigarette smoking
Men who smoke a pack of cigarettes daily run more than twice the risk of developing cardiac disease than nonsmoking men. Men who smoke two or more packs a day are four times as likely to get the disease. Women smokers also increase their risk of cardiac disease. Regardless of sex, the more a client smokes, the greater the risk. However, the effects of cigarette smoking seem reversible. Smokers who quit eventually return to the same risk level as people who have never smoked.

Hyperlipidemia
Hyperlipidemia refers to elevated lipid concentrations in plasma. Normally, total cholesterol (a component of lipoproteins) levels range from 160 to 180 mg/dl; a level above 180 mg/dl doubles the risk of cardiac disease. More men than women have abnormally high cholesterol levels. Serum cholesterol travels in lipoprotein fractions, including high-density lipoproteins (HDLs), which help remove cholesterol from the body, and low-density lipoproteins (LDLs), which promote cholesterol deposits in the body. Hyperlipidemia usually can be controlled with a low-fat diet, exercise, and antilipemic agents.

Diabetes mellitus
At age 45, diabetic men run twice the risk of cardiac disease as nondiabetic men; premenopausal diabetic women have six times the rate of cardiac disease as premenopausal nondiabetic women. Diabetes usually can be controlled with diet, insulin, and exercise.

Contributing factors

Obesity
Obesity doubles the risk of congestive heart failure and cerebrovascular accident. It slightly increases the risk of coronary artery disease, probably because many obese individuals also have increased serum cholesterol and glucose levels as well as elevated blood pressure.

Inactivity
Lack of exercise seems to decrease HDL levels and promote atherosclerosis. Regular exercise increases HDL levels, lowers the resting heart rate, and may improve myocardial oxygenation.

Stress
Clients with type A personalities run twice the risk of cardiac disease as their more relaxed type B counterparts. Type A personalities typically exhibit chronic overreaction to stress; an exaggerated sense of urgency; excessive aggressiveness, competitiveness, and hostility; and compulsive striving for achievement. Stress contributes to cardiac disease by elevating catecholamine levels, which increase blood pressure and myocardial oxygen consumption. It can also lead to overeating and lack of exercise.

Diet
A diet high in cholesterol and saturated fats may promote hypertension and hyperlipidemia. High caffeine intake (more than the amount in six cups of coffee a day) may contribute to hypertension and dysrhythmias. Moderate alcohol consumption (one or two drinks a day) may reduce the risk of cardiac disease.

Risk factors of cardiac disease continued

Other risk factors

Left ventricular hypertrophy (LVH)
A client with LVH greatly risks cardiac disease. Nearly half of all clients who die from cardiovascular disease first show signs of LVH.

Oral contraceptive use
In women who use oral contraceptives, the risk of hypertension is double or triple that of nonusers. Such women also have a higher risk of myocardial infarction, which increases with age, duration of oral contraceptive use, and smoking.

Gout
Twice as many men with gout develop cardiac disease as do men without gout. The higher risk may result from hyperlipidemia, hypertension, obesity, and glucose intolerance—common effects of gout.

Environmental factors
Cold, snowy regions have a higher mortality from cardiac disease. High-altitude regions and those with "hard" drinking water have a lower mortality.

Dyspnea also may result from pulmonary disorders as well as other cardiovascular disorders, such as coronary artery disease, myocardial ischemia, and myocardial infarction. Dyspnea may occur with mild, moderate, or extreme exertion; at rest; or even during sleep, when episodes of coughing and breathing difficulty may awaken the client [paroxysmal nocturnal dyspnea]. Suggest that the client can help prevent dyspnea at night by sleeping on several pillows.)

Do you ever feel dizzy when you change positions?
(RATIONALE: Syncope develops when reduced cardiac output or vascular insufficiency deprives the brain of blood. It can accompany various cardiovascular problems, such as aortic stenosis [valve narrowing], mitral stenosis, certain dysrhythmias, and pacemaker failure.)

Do your shoes or rings feel tight? Do your ankles or feet feel swollen? If so, how long have you felt this way?
(RATIONALE: Swelling in the extremities signals edema, a common sign of cardiac disease. Edema indicates interstitial fluid collection and can occur when the heart fails to pump blood adequately, as in cardiac failure.)

Does your heart ever feel like it is pounding, racing, or skipping beats?
(RATIONALE: Palpitations may result from a dysrhythmia or from vigorous exercise.)

Do you tire more easily than you used to? What type of activity causes you to feel fatigued? How long can you perform this activity before you feel fatigued? Does rest relieve the fatigue?
(RATIONALE: Fatigue and weakness on mild exertion, especially if relieved by rest, may indicate early heart failure. In this disorder, the heart cannot provide enough blood to meet the slightly increased metabolic needs of the cells. However, few clients recognize fatigue as a cardiac symptom. When they feel fatigued during an activity, they stop and rest, preventing the occurrence of more obvious cardiac symptoms.)

What prescription or over-the-counter medications do you take routinely? What medications do you take periodically? For what disorders do you take these medications? What is the dosage for each medication? How does each one make you feel?
(RATIONALE: Cardiac and noncardiac medications can affect cardiovascular function, especially in elderly clients who are at increased risk for adverse reactions and toxicity. For more information, see *Adverse drug reactions*, page 299.)

Do you have any ulcers or sores on your legs? If so, are they healing? Do you notice any change in the feeling in your legs?
(RATIONALE: Decreased circulation to the lower extremities can cause ulcers that do not heal and can decrease sensation. Often, these changes occur so slowly that the client does not perceive them as a problem. In fact, the client may not offer information about these changes unless questioned.)

Past health status

During this part of the health history, ask the following questions to explore the client's medical history for additional information related to the cardiovascular system:

(Text continues on page 298.)

Evaluating chest pain

If a client reports chest pain, the nurse should ask about its provocative (aggravating) factors and palliative (alleviating) actions, quality or quantity, region and radiation, severity, and timing. By using the PQRST method of symptom analysis, the nurse can determine if the pain is caused by cardiac, pulmonary, or gastroesophageal disorders.

PROVOCATIVE FACTORS AND PALLIATIVE ACTIONS	QUALITY OR QUANTITY	REGION AND RADIATION	SEVERITY	TIMING
Cardiac cause: Angina				
Provocative factors: emotional stress, extreme weather, heavy meal, hot bath or shower, physical exertion, sexual intercourse, spontaneous (no apparent cause) *Palliative actions:* nitroglycerin, rest, high Fowler's position	Crushing or squeezing sensation; feeling of heaviness, pressure, or tightness; dull ache; or indigestion	Substernal region; radiation to left shoulder, jaw, neck, arm, elbow, or wrist	Mild to severe	Gradual or sudden onset; 5 to 10 minutes duration
Cardiac cause: Myocardial infarction				
Provocative factors: Same as above *Palliative actions:* morphine, nitroglycerin	Crushing or squeezing sensation; feeling of heaviness, pressure, or tightness; dull ache; or indigestion	Substernal region; radiation to left shoulder, jaw, neck, arm, elbow, wrist, or fingers	Asymptomatic to severe	Gradual or sudden onset; constant duration during episode
Cardiac cause: Postmyocardial syndrome				
Provocative factors: coughing, deep breathing, laughing, movement *Palliative actions:* aspirin, high Fowler's position, indomethacin (Indocin), nitroglycerin	Knifelike, sharp, or stabbing sensation	Substernal region or at left sternal border; radiation to shoulders (but not down arms)	Severe	Sudden onset (typically occurs 1 week to 1 year after myocardial infarction; tends to recur); constant duration
Cardiac cause: Pericarditis				
Provocative factors: coughing, deep breathing, laughing, lying down, movement *Palliative actions:* high Fowler's position, leaning forward	Knifelike, sharp, or stabbing sensation	Substernal region; radiation to back, neck, left shoulder, or arm	Mild to severe	Sudden onset; constant duration
Cardiac cause: Dissecting aortic aneurysm				
Provocative factors: lifting heavy weight, spontaneous *Palliative actions:* narcotic analgesic, surgery	Ripping or tearing sensation, throbbing of chest with heartbeat	Upper back (or upper anterior chest) region; radiation through back, abdomen, or thighs	Severe (especially at onset)	Sudden onset; few hours to days duration
Pulmonary cause: Pulmonary artery hypertension				
Provocative factors: anemia, carbon monoxide, chronic hypoxemia (acute flare-up), high altitude *Palliative action:* oxygen	Crushing or gripping sensation	Substernal region; does not radiate	Severe	Sudden onset; intermittent, nocturnal, or constant duration

Evaluating chest pain continued

PROVOCATIVE FACTORS AND PALLIATIVE ACTIONS	QUALITY OR QUANTITY	REGION AND RADIATION	SEVERITY	TIMING
Pulmonary cause: Pulmonary embolism				
Provocative factors: coughing, deep breathing, immobility *Palliative actions:* high Fowler's position, splinting of chest, position change	Gripping or stabbing sensation that worsens with deep breathing, or sensation of the inability to take a breath	Affected region; may radiate to neck or shoulder	Mild to severe	Sudden onset; few minutes to days duration
Pulmonary cause: Pneumothorax				
Provocative factors: coughing, exertion, Valsalva maneuver, spontaneous (no apparent cause) *Palliative action :* chest tube insertion	Often described as sharp or tearing sensation	Lateral thorax; radiation to ipsilateral shoulder	Mild to severe	Sudden onset; few hours duration
Pulmonary cause: Pneumonia				
Provocative factors: aspiration, hypoventilation (secondary to other disorders) *Palliative actions:* analgesic, rest	Burning, stabbing, or tearing sensation	Retrosternal region; usually does not radiate	Mild to severe	Gradual or sudden onset; days to weeks duration
Pulmonary cause: Rib fracture				
Provocative factors: chest compression during cardiopulmonary resuscitation, coughing, deep breathing, laughing, movement *Palliative actions:* analgesic, heat	Sore, stabbing, or sticking sensation	Affected area (rib, sternum, or costochondral joint); does not radiate	Mild to severe	Gradual or sudden onset; few weeks duration
Gastroesophageal cause: Esophageal reflux				
Provocative factors: alcohol, aspirin, caffeine, constipation, spicy meal, lying down after meal, lifting heavy weight, obesity, smoking, straining, wearing clothing too tight at waist *Palliative actions:* antacid, food	Heartburn or dull, burning, or squeezing sensation	Epigastric and retrosternal region; mimics angina but rarely radiates to left shoulder, jaw, neck, arm, elbow, or wrist	Mild to severe	Onset during or after meal; intermittent duration (usually 10 minutes to 1 hour)
Gastroesophageal cause: Esophageal spasm				
Provocative factors: cold liquids, exercise, swallowing, spontaneous (no apparent cause) *Palliative action:* nitroglycerin	Dull, burning, crushing, gripping, or squeezing sensation or feeling of pressure	Retrosternal region and area across chest; radiation to left arm, neck, jaw, or back	Mild to severe	Sudden onset; seconds to minutes duration (with lingering ache); tends to recur
Gastroesophageal cause: Esophageal rupture				
Provocative factors: alcohol, coughing, external trauma, heavy meal, swallowing, vomiting *Palliative action:* surgery	Tearing or crushing sensation	Epigastric and retrosternal region; radiation to lower thoracic spine	Severe	Sudden onset; constant duration

Were you born with a heart problem? If so, when and how was it treated?
(RATIONALE: Problems related to congenital heart disorders, such as tetralogy of Fallot and ventricular septal defect, may persist even after treatment or surgical correction.)

Have you had rheumatic fever? If so, when? Have any heart problems resulted from the rheumatic fever?
(RATIONALE: Rheumatic fever can lead to rheumatic heart disease, eventually causing valvular stenosis or insufficiency.)

Have you had a heart murmur? If so, who told you about it and when?
(RATIONALE: Many people have innocent, or functional, murmurs that are unrelated to structural heart disease. Other people have murmurs that are caused by permanent structural problems, such as septal defects or valvular stenosis or insufficiency caused by rheumatic fever.)

Do you have high blood pressure, high cholesterol, or diabetes mellitus? If so, when was the disorder first diagnosed? How do you manage it? Has it affected your life-style? If so, how?
(RATIONALE: Hypertension, hyperlipidemia, and diabetes mellitus are major risk factors of cardiac disease. Information about current management and life-style may affect nursing interventions that can help the client reduce the effects of these disorders, such as modifying the diet, increasing activity levels, and decreasing stress.)

Have you experienced chest pain, shortness of breath, fainting or dizziness, foot or ankle swelling, palpitations, or a bluish discoloration of your skin?
(RATIONALE: These are all major signs and symptoms of heart disease.)

Have you experienced confusion?
(RATIONALE: Confusion may be a sign of cardiac disease, especially in an elderly client. It typically results when a dysrhythmia decreases cardiac output. The decreased output, in turn, causes cerebrovascular insufficiency—and confusion.)

Have you felt fatigued in the past few months? What was the cause? How frequently has fatigue occurred?
(RATIONALE: Fatigue is a common symptom of heart disease. The frequency of fatigue and the circumstances surrounding it may provide clues to the severity of the heart disease. For example, fatigue at rest suggests a more severe disorder than fatigue after exertion.)

Have you had dental work done or undergone an invasive procedure, such as cystoscopy or endoscopy, within the last few weeks? If so, which procedure and when?
(RATIONALE: Invasive procedures can create an entry for organisms that can cause infective endocarditis, an endocardial infection from such bacteria as *Streptococcus, Pneumococcus,* or *Staphylococcus.*)

Have you ever had an allergic reaction to a medication? If so, which one? How would you describe the reaction?
(RATIONALE: Knowledge of a previous allergic reaction can prevent prescription of the causative drug—and serious adverse reactions. Description of the reaction will help differentiate between a side effect, which may be managed by a dosage change, and a true allergic response.)

For a female client, pose additional questions. (See *Sex-specific questions,* page 300.)

Family health status

Next, investigate the cardiovascular status of the client's family by asking the following questions:

Has anyone in your family been treated for heart disease? If so, how was the person related to you? What was the disorder? At what age did it occur?
(RATIONALE: The incidence of cardiac disease in a blood relative increases the risk of cardiac disease in the client.)

Has anyone in your family died suddenly of an unknown cause?
(RATIONALE: The family member may have died from cardiac arrest. If so, this puts the client at a greater risk of cardiac disease.)

Does anyone in your family have high blood pressure, high cholesterol, or diabetes mellitus? If so, at what age did the disease develop? How is it treated?
(RATIONALE: The incidence of cardiac disease is higher in clients with a family history of hypertension, hyperlipidemia, or diabetes mellitus.)

Developmental considerations

A pediatric, pregnant, or elderly client will require additional health history questions to investigate developmental status.

Pediatric client. Try to involve the child in the interview along with the parent or guardian. The child's age will determine the degree of involvement and the terminology

Adverse drug reactions

When obtaining a health history to assess a client's cardiovascular system, the nurse should ask about current drug use. Many drugs affect cardiovascular function; some can cause severe problems, such as heart block and myocardial infarction. The commonly used drugs listed below may cause adverse reactions affecting the cardiovascular system.

DRUG CLASS	DRUG	POSSIBLE ADVERSE REACTIONS
Antidepressants	trazodone hydrochloride	Hypotension, hypertension, syncope, chest pain, tachycardia, palpitations, EKG changes
	tricyclic antidepressants	Postural hypotension, hypertension, EKG changes, dysrhythmias, syncope, thrombosis, thrombophlebitis, congestive heart failure (CHF)
Antineoplastics	daunorubicin hydrochloride, doxorubicin hydrochloride	Dose-dependent cardiomyopathy manifested by CHF, EKG changes, dysrhythmias
Antipsychotics	phenothiazines	Hypotension, postural hypotension, tachycardia, syncope, EKG changes, dysrhythmias
Anxiolytics	diazepam	Hypotension, bradycardia, cardiac arrest, dysrhythmias (with I.V. route)
	midazolam hydrochloride	Hypotension, cardiorespiratory arrest
Cerebral stimulants	amphetamine sulfate	Tachycardia, palpitations, dysrhythmias, hypertension, hypotension
	caffeine	Tachycardia
Hormones	oral contraceptives	Hypertension, fluid retention, increased risk of cerebrovascular accident, myocardial infarction, thromboembolism
	conjugated estrogens, chlorotrianisene, diethylstilbestrol	Hypertension, thromboembolism, thrombophlebitis
	vasopressin	Angina in clients with vascular disease; in large doses, hypertension, bradycardia, minor dysrhythmias, myocardial infarction
Nonsteroidal anti-inflammatory agents	indomethacin	CHF, tachycardia, chest pain, hypertension, edema
	phenylbutazone	Hypertension, CHF, pericarditis, myocarditis, pericardial effusion
Spasmolytics	aminophylline, theophylline	Palpitations, sinus tachycardia, extrasystoles, ventricular dysrhythmias, hypotension
Miscellaneous agents	bethanechol chloride	Hypotension, reflex tachycardia
	hydralazine hydrochloride	Tachycardia, angina pectoris, EKG changes
	levodopa-carbidopa	Orthostatic hypotension
	levothyroxine	With excessive doses, angina pectoris, dysrhythmias, tachycardia, hypertension
	phenytoin sodium	Hypotension, ventricular fibrillation (with I.V. route)

Sex-specific questions

The following questions will help evaluate the cardiovascular status of a female client.

Have you had any problem pregnancies? If so, how would you describe the problem?
(RATIONALE: Women who have had toxemia of pregnancy have an increased risk of developing postpartum cardiomyopathy, a myocardial weakness that impairs cardiac muscle contraction.)

Do you use a contraceptive? If so, which one?
(RATIONALE: Women who use birth control pills and smoke cigarettes run a six times greater risk of having a cerebrovascular accident, or stroke, than nonsmokers who use other forms of contraception. Women who use intrauterine devices [IUDs] have a higher risk of developing pelvic inflammatory disease than nonusers. If this disorder becomes systemic, it may cause endocarditis.)

to use. For a thorough cardiovascular assessment of a child, ask the following questions:

Has the child experienced any growth delay?
(RATIONALE: Slow growth may result from impaired cardiac output.)

Does the child have any problems with coordination?
(RATIONALE: A poorly coordinated child who is unusually tall and thin may have Marfan's syndrome, a congenital disorder characterized by musculoskeletal disturbances, such as bone elongation and incoordination, and by cardiovascular abnormalities that may affect the aorta, aortic valve, and myocardium.)

Does the child turn blue when crying?
(RATIONALE: The bluish skin color signals cyanosis, which may indicate a congenital heart disease.)

Does the child stop frequently during play to sit or squat?
(RATIONALE: Frequent rest breaks during play suggest exercise intolerance, which frequently accompanies congenital cardiac disorders.)

Does the child have difficulty feeding?
(RATIONALE: Feeding difficulty may result from congestive heart failure or a congenital heart disease that causes dyspnea. In such a child, the heart cannot increase its work load enough to provide the extra energy required during eating.)

Does the child tire easily or sleep excessively?
(RATIONALE: Poor exercise tolerance and fatigue may indicate congenital heart disease or congestive heart failure.)

Does the child frequently develop strep throat infections or a sore throat accompanied by fever?
(RATIONALE: Streptococcal infections may lead to rheumatic fever and rheumatic heart disease. To help prevent such infections, teach the parents to keep the child away from infected people and to see that the child practices good dental hygiene to prevent gingivitis [gum infection], which can lead to throat infection. To help prevent rheumatic heart disease, teach the parents to recognize and immediately report signs of infection: sore throat, fever, pain upon swallowing, and enlarged lymph glands in the neck.)

Pregnant client. Pregnancy causes many physiologic changes. The following additional questions help assess for these effects:

During this pregnancy, has any health care professional said that you have a heart murmur?
(RATIONALE: The increased blood volume associated with pregnancy can create an innocent, physiologic murmur. However, any murmur requires further study to exclude a pathologic cause.)

Do you ever feel dizzy when you change positions?
(RATIONALE: Early in pregnancy, vasodilation normally causes blood pressure to fall, which may result in syncope, especially with position changes.)

Has your blood pressure been elevated during this pregnancy?
(RATIONALE: Blood pressure elevation can be a sign of toxemia of pregnancy, an abnormal—and potentially fatal—condition characterized in its early stages by hypertension, proteinuria, and edema.)

Have you noticed any swelling in your feet or ankles? Have you developed varicose veins in your legs or genitals? Have you developed hemorrhoids?
(RATIONALE: During pregnancy, increased venous pressure and venous pooling can result in edema and varicosities, including hemorrhoids. These effects usually subside after delivery.)

Elderly client. The cardiovascular system undergoes many physiologic changes with age, which makes it more susceptible to disorders. To uncover potential problems in an elderly client, ask the following health history questions:

Does your heart pound after stress or exertion?
(RATIONALE: As the heart loses elasticity and muscle strength with age, it becomes less responsive to the body's increased oxygen demands caused by stress or exertion. Because of this, the heart seems to pound and takes longer to return to its normal rate.)

Do you ever feel dizzy when changing position or exerting yourself?
(RATIONALE: Tortuous carotid arteries, a thickened endothelium, and a conduction system that has developed fibrosis can reduce an elderly client's blood supply to the brain, which can cause syncope.)

Do you suffer from shortness of breath? If so, is it ever accompanied by coughing or wheezing?
(RATIONALE: In an elderly client, a myocardial infarction or an ischemic episode may cause dyspnea, but no pain. A nonproductive cough, wheezing, or hemoptysis [coughing up of blood] may accompany the dyspnea.)

Health promotion and protection patterns

To determine how the client provides for or maintains health, the nurse should investigate health promotion and protection behaviors.

Personal habits

Personal habits can affect health positively or negatively. To assess the client's personal habits, pose the following questions:

Do you smoke cigarettes, cigars, or a pipe or chew tobacco? If so, how long have you smoked? How many cigarettes, cigars, or pipes of tobacco do you smoke per day? Did you ever stop smoking? How long did it last? What method did you use to stop? Do you remember why you started smoking again? If you do not use tobacco now, have you smoked or chewed tobacco in the past? If you stopped, what influenced you to do so?
(RATIONALE: Smoking, especially cigarette smoking, is a major risk factor of cardiac disease. Because smoking and chewing tobacco are addictions, the client may become defensive about this behavior, so remain nonjudgmental during the health history. Later, discuss the importance of stopping smoking or chewing tobacco and suggest methods that can be used. Report the smoking history in pack years by multiplying the number of years of smoking by the number of packs smoked per day. For periods when pack use differed, calculate the pack years for each period and add these subtotals to obtain the number of pack years.)

Do you drink alcoholic beverages? If so, what type? How often do you drink? How many drinks? Spread over how much time?
(RATIONALE: In small amounts, alcohol may benefit some individuals because it is a vasodilator—it opens the vessels and increases the blood flow. However, alcohol can be habit-forming or addictive and can cause cardiomyopathy as well as problems in other body systems. Usually, clients who are defensive about alcohol use respond best when asked direct questions in a nonjudgmental manner.)

Sleep and wake patterns

Cardiovascular problems can interfere with sleep and rest. The following questions investigate such problems:

How long do you sleep each night?
(RATIONALE: Abnormally long sleep for the client's age may indicate a cardiovascular problem, such as a cardiomyopathy. To determine if the amount of sleep is abnormal for the client's age, see Chapter 5, Activities of Daily Living and Sleep Patterns.)

Do you feel rested each morning? Do you feel tired later in the day? Do you take naps?
(RATIONALE: Recently developed tiredness at any time of day and regular napping suggest fatigue, a common symptom of low cardiac output.)

Have you been told that you snore during sleep?
(RATIONALE: Snoring may be associated with sleep disorders, such as obstructive sleep apnea, that lead to dysrhythmias because they reduce the oxygen supply to the heart.)

Do you awaken during the night to urinate?
(RATIONALE: Nocturia may occur in a client with low cardiac output. In such a client, the cardiac output may not be high enough to perfuse the kidneys properly during the day. At night, however, when the rest of the body has lower metabolic needs, the heart may be able to perfuse the kidneys better. This may lead to increased urine formation at night—and nocturia.)

Do you experience episodes of shortness of breath or coughing during the night? If so, when and how frequently do they occur?
(RATIONALE: Episodes of dyspnea and coughing at night are signs of paroxysmal nocturnal dyspnea, which results from congestive heart failure and interstitial pulmonary congestion.)

Do you become short of breath when you lie flat? How many pillows do you use at night? Has this number changed recently?
(RATIONALE: Orthopnea, or shortness of breath that occurs in the supine position, may result from the pulmonary congestion that accompanies congestive heart failure.)

Exercise and activity patterns

Although aerobic exercise is the best cardiac conditioner, any regular exercise or activity can help prevent cardiovascular problems. The following questions investigate the client's exercise and activity levels:

Do you exercise routinely? If so, what exercises do you perform? How would you describe the frequency, intensity, and length of time that you exercise?
(RATIONALE: At rest, the heart rate and blood pressure provide the cardiac output needed to maintain adequate system function. With activity or exercise, the body's needs increase, requiring a higher cardiac output. Cardiac output, heart rate, systolic blood pressure, respiratory rate, and oxygen consumption increase as the intensity of the exercise increases. The degree of exercise tolerance reveals the client's cardiovascular response to increased metabolic demands.)

Did a health care professional prescribe your exercise plan? If so, who?
(RATIONALE: The client may be taking part in a cardiac rehabilitation program based on metabolic equivalents of a task [METs]. If so, document the client's level of activity. For information about the metabolic demands of specific activities, see *MET measurements,* pages 304 and 305.)

Do environmental factors, such as temperature extremes, humidity, or pollution, affect your ability to exercise or the way you feel after exercise?
(RATIONALE: Because environmental factors normally decrease exercise tolerance slightly, symptoms may appear only under these conditions when the cardiac output cannot meet the increased demand.)

Has your exercise level changed from that of 6 months, 1 year, or 5 years ago? What caused this change?
(RATIONALE: Exercise intolerance and a decreased activity level may be the first signs that the cardiac output cannot meet the increased metabolic demands caused by exercise. These signs may indicate decreased cardiac output from a disorder such as coronary insufficiency or coronary artery disease.)

Have you noticed any change in your ability to perform the usual activities of daily living?
(RATIONALE: For an elderly or sedentary client, an inability to perform the activities of daily living may be the first sign that the cardiac output cannot meet the metabolic demands caused by low-level activities.)

Do you participate in any recreational activities, such as hobbies or sports? If so, how frequently do you engage in them? How do you feel after these activities? Has your level of involvement in these activities changed recently? If so, what caused this change?
(RATIONALE: The energy expenditure for recreational activities provides information about cardiac function. A decrease in frequency or level of involvement in recreational activities may suggest decreased cardiac output from coronary insufficiency, coronary artery disease, or some other heart disorder.)

When you walk or exercise, do you experience leg pain?
(RATIONALE: Leg pain may result from narrowed arteries that cannot provide the increased blood and oxygen needed.)

Nutritional patterns

Because diet is important to cardiovascular health, investigate this area by asking the following questions:

What have you eaten during the past 3 days?
(RATIONALE: A 3-day diet recall may reveal patterns that contribute to the risk of cardiac disease, such as regular consumption of high-cholesterol foods or excessive caffeine intake. It can also indicate the need for nutritional teaching.)

Do you follow any special diet? If so, did a health care professional prescribe this diet for you?
(RATIONALE: The client may restrict the intake of specific foods because of religious beliefs or personal preferences. If the client's diet is harmful, gently explain why and suggest ways to modify it.)

Do you eat at fast-food restaurants? How often? What items do you usually order?
(RATIONALE: Many fast-food items contain empty calories as well as high levels of sodium and fat, which can contribute to cardiac disease. If the client eats such foods frequently, teach about the risk factors of cardiac disease and suggest healthier fast-food items.)

Does your ethnic or cultural background influence your diet? Does your religion restrict, or otherwise affect, what you eat?

(RATIONALE: A client's religious, ethnic, or cultural background can affect dietary habits and, ultimately, the client's cardiovascular health.)

Have you gained any weight recently?
(RATIONALE: A weight increase of 2 to 3 lb in 48 hours may signal fluid retention, which can lead to congestive heart failure.)

Stress and coping patterns

Examining stress and coping patterns provides information about the client's personality type and aids in planning nursing interventions. The following questions investigate these concerns:

What causes you to feel stressed? How often does this occur? What physical feelings do you have when you are stressed?
(RATIONALE: A risk factor of cardiac disease, stress increases the heart rate and blood pressure without providing an outlet for these responses. [In contrast, exercise produces the same physical effects, but dissipates them through activity.] Habitual stress frequently increases the heart rate and blood pressure, causing progressive changes in the heart and vessels and eventually leading to cardiac disease. In a client with coronary artery disease, stress can lead to chest pain and dyspnea, symptoms of myocardial ischemia.)

Do you feel pressured to complete tasks in a short time? Do you rush from one job or task to another?
(RATIONALE: Positive answers to these questions may classify the client as a type A personality. Research suggests that type A personalities have a higher incidence of myocardial infarction and coronary artery disease than other personality types. However, they may have a better chance for survival after a myocardial infarction. During the health history, certain client behaviors may support the type A classification: speaking quickly, acting impatiently, answering questions before they are completed, checking the clock frequently, and squirming or acting restless instead of sitting quietly.)

How do you cope with stress in your life?
(RATIONALE: If the client has found successful ways to manage stress, incorporate them into the care plan. If not, avoid previously unsuccessful strategies and help determine which strategies to try in the future.)

Other health promotion and protection patterns

Other factors can affect a client's health promotion and protection behaviors, such as economic influences, environmental and occupational health patterns, and daily activities. To assess these factors, ask the following questions:

Do your financial resources and insurance adequately cover your medical needs and preventive measures?
(RATIONALE: Without adequate health insurance and financial resources, the client may not be able to obtain necessary medical services and prescribed medications. Many health insurance plans do not reimburse preventive measures, such as exercise, smoking cessation, weight reduction, or stress management programs. Although such health promotion programs may reduce the need for medical attention, the expense may prevent the client from participating.)

How is your house or apartment laid out physically? Must you climb steps to get inside? Must you climb steps to get from room to room? If so, how many? On which level are the bathroom, bedroom, and kitchen?
(RATIONALE: The physical layout of the client's house or apartment can provide an estimate of the energy needed to get around it. If the client develops chest pain and dyspnea when climbing steps, discuss ways to limit their use or to rearrange the house based on the number of steps used.)

Do certain weather conditions affect your symptoms? If so, what conditions and how do they affect your symptoms?
(RATIONALE: On extremely cold, windy, or hot days, a client may experience increased chest pain and dyspnea because the heart must work harder to regulate the body temperature. Teach the client to avoid being outdoors during these weather conditions.)

What is your occupation? Are you currently employed in that field?
(RATIONALE: A client may not be able to work at the usual occupation because of cardiovascular limitations. For example, a cardiovascular disorder may prohibit a mail carrier from lifting heavy mail bags, which is required on the job.)

How many hours do you work per day? How many days do you work per week? What are your responsibilities? What are the physical demands of the job? How much lifting do you do? How much walking?
(RATIONALE: The answers to these questions help determine the client's cardiovascular work load during a routine work day. They also will aid in developing an appropriate activity plan, whether the client works at a desk or stands and walks for 8 hours a day.)

Do you work in a hot, cold, humid, dusty, smoky, noisy, or outdoor environment?
(RATIONALE: Cardiovascular symptoms can result from environmental hazards in the workplace. For example,

MET measurements

For a client undergoing cardiac rehabilitation or a client with cardiovascular signs and symptoms, the nurse should evaluate the client's activity level by using metabolic equivalents of a task (METs). MET measurements provide an estimate of the amount of energy—and the cardiovascular work load—required by different activities.

One MET of energy equals consumption of about 3.5 ml of oxygen per kilogram of body weight each minute. Higher MET levels represent multiples of this energy consumption level. This chart shows how many METs various activities use.

1 MET

- Bed rest
- Sitting
- Eating
- Reading
- Sewing
- Watching television

1 to 2 METs

- Dressing
- Shaving
- Brushing teeth
- Washing at sink
- Making bed
- Desk work
- Driving car
- Playing cards
- Knitting
- Typing (electric typewriter)
- Walking 1 mph (1.6 km/hr) on level ground

2 to 3 METs

- Tub bathing
- Cooking
- Waxing floor
- Riding power lawn mower
- Playing piano
- Driving small truck
- Using hand tools
- Typing (manual typewriter)
- Repairing car
- Walking 2 mph (3.2 km/hr) on level ground
- Bicycling 5 mph (8 km/hr) on level ground
- Playing billiards
- Fishing
- Bowling
- Golfing (with motor cart)
- Operating motorboat
- Riding horseback (at walk)

3 to 4 METs

- General housework
- Cleaning windows
- Light gardening
- Pushing light power mower
- Sexual intercourse
- Assembly-line work
- Driving large truck
- Bricklaying
- Plastering
- Walking 3 mph (4.8 km/hr)
- Bicycling 6 mph (9.7 km/hr)
- Sailing
- Golfing (pulling hand cart)
- Pitching horseshoes
- Archery
- Badminton (doubles)
- Horseback riding (at slow trot)
- Fly-fishing

4 to 5 METs

- Heavy housework
- Heavy gardening
- Home repairs, including painting and light carpentry
- Raking leaves
- Painting
- Masonry
- Paperhanging
- Calisthenics
- Table tennis
- Golfing (carrying bag)
- Tennis (doubles)
- Dancing
- Slow swimming

a mail carrier may develop dyspnea and chest pain from working in hot, humid air; a factory worker may feel dyspneic in a closed, smoky environment.)

How would you describe your typical day? Do your daily activities vary on weekends? If so, how?
(RATIONALE: The answers to these questions establish the client's activity level and tolerance for routine and less routine activities. They also provide an opportunity to teach the client how to prevent cardiovascular problems by pacing activities better and by trying alternative, less tiring activities.)

Role and relationship patterns

Cardiovascular disorders can affect many role and relationship patterns. To discover the extent of this effect, ask the client these questions:

Do you think of yourself as a healthy or sick person? What makes you feel this way? Do you feel that your health problem has changed your life?
(RATIONALE: Because many people think the heart is the seat of emotions, a cardiovascular dysfunction can negatively affect the client's sense of identity and self-esteem.)

What are your typical responsibilities at home? What are the usual responsibilities of your spouse and children? Have your responsibilities at home changed since you developed a health problem? If so, how do you feel about these changes?
(RATIONALE: Family members typically feel protective of a loved one with a cardiac disease. This feeling may lead to changes in usual family responsibilities and relationships, possibly decreasing the client's self-esteem and upsetting the client's self-concept.)

Has your usual pattern of sexual activity changed in any way? If so, how would you describe this change? How do you feel about it?
(RATIONALE: Some clients with cardiac disease or their spouses may avoid sexual activity because they fear that it will cause further heart damage. In reality, they may not need to avoid sex, but simply pace themselves care-

5 to 6 METs	6 to 7 METs	7 to 8 METs	8 to 9 METs	10 or more METs
• Sawing softwood • Digging garden • Shoveling light loads • Using heavy tools • Lifting 50 lb • Walking 4 mph (6.4 km/hr) • Bicycling 10 mph (16.1 km/hr) • Skating • Fishing with waders • Hiking • Hunting • Square dancing • Horseback riding (at brisk trot)	• Shoveling snow • Splitting wood • Mowing lawn with hand mower • Walking or jogging 5 mph (8 km/hr) • Bicycling 11 mph (17.7 km/hr) • Tennis (singles) • Waterskiing • Light downhill skiing	• Sawing hardwood • Digging ditches • Lifting 80 lb • Moving heavy furniture • Paddleball • Touch football • Swimming (backstroke) • Basketball • Ice hockey	• Lifting 100 lb • Running 5.5 mph (8.9 km/hr) • Bicycling 13 mph (20.9 km/hr) • Swimming (breaststroke) • Handball (noncompetitive) • Cross-country skiing • Fencing	• Running 6 mph (9.7 km/hr) or faster • Handball (competitive) • Squash (competitive) • Gymnastics • Football (contact)

fully and use less strenuous positions. Other clients with cardiac disease may experience impotence, which may result from psychological factors, such as fear, or from adverse reactions to antianginal or antihypertensive medications.)

Physical assessment

Before assessing the client's cardiovascular system, the nurse must evaluate various client factors that may reflect cardiovascular function, including general appearance, body weight, vital signs, and related body structures.

Preparing for cardiovascular assessment

To prepare for a thorough physical assessment of the cardiovascular system, follow these guidelines. After washing your hands, gather the necessary equipment: a stethoscope, a sphygmomanometer with inflatable cuff, scales, a ruler, and a gown and drapes to cover the client.

Then prepare the environment. Select a setting that affords privacy. Adjust the thermostat, if necessary, to create a warm environment. (A cool environment may alter the client's skin temperature and color, heart rate, and blood pressure.) Also, make sure the environment is quiet, particularly during auscultation of heart sounds. If possible, close the door and windows to shut out extraneous noises, and turn off radios and noisy equipment.

Physical assessment of the cardiovascular system requires evaluation of the vital signs—temperature, pulse rate, respiration rate, and blood pressure. It also involves the basic techniques of inspection, palpation, percussion, and auscultation. However, the assessment does not have to be performed in this exact order. Combine parts of the assessment, as needed, to conserve time and the client's energy. For example, combine chest inspection, palpation, and auscultation to reduce the amount of time that the client is disrobed. Alter the order of assessment tasks, as needed, if a client experiences cardiovascular difficulties during the assessment. For example, if a client develops chest pain and dyspnea during the assessment, quickly check the vital signs and then auscultate the heart.

Because cardiovascular assessment requires exposure of the chest, a female client may be embarrassed. To help minimize this feeling, explain each assessment step beforehand, use drapes appropriately throughout the assessment, and expose only the area being assessed at the time.

General appearance, body weight, and vital signs

To begin the physical assessment, observe the client's general appearance, particularly noting weight and muscle composition. The client should appear well developed, well nourished, alert, and energetic. Document any departures from the norm, such as if the client appears older or younger than his or her chronologic age or if the client appears tired or moves slower than most people of the same age.

Body weight. Accurately measure and record the client's height and body weight. These anthropometric measurements will help guide treatment plans, determine medication dosages, assist with appropriate nutritional counseling, and detect fluid overload. Increases or decreases in weight may be significant, especially if extreme. A weight gain of several pounds overnight commonly occurs in a client who is developing congestive heart failure.

Next, assess the client for cardiac cachexia (weakness and muscle wasting) by observing the amount of muscle bulk in the upper arms, thighs, and chest wall. For a more precise measurement of cachexia, calculate the percentage of body fat using anthropometric measurements. For men, the percentage of body fat normally averages 14% to 18%; for women, it ranges from 20% to 25%. Many clients with chronic cardiac disease develop cardiac cachexia, losing body fat and muscle mass. Loss of the body's energy stores reduces healing capacity and immune system effectiveness.

Vital signs. Measure the body temperature to obtain valuable information about the client's cardiovascular system. An elevated body temperature can indicate a cardiovascular inflammation or infection. A mild to moderate temperature elevation usually occurs 2 to 5 days after a myocardial infarction as the healing infarct passes through the inflammatory stage. Acute pericarditis may cause a similar temperature elevation. Higher elevations accompany infections, such as infective endocarditis, which causes fever spikes (unusually high temperatures).

Whatever the cause, a temperature elevation always occurs with an increase in metabolism, which increases the cardiac work load. That explains why a feverish client with known heart disease requires observation for other signs of increased cardiac work load, such as an increased heart rate.

Next, assess the client's blood pressure. To measure it accurately, first palpate and then auscultate the blood pressure in an arm or a leg. Wait 3 to 5 minutes between measurements. (For an illustrated procedure, see *Measuring blood pressure* in Chapter 4, Physical Assessment Skills.) Normally, blood pressure measures less than 140/90 mm Hg in a resting adult and 78 to 114/46 to 78 mm Hg in a young child.

Elevated blood pressure may result from hypertension or emotional stress associated with physical assessment. If the client's blood pressure is elevated, repeat the measurement in 5 to 10 minutes (after allowing the client to relax) to determine if the elevation is stress-related. According to the American Heart Association, hypertension is present when the blood pressure is elevated above 140/90 mm Hg on several successive readings. (The diagnosis is not made on one reading alone.)

When assessing a client's blood pressure for the first time, take measurements in both arms. A difference of 10 mm Hg or more between the arms may indicate thoracic outlet syndrome—compression of the arterial flow to one arm produced by pressure from the clavicle or first rib—or other forms of arterial obstruction.

If the blood pressure is elevated in both arms, measure the pressure in the thigh. Wrap a large cuff around the client's upper leg at least 1" above the knee. Place the stethoscope over the popliteal artery, located on the posterior surface slightly above the knee joint. Listen for sounds when the bladder of the cuff is deflated, as for an arm pressure. Blood pressure that is abnormally high in the arms, but normal or low in the legs, suggests aortic coarctation (narrowing).

After measuring the client's blood pressure, calculate the pulse pressure (the difference between the higher, systolic pressure and the lower, diastolic pressure). The pulse pressure, which reflects arterial pressure during the resting phase of the cardiac cycle, normally ranges from 30 to 50 mm Hg.

The pulse pressure increases when the stroke volume (output of each ventricle at every contraction) increases, as in exercise, anxiety, or bradycardia (heart rate of less than 60 beats/minute). It also increases when the peripheral vascular resistance or aortic distensibility decreases, as in anemia, hyperthyroidism, fever, hypertension, aortic coarctation, or aging.

The pulse pressure decreases when a mechanical obstruction exists, such as mitral or aortic stenosis; when the peripheral vessels constrict, as in shock; or when the stroke volume decreases, as in heart failure, hypovolemia, or tachycardia.

As part of vital sign measurements, assess the radial pulse to determine the client's heart rate. For a client with suspected cardiac disease, be sure to palpate for a full minute to detect any dysrhythmias. Normally, an adult's pulse ranges from 60 to 100 beats/minute. Its rhythm should feel regular, except for a subtle slowing on expiration, which is caused by nonpathologic sinus dysrhythmia.

Count the client's respirations, observing for eupnea—a regular, unlabored, and bilaterally equal breathing pattern. Tachypnea (rapid respirations) may indicate a low cardiac output. Dyspnea, which may indicate congestive heart failure, may not be evident at rest but may occur with speaking. So note if the client must pause after only a few words to take a breath. A Cheyne-Stokes respiratory pattern (breathing that gradually becomes faster and deeper than normal and then slower, alternating with periods of apnea) may accompany severe heart failure, although it is more commonly associated with coma.

Assessing related body structures

Because the cardiovascular system affects many other body systems, a client with a cardiovascular disorder may exhibit signs of illness in other parts of the body. The nurse should include these areas in the physical inspection.

Skin, hair, and nails. Because of racial and genetic differences, normal skin color can vary widely from client to client. Ask the client if the present skin tone is the normal color.

Then inspect the skin color, particularly noting any cyanosis. If cyanosis is present, determine whether it is central or peripheral. (For more information, see Chapter 10, Respiratory System.) Examine the underside of the tongue, buccal mucosa, and conjunctiva for signs of central cyanosis. Inspect the skin of the extremities and the nail beds for signs of peripheral cyanosis.

To detect cyanosis in a dark-skinned client, inspect the oral mucous membranes, such as the lips and gingivae (gums), which normally appear pink and moist, but will be ashen gray if cyanotic. In a dark-skinned client, these areas provide a better way to assess skin color because the color range for normal mucous membranes is narrower than that for the skin. (For more information about mucous membrane assessment, see Chapter 8, Head and Neck.)

Central cyanosis suggests reduced oxygen intake or transport from the lungs to the bloodstream, conditions that may occur with congestive heart failure. Peripheral cyanosis suggests constriction of peripheral arterioles, which can occur as a natural response to cold or anxiety or can result from hypovolemia, cardiogenic shock, or a vasoconstrictive disease that reduces, slows, or restricts peripheral blood flow.

When evaluating the client's skin color, also observe for flushing (a reddish discoloration caused by vasodilation) and pallor (an unusual paleness or absence of skin color). Flushing can result from medications, excess heat, or autonomic nervous system stimulation by anxiety or fear. Pallor can result from anemia or increased peripheral vascular resistance caused by atherosclerosis.

Next, assess the client's perfusion by evaluating the arterial flow adequacy. To assess arterial blood flow and perfusion, perform this test using the following guidelines. With the client lying down, elevate one of the client's legs 12″ (30 cm) above heart level for 60 seconds. Next, tell the client to sit up and dangle both legs. Compare the color of both legs over the edge of the bed. The leg that was elevated should show mild pallor compared to the other leg.

The original color should return to the pale leg in about 10 seconds, and the veins should refill in about 15 seconds. Significant arterial insufficiency may be present if the client's foot shows marked pallor, delayed color return that ends with a mottled appearance, or delayed venous filling, or if the leg shows marked redness.

Touch the client's skin, which should feel warm and dry. Cool, clammy skin results from vasoconstriction, which occurs when the cardiac output is low, as in shock. Warm, moist skin results from vasodilation, which occurs when the cardiac output is high, as during exercise.

Next, evaluate the client's skin turgor (resiliency) by grasping and raising the skin between two fingers and then letting it go. Normally, the skin returns immediately to its original position. Taut, shiny skin that cannot be grasped and raised may result from ascites or the marked edema that accompanies congestive heart failure. Skin that does not return immediately to the original position exhibits tenting, a sign of decreased skin turgor, which may result from dehydration, especially if the client takes diuretics. It also may result from age, malnutrition, or an adverse reaction to steroid treatment.

Next, observe the skin for signs of edema (swelling caused by abnormal fluid accumulation in the interstitial spaces). To detect edema, inspect the client's arms and legs for symmetrical swelling. Because edema usually affects lower or dependent areas of the body first, be especially alert when assessing the arms, hands, legs, feet, and ankles of an ambulatory client or the buttocks and sacrum of a bedridden client. If edema is present, determine its type (pitting or nonpitting), location, extent, and symmetry (unilateral or symmetrical). If the client has pitting edema, assess the degree of pitting. (For more information, see *Evaluating pitting edema* in Chapter 14, Urinary System.)

Edema can result from congestive heart failure or venous insufficiency, which may be caused by varicosities or thrombophlebitis. Chronic right heart failure may even cause ascites (fluid effusion into the peritoneal cavity), which leads to generalized edema and abdominal distention. Venous compression in a specific area may result in localized edema along the path of the compressed vessel.

While inspecting the client's skin, note the location, size, number, and appearance of any lesions. Certain types of lesions may indicate cardiovascular disorders. For example, dry, open lesions on the lower extremities accompanied by pallor, cool skin, and lack of hair growth signify arterial insufficiency as seen with arterial peripheral vascular disease. Wet, open lesions with red or purplish edges that appear on the legs may result from the venous stasis associated with venous peripheral vascular disease.

Inspect the hair on the client's arms and legs. Although genetic factors determine hair distribution and density for an individual client, hair should be distributed symmetrically and should grow thicker on the anterior surface of the arms and legs in all clients. Lack of normal body hair on the arms and legs may indicate diminished arterial blood flow to these areas.

While examining the arms and legs, note whether their length is proportionate to the length of the trunk. Long, thin arms and legs may be a sign of Marfan's syndrome, a congenital disorder that also causes cardiovascular problems, such as aortic dissection, aortic valve incompetence, and cardiomyopathy.

Inspection of the nails can provide important information about the client's cardiovascular system. Fingernails normally appear smooth, rounded, and pinkish and have no markings. A bluish color in the nail beds indicates peripheral cyanosis.

Assess the capillary refill in the fingernails to estimate the rate of peripheral blood flow. To evaluate capillary refill, follow these steps. Apply pressure to the client's fingernail for 5 seconds. The area under pressure should blanch. Then remove the pressure and observe how rapidly the normal color returns to the fingernail. In a client with a good arterial supply, the color should return briskly, in less than 3 seconds. If capillary refill is delayed, note how many seconds it takes for the color to return to the nail. Delayed capillary refill suggests reduced circulation to that area, which can occur with low cardiac output and may lead to arterial insufficiency.

Assess the angle between the nail and the cuticle, which should be less than 180 degrees. An angle of 180 degrees or greater indicates finger clubbing, which may be accompanied by enlarged finger tips with spongey, slightly swollen nail bases. Finger clubbing commonly indicates chronic tissue hypoxia. (For more information, see *Finger clubbing* in Chapter 10, Respiratory System.)

Also inspect the shape of the nails, which should be smooth and rounded. A concave depression in the middle of a thin nail indicates koilonychia (spoon nail), a sign of iron-deficiency anemia. This disorder can affect the heart by reducing the ability of the blood to carry oxygen.

Finally, check for splinter hemorrhages—small, thin, red or brown lines that run from the base to the tip of the nail. Splinter hemorrhages develop in clients with bacterial endocarditis.

Eyes. The eyes should be clear and bright, and the eyelids free of lesions. Inspect the eyelids for xanthelasmas—small, slightly raised, yellowish plaques that usually appear around the inner canthus. Because these plaques result from lipid deposits, they may signal severe hyperlipidemia, a risk factor of cardiac disease.

Observe the color of the sclerae, which normally appear white. Yellowish sclerae may be the first sign of jaundice, which typically results from a liver disorder but also may result from liver congestion caused by right heart failure. Next, inspect the eyes for arcus senilis—a thin grayish ring around the edge of the cornea. Although arcus senilis is a common effect of aging that normally appears in elderly clients, it can indicate hyperlipidemia in clients under age 65.

Using an ophthalmoscope, examine the retinal structures, including the retinal vessels and background. The retina should be light yellow to orange and the background free from hemorrhages and exudates. Structural changes, such as narrowing or blocking of a vein where an arteriole crosses over, indicate hypertension. Soft exudates may suggest hypertension or subacute bacterial endocarditis. (For more information, see *Advanced assessment skills: Ophthalmoscopic examination* in Chapter 9, Eyes and Ears.)

Also note the client's ability to hold the head still. A slight, rhythmic bobbing of the head in time with the heartbeat is Musset's sign, which may accompany the high back pressure caused by aortic insufficiency or aneurysm.

Inspection

After evaluating related body structures, assess the cardiovascular system. Guidelines for inspection are described in the following paragraphs, beginning with a general inspection of the chest and thorax. Expose the client's anterior chest and observe its general appearance. Normally, the lateral diameter is twice the anteroposterior diameter. Note any deviations from the typical chest shape.

Jugular veins

Next, inspect the neck for jugular vein distention. When the client is supine, the neck veins normally protrude; when the client stands, they normally lie flat. When the client sits at a 45-degree angle in semi-Fowler's position, the jugular vein will appear distended only if the client has right heart dysfunction. To check for jugular vein distention, place the client in semi-Fowler's position with the head turned slightly away from the side being examined. Use tangential lighting (lighting from the side) to cast small shadows along the neck, which allow you to see pulse wave movement better.

If distention is present, characterize it as mild, moderate, or severe. Determine the level of distention in fingerbreadths above the clavicle or in relation to the jaw or clavicle. Also, note the amount of distention in relation to the head elevation.

Next, evaluate central venous pressure. The jugular vein demonstrates right heart pressure just as the mercury in a sphygmomanometer column demonstrates blood pressure. Because of this relationship, jugular vein distention can provide a rough estimate of central venous pressure. (For an illustrated procedure, see *Estimating central venous pressure,* page 310.)

Precordium

Before inspecting the precordium (the area over the heart), place the client supine with the head flat or elevated for respiratory comfort. Stand to the right of the client. Then identify the necessary anatomic landmarks. (For an illustration, see *Precordium inspection and palpation,* page 311.)

Using tangential lighting to cast shadows across the chest, watch for chest wall movement, visible pulsations, and exaggerated lifts or heaves (strong outward thrusts palpated over the chest during systole) in all six areas of the precordium: sternoclavicular, aortic, pulmonic, right ventricular, left ventricular, and epigastric. If pulsations are difficult to see in an obese client or a client with large breasts, perform inspection with the client sitting. This position brings the heart closer to the anterior chest wall and makes pulsations more noticeable.

Inspection normally reveals pulsations at the point of maximum impulse (PMI) of the apical impulse. The apical impulse (pulsations at the apex of the heart) normally appears in the fifth intercostal space at or just medial to the midclavicular line. This impulse reflects the location and size of the heart, especially of the left ventricle. A slight sternal movement and pulsations over the pulmonary arteries or the aorta may be normal in thin adults and in children. Visible pulsations in the epigastric area also may be normal in these clients.

Abnormal findings

On inspection, the chest shape may reveal an abnormality, such as barrel chest (rounded thoracic cage caused by chronic obstructive pulmonary disease), pectus excavatum (depressed sternum), scoliosis (lateral curvature of the spine), or kyphosis (convex curvature of the thoracic spine). If severe enough, these conditions can impair cardiac output by preventing chest expansion and inhibiting heart muscle movement.

Retractions (visible indentations of the soft tissue covering the chest wall) or the use of accessory muscles to breathe typically results from a respiratory disorder but may also be caused by a cardiovascular disorder that affects the respiratory system, such as a congenital heart defect or congestive heart failure.

Jugular vein distention occurs when the right atrial pressure is above normal. It reflects an increase in fluid volume caused by right heart dysfunction.

During precordium inspection, any visible pulsation to the right of the sternum is abnormal and may indicate an aortic aneurysm. A pulsation in the sternoclavicular or epigastric area also may indicate an aortic aneurysm. A sustained, forceful apical impulse suggests left ventricular hypertrophy, which increases blood pressure and may cause cardiomyopathy and mitral regurgitation. A laterally displaced apical impulse may be a sign of left ventricular hypertrophy.

Estimating central venous pressure

The nurse can estimate a client's central venous pressure indirectly by determining the height from the right atrium to the highest level of visible pulsation in the jugular vein. To begin, place the client at a 45-degree angle and use tangential lighting to observe the internal jugular vein. Note the highest level of visible pulsation.

Next, locate the angle of Louis, or sternal angle. To do this, palpate the clavicles where they join the sternum (the suprasternal notch). Place two of your fingers on the suprasternal notch and slide them down the sternum until they reach a bony protuberance. This is the angle of Louis. The right atrium lies about 2" (5 cm) below this point.

To estimate central venous pressure, measure the vertical distance between the highest level of visible pulsation and the angle of Louis. Normally, this distance is less than 1⅛" (3 cm). Add 2" (5 cm) to this figure to estimate the total distance between the highest level of pulsation and the right atrium. A total that exceeds 4" (10 cm) may indicate elevated central venous pressure and right ventricular failure.

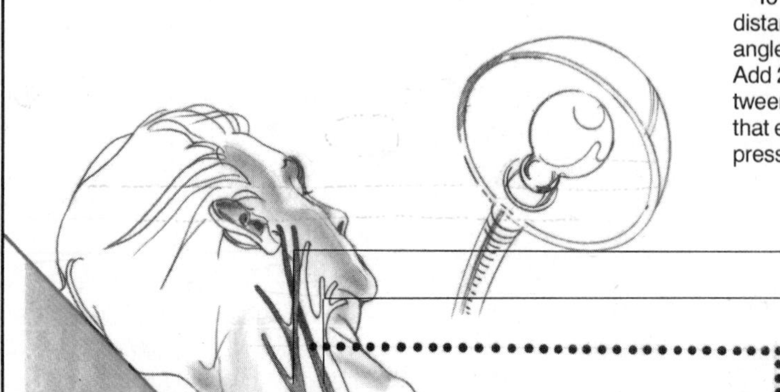

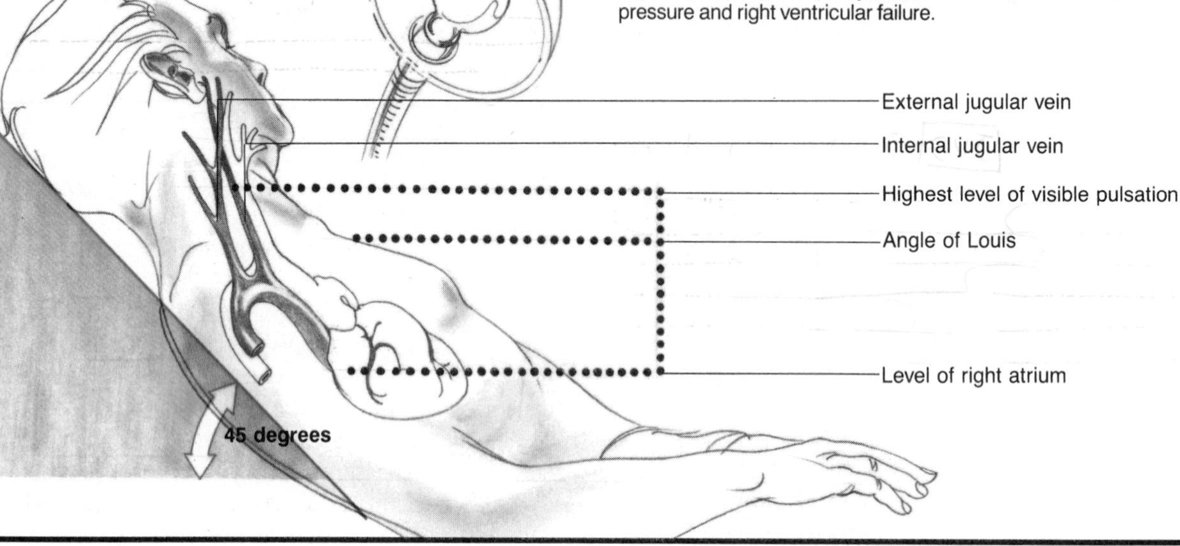

Palpation

To continue the physical assessment, palpate the peripheral pulses and precordium according to the following guidelines. To aid palpation, ensure that the client is positioned comfortably, draped appropriately, and kept warm. Also, be sure to warm your hands and use gentle to moderate pressure for palpation.

Pulses

While assessing the client's vital signs, you palpated the radial pulse to assess the heart rate quickly. Now palpate the other major pulse points to assess blood flow to the tissues. The larger central arteries (the carotids) lie closer to the heart and have slightly higher pressures than the smaller peripheral arteries. Because of this, the central arteries demonstrate pulsations before the peripheral arteries and are easier to palpate.

Palpate the carotid, brachial, radial, femoral, popliteal, dorsalis pedis, and posterior tibial pulses. These arteries are close to the body surface and lie over bones, making palpation easier. (For illustrations of these pulse sites, see *Palpating arterial pulses,* pages 312 and 313.)

Be sure to press gently over the pulse sites; excess pressure can obliterate the pulsation, making the pulse appear absent when it is not. Also, palpate only one carotid artery at a time; simultaneous palpation can slow the pulse or decrease the blood pressure, causing the client to faint.

During palpation, identify the pulse rate, rhythm, symmetry, contour, and strength at each site. The normal pulse rate varies with age and other factors but usually ranges from 60 to 100 beats/minute in adults. The pulses should feel regular in rhythm and equal in strength bilaterally. Their contour should include a smooth upstroke and downstroke. Pulses with a normal amplitude are easily palpable and obliterated only with strong finger pressure. (For more information, see *Identifying normal and abnormal pulses,* pages 314 and 315.)

Grade the pulse amplitude bilaterally at each site, using the pulse rating scale required by the health care facility. (For an example of a commonly used rating scale, see *Documenting pulse amplitude* in Chapter 4, Physical Assessment Skills.) Also be sure to document any variations in rate, rhythm, contour, symmetry, and strength.

Precordium inspection and palpation

To detect normal and abnormal pulsations over the precordium, the nurse should inspect and palpate six different areas according to the following guidelines.

1 Locate the six precordial areas by using the anatomic landmarks named for the underlying structures.

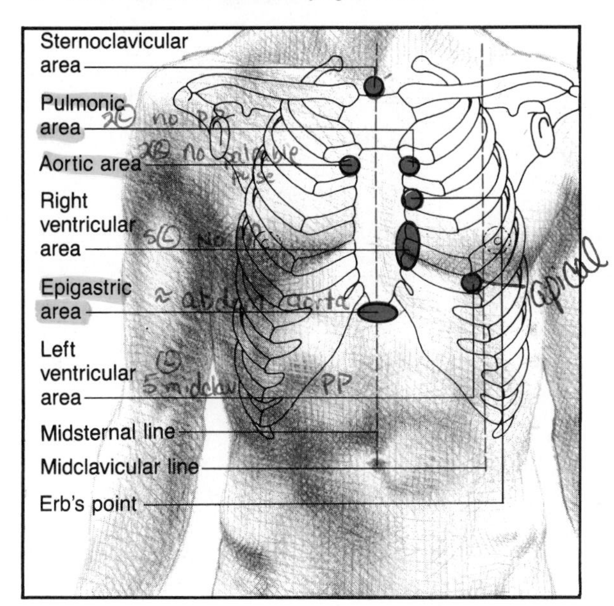

2 Then palpate (or inspect) the *sternoclavicular area,* which lies at the top of the sternum at the junction of the clavicles. Move to the *aortic area* located in the second intercostal space on the right sternal border. Next, assess the *pulmonic area* found in the second intercostal space on the left sternal border. Follow this with palpation at the point where the fifth rib joins the left sternal border—the *right ventricular area.* Then assess the *left ventricular area (apical area),* as illustrated, which falls at the fifth intercostal space at the midclavicular line. Finally, palpate the *epigastric area* at the base of the sternum between the cartilage of the left and right seventh ribs.

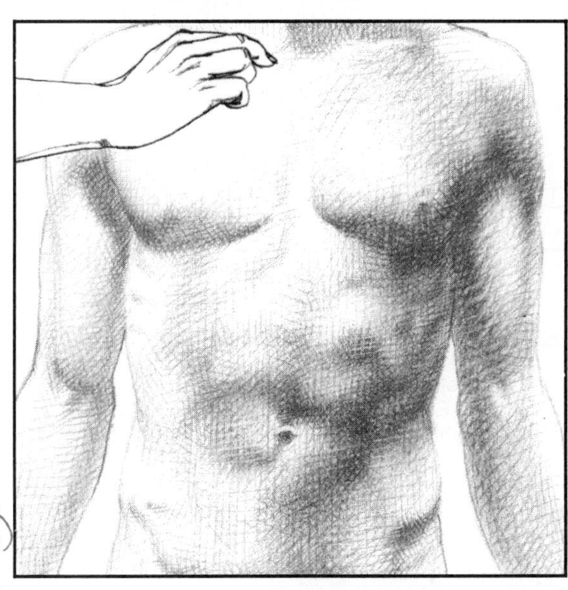

Precordium

When palpating the precordium, use the pads of the fingers because they are especially sensitive to vibrations and can effectively assess large pulse sites. Be sure to follow a systematic palpation sequence that covers the sternoclavicular, aortic, pulmonic, right ventricular, left ventricular (apical), and epigastric areas. (For an illustration, see *Precordium inspection and palpation.*) Most health care professionals start at the sternoclavicular area and move methodically through the palpation sequence down to the epigastric area. At the sternoclavicular area, you may feel pulsation of the aortic arch, especially in a thin or average-build client. In the epigastric area, you may palpate the abdominal aorta pulsation in a thin client.

To locate the apical impulse, place your fingers over the apical area—a spot at the midclavicular line in the fifth intercostal space. For most clients, this is the PMI, the place where pulsations are felt best. In fact, the apical area is commonly the only place where pulsations are palpable; light palpation should reveal a tap with each heartbeat over a space that is roughly ¾" (2 cm) in diameter. Moderately strong, the normal apical impulse demonstrates a swift upstroke and downstroke early in systole, caused by the left ventricular movement. The duration of the normal pulse is about one third that of the cardiac cycle, if the heart rate is less than 100 beats/minute. It should correlate with the first heart sound and carotid pulsation. Normally, pulsations should not be palpable over the aortic, pulmonic, or right ventricular area.

(Text continues on page 315)

Palpating arterial pulses

The arteries that are close to the surface and over bone are the easiest to palpate. To palpate the arterial pulses, apply pressure with the index and middle fingers. Palpate gently, or you may obliterate the pulses, especially those in the legs, which are farthest from the heart and therefore have the lowest pressure. As you palpate, proceed systematically from head to toe, noting the pulse rate, rhythm, symmetry, contour, and strength at each site. (To determine symmetry, compare the pulse on one side of the body to that on the other side of the body.)

Carotid pulse
Lightly place your fingers just medial to the trachea and below the jaw angle.

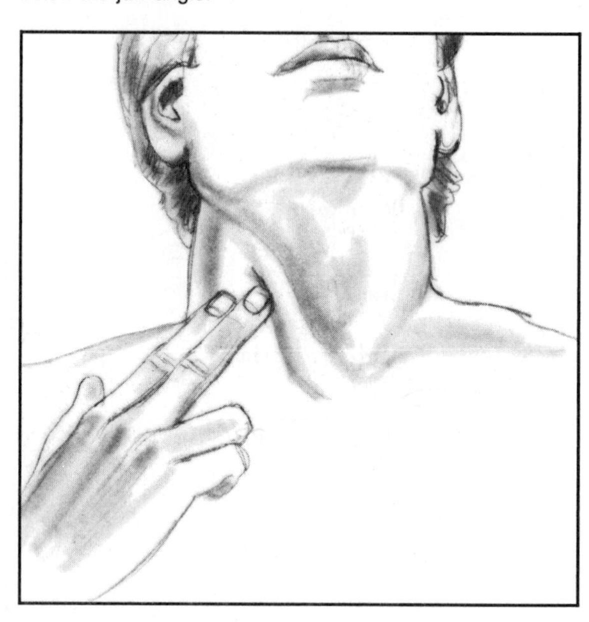

Femoral pulse
Press relatively hard at a point inferior to the inguinal ligament. For an obese client, palpate in the crease of the groin halfway between the pubic bone and the hip bone.

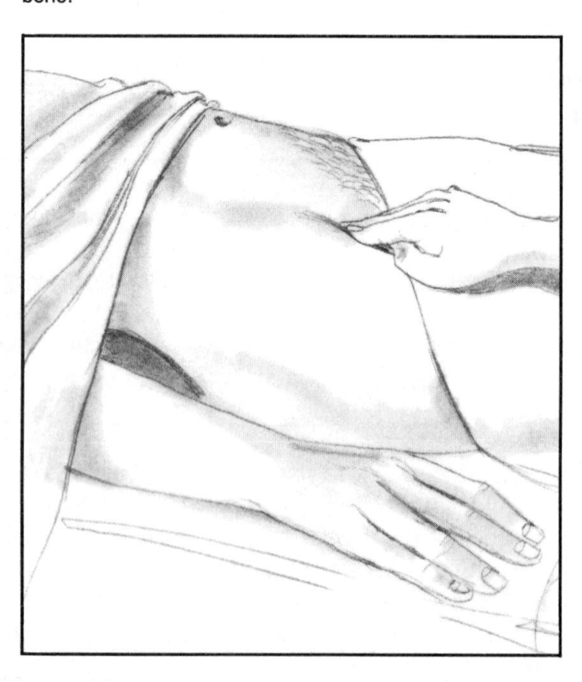

Popliteal pulse
Press firmly against the popliteal fossa at the back of the knee.

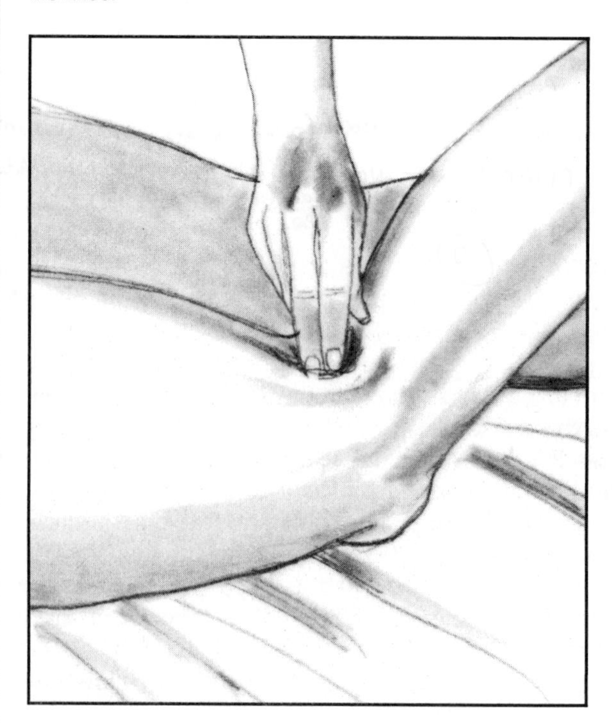

Brachial pulse
Position your fingers medial to the biceps tendon.

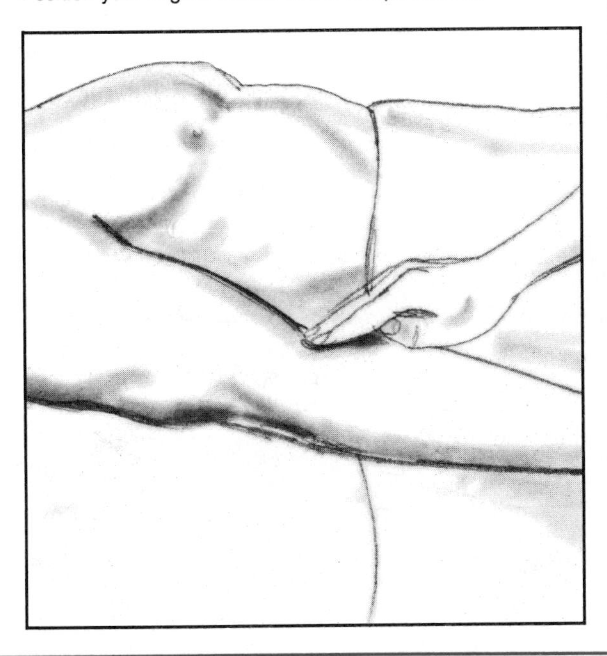

Radial pulse
Apply gentle pressure to the medial and ventral side of the wrist just below the thumb.

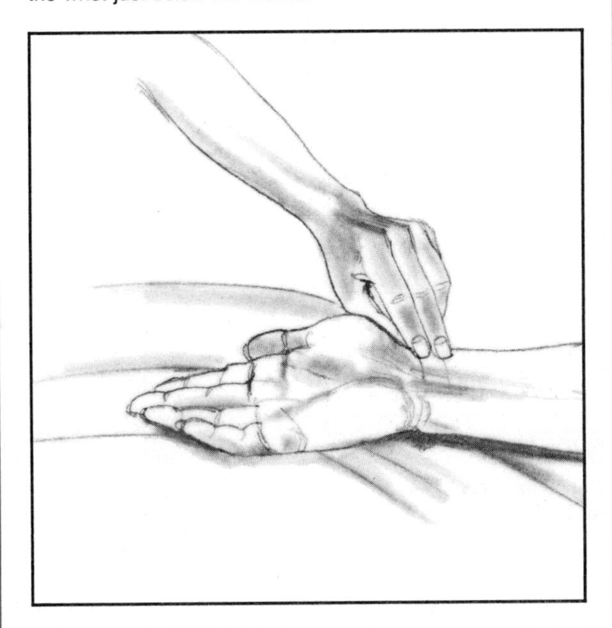

Dorsalis pedis pulse
Place your fingers on the medial dorsum of the foot while the client points the toes down. In this site, the pulse is difficult to palpate and may seem to be absent in some healthy clients.

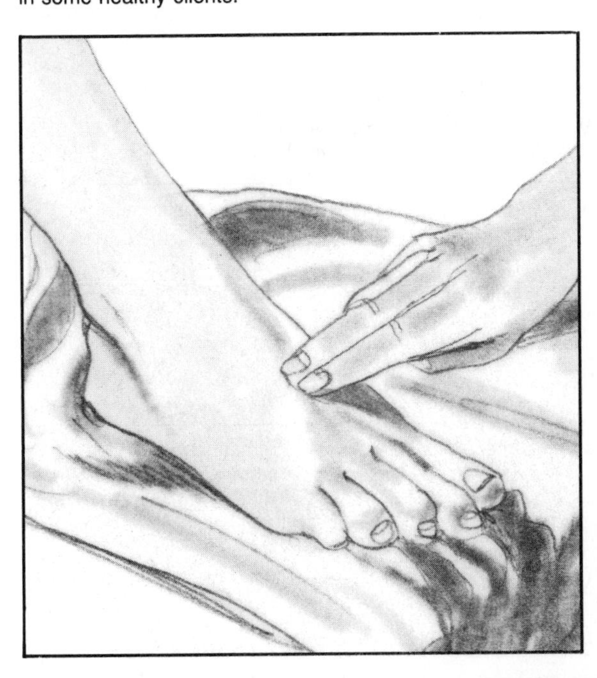

Posterior tibial pulse
Apply pressure behind and slightly below the malleolus of the ankle.

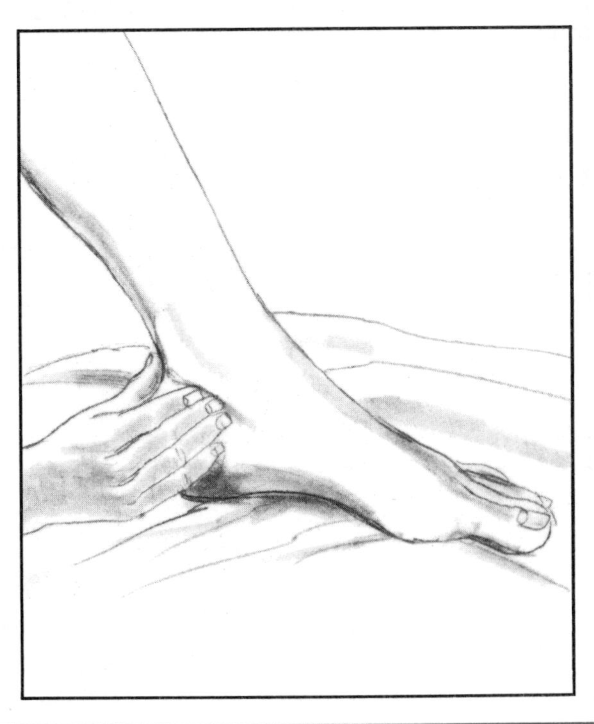

Identifying normal and abnormal pulses

To identify various pulse abnormalities, the nurse should compare the client's peripheral pulse wave to the normal pulse wave shown here. Several common pulse abnormalities are associated with cardiovascular disorders, as described in the chart below.

NORMAL PULSE

As shown in this illustration, a normal pulse has two components: systole and diastole. Indicated by the initial upstroke, systole signifies the arterial pressure during ventricular contraction. Diastole, the downstroke, indicates the arterial pressure during ventricular relaxation when the heart fills.

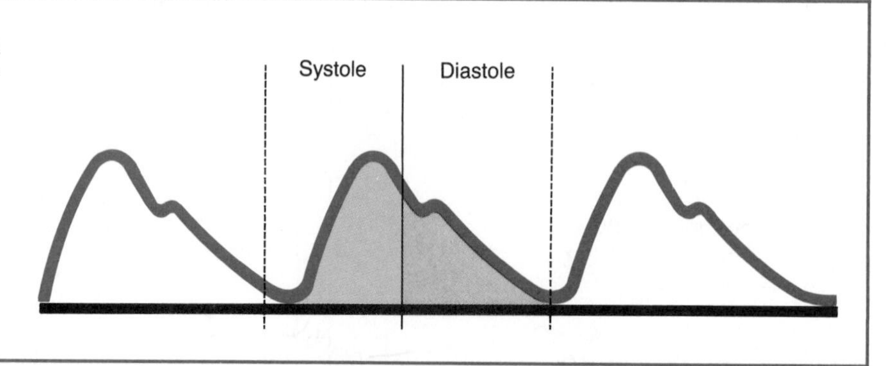

ABNORMAL PULSES

PULSE ABNORMALITY	DESCRIPTION	POSSIBLE CAUSE
Corrigan's pulse (water hammer pulse)	Increased pulse pressure with a rapid upstroke and downstroke and a shortened peak 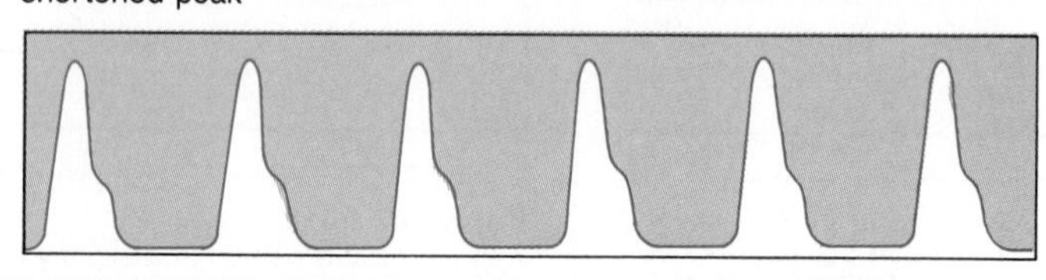	Aortic regurgitation, patent ductus arteriosus, systemic arteriosclerosis
Large, bounding pulse	Bounding pulse in which a great surge precedes a sudden absence of force or fullness 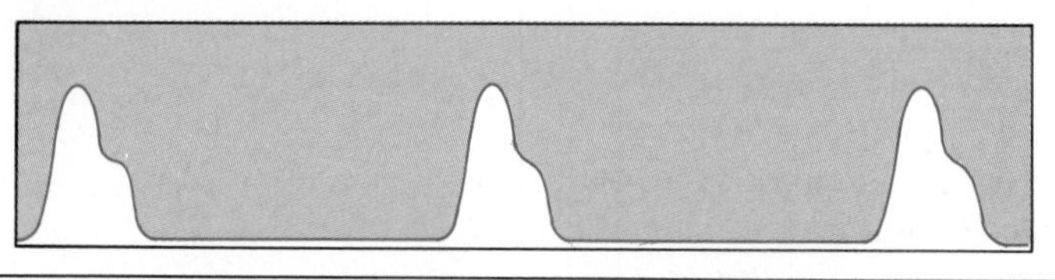	Increased stroke volume, as in aortic regurgitation; increased stiffness of arterial walls, as in atherosclerosis or normal aging; exercise; anxiety; fever; hypertension
Pulsus alternans	Regular pulse rhythm with alternation of weak and strong beats (amplitude or volume) 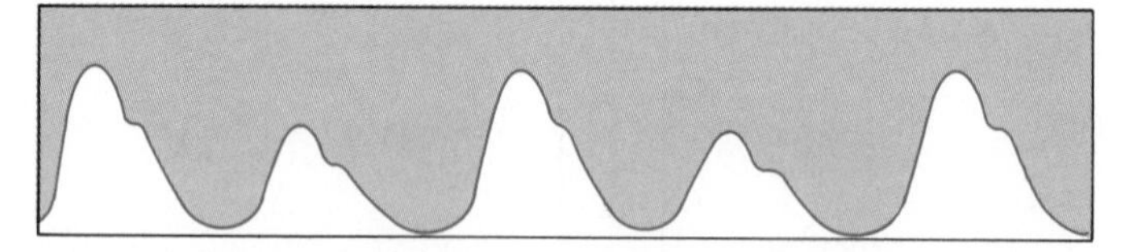	Left ventricular failure
Pulsus bigeminus	Irregular pulse rhythm in which premature beats alternate with sinus beats 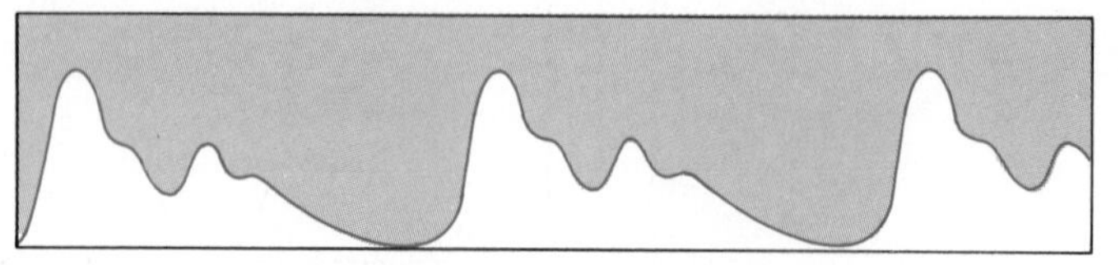	Premature ventricular beats caused by heart failure, hypoxia, or other condition

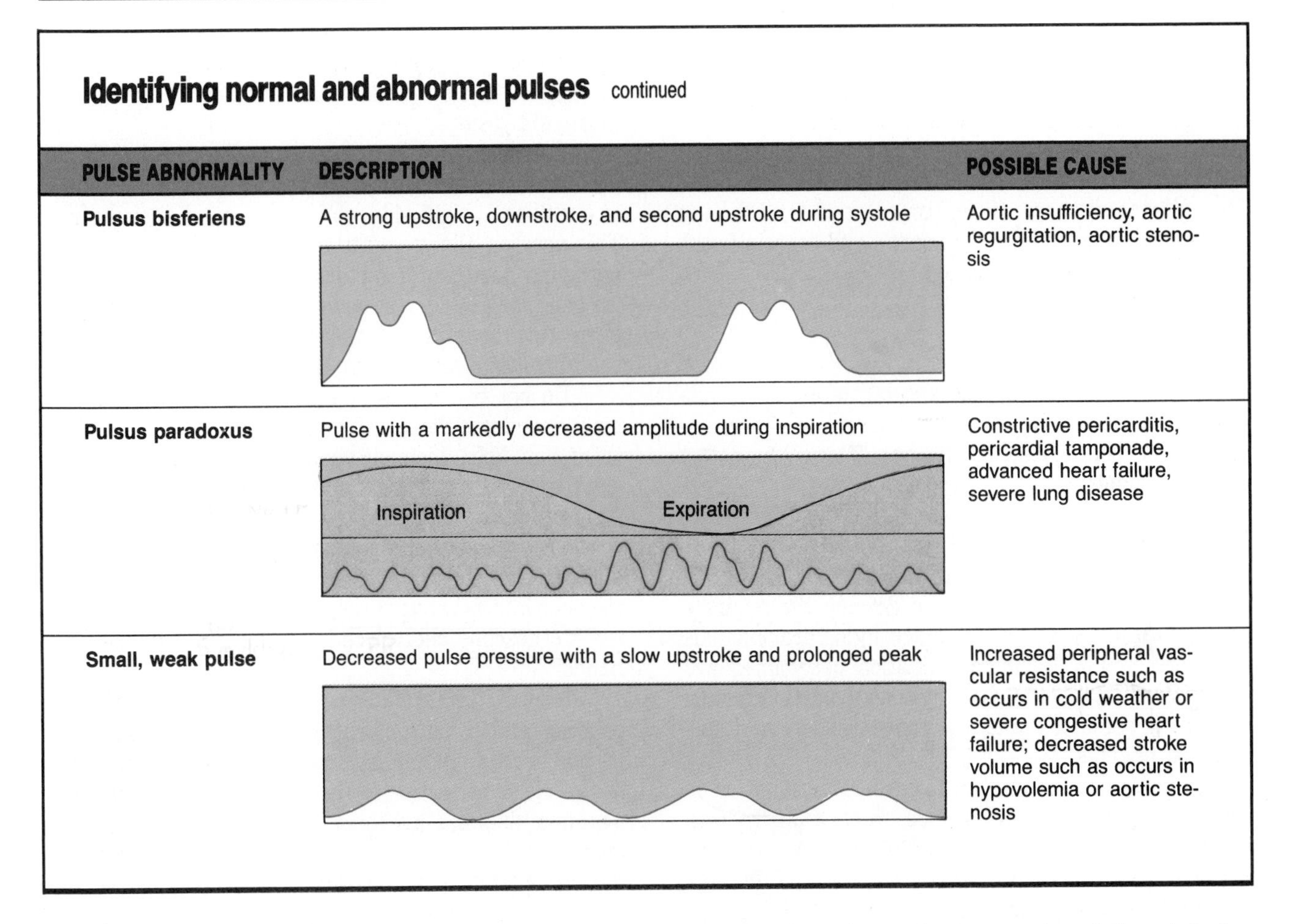

Identifying normal and abnormal pulses continued

PULSE ABNORMALITY	DESCRIPTION	POSSIBLE CAUSE
Pulsus bisferiens	A strong upstroke, downstroke, and second upstroke during systole	Aortic insufficiency, aortic regurgitation, aortic stenosis
Pulsus paradoxus	Pulse with a markedly decreased amplitude during inspiration	Constrictive pericarditis, pericardial tamponade, advanced heart failure, severe lung disease
Small, weak pulse	Decreased pulse pressure with a slow upstroke and prolonged peak	Increased peripheral vascular resistance such as occurs in cold weather or severe congestive heart failure; decreased stroke volume such as occurs in hypovolemia or aortic stenosis

Abnormal findings

A weak pulse indicates either low cardiac output or increased peripheral vascular resistance, as in arterial atherosclerotic disease. Weak pedal pulses are common in elderly clients; however, absence of a pulse in a warm foot with normal color carries little significance. A strong bounding pulse occurs in clients with hypertension and in high cardiac output states such as exercise, pregnancy, anemia, and thyrotoxicosis.

A more forceful and longer apical impulse (lasting longer than one third of the cardiac cycle) may indicate increased cardiac output; a displaced or diffuse impulse may indicate left ventricular hypertrophy. A pulsation in the aortic, pulmonic, or right ventricular area can result from chamber enlargement or valvular disease. A pulsation in the sternoclavicular or epigastric area suggests an aortic aneurysm.

A palpable thrill (fine vibration) indicates blood flow turbulence, usually related to valvular dysfunction. If a thrill is present, determine how far it radiates. Make a mental note to listen for a murmur at this site during auscultation. A heave (a strong outward thrust during systole) along the left sternal border may indicate right ventricular hypertrophy; over the left ventricular area, a ventricular aneurysm. In a thin client, a heave may occur when cardiac output is increased and contraction is more forceful, such as with exercise, fever, or anxiety. A displaced PMI suggests left ventricular hypertrophy caused by volume overload from a disorder, such as mitral or aortic stenosis, a septal defect, or acute myocardial infarction. DO NOT Palpate over visible epigastric pulse.

Percussion

The nurse may percuss the borders of the heart to estimate its size. However, most clients with cardiovascular signs and symptoms receive chest X-rays, which eliminate the need for percussion by providing more exact information about the heart. Also, many clients with cardiovascular disorders exhibit related lung problems, which reduce the accuracy of percussion.

As part of the complete cardiovascular assessment, use mediate percussion to identify the size of the heart. Beginning at the anterior left axillary line, percuss toward the sternum in the fifth intercostal space. The percussion note changes from resonance to dullness at the left border of the heart, usually near the PMI. On the right, the border of the heart lies under the sternum and cannot be percussed. Percussion should locate the left border of the heart at the midclavicular line in the fifth intercostal space. If the border extends to the left of the midclavicular line, the heart—and especially the left ventricle—may be enlarged.

Auscultation

To complete the basic cardiovascular assessment, auscultate the precordium to detect heart sounds, and auscultate the central and peripheral arteries to detect vascular sounds.

Precordium

The cardiovascular system requires more auscultation than any other body system. To develop the requisite skill, practice auscultating and identifying heart sounds in the precordium. During auscultation, use your knowledge of cardiac anatomy and physiology and information from other parts of the assessment to understand auscultation findings.

Initially, gain experience in cardiac auscultation on clients with normal heart sounds, rates, and rhythms. Then move to clients with known abnormal sounds, seeking help from experts to identify auscultation findings. Remember that you must know how to identify normal findings before you can detect abnormal ones. So concentrate first on hearing the normal sounds rather than trying to identify abnormalities.

Auscultation of heart sounds can be difficult. Even with a stethoscope, you will find that the amount of tissue between the source of the sound and the outer chest wall can affect which sounds you can hear. Fat, muscle, and air tend to reduce sound transmission. Thus, if a client is obese or has a muscular chest wall or hyperinflated lungs, the sounds may seem more distant and difficult to hear. These natural limitations require the nurse to control the environment as much as possible during auscultation.

To prepare to auscultate a client's cardiovascular system, make sure that the room is as quiet as possible. If the client has special equipment, such as an oxygen nebulizer or suction device, try to schedule auscultation for a time when the equipment can be turned off temporarily.

Next, select a stethoscope with a chestpiece that is sized appropriately for the client's chest. If necessary, choose a pediatric chestpiece for a thin adult. Use the diaphragm of the stethoscope to detect high-pitched heart sounds, such as the normal S_1 and S_2 sounds. Use the bell to identify low-pitched sounds, such as mitral murmurs and gallops.

Help the client into a supine position, either flat or at a comfortable elevation. If you are right-handed, stand at the client's right side while performing auscultation. This position allows you to manipulate the stethoscope with your dominant hand and assist the client with your nondominant hand. Use alternate positions, as needed, to improve heart sound auscultation. (For illustrations, see *Positioning the client for cardiac auscultation.*)

Do not try to auscultate through clothing or surgical dressings; these will muffle heart sounds or make them inaudible. Instead, open the front of the client's gown and drape the client appropriately to limit the area exposed during auscultation.

Then explain the procedure to the client, and instruct the client to breathe normally, inhaling through the nose and exhaling through the mouth. Finally, warm the stethoscope chestpiece by rubbing it between your hands.

Identify the cardiac auscultation sites. Because the opening and closing of the heart valves create most normal heart sounds, auscultation sites lie close together in the chest behind or to the left of the sternum. Auscultation sites are not located directly over the valves, but lie over the pathways the blood takes as it flows through chambers and valves. (For an illustration, see *Cardiac auscultation*, page 318.)

Now auscultate, listening selectively for each cardiac cycle component. Move the stethoscope slowly and methodically over the four main auscultation sites. Remember to follow the same auscultation sequence during every cardiovascular assessment.

Concentrate to hear the relatively quiet heart sounds. Closing your eyes while you listen for specific sounds may help you concentrate. Remember that stethoscope movement, especially over chest hair, or client movement or shivering creates noise that will interfere with your hearing cardiac sounds clearly. So keep your hand steady, and ask the client to remain as still as possible.

To assess heart sounds, begin by listening for a few cycles to become accustomed to the rate and rhythm of the sounds. Two sounds normally occur: the first heart sound (S_1) and the second heart sound (S_2), which are separated by a silent period.

During auscultation, characterize heart sounds by their pitch (frequency), intensity (loudness), duration, and timing in the cardiac cycle. Normal heart sounds have a brief duration (a fraction of a second) and are

Positioning the client for cardiac auscultation

During auscultation, the nurse usually stands to the right of the client, who is in a supine position. The client may lie flat or at a comfortable elevation.

If heart sounds seem faint or undetectable, try repositioning the client. Alternate positioning may enhance the sounds or make them seem louder by bringing the heart closer to the surface of the chest. Common alternate positions include a seated, forward-leaning position and the left-lateral recumbent position.

Forward-leaning position

This position is best for hearing high-pitched sounds related to semilunar valve problems, such as aortic and pulmonic valve murmurs. To auscultate these sounds, help the client to the forward-leaning position and place the diaphragm of the stethoscope over the aortic and pulmonic areas in the right and left second intercostal space.

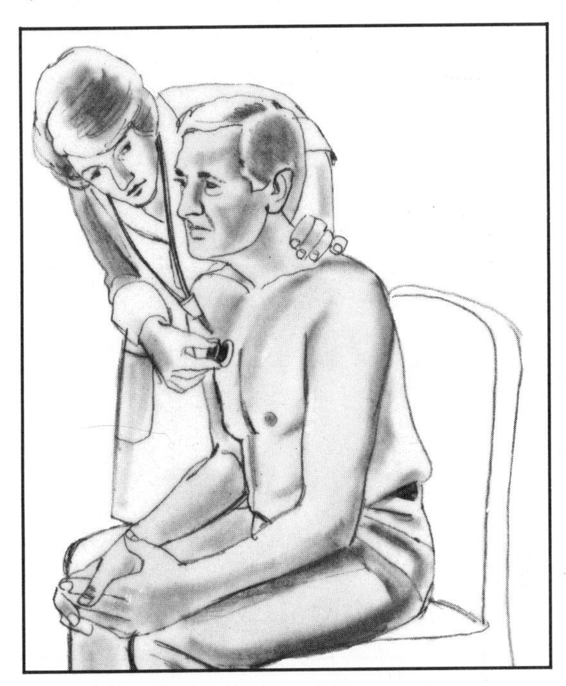

Left-lateral recumbent position

This position is best for hearing low-pitched sounds related to atrioventricular valve problems, such as mitral valve murmurs and extra heart sounds. To auscultate these sounds, help the client to the left-lateral recumbent position and place the bell of the stethoscope over the apical area. If these positions do not enhance heart sounds, try auscultating with the client standing or squatting.

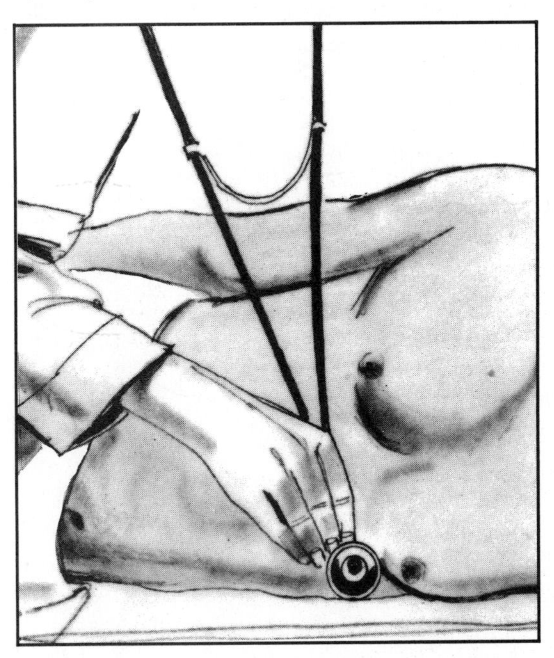

followed by slightly longer periods of silence. The timing of heart sounds in relation to the cardiac cycle is particularly important. (For more information, see *Events in the cardiac cycle,* page 292.)

The first heart sound—the *lub* of *lub-dub*—marks the beginning of systole. It occurs as the mitral and tricuspid valves close. This event immediately precedes the increase in ventricular pressure, aortic and pulmonic valve opening, and the ejection of blood into the circulation. All of these events occur within one third of a second. The mitral valve actually closes slightly before the tricuspid valve. An experienced examiner may be able to discriminate the sound of each valve closing, which sounds somewhat like *li-lub*. This occurrence is called a split S_1. However, an inexperienced examiner could confuse a split S_1 with an abnormal extra sound occurring just before S_1. The first heart sound is louder in the mitral and tricuspid listening areas (*LUB-dub*) and softer in the aortic and pulmonic areas (*lub-DUB*).

Carefully compare the loudness of the normal heart sounds at each site; this will help you differentiate systole from diastole. Identifying the phases of the cardiac cycle is necessary to time any abnormal sounds that

Cardiac auscultation

Auscultation is the most important technique used to assess the cardiovascular system. To perform cardiac ausculation, follow these guidelines.

1. Locate the four different auscultation sites, as illustrated. The shaded areas indicate the auscultation sites; the arrows show the direction of the blood flow from the valve creating the sound. In the aortic area, blood moves from the left ventricle during systole, crossing the aortic valve and flowing through the aortic arch. In the pulmonic area, blood ejected from the right ventricle during systole crosses the pulmonic valve and flows through the main pulmonary artery. In the tricuspid area, sounds reflect blood movement from the right atrium across the tricuspid valve, filling the right ventricle during diastole. In the mitral, or apical, area, sounds represent blood flow across the mitral valve and left ventricular filling during diastole.

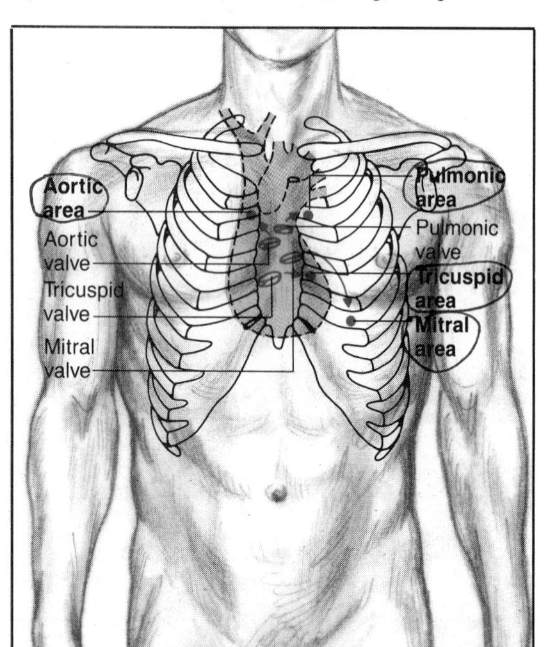

2. Then begin auscultation in the aortic area, placing the stethoscope in the second intercostal space along the right sternal border, as shown. Continue auscultation by moving to the pulmonic area, located in the second intercostal space at the left sternal border. Then assess in the third auscultation site, the tricuspid area, which lies in the fourth intercostal space along the left sternal border. Finally, listen in the mitral area, located in the fifth intercostal space near the midclavicular line. (If the client's heart is enlarged, the mitral area may be closer to the anterior axillary line.)

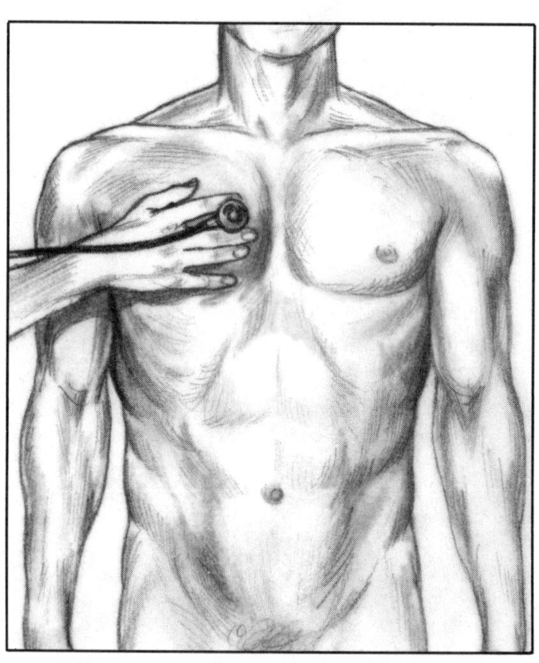

can occur. You also can identify the S_1 by palpating the carotid pulse during auscultation. The pulse upstroke occurs almost simultaneously with the first heart sound.

The second heart sound—the *dub* of *lub-dub*—occurs at the beginning of diastole. Because closing of the aortic and pulmonic valves produces the S_2 sound, this sound is louder in the aortic and pulmonic areas of the chest. At these sites, the sequence sounds like *lub-DUB*. The second heart sound coincides with the pulse downstroke. At normal rates, the diastolic pause between S_2 and the next S_1 exceeds the systolic pause between S_1 and S_2.

During auscultation, S_2 may have a split sound, like that of a broken syllable. This sound may be normal because the aortic and pulmonic valves that produce the sound do not close at exactly the same time. A normal S_2 occurs during inspiration but disappears with expiration. This type of split S_2 commonly occurs in healthy children and young adults.

At each auscultatory site, use the diaphragm to listen closely to S_1 and S_2 and then compare them. Next, listen to the systolic period between S_1 and S_2 and the diastolic period between S_2 and the next S_1. Then, auscultate again, using the bell of the stethoscope. Both periods should be silent. If you hear any sounds during these periods, or any variations in the first and second heart sounds, document the characteristics of the sound, particularly noting the auscultatory site and the part of the cardiac cycle in which it occurred.

Arteries

The nurse should auscultate the carotid, femoral, and popliteal arteries as well as the abdominal aorta. (For an illustrated procedure, see *Arterial auscultation.*) Over the carotid, femoral, and popliteal arteries, auscultation should reveal no sounds; over the abdominal aorta, it may detect bowel sounds, but no vascular sounds.

Abnormal findings

Auscultation may detect first and second heart sounds that are accentuated, diminished, or inaudible. These abnormalities may result from pressure changes, valvular dysfunctions, and conduction defects. Auscultation also may reveal a prolonged, persistent, or reversed split sound, which may result from a mechanical or electrical problem. (For more information, see *Implications of abnormal heart sounds*, page 320.)

During auscultation of the central and peripheral arteries, the nurse may notice a bruit—a continuous sound caused by turbulent blood flow. A bruit over the carotid artery usually indicates atherosclerosis; over the femoral or popliteal arteries, narrowed vessels; over the abdominal aorta, an aneurysm (weakness in the arterial wall that allows a sac to form) or a dissection (a tear in the layers of the arterial wall). (For some common disorders associated with abnormal findings, see *Integrating assessment findings*, pages 321 and 322.)

Developmental considerations

The nurse must adjust the usual assessment techniques for pediatric, pregnant, and elderly clients. The nurse also needs to evaluate abnormal findings differently for these clients.

Pediatric client. Assess the developmental stage of the child. Height, weight, growth pattern, and motor and cognitive ability are important to assess, because cardiovascular dysfunction can retard their development.

Arterial auscultation

To assess the arteries, auscultate the carotid, femoral, and popliteal arteries and the abdominal aorta by following these steps.

First, ask the client to hold his or her breath while you auscultate. Then assess the carotid arteries by auscultating with the bell of the stethoscope bilaterally on both sides of the trachea, as shown. To evaluate the femoral and popliteal arteries, place the bell of the stethoscope over the pulse sites that were palpated earlier in the assessment. Finally, auscultate the abdominal artery by listening to the epigastric area. Normally, auscultation should detect no vascular sounds. This procedure may, however, detect a bruit (continuous vibrating, blowing, or rumbling noise), an abnormal sound caused by turbulent blood flow in the vessels.

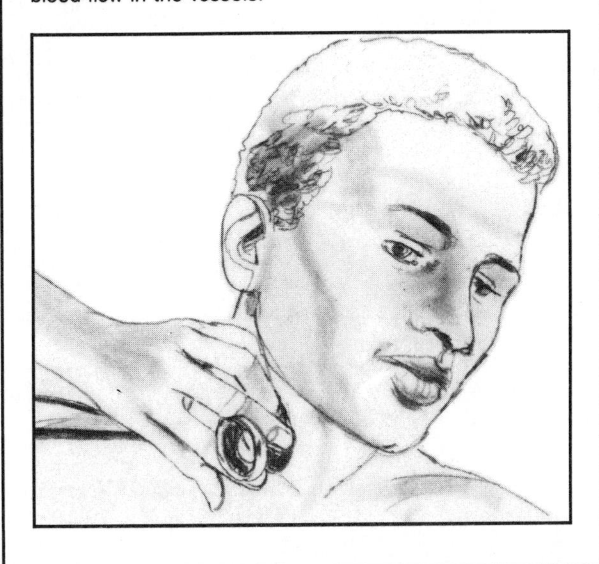

A neonate's pulse rate may range from 70 to 190—much faster than an adult's. As the child ages, the pulse rate gradually decreases to adult levels. A neonate's blood pressure is normally much lower than that of an adult and gradually increases to adult levels with age. (For more information, see *The effect of age on vital signs* in Chapter 4, Physical Assessment Skills.)

In many normal, healthy children and young adults, auscultation reveals a split S_2. Splitting occurs during inspiration, when right ventricular ejection takes slightly longer than left ventricular ejection and causes a slight delay in the pulmonic valve closing. Inspiration decreases intrathoracic pressure, enhancing ventricular filling and increasing the delay, so the split normally occurs during inspiration. The inspiratory delay is long enough to allow the nurse to discriminate two separate components of S_2, which sound like *di-dub* and reflect the aortic and pulmonic valve closings. Splitting is less likely to occur

Implications of abnormal heart sounds

Whenever basic or advanced auscultation reveals an abnormal heart sound, the nurse must accurately identify the sound as well as its location and timing in the cardiac cycle. The location will provide baseline information; the other characteristics can help identify the possible cause of the sound, as shown in the chart below.

ABNORMAL HEART SOUND	TIMING	POSSIBLE CAUSES
Basic auscultation		
Accentuated S_1	Beginning of systole	Mitral stenosis; fever
Diminished S_1	Beginning of systole	Mitral regurgitation; severe mitral regurgitation with calcified immobile valve; heart block
Split S_1	Beginning of systole	Right bundle branch block
Accentuated S_2	End of systole	Pulmonary or systemic hypertension
Diminished or inaudible S_2	End of systole	Aortic or pulmonary stenosis
Persistent S_2 split	End of systole	Delayed closure of the pulmonic valve, usually from overfilling of the right ventricle, causing prolonged systolic ejection time
Reversed or paradoxical S_2 split that appears in expiration and disappears in inspiration	End of systole	Delayed ventricular stimulation; left bundle branch block or prolonged left ventricular ejection time
Advanced auscultation		
S_3 (ventricular gallop)	Early diastole	Normal in children and young adults; overdistention of ventricles in rapid-filling segment of diastole; mitral insufficiency; ventricular failure
S_4 (atrial gallop or presystolic extra sound)	Late diastole	Forceful atrial contraction from resistance to ventricular filling late in diastole; left ventricular hypertrophy, pulmonary stenosis, hypertension, coronary artery disease, and aortic stenosis
Pericardial friction rub (grating or leathery sound at left sternal border; usually muffled, high pitched, and transient)	Throughout systole and diastole	Pericardial inflammation

during expiration, because the semilunar valves close more synchronously, but it can occur with dysrhythmias, septal defects, and pulmonary disease. A displaced PMI in a child suggests coarctation of the aorta.

Pregnant client. In a pregnant client, heart sounds may seem loud and the PMI may be shifted slightly to the left. These normal physiologic findings occur as the enlarged uterus displaces the heart. During palpation of the pulses, the nurse may detect edema and varicosities, especially in the legs.

Elderly client. With age, the heart rate slows and the normal blood pressure may increase. Although the systolic and diastolic blood pressures both increase, the systolic pressure rise is greater because of the increased rigidity of the vascular tree.

During inspection of the sternoclavicular area, the nurse may detect obvious pulsations caused by calcification and dilation of the aorta. The superficial vessels of the forehead, neck, and extremities may feel prominent and ropelike during palpation.

Auscultation may be difficult in an elderly client because the chest is more likely to be barrel shaped,

Integrating assessment findings

Sometimes, a cluster of assessment findings will strongly suggest a particular cardiovascular disorder. In the chart below, column one shows groups of presenting signs and symptoms—the ones that make the client seek medical attention. Column two presents related assessment findings that the nurse may discover during the health history and physical assessment. The client may have one or more of these findings. Column three shows the possible disorder indicated by a cluster of these findings.

PRESENTING SIGNS AND SYMPTOMS	RELATED ASSESSMENT FINDINGS	POSSIBLE DISORDER
Dull or burning chest pain or a feeling of pressure, tightness, or heaviness that builds and fades gradually and that may radiate to the abdomen or to the jaw, teeth, face, or left arm; dyspnea, possibly with a sense of constriction around the larynx or upper trachea; palpitations or skipped beats	Family or personal history of coronary artery disease, atherosclerotic heart disease, cerebrovascular accident (CVA), diabetes, gout, or hypertension History of obesity caused by excessive carbohydrate and saturated fat intake; smoking; lack of exercise; stress (type A personality) Male client over age 40 Precipitating factors, such as exertion, stress, hot or cold weather, and emotions Anxiety Diaphoresis Tachycardia Blood pressure changes, possibly hypertension, particularly during episode of chest pain Transient crackles Paradoxical splitting of S_2	Angina pectoris
Constricting, crushing, heavy-weight-like chest pain that occurs suddenly and may build to maximum intensity in a few minutes and that usually affects the central and substernal areas but is not relieved by nitroglycerin; dyspnea, possibly accompanied by orthopnea, cough, and wheezing; fatigue and weakness; palpitations or skipped beats	Family or personal history of coronary artery disease, CVA, diabetes mellitus, gout, or hypertension History of obesity, smoking, lack of exercise, stress History of episodes of angina pectoris Anxiety, tenseness, sense of impending doom Nausea and vomiting Diaphoresis Pallor or cyanosis Tachycardia or bradycardia and weak pulse Normal or decreased blood pressure Distant-sounding gallop rhythm Pericardial friction rub Crackles	Acute myocardial infarction
Dyspnea with exertion accompanied by cough; orthopnea; paroxysmal nocturnal dyspnea; dyspnea at rest (in advanced disease); fatigue on exertion, accompanied by weakness; rapid heart rate and skipped beats	Use of pillows to improve breathing during sleep Wheezing on inspiration and expiration, daytime oliguria, nighttime polyuria, anorexia, progressive weight gain, generalized edema, fatigue Profuse diaphoresis Pallor or cyanosis Frothy white or pink sputum Heaving apical impulse Dullness at lung bases and basilar crackles S_3 and S_4 heart sounds Decreased or absent breath sounds	Left ventricular failure
Dyspnea; fatigue, in severe cases accompanied by weakness and confusion; irregular heartbeat; dependent edema that begins in ankles and progresses to the legs and genitalia (initially subsides at night, later does not); weight gain	Anorexia, right upper abdominal pain or discomfort on exertion, nausea, and vomiting History of left ventricular failure, mitral or pulmonic valve stenosis, tricuspid regurgitation, pulmonary hypertension, or chronic obstructive pulmonary disease Lower left sternal heave independent of apical impulse Enlarged, tender, pulsating liver Tricuspid regurgitation murmur Abdominal fluid wave and shifting dullness Jugular vein distention Tachycardia Right ventricular S_3 sound	Acute right ventricular failure

continued

Integrating assessment findings continued

PRESENTING SIGNS AND SYMPTOMS	RELATED ASSESSMENT FINDINGS	POSSIBLE DISORDER
Paroxysmal nocturnal dyspnea accompanied by orthopnea; fatigue; palpitations; dry skin; pain in arms and legs; possibly edema and ascites	Fever Signs of right or left heart failure, such as peripheral edema, basilar crackles, dyspnea, and tachycardia Cardiac impulse displaced to the left Systolic murmur S_3 heart sound Orthostatic hypotension	Cardiomyopathies
Chest pain; dyspnea; fatigue or malaise; weight loss; redness or swelling	Recent history of acute infection, surgery, instrumentation, dental work, drug abuse, abortion, or transurethral prostatectomy History of rheumatic, congenital, or atherosclerotic heart disease Daily fever Petechiae on conjunctivae and buccal mucosa Splinter hemorrhages beneath nails Pallor or yellow-brown skin color Splenomegaly Change in existing heart murmur or development of new murmur	Subacute or acute bacterial endocarditis
Dyspnea; fatigue, usually severe; dependent peripheral edema	Female client History of mitral valve disease Olive-colored skin Mid-diastolic thrill between lower left sternal border, apical impulse, and diastolic rumbling Murmur along lower left sternal border Cyanosis during crying, poor feeding, and poor activity tolerance in a child	Tricuspid stenosis
Dyspnea on exertion or at rest; orthopnea; paroxysmal nocturnal dyspnea; hemoptysis; fatigue that increases as exercise tolerance decreases; pain in extremities	Female client under age 45 Recent bronchitis or upper respiratory tract infection that may worsen symptoms History of rheumatic fever, congenital valve disorder, or tumor (myxoma) Flushed cheeks Precordial bulge and diffuse pulsation in young client Tapping sensation over normal area of apical impulse Mid-diastolic or presystolic thrill (or both) at apex Small, weak pulse Localized, delayed, rumbling, low-pitched murmur at or near apex	Mitral stenosis
Dyspnea on exertion; fatigue; possible peripheral edema	History of congenital stenosis or rheumatic heart disease associated with other congenital heart defects, such as tetralogy of Fallot Jugular vein distention Hepatomegaly Systolic murmur at left sternal border Split S_2 with delayed or absent pulmonic component Cyanosis during crying, poor feeding, and poor activity tolerance in a child	Pulmonic stenosis

which distances cardiac sounds. To increase the intensity of heart sounds, have the client sit up or lean forward during auscultation.

Advanced assessment skills

During a complete assessment of the cardiovascular system, the nurse should employ two advanced skills: inspection of the client's jugular venous pulse and auscultation of extra heart sounds (gallops), murmurs, clicks, snaps, and rubs.

Recognition of normal heart sounds requires a great deal of practice and skill. Recognition of abnormal sounds requires an even higher degree of skill. The nurse should attempt advanced auscultatory skills only after mastering the recognition of S_1, S_2, and splitting. The following paragraphs describe guidelines for performing the advanced assessment.

Inspection of the jugular venous pulse

Assessment and analysis of the jugular venous pulse can provide information about right heart dynamics. To do this, inspect the client's right internal jugular vein and observe its pulsations, which constitute the jugular venous pulse. While inspecting the jugular vein, use the carotid pulse or heart sounds to time the venous pulsations with the cardiac cycle. Then plot the venous waveform. (For more information, see *Advanced assessment skills: Assessing the jugular venous pulse*.)

Abnormal pulsations of the jugular vein may signal a dysrhythmia. For example, an exaggerated *a* wave may indicate pulmonic or tricuspid stenosis—conditions that elevate right atrial pressure. A giant *a* wave, or cannon wave, may signal serious conduction defects.

Auscultation of extra heart sounds

Before performing advanced auscultation, prepare the environment, the equipment, and the client as for the basic assessment. During auscultation, follow the four-part auscultation sequence, moving the stethoscope slowly between cardiac auscultation sites. Auscultation may reveal a third heart sound, a fourth heart sound, or both. (For an illustration, see *Extra heart sounds and the cardiac cycle*, page 324.)

Third heart sound. Also known as S_3 or a ventricular gallop, the third heart sound is a low-pitched noise heard best with the bell of the stethoscope. Its rhythm resembles that of a horse galloping, and its cadence sounds like that of the word "Ken-tuc-ky" (*lub-dub-by*). Listen for S_3 with the client in the left lateral decubitus position or in the supine position.

ADVANCED ASSESSMENT SKILLS

Assessing the jugular venous pulse

As part of the advanced cardiovascular assessment, the nurse can evaluate the jugular venous pulse by observing the client's right internal jugular vein. The jugular venous pulse consists of five components called waves: three positive, or ascending, waves (*a, c,* and *v*) and two negative, or descending, waves (*x* and *y*). The following pulsations of the positive waves occur ⅜" to ¾" (1 to 2 cm) above the clavicle, just medial to the sternocleidomastoid muscle:

- The *a* wave marks the initial pulsation of the jugular vein. It occurs just before the first heart sound and is produced by right atrial contraction and transmission of pressure to the jugular veins.
- The *c* wave occurs shortly after the first heart sound. It results from tricuspid valve closing at the beginning of ventricular systole.
- The *v* wave peaks as the tricuspid valve closes. It results from passive atrial filling.

Although the negative waves are not visible as pulsations, they help define the ascending pulses and are shown when the jugular venous pulse is recorded as a wave form. The negative waves occur as follows:

- The *x* descent follows the *a* and *c* waves. It results from right atrial relaxation as well as from pressure on the tricuspid valve during ventricular systole, reducing right atrial pressure.
- The *y* descent follows the *v* wave and is produced by the opening of the tricuspid valve. It occurs as the atria empty rapidly into the ventricles during early diastole.

Five waves of the jugular venous pulse

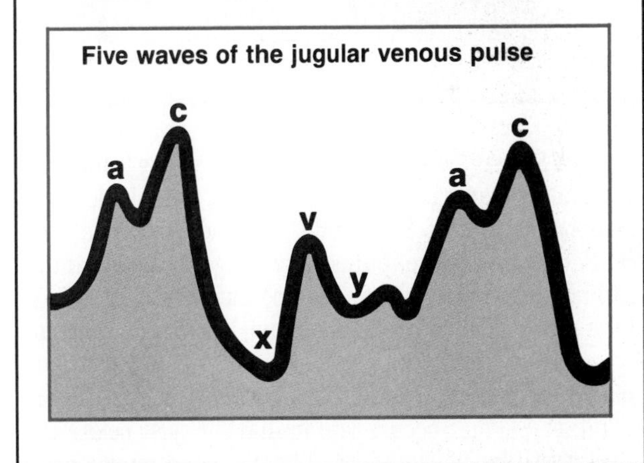

S_3 typically occurs during early to mid-diastole, at the end of the passive filling phase of either ventricle. It may signify that the ventricle is not compliant enough to accept the filling volume without additional force. If the right ventricle is noncompliant, the sound will occur in the tricuspid area; if the left ventricle is noncompliant, in the mitral area. A heave may be palpable when the sound occurs.

Extra heart sounds and the cardiac cycle

The timing of an extra heart sound in the cardiac cycle can help the nurse identify it. The illustrations below show the normal heart sounds S_1 and S_2 (top) and the extra heart sounds S_3 and S_4 (bottom). Compare the illustrations to understand where the extra heart sounds fall in relation to systole, diastole, and the normal heart sounds.

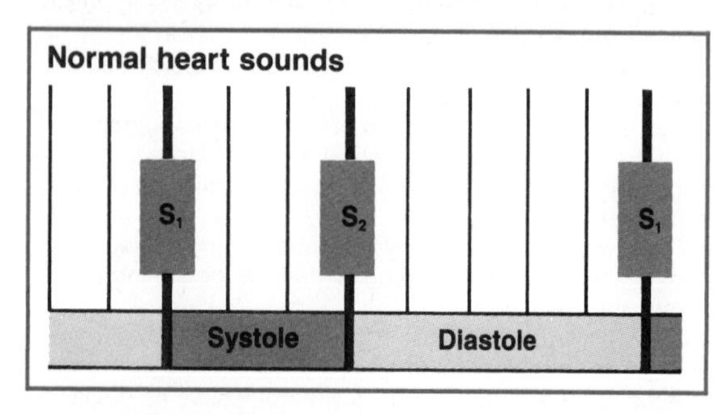

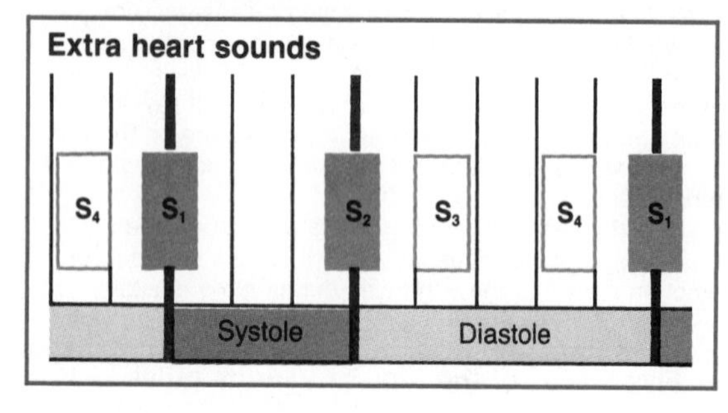

An S_3 may be normal in a child or young adult, but in a client over age 30 it is usually a pathologic sign. Common causes of S_3 include right-side heart failure, left-side heart failure, pulmonary congestion, and intracardiac shunting of blood. Less common causes include acute myocardial infarction, anemia, and thyrotoxicosis.

Fourth heart sound. Auscultation may reveal a fourth heart sound, or S_4, that occurs late in diastole, just before the pulse upstroke. This abnormal heart sound immediately precedes the S_1 of the next cycle and is associated with acceleration and deceleration of blood entering a chamber that resists additional filling. S_4 is known as the atrial or presystolic gallop, because it occurs during atrial contraction.

The fourth heart sound has the same cadence as the word "Ten-nes-see" (*le-lub-dub*). Heard best with the bell of the stethoscope and with the client supine, S_4 may occur in the tricuspid or mitral area, depending on which ventricle is dysfunctional.

Although rare, S_4 may be a normal sound in a young client with a thin chest wall. More typically, however, S_4 indicates cardiovascular disease. It accompanies myocardial infarction during the acute period. If the sound persists, it may indicate impaired ventricular compliance and, at times, volume overload. Other conditions that may cause an S_4 include hypertension, coronary artery disease, cardiomyopathy, angina, anemia, elevated left ventricular pressure, and aortic stenosis. An S_4 frequently appears in elderly clients because of age-related systolic hypertension and aortic stenosis.

Third and fourth hearth sounds. Occasionally, a client may have a third and a fourth heart sound. In such a client, auscultation may reveal two separate abnormal heart sounds and two normal sounds (quadruple rhythm). Because diastole shortens as the heart rate increases, S_3 and S_4 occur so close together that they appear to be one sound—a summation gallop.

Auscultation of murmurs

Advanced cardiac auscultation may reveal a murmur—a vibrating, blowing, or rumbling noise that is longer than a heart sound. Turbulent blood flow produces this abnormal heart sound.

If a murmur is present, identify the location where it is loudest, pinpoint the time when the murmur occurs during the cardiac cycle, and describe its pitch (frequency), pattern, quality, and intensity (loudness). This information will help determine the cause of the murmur.

Location and timing. Murmurs can occur in any cardiac auscultatory site. They also can radiate from one site to another. To identify the radiation area, auscultate from the site where the murmur is heard best to the farthest site where the sound is still heard. Then note the anatomic landmark of this farthest site.

When timing a murmur, determine if it occurs during diastole or systole. A murmur that occurs between S_1 and S_2 is a systolic murmur; between S_2 and the next S_1, a diastolic murmur. Also determine at which point in systole or diastole the murmur occurs—for example, mid-diastole or late systole. In some clients, murmurs may occur during both portions of the cardiac cycle, creating a continuous murmur.

Pitch, pattern, and quality. The rate and pressure of blood flow determine the pitch of a heart murmur. The pitch may be high, medium, or low. If you can hear a murmur with the bell of the stethoscope, but not with the diaphragm, it is a low murmur; with the diaphragm, but not with the bell, a high murmur; with both, a medium murmur.

Different intensities can form an identifiable pattern. When the velocity of blood flow increases, the murmur becomes louder, creating a pattern known as crescendo; when velocity decreases, the murmur becomes quieter, creating a pattern known as decrescendo. A murmur with increasing loudness followed by increasing softness has a crescendo-decrescendo pattern.

Many factors affect the quality of a murmur, including the volume of blood flow, the force of the contraction, and the degree of valve compromise. Heart murmur quality can be described as musical, blowing, harsh, rasping, rumbling, or machinelike.

Intensity. Use a standard, six-level grading scale to describe the intensity of the murmur. (For more information, see *Advanced assessment skills: Grading murmur intensity.*)

Causes of murmurs. A murmur can be innocent (nonpathologic) or a sign of a cardiac problem (pathologic). An innocent, or functional, murmur may appear in a client without heart disease. It occurs early in systole, seldom exceeds grade II in intensity, and usually is heard best in the pulmonic area. When the client changes from a supine to a sitting position, this type of murmur may disappear. When the client's cardiac output increases, as in fever, exercise, anemia, anxiety, or pregnancy, the murmur may increase in intensity.

Innocent murmurs affect up to 25% of all children but usually disappear by adolescence. Another type of nonpathologic murmur commonly affects elderly clients who experience changes in the aortic valve structures and the aorta. These clients frequently exhibit insignificant short systolic murmurs heard best at the left sternal border or in the aortic area.

Pathologic murmurs can occur during systole or diastole and can affect any heart valve. They can result from valvular stenosis (inability of the heart valves to open properly), valvular insufficiency (inability of the heart valves to close properly, allowing regurgitation of blood), or a septal defect (a defect in the septal wall separating two heart chambers). (For more information, see *Advanced assessment skills: Heart murmur identification*, page 328.)

Auscultation of other abnormal heart sounds

During auscultation, three other abnormal sounds may occur: clicks, snaps, and rubs.

Clicks. Clicks (high-pitched abnormal heart sounds auscultated at the apex during mid- to late systole) result from tensing of the chordae tendineae structures and mitral valve cusps. Initially, the mitral valve closes securely, but a large cusp prolapses into the left atrium. The click usually precedes a late systolic murmur caused by regurgitation of a little blood from the left ventricle into the left atrium. Mitral valve prolapse and these classic auscultatory findings occur in 5% to 10% of young adults and affect more women than men.

To detect the high-pitched click of mitral valve prolapse, place the stethoscope diaphragm at the apex and listen during mid- to late systole. To enhance the sound, change the client's position to sitting or standing, and listen along the lower left sternal border.

Snaps. Auscultation may detect an opening snap immediately after S_2. The snap resembles the normal S_1 and S_2 in quality and is heard medial to the apex along the lower left sternal border. Its high pitch helps differentiate it from an S_3. Because the opening snap may accompany mitral or tricuspid stenosis, it usually precedes a mid- to late diastolic murmur—a classic sign of stenosis. It results from the stenotic valve attempting to open.

(Text continues on page 328.)

ADVANCED ASSESSMENT SKILLS

Grading murmur intensity

The intensity of murmurs varies greatly. To grade murmur intensity, the nurse can use this standard scale, which ranks murmurs from I to VI.

Grade I
Very faint; barely audible even to the trained ear

Grade II
Soft and low; easily audible to the trained ear

Grade III
Moderately loud; about equal to the intensity of normal heart sounds

Grade IV
Loud with a palpable thrill at the murmur site

Grade V
Very loud with a palpable thrill; audible with the stethoscope in partial contact with the chest

Grade VI
Extremely loud with a palpable thrill, audible with the stethoscope over—but not in contact with—the chest

Applying the nursing process

Assessment findings form the basis of the nursing process. Using them, the nurse formulates the nursing diagnoses and develops appropriate planning, implementation, and evaluation of the client's care.

The table below shows how the nurse can use cardiovascular system assessment data in the nursing process for the client described in the case history (shown at right). In the first column, history and physical assessment data appear, followed by a paragraph of mental notes. These notes help the nurse make important mental connections among assessment findings, aiding in development of the nursing diagnoses and planning.

The second column presents several appropriate nursing diagnoses; however, the information in the remaining three columns is based on the *first* nursing diagnosis. Although it is not part of the nursing process, documentation appears in the last column because of its importance. Documentation consists of an initial note using all components of the SOAPIE format and a follow-up note using the appropriate SOAPIE components.

ASSESSMENT	NURSING DIAGNOSES	PLANNING	IMPLEMENTATION
Subjective (history) data • Client states: "I get so tired and weak from doing absolutely nothing. I even get short of breath! I don't see how I'll ever manage my house, let alone go back to work in a few weeks." • Client reports no dizziness or palpitations on standing, no chest pain on exertion. • Client states: "I still can't believe I had a heart attack. I always thought men had heart attacks, not women. I don't understand this cholesterol stuff Dr. Thomas was talking about. I like to eat real food." • Client reports that she eats three meals a day plus snacks. She does not eat dessert but has cookies after work. • Client states that she does not smoke cigarettes. She used birth control pills for about 7 years. **Objective (physical) data** • Height 5′3″, weight 156 lb • Vital signs: blood pressure 140/90 supine and sitting, 132/90 standing; temperature 97.8° F.; pulse 84 at rest, 96 after mild exertion, regular rhythm; respirations 18 at rest, 24 after mild exertion. Pulse and respirations return to normal within 5 minutes after exertion. • Skin turgor and color normal, no pallor on standing. • Cardiac enzyme results: CPK-MB and SGOT elevations now almost normal; LDH_1, LDH_2, and HBD remain high. Total cholesterol (300 mg/dl), triglyceride (180 mg/dl), and LDL-cholesterol (190 mg/dl) levels are elevated. **Mental notes** *The MI may have decreased the client's cardiac output, which would also reduce exercise tolerance. Her excess weight may also contribute to exercise intolerance. A gradual increase in activity should help lessen the deconditioning and provide an opportunity to assess her response and teach her how to increase the exercise safely. Client's lack of knowledge about risk factors of cardiac disease and necessary dietary changes put her at risk for further problems. The high cholesterol and LDL levels probably indicate a need to reduce saturated fat intake. Hospital meals don't match her home meal plan in amount of food or timing. She should receive dietary counseling.*	• Activity intolerance related to decreased cardiac output. • Knowledge deficit related to heart disease, risk factors, and required dietary regimen. • Potential disturbance in self-concept related to concerns about mortality. • Potential alteration in sexuality patterns related to fear of further cardiac injury.	**Goals** By discharge, the client will: • be able to manage activities at 3 to 4 metabolic equivalents of a task (METs) without distress. By the end of the 4-week recuperative period, the client will: • attend cardiac rehabilitation sessions three times a week • be able to manage activities at 5 to 6 METs without distress.	• Institute low-level (1 to 2 MET level) activities, such as walking and range-of-motion exercises, and exercise plan for cardiac rehabilitation. • Assess the client's heart rate, heart rhythm, blood pressure, heart sounds, and lung sounds before, during, and after exercise. • Teach the client to conserve energy by resting between activities, sitting to perform tasks, and stopping an activity if fatigue occurs or if pulse or respiration rate exceeds the prescribed limits. • Teach the client to monitor home activity by checking her pulse rate at rest, immediately after activity, and 3 minutes after activity. • Instruct the client to report dyspnea, chest pain, palpitations, or a pulse rate that decreases with activity, exceeds 110 beats/minute, becomes irregular, or does not return to normal after 3 minutes.

CASE HISTORY

Mrs. Sally Tate, age 52, was admitted to the coronary care unit (CCU) after experiencing the classic pain and dyspnea associated with a myocardial infarction (MI). During her stay in the CCU, her pain was controlled with morphine and oxygen therapy. Mrs. Tate is now in the stepdown telemetry unit. If her progress continues, she will be discharged to home care after 72 hours.

EVALUATION	DOCUMENTATION BASED ON NURSING PROCESS DATA			
		Initial		**Follow-up**
During hospitalization, the client will: • gradually increase from 2 to 3 to 4 METS without demonstrating fatigue or dyspnea and with vital signs that return to normal 5 minutes after activity. After 4 weeks of convalescence, the client will: • exercise to the target heart rate without fatigue, chest pain, or ischemic EKG changes as measured by the stress test. • walk 3 miles over a flat course in less than 1 hour.	**S**	Client states: "I get so weak and tired when I do anything. I even get short of breath." Client denies chest pain, dizziness, or palpitations with position change or activity. Client states: "I always thought men had heart attacks, not women. I don't understand this cholesterol stuff. I like to eat real food."	**S**	Client reports doing normal housework and walking 3 miles three times a week with spouse or friend at high school track or mall. Walks distance in less than 1 hour at track; mall takes longer. Requests return to work, bored at home. Client states that she is nervous before stress test and somewhat fatigued afterward.
	O	Blood pressure 140/90 supine and sitting, 132/90 standing; temperature 97.8° F.; pulse 84 at rest, 96 after mild exertion, regular rhythm; respirations 18 at rest, 24 after mild exertion. Pulse and respirations return to normal within 5 minutes. Skin color and turgor normal. No pallor with standing or activity.	**O**	During stress test, client exercised to target rate without ischemic changes. Pulse, respirations, and blood pressure returned to normal limits within 5 minutes after test.
	A	Activity intolerance related to decreased cardiac output. Laboratory values show high cholesterol and LDL-cholesterol levels.	**A**	Improvement shown; exercise tolerance increased.
	P	Institute low-level (1 to 2 MET level) activities and exercise plan for cardiac rehabilitation, progressing to 3 to 4 MET level by discharge, and evaluate response. Teach client about energy conservation and home rehabilitation program: activities, restrictions, reportable occurrences. Expect to arrange for low-level stress test before discharge and stress test 4 weeks after discharge.	**P**	Client will continue cardiac rehabilitation program under department supervision.
	I	Taught client active range-of-motion exercises. Helped client walk to bathroom and sit at sink to wash. Returned client to bed to rest.	**I**	Client can describe reportable symptoms, denies experiencing any after exercise.
	E	Blood pressure, pulse, and respirations within normal limits 5 minutes after client returned to bed. Fatigue gone after short rest period. Client asked to learn what comes next.		

ADVANCED ASSESSMENT SKILLS

Heart murmur identification

An advanced skill, heart murmur identification takes a great deal of practice to perfect. To develop this ability, the nurse should listen closely to a murmur to identify its timing in the cardiac cycle. Then the nurse can determine its other characteristics one at a time, including its quality, pitch, location, and radiation. All of these characteristics will help identify the underlying condition, as shown in the chart below.

TIMING	QUALITY	PITCH	LOCATION	RADIATION	CONDITION
Midsystolic (systolic ejection)	Harsh, rough	Medium to high	Pulmonic	Toward left shoulder and neck	Pulmonic stenosis
	Harsh, rough	Medium to high	Aortic and suprasternal notch	Toward carotid arteries or apex	Aortic stenosis
Holosystolic (pansystolic)	Harsh	High	Tricuspid	Precordium	Ventricular septal defect
	Blowing	High	Mitral, lower left sternal border	Toward left axilla	Mitral insufficiency
	Blowing	High	Tricuspid	Toward apex	Tricuspid insufficiency
Early diastolic	Blowing	High	Mid-left sternal edge (not aortic area)	Toward sternum	Aortic insufficiency
	Blowing	High	Pulmonic	Toward sternum	Pulmonic insufficiency
Mid- to late diastolic	Rumbling	Low	Apex	Usually none	Mitral stenosis
	Rumbling	Low	Tricuspid, lower right sternal border	Usually none	Tricuspid stenosis

Rubs. To detect a pericardial friction rub, use the diaphragm of the stethoscope to auscultate at the third left intercostal space along the lower left sternal border. Listen for a harsh, scratchy, scraping, or squeaking sound that can occur throughout systole, diastole, or both . To enhance the sound, have the client sit upright and lean forward or exhale. A rub usually indicates pericarditis (inflammation of the pericardium).

Documentation

Before documentation begins, review the assessment findings to determine what they may indicate. To do this, thoughtfully consider the physical assessment data about the client's cardiovascular system, related body structures, general appearance, body weight, and vital signs. Also review the client's health history data.

As the final step of the cardiovascular assessment, evaluate results of the client's laboratory studies. (For a summary of frequently used laboratory studies and their significance, see *Common laboratory studies*.) Also consider the results of any other diagnostic tests that may be ordered. Common cardiovascular diagnostic tests include the chest X-ray, the electrocardiogram (EKG), the exercise EKG, and the echocardiogram. A chest X-ray may be done to assess the size and position of the heart and to detect structural abnormalities, such as aortic dissection and valvular calcification. The most frequently performed cardiac diagnostic test, an EKG may be or-

Common laboratory studies

For a client with cardiovascular signs and symptoms, various laboratory studies can provide valuable clues to the possible cause, as shown in the chart below. (*Note:* Keep in mind that abnormal findings may stem from a problem unrelated to the cardiovascular system.) Remember that values differ among laboratories, so check the normal value range for the specific laboratory.

TEST AND SIGNIFICANCE	NORMAL VALUES OR FINDINGS	ABNORMAL FINDINGS	POSSIBLE CARDIOVASCULAR OR RELATED CAUSES OF ABNORMAL FINDINGS
Blood tests			
Creatinine phosphokinase (CPK) This enzyme reflects tissue catabolism. Its isoenzyme, CPK-MB, is specific to cardiac tissue.	Total CPK *Males:* 23 to 99 u/liter *Females:* 15 to 57 u/liter CPK-MB Less than 5% of total CPK	Above-normal level Above-normal level	Myocardial infarction Myocardial infarction
Lactic dehydrogenase (LDH) This enzyme reflects cellular damage. Two of its five isoenzymes are specific to cardiac tissue: LDH_1 and LDH_2.	Total LDH: 48 to 115 IU/liter LDH_1: 18% to 29% of total LDH LDH_2: 29.4% to 37.5% of total LDH	Above-normal level	Myocardial infarction, rheumatic carditis, myocarditis
Serum glutamic-oxaloacetic transaminase (SGOT) Also known as aspartate aminotransferase, this enzyme also reflects cellular damage but is less specific than LDH.	8 to 20 u/liter	Above-normal level	Myocardial infarction
Hydroxybutyric dehydrogenase (HBD) Also known as alpha-hydroxybutyric dehydrogenase, this enzyme reflects LDH_1, LDH_2, and LDH_5 activity.	114 to 290 u/liter	Above-normal level	Myocardial infarction
Triglycerides This test provides a quantitative analysis of stored lipids.	Below 200 mg/dl	Above-normal level	Increased risk of coronary artery disease
Total cholesterol This test measures the circulating levels of free cholesterol and cholesterol esters.	Below 200 mg/dl	Above-normal level	Increased risk of coronary artery disease
Lipoprotein cholesterol fractionation This test measures high-density lipoproteins (HDLs) and low-density lipoproteins (LDLs).	HDL: greater than 50 mg/100 ml LDL: less than 130 mg/100 ml	Above-normal level Above-normal level	Decreased risk of coronary artery disease Increased risk of coronary artery disease

dered to obtain a graphic record of the electrical activity of the heart. This test can locate a myocardial infarction and can detect chamber enlargement, ischemia, conduction defects, and dysrhythmias. An exercise EKG may be performed to assess the cardiac response to physical stress. In this test, the client exercises on a treadmill or stationary bicycle while an EKG is recorded along with the client's blood pressure. This test provides information that cannot be obtained from a resting EKG alone. Echocardiography may be performed to assess the size, shape, and motion of cardiac structures. This widely used, noninvasive test helps evaluate clients with chest pain, enlarged cardiac silhouettes on X-ray films, EKG changes, and abnormal heart sounds on auscultation.

Other cardiovascular tests may include such studies as thallium imaging, which evaluates myocardial blood flow and myocardial cell status after intravenous injection of a radioisotope; and cardiac catheterization, which determines blood pressure and flow in the cardiac chambers by passing a catheter into the right or left side of the heart.

After reviewing all of the assessment data, the nurse should be able to formulate appropriate nursing diagnoses and then use them to plan, implement, and evaluate the client's nursing care. (For a case study that shows how to apply the nursing process to a client with a cardiovascular disorder, see *Applying the nursing process*, pages 326 and 327.)

When the assessment is complete, document the data completely, including normal and abnormal findings. The following example shows how to document some normal physical assessment findings:

> *Weight:* 165 lb
> *Height:* 5′9″
> *Vital signs:* Blood pressure 126/72 right arm and 120/76 left arm with a 4 mm Hg systolic drop when moving from supine to standing position; temperature 98.4° F.; pulse 64 and regular; respirations 14 and regular.
>
> Muscles well defined. Muscle strength and gait normal. Skin color normal. Mucous membranes pink and moist. Skin turgor normal. Lower extremity exhibits normal perfusion with color return in less than 10 seconds and venous refill in 15 seconds. Capillary refill brisk. No neck veins visible with client at a 45-degree angle. All pulses palpated, bilaterally equal +2. PMI palpated in the fifth intercostal space at the midclavicular line. No thrills or heaves palpated. Auscultation reveals normal S_1 and S_2 with no murmurs, gallops, clicks, snaps, rubs, or bruits.

The following example shows how to document some abnormal physical assessment findings:

> *Weight:* 102 lb
> *Height:* 5′6″
> *Vital signs:* Blood pressure 100/80 in both arms with a 10 mm Hg systolic and diastolic drop when moving from supine to sitting position; temperature 99.5° F.; pulse 104 and irregular; respirations 28 and labored with an audible inspiratory wheeze.
>
> Client appears thin and weak. Skin color: generalized pallor with purplish discoloration from toes to 3″ above the ankles and a 2-cm-diameter lesion on the right inner aspect of the left ankle. Lower extremity perfusion delayed with color return in 20 seconds. Skin turgor poor. No hair growth bilaterally below the knees. +3 pedal edema bilaterally at the ankles diminishes to +1 just below the knee. Capillary refill sluggish. Neck veins distended 6 cm with client at a 45-degree angle. Pedal and popliteal pulses +1; all other pulses bilaterally equal +2. PMI palpated in the fifth intercostal space at the anterior axillary line. Auscultation reveals a third heart sound, bilateral carotid bruits, and a Grade III holosystolic murmur heard best in the aortic area with radiation to the neck.

The nurse must also document the other nursing process steps—nursing diagnosis, planning, implementation, and evaluation—when applying them to the care plan for the client with a cardiovascular disorder.

Chapter summary

To assess the client's cardiovascular system effectively, the nurse must gather health history data, physical assessment findings, and laboratory study results. Then the nurse evaluates this information by applying a knowledge of cardiovascular anatomy and physiology. Chapter 11 describes how to gather and evaluate assessment information. Here are the chapter highlights:

• The cardiovascular system includes the heart and five types of blood vessels: arteries, arterioles, capillaries, venules, and veins. Its two basic functions are to deliver oxygenated blood to body tissues and to remove waste substances from them.

- The heart consists of four chambers and four valves. The four chambers include two atria and two ventricles. The four valves include two atrioventricular (AV) valves, known as the tricuspid and mitral valves; and two semilunar (SL) valves, known as the pulmonic and aortic valves. All of the chambers and valves work together to keep the blood flowing in one direction through the heart.
- The heart is the center of the circulatory system, a vast network of blood vessels that nourish all functioning body cells. This network can be divided into two branches: the pulmonary circulation, which routes blood through the lungs to pick up oxygen and liberate carbon dioxide; and the systemic circulation, including the coronary circulation, which takes blood to all active cells to exchange oxygen and nutrients for waste products.
- The cardiac conduction system has two main parts: the extrinsic conduction system, which includes the autonomic nervous system; and the intrinsic conduction system, which includes the sinoatrial node, the atrioventricular node, and other specialized nerves and fibers in the heart. Both parts of the conduction system work together to stimulate heart muscle contraction—and the pumping action of the heart—at a pace that meets the body's metabolic needs.
- The cardiac cycle is divided into two main parts: systole (ventricular contraction) and diastole (ventricular relaxation). Atrioventricular valve closing creates the first heart sound (S_1) and signals the start of systole. Semilunar valve closing produces the second heart sound (S_2) and marks the beginning of diastole.
- The cardiovascular health history should include questions about the client's risk factors for cardiac disease, such as heredity, sex, race, age, hypertension, cigarette smoking, hyperlipidemia, diabetes, and other factors. It also should investigate the presence of cardiovascular signs and symptoms, such as chest pain, dyspnea, cough, dizziness, edema, palpitations, fatigue, and cyanosis.
- During the health history, the nurse asks about the client's health beliefs and any health promotion practices, the client follows. Additional questions should evaluate the client's current and past use of prescription and over-the-counter medications.
- Health history questions help the client describe a normal day's activities, including sleep and wake patterns, nutritional patterns, exercise and activity patterns, and stress and coping patterns. They also investigate role and relationship patterns.
- Before beginning the full cardiovascular physical assessment, the nurse measures the client's height and weight and obtains the vital signs, paying particular attention to the pulse and blood pressure.
- Then the nurse assesses related body structures by evaluating the color, temperature, and turgor of the skin and assessing it for lesions and peripheral edema; noticing the pattern of peripheral hair growth; assessing the speed of capillary refill; checking the shape of the fingernails; and looking for cardiovascular effects in the eyes.
- Cardiovascular inspection should begin with assessment of chest configuration and respiratory movements. Then the nurse evaluates neck veins for distention and the precordium for pulsations, heaves, or lifts.
- To palpate the cardiovascular system, the nurse begins with the central and peripheral pulses, noting their strength and contour using a standard grading scale. Then the nurse continues with palpation of the precordium for vibrations and the apical impulse or other pulsations over the aortic, pulmonic, right ventricular, left ventricular (apical), and epigastric areas. All palpable impulses should be described by their size and location.
- Heart sound auscultation requires use of the diaphragm and the bell of the stethoscope. S_1 normally sounds louder at the mitral and tricuspid sites; S_2, at the aortic and pulmonic sites. The nurse should identify any abnormal heart sound by its timing in the cardiac cycle, the location where it is the loudest, and any other descriptive characteristics that apply, such as quality and pitch. The nurse also auscultates the carotid arteries for bruits (continuous, murmurlike sounds).
- Advanced assessment skills include auscultation and identification of extra heart sounds, murmurs, clicks, snaps, and rubs. The low-pitched extra heart sounds (S_3 and S_4), or gallops, occur in the mitral or tricuspid sites early or late in diastole. Murmurs (longer abnormal sounds) may appear in any cardiac auscultatory site in early, mid-, or late systole or diastole. Clicks and snaps are both high-pitched abnormal sounds, but clicks usually occur during mid- to late systole, whereas snaps occur immediately after S_2. A rub is a harsh, scratchy, or creaking sound that can be heard at various times during the cardiac cycle.
- To complete the cardiovascular assessment, the nurse reviews the history and physical assessment findings along with the results of any laboratory tests, such as cardiac enzyme studies and total cholesterol counts.
- The nurse documents all assessment findings and uses them to formulate nursing diagnoses. Then the nurse can plan, implement, and evaluate the client's care.

Study questions

1. Mr. Jenkins, age 56, comes to the ambulatory care center complaining of two 3-minute episodes of chest pain that were accompanied by shortness of breath and sweating. He says that he has felt more tired than usual for the past 2 months. His risk factors of cardiac disease include family history (father died of a heart attack at age 60), cigarette smoking (1 pack per day for 40 years), hypertension, and inactivity.

His pulse is 92 and irregular; blood pressure, 156/94; temperature, 98° F.; and respirations, 16 and unlabored. He is 5′8″ tall and weighs 205 lb. His color appears normal, and his skin feels warm and dry. His neck veins exhibit no distention while he is seated. All pulses are palpable, equal, and +2. During auscultation, his lungs sound clear and his first and second heart sounds are normal with no gallops, murmurs, or rubs.

Just as you are about to leave the room, Mr. Jenkins develops substernal chest pain that radiates down his left arm. Auscultation reveals a third heart sound, and Mr. Jenkins develops dyspnea and diaphoresis. His chest pain subsides after 3 minutes.

How would you describe the following information related to your nursing assessment of Mr. Jenkins?
- history (subjective) assessment data
- physical (objective) assessment data
- assessment techniques and equipment
- two appropriate nursing diagnoses
- documentation of your findings.

2. What are the usual differences in physical assessment findings for a client with arterial peripheral vascular disease and a client with venous peripheral vascular disease?

3. Mr. Young, age 55, was admitted to the hospital with a diagnosis of myocardial infarction. While caring for Mr. Young, you perform a physical assessment. What areas will you focus on to provide information about his cardiovascular status?

4. Mrs. Schaeffer, age 73, has a history of congestive heart failure. As a public health nurse, you see her every week to assess her cardiovascular status. During the assessment, which areas should you focus on and why?

5. Whether you work in a hospital or outpatient setting, all clients require heart sound auscultation. What are the four cardiac auscultatory sites? Where are they located? What mechanical and electrical events occur during the two normal heart sounds?

Selected references

Andreoli, K., Zipes, D., Wallace, A., Kinney, G., Fowkes, V. (1987). *Comprehensive cardiac care* (6th ed.). St. Louis: Mosby.

Bondy, B. (1987). An overview of arterial disease. *Journal of Cardiovascular Nursing,* 1(2), 1-11.

Braddy, P. (1989). Cardiac assessment tool. *Critical Care Nurse,* 9(9), 71-81.

Brandenburg, R. (1987). *Cardiology: Fundamentals and practice.* Chicago: Year Book.

Braunwald, E. (1988). *Heart disease: A textbook of cardiovascular medicine.* Philadelphia: Saunders.

Burke, L. (1987). Risk-factor modification in the prevention of coronary heart disease. *Journal of Cardiovascular Nursing,* 1(4), 67-75.

Calloway, C. (1990). Zeroing in on chest pain. *Nursing90,* 20(4), 44-45.

Cardiac Problems. (1989). NurseReview Series. Springhouse, PA: Springhouse Corp.

Carlson, K. (1989). Assessing a child's chest. *RN,* 52(11), 26-32.

Diagnostics (2nd ed.). (1986). Nurse's Reference Library. Springhouse, PA: Springhouse Corp.

Durham, C. (1988). The no-fault way to assess carotid arteries. *Nursing88,* 18(11), 65-67.

Guyton, A. (1991). *Textbook of medical physiology* (8th ed.). Philadelphia: Saunders.

Harrell, J., Champagne, M., Jarr, S., and Miyaya, M. (1990). Teaching cardiovascular assessment. *Journal of Continuing Education in Nursing,* 21(6), 241-244.

Henry, J. (1991). *Clinical diagnosis and management by laboratory methods* (18th ed.). Philadelphia: Saunders.

Horwitz, L., and Graves, B. (1985). *Signs and symptoms in cardiology.* Philadelphia: Lippincott.

Hudak, C., Gallo, B., and Benz, J. (1990). *Critical care nursing: A holistic approach* (5th ed.). Philadelphia: Lippincott.

Hurst, W., Schlant, R., Rackley, C., Sonneblick, E., and Wenger, N. (Eds.). (1990). *The heart* (6th ed.). New York: McGraw-Hill.

Kadota, L. (1985). Theory and application of thermodilution cardiac output measurement: A review. *Heart & Lung,* 14(6), 605-616.

Kenner, C., Guzetta, C., and Dossey, B. (1985). *Critical care nursing: Body-mind-spirit* (2nd ed.). Philadelphia: Lippincott.

Konick-McMahan, J. (1989). Jugular vein distension: Trouble in the heart's right side. *Nursing89,* 19(2), 100-102.

McEvoy, G. (Ed.). (1992). *American Hospital Formulary Service drug information.* Bethesda, MD: American Society of Hospital Pharmacists.

Persons, C. (1987). *Critical care procedures and protocols: A nursing process approach.* Philadelphia: Lippincott.

Sokolow, M., McIlroy, M., and Cheitlin, M. (1990). *Clinical cardiology* (5th ed.). East Norwalk, CT: Appleton & Lange.

Yee, B., and Zorb, S. (1986). *Cardiac critical care nursing.* Boston: Scott-Foresman.

Nursing research

Blackburn, S., and Patteson, D. (1991). Effects of cycled light activity state and cardiorespiratory function in preterm infants. *Journal of Perinatal and Neonatal Nursing,* 4(4), 47-54.

Fagan, M. (1988). Relationship between nurses' assessments of perfusion and toe temperature in pediatric patients with cardiovascular disease. *Heart & Lung,* 17(2), 157-165.

Gilliss, C., Neuhaus, J., and Hauck, W. (1990). Improving family functioning after cardiac surgery: A randomized trial. *Heart & Lung,* 19(6), 648-654.

Glick, M. (1986). Caring, touch and anxiety of myocardial infarction patients in the intermediate cardiac care unit. *Intensive Care Nursing,* 2(2), 61-66.

Liddy, K., and Crowley, C. (1987). Do M.I. patients have the information they need for the recovery phase at home? *Home Healthcare Nurse,* 5(3), 19-22, 24-5.

Murdaugh, C., and Verran, I. (1987). Theoretical modeling to predict physiological indicators of cardiac preventative behaviors. *Nursing Research,* 36(5), 284-291.

Nyamathi, A. (1987). The coping responses of female spouses of patients with myocardial infarctions. *Heart & Lung,* 16(1), 86-92.

Prentice, J., Hooper, N., MacLean, D., and Calcott, R. (1990). Baseline assessment: Report of a companywide risk factor survey. *AAOHN Journal,* 38(9), 403-408.

Storm, D., Metzger, B., and Therrien, B. (1989). Effects of age on autonomic cardiovascular responsiveness in healthy men and women. *Nursing Research,* 38(6), 326-330.

Sutterer, J., et al. (1989). Risk factor knowledge, status, and change in a community screening project. *Journal of Community Health,* 14(3), 137-147.

Thomas, S., and Friedmann, E. (1990). Type A behavior and cardiovascular responses during verbalization in cardiac patients. *Nursing Research,* 39(1), 48-53.

12

Female and Male Breasts

Objectives

After reading and studying this chapter, you should be able to:

1. Name, describe, and locate the parts of the human breast and axillary nodes.
2. Discuss the physiologic function of the human breast.
3. Describe female breast changes that occur at puberty, during menstruation, during pregnancy, during lactation, and at menopause.
4. Explain the purpose of breast-related health history data.
5. Identify representative adverse reactions to drugs that affect the breast.
6. Identify developmental changes that are important to breast assessment.
7. Describe how to inspect and palpate the breast and axilla.
8. Teach breast self-examination to a female client.
9. Differentiate between normal and abnormal findings during physical assessment of the breast.
10. Use the nursing process to document breast assessment findings.

Introduction

This chapter describes the anatomy and physiology of the female and male breasts and axillae, emphasizes important breast structures and functions, and identifies normal changes associated with breast maturation. It presents appropriate health history questions to ask during a breast assessment and offers rationales to help the nurse understand the significance of the collected data.

The chapter also describes the steps of a breast physical assessment, including inspection and palpation of the breasts and axillae; psychological preparation of the client; and breast self-examination techniques.

Because of its devastating effects, breast cancer is discussed at length. The second leading cause of death in women, breast cancer currently affects one in ten women in the United States; only 1% of all breast cancers occur in men.

Most breast tumors and related problems are not cancer, although they require careful assessment to rule out malignant conditions. A nurse can be a frontline promoter of breast care, teaching a client breast self-examination and encouraging routine breast assessment and mammography, when appropriate.

In the past, a woman with breast cancer had only one option: radical mastectomy (surgical removal of the breast, axillary lymph nodes, and pectoral muscles). Today, she has several treatment options. Growing data support the efficacy of treating selected breast cancers with lumpectomy (surgical removal of diseased tissue only) and radiotherapy or chemotherapy. Refinements in reconstructive surgery offer the client the opportunity to avoid disfigurement if radical surgery is required.

Besides discussing breast cancer, this chapter also describes developmental concerns related to the breast, how to document information obtained during breast assessment, and how to develop an individualized nursing care plan.

Glossary

Areola mammae: pigmented circular area surrounding the nipple of each breast, commonly called the areola.

Colostrum: fluid secreted by the breast during pregnancy and the first few days postpartum, before lactation begins. It is a thin, yellowish, serous fluid consisting of immunologically active substances, white blood cells, water, protein, fat, and carbohydrates.

Dimpling: breast skin puckering or depression possibly caused by an underlying growth; also called retraction.

Gynecomastia: enlargement of one or both male breasts, usually secondary to hormonal changes during puberty.

Lactation: process of synthesis and secretion of breast milk during nourishment of an infant or child.

Lumpectomy: surgical removal of only diseased breast tissue.

Mammogram: breast X-ray.

Nipple: pigmented spherical protuberant nub of erectile tissue surrounded by the areola on each breast. The lactiferous ducts (channels carrying milk from the breast lobes) open into the nipple.

Nipple inversion: inturning or depression of the central portion of the nipple.

Peau d'orange: orange-peel-like appearance of breast skin caused by edema.

Supernumerary breast: one or more extra breasts consisting of a nipple or breast tissue, or both, located along the milk lines (embryonic ridges that extend from the axilla to the groin).

Tail of Spence: extension of breast tissue, which projects from the upper outer quadrant of the breast toward the axilla; also called axillary tail.

Anatomy and physiology review

The breasts are similar in both sexes until puberty, when the ovaries secrete the hormones estrogen and progesterone, causing breast enlargement in females. Unstimulated by hormones, the male breast retains preadolescent characteristics.

Estrogen secretion causes duct tissue growth and fat deposits; progesterone stimulates glandular development. (For a description of breast anatomy and physiology, see *The breasts*, pages 336 and 337.)

Developmental changes

Breast size and composition change with the client's age. Endocrine changes, such as those occurring during pregnancy or menstrual cycle phases, and genetic factors also affect breast size and composition.

Puberty

Except for a small amount of primary duct branching, the breasts lie dormant during childhood and preadolescence. An early sign of puberty, breast development (thelarche) begins between ages 8 and 13 (age 11 is average) when breast buds appear. Usually, the time span from beginning of breast buds to onset of menses is 2 to 3 years. (For illustrations, see *Female breast development*, page 338.)

Young adolescent boys may have some temporary stimulation of breast tissue. Estrogen is produced in both sexes, as is testosterone, and until testosterone is produced in sufficient quantity to override the estrogen in the young male, some breast enlargement (gynecomastia) of one or both breasts may occur.

Pregnancy and lactation

During pregnancy, the breasts enlarge several times normal size from proliferation and hypertrophy of the acini cells and lactiferous (milk) ducts. These changes occur in response to the hormones from the corpus luteum and the placenta. Colostrum (mammary gland fluid secreted before lactation begins) is produced in the acini cells as epithelial secretory activity increases in the third trimester.

Withdrawal of placental and luteal sex hormones and the infant's sucking suppress the prolactin-inhibiting factor or hormone (PIH), thus preparing the breast for postpartum lactation. Secreted by the anterior pituitary, prolactin then stimulates milk production. Alveoli-to-duct milk release (the let-down reflex) occurs when oxytocin, secreted from the posterior pituitary, causes myoepithelial cell contraction. Tactile (such as occurs with suckling), autonomic, and sensory stimuli

(Text continues on page 338.)

The breasts

Normally occurring in pairs, the breasts are located vertically between the second or third and the sixth or seventh ribs on the anterior chest wall over the pectoralis major and the serratus anterior muscles; horizontally, they lie between the sternal border and the midaxillary line.

The female breast

A modified sebaceous gland, the female breast is composed of a centrally located nipple of pigmented erectile tissue surrounded by an areola of pink to brown pigment that is darker than the adjacent breast tissue. Called Montgomery's tubercles, sebaceous glands appear irregularly on the areolar surface as elevated, small, round papules. Hair follicles are normally seen around the periphery of the areola.

The female breasts are composed of glandular, fibrous, and fatty (adipose) tissue. A small triangle of breast tissue called the tail of Spence, or axillary tail, projects into the axilla. Around each breast are 12 to 25 glandular lobes. Each lobe is composed of 20 to 40 lobules that contain the acini cells (or alveoli), the milk-producing breast structures. These cells empty into the lactiferous ducts, which carry milk from each lobe to the nipple.

Fibrous tissue bands (Cooper's ligaments), attached to the chest wall musculature, support each breast. Fat makes up the remainder of the breast, and lies primarily behind and above the glandular lobes.

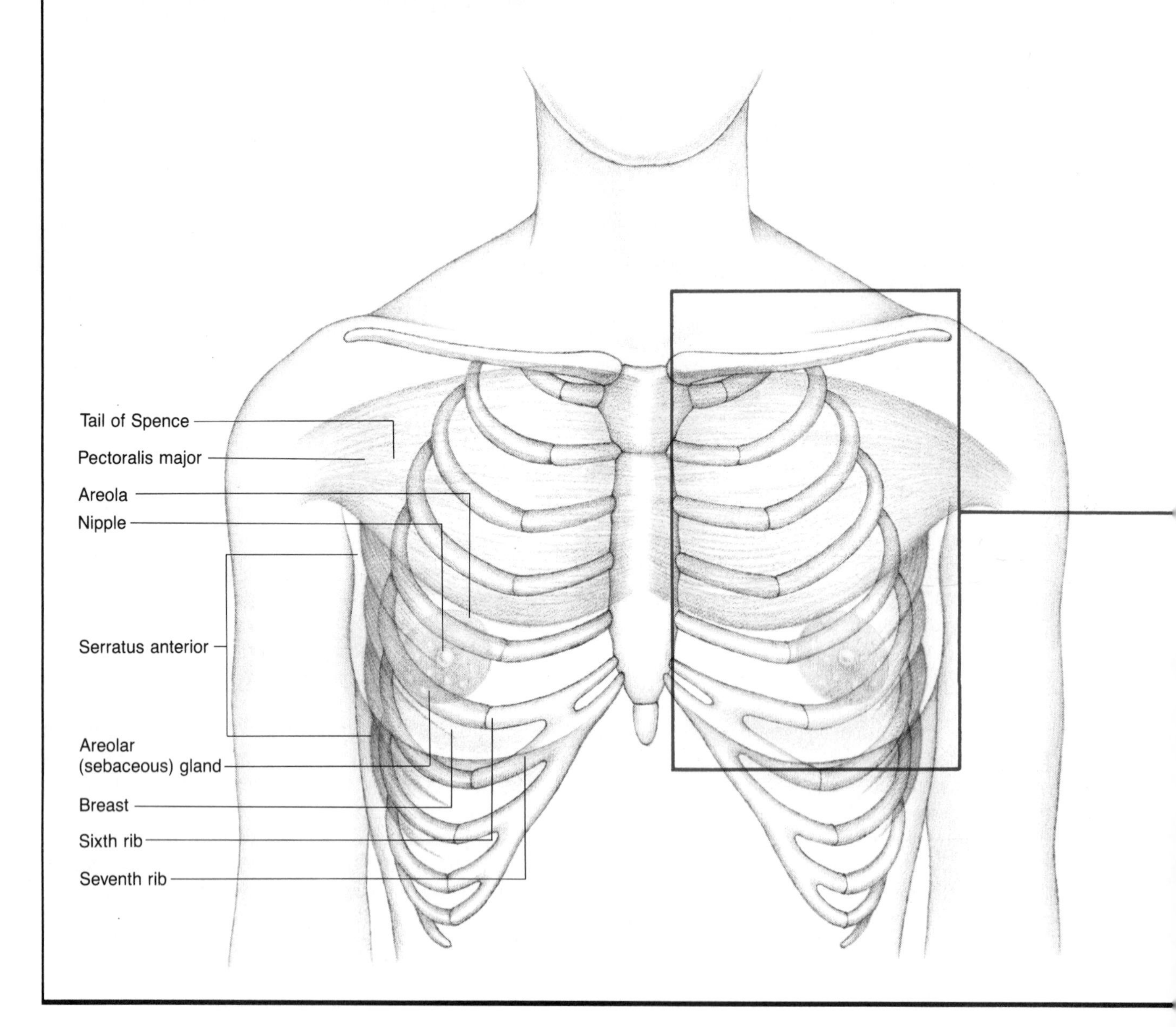

The male breast

The male breast is composed of a nipple, the surrounding areola, and a flat body of breast tissue that usually is not palpably distinguishable from the adjacent chest tissue.

Lymphatic drainage of the breasts

In females and males, each breast contains a lymphatic network that drains the breast of lymph and returns it to the blood.

The *pectoral (anterior)* lymph nodes, located along the lower border of the pectoralis major inside the anterior axillary fold, drain most of the breast and the anterior chest wall.

The *brachial (lateral)* nodes, located along the upper humerus, drain most of the arm.

The *subscapular (posterior)* nodes, located along the lateral scapular border deep within the posterior axillary fold, drain a part of the arm and the posterior chest wall.

The *midaxillary (central axillary)* nodes are close to the ribs and the serratus anterior, high in the axilla. The pectoral, brachial, and subscapular nodes drain into the midaxillary nodes.

Deeper internal mammary nodes that are inaccessible to palpation drain the mammary lobules, whereas the superficial lymphatic vessels drain the skin. Thus, breast cancer may spread through the lymphatic system to the infraclavicular or supraclavicular nodes, to nodes deep in the chest or abdomen, or to the opposite breast, depending on the primary lesion location.

Lateral cross section of female breast

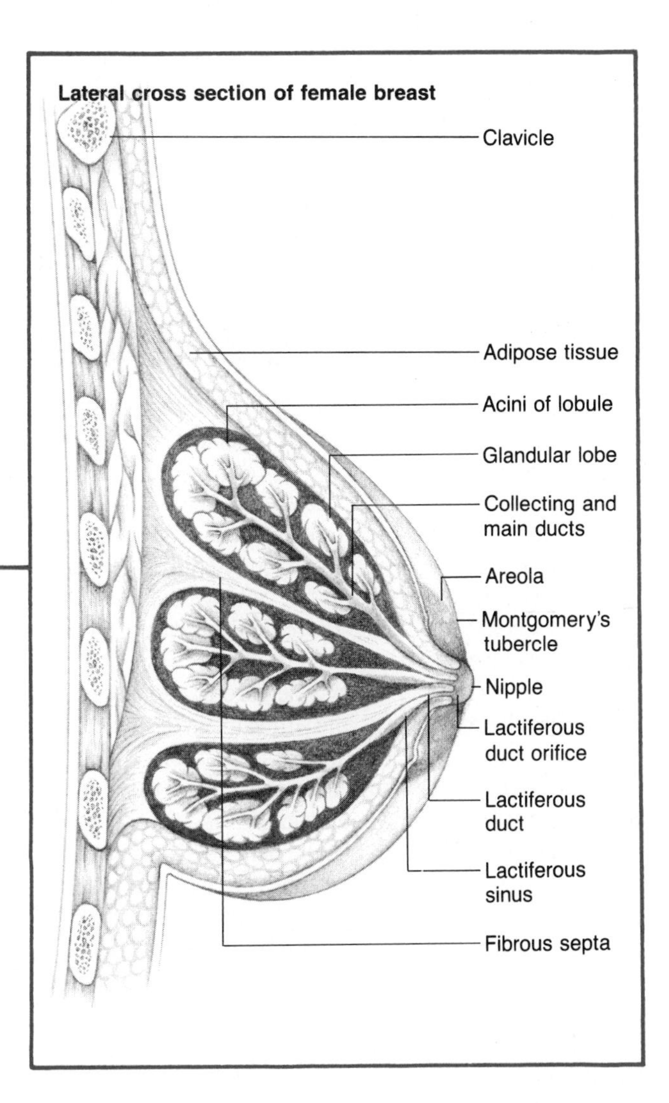

Lymph nodes

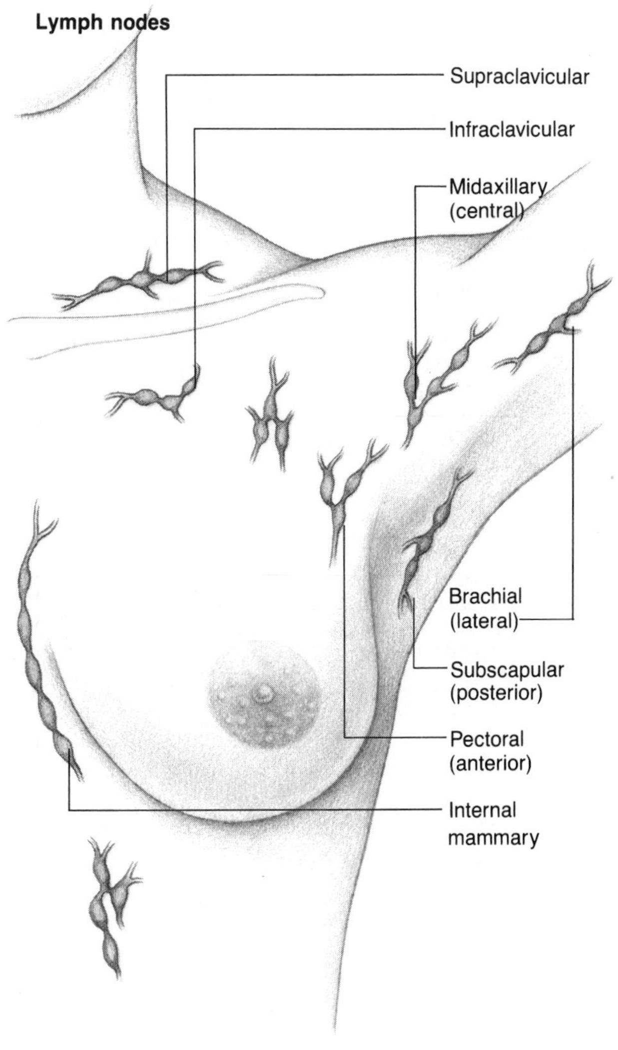

Female breast development

This chart shows the sexual maturity stages of breast development in females.

Stage 1: Preadolescent
Nipple elevation begins.

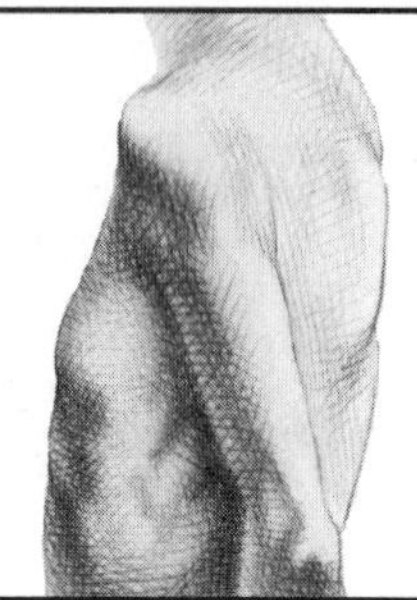

Stage 2: Breast budding
Breast and nipple elevation appears as a small mound with areolar enlargement.

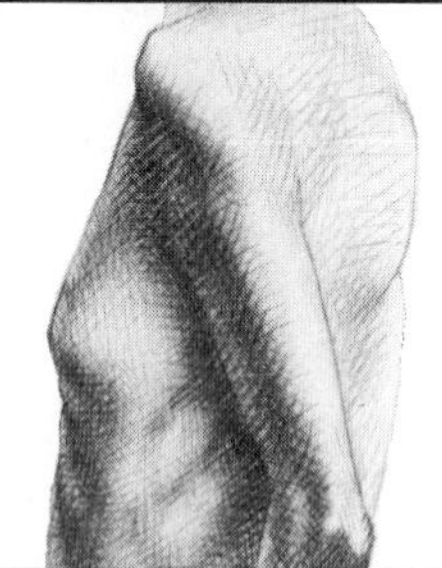

Stage 3: Continued enlargement
The breast and areola enlarge without distinct evidence of separation between them.

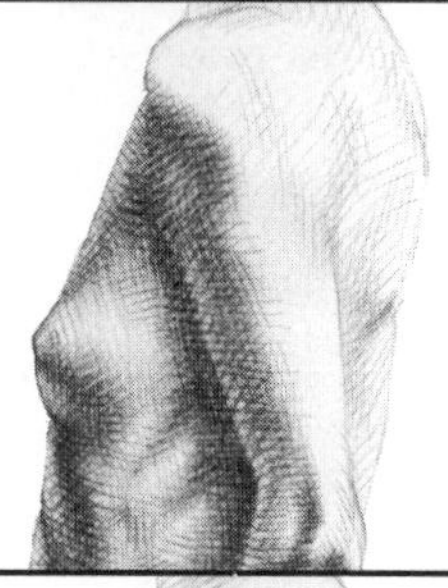

Stage 4: Secondary mound
A secondary mound forms beyond the original breast mound as the areola and nipple project.

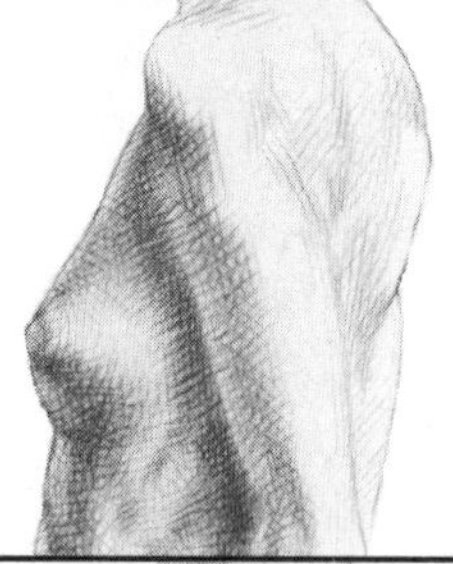

Stage 5: Breast maturity
The nipple projects and the areola becomes part of the breast contour.

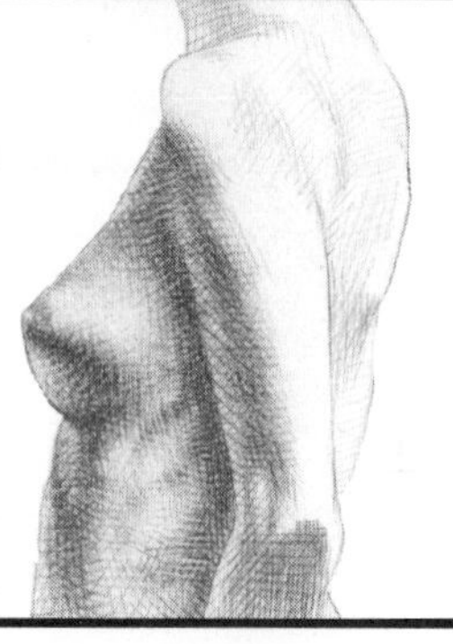

Adapted with permission of the publisher from Tanner, J.M., *Growth at Adolescence*, 2nd ed., Oxford: Blackwell Scientific Publications, Ltd., 1962.

can cause contraction of the circular and longitudinal smooth muscle fibers in the nipple epithelium, resulting in nipple erection and milk flow from the lactiferous ducts.

The breast alveoli (acini cells) and lactiferous ducts become engorged from milk and edema, making them tender and full. Once the infant's need for milk and the mother's milk supply become harmonious, the extreme tenseness and tenderness of early engorgement pass. When lactation ends, the breasts return to pregestational size (involute) in about 3 months.

Maturity

As women reach menopause, estrogen secretion declines, causing glandular tissue to atrophy and be replaced with fatty deposits. A reduction in breast size results. The breasts become flabbier and hang more loosely from the chest as ligaments relax. The ducts around the nipples may become palpable as firm strings, and the nipples flatten, losing some erectile quality.

Health history

The nurse should prepare the client for the health history by explaining the purpose of the interview. Use the following guidelines.

Discussing the breast may be embarrassing and difficult for a female client, so ensure a comfortable interview environment that offers privacy and freedom from interruptions. Perform the interview before the physical assessment while the client is sitting up and dressed or covered with a gown.

During the health history, be sure to ask questions about the client's health and illness patterns, health promotion and protection patterns, and role and relationship patterns. Although the health history will focus on the breast, inquire about the status of other body structures and systems. In the female, the breast is commonly assessed as part of the reproductive system, so expect some breast questions to elicit answers about the reproductive system. For example, breast tenderness often occurs during a specific time of the menstrual cycle.

Most of the questions in this section relate to women, because few breast disorders occur in men. Ask questions that relate to male breast history as applicable.

Health and illness patterns

To assess important health and illness patterns, explore the client's current, past, and family health status, as well as developmental considerations.

Current health status

A woman about to undergo breast assessment probably will be concerned about her current health status, especially if she has noticed a change or lump in her breast. If she has, carefully document the chief complaint, using the client's own words. Using the PQRST method, ask the client to describe completely this complaint and any others. (For a detailed explanation of the PQRST method, see *Symptom analysis* in Chapter 3, The Health History.) Ask the following questions to learn more about the client's current health status:

How old are you?
(RATIONALE: Because approximately 80% of breast cancers occur in women over age 40, age is important in breast assessment.)

What changes, if any, have you noticed in your breasts?
(RATIONALE: Breast changes may be menstrual-cycle related, or they may indicate cancer or benign breast disease, such as fibrocystic disease, which causes multiple, benign cysts of the breast.)

How would you describe the change?
(RATIONALE: A breast lump may indicate a benign cyst, a fibroadenoma, or a malignant tumor. Lumpy breasts may indicate fibrocystic disease, which occurs in about 58% of American women. The relationship between fibrocystic disease and breast cancer is uncertain. However, most researchers believe that fibrocystic disease is not a breast cancer precursor, unless the client shows evidence of epithelial hyperplasia [abnormal increase in epithelial cells], also called florid fibrocystic disease. An inverted nipple, skin swelling, skin dimpling, and superficial veins that are more prominent on one breast than the other may indicate cancer.)

Have you noticed any changes in your underarm (axillary) areas?
(RATIONALE: Any progressive swelling may indicate cancer. Dark pigmentation and a velvety-textured axilla also may indicate cancer.)

If you have noticed a change, how long ago did you notice it?
(RATIONALE: Some changes relate to the menstrual cycle or to activities that involve strenuous chest movement.)

Has the change become more pronounced lately?
(RATIONALE: The client's answer may indicate how rapidly the lump, or lesion, is growing.)

Do you have breast pain or tenderness?
(RATIONALE: Breast pain or tenderness is usually menstrual-cycle related.)

Have you noticed any nipple discharge?
(RATIONALE: Data about the discharge color and consistency, the number of ducts involved, and whether the discharge occurs spontaneously or manually or from one or both nipples can help diagnose the problem. Any discharge unrelated to obstetric delivery or lactation needs evaluation.)

Do you have any rash or eczema on either nipple?
(RATIONALE: Paget's disease, a cancer of the nipple and areola that is usually associated with cancer in deeper breast structures, looks like eczema when it begins.)

Do you currently take any over-the-counter or prescription medications (including birth control pills or estrogen)? If so, which ones and how often do you take them?
(RATIONALE: Some medications can cause breast changes. Oral contraceptives may cause breast enlargement, tenderness, or discharge. Sometimes prescribed to alleviate postmenopausal symptoms, prolonged estrogen therapy without progesterone, is associated with uterine cancer. For additional information, see *Adverse drug reactions,* page 340.)

Past health status

During this part of the health history, ask the following questions to explore the client's medical history for breast-related information:

Have you ever had breast surgery? If so, when and why?
(RATIONALE: Previous breast surgery could have been for cancer or benign fibroadenomas. If the client had breast cancer, breast changes could indicate another malignant lesion.)

At what age did you begin to menstruate?
(RATIONALE: Onset of menses [menarche] before age 12 increases breast cancer risk because the breast is exposed to estrogen for a longer-than-normal time.)

If you have children, at what age did you bear them?
(RATIONALE: Having the first child before age 18 decreases a woman's risk of breast cancer; childlessness or bearing a first child after age 30 increases the risk.)

Adverse drug reactions

When obtaining a health history to assess a client's breast, the nurse should ask about current drug use. Many drugs cause breast changes, such as enlargement or tenderness, and the chart below presents some of them.

DRUG CLASS	DRUG	POSSIBLE ADVERSE REACTIONS
Androgens	danazol, fluoxymesterone, methyltestosterone, testosterone	*Female:* decreased breast size *Male:* gynecomastia
Antidepressants	tricyclic antidepressants	*Female:* breast engorgement and galactorrhea (spontaneous milk flow) *Male:* gynecomastia
Antipsychotics	chlorpromazine hydrochloride, fluphenazine, haloperidol, perphenazine, prochlorperazine maleate, thioridazine, thiothixene	*Female:* galactorrhea, moderate engorgement of the breast with lactation, mastalgia (breast pain) *Male:* gynecomastia, mastalgia
Cardiac glycosides	digitoxin, digoxin	*Male:* gynecomastia
Estrogens	chlorotrianisene, conjugated estrogens, esterified estrogens, estradiol, estrone, ethinyl estradiol	*Female:* breast changes, tenderness, enlargement, secretions *Male:* breast changes, tenderness, gynecomastia
	dienestrol	*Female:* breast tenderness
	diethylstilbestrol	*Female:* breast tenderness, enlargement *Male:* breast tenderness, gynecomastia
Oral contraceptives	estrogen-progesterone combinations	*Female:* breast changes, tenderness, enlargement, secretions
Progestins	hydroxyprogesterone caproate, medroxyprogesterone acetate, norethindrone, norethindrone acetate, norgestrel, progesterone	*Female:* breast tenderness or galactorrhea
Miscellaneous agents	isoniazid	*Male:* gynecomastia
	reserpine	*Female:* breast engorgement, galactorrhea *Male:* gynecomastia
	spironolactone	*Female:* breast tenderness *Male:* painful gynecomastia
	cimetidine	*Female:* galactorrhea *Male:* gynecomastia

If you have children and did not breast-feed, did you take any medications to suppress lactation?
(RATIONALE: The use of estrogens or androgens to suppress lactation is no longer recommended. These drugs have been implicated in endometrial cancer.)

If you have gone through menopause, at what age did this occur?
(RATIONALE: Menopause [cessation of menses] after age 55 increases the risk of breast cancer because it exposes the breast to estrogen for a longer-than-normal time.)

Did you gain excess weight after menopause?
(RATIONALE: Postmenopausal weight gain increases estrogen levels, which increases breast cancer risk.)

Have you ever had a mammogram (breast x-ray)? If so, when?
(RATIONALE: Breast exposure to excessive ionizing radiation [such as that produced by early mammography machines] increases breast cancer risk.)

Have you had cancer, such as cancer of the uterine lining?
(RATIONALE: Previous or concurrent cancers, especially endometrial cancer, increase breast cancer risk.)

Have you had your uterus or ovaries removed, or have you had radiotherapy of your ovaries or uterus?
(RATIONALE: Breast cancer risk is decreased in women who have undergone any of these procedures.)

Family health status

Investigate the client's family history of breast disease by asking these questions:

Did your mother or any siblings have breast cancer?
(RATIONALE: Breast cancer risk increases for a client who has a mother or sibling with a breast cancer history, especially if the cancer developed before menopause.)

If your mother or sibling had breast cancer, was it in one breast or both?
(RATIONALE: The risk of breast cancer increases further for a person whose mother or sibling had bilateral breast cancer.)

Developmental considerations

For a female pediatric, pregnant, or elderly client, the following questions help investigate developmental status.

Pediatric client. If the child is over age 10, ask:

How you think your breasts will change as you get older?
(RATIONALE: The premenarchal child needs to know what growth and development to expect so that sexual maturity changes will not be frightening. Present an illustrated, matter-of-fact introduction to expected changes to help alleviate the child's potential fears.)

Pregnant client. Help alleviate the pregnant client's concerns by asking:

Do you wear a supportive brassiere?
(RATIONALE: Wearing a well-fitting, supportive brassiere can help prevent breast tone loss that may cause pendulous breasts later in life.)

Do you plan to breast-feed?
(RATIONALE: If the client plans to breast-feed, teach her how to roll the nipple gently between her thumb and index finger about 10 times twice a day to toughen it, and thereby decrease potential discomfort.)

Do you have any concerns about breast-feeding?
(RATIONALE: Many women are afraid that their breasts will be smaller when they stop breast-feeding. Reassure the client that the decrease in size after breast-feeding seems great only because the lactating breast enlarges so dramatically.)

Elderly client. The elderly client also needs breast-care assessment. Ask the client:

Do you wear a well-fitting, supportive brassiere?
(RATIONALE: Because breasts tend to sag with age, a good suppportive brassiere can prevent breast pain and discomfort.)

Health promotion and protection patterns

To continue the health history, ask the following questions to assess the client's personal health habits, exercise patterns, nutritional practices, stress patterns, economic situation, and environmental and occupational patterns.

Do you perform breast self-examination? If so, how often?
(RATIONALE: The answer indicates the client's knowledge about breast care. If the client does not examine her breasts monthly, explain that breast self-examination is essential to early detection of cancer. For teaching guidelines, see *Teaching breast self-examination,* page 342.)

Would you please demonstrate how you perform breast self-examination?
(RATIONALE: A demonstration ensures that the client knows the correct technique, which is essential for maximum effectiveness.)

When do you perform breast self-examination?
(RATIONALE: The client should perform her breast self-examination on the 5th to 7th day after the first day of the menstrual period, when the hormonal effect, which can cause breast tenderness or lumpiness, is reduced. A postmenopausal client should choose a regular time each month to examine her breasts. If a client is on cyclical estrogen therapy, the last day the client is off the medication is best for self-examination.)

When was your last mammogram?
(RATIONALE: A client age 35 to 40 should have a baseline screening mammogram. A client age 40 to 49 should have one every 1 to 2 years; a client over age 50, once a year. A client with a family history of breast cancer may need mammography more frequently, as determined by the physician.)

Teaching breast self-examination

Breast self-examination (BSE) is one of the most important health habits to teach the client. The nurse can teach BSE during the palpation phase of assessment. (If the client already performs BSE, check to make sure her technique is correct.) Follow the steps below.

1 First, teach the client how to look at herself in a mirror and, with her arms at her sides, check for any visible abnormalities. She should observe for dimpling, retraction, or breast flattening as she first elevates her arms slowly, then presses her hands against her hips, and finally, bends forward.

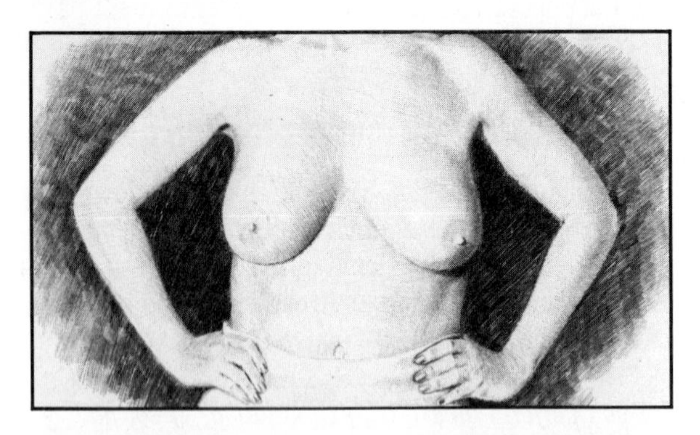

2 Next, by placing your hand over the client's, show her how to use the pads of the middle three fingers of the opposite hand to palpate the breast systematically by compressing the breast tissue against the chest wall. She should palpate all portions of the breast, areola, nipple, tail of Spence, and axilla when she is in the shower or standing before a mirror. She should repeat the procedure lying down with a pillow or folded towel under the shoulder of the side she is examining.

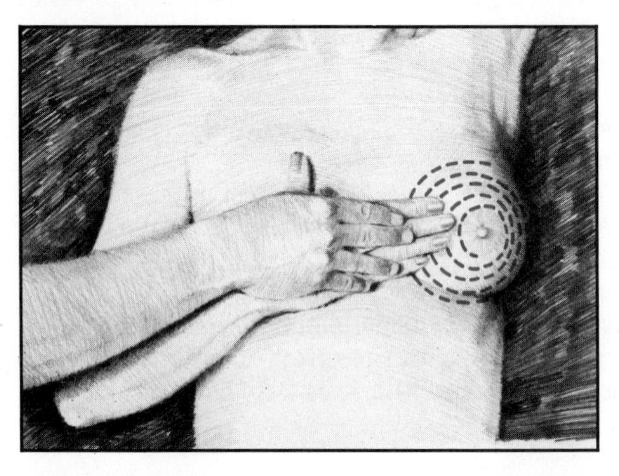

3 Next, show her how to compress the nipple gently between the thumb and index finger as she observes for any discharge.

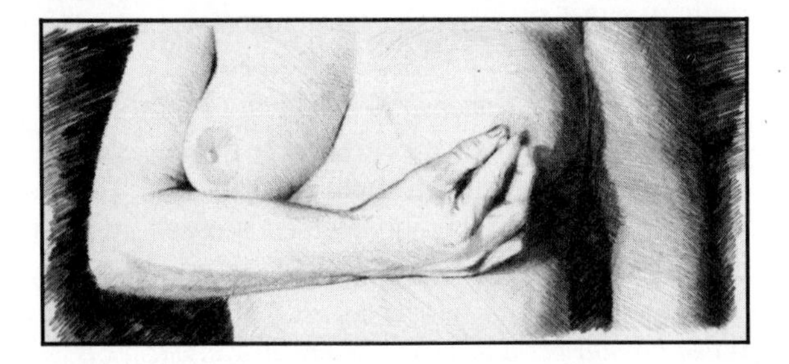

4 Finally, explain that she should report any redness or inflammation, swelling, masses, flattening, puckering, dimpling, retraction, sunken areas, asymmetrical nipple direction, discharge, bleeding, lesions, or eczematous nipple changes to her physician.

If you have a breast change, can you relate it to a change in the type of brassiere you wear or a sudden blow to your breast?
(RATIONALE: Some breast changes are caused by constant irritation from a poorly fitting wire brassiere or other trauma, such as a blow to the breast.)

Have you recently changed your routine activities—for example, have you begun a new job or engaged in a new sport?
(RATIONALE: Activities that strain the chest structures, such as tennis or physical tasks required in certain jobs, can cause breast changes. Jogging or increased sexual manipulation of the breast can cause nipple pain or irritation.)

How much fat do you consume in your diet?
(RATIONALE: A high dietary intake of fat increases breast cancer risk.)

Have you experienced high stress levels for a long time?
(RATIONALE: Chronic psychological stress increases breast cancer risk.)

Role and relationship patterns

In the United States, female breasts are significantly associated with sexuality. Consequently, any threat to the breast can threaten a woman's body image and feelings of personal worth, directly affecting relationships with others, especially men. When assessing role and relationship patterns, ask these questions:

How important are your breasts to a positive view of yourself?
(RATIONALE: If a client has a breast lump that may need surgery, she may fear disfigurement, perhaps even more than the threat of cancer. This question will help the client express her feelings about impending breast assessment or treatment.)

If you have breast tenderness or pain related to lumpy breasts, how does it affect your sex life?
(RATIONALE: If breast pain or tenderness caused by fibrocystic disease affects a client's sexual relationships, suggest treatments to relieve the pain. Such treatments include mild analgesics, warm compresses, or sleeping bras; a low-salt diet, especially in the latter half of the menstrual cycle; restricted intake of caffeine-containing foods and drinks, such as chocolate, coffee, and colas; or use of vitamin E supplements.)

Physical assessment

Because a breast assessment may be embarrassing for a client, the nurse must anticipate the need for privacy. Although the female client frequently feels uncomfortable totally exposed from the waist up, the assessment will be inaccurate if both breasts cannot be compared. A sensitive nursing approach will help the client accept the need to disrobe. The nurse also should reassure the client that she can cover herself as soon as possible, and remind the client that teaching or reviewing breast self-examination with her is necessary to check her technique.

The male client may question the need to assess his breasts and axillae. To help him understand the need for this assessment, explain that breast cancer occasionally occurs in men.

Gentleness, privacy, warm hands, an objective approach, and explanations all contribute to client comfort during physical assessment.

To prepare for a thorough breast assessment, obtain a flashlight; a small pillow, folded sheet, or towel; a ruler; and a cytologic fixative and slide for nipple discharge. Plan to use inspection and palpation techniques.

Be sure to have good lighting to help you detect subtle skin changes. For a supine examination, place a small pillow or folded towel under the client's back on the side being assessed. This allows the breast tissue to spread more evenly across the chest wall for examination. Use a ruler to measure lesions, and a flashlight (equipped with a transilluminator, if possible) to augment lighting when you inspect suspicious-looking skin or subcutaneous lesions.

Position the examination table so that you have easy access to the client. Then, allow sufficient time for a thorough assessment. Proceed systematically, examining all breast areas.

Inspection

Begin the assessment with the client seated, disrobed to the waist and with the arms resting at each side.

First inspect the breasts for size and symmetry. In women, the breasts are normally symmetrical, convex, and similar in appearance. Usually, however, one breast is smaller than the other. The male breast usually is not convex unless the client is overweight.

Look for obvious masses, flattening of the breast on one side, or retraction or dimpling (a depression in a localized breast surface area). To inspect for hidden dimpling, ask the client to place her hands against her hips. Then, ask her to raise her arms slowly over her head. Inspect for equal and free breast movement without signs of dimpling. Repeat if necessary.

Ask the client with large or pendulous breasts to stand and lean forward with her hands or arms outstretched. Support the client's arms or use a chair or table. Both breasts should swing forward freely. Next, evaluate skin texture; it should look smooth and soft. The venous pattern on the skin should be similar bilaterally. Pronounced bilateral venous patterns are normal in obese or fair-skinned people.

Do not be concerned with unchanged, nontender, and long-standing surface skin lesions, such as nevi (pigmented congenital skin blemishes), but do examine recent changes closely. Purple striations, which turn silver over time, may be seen if the client has been pregnant or has gained weight.

Inspect the nipples and areolae for size, shape, and color. The nipples and areolae should be similarly round or oval, of equal size, and free of rashes, fissures, or ulcerations. The nipples usually point in the same direction—outward, slightly upward, and lateral. Inspect the nipples for a discharge. A manually expressed discharge can normally occur, but a spontaneous discharge should not. Montgomery's tubercles (sebaceous glands that secrete a waxy substance) normally appear on male and female areolae.

Check the axillae for rashes, signs of infection such as boils, and unusual pigmentation. The axillae should be free of rashes or lesions and have hair growth if the client is past puberty.

Abnormal findings

Masses, dimpling, or flattening may indicate an abnormality, possibly cancer. Dimpling results from a tumor shortening fibrotic breast areas or immobilizing Cooper's ligaments. Edema, skin thickening, and an orange peel appearance (peau d'orange) may result from a cancer that blocks lymph drainage.

A reddish color may signify infection and inflammation. A red, scaly, eczema-like area over one nipple and areola could be Paget's disease. A unilateral venous pattern may indicate dilated veins from an underlying disease. Although some women normally have bilaterally inverted nipples, one inverted nipple (unless long present) should arouse suspicion. View any eczematous lesion as possible cancer and assess further.

Although uncommon, some women have an extra nipple, an extra breast with a nipple, or extra breast tissue along the milk lines—embryonic ridges that extend from the axilla to the groin. (For an illustration, see *Milk lines.*) Called supernumerary breasts or nipples, these congenital anomalies are small, visible, palpable masses. Milk lines normally atrophy during fetal development, except where the breasts develop. However, in some women, the ridges persist in part or in their entirety.

Malignant acanthosis nigricans, a rare cancer, is associated with dark pigmentation and velvety skin texture in the axilla.

Milk lines

Supernumerary breasts or nipples may develop anywhere along the milk lines, embryonic ridges that extend from the axilla to the groin.

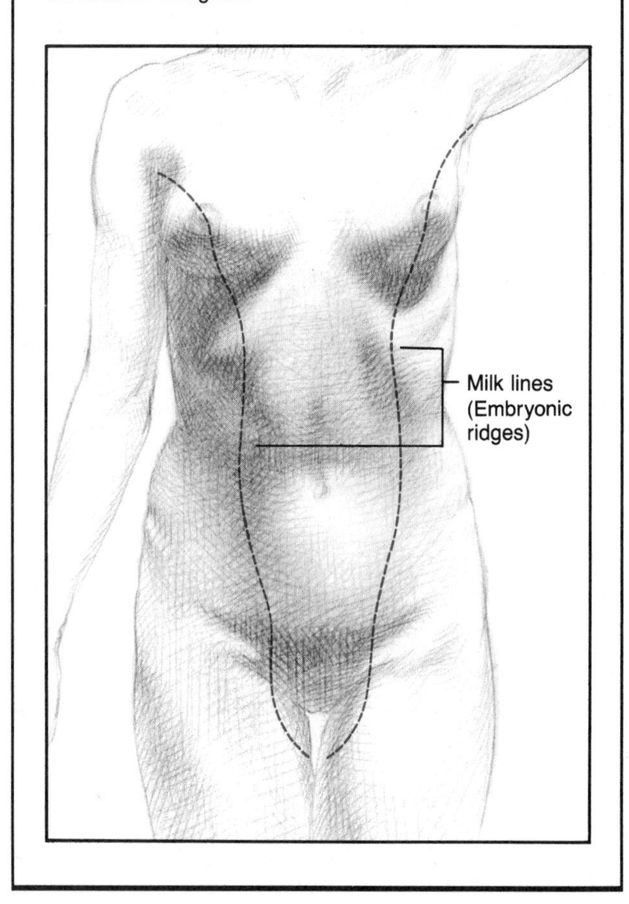

Palpation

To facilitate breast palpation, ask the client to lie supine; for axillary palpation, ask the client to sit up. (For an illustrated description of the procedure, see *Palpating the axillae and breasts.*)

For assessment purposes, mentally divide the breasts into four quadrants and a fifth segment, the tail of Spence. Findings can be described easily according to a quadrant or segment. Think of the breast as a clock, with the nipple in the center. Then, localize lesions according to time (2 o'clock, for example) and distance in centimeters from the nipple. (For an illustration, see *Describing the location of abnormalities,* page 352.)

Abnormal findings

Any palpable mass, induration, tenderness associated with a mass, or inflammation found in the breast or axilla is abnormal. Cancerous nodules are likely to be hard, irregularly shaped, fixed, nontender, and poorly circumscribed. If you palpate a mass, note the size in centimeters, the shape (oval, round, or irregular), consistency (firm, cystic, hard, or rubbery), circumscription (delineation from the surrounding tissue), mobility (whether fixed to the underlying tissue or freely movable), tenderness, and location by distance in centimeters from the nipple, by location on the clock, or by quadrant. Abnormal findings require further evaluation by a physician using specific diagnostic tests.

Because spontaneous nipple discharge may indicate a cancer, refer the client to a physician for further evaluation. At the same time, note the color, consistency, and location (one or both nipples, one or more ducts). Other abnormal findings requiring referral to a physician include fissures, nodules, or masses in the areola. (For some common abnormal assessment findings associated with the breast, see *Integrating assessment findings,* page 349.)

(Text continues on page 348.)

Palpating the axillae and breasts

Palpate the male or female axillae with the client sitting or lying down. However, the sitting position provides easier access for palpation.

1 Begin with the client's right axilla. Ask the client to relax the right arm while you use your left hand to support the client's elbow or wrist. With your right middle three fingers cupped, reach high into the central axilla. Sweep the fingers downward and against the ribs and serratus anterior to try to feel the central nodes. Palpating one or two small, nontender, freely movable nodes is normal.

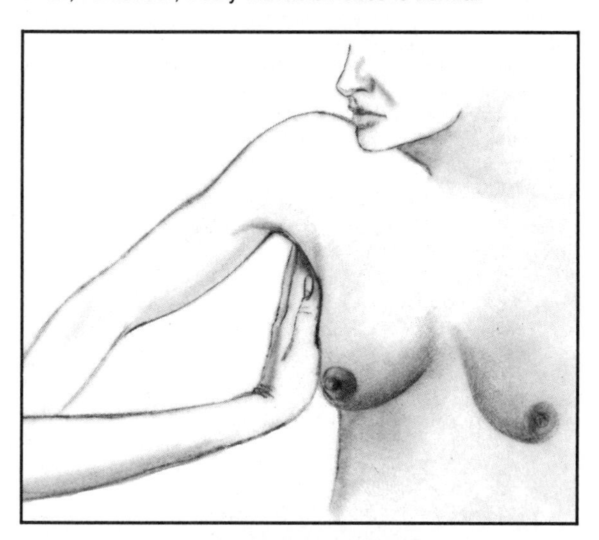

2 Assess the anterior nodes by palpating with both hands along the anterior axillary fold.

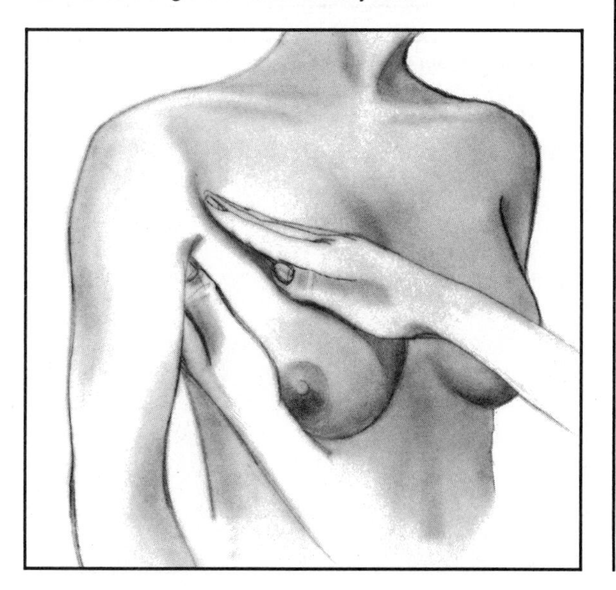

3 Assess the posterior nodes by palpating along the posterior axillary fold.

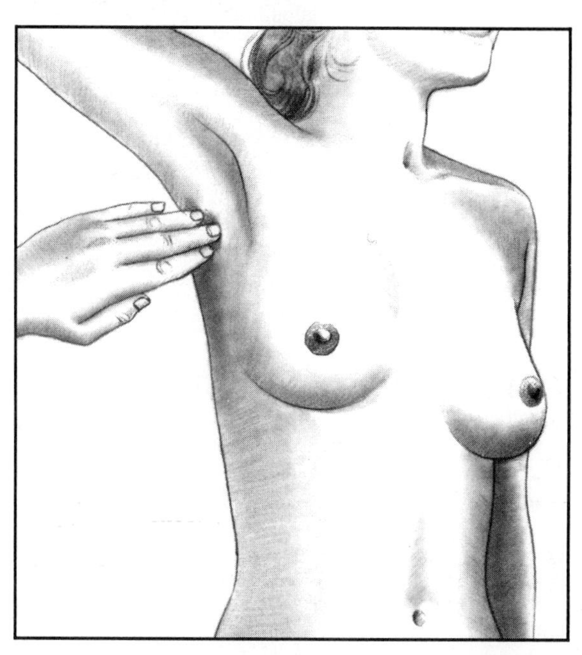

4 Palpate the lateral nodes by pressing your fingers along the upper inner arm, trying to compress these nodes against the humerus. Repeat the assessment on the client's left side. Assess the infraclavicular and supraclavicular nodes if any axillary node findings appear abnormal. (See Chapter 19, Immune System and Blood.)

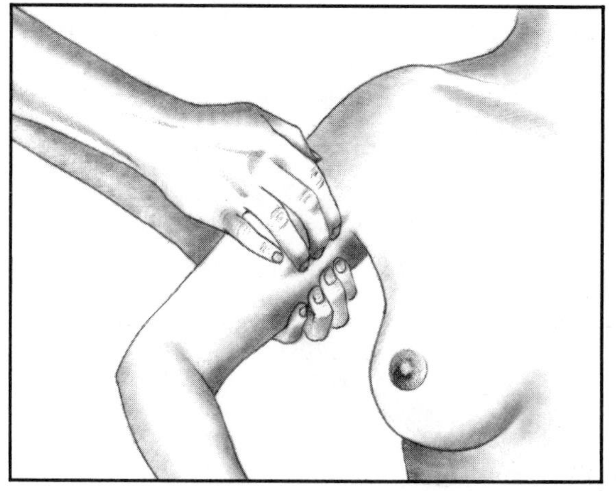

continued

Palpating the axillae and breasts continued

5 To palpate the breast, ask the client to lie supine with a small pad or pillow placed under the shoulder of the side being examined and with the arm on that same side placed above the client's head. This position allows the breast tissue to spread out evenly, facilitating the examination. Palpate a woman with large breasts in the supine and seated positions.

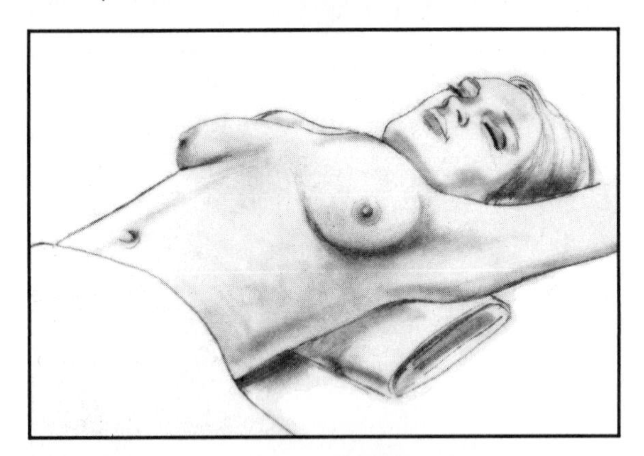

6 Using the middle three finger pads, palpate the breast in a systematic pattern, rotating the fingers gently against the chest wall. Palpate circularly from the center out or from the periphery in, making sure you palpate the tail of Spence.

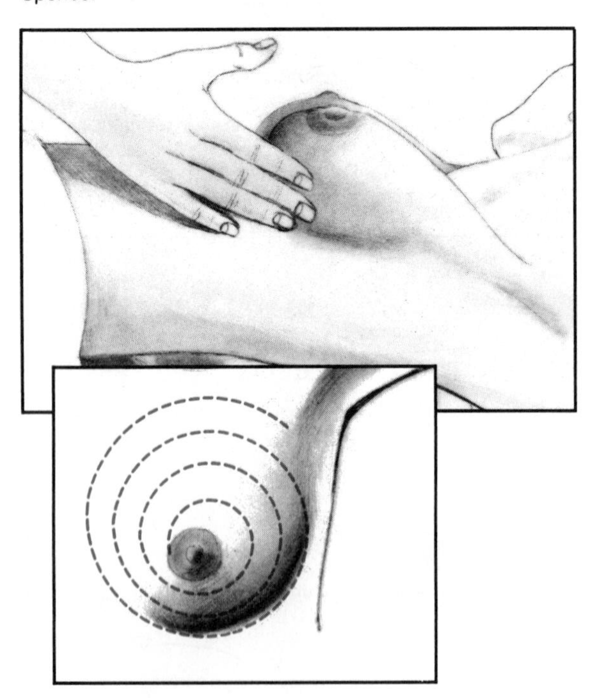

7 Choosing to palpate across or down the breast is also satisfactory, especially on a client with pendulous breasts. This is best done with the client seated.

As you palpate, feel for masses or areas of induration (hardness). If a mass is suspected, move or compress the breast gently to look for dimpling. Also palpate for consistency and elasticity. The youthful breast is firmly elastic, with the glandular tissue feeling like small lobules. The mature breast may feel more granular or stringy. More nodularity and fullness may occur premenstrually. The normal inframammary ridge at the lower edge of the breast is firm and may be mistaken for a tumor.

Also assess for tenderness, which will depend on the time in the menstrual cycle that the assessment is performed. The breasts are frequently tender the week before the menstrual period. Note where the client is in the menstrual cycle when breast assessment data are recorded and interpreted.

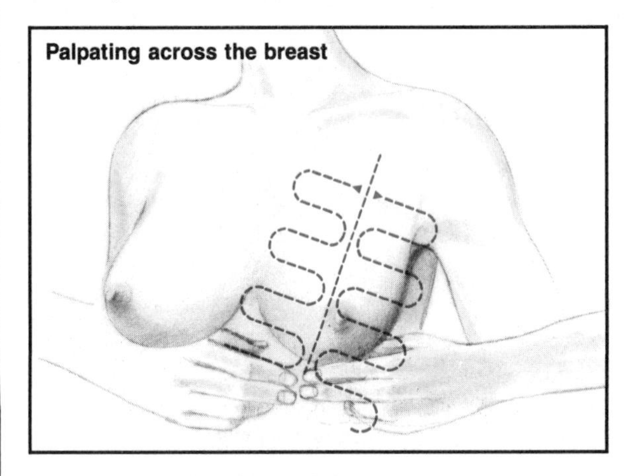

Palpating across the breast

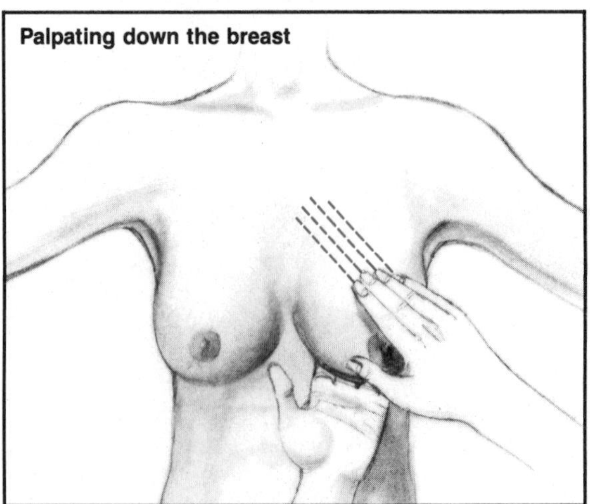

Palpating down the breast

Palpating the axillae and breasts continued

8 Palpate the areola and nipple of male and female clients alike. Palpate the nipple by gently compressing it between your thumb and index finger. The nipple will become erect and the areola will pucker normally from the tactile stimulation.

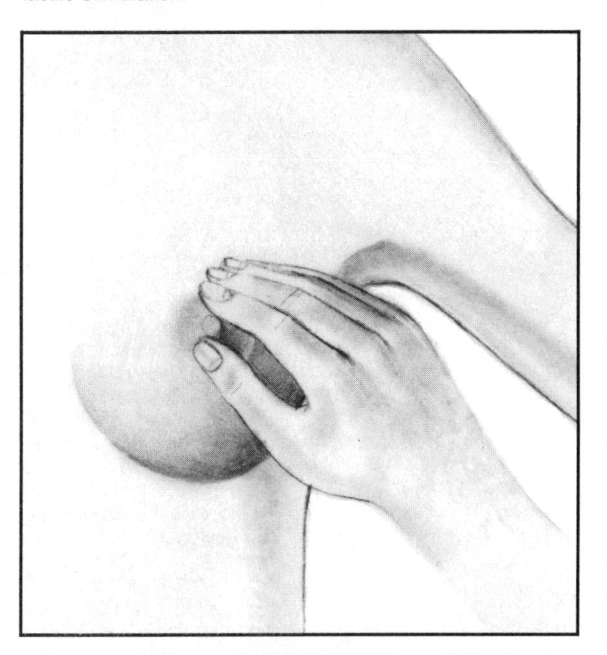

9 Gently milk the nipple for discharge by compressing it between the thumb and index finger. If discharge occurs, note the duct or ducts through which it appears.

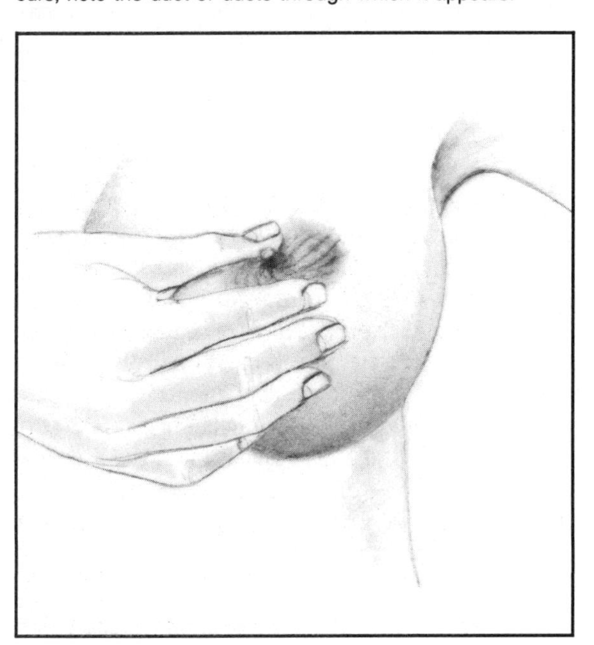

10 Make a cytologic smear of any discharge not explained by pregnancy or lactation. Place a glass slide over the nipple, smear the discharge on it, and spray with fixative immediately.

Some experts no longer check for discharge by squeezing the nipples because many women normally have a benign discharge on palpation. However, a spontaneous discharge is significant and needs physician referral.

Making a smear of discharge

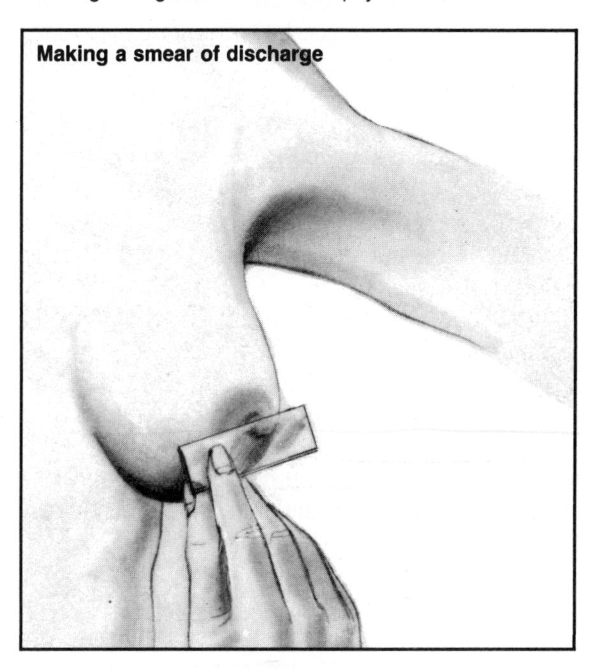

Spraying slide with fixative

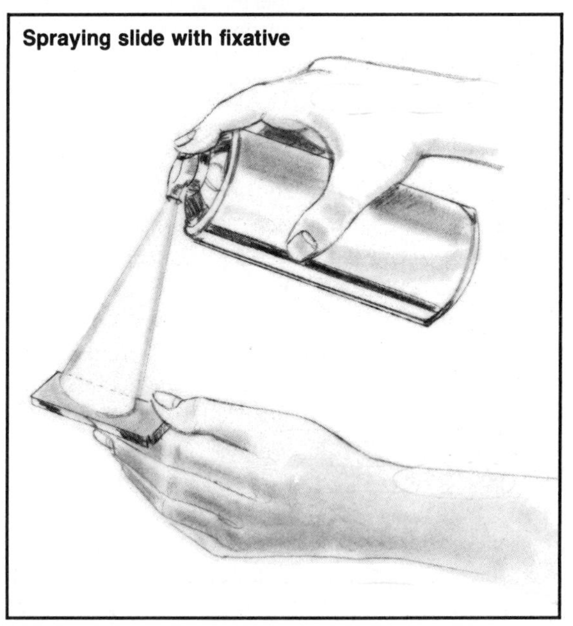

Developmental considerations

Breast appearance changes during life-cycle stages, which makes the nurse's familiarity with the changes essential to accurate breast assessment.

Infants. Male and female neonates may exhibit breast enlargement caused by maternal estrogen transferred at birth. This enlargement, which may be as great as ⅝" (1.5 cm), is palpable behind the nipple and is transitory, usually disappearing within 2 weeks. It seldom lasts for more than 3 months. In some infants, a white, milky fluid known as witch's milk may be expressed from the enlarged breast.

Adolescents. Assess the sexual maturity level of the female adolescent. If a female client expresses concern that her breasts are developing asymmetrically, reassure her that this is normal. The breasts will become fairly equal with full development.

Gynecomastia commonly occurs in young adolescent males and usually disappears within a year. Bilateral or unilateral, the condition may embarrass the young man and concern his parents or guardians. Reassure these clients that gynecomastia is temporary and will disappear with maturation. Explain that the swelling affects the tissue under the areola, sometimes making the breast tender or painful.

Pregnant and lactating clients. As the breasts enlarge during pregnancy, a female client may need to change her brassiere size and style for better support. Tingling, fullness, and tenderness are normal complaints. Darkened nipples and areolae are normal; purplish linear streaks (striae gravidarum) may develop on the breast mounds as they increase in size.

After the 6th gestational week, colostrum may flow and dry on the nipple. Because the alveoli enlarge, the breasts feel nodular. The venous pattern becomes bilaterally prominent, and vascular spiders, resulting from elevated estrogen levels, may develop on the upper trunk.

In a lactating client, examine the breasts for engorgement. If engorged, the breasts feel hard and warm, and the skin will appear red and shiny. The client usually complains of pain. Check the nipples for irritation, such as cracks, fissures, bleeding, redness, tenderness, blisters, and petechiae if the client is breast-feeding.

Elderly clients. The breasts of an elderly female client normally feel more granular and the tissues less firm and elastic. The inframammary ridge (cartilage below the breast) thickens as a woman matures; do not mistake it for a mass.

Gynecomastia in an elderly male client may be bilateral (the result of estrogen-secreting tumors or estrogen treatment for cancer) or unilateral (most commonly caused by prednisone therapy, although phenothiazines and digitalis also may cause it). Be concerned by unilateral gynecomastia, which could indicate a malignant condition. In the case of drug-induced gynecomastia, however, the enlarged tissue lacks normal breast tissue quality, feeling like a firm disc around the areola above the glandular lobes. Extreme enlargement may require surgical correction for psychological or cosmetic reasons.

Diagnosing breast lesions

The following techniques are currently used to diagnose and evaluate breast lesions.

Mammography
This procedure usually requires two low-dose-radiation X-ray exposures of each breast—anterior and oblique views. The breast is compressed to reduce tissue thickness, allowing better detection of small tumors. Early detection enhances cure chances if a malignant lesion exists. Mammography detects lumps as small as 4 mm and even 1-mm calcium deposits—sometimes a sign of cancer. A 30% decrease in mortality is estimated in one report on mammography screening—or 10,000 lives saved per year.

The American Cancer Society and the American College of Radiology recommend a baseline mammogram for all women age 35 to 40, once every 1 to 2 years for women age 40 to 49, and once yearly for all women over age 50. Radiation exposure at these intervals and low dosages is minimal. Because about 10% to 15% of tumors are missed by mammography, regular physical examinations and breast self-examinations are essential.

Thermography
This procedure identifies heat patterns from increased metabolism of malignant tumors. However, small or deep cancers may be missed, making thermography less comprehensive than mammography. Thermography is being replaced by ultrasonography and low-dose mammography.

Transillumination
Also known as diaphanography or light scanning, transillumination projects infrared light through breast tissue. A video camera photographs the light, which a computer transforms into images on a video screen. Lesions or areas of increased vascularity appear darker than surrounding tissue. Currently a popular supplement to mammography, this quick, safe, and painless procedure emits no radiation, making it useful for showing tumor changes without repeatedly exposing the client to radiation.

Integrating assessment findings

Sometimes, a cluster of assessment findings will strongly suggest a particular breast disorder. In the chart below, column one shows groups of presenting signs and symptoms—the ones that make the client seek medical attention. Column two shows related assessment findings that the nurse may discover during the health history and physical assessment. The client may have one or more of these findings. Column three shows the possible disorder indicated by a cluster of these findings.

PRESENTING SIGNS AND SYMPTOMS	RELATED ASSESSMENT FINDINGS	POSSIBLE DISORDER
Thickened, nodular areas in breast (usually bilateral); may be slight; pain and tenderness possible, especially premenstrually	Female client in childbearing years Exacerbated by caffeine intake Single or multiple breast masses; usually bilateral, mobile, well-defined, tender, in upper outer quadrant Cystic fluid (typically gray-green) from aspirated cysts	Fibrocystic disease (mammary dysplasia, cystic adenosis, chronic cystic disease, cystic mastitis)
Nipple discharge accompanied by nipple retraction; pain in affected areas; itching around nipple	Female client in early-stage menopause Subareolar ducts that feel like rubbery lesions filled with a pastelike material Enlarged regional lymph nodes possible	Mammary duct ectasia (dilatation)
Nipple discharge, usually bloody; breast lump	Caucasian female client of middle or upper socioeconomic class, over age 35, with a family history of breast cancer, a personal history of long menstrual cycles, early menses, late menopause, or a first pregnancy after age 35 History of endometrial or ovarian cancer Enlarged, shrunken, or dimpled breast with no pain Nipple erosion, retraction, or discharge Nontender, firm or hard lump that is irregularly shaped and fixed to skin or underlying tissues Enlarged surrounding lymph nodes	Breast cancer
Well-defined mass or masses in breast; no pain	Female client in teens or early 20s Round, firm, discrete, movable mass, ⅜" to 2" (1 to 5 cm) in diameter; usually solitary but may be multiple and bilateral	Fibroadenoma of breast
Pain accompanied by tenderness in breast; hard, reddened breast	Female client in third or fourth week postpartum History of cracked nipples Breast abscess Painful, enlarged, axillary lymph nodes Firm, tender, warm, and reddened area in affected breast	Mastitis
Serous or serosanguineous discharge from one nipple duct unilaterally; moderate pain	Female client age 35 to 55 No palpable tumor or mass, or a soft mass that is difficult to distinguish from surrounding tissue	Interductal papilloma

Documentation

To document assessment findings accurately, first evaluate all findings. Then look for relationships between health history and physical assessment data. Also review the results of any diagnostic studies that were ordered. (For more information, see *Diagnosing breast lesions.*)

Consider assessment data the first nursing process step. The foundation for appropriate nursing diagnoses, these data allow planning, implementation, and evaluation of the client's nursing care. (For a case study that shows how to apply the nursing process to a client with a breast disorder, see *Applying the nursing process,* pages 350 and 351.)

After completing the assessment, document all data completely, including normal and abnormal findings.

(Text continues on page 352.)

Applying the nursing process

Assessment findings form the basis of the nursing process. Using them, the nurse formulates nursing diagnoses and develops appropriate planning, implementation, and evaluation of the client's care.

The table below shows how the nurse can use breast assessment data in the nursing process for the client described in the case history (shown at right). In the first column, history and physical assessment data are followed by a paragraph of mental notes. These notes help the nurse make important mental connections among assessment findings, aiding in development of the nursing diagnoses and planning.

The second column presents several appropriate nursing diagnoses; however, the information in the remaining three columns is based on the *first* nursing diagnosis. Although it is not part of the nursing process, documentation appears in the last column because of its importance. Documentation consists of an initial note using all components of the SOAPIE format and a follow-up note using the appropriate SOAPIE components.

ASSESSMENT	NURSING DIAGNOSES	PLANNING	IMPLEMENTATION
Subjective (history) data • Client states, "My husband felt a lump in my right breast, but I can't feel it. I feel some tenderness, though." • Client says her last menstrual period was 3 weeks ago, and she's never quite sure about when it will occur. • Client says, "I don't examine my breasts because I don't know how. I've never had a mammogram." • Client says she has taken oral contraceptives for 2 years. • Client states, "I'm afraid of getting cancer because my maternal aunt had a mastectomy for cancer when she was 40." • Client says her job involves tight deadlines and is very stressful. **Objective (physical) data** • Right breast slightly larger than left breast. • Left nipple inverted but easily everted by gentle palpation. • No masses palpated. • No retraction or breast tissue dimpling with client's arms raised or at her side. • No breast flattening or induration. • No spontaneous discharge noted from nipples; no discharge on palpation. **Mental notes** *Although Ms. Moore has a family history of breast cancer, she is in a low-risk category (by age) for the disease. Breast palpation reveals no masses. Her husband felt the mass when Ms. Moore was premenstrual, so it could have been related to premenstrual breast fullness. Breast lumpiness could also result from oral contraceptives. Client needs information about breast cancer risk factors (such as chronic stress) and breast self-examination.*	• Knowledge deficit related to normal female physiology. • Anxiety related to family breast cancer history. • Knowledge deficit related to breast self-examination. • Disturbance in self-concept related to potential for deformity. • Knowledge deficit related to breast cancer risk factors.	**Goals** Before leaving the clinic today, the client will: • describe how to keep a symptom record of her menstrual cycle for 2 months. • explain the hormonal effects of estrogen and progesterone on the normal ovulation-menstruation cycle. • discuss the effects of hormonal contraceptive drugs on the breasts. • identify potential differences between normal and abnormal breast changes. • demonstrate breast self-examination.	• Use illustrations to review breast anatomy and physiology and explain the hormonal influences of menstruation. • Discuss normal body changes that the client notices before, during, and after her menstrual cycle. • Tell the client about potential adverse effects that oral contraceptives may have on the breast. • Define examples of breast abnormalities, comparing them to normal breast changes. For example, bilateral tenderness during the menstrual cycle may be normal in the client who uses oral contraceptives, but persistent tenderness of one breast may be abnormal. • Teach the client how to keep a calendar of menstrual-cycle-related signs and symptoms. • Teach the client breast self-examination.

CASE HISTORY

Ms. Maria Moore, a 24-year-old copy editor, is a Native American whose clinic visit was prompted when her husband discovered a tender lump in her right breast last month.

EVALUATION		DOCUMENTATION BASED ON NURSING PROCESS DATA		
At the next follow-up visit, the client: • brought a 2-month record of her menstrual cycle, including related breast signs and symptoms. • explained the reasons for breast changes she experienced during the menstrual cycle. • described the differences between normal and abnormal breast changes.		**Initial**		**Follow-up**
	S	Client states, "I cannot feel the lump my husband found last month, but I am afraid of cancer because my aunt had a mastectomy when she was 40." Client says she has taken oral contraceptives for 2 years; admits she knows little about breast anatomy and physiology or the menstrual cycle; recalls her last menstrual period was 3 weeks ago.	**S**	Client states, "I have been examining my breasts and notice lumpiness during my menstrual cycle." Client also brought menstrual-cycle calendar to clinic and explained changes she noted and how they relate to the menstrual cycle.
	O	Right breast slightly larger than left. Left nipple inverted but easily everted by gentle palpation. No masses or indurations felt. No breast dimpling or tissue retraction with arms lowered at side or raised overhead. No spontaneous discharge from nipple; no discharge on palpation.	**O**	No masses felt. Right breast slightly larger than left. No breast dimpling or tissue retraction with arms elevated or at side.
	A	Knowledge deficit related to normal female physiology. Client shows an interest in learning by asking questions.	**A**	Client complied with suggestion to keep a menstrual-cycle calendar. Client understands normal and abnormal breast changes.
	P	Review normal female anatomy and physiology and the influence of menstruation and oral contraceptives on breasts. Teach breast self-examination.		
	I	Reviewed normal breast anatomy and physiology and discussed menstruation as well as breast changes related to it. Taught client how to keep a menstrual-cycle calendar and to record breast changes associated with menstruation. Taught client breast self-examination.		
	E	Client explained how to keep menstrual-cycle calendar and discussed general breast changes related to the menstrual cycle.		

Describing the location of abnormalities

Mentally divide the breast into four sections: the upper outer, upper inner, lower outer, and lower inner quadrants. The upper outer quadrant includes the tail of Spence. Then, picture the breast as a clock with the nipple as the center; describe the location of dimpling, induration, or a mass by its location on the clock. This lesion appears at 2 o'clock.

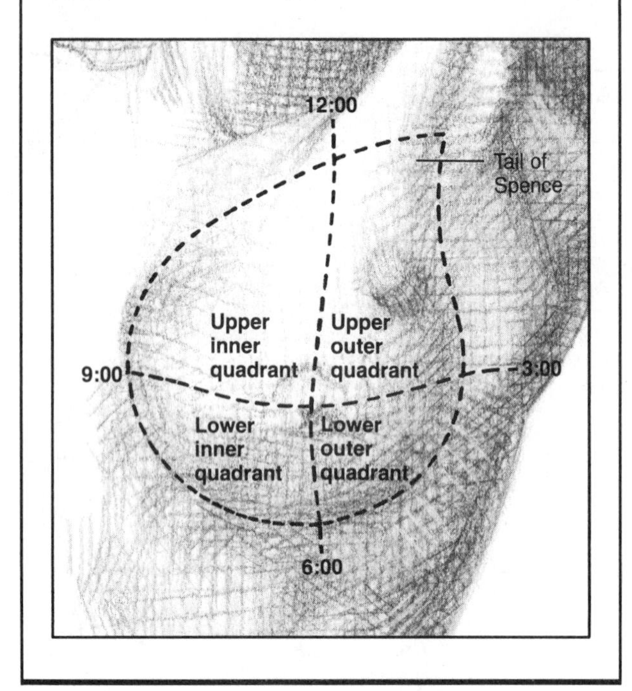

The following example shows how to document normal physical assessment findings for the breast:

> Breasts and nipples symmetrical in shape with left breast slightly larger than right. No dimpling, retractions, skin lesions, nodules, inflammation, or tenderness. Nipples erect and point in same direction. Breasts move symmetrically when client raises arms. No nipple discharge spontaneously or on palpation. Axillae have no masses, tenderness, unusual pigmentation, or lesions. A few mobile, nontender nodes less than 1 cm in diameter on the right anterior axillary fold.

The following example shows how to document abnormal physical assessment findings for the breast:

> Left breast has no dimpling, retractions, skin lesions, nodules, inflammation, or tenderness. Right breast has area of irregular thickening, tenderness, and inflammation in the upper outer quadrant (see drawing) at 10 o'clock that is 5 to 6 cm in diameter and 3 cm long. Area is warm to touch and slightly elevated. Three nodes in right anterior axillary area are tender and enlarged (about 1.5 cm). The nodes are firm, oval, and mobile.

Be sure to document the remaining nursing process steps—nursing diagnoses, planning, implementation, and evaluation—as applied to the care plan for the client with a breast disorder.

Chapter summary

A nurse relies on health history data and physical assessment findings to assess the breast. This chapter tells which health history questions to ask to elicit the necessary information about the client's breast status. Although breast assessment is usually associated with female clients, male breast assessment is also important. Here are the chapter highlights:

- The human breasts are modified sebaceous glands located as a pair on the anterior chest. Each has a central nipple with surrounding areola.
- Female breasts have 12 to 25 glandular lobes containing milk-producing alveoli. Hormones control breast tissue growth and lactation. Four major lymph node groups provide lymphatic drainage of the breast.
- Maturational changes at puberty affect the breasts. Sexual maturity ratings provide a general time reference for adolescent female breast development. Adolescent males may experience temporary breast changes.
- The health history should include questions that detect breast cancer risk factors in females, including age, parity (number of pregnancies), and family history of breast cancer.
- The health history also should assess the client's drug use because many drugs can cause such breast changes as tenderness, pain, and fibrocystic disease.
- The comprehensive breast assessment includes breast inspection and palpation with the client seated and supine, and disrobed from the waist up. Deviations in size, symmetry, contour, sensitivity, and skin characteristics of the nipples, breasts, and axillae may indicate abnormalities. Position changes may elicit dimpling or retraction.
- Breast assessment provides an ideal opportunity to instruct the client in breast self-examination techniques.
- Accurate documentation of assessment findings are an essential component of the client's care plan.

Study questions

1. Alice Rogers, age 68, comes to the clinic because her right breast has developed a sunken area above the areola. Which 10 pertinent health history questions would you ask Ms. Rogers when gathering subjective data?

2. Jimmy Allen, age 12, is brought to the clinic by his father. Mr. Allen and Jimmy are concerned because Jimmy has enlarged breasts. After performing an assessment, what would you probably tell them?

3. Elisa Howell, age 18, goes to her college health clinic for a routine checkup. You note that she has large, pendulous breasts. Which four specific breast assessment steps should you perform to ensure a thorough breast assessment for Ms. Howell?

4. Phyllis Anderson, a 35-year-old secretary, comes to the physician's office with the complaint of lumpy, tender breasts for the past 6 months. She says that the lumps are located in the upper outer areas of her breasts and the tenderness is worse before her menstrual period, which is due in 5 days. Because of job stress, Ms. Anderson drinks at least 5 cups of coffee daily. She has noticed no discharge from either nipple and no discharge occurs during palpation. Physical assessment reveals no masses, but several mobile, fairly well-defined tender cystic nodules exist in both breasts in the upper outer quadrants. You find no other abnormalities. Ms. Anderson examines her breasts monthly and takes no medications.

How would you document the following information related to your nursing assessment of Ms. Anderson?

- subjective (history) assessment data
- objective (physical) assessment data
- assessment techniques and equipment
- two appropriate nursing diagnoses
- documentation of your findings

5. During a regular prenatal visit, Mrs. Hammersmith, age 25, mentions that her breasts have grown larger during pregnancy. She asks you what she can expect during the remainder of her pregnancy and when she breast-feeds the new baby. How do you respond?

Selected references

Cancer statistics. (1991). New York: American Cancer Society.

Daniel, W. (1985). Growth at adolescence: Clinical correlates. *Seminars in Adolescent Medicine,* 1(1), 15-24.

Donegan, W. (1990). Diseases of the breast. In D. Danforth and J. Scott (Eds.), *Danforth's obstetrics and gynecology* (6th ed.). Philadelphia: Lippincott.

Dupont, W., and Page, D. (1985). Risk factors for women with proliferative breast disease. *New England Journal of Medicine,* 213(3), 146-151.

Funch, D. (1986). Socioeconomic status and survival for breast and cervical cancer. *Women's Health,* 11(3-4), 37-54.

Kister, S. (1991). Diseases of the breast. In R. Rokel (Ed.), *Conn's current therapy.* Philadelphia: Saunders.

Kopans, D. (1985). Use of mammography to detect cancer earlier. *Contemporary OB/GYN,* 26, 170-179.

Levinson, W., and Dunn, P. (1986). Nonassociation of caffeine and fibrocystic breast disease. *Archives of Internal Medicine,* 146(9), 1773-1775.

Lubin, F., Ron, E., and Wax, Y. (1985). A case control study of caffeine and methylxanthines in benign breast disease. *JAMA,* 253(16), 2388-2392.

Sloane, E. (1985). *Biology of women.* Albany, NY: Delmar.

Tanner, J. (1962). *Growth at adolescence* (2nd ed.). Oxford: Blackwell Scientific.*

Nursing research

Bottorff, J., and Morse, J. (1990). Mothers' perceptions of breast milk. *JOGNN,* 19(6), 518-527.

Lauver, D., and Keenan, C. (1990). Identifying women's descriptions of breast tissue for the promotion of breast self-examination. *Health Care for Women International,* 12(1), 73-83.

Morse, J., Jehle, C., and Gamble, D. (1990). Initiating breastfeeding: A world survey of the timing of postpartum breastfeeding. *International Journal of Nursing Studies,* 27(3), 303-313.

*Landmark publication

13

Gastrointestinal System

Objectives

After reading and studying this chapter, you should be able to:

1. Describe the organs of the gastrointestinal (GI) system, including the alimentary canal and accessory GI organs.
2. Explain the GI processes of digestion and elimination.
3. Discuss the relationship of the liver, gallbladder, and pancreas to GI function.
4. Discuss important health history components that provide information about GI system status.
5. Demonstrate how to perform an abdominal assessment on an adult, a child, an elderly client, and a pregnant client.
6. Differentiate between normal and abnormal findings detected on physical assessment of the GI system.
7. Describe the most important laboratory tests used to evaluate GI function.
8. Identify representative adverse reactions caused by drugs that affect GI function.
9. Document GI system assessment findings correctly.
10. Use the nursing process to develop a nursing care plan for a client with a GI problem.

Introduction

Virtually everyone experiences some type of GI system problem at one time or another. Besides being common, GI disorders have wide-ranging metabolic implications. For example, untreated vomiting and diarrhea can affect acid-base balance (the stable concentration of hydrogen ions in body fluids), and numerous disorders can interfere with nutritional status and normal body processes. For these reasons, the nurse should take a holistic approach to GI system assessment.

This chapter begins with a review of the anatomy and physiology of the GI system, including the alimentary canal and accessory GI organs— liver, gallbladder and bile ducts, and pancreas. It then describes how to conduct a health history interview to obtain information about the client's problem. Next, the chapter discusses how to perform a systematic physical assessment of the GI system, covering the basic techniques of abdominal examination—inspection, auscultation, percussion, and palpation—as well as more advanced assessment skills, including percussing and palpating the liver, performing a rectal examination, and eliciting abdominal pain. This section of the chapter also presents normal and abnormal assessment findings and the possible implications of abnormal findings. It also discusses special considerations applying to pediatric, pregnant, and elderly clients. The chapter concludes with examples of how to document assessment findings correctly.

Anatomy and physiology review

The GI system consists of two major components: the alimentary canal and the accessory GI organs. The alimentary canal (also referred to as the GI tract) consists

Glossary

Abdominal distention: visible enlargement of the abdominal cavity commonly caused by liquid, gas, or tumors.
Ascites: collection of fluid in the abdominal cavity.
Borborygmi: audible abdominal sounds produced by hyperperistaltic movements, usually caused by hunger.
Chyme: thick, nearly liquid food bolus that forms in the stomach from the digestive process.
Constipation: retention of feces associated with bowel hypoactivity.
Deglutition: process of swallowing.
Diarrhea: frequent elimination of loose stool.
Diastasis recti: failure of the rectus abdominis muscles to join in utero, causing a midline protrusion from the xiphoid to the umbilicus or pubic symphysis.
Digestion: breakdown of food and fluid into simple chemicals that can be absorbed into the bloodstream and transported throughout the body.
Dyspepsia: indigestion.
Dysphagia: difficulty swallowing.
Encopresis: fecal incontinence.
Fat emulsification: breakdown of large fat particles in the intestine to smaller particles, largely through the action of bile acids.
Flatus: intestinal air or gas passed through the rectum.
Hematemesis: vomiting of bright red blood commonly caused by a bleeding ulcer or esophageal bleeding.
Mastication: the process of chewing.
Melena: abnormal black, tarry stool containing digested blood, usually caused by upper GI tract bleeding.
Peristaltic movements: contractions that move GI contents distally toward the large intestine.
Projectile vomiting: forceful vomiting that is propelled away from the body.
Referred pain: pain that spreads or radiates to another anatomic location.
Segmenting movements: localized ring contractions in the bowel that result in the mixing of the intestinal contents.
Striae: lines resulting from rapid or prolonged skin stretching.

primarily of a hollow muscular tube beginning in the mouth and extending to the anus and including the pharynx, esophagus, stomach, small intestine and large intestine. (For a discussion of oral cavity anatomy and physiology, see Chapter 8, Head and Neck.) Accessory organs that aid GI function include the liver, the biliary duct system (gallbladder and bile ducts), and the pancreas. (For an anatomic review of these structures, see *Gastrointestinal system,* pages 356 and 357.)

Together, the GI and accessory organs serve two major functions: digestion, the breaking down of food and fluid into simple chemicals that can be absorbed into the bloodstream and transported throughout the body; and elimination of waste products from the body through excretion of feces.

Digestion and elimination

The digestive process begins in the oral cavity where chewing (mastication), salivation, the beginning of starch digestion, and swallowing (deglutition) all take place.

When the food bolus is swallowed and leaves the oral cavity, the upper esophageal (hypopharyngeal) sphincter relaxes, allowing food to enter the esophagus. In the esophagus, peristaltic waves activated reflexively by the glossopharyngeal nerve propel the food down toward the stomach. As the food moves through the esophagus, glands in the esophageal mucosal layer secrete mucus that lubricates the bolus, promoting its passage, and also protects the esophageal mucosal layer from damage from poorly chewed foods.

Before food enters the stomach from the esophagus, the cephalic phase of digestion has already begun. In this stage, the stomach secretes digestive juices (hydrochloric acid and pepsin) in response to the person's smelling, tasting, chewing, or thinking of food. Food entering the stomach through the cardiac sphincter causes stomach wall distention, initiating the gastric phase of digestion. In this phase, stomach wall distention stimulates the antral mucosa of the stomach to release gastrin. A polypeptide hormone, gastrin in turn stimulates the motor functions of the stomach and gastric juice secretion by the gastric glands. These highly acidic digestive secretions (pH of 0.9 to 1.5) consist mainly of pepsin, hydrochloric acid, intrinsic factor, and proteolytic enzymes. Foods with particular chemical makeups (secretagogues)—such as protein, spices, caffeine, and alcohol—are particularly strong stimulants of gastric secretions, as are histamines and vagal nerve responses.

The stomach has three major motor functions: food storage, food mixing with gastric juices, and slow food release into the small intestine for further digestion and

(Text continues on page 358.)

Gastrointestinal system

The GI system consists of the alimentary canal and accessory organs. The following illustrations and descriptions provide information on these structures.

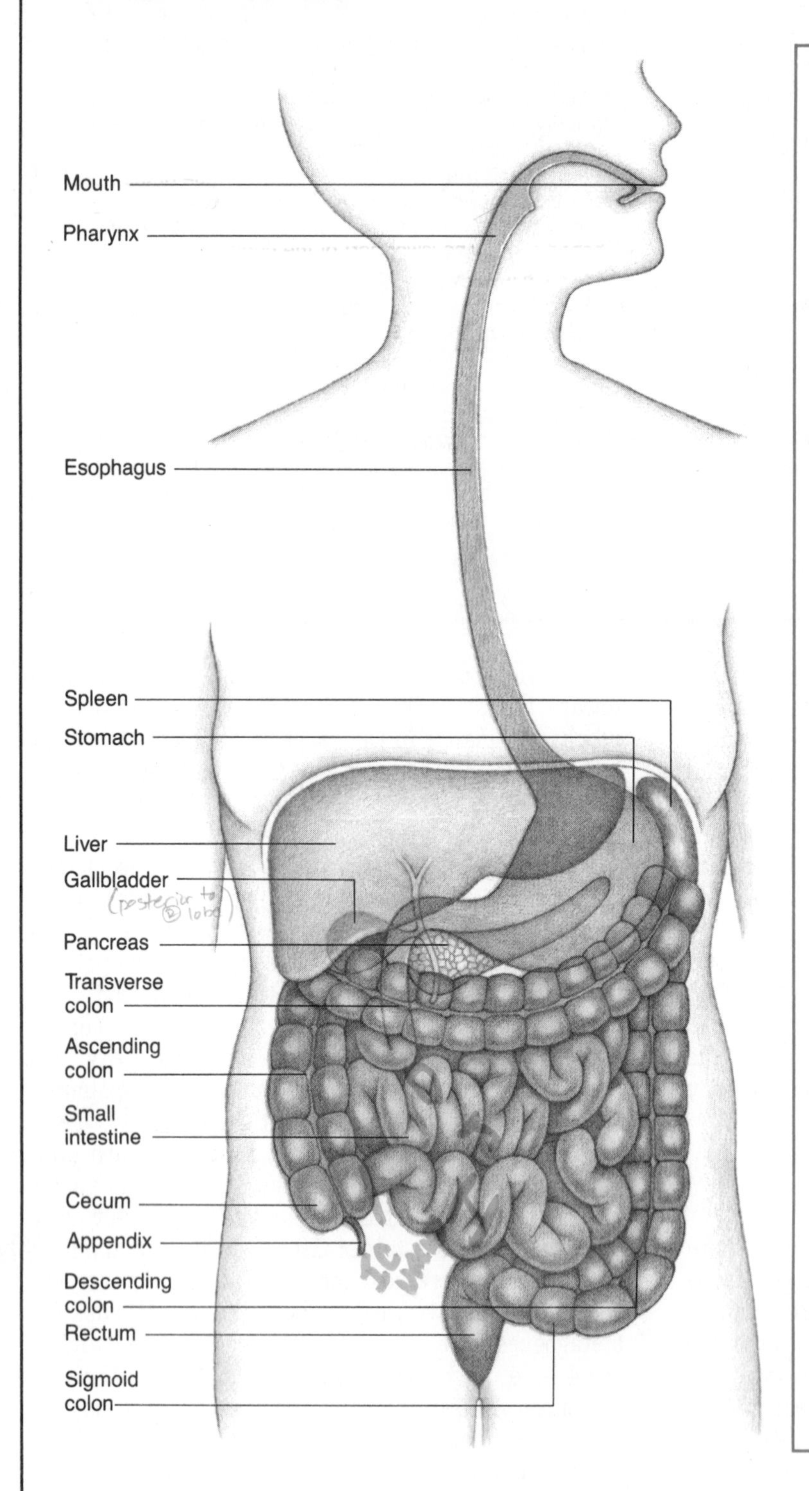

Alimentary canal walls

The walls of all the organs in the alimentary canal contain four basic tissue layers: a mucosal lining, a submucosal coat, a muscular coat, and a fibroserous coat. The innermost layer—the thin, smooth, moist mucosal lining—varies in structure at points along the canal. In the small intestine, for example, it contains villi—fingerlike projections that increase absorption. In some areas—mainly the stomach and small intestine—glandular cells of this layer secrete digestive juices; all along the canal, the layer secretes mucus, which helps protect the canal walls and aids propulsion of food through the canal.

The next layer, the submucosal coat, consists of connective tissue supplied by complex blood vessel, lymphatic, and nerve networks.

The muscular coat consists of smooth muscle fibers in inner and outer layers. The inner layer contains circular muscle fibers that narrow the lumen of the canal when they contract. The outer layer contains longitudinal muscle fibers that shorten the canal lumen when they contract.

The fibroserous coat, also known as the visceral peritoneum, covers the outer walls of the alimentary canal. Between this layer and the parietal peritoneum, which lines the abdominal wall, lies the peritoneal cavity. A portion of the parietal peritoneum, the mesentery, anchors the small intestine to the posterior wall of the abdomen. Another portion, the greater omentum, hangs loosely over the intestines. The lesser omentum attaches the liver to the lesser curve of the stomach and part of the duodenum.

Schematic of alimentary canal wall

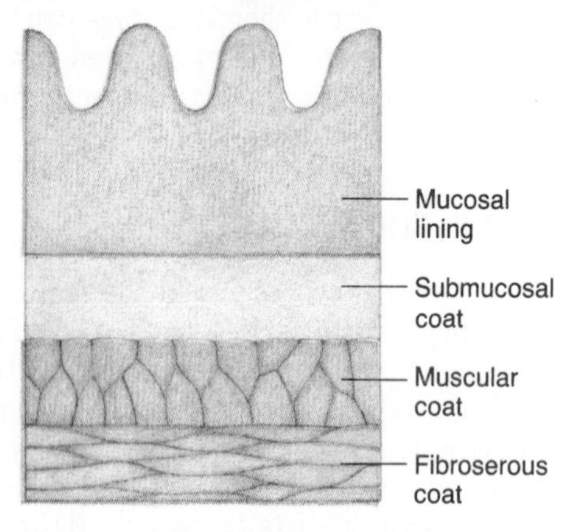

Alimentary canal structures

The alimentary canal is a musculomembranous tube, about 30′ (9 m) long, extending from the mouth to the anus. It includes the mouth and pharynx, esophagus, stomach, small intestine, and large intestine.

Mouth and pharynx

At the beginning of the alimentary canal lie the mouth and pharynx. Together with the other oral cavity structures, the mouth and pharynx prepare food for digestion and passage through the rest of the alimentary canal.

Esophagus

A muscular tube about 9″ (23 cm) long, the esophagus propels food from the pharynx to the stomach. It extends from the cricoid cartilage to the cardiac sphincter of the stomach, passing behind the trachea and heart and through the diaphragm.

Stomach

An elongated, J-shaped pouch, the stomach lies under the diaphragm, roughly between the liver and spleen, and in front of the pancreas. It consists of three sections: the fundus, the body (or corpus), and the antrum (or pylorus). Food enters the fundus through the cardiac sphincter at the proximal end, passes through the body to the antrum, then exits through the pyloric sphincter at the distal end.

The interior wall of the stomach is lined with rugae, mucosal folds containing glands that secrete gastric juice. Loose in nature, the rugae allow the stomach to distend when filled with food and to contract when empty.

Small intestine

A coiled tube approximately 21′(6.4 m) long and extending from the pyloric sphincter to the ileocecal valve, the small intestine is situated in the central and caudal part of the abdominal cavity, surrounded by the large intestine, and consists of three sections. The duodenum, the uppermost and smallest section, measures about 1′ (30.5 cm); the jejunum, the middle section, about 8′ (2.4 m); and the ileum, the lowermost and largest section, about 12′ (3.6 m).

The extensive mucosal layer of the small intestine aids fluid and nutrient absorption during digestion.

Large intestine

A tube approximately 2½″ (6.4 cm) in diameter and 6′ (1.8 m) in length extending from the ileocecal valve to the anus, the large intestine consists of three sections: the cecum, the colon, and the rectum.

The cecum is a blind pouch, about 2″ to 3″ (5 to 7.5 cm) long, extending below the ileocecal valve and ending in the vermiform appendix, a rudimentary organ that has no intestinal function but often holds great clinical significance.

The colon consists of ascending, transverse, descending, and sigmoid segments. The ascending colon begins at the ileocecal valve and extends along the right side of the abdomen, up to the lower border of the liver at the hepatic flexure. This flexure marks the junction of the ascending colon and the transverse colon, which extends horizontally across the abdomen, below the liver and stomach and above the small intestine. The transverse colon ends at the splenic flexure, at which point the descending colon begins. This segment extends down along the left side of the abdomen to the level of the iliac crest. The sigmoid colon begins at the level of the iliac crest and courses downward in an S-shaped curve. The lower part of the curve bends toward the left as it joins the rectum, the last portion of the alimentary canal. About 7″ to 8″ (18 to 20.5 cm) long, the rectum begins at the sigmoid colon and extends to the anus. The terminal portion of the rectum, the anal canal, contains the internal and external anal sphincters, which open to permit defecation.

Accessory GI organs

Accessory organs that aid GI function include the liver, biliary system (gallbladder and bile ducts), and pancreas.

Liver

The body's largest gland (weighing 3 to 4 lb [1.5 to 2 kg]) and one of its most complex organs, the liver lies in the upper right abdominal quadrant, encased (except for the lower margin) by the rib cage. It consists of four lobes: right lobe, caudate lobe, quadrate lobe, and left lobe. (The caudate and quadrate lobes are sometimes considered part of the right lobe.) Each lobe is divided into numerous lobules—the functional units of the liver composed of polyhedral hepatic cells (hepatocytes).

Biliary system

The gallbladder, a small, pear-shaped organ attached to the liver under the right lobe, measures about 3″ (8 cm) long by 1″ (2.5 cm) wide at its thickest part. Composed of folds and rugae, the gallbladder distends to receive bile from the liver; fully distended, it can hold up to 70 ml of bile. Bile leaves the liver via the hepatic duct, which joins the cystic duct of the gallbladder. These ducts form the common bile duct, which empties into the duodenum.

Pancreas

A slender organ measuring about 6″ (15.5 cm) long and 1½″ (3.8 cm) wide, the pancreas lies horizontally across the posterior abdomen behind the stomach, extending roughly from the duodenum to the spleen. It consists of three major segments: head, body, and tail. Within the pancreas, exocrine cells known as acinar cells release digestive enzymes into numerous small ducts that eventually merge into the main pancreatic duct. The pancreas also produces insulin and glucagon, which regulate glucose levels.

Food ↓ (in fundus + body) ↓ chyme

absorption. Except for alcohol, little food absorption normally takes place in the stomach. Food is mixed by tonic and peristaltic contractions of the fundus and body of the stomach. These contractions churn the food into tiny particles and mix it with gastric juices, forming a thick, almost liquid food bolus known as chyme. After mixing occurs, stronger peristaltic waves move the chyme into the antrum of the stomach, where it backs up against the pyloric sphincter before its release into the duodenum.

The rate of stomach emptying depends on a complex interplay of factors that promote and inhibit the process. Promoting factors include gastrin release and neural signals caused by stomach wall distention. Inhibiting factors include a neural response in the duodenum—the enterogastric reflex—and the response of duodenal chemoreceptors to the volume and chemical composition of chyme. In this reaction, the duodenum releases secretin and gastric-inhibiting peptides, and the jejunum secretes cholecystokinin—all of which act to decrease gastric motility. Together, these contrasting mechanisms adjust the rate of stomach emptying to correspond to small intestine capabilities.

Most food digestion and absorption occurs in the small intestine, where intestinal contractions and various digestive secretions break down carbohydrates, proteins, and fats and enable the intestinal mucosa to absorb these nutrients, along with water and electrolytes, into the bloodstream for use by the body.

Small intestine contractions can be classified into two types of movements: segmenting and peristaltic. Segmenting movements, localized ringlike contractions spaced at short intervals along the small intestine, mix chyme with intestinal secretions to aid absorption. Stronger peristaltic movements propel chyme through the small intestine toward the ileocecal valve for passage into the large intestine. At the ileocecal valve, resistance to emptying (controlled by neural and hormonal factors) prolongs the time that chyme remains in the small intestine, enhancing absorption. By the time chyme passes through the ileocecal valve and enters the colon, it consists chiefly of nondigestible substances.

The colon has three major functions: absorption of remaining nutrients, water, and electrolytes; synthesis of vitamins; and elimination of waste products (feces). Most absorption occurs in the proximal half of the colon. The distal half mainly stores feces for elimination. Activity of resident bacterial flora—mainly *Bacteroides fragilis* and *Escherichia coli*—promote synthesis of various vitamins, including folic acid, riboflavin, vitamin K, and nicotinic acid. Of these, vitamin K synthesis is most important, because the amount of vitamin K received from ingested foods normally is insufficient for maintenance of blood coagulation.

In the lower colon, long, relatively sluggish contractions cause propulsive waves known as mass movements. These movements, which normally occur several times a day, propel intestinal contents into the rectum and produce the urge for elimination, or defecation. Defecation normally results from the defecation reflex, a sensory and parasympathetic nerve-mediated response, along with the person's relaxation of the external anal sphincter.

Accessory organ functions

The liver, biliary duct system, and pancreas aid digestion and perform other functions to enhance the body's nutritional status.

The liver performs complex and important functions related to digestion and nutrition. It plays an important role in carbohydrate metabolism; detoxifies various endogenous and exogenous toxins in plasma; synthesizes plasma proteins, nonessential amino acids, and vitamin A; stores essential nutrients (vitamins K, D, and B_{12} and iron); removes ammonia from body fluids and converts it to urea for excretion in urine; and secretes bile. Bile, a greenish liquid composed of water, cholesterol, bile salts, electrolytes, and phospholipids, figures prominently in fat emulsification (breakdown) and intestinal absorption of fatty acids, cholesterol, and other lipids. When bile salts are absent from the intestinal tract, lipids are excreted and fat-soluble vitamins are absorbed poorly. Bile also aids in excretion of conjugated bilirubin (an end product of hemoglobin degradation) from the liver and thereby prevents jaundice.

The gallbladder concentrates and stores bile and releases it into the biliary duct system for transportation to the duodenum.

The pancreas functions as an endocrine gland and an exocrine gland. (For information about endocrine functions, see Chapter 20, Endocrine System.) Exocrine functions involve secretion of pancreatic digestive enzymes, which aid intestinal absorption of proteins, fats, and carbohydrates.

Abdominal muscles and blood supply

Major abdominal supporting muscles include the rectus abdominis and the oblique muscles of the abdomen. A pair of bandlike muscles, the rectus abdominis compresses the abdomen and assists trunk flexion. The sheetlike oblique muscles are in two pairs. The internal obliques help compress the abdomen, flex the thorax, and aid expiration. The external obliques also help compress the abdomen and flex the thorax, and they aid expulsion of stomach contents during vomiting.

Blood is supplied to GI organs through three main arteries. The celiac branches of the descending aorta supply blood to the esophagus, stomach, duodenum, gallbladder, and spleen. The superior mesenteric artery supplies the jejunum, ileum, cecum, ascending colon, and part of the transverse colon. The inferior mesenteric artery supplies the transverse, descending, and sigmoid colon and rectum.

The portal vein collects blood from venous drainage of the GI tract and delivers it to the liver. Emerging from the liver, the portal vein network unites to form the hepatic vein, which empties into the inferior vena cava.

Health history

A complete and accurate GI system assessment depends on the nurse asking the right health history questions, then relating the client's responses to physical assessment findings. Whether or not the client has an overt GI problem, questions should cover dietary intake, appetite, digestion, bowel elimination patterns, medication use, and history of past and present GI disorders. (For health history questions on dietary intake and appetite, see Chapter 6, Nutritional Status.) When performing a GI system assessment, keep the following guidelines in mind.

Fully explore all GI complaints, even vague or seemingly mild ones, such as "heartburn," "upset stomach," and "too much gas." Although the client may dismiss them as unimportant, such complaints may signal a serious underlying problem.

Also remember that many clients consider GI function—particularly elimination—a private matter and may feel uncomfortable discussing it. To encourage honest and complete client responses to GI questions, conduct the health history interview in private.

Ask only those detailed questions that apply to the client's condition. For example, ask a client with abdominal pain detailed questions about the pain and related symptoms. However, if the client does not report vomiting, skip the detailed questions about this symptom.

Health and illness patterns

To assess important health and illness patterns, use the following guidelines to explore the client's current, past, and family health status, as well as the developmental status.

Current health status

Because current health status is foremost in the client's mind, begin the interview by exploring this topic. Carefully document the chief complaint in the client's own words. Using the PQRST method, ask the client to describe this complaint and any others completely. (For a detailed explanation of this method, see *Symptom analysis* in Chapter 3, The Health History.) To investigate the client's current health status further, ask the following questions about GI function:

Do you have any pain in your mouth, throat, abdomen, or rectum? If so, how would you describe it?
(RATIONALE: Pain is one of the most common GI symptoms; abdominal pain may signal a serious GI problem. GI pain is usually described as burning, squeezing, or dull, or as a sensation of the stomach being tied in knots.)

Can you walk in an upright position?
(RATIONALE: A client with an "acute abdomen," as in appendicitis or bowel perforation, typically cannot stand upright and keeps the trunk flexed even when walking.)

Were you drinking alcohol before the stomach pain began?
(RATIONALE: Bouts of pancreatitis often occur or recur after weddings, holidays, and other celebrations where the client may have consumed a large amount of alcohol. Alcohol will also exacerbate an ulcer.)

What, if anything, reduces the pain?
(RATIONALE: Ulcer pain is often relieved by ingestion of food or antacids.)

Is the pain confined to one area, or does it affect other parts of the abdomen?
(RATIONALE: Pain in an abdominal organ often radiates to other areas. For more information, see *Understanding referred pain,* page 360.)

If you have abdominal pain, when does it occur in relation to eating?
(RATIONALE: Peptic ulcer pain usually begins 2 hours after meals or when the stomach is empty. Insufficient blood flow to the bowel usually causes pain within 30 minutes after a meal.)

What other symptoms accompany this pain?
(RATIONALE: Fever, malaise, nausea, vomiting, redness, and swelling [such as in the mouth] may indicate a GI tract infection or inflammation.)

Understanding referred pain

Referred pain, felt at a site different from that of the injured or diseased organ, occurs because some nerves that supply the organ also supply the body surface. These nerves transmit pain impulses along common pathways. The pain may occur relatively near the affected organ or some distance from it. Organ pain usually feels more diffuse than surface pain.

This chart identifies common areas to which specific organ pain is referred.

ORGAN	REFERRED PAIN AREA
Gallbladder	• Right upper quadrant • Right posterior infrascapular area
Diaphragm	• Posterior neck • Posterior shoulder area
Duodenum	• Midline of the abdominal wall just above the umbilicus (usually)
Appendix	• Umbilicus • Parietal peritoneal involvement, right lower quadrant
Ureter	• Inguinal region • Either side of the spinal column above the hip bones

Do you have heartburn or indigestion?
(RATIONALE: These conditions usually are associated with ingestion of spicy foods. Dyspepsia also may occur in hiatal hernia, GI cancer, or as an adverse reaction to certain medications. (For a list of common drugs that cause GI effects, see *Adverse drug reactions,* pages 362 and 363.)

Have you had nausea and vomiting along with the pain?
(RATIONALE: This may indicate appendicitis.)

If so, did you notice any blood in the vomit?
(RATIONALE: Hematemesis [vomiting of bright red blood] may indicate bleeding ulcer or esophageal bleeding.)

Did the vomited material have a fecal odor?
(RATIONALE: This may indicate a small-bowel obstruction.)

Is the pain related to constipation and swelling in the abdomen?
(RATIONALE: Such findings may indicate intestinal obstruction.)

Do any GI symptoms, such as cramping or pain, ever waken you?
(RATIONALE: Ulcer pain often occurs in the predawn hours when the stomach is empty, disrupting normal sleep patterns.)

Have you had other problems, such as fever, at the same time?
(RATIONALE: Certain serious abdominal problems, such as appendicitis and pancreatitis, are often accompanied by fever.)

Do you have any difficulty swallowing?
(RATIONALE: Dysphagia may indicate a partial obstruction or neurologic disease causing loss of motor coordination.)

When did you last have a bowel movement or pass gas?
(RATIONALE: Inability to pass feces or gas [flatus] may indicate an obstruction. Diarrhea may indicate infection or inflammation.)

How often do you have bowel movements? Have you noticed any change in your normal pattern of bowel movements?
(RATIONALE: Normal bowel movement frequency ranges from three times a day to three times a week. A change in pattern needs to be explored; it could occur from bowel cancer, infection, or many other disorders.)

Are the stools formed or loose? If formed, are they soft or hard?
(RATIONALE: Hard stools may indicate constipation; loose stools, diarrhea.)

Do you have difficulty passing stools?
(RATIONALE: An affirmative answer may indicate constipation.)

What color are your stools?
(RATIONALE: Clay-colored or very lightly pigmented stools may indicate a liver or biliary tract problem. Black stools may indicate GI bleeding or may result from the use of iron supplements. Green stools may result from eating green vegetables.)

Have you recently had an unintentional weight loss, appetite loss, unexplained fatigue, or recurrent fever?
(RATIONALE: These symptoms may indicate malabsorption, GI cancer, infection, or inflammation in the GI tract.)

Have you been depressed or felt anxious recently?
(RATIONALE: Emotional distress can cause symptoms of GI distress, such as diarrhea, nausea, and anorexia.)

Do you have eye pain, tearing, redness, or a poor tolerance for light?
(RATIONALE: These symptoms suggest uveitis, which sometimes accompanies ulcerative colitis or Crohn's disease.)

Do you have any difficulty breathing? Have you noticed a change in the size of your abdomen (stomach area)?
(RATIONALE: Increased abdominal girth from ascites [collection of fluid in the abdominal cavity] or tumor can reduce chest expansion.)

Do you have any difficulty with body movement or pain in your joints?
(RATIONALE: These symptoms signal arthritis, which may occur with ulcerative colitis or Crohn's disease. Impaired mobility can lead to constipation.)

Have you noticed any swelling in your neck, underarms, or groin?
(RATIONALE: Enlarged lymph glands may cause swelling in those areas and may point to a GI infection or cancer.)

Past health status

During this part of the health history, ask the following questions to explore the client's medical history for additional GI information:

Have you had any problems with your mouth, throat, abdomen, or rectum that have lasted for a long time?
(RATIONALE: Many GI problems are chronic. Long-term GI problems, such as chronic ulcerative colitis or GI polyposis, may predispose a client to colorectal cancer.)

Have you had any nerve problems, such as weakness or numbness in your hands and fingers?
(RATIONALE: Many neurologic conditions, such as cerebrovascular accident, myasthenia gravis, and peripheral nerve damage, can also affect nervous innervation of the GI tract and alter GI function by slowing motility.)

Have you ever had surgery on your mouth, throat, abdomen, or rectum?
(RATIONALE: Surgery may cause adhesions that can lead to strictures and altered GI function.)

Do you have any allergies such as to milk products?
(RATIONALE: Allergic reactions to foods or medications may cause various GI symptoms.)

Do you use laxatives or enemas? If so, how often?
(RATIONALE: Laxatives and frequent enemas affect intestinal motility. Chronic use may cause constipation or diarrhea.)

Do you take any prescription or over-the-counter medications? If so, which drugs and at what dosages?
(RATIONALE: Many different medications alter GI function or produce adverse GI reactions.)

Family health status

Next, investigate the GI status of the client's family by asking the following questions:

Has anyone in your family had colorectal cancer or polyps?
(RATIONALE: A family history of either disorder increases the client's risk for developing colorectal cancer.)

Has anyone in your family had colitis?
(RATIONALE: A family history of colitis increases the client's risk for colitis.)

Developmental considerations

If the client is young, pregnant, or elderly, be sure to investigate developmental status by exploring the following areas:

Pediatric client. When assessing a pediatric client, try to involve the child and the parent or guardian in the interview. For any child who can speak, encourage participation in the interview, and use age-appropriate words. To help assess a child thoroughly, ask the following questions (directed to the parent or guardian):

What is the color, consistency, and number of your newborn's stools?
(RATIONALE: During the first 5 to 6 days after birth, the neonate's stool normally changes from greenish black to greenish yellow, then to pasty yellow for the formula-fed infant and mushy yellow for the breast-fed infant. The number of stools the first 5 days is usually 4 to 6, decreasing to 1 or 2 a day.)

What special words does your child use for having a bowel movement?
(RATIONALE: Learning the special words for elimination will help ease the hospital adjustment.)

At what age was your child toilet trained? Did any problems occur?
(RATIONALE: Achievement of independent toileting is a developmental milestone indicating a level of physical maturity.)

Does your child seem to have more "accidental" bowel movements when ill?
(RATIONALE: Regression in bowel elimination habits is fairly common during a child's illness and hospitalization.)

Adverse drug reactions

When obtaining a health history to assess a client's GI system, the nurse must ask about current drug use. Many drugs affect GI function. For example, many antibiotics can cause nausea, vomiting, and diarrhea. The commonly used drugs listed below may cause adverse reactions affecting the GI system.

DRUG CLASS	DRUG	POSSIBLE ADVERSE REACTIONS
Analgesics	acetaminophen	Hepatic necrosis with high (toxic) doses
	aspirin	GI disturbances, GI bleeding, ulceration
Antacids	aluminum hydroxide	Constipation
	calcium carbonate	Constipation, gastric hypersecretion, acid rebound
	magnesium hydroxide	Diarrhea
Anticholinergic agents	All anticholinergics	Nausea, vomiting, constipation, xerostomia (dry mouth), bloated feeling, paralytic ileus
Antidepressants	amitriptyline hydrochloride, nortriptyline hydrochloride	Constipation, adynamic ileus, elevated liver enzyme concentrations, jaundice, hepatitis
Antidiabetic agents	acetohexamide	Nausea, vomiting, diarrhea, heartburn (pyrosis), jaundice
	chlorpropamide	Nausea, vomiting, heartburn, cholestatic jaundice
Anti-infectives	ampicillin	Diarrhea, nausea, vomiting, pseudomembranous colitis
	clindamycin hydrochloride	Nausea, vomiting, diarrhea, tenesmus (straining at stool), pseudomembranous and nonspecific colitis
	erythromycin	Abdominal pain and cramping, nausea, vomiting, diarrhea, hepatic dysfunction, jaundice
	metronidazole	Taste disturbances, abdominal discomfort, diarrhea, nausea, vomiting
	sulfonamides	Nausea, vomiting, hepatic changes
	tetracycline hydrochloride	Nausea, vomiting, diarrhea, stomatitis
Antihypertensives	clonidine hydrochloride	Nausea, vomiting, constipation
	guanethidine sulfate	Increased frequency of bowel movements, explosive diarrhea
	methyldopa	Elevated liver function tests
Antineoplastic agents	All antineoplastics	Nausea, vomiting, stomatitis
Antituberculosis agents	isoniazid	Increased liver enzyme concentrations
	rifampin	Heartburn, nausea, vomiting, diarrhea, increased liver enzyme concentrations

Adverse drug reactions continued

DRUG CLASS	DRUG	POSSIBLE ADVERSE REACTIONS
Cardiac agents	digoxin	Nausea, vomiting, diarrhea, anorexia with high (toxic) doses
	quinidine sulfate	Nausea, vomiting, diarrhea, abdominal cramps, colic
Narcotic analgesics	codeine, meperidine hydrochloride, methadone hydrochloride, morphine sulfate, oxycodone	Nausea, vomiting, constipation, biliary spasm or colic
Nonsteroidal anti-inflammatory agents	ibuprofen, indomethacin, salicylates	Nausea, vomiting, dyspepsia, GI bleeding, peptic ulcer
Phenothiazines	prochlorperazine maleate, thioridazine hydrochloride	Constipation, dyspepsia, paralytic ileus, cholestatic jaundice (hypersensitivity reaction)
Miscellaneous agents	allopurinol	Altered liver function, nausea, vomiting, diarrhea
	aminophylline, theophylline	GI irritation, epigastric pain, nausea, vomiting, anorexia
	barium sulfate	Cramping, diarrhea
	colchicine	Diarrhea, nausea, vomiting, abdominal pain
	estrogen-progestin combinations	Nausea, vomiting, diarrhea, abdominal cramps, altered liver function tests, cholestatic jaundice
	ferrous sulfate	Constipation, nausea, vomiting, black stools
	gold sodium thiomalate, auranofin	Changes in bowel habits, diarrhea, abdominal cramping, nausea, vomiting
	griseofulvin	Nausea, vomiting, diarrhea, flatulence
	levodopa	Nausea, vomiting, anorexia
	phenytoin sodium	Nausea, vomiting, constipation, dysphagia
	potassium supplements	Nausea, vomiting, diarrhea, abdominal discomfort, small-bowel ulceration (with enteric-coated tablets)
	prednisone	Epigastric pain, gastric irritation, pancreatitis

Are your child's underpants often stained with stool?
(RATIONALE: This may indicate encopresis [fecal incontinence].)

Do you suspect that your child sometimes deliberately holds back stool?
(RATIONALE: This may indicate the cause of constipation. A children may sometimes use bowel function as a weapon in power struggles with parents.)

Do your the child's stools ever appear large, bulky, and frothy and float in the toilet bowl? Are they especially malodorous?
(RATIONALE: This may indicate a malabsorptive state, such as celiac disease or cystic fibrosis.)

Is your child currently under any unusual stress?
(RATIONALE: Stress may be expressed by bowel problems in the early school-age child.)

Does your infant have projectile vomiting (forceful vomiting that is propelled away from the body) but continually wants to eat?
(RATIONALE: Projectile vomiting may indicate pyloric stenosis or gastroesophageal reflux. An infant with such a disorder will be constantly hungry but cannot retain food.)

Pregnant client. When assessing a pregnant client, be aware that pregnancy normally displaces the colon, decreasing peristaltic activity. This commonly leads to GI problems such as constipation. Hemorrhoids result from pelvic vein compression by the expanding uterus. To assess the pregnant client, ask the following questions:

Do you ever experience nausea and vomiting? If so, does it occur at a specific time or throughout the day?
(RATIONALE: "Morning sickness" with early-morning nausea and vomiting—although afternoon or evening episodes also may occur—is common during the first trimester of pregnancy. However, continual nausea and vomiting throughout the day may indicate a more serious GI problem.)

How have your bowel habits changed since you became pregnant?
(RATIONALE: Constipation is common in pregnancy because of pressure on the bowel from the expanding uterus.)

Have you experienced abdominal pain?
(RATIONALE: Abdominal pain before the expected delivery date may indicate ectopic pregnancy, abruptio placentae, or uterine rupture. Conditions unrelated to pregnancy, such as appendicitis, sometimes can occur.)

Have you experienced heartburn?
(RATIONALE: Heartburn, caused by abnormal gastroesophageal sphincter activity from diaphragmatic pressure from the expanded uterus, commonly occurs during pregnancy.)

How do you feel about your pregnancy?
(RATIONALE: Negative feelings, depression, fear, and anxiety can produce a wide variety of GI symptoms.)

Elderly client. When assessing an elderly client, keep in mind that aging alters intestinal motility and liver size and decreases digestive enzyme secretions. These changes may lead to decreased digestive function and increased food intolerance. Also, an elderly client may not metabolize certain drugs as well as a younger client. To assess for these potential problems, ask the following questions:

Do you ever lose control of your bowels?
(RATIONALE: Fecal incontinence in an elderly client may result from loss of sphincter tone or leakage of liquid stool around a fecal impaction.)

Do you experience constipation regularly? Does this represent a change in your normal bowel elimination habits?
(RATIONALE: Constipation may result from decreased intestinal motility with aging; however, sudden onset may herald colorectal cancer.)

Do you experience diarrhea after ingesting certain foods?
(RATIONALE: Diarrhea may result from a food intolerance, to which an elderly client may have increased susceptibility.)

Do you need assistance at home to go to the bathroom?
(RATIONALE: Decreased mobility or other problems associated with aging may interfere with the client's ability to use the bathroom effectively, possibly leading to constipation or incontinence.)

Health promotion and protection patterns

To determine the client's emphasis on health, ask the following questions about health care habits, which may identify potential GI system problems:

Do you smoke? If so, how much and for how many years?
(RATIONALE: Heavy smoking can aggravate an ulcer and may predispose the client to oral cancer.)

Do you drink alcohol? If so, how much and how often? How long have you maintained this pattern?
(RATIONALE: Alcohol irritates the stomach lining and can precipitate hepatic and pancreatic disease.)

Do you drink coffee, tea, or cola, or use any other caffeine-containing products?
(RATIONALE: Caffeine irritates the stomach lining and increases intestinal motility.)

How do you care for your teeth and gums?
(RATIONALE: Poor dental hygiene can lead to gingivitis or other gum disease, and loss of teeth.)

How do you spend a normal day? Do you participate in any regular exercise program?
(RATIONALE: A sedentary life-style can contribute to constipation.)

What do you do for a living? How do you feel about your job?
(RATIONALE: The answers to these questions may identify unusual stressors or circumstances that may trigger GI problems. For example, an air-traffic controller or a single mother of teenagers may be predisposed to gastritis or diarrhea from stress. A sedentary job may predispose a client to constipation. A job that requires shift rotations may cause a worker to skip meals, or eat at odd hours, causing GI upset.)

Role and relationship patterns

Conclude the history by inquiring about the role and relationship patterns that can be affected by GI system disorders. To discover the extent of this influence, ask the client the following questions:

Have you lived in or traveled to a foreign country? If so, when and where?
(RATIONALE: A client who has recently immigrated or returned from traveling abroad may have a GI ailment endemic to the foreign country, such as intestinal parasites.)

In your family, who does the food shopping and who prepares the meals? Does the entire family usually eat together? Have these routines changed recently?
(RATIONALE: Illness can disrupt family roles and relationships, increasing stress and exacerbating GI symptoms.)

Have you recently lost a loved one, experienced a breakup of a relationship, or undergone a similar stressful event?
(RATIONALE: Depression, loss, and life changes can affect eating and elimination patterns and produce various GI symptoms.)

Physical assessment

Physical assessment of the GI system usually includes evaluation of the mouth, abdomen, and rectum. This section discusses how the nurse assesses the abdomen and rectum; for information on mouth assessment, see Chapter 8, Head and Neck.

To perform a thorough abdominal and rectal assessment, gather the following equipment: gloves, stethoscope, flashlight, measuring tape, felt-tip pen, and a gown and drapes to cover the client. Make sure that the examination room is private, quiet, warm, and well lit.

Before beginning, explain the steps and reassure the client that the assessment should not be painful, although it may be uncomfortable at times. Then, ask the client to urinate, undress and put on a gown, and lie supine on the examination table with arms at sides and head supported comfortably on a pillow (to prevent abdominal muscle tensing). Drape the genital area and raise the gown to bare the abdomen, making sure to keep a female client's breasts covered.

To assess the abdomen, perform the four basic steps in the following sequence: inspection, auscultation, percussion, and palpation. (For more information on these techniques, see Chapter 4, Physical Assessment Skills.) Unlike other body systems in which auscultation is performed last, the GI system requires abdominal auscultation *before* percussion and palpation, which can alter intestinal activity and bowel sounds.

To ensure more accurate assessment findings and consistent documentation of your findings, mentally divide the client's abdomen into regions, using either the quadrant or the nine region method. (For illustrations, see *Identifying abdominal landmarks,* page 366.) When assessing a client with abdominal pain, always perform auscultation, percussion, and palpation in the painful quadrant last. If you touch the painful area first, the client may tense the abdominal muscles, making assessment difficult.

Inspection

Begin the abdominal assessment by inspecting the client's entire abdomen, noting overall contour and skin integrity, appearance of the umbilicus, and any visible pulsations. Assess abdominal contour from the foot of the bed and the client's side, stooping so that the abdomen is at eye level. With the client supine, the abdomen normally appears slightly rounded, with gently curved, symmetric lateral borders. Be aware of variations in contour depending on body type. A slender person may have a flat or slightly concave abdomen; an obese person, a protruding abdomen. Note any localized distention or irregular contours for further assessment.

Next, inspect the abdominal skin, which normally appears smooth and intact, and has varying amounts of hair. Look for areas of discoloration, striae (lines resulting from rapid or prolonged skin stretching), rashes or other lesions, dilated veins, and scars. Document the location and character of these findings.

Observe the entire abdomen for movement from peristalsis or arterial pulsations. Normally, peristalsis is not

Identifying abdominal landmarks

To aid accurate abdominal assessment and documentation of findings, the nurse can mentally divide the client's abdomen into regions. The quadrant method, the easiest and most commonly used, divides the abdomen into four equal regions by two imaginary lines crossing perpendicularly at the umbilicus. The nine regions method provides more precise location identification. The diagrams below show how the underlying abdominal organs relate to these two methods of identifying abdominal landmarks.

QUADRANT METHOD

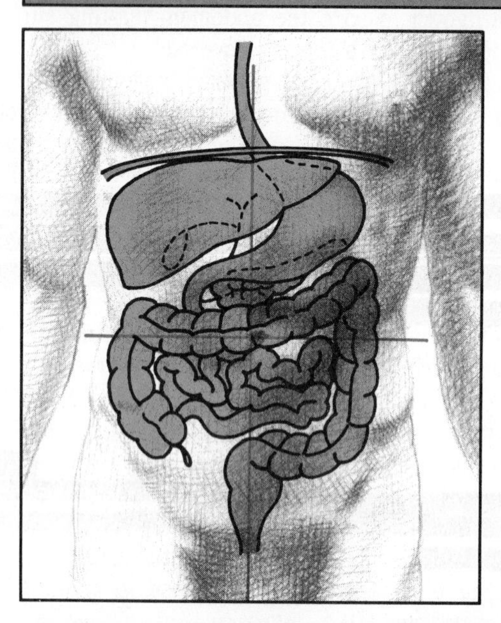

Right upper quadrant (RUQ)	Left upper quadrant (LUQ)
Liver and gallbladder Pylorus Duodenum Head of pancreas Hepatic flexure of colon Portions of ascending and transverse colon	Left liver lobe Stomach Body of pancreas Splenic flexure of colon Portions of transverse and descending colon
Right lower quadrant (RLQ)	**Left lower quadrant (LLQ)**
Cecum and appendix Portion of ascending colon	Sigmoid colon Portion of descending colon

NINE REGIONS METHOD

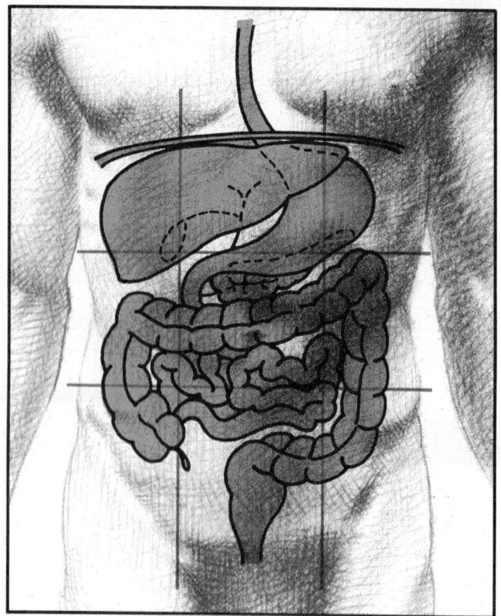

Right hypochondriac	Epigastric	Left hypochondriac
Right liver lobe Gallbladder	Pyloric end of stomach Duodenum Pancreas Portion of liver	Stomach Tail of pancreas Splenic flexure of colon
Right lumbar	**Umbilical**	**Left lumbar**
Ascending colon Portion of duodenum and jejunum	Omentum Mesentery Lower part of duodenum Jejunum and ileum	Descending colon Portions of jejunum and ileum
Right inguinal	**Suprapubic or hypogastric**	**Left inguinal**
Cecum Appendix Lower end of ileum	Ileum	Sigmoid colon

visible. In some clients, aortic pulsations may be seen in the epigastric area.

To detect any umbilical or incisional hernias, have the client raise the head and shoulders while remaining supine. True umbilical or incisional hernias may protrude during this maneuver. Finally, inspect the umbilicus for position, contour, and color. The umbilicus should be midline, concave, and consistent with the color of the rest of the abdomen.

Abnormal findings

A concave (scaphoid) abdominal contour may indicate malnutrition. Abdominal distention may point to a tumor, excessive fluid or gas accumulation, or, less commonly, severe malnutrition.

Visible skin abnormalities often provide valuable clues to underlying abdominal problems. Bulging around old scars may indicate an incisional hernia. Striae commonly result from obesity or pregnancy, but also may indicate an abdominal tumor or other disorder, such as Cushing's syndrome, which characteristically causes purplish striae. Recently developed striae usually appear pink or blue; older striae, white or silver. In a dark-skinned client, striae may appear lighter than the surrounding skin. Tense, glistening skin may indicate ascites. Dilated, tortuous superficial abdominal veins may point to inferior vena caval obstruction. Cutaneous angiomas (tumors composed of blood or lymph vessels) may indicate liver disease.

An everted umbilicus is normal in some clients; in others, however, it may indicate increased intra-abdominal pressure. A bluish tinge around the umbilicus may point to intra-abdominal bleeding.

Strong visible peristaltic waves often indicate intestinal obstruction. Abdominal aortic pulsations may become more pronounced and obvious from increased intra-abdominal pressure, as from a tumor or ascites.

To help document assessment findings, draw a diagram of the client's abdominal quadrants and record the location, size, and color of any abnormalities.

Auscultation

Auscultation provides information on bowel motility and the underlying vessels and organs. (For illustrations, see *Auscultating the abdomen*.) After inspecting the client's

Auscultating the abdomen

Before using a stethoscope to auscultate the abdomen, warm your hands and the stethoscope to prevent muscular contraction, which can alter auscultatory findings. The nurse auscultates for bowel sounds throughout all four quadrants, using the diaphragm of the stethoscope, as shown. Then using the bell of the stethoscope, listen for vascular sounds in the sites shown.

Stethoscope placement for auscultation

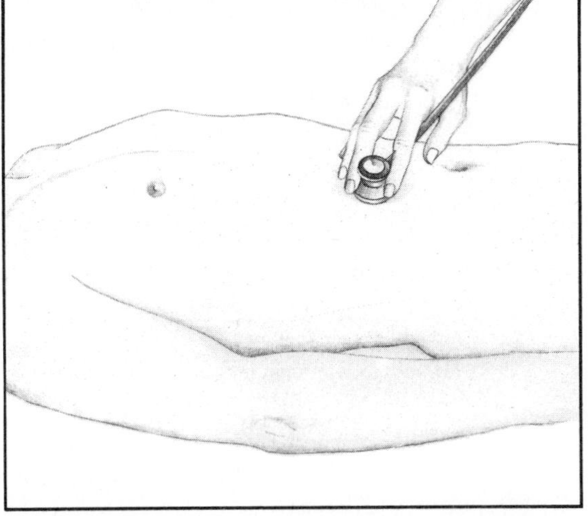

Auscultation sites for vascular sounds

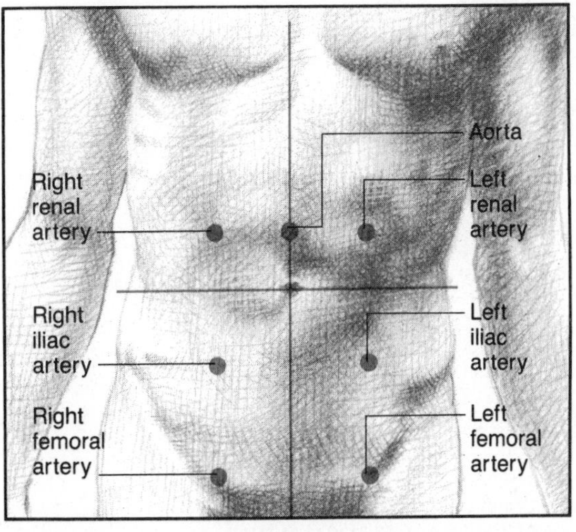

abdomen, use a stethoscope to auscultate for bowel and vascular sounds. To auscultate bowel sounds, lightly press the stethoscope diaphragm on the abdominal skin in all four quadrants. Normally, air and fluid moving through the bowel by peristalsis create soft, bubbling sounds with no regular pattern, often with soft clicks and gurgles interspersed, every 5 to 15 seconds. A hungry client normally may have a familiar "stomach growl," a condition of hyperperistalsis called borborygmi. Rapid, high-pitched, loud, and gurgling bowel sounds are *hyperactive*, which may occur normally in a hungry client. Sounds occurring at a rate of one every minute or longer are *hypoactive* and normally occur after bowel surgery or when the colon is feces filled.

Before reporting absent bowel sounds, be sure the client has an empty bladder; a full bladder may obscure the sounds. Gently pressing on the abdominal surface may initiate peristalsis and audible bowel sounds, as will having the client eat or drink something.

Next, use the bell of the stethoscope to auscultate for vascular sounds. Normally, you should detect no vascular sounds. (For information about abnormal bowel and vascular sounds and their implications, see *Abnormal abdominal sounds*.)

Percussion

Abdominal percussion helps determine the size and location of abdominal organs and detects excessive accumulation of fluid and air in the abdomen. To perform this technique, percuss in all four quadrants, keeping approximate organ locations in mind as you progress. (For more information, see *Percussing the abdomen*.) Percussion sounds vary depending on the density of underlying structures; usually, you will detect dull notes over solids and tympanic notes over air. The predominant abdominal percussion sound is tympany, created by percussing over an air-filled stomach or intestine. Dull sounds normally occur over the liver and spleen, a lower intestine filled with feces, and a bladder filled with urine. (For more information on liver percussion, see "Advanced assessment skills," pages 374 and 375.) Distinguishing abdominal percussion notes may be difficult in an obese client.

Note: Keep in mind that abdominal percussion or palpation is contraindicated in clients with suspected abdominal aortic aneurysm or those who have received abdominal organ transplants, and should be performed cautiously in clients with suspected appendicitis.

Abnormal abdominal sounds

Abdominal auscultation may reveal several abnormal sounds, including bowel sound alterations, systolic bruits, venous hum, and friction rub. This chart describes each of these sounds, lists the best places to listen for them, and explains what they may indicate.

SOUND AND DESCRIPTION	LOCATION	POSSIBLE INDICATION
Bowel sounds Sounds created by air and fluid movement through the bowel	All four quadrants	• Hyperactive sounds unrelated to hunger: diarrhea or early intestinal obstruction • Hypoactive, then absent, sounds: paralytic ileus or peritonitis • High-pitched "tinkling" sounds: intestinal fluid and air under tension in a dilated bowel • High-pitched "rushing" sounds coinciding with an abdominal cramp: intestinal obstruction
Systolic bruits Vascular "blowing" sounds resembling cardiac murmurs	Abdominal aorta Renal artery Iliac artery	• Partial arterial obstruction or turbulent blood flow, as in dissecting abdominal aneurysm • Renal artery stenosis • Hepatomegaly
Venous hum Continuous, medium-pitched tone created by blood flow in a large, engorged vascular organ such as the liver	Epigastric and umbilicus	• Increased collateral circulation between portal and systemic venous systems, as in hepatic cirrhosis
Friction rub Harsh, grating sound resembling two pieces of sandpaper rubbing together	Hepatic	• Inflammation of the peritoneal surface of an organ, as from a liver tumor

Percussing the abdomen

The nurse should percuss the abdomen systematically, starting with the right upper quadrant and moving clockwise to the percussion sites in each quadrant. However, if the client complains of pain in a particular quadrant, adjust the percussion sequence to percuss that quadrant last. Remember when tapping to move your right finger away quickly so you do not inhibit vibrations.

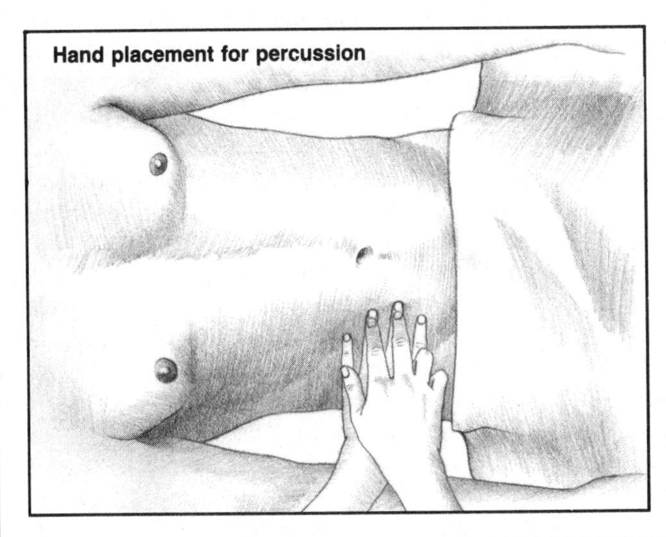

Hand placement for percussion

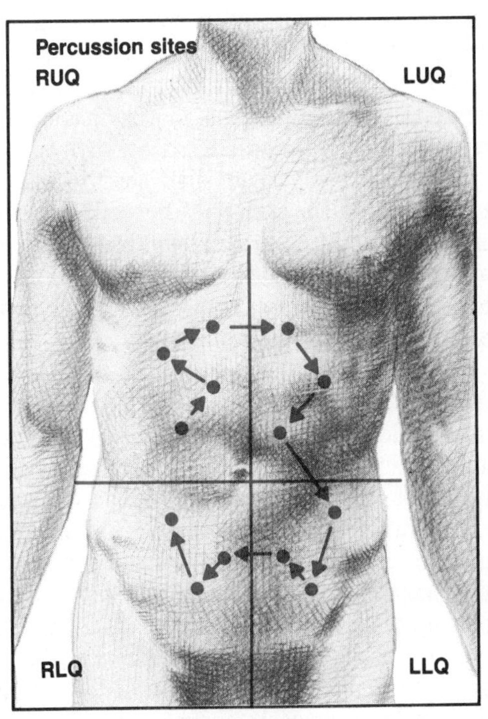

Percussion sites

Abnormal findings

Abnormal percussion findings usually occur in clients with abdominal distention from air accumulation, ascites, or masses. Extremely high-pitched tympanic notes may indicate gaseous bowel distention. Ascites produces shifting dullness (a shift in the point where the percussion note changes from tympany to dullness when the client changes position), caused by fluid shifting to dependent areas.

If the client has abdominal distention, assess its progression by taking serial measurements of abdominal girth. To do so, wrap a tape measure around the client's abdomen at the level of the umbilicus and record the measurement. Be sure to mark the point of measurement with a felt-tip pen to ensure that subsequent readings are taken at the same point.

Palpation

Abdominal palpation provides useful clues about the character of the abdominal wall; the size, condition, and consistency of abdominal organs; the presence and nature of any abdominal masses; and the presence, degree, and location of any abdominal pain. Commonly used techniques for abdominal palpation include light palpation, deep palpation, and ballottement. (For detailed information about these procedures, see Chapter 4, Physical Assessment Skills.)

To perform light palpation, gently press your fingertips about ½" to ¾" (1 to 2 cm) into the abdominal wall. The light touch helps relax the client. The client who finds the sensation disagreeable or ticklish can place his or her hand atop yours and follow along. This usually relaxes the client and decreases involuntary muscle contractions in response to touch. To perform deep palpation, press the fingertips of both hands about 1½" (4 cm) into the abdominal wall. Move your hands in a slightly circular fashion, so that the abdominal wall moves over the underlying structures. When palpating the abdomen, systematically cover all four quadrants, assessing for organ location, masses, and areas of tenderness or increased muscular resistance. If a mass is detected on light or deep palpation, note its location, size, shape, consistency, type of border, degree of tenderness, presence of pulsations, and degree of mobility (fixed or mobile).

Ballottement involves the light, rapid bouncing or tapping of the fingertips against the abdominal wall. Use this technique to help elicit abdominal muscle resistance or guarding that can be missed with deep palpation, or to detect the movement or bounce of a freely movable mass. Your fingers should also bounce at the underlying dense liver tissue in the upper right quadrant. If the client has ascites, you may need to use deep ballottement. To do so, push your fingertips deeply inward in a rapid motion, then quickly release the pressure, maintaining fingertip contact with the abdominal wall. You should feel the movement of an underlying organ or a movable mass toward your fingertips.

Abnormal findings

Abnormal abdominal palpation findings include increased abdominal wall resistance, tenderness or guarding (flexion of the abdominal muscles), and masses. Tenderness, guarding, and complaints of abdominal pain may indicate appendicitis. Deep palpation may evoke rebound tenderness when you suddenly withdraw your fingertips, a possible sign of peritoneal inflammation. A client who complains of generalized tenderness may make accurate evaluation of palpation findings difficult. To assess tenderness accurately in such a client, place your stethoscope on the abdomen and pretend to auscultate, but actually press into the abdomen with the stethoscope as you would with your hands and see if the client still complains of pain.

Caution: Do not palpate a pulsating midline mass; it may be a dissecting aneurysm, which can rupture under the pressure of palpation. Report such a mass to the physician immediately.

An inexperienced nurse may easily mistake certain normal abdominal structures for masses: the uterus, palpated midline in the lower abdomen; a feces-filled colon, usually palpated in the left lower quadrant; and the sacral promontory in a thin client, palpated as a deep bony mass below the level of the umbilicus. With experience, you will distinguish accurately between normal and abnormal palpation findings. (For information about common selected disorders and their associated findings, see *Integrating assessment findings*, pages 372 and 373.)

Developmental considerations

Consider the following differences in assessment techniques and findings when assessing a pediatric, pregnant, or elderly client.

Pediatric client

When preparing a child for an abdominal examination, explain the procedure in age-appropriate terms (for example, "I'll be checking your tummy."). Reassure the child that the parent or guardian can stay in the examination room throughout the assessment. To put the child more at ease, allow touching of the equipment and asking of questions about what you are doing. Demonstrate the techniques on a doll or stuffed toy.

Positioning for the assessment depends on the child's age and level of cooperation. An older child may lie supine on the examination table as an adult would. When examining a young child or infant, place the child across a parent's lap, or lay the child's buttocks and legs across your lap and the child's head on the parent's lap.

The assessment sequence for a pediatric client also depends on the child's age and cooperation level. You may need to perform certain steps out of the normal assessment sequence. For example, if the child has remained quiet for auscultation of heart and lung sounds, you may want to auscultate the abdomen at once. Because percussion and palpation involve touching the child, defer these until the end of the examination, when the child has developed some trust in you and is more likely to cooperate with you.

Do not perform a rectal examination on a child, unless a specific sign or symptom, such as constipation, encopresis, or bleeding, is present. Even then, expect a pediatric nurse practitioner or a physician to perform this examination.

Inspect a child's abdomen as you would an adult's, keeping in mind the differences in normal and abnormal findings among age-groups. During inspection, the contour of a child's abdomen may be the first clue to a possible GI disorder. In a child under age 4, a mild potbelly (distention) when the child stands or sits is a normal finding. In a child between ages 4 and 13, a mildly protruding abdomen is normal only when the child stands. An extreme potbelly may result from enlargement of the viscera, ascites, neoplasm, abdominal wall defects, or starvation; a depressed or concave abdomen may indicate a diaphragmatic hernia, especially when accompanied by localized swelling. Note any scars or abdominal vascularity. In contrast to an adult, superficial veins normally are readily visible in an infant.

To inspect an infant's abdomen, stand at the foot of the table and direct a light across the abdomen from the infant's right side. Observe for peristaltic waves, which are normally invisible. Visible peristaltic waves may indicate intestinal obstruction. Reverse (left-to-right) peristaltic waves commonly point to pyloric stenosis; other possible causes include bowel malrotation, duodenal ulcer, and duodenal stenosis.

When inspecting a child's abdomen, keep in mind that a child's respiratory movements are primarily abdominal; costal respiratory movements may indicate peritonitis, obstruction, or accumulation of ascitic fluid. The transition from abdominal to costal respirations is gradual with age. Usually a child breathes abdominally until age 6 or 7.

Also observe a young child for diastasis recti abdominis (separation of the two rectus abdominis muscles with a protrusion in the separation). This benign condition, especially common in Black infants, usually disappears during the preschool years. At the same time, inspect for umbilical hernia. (For the best view, wait until the child cries, which increases intra-abdominal pressure and makes herniation more apparent.)

Auscultate a child's abdomen as you would an adult's. In a child with a disorder, auscultation may reveal one of several abnormal findings. For example, it may detect an abdominal murmur, possibly indicating coarctation of the aorta; a venous hum, suggesting portal hypertension; or a double "pistol shot" sound in the femoral artery, possibly signaling aortic insufficiency. In addition to these vascular sounds, auscultation may reveal high-pitched bowel sounds, suggesting gastroenteritis or impending intestinal obstruction; or absent bowel sounds, a sign of paralytic ileus or peritonitis; or a hepatic friction rub, which usually indicates inflammation.

A child's underdeveloped abdominal wall should make palpation easier than in an adult. But this part of an abdominal examination is subjective, and requires the child's cooperation in reporting symptoms truthfully. Because the child may be more ticklish and tense than an adult, distract the child during palpation, perhaps by starting a discussion or asking the child to count or recite the alphabet. Get a preschool child to cooperate by playing a game ("Let me feel your tummy and guess what you had for breakfast. A watermelon? A box of candy?"). Having an infant suck on a pacifier (not a bottle of milk, which may cause regurgitation) may help relax the abdomen and enhance palpation. To minimize ticklishness and give the child some sense of control over the situation, palpate the abdomen with the child's hand under your own. (Although this technique can identify localized pain, it is not sufficiently sensitive to detect most palpable findings.)

To augment the child's verbal descriptions of pain, look for visible clues as you palpate. A child may use abdominal guarding more than an adult in response to abdominal pain. Other clues to a child's pain include grimacing, sudden protective movement with an arm or leg, and a change in the pitch of the cry. Palpation in a quadrant other than the painful quadrant should reveal a soft, nontender abdomen. If not, the child is still tense. To avoid inaccurate findings, try to relax the child before proceeding. A slightly tender descending colon may be caused by stool. Tenderness in the right lower quadrant may indicate an inflamed appendix. Generalized tenderness and rigidity in the affected quadrant often points to peritoneal irritation. If these findings are present, ask the child to cough; a reduced or withheld cough may confirm peritoneal irritation. These findings contraindicate palpating for rebound tenderness, a potentially painful procedure for a child.

Palpate the infant's abdomen for umbilical hernia. (Commonly present at birth and often not visible, umbilical hernias usually increase in size until age 1 month and then gradually decrease until about age 1.) To do so, press down on the infant's umbilicus. If you can insert one fingertip, the infant has a small hernia. Treatment usually consists of letting the hernia close by itself without surgery. Any hernia larger than ¾" (2 cm) or one that increases in size after age 1 month requires further assessment.

Because a child commonly swallows air during eating and crying, percussion may reveal louder tympanic notes than those normally found in an adult. Tympany along with abdominal distention may result from ascites or solid masses. In a neonate, ascites usually results from GI perforation; in an older child, from congestive heart failure, cirrhosis, or nephrosis.

Pregnant client

Vary the assessment position for a pregnant client depending on the stage of the pregnancy. In the final weeks, for example, a client may find the supine position uncomfortable because it can impair respiratory excursion and blood flow. To enhance comfort, place her in a side-lying or semi-Fowler's position.

When assessing a pregnant client's abdomen, keep in mind the normal variations in assessment findings associated with pregnancy. Common findings include increased pigmentation of the abdominal midline (linea nigra), striae, upward displacement of the umbilicus and diastasis recti abdominis.

Elderly client

Positioning of an elderly client for abdominal assessment depends on the client's physical condition. For example, an elderly client with orthopnea (difficulty breathing while lying down) cannot recline. Position such a client with the head and trunk raised and knees slightly flexed to help relax the abdomen.

Abdominal assessment in an elderly client follows the same pattern as that for any adult client, with several differences. Because the abdominal wall usually thins

(Text continues on page 374.)

Integrating assessment findings

Sometimes, a cluster of assessment findings will strongly suggest a particular GI disorder. In the chart below, column one shows groups of presenting signs and symptoms—the ones that make the client seek medical attention. Column two shows related assessment findings that the nurse may discover during the health history and physical assessment. The client may exhibit one or more of these findings. Column three shows the possible disorder indicated by a cluster of these findings.

PRESENTING SIGNS AND SYMPTOMS	RELATED ASSESSMENT FINDINGS	POSSIBLE DISORDER
Failure to pass meconium within 24 hours after birth, vomiting	Infant, several days old History of other GI, cardiac, or esophageal congenital defects Inability to insert finger into anus on rectal examination Absence of anal opening or the thin translucent membrane of rectal atresia	Imperforate anus
Severe, possibly projectile, vomiting	Infant, several weeks old Visible left-to-right peristaltic waves Palpable mass at the right costal margin of the epigastrium History of chronic regurgitation since birth or first few weeks of life	Pyloric stenosis
Heartburn, nausea, vomiting, possibly dysphagia and abdominal pain	Elderly female client Increased intra-abdominal pressure caused by straining, obesity, ascites, or coughing	Hiatal hernia
Gnawing, burning abdominal pain that worsens about 1 hour after meals and is relieved—or sometimes exacerbated—by eating; nausea and possibly hematemesis; constipation or diarrhea; melena (black, tarry stools)	Use of drugs that irritate the GI tract History of regular recurrence and disappearance of signs and symptoms Caffeine overuse Cigarette smoking Abdominal tenderness on palpation	Peptic ulcer
Epigastric pain slightly left of midline, indigestion, nausea, vomiting, possibly hematemesis, constipation or diarrhea, melena	Use of drugs that irritate the GI tract Ingestion of irritating foods Alcoholism Pernicious anemia Severe stress Burns Surgery Trauma Sepsis Abdominal tenderness on palpation	Gastritis
Mild constant pain in right upper quadrant; nausea; vomiting; constipation or diarrhea; clay-colored stools	History of ingestion of contaminated food or water, or contact with infected person or secretions I.V. drug user or sexually exposed to hepatitis-infected individual Headache Cough Coryza (nasal discharge and mucosa swelling) Anorexia Fatigue Arthralgia (joint pain), myalgia (muscle pain) Recent blood transfusion Fever and chills Abdominal tenderness in right upper quadrant Hepatomegaly, jaundice, possibly splenomegaly, and cervical adenopathy (second stage)	Viral hepatitis A or B

Integrating assessment findings continued

PRESENTING SIGNS AND SYMPTOMS	RELATED ASSESSMENT FINDINGS	POSSIBLE DISORDER
Mild right upper quadrant pain, increasing as disease progresses; nausea; vomiting; constipation or diarrhea	Alcoholism Hepatitis Heart failure Hemochromatosis (iron metabolism disorder) Malaise and fatigue Anorexia and weight loss Pruritus Dark urine Bleeding tendencies Palpable liver and possibly spleen Jaundice Spider angiomas Peripheral edema Ascites as disease progresses	Cirrhosis
Constant epigastric pain that may radiate to the back and is worsened by lying down; nausea; bilious vomiting	Alcoholism History of cholelithiasis Peptic ulcer Use of irritating drugs such as azathioprine Pain aggravated by food or alcohol ingestion Restlessness Mild fever Tachycardia Hypotension Abdominal distention and tenderness Decreased bowel sounds Abdominal rigidity and crackles auscultated at lung base (in severe disease)	Pancreatitis (acute or chronic)
Severe, cramping pain in epigastrium or right upper quadrant that may be referred to back of right scapula, usually of sudden onset and subsiding after about an hour followed by a dull ache; nausea; vomiting	Obese, multiparous woman over age 40 Intolerance to fatty foods Indigestion, flatulence, and belching Fever Abdominal tenderness in right upper quadrant Abdominal rigidity with guarding Palpable liver and gallbladder Jaundice Tachycardia	Cholecystitis
Occasional left lower quadrant pain; mild nausea, usually without vomiting; constipation with onset of pain	Diet low in roughage and fiber Low-grade fever Abdominal tenderness in severe disease	Diverticulitis
Cramping, right lower quadrant pain; nausea, usually without vomiting; mild, urgent diarrhea	Family history of disease Emotional stress Flatulence Weight loss Weakness, malaise Altered immune function Uveitis Low-grade fever Abdominal tenderness Palpable mass in right lower quadrant	Crohn's disease
Occasional pain on defecation; severe pain if thrombosed	Prolonged sitting Multiple pregnancies Visible external hemorrhoids Palpable internal hemorrhoids Bright red blood in stool	Hemorrhoids

(from muscle wasting and loss of fibroconnective tissue) and abdominal muscle tone becomes more relaxed with aging, abdominal palpation may be easier and the results more accurate in an elderly client. For these same reasons, abdominal rigidity—in a younger client, an important sign of peritoneal inflammation—occurs much less often in an elderly client; abdominal distention, more often.

Advanced assessment skills

After mastering the skills required to perform a basic abdominal assessment, you may develop more advanced physical assessment techniques: percussion and palpation of the liver, rectal examination, and specific maneuvers to elicit abdominal pain.

Liver assessment

You can estimate the size and position of the liver through percussion and palpation. (For an illustrated procedure, see *Advanced assessment skills: Assessing the liver.*)

On percussion, several conditions may distort or obscure the dull percussion sounds that identify liver borders. The upper border of liver dullness can be obscured by lung consolidation or a right pleural effusion; the lower border of dullness, by gas in the colon.

Use a technique known as fist percussion (or blunt percussion) to detect tenderness, a common sign of gallbladder or liver disease or inflammation. To perform this maneuver, place one hand flat over the client's lower right rib cage along the midclavicular line, then strike the back of this hand with your other hand clenched in a fist. Client discomfort and muscle guarding indicate tenderness. *Note:* Use this maneuver only on a client with unconfirmed but suspected inflammation or hepatomegaly, and defer it until the end of the abdominal assessment. If the client complains of any pain or discomfort during the assessment—particularly over the spleen—do not perform this maneuver.

If locating the inferior border of the liver through percussion is difficult or impossible, try the "scratch test." To perform this test, lightly place the diaphragm of the stethoscope over the approximate location of the lower border of the liver. Auscultate while stroking the client's abdomen lightly with your right index finger (from well below the level of liver dullness) in the pattern used for locating the lower border of the liver through percussion. Start the stroke along the midclavicular line at the right iliac crest and move upward. Because the liver transmits sound waves better than the air-filled ascending colon, the scratching noise heard through the stethoscope becomes louder over the solid liver.

Usually, palpating the liver is impossible in an adult client. However, if palpable, the liver border normally feels smooth and firm, with a rounded, regular edge. A palpable liver may indicate hepatomegaly; it also may occur in an extremely thin client or in the following variations. In a child, the liver is proportionately larger, with palpation 1 to 2 finger breadths below the ribs considered normal. A low diaphragm, as occurs in emphysema, will displace a normal-sized liver downward, making it easily palpable below the costal margin. In a normal variation known as Riedel's lobe, the right lobe is elongated down toward the right lower quadrant and is palpable below the right costal margin.

Rectal examination

Usually, routine rectal examination is performed only for a client over age 40; however, it may also be performed for a client of any age with a history of bowel elimination changes or anal area discomfort and for an adult male of any age with a urinary problem.

The client may find rectal examination uncomfortable, both physically and psychologically. Help the client relax by explaining the procedure before proceeding and reassuring that the examination should not be painful, although it may produce some discomfort. Normally, perform the rectal examination at the end of the physical assessment.

Client positioning for rectal examination depends on several factors: client mobility, age, or pregnancy, and the availability of an examination table or client bed. Have an ambulatory client stand with the toes pointed inward and bend forward over the examination table. The knee-chest position, an excellent alternative position for a client in bed, is not suitable usually for an ill, elderly, or pregnant client. Instead, position such a client in a left lateral Sims' position, with the knees drawn up and the buttocks near the edge of the bed or examination table.

Begin the rectal examination with inspection. Spread the client's buttocks to expose the anus and surrounding area. The skin of the anal area should appear intact and darker than surrounding skin. Inspect for breaks in the skin, fissures, discharge, inflammation, lesions, scars, rectal prolapse, skin tags, and external hemorrhoids. (Skin tags often occur in clients with inflammatory bowel disease.) Ask the client to strain as though defecating. This maneuver can make visible internal hemorrhoids, polyps, rectal prolapse, and fissures.

Next, palpate the external rectum. Put on a glove and apply lubricant to your index finger. As the client strains again, palpate for any anal outpouchings or bulges, nodules, or tenderness. Then, palpate the internal rectum. Before beginning, explain to the client that

ADVANCED ASSESSMENT SKILLS

Assessing the liver

To assess the liver, the nurse should percuss and attempt to palpate or hook the liver.

Liver percussion

1 To percuss the client's liver, begin percussing the abdomen along the right midclavicular line, starting below the level of the umbilicus. Move upward until the percussion notes change from tympany to dullness, usually at or slightly below the costal margin. Mark the point of change with a felt-tip pen.

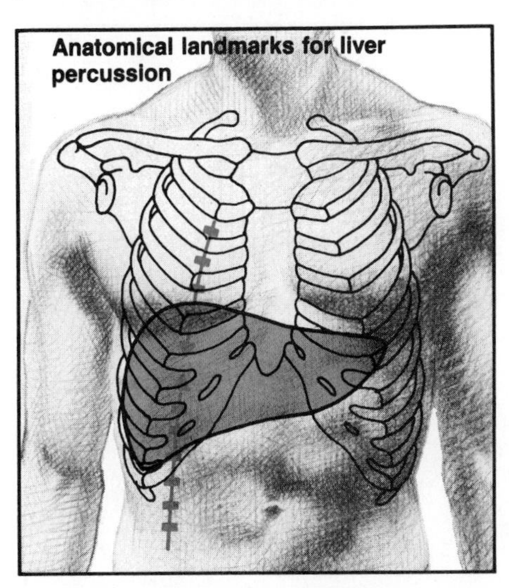

2 Percuss along the right midclavicular line starting above the nipple. Move downward until percussion notes change from normal lung resonance to dullness, usually at the 5th to 7th intercostal space. Again, mark the point of change with a felt-tip pen. Estimate liver size by measuring the distance between the two marks.

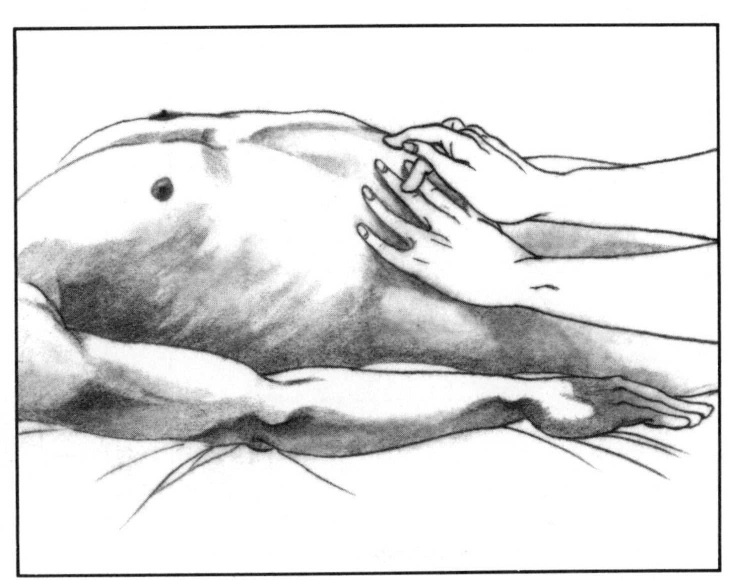

Liver palpation

To palpate the liver, place one hand on the client's back at the approximate height of the liver. Place your other hand below your mark of liver dullness on the right lateral abdomen. Point your fingers toward the right costal margin and press gently in and up as the client inhales deeply. This maneuver may bring the liver edge down to a palpable position.

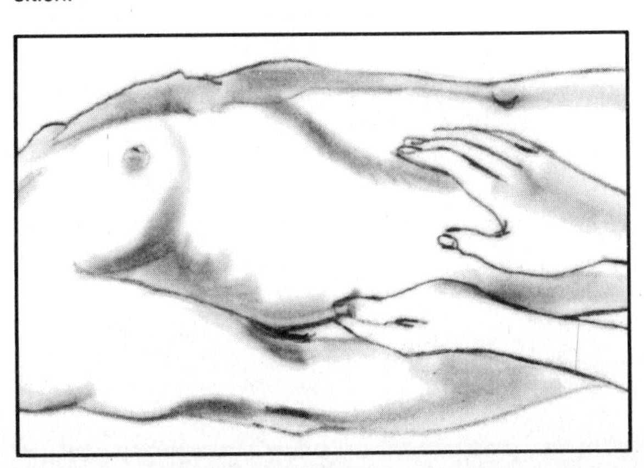

Liver hooking

If liver palpation is unsuccessful, try hooking the liver. To do so, stand on the client's right side at about shoulder level. Place your hands, side by side, below the area of liver dullness. As the client inhales deeply, press your fingers in and upward, attempting to feel the liver with the fingertips of both hands.

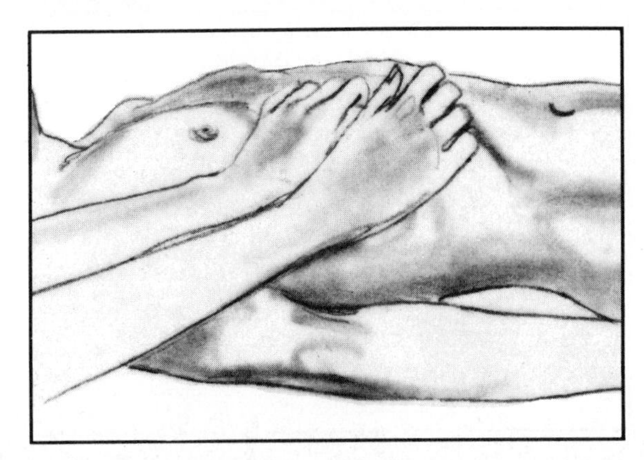

ADVANCED ASSESSMENT SKILLS

Eliciting abdominal pain

Rebound tenderness and the iliopsoas and obturator signs can indicate conditions such as appendicitis or peritonitis. The nurse can elicit these signs of abdominal pain.

Rebound tenderness

1 Position the client supine, with the knees flexed to relax the abdominal muscles. Place your hands gently on the right lower quadrant at McBurney's point—located about midway between the umbilicus and the anterior superior iliac spine.

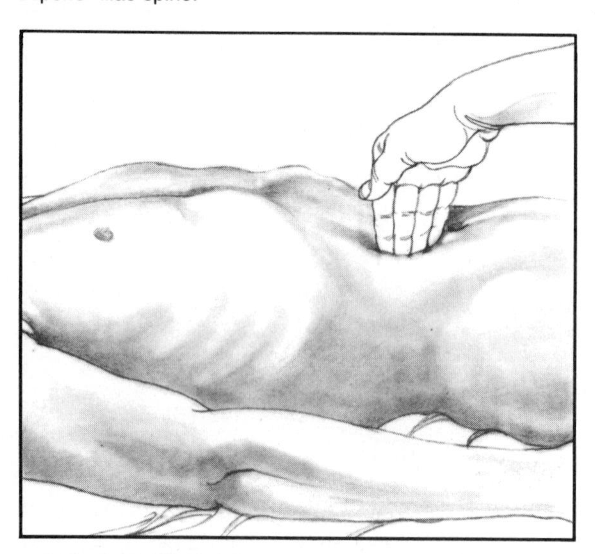

2 Slowly and deeply dip your fingers into the area, then release the pressure in a quick, smooth motion. Pain on release—rebound tenderness—is a positive sign. The pain may radiate to the umbilicus. *Caution:* Do not repeat this maneuver, to minimize the risk of rupturing an inflamed appendix.

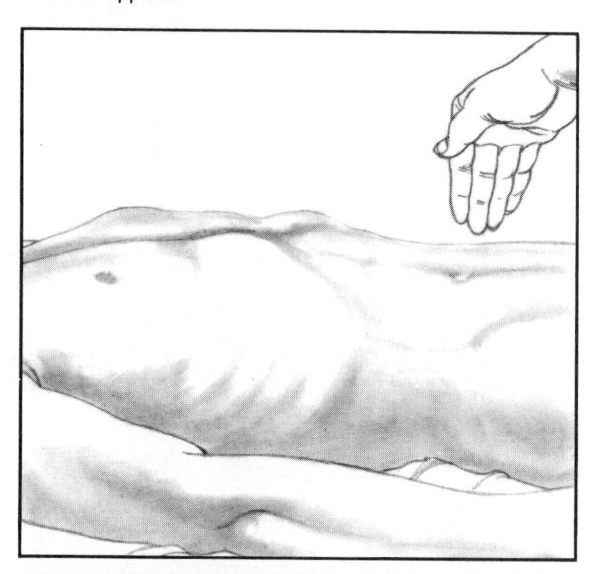

Iliopsoas sign

Position the client supine with the legs straight. Instruct the client to raise the right leg upward as you exert slight pressure with your hand.

Repeat the maneuver with the left leg. With testing on either leg, increased abdominal pain is a positive result, indicating irritation of the psoas muscle.

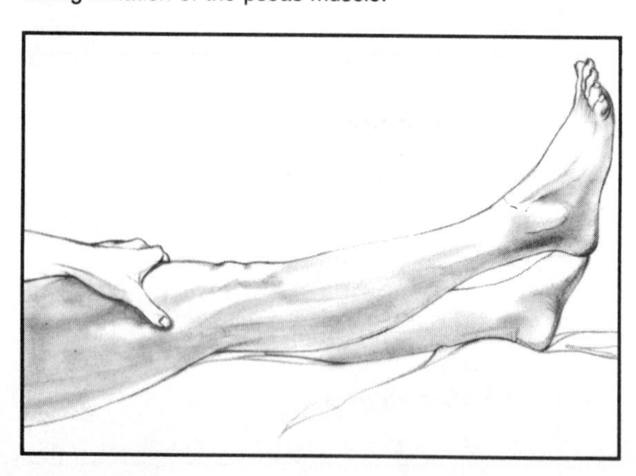

Obturator sign

Position the client supine with the right leg flexed 90 degrees at the hip and knee. Hold the client's leg just above the knee and at the ankle, then rotate the leg laterally and medially. Pain in the hypogastric region is a positive sign, indicating irritation of the obturator muscle.

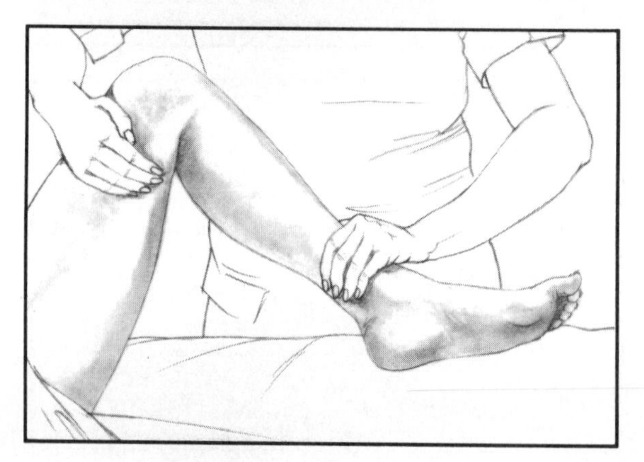

you will insert your gloved, lubricated finger a short distance into the rectum and that this maneuver will cause a feeling of pressure similar to that produced by the urge to defecate. Have the client breathe through the mouth and relax. When the anal sphincter is relaxed, gently insert your finger approximately 2½" to 4" (6 to 10 cm), angling it toward the umbilicus. (*Note:* Do not attempt to force entry through a constricted anal sphincter. Wait with your fingertip resting lightly on the sphincter until the sphincter relaxes.) Once you have inserted your finger, rotate it systematically to palpate all aspects of the rectal wall for nodules, tenderness, irregularities, and fecal impaction. The rectal wall should feel smooth and soft. In a female client, try to feel the posterior side of the uterus through the anterior rectal wall. (For more information, see Chapter 15, Female Reproductive System.) In a male client, assess the prostate when palpating the anterior rectal wall; the prostate should feel firm and smooth. (For more information, see Chapter 16, Male Reproductive System.)

With your finger fully inserted, ask the client to bear down again; this may cause any lesions higher in the rectum to move down to a palpable level. To assess anal sphincter competency, ask the client to tighten the anal muscles around your finger. Finally, withdraw your finger and examine it for blood, mucus, or stool. If stool is present, note its color and test a sample for occult blood.

Developmental considerations. In an infant or young child, perform rectal palpation only when significant symptoms are present. (Usually a pediatric nurse practitioner or physician performs this assessment.) The preferred position for an infant is supine with the legs drawn up, or across the parent's lap face down with buttocks up. Slight bleeding and protrusion of the rectal mucosa may occur after you withdraw the examining finger.

When inspecting a child's rectum, be alert for signs of tearing, irritation, or discharge in the perianal area. Such findings may be signs of an incompetent sphincter or sexual abuse.

A pregnant client commonly develops hemorrhoids at some point during pregnancy. An elderly client may experience loss of sphincter tone and fecal incontinence with aging, and may be more susceptible to colon cancer and rectal prolapse.

Techniques to elicit abdominal pain

Advanced techniques used to determine the presence and nature of abdominal pain and help detect appendicitis include eliciting rebound tenderness, the iliopsoas sign, and the obturator sign. Rebound tenderness, a classic indicator of localized peritoneal irritation in appendicitis, can be elicited by palpating the right lower quadrant over McBurney's point (located about 2" [5 cm] below the right anterior superior spine of the ilium, on a line between the ilium and the umbilicus). The techniques for eliciting the iliopsoas and obturator signs may be used to elicit right lower quadrant tenderness in a client with suspected appendicitis and diffuse pain. (For illustrated procedures, see *Advanced assessment skills: Eliciting abdominal pain*.)

Developmental considerations. A young child may experience the pain of appendicitis as diffuse or centered around the umbilicus, although it may localize later. Asking the supine child to try to raise the head while you push back against the child's forehead will sometimes elicit pain in the right lower quadrant.

Documentation

To understand the significance of assessment findings and form a clear picture of the client's GI status, the nurse must carefully review physical assessment findings and health history information, as well as laboratory study results. (For a summary of frequently used laboratory studies and their significance, see *Common laboratory studies*, pages 380 to 382.) Based on these data, the nurse can formulate appropriate nursing diagnoses, which determine how best to plan, implement, and evaluate the client's nursing care. (For an example of how to apply the nursing process to a client with a GI disorder, see *Applying the nursing process*, pages 378 and 379.)

Proper documentation is an essential element in organizing assessment data and making it available to other members of the health care team. After completing the assessment, document the data completely, including normal and abnormal findings.

The following sample illustrates the proper way to document normal physical assessment findings in the GI system:

> Weight: 148 lb
> Height: 5′ 8″
> Abdomen slightly convex, no skin lesions, no herniations, no pulsations. Normal bowel sounds aus-

(Text continues on page 382.)

Applying the nursing process

Assessment findings form the basis of the nursing process. Using them, the nurse formulates the nursing diagnoses and develops appropriate planning, implementation, and evaluation of the client's care.

The table below shows how the nurse can use GI system assessment data in the nursing process for the client described in the case history (shown at right). In the first column, history and physical assessment data appear, followed by a paragraph of mental notes. These notes help the nurse make important mental connections among assessment findings, aiding in development of the nursing diagnoses and planning.

The second column presents several appropriate nursing diagnoses; however, the information in the remaining three columns is based on the *first* nursing diagnosis. Although it is not part of the nursing process, documentation appears in the last column because of its importance. Documentation consists of an initial note using all components of the SOAPIE format and a follow-up note using the appropriate SOAPIE components.

ASSESSMENT	NURSING DIAGNOSES	PLANNING	IMPLEMENTATION
Subjective (history) data • Client states, "I have a lot of cramps in my stomach and diarrhea." • Client reports she has had intermittent bouts of diarrhea for 3 months since her son was killed in an auto accident. She has obtained temporary relief through the use of a liquid diet and Kaopectate. • Client states she has been losing weight steadily. • Client says she came to the hospital today when she noticed blood in her stool and had two episodes of vomiting. • Client also reports having 10 to 15 watery stools during the past 24 hours and is feeling "weak." **Objective (physical) data** • Vital signs: temperature 100.8° F. (38.1° C.), pulse 112/min. and regular, respirations 30/min. and regular, blood pressure (BP) 100/66. • Abdominal inspection shows abdomen to be slightly convex with no hernias or pulsations. Four-inch, well-healed surgical scar present in LUQ. • Auscultation reveals frequent, hyperactive bowel sounds. • Percussion reveals increased tympany in all four quadrants. • Palpation causes abdominal rigidity and guarding in LLQ. • Rectal examination shows excoriation of perianal area and semiliquid stool in anal canal. Stools are brown, mucoid, semiliquid, and positive for occult blood. • Client has I.V. in cephalic vein of left hand of 1,000 ml 5% dextrose in ½ normal saline infusing at 150 ml/hr via infusion pump. **Mental notes** *Considered along with assessment and laboratory findings, the client's complaints suggest ulcerative colitis. Effectiveness of liquid diet and Kaopectate, common home remedies for GI upset, will diminish as ulceration advances. Anxiety and strong emotions exaggerate ulceration process.*	• Fluid volume deficit related to bowel hypermotility. • Alteration in comfort: cramping, related to increased bowel activity. • Alteration in bowel elimination: diarrhea, related to inflammatory process. • Knowledge deficit related to self-management of illness. • Alteration in nutrition: less than body requirements, related to decreased absorption.	**Goals** Within 24 hours, the client will: • show marked improvement in skin turgor • have normal urine output and urine specific gravity • have marked reduction in watery stools. By the end of the week, the client will: • maintain stable weight.	• Observe and record frequency, amount, and character of diarrhea, along with any precipitating factors. • Encourage frequent rest periods during acute phase. • Monitor intake and output, daily weights, and urine specific gravity. • Monitor skin turgor daily. • Monitor serum electrolytes. • Note any muscle weakness or cardiac dysrhythmias. • Start I.V. hydration, as prescribed. • Encourage oral fluids in amounts necessary to maintain hydration (up to 2,500 ml per day unless contraindicated)—especially fluids with electrolytes, such as boullion and Gatorade. • Provide mouth care every 3 to 4 hours to keep membranes moist.

CASE HISTORY

Mrs. Maria Cortes, age 41, a married woman who works part-time as a sales clerk in a department store, was admitted to the hospital with a preliminary medical diagnosis of ulcerative colitis.

EVALUATION	DOCUMENTATION BASED ON NURSING PROCESS DATA			
		Initial		**Follow-up**
After 24 hours, the client: • had normal skin turgor • passed two large watery stools • exhibited pink, moist oral mucous membranes • had serum electrolytes within normal limits • had a urine specific gravity of 1.020. After 1 week, the client: • reported passing one formed brown stool every 24 hours • noted no weight loss.	**S**	Client states, "I have a lot of cramps in my stomach and diarrhea," and "I feel so weak." Client says she sought medical attention after noticing blood in her stool and vomiting twice in one day. Client reports having 10 to 15 watery stools during the past 24 hours.	**S**	Client states, "I haven't had a bowel movement in 6 hours. What a relief! My bottom still hurts, though."
	O	Client resting in bed with eyes closed, side rails up. Responds appropriately when roused. Pulse 112, sinus tachycardia noted on cardiac monitor, respirations 30 and regular, BP 100/66. Skin dry; skin turgor poor. Movement in all extremities; no tremors. Oral liquids taken in small amounts through straw. 1,000 ml 5% dextrose in ½ normal saline (5% D½NS) infusing at 150 ml per hour via infusion pump to cephalic vein of left hand. No swelling or redness at infusion site. Bowel sounds hyperactive in all four quadrants; abdomen soft. One large diarrheal stool passed in bedpan: liquid, brown, no visible blood but Hemetest positive for occult blood. Perianal area superficially excoriated.	**O**	Client sitting up in bed, pulse 76 and regular, respirations 20 and regular, BP 112/76. 1,000 ml of 5% D½NS infusing at 150 ml per hour via infusion pump in cephalic vein of left hand. Auscultation reveals normal bowel sounds. Abdomen soft on palpation. Skin turgor improved, showing rapid response. Perianal area excoriated.
	A	Fluid volume deficit related to bowel hypermotility. Client fatigued from numerous loose watery stools.	**A**	Hydration improved. Bowel movements less frequent, last one occurring 6 hours ago.
	P	Continue bed rest and fluid and electrolyte replacement. Monitor intake and output, serum electrolytes, and vital signs; provide skin care.	**P**	Continue I.V. hydration. Continue zinc oxide application to perianal area. Monitor intake and output and electrolyte levels.
	I	1,000 ml 5% D½NS with 30 mEq KCl, 2 ml multivitamins started in cephalic vein of left hand using #20 Jelco. Perianal area cleansed; zinc oxide applied. Oral mucous membranes moistened.		
	E	Client weak, in bed with I.V. absorbing without difficulty. Liquid bowel movements continue.		

Common laboratory studies

For a client with GI signs and symptoms, various laboratory studies can provide valuable clues to the possible cause, as shown in the chart below. (*Note:* Keep in mind that abnormal findings may stem from a problem unrelated to the GI system.) Remember that values differ among laboratories, and check the normal value range for the specific laboratory.

TEST AND SIGNIFICANCE	NORMAL VALUES OR FINDINGS	ABNORMAL FINDINGS	POSSIBLE GI OR RELATED CAUSES OF ABNORMAL FINDINGS
Blood tests			
Alkaline phosphatase Measuring this enzyme helps detect focal hepatic lesions.	1.5 to 4 Bodansky units/dl	Above-normal level	Liver disease, obstructive biliary disease
Alpha-fetoprotein Detecting this glycoprotein in a nonpregnant client may indicate hepatocellular carcinoma.	No alpha-fetoprotein	Presence of alpha-fetoprotein	Primary liver cancer
Amylase and lipase Measuring these pancreatic enzymes is the most valuable indicator of pancreatic function.	*Amylase:* 60 to 80 Somogyi units/dl *Lipase:* 32 to 80 units/liter	Above-normal level	Pancreatic inflammation or obstruction, GI ulceration
Bilirubin Measuring direct (prehepatic) and indirect (posthepatic) bilirubin helps evaluate hepatobiliary and erythropoietic functions.	*Direct:* 0.5 mg/dl or less *Indirect:* 1.1 mg/dl or less *Neonates:* 1 to 12 mg/dl (total)	Above-normal level	Hepatitis, biliary tract obstruction (direct and indirect); fasting (total and direct); hemolytic disease (indirect)
Carcinoembryonic antigen (CEA) Normally, production of this glycoprotein halts shortly after birth; it may begin again later if a neoplasm develops.	5 ng/dl	Above-normal level	Colorectal cancer
Cholesterol This test reflects the body's fat metabolism.	120 to 220 mg/dl	Above-normal level	Obstructive biliary disease, fatty liver degeneration
		Below-normal level	Chronic liver disease
Electrolytes These tests provide a quantitative analysis of major extracellular electrolytes (sodium, calcium, chloride, and bicarbonate) and major intracellular electrolytes (potassium, magnesium, and phosphate).	*Sodium* 135 to 145 mEq/liter	Above-normal level	Dehydration as in massive diarrhea, intestinal obstruction
	Calcium 4.5 to 5.5 mEq/liter	Above-normal level	Metabolic alkalosis
		Below-normal level	Malabsorption diarrhea
	Chloride 100 to 108 mEq/liter	Above-normal level	Dehydration
		Below-normal level	Vomiting, diarrhea, intestinal obstruction
	Bicarbonate 22 to 26 mEq/liter	Above-normal level	Metabolic alkalosis caused by massive loss of gastric acids from vomiting or gastric drainage
		Below-normal level	Metabolic acidosis caused by persistent diarrhea

Common laboratory studies *continued*

TEST AND SIGNIFICANCE	NORMAL VALUES OR FINDINGS	ABNORMAL FINDINGS	POSSIBLE GI OR RELATED CAUSES OF ABNORMAL FINDINGS
Electrolytes (continued)	*Phosphate* 1.8 to 2.6 mEq/liter	Above-normal level	High intestinal obstruction
		Below-normal level	Malnutrition; malabsorption syndromes
	Potassium 3.8 to 5.5 mEq/liter	Below-normal level	Loss of body fluids through upper or lower GI tract
	Magnesium 1.5 to 2.5 mEq/liter	Below-normal level	Chronic diarrhea
Gamma glutamyl transpeptidase (GGT) This test detects increased activity of GGT, which reflects liver function.	*Males:* 6 to 47 units/liter *Females under 45 years:* 5 to 27 units/liter *Females over 45 years:* 6 to 37 units/liter	Above-normal level	Liver disease, alcoholism
pH (hydrogen ion concentration) This test reflects the acid-base balance of the blood.	7.35 to 7.42	Above-normal level	Metabolic alkalosis from vomiting, gastric drainage, or other GI fluid losses
		Below-normal level	Metabolic acidosis from persistent diarrhea
Phosphorus Blood concentration of phosphorus is affected by the action of vitamin D and intestinal absorption of calcium.	3 to 4.5 mg/dl	Below-normal level	Malabsorption, cirrhosis, starvation, antacid overdose
Serum glutamic-pyruvic transaminase (SGPT), serum glutamic-oxaloacetic transaminase (SGOT) Blood levels of these enzymes increase in response to cellular injury.	*SGPT* *Males:* 10 to 32 units/liter *Females:* 9 to 24 units/liter *SGOT:* 8 to 20 units/liter	Above-normal levels of SGPT and SGOT	Hepatocellular damage
		Above-normal levels of SGOT	Pancreatic inflammation
Total protein This test reflects the sum of albumin and globulin fractions in serum.	6.6 to 7.9 g/dl	Above-normal level	Liver disease, dehydration
		Below-normal level	Chronic hepatic insufficiency
Urine tests			
Bilirubin This test detects bile pigments in urine.	No bilirubin	Presence of bilirubin	Biliary obstruction
Urobilinogen This test detects impaired liver function.	*Males:* 0.3 to 2.1 Ehrlich units/2 hr; *females:* 0.1 to 1.1 Ehrlich units/2 hr;	Above-normal level	Impaired liver function
		Below-normal level	Total biliary obstruction

continued

Common laboratory studies continued

TEST AND SIGNIFICANCE	NORMAL VALUES OR FINDINGS	ABNORMAL FINDINGS	POSSIBLE GI OR RELATED CAUSES OF ABNORMAL FINDINGS
Fecal tests			
Fecal occult blood test This test measures occult (concealed) blood in stool samples.	2 to 2.5 ml/day	Above-normal level	GI bleeding, colorectal cancer
Stool culture Bacteriologic examination of stool sample detects pathogenic organisms causing GI disease.	No pathogens	Presence of pathogens	Bacterial, viral, or fungal GI infection
Stool examination for ova and parasites This test confirms or rules out intestinal parasitic infestation and disease.	No parasites or ova in stool	Presence of parasites or ova	Parasitic infestation and possible infection

cultated every 10 seconds, all four quadrants. No bruits. No tenderness or masses. Percussion reveals liver edge at costal margin, liver palpated as firm, smooth, nontender.

The following sample shows how to document abnormal physical assessment findings in the GI system:

Weight: 204 lb
Height: 5′ 7″
Abdomen distended. Visible dilated vein over periumbilical area and abdominal wall. Protruding umbilicus. Abdominal girth 94 cm, measured at level of umbilicus. Normal bowel sounds auscultated every 6 seconds. No bruits or friction rubs detected. Upper and lower borders of liver dullness percussed in midclavicular line; estimated height of liver 17 cm. Diminished tympany over suprapubic area; shifting dullness present. Blunt, nontender liver edge palpated 9 cm below right costal margin. No other organs palpated. Fluid wave present. No abdominal tenderness.

Along with assessment findings, document the other nursing process steps—nursing diagnosis, planning, implementation, and evaluation—as you use them to care for a client with a GI disorder.

Chapter summary

To assess a client's GI system effectively, the nurse must rely on health history data, physical assessment findings, and laboratory results. Chapter 13 describes how to gather and integrate this information. Here are the highlights of the chapter:

- The GI system consists of the alimentary canal and accessory organs. A musculomembranous tube, the alimentary canal extends from the mouth to the anus. It includes the mouth, pharynx, esophagus, stomach, small intestine, and large intestine.
- Accessory GI organs include the liver, which lies in the right upper abdominal quadrant; the biliary system, which consists of the gallbladder and bile ducts and is attached to the liver; and the pancreas, which lies horizontally across the posterior abdomen behind the stomach.
- The GI tract has two major functions: digestion, the breakdown of food and fluid into simple chemicals that can be absorbed into the bloodstream and transported throughout the body, and elimination of waste products from the body through excretion of feces.
- When obtaining the health history, establish a comfortable interview environment and use terms familiar

to the client. Because GI complaints may result from other problems in the body, maintain a holistic approach by investigating complaints associated with related body structures.

- During the health history, the nurse explores the client's medication use. Such information may reveal whether the client is receiving treatment for a GI dysfunction or may suggest that an adverse drug reaction may have caused the dysfunction.
- When physically assessing the client's abdomen, the nurse uses inspection, auscultation, percussion, and palpation. In the abdominal assessment, auscultation precedes palpation and percussion because these techniques can change intestinal activity, which will interfere with bowel sound auscultation.
- During inspection, the nurse examines the abdominal contour for symmetry; the skin for lesions, scars, or discolorations; and the umbilicus for position, irritation, protrusion, and pulsations.
- Auscultation allows the nurse to assess bowel sounds and abdominal blood vessel sounds. Bowel sounds are best heard with the diaphragm of the stethoscope; vascular sounds, with the bell. Auscultation should be done in all four abdominal quadrants.
- Percussion of the abdomen provides information about the size and location of the internal abdominal organs and detects excessive accumulation of fluid and air in the abdomen. Percussion should be performed systematically, starting with the right upper quadrant (unless the client is experiencing pain there) and moving clockwise through percussion sites in each quadrant.
- Palpation of the abdomen helps to substantiate previous findings and provides useful information about the nature of the abdominal wall; the size, condition, and consistency of organs; the presence and character of any masses; and the presence, location, and degree of any pain or tenderness.
- Advanced GI assessment skills used in abdominal assessment include liver percussion, palpation, and hooking; rectal examination; and techniques to elicit abdominal pain, including eliciting rebound tenderness, the iliopsoas sign, and the obturator sign.
- To complete the GI assessment, the nurse reviews the results of any laboratory studies ordered to assess GI function. Commonly ordered tests include stool analysis for occult blood, bacteria, and ova and parasites; blood tests for alkaline phosphatase, alpha-fetoprotein, amylase and lipase, bilirubin, carcinoembryonic antigen, cholesterol, electrolytes, gemma glutamyl transpeptidase, pH, phosphorus, serum glutamic-pyruvic transaminase and serum glutamic-oxaloacetic transaminase and total protein; and urine studies evaluating bilirubin and urobilinogen.
- The nurse documents all assessment findings—both normal and abnormal—and uses them in the nursing process to plan, implement, and evaluate the client's care.

Study questions

1. What subjective and objective findings would you most often see in a client with diverticulitis? How do these contrast with the most likely findings in Crohn's disease?

2. During the health history, a 32-year-old male client reports a history of bleeding hemorrhoids. You note that he has a hemoglobin of 12.2 g/dl and melena. Are these objective findings consistent with the client's history? What further assessment steps should you take?

3. Mrs. Cavanaugh brings her 7-month-old daughter to the clinic, stating that the child has had 9 to 10 loose, liquid stools a day for 3 days and that she is taking her bottle poorly. What health history questions and physical assessment procedures will be most useful for this client?

4. Which three types of clients are at greatest risk for constipation, and why?

5. Mrs. Stevens, a 71-year-old widow, comes to the outpatient clinic complaining of "constipation." She also complains of lack of appetite and occasional nausea, especially at bedtime. She states that since her husband died, she no longer cares to cook and no longer takes the long daily walks the couple used to share.

In the following categories, what information would you record regarding the nursing assessment of Mrs. Stevens?

- history (subjective) assessment data
- physical (objective) assessment data
- assessment techniques and equipment
- two appropriate nursing diagnoses
- documentation of findings.

Selected references

Assessment. (1986). Nurse's Reference Library. Springhouse, PA: Springhouse Corp.

Barisonek, K., Newman, E., and Logio, T. (1984). Assessment under pressure: When your patient says 'My stomach hurts.' " *Nursing84,* 14(11), 34-42.

Diagnostics (2nd ed.). (1986). Nurse's Reference Library. Springhouse, PA: Springhouse Corp.

Doenges, M., Jeffries, M., and Moorhouse, M. (1989). *Nursing care plans: Guidelines for planning patient care* (2nd ed.). Philadelphia: Davis.

Gastrointestinal Problems. (1986). NurseReview Series. Springhouse, PA: Springhouse Corp.

Guyton, A. (1991). *Textbook of medical physiology* (8th ed.). Philadelphia: Saunders.

Henry, J. (1991). *Clinical diagnosis and management by laboratory methods* (18th ed.). Philadelphia: Saunders.

Jacobs, D., and Strober, W. (1984). Gastrointestinal infections in the immunocompromised host. *Hospital Medicine,* 20(11), 51-83.

Lind, C., and Cerda, J. (1987). Diagnosis: GI complaints in the geriatric patient (parts 1 and 2). *Hospital Medicine,* 23(10), 183-199; 23(11), 21-39.

Lindsey, M. (1989). Abdominal assessment. *Orthopedic Nursing,* 8(4), 34-38.

Lloyd, R., Scali, V., Ferko, J. III, Gonzales, E., Rippert, J., and Stout, S. (1989). Assessing abdominal pain. *Emergency,* 21(10), 31, 33, 38+.

McConnell, E. (1990). Assessing abdominal pain in a postoperative patient. *Nursing90,* 20(3), 86-88.

McConnell, E. (1990). Assessing severe abdominal pain. *Nursing90,* 20(6), 76, 79.

McConnell, E. (1990). Auscultating bowel sounds. *Nursing90,* 20(5), 106.

McEvoy, G. (Ed.). (1992). *American Hospital Formulary Service drug information.* Bethesda, MD: American Society of Hospital Pharmacists.

O'Toole, M. (1990). Advanced assessment of the abdomen and gastrointestinal problems. *Nursing Clinics of North America,* 25(4), 771-776.

Schroeder, S., Krupp, M., Tierney, L., and McPhee, S. (Eds.). (1991). *Current medical diagnosis and treatment.* East Norwalk, CT: Appleton & Lange.

Smith, C. (1985). Detecting acute abdominal distention. *Nursing85,* 15(9), 34-39.

Nursing research

Candy, C. (1987). Recent advances in the care of children with diarrhea: Giving responsibility to the nurse and parents. *Journal of Advanced Nursing,* 12(1), 95-99.

Reynolds, S., and Jaffe, D. (1990). Quick triage of children with abdominal pain. *Emergency Medicine,* 22(14), 39-40, 42.

Ricci, J. (1987). Alcohol-induced upper GI hemorrhage: Case studies and management. *Critical Care Nurse,* 7(1), 56-63.

14

Urinary System

Objectives

After reading and studying this chapter, you should be able to:

1. Identify the anatomic location of urinary system structures.
2. Discuss the main functions of the kidneys and their basic functional units.
3. Give examples of appropriate health history questions to ask the client when assessing the urinary system.
4. Describe normal urine characteristics.
5. Locate the costovertebral angle.
6. Differentiate between normal and abnormal findings during physical assessment of the kidneys, bladder, and urethral meatus.
7. Describe the most important laboratory tests used to evaluate kidney function.
8. Describe representative adverse effects of drugs on the urinary system.
9. Document urinary system assessment findings using the nursing process.

Introduction

This chapter reviews the anatomy and physiology of the urinary system, describes urine formation, and explains the relationship between hormones and the urinary system. Then it discusses the tools used to evaluate a client's urinary system, including the health history and physical assessment. It presents normal and abnormal history and physical findings and includes information about relevant laboratory studies. The chapter concludes with a case study that shows how to document urinary assessment findings using the nursing process.

Certain urinary signs and symptoms—for example, hematuria, cloudy urine, incontinence, frequency, hesitancy, and urgency—should immediately indicate the need for a urinary system assessment. Other findings, such as abdominal pain and edema, also may warrant a complete urinary system assessment, even though their connection to this system may seem less obvious.

The kidneys keep useful materials and excrete waste, foreign, or excessive materials. Through this basic function, the kidneys have profound effects on other body systems and on the client's overall health. Because the kidneys play a key role in acid-base balance (the stable concentration of hydrogen ions in body fluids) and homeostasis (chemical and physical equilibrium of fluids in the body's internal environment), a urinary system assessment may uncover clues to possible problems in any body system.

Because of the interactions between the urinary system and other body systems, a disorder originating in another system can disrupt urinary function. For example, the cardiovascular system must deliver blood to the kidneys at a pressure adequate for filtration. The kidneys, in turn, regulate fluid balance, which maintains the circulating volume and electrolyte balance necessary for myocardial function.

Interacting with the nervous system, the kidneys help regulate blood pressure and control urination. Interacting with the endocrine system, they help maintain sodium and water balance by responding to aldosterone and antidiuretic hormone (ADH). The kidneys synthesize several prostaglandins (hormonelike unsaturated fatty acids that help regulate blood pressure) and produce the biologically active form of vitamin D, which helps maintain normal calcium levels.

Glossary

Acid-base balance: stable concentration of hydrogen ions in body fluids.

Active transport: movement of materials across cell membranes via chemical activity, permitting entry of larger molecules than could otherwise enter.

Albuminuria: albumin in the urine (as in glomerulonephritis).

Aldosterone: mineralocorticoid produced by the adrenal cortex that regulates the sodium and potassium balance in the blood.

Antidiuretic hormone (ADH): hormone secreted by the hypothalamus and stored in the posterior lobe of the pituitary gland; reduces urine production by increasing the water reabsorption in the renal tubules.

Calculus: pathologic stone, formed of mineral salts, usually found in a hollow organ or duct, such as the ureter. A calculus may cause inflammation or obstruction.

Diffusion: movement of molecules in a solution from an area of greater concentration to one of lesser concentration; results in even particle distribution.

Elimination: removal of the body's waste products by the skin, kidneys, lungs, and intestines; final excretion phase.

Enuresis: involuntary urination during sleep; bedwetting.

Excretion: process of removing or shedding substances by body organs or tissues during natural metabolic activity; usually begins at the cellular level.

Glomerular filtrate: fluid lacking proteins and red blood cells that has been filtered by glomerular capillaries; passes into the proximal convoluted tubules of the nephrons.

Homeostasis: state of chemical and physical equilibrium of fluids in the body's internal environment.

Hydrostatic pressure: pressure exerted by a fluid.

Hypercalciuria: elevated urine calcium level.

Hypertonic solution: solution having a greater concentration of dissolved particles than another solution, hence exerting greater osmotic pressure than that solution. For example, a saline solution whose salt content exceeds that of intracellular and extracellular fluid is hypertonic.

Hypotonic solution: solution having a lesser concentration of dissolved particles than another solution, hence exerting less osmotic pressure than that solution. For example, a saline solution containing less salt than that found in intracellular and extracellular fluid is hypotonic.

Incontinence: inability to control urination or defecation. Urinary incontinence may result from infection, a spinal cord lesion, or a sphincter injury. Coughing, sneezing, or heavy lifting may precipitate stress incontinence.

Insensible fluid loss: water lost from the body through evaporation, for example, that lost from the lungs during expiration.

Isotonic solution: solution having the same concentration of dissolved particles as another solution, hence exerting the same osmotic pressure. For example, a saline solution containing the same amount of salt found in intracellular and extracellular fluid is isotonic.

Micturition: urination; the act of voiding, emptying, or evacuating urine from the body.

Nephritis: kidney (renal) disease characterized by kidney inflammation and dysfunction.

Nephrolithiasis: Kidney stone, urinary calculi.

Nocturia: excessive urine excretion at night; may stem from renal disease or excessive fluid consumption shortly before bedtime.

Oliguria: diminished capacity to form and eliminate urine; may result from a fluid or electrolyte imbalance, a renal lesion, or urinary tract obstruction.

Osmolality: osmotic pressure of a solution; expressed in milliosmols (mOsm), a unit of measure representing the concentration of particles in a solution per kilogram of water. Osmolality of body fluids ranges from 280 to 294 mOsm/kg.

Osmosis: movement of a pure solvent, such as water, through a semipermeable membrane from a solution of lesser concentration of solute to one of greater concentration of solute, balancing the concentration in both areas.

Osmotic pressure: pressure exerted on a semipermeable membrane separating a solution from a solvent, when only the solvent, not the solutes, can permeate the membrane.

Passive transport: movement of small molecules across a cell membrane by diffusion; occurs when the concentration of chemicals outside a cell increases and molecules start moving into the cell, changing the intracellular equilibrium.

pH: hydrogen ion concentration, reflecting a solution's acidity or alkalinity on a scale of 1 to 14. Normal urine pH, for example, ranges from 4.5 to 8.0.

Polydipsia: excessive thirst, characteristically accompanying diabetes mellitus.

Polyuria: excretion of an abnormally large urine volume; may result from diuretics, diabetes mellitus, diabetes insipidus, alcohol intake, or excessive fluid intake.

Pyuria: pus in the urine.

Glossary

Secretion: discharge of a substance into a cavity, vessel, or organ or onto the skin surface.
Solute: substance dissolved in a solution.
Solvent: liquid in which another substance can be dissolved.
Specific gravity: relative weight of a fluid compared to the weight of an equal amount of water, determined by the amount of solids in the fluid. For example, urine with a specific gravity of 1.010 is 1.010 times heavier than water.
Tubular reabsorption: movement of selective substances, such as sodium, out of the glomerular filtrate into the blood.
Tubular secretion: movement of certain substances (for example, potassium and hydrogen) out of the blood and into the glomerular filtrate.
Uremic frost: pale, frostlike deposit of white or yellow urate crystals on the skin. Sometimes accompanying renal failure and uremia, uremic frost forms when urea compounds and other metabolic waste products cannot be excreted by the kidneys into the urine and instead are excreted through small superficial capillaries to the skin, where they collect on the surface.
Urinary hesitancy: decrease in the force of the urine stream, commonly accompanied by difficulty starting the urine flow. It usually results from an obstruction or a stricture between the bladder and urethral meatus.
Urinary frequency: abnormally frequent urination, or urge to urinate, without an increase in total daily urine output.
Urinary urgency: sudden powerful urge to urinate, commonly caused by urinary tract infection.
Urinary catheter: hollow, flexible tube inserted through the urethral meatus into the bladder to drain urine.
Void: to eliminate waste matter from the body, as in evacuation of urine from the bladder.

For these reasons, the nurse must always assess for signs and symptoms of urinary system disorders—even if the client's chief complaint seems unrelated. The assessment should include a detailed health history, a thorough physical assessment, and an analysis of laboratory test results (such as routine urinalysis findings, serum creatinine levels, and blood urea nitrogen [BUN] values). Information obtained then serves as the foundation for the remaining nursing process steps and helps the nurse develop an individualized care plan.

Anatomy and physiology review

The urinary system consists of two kidneys, two ureters, one bladder, and one urethra. (For information about these structures, see *The urinary system,* pages 388 and 389.) Working together, these structures remove wastes from the body and regulate acid-base balance by retaining or excreting hydrogen ions.

Urine formation

Three processes—glomerular filtration, tubular mineralocorticoid reabsorption, and tubular secretion—take place in the nephrons, ultimately leading to urine formation. (For more information, see *Functional anatomy of the nephron,* page 390.)

The kidneys can vary the amount of substances reabsorbed and secreted in the nephrons, changing the composition of excreted urine. Normal urine constituents include sodium, chloride, potassium, calcium, magnesium, sulfates, phosphates, bicarbonates, uric acid, ammonium ions, creatinine, urobilinogen, a few leukocytes and red blood cells (RBCs), and, in the male, possibly a few sperm. Urine also may contain drugs if the client is receiving drugs that undergo urinary excretion.

Varying with fluid intake and climate, total daily urine output averages 720 to 2,400 ml. For example, after a client ingests a large volume of fluid, urine output increases as the body rapidly excretes excess water. During a client's water deprivation or excess intake of such solutes as sodium, urine output decreases as the body retains water to restore normal fluid concentration.

Hormones and the kidneys

Hormones help regulate tubular reabsorption and secretion. For example, ADH acts in the distal tubule and collecting ducts to increase water reabsorption and urine concentration. ADH deficiency decreases water reab-

(Text continues on page 391.)

The urinary system

As this frontal view suggests, the kidneys constitute the major portion of the urinary system. The rest of this system consists of ureters, the bladder, and the urethra.

Kidneys

Bean-shaped, the kidneys measure approximately 4½″ (11.4 cm) long and 2½″ (6.4 cm) wide. Located retroperitoneally, they lie on either side of the vertebral column, between the 12th thoracic and 3rd lumbar vertebrae. Here, the kidneys lie protected, behind the abdominal contents and in front of the muscles attached to the vertebral column. A perirenal fat layer offers further protection.

Crowded by the liver, the right kidney extends slightly lower than the left. Atop each kidney (suprarenal) lies an adrenal gland. At the hilus—an indentation in the medial aspect of each kidney—the renal artery, renal vein, lymphatic vessels, and nerves enter the kidney. The renal pelvis, a funnel-shaped ureter extension, also enters here.

Highly vascular organs, the kidneys regulate fluid and electrolyte balance through glomerular filtration, reabsorption, and secretion; via urine excretion, they rid the body of waste products.

A cross-section of the kidney reveals the outer renal cortex, central renal medulla, internal calyces, and renal pelvis. At the microscopic level, the nephron serves as the functional unit of the kidneys.

Each kidney contains approximately 1 million nephrons. A nephron, in turn, consists of a glomerulus (a capillary network), Bowman's capsule (a cup-shaped structure that surrounds and supports the glomerulus), proximal convoluted tubule, loop of Henle, distal convoluted tubule, and collecting tubule.

Blood enters the glomerulus via afferent arterioles (tiny arterial branches proceeding toward the glomerulus) and leaves via efferent arterioles (similar arterial branches directed away from the glomerulus). The glomerulus, Bowman's capsule, and proximal and distal tubules lie in the outer renal cortex; the loop of Henle and related blood vessels and collecting tubules descend into the central renal medulla, forming the renal pyramids. Tapered portions of the pyramids empty into the cuplike internal calyces, which channel urine into the renal pelvis.

Ureters

As ducts allowing urine to pass from the kidneys to the bladder, the ureters measure about 10″ to 12″ (25 to 30 cm) long in adults. Ureter diameter varies from 2 to 8 mm, with the narrowest portion at the ureteropelvic junction. Because

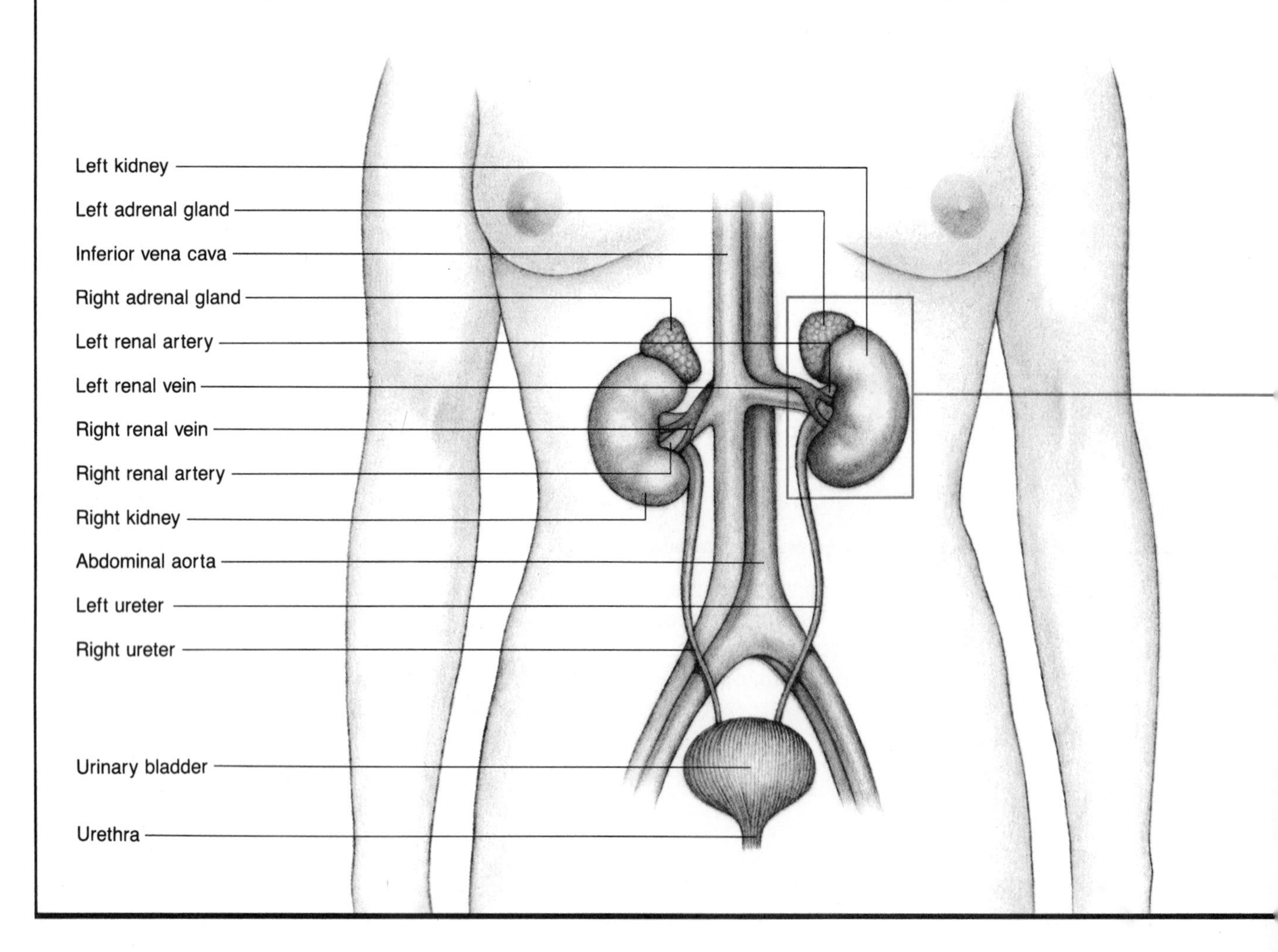

the left kidney is higher than the right kidney, the left ureter typically is slightly longer than the right ureter.

Originating in the ureteropelvic junction of the kidneys, the ureters travel obliquely to the bladder, channeling urine via peristaltic waves occurring at a rate of approximately 1 to 5 per minute.

Bladder

A hollow, spherical, muscular organ in the pelvis, the bladder serves as the body's urine storage site. It lies anterior and inferior to the pelvic cavity and posterior to the symphysis pubis. Bladder capacity ranges from 500 to 600 ml in a normal adult, less in children and elderly persons. If the amount of stored urine exceeds bladder capacity, the bladder distends above the symphysis pubis.

The base of the bladder contains three openings that form a triangular area called the trigone. Two ureteral orifices act as the posterior boundary of the trigone; one urethral orifice forms its anterior boundary.

Urination results from involuntary (reflex) and voluntary (learned or intentional) processes. When urine distends the bladder, the involuntary process begins: parasympathetic nervous system fibers transmit impulses that make the bladder contract and the internal sphincter (located at the internal urethral orifice) relax. Then, the cerebrum stimulates voluntary relaxation and contraction of the external sphincter (located about ¾″ [2 cm] beyond the internal sphincter).

Urethra

A small duct, the urethra channels urine outside the body from the bladder. It has an exterior opening termed the urinary (urethral) meatus. In the female, the urethra ranges from 1″ to 2″ (3 to 5 cm) long, with the urethral meatus located anterior to the vaginal opening. In the male, the urethra is approximately 8″ (20 cm) long, with the urethral meatus located at the end of the glans penis. The male urethra serves as a passageway for semen as well as urine. (For a discussion of urinary system characteristics specific to the male client, see Chapter 16, Male Reproductive System.)

Kidney cross section

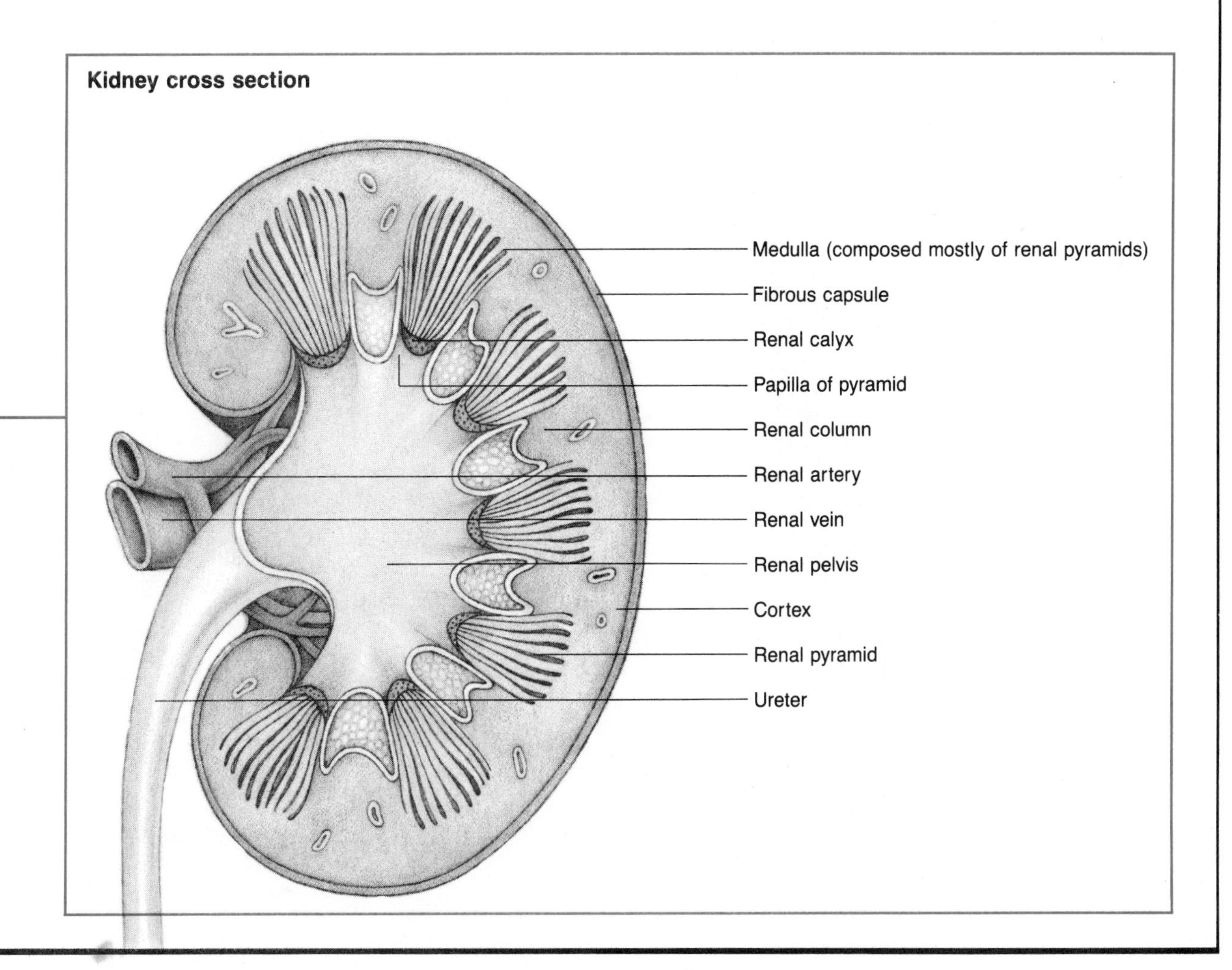

Functional anatomy of the nephron

The basic functional unit of the kidney, the nephron consists of a glomerulus (located inside Bowman's capsule), distal and proximal convoluted tubules, a collecting tubule, and the loop of Henle. Each nephron performs three main activities. It:

- mechanically filters fluids, wastes, electrolytes, acids, and bases into the tubular system
- reabsorbs selected molecules
- secretes selected molecules.

Filtration occurs in the glomerulus, where high hydrostatic pressure forces fluid and small molecules to move through glomerular capillary walls into Bowman's capsule. The resulting fluid, called glomerular filtrate, passes into the proximal convoluted tubule, loop of Henle, and distal convoluted tubule before reaching the collecting duct.

Secretion and reabsorption occur throughout the tubular system. Via active and passive transport, substances pass from the circulation into the tubules (secretion), then from the tubules back into the circulation (reabsorption). (In the illustration, arrows indicate these processes.) Along the way, selective secretion and reabsorption convert the glomerular filtrate into urine.

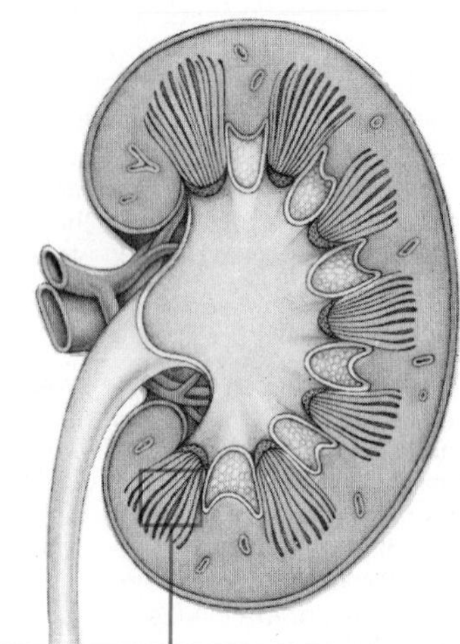

Schematic of a nephron

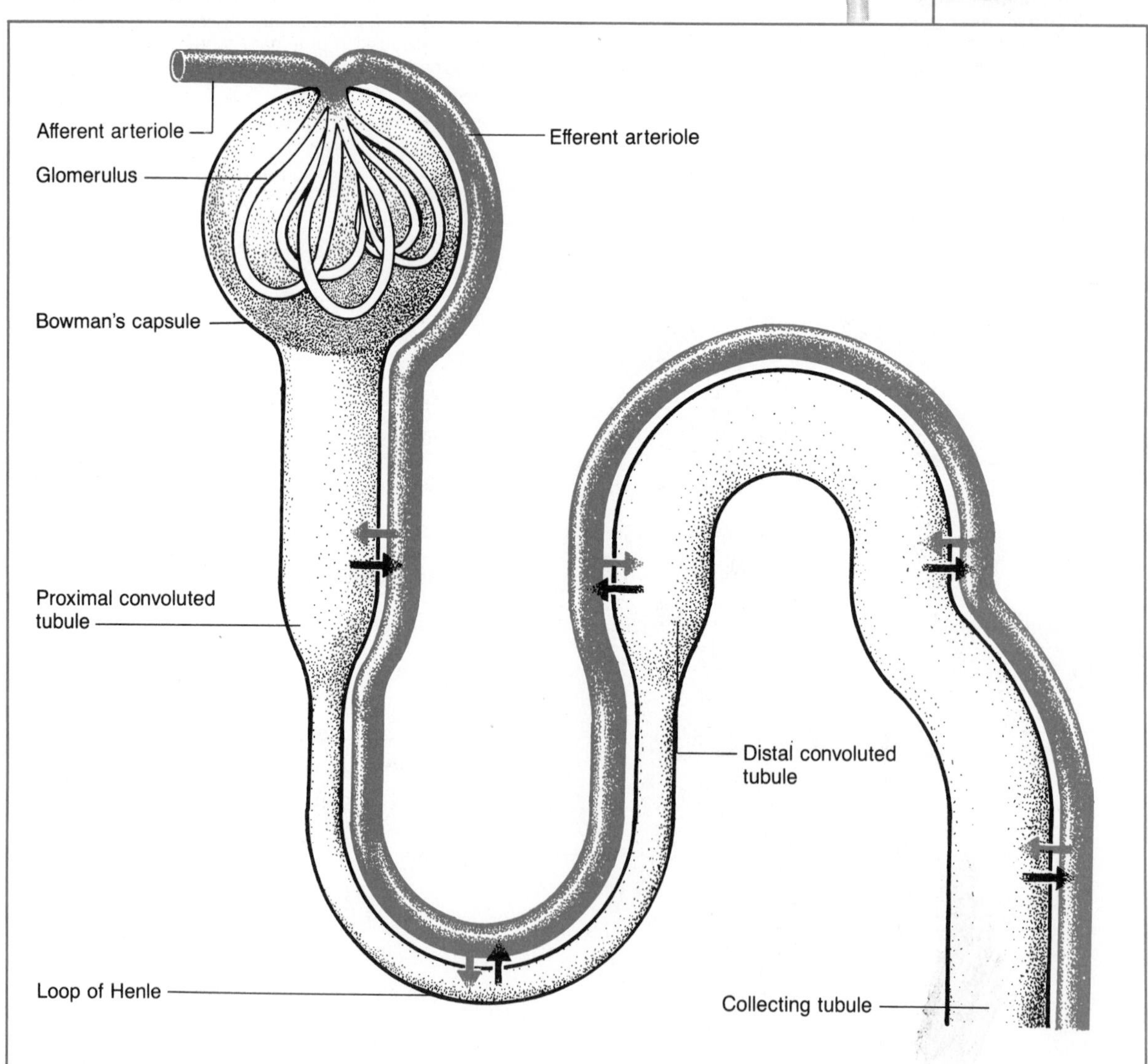

sorption, causing dilute urine to form. Aldosterone affects tubular reabsorption by regulating sodium retention and helping to control potassium secretion by tubular epithelial cells.

By secreting the hormone renin, a proteolytic enzyme, the kidneys play a crucial role in blood pressure and fluid volume regulation. Sodium concentration in the renal tubules stimulates renin secretion; renin then converts the plasma protein angiotensinogen to the polypeptide angiotensin I. In the lungs, angiotensin I is converted to angiotensin II, a potent vasoconstrictor that stimulates aldosterone secretion from the adrenal cortex. This leads to an elevated aldosterone level, which in turn triggers sodium reabsorption from the distal tubules and collecting ducts. Passively attracted to sodium, water moves with sodium into the blood for reabsorption. Here, it increases blood volume and pressure, ensuring adequate glomerular function.

The distal tubules of the kidneys regulate potassium excretion. Responding to an elevated serum potassium level, the adrenal cortex increases aldosterone secretion. Through a poorly understood mechanism, aldosterone also affects the potassium-secreting capacity of distal tubular cells.

The other hormonal functions of the kidneys include secretion of the hormone erythropoietin and regulation of calcium and phosphorus balance. In response to low arterial oxygen tension, the kidneys produce erythropoietin, which travels to the bone marrow, where it stimulates increased RBC production. To help regulate calcium and phosphorus balance, the kidneys filter and reabsorb approximately half of unbound serum calcium and activate vitamin D_3, a compound that promotes intestinal calcium absorption and regulates phosphate excretion.

Health history

Before collecting health history information about a client's urinary system, the nurse will prepare for the interview by following these three important steps:

• Establish a comfortable interview environment. To do this, ensure the client's privacy and conduct the interview at a comfortable pace without interruptions. Otherwise, the client may feel rushed or uncomfortable and may omit important details.

• Use terms familiar to the client. If you must use such medical terms as *void, urinate, catheter,* or *enuresis,* make sure the client understands them.

• Even though the health history will focus on the urinary system, maintain a holistic approach by inquiring about the status of other body systems. Urinary problems may result from—or cause—problems in other body systems. In some cases, urinary problems impair other aspects of the client's life. For example, a client with stress incontinence may refuse to take a long car trip. This reluctance to travel could disrupt the client's social and family life.

Health and illness patterns

A health and illness pattern assessment requires an exploration of the client's current, past, and family health status and any developmental considerations. To accomplish this, the nurse should follow the steps described below.

Current health status

Because current health status is foremost in the client's mind, begin the interview by exploring this topic. Carefully document the chief complaint in the client's own words. Using the *PQRST* method, ask the client to completely describe this complaint and any others. (For a detailed explanation of this method, see *Symptom analysis* in Chapter 3, The Health History.) To investigate the client's current health status further, ask the following questions about urinary function:

Do you ever have trouble starting or maintaining a urine stream?
(RATIONALE: Urinary hesitancy, or difficulty starting a urine stream, may result from a urethral stricture, such as from an enlarged prostate gland or from a partial obstruction from a kidney stone.)

Have you noticed a change in the size of your urine stream? If so, can you describe it?
(RATIONALE: Decreased stream size may indicate a partial urethral obstruction, such as from a renal calculus that has descended into the urethra or an enlarged prostate.)

Do you ever experience urinary urgency—the feeling that you must urinate immediately? If so, do you ever experience this without urinating?
(RATIONALE: Urinary urgency—with or without urination—suggests a bladder dysfunction or lower urinary tract infection. A client with urgency accompanied by urination may need to be near a bathroom or commode at all times.)

Evaluating urine color

To help assess the client's current health status, the nurse must ask about any urine color changes. As the table below shows, a change from the normal amber or straw color can result from fluid intake, medications, and dietary factors as well as from various disorders.

URINE APPEARANCE	POSSIBLE CAUSES
Blue-green	Methylene blue
Cloudy	Infection, inflammation, glomerular nephritis, vegetarian diet
Colorless or pale straw color (dilute urine)	Excess fluid intake, anxiety, chronic renal disease, diabetes insipidus, diuretic therapy
Dark brown or black	Acute glomerulonephritis, drugs (such as nitrofurantoin and chlorpromazine)
Dark yellow or amber (concentrated urine)	Low fluid intake, acute febrile disease, vomiting or diarrhea causing large fluid loss
Green-brown	Bile duct obstruction
Orange-red to orange-brown	Urobilinuria, drugs (such as phenazopyridine), obstructive jaundice (tea-colored urine)
Red or red-brown	Porphyria, hemorrhage, drugs (such as phenazopyridine hydrochloride)

Does your bladder feel full after you urinate?
(RATIONALE: A full bladder sensation after voiding may indicate retention caused by bladder dysfunction or infection.)

Do you ever feel a burning sensation when you urinate? If so, how often?
(RATIONALE: A burning sensation during urination may result from a lower urinary tract infection.)

Do you ever have pain when you urinate? If so, how often?
(RATIONALE: Painful urination suggests a lower urinary tract infection or obstruction.)

What color is your urine? Does it appear dark yellow and cloudy? Does it ever look red, brown, or black?
(RATIONALE: Urine normally appears amber or straw-colored. Abnormal urine colors, which range from dark yellow to black, may result from a urinary disorder, a change in fluid intake or diet, or administration of certain drugs. For detailed information, see *Evaluating urine color.*)

Do you ever pass gas in your urine?
(RATIONALE: Passage of gas in the urine can stem from urinary tract infection by certain gas-producing bacteria.)

Do you ever have pain in your side that radiates around to your back or into your lower abdomen? If so, do position changes relieve the pain or make it worse?
(RATIONALE: Flank pain may indicate renal colic; lower abdominal pain may signal obstruction or infection. Pain relieved by lying down suggests inflammation from infection; pain unrelieved by position changes may mean renal colic.)

Do you ever have pain around the costovertebral angle? (Point out this area to the client.)
(RATIONALE: Pain around the costovertebral angle suggests kidney infection.)

Do you ever have a urethral discharge? If so, how would you characterize its color and odor? How long have you had this discharge? How would you describe the amount? Has the amount of the discharge increased or decreased?

Sex-specific questions

The following questions will help evaluate a male or female client's current health status.

Questions for a male client

Have you been circumcised? If not, do you have any difficulty retracting the foreskin?
(RATIONALE: Difficulty retracting the foreskin suggests phimosis—foreskin constriction over the glans—usually from a previous infection.)

Questions for a female client

Do you ever leak urine when you laugh, cough, sneeze, or exercise or when you bend to pick something up, rise from a sitting position, or sit from a standing position? Does leakage occur when you strain at stool or immediately after you feel the urge to urinate?
(RATIONALE: Positive responses to these questions suggest bladder dysfunction, such as that occurring in women who have had multiple births.)

Have you ever been pregnant or given birth? If so, how many times? Have you had any forceps deliveries?
(RATIONALE: Pregnancy may weaken bladder control by resulting in fetal pressure on the bladder; delivery may weaken bladder control by causing stretching of pelvic floor muscles. A forceps delivery may injure urinary and genital structures.)

(RATIONALE: Urethral discharge frequently accompanies a lower urinary tract infection or, in a male client, a sexually transmitted disease, such as gonorrhea. Discharge color, odor, and amount help identify the infection type.)

Pose additional history questions based on the client's sex. (For further information, see *Sex-specific questions.*)

Past health status

During this part of the health history, ask the following questions to explore the client's medical history for additional information related to the urinary system:

Have you ever had a kidney or bladder problem, such as a urinary tract infection? If so, describe the problem and tell when it first occurred.
(RATIONALE: A history of kidney or bladder problems increases the risk of recurrence or urinary system complications.)

Have you ever been hospitalized for a kidney or bladder problem?
(RATIONALE: Hospitalization indicates that the kidney or bladder problem was serious and acute.)

Have you ever had kidney or bladder stones? If so, when? How were they treated?
(RATIONALE: Kidney or bladder stones [calculi] can recur. Determining how the problem was treated provides information that can help focus the nursing care plan.)

Have you ever had a kidney or bladder injury? If so, when and how was it treated?
(RATIONALE: Trauma can alter kidney or bladder structure or function.)

Have you ever worn an external drainage device? If so, when and why?
(RATIONALE: A positive response means that the client has undergone urinary diversion surgery. Find out the type of surgery and why it was performed.)

Have you ever been catheterized? If so, why?
(RATIONALE: A history of catheterization indicates that the client could not urinate or experienced urinary retention or inhibited bladder emptying. In a few cases, however, catheterization is performed to collect a urine specimen.)

Have you ever had syphilis, gonorrhea, or another sexually transmitted disease? If so, how long ago and how was it treated?
(RATIONALE: Sexually transmitted diseases can cause urinary and genital dysfunction.)

Do you currently take any prescribed or over-the-counter medications? If so, which ones do you take and how frequently do you take them?
(RATIONALE: Some medications can affect urinary function or alter urine appearance. For additional information, see *Adverse drug reactions,* pages 394 and 395.)

Are you allergic to any medications? If so, which ones?
(RATIONALE: Some allergic reactions can cause tubular damage; severe anaphylactic reactions can produce temporary renal failure and permanent tubular necrosis.)

If you have had an allergic reaction to a medication, how would you describe it?
(RATIONALE: Some clients confuse an adverse drug reaction, which commonly causes nausea or diarrhea, with an allergic reaction, which typically causes hives or throat constriction. Having the client describe exactly what occurred can help determine the specific reaction.)

Are you currently receiving treatment for a medical problem, such as diabetes mellitus or high blood pressure?
(RATIONALE: Diabetes mellitus can increase the risk of urinary tract infection; both diabetes mellitus and hypertension can lead to nephropathy.)

Family health status

Next, investigate the urinary system status of the client's family by asking the following questions:

Has anyone in your family ever been treated for kidney problems?
(RATIONALE: Polycystic kidney disease and all types of hereditary nephritis are genetically transmitted.)

Has anyone in your family ever had kidney or bladder stones?
(RATIONALE: Kidney and bladder calculi have a familial tendency.)

Has anyone in your family ever had hypertension, diabetes mellitus, gout, or coronary artery disease?
(RATIONALE: These disorders, which may have a familial tendency, can alter renal function.)

Adverse drug reactions

When obtaining a health history to assess a client's urinary system, the nurse must ask about current drug use. Many drugs affect urinary system function; some can cause permanent renal damage. For example, certain antiarrhythmics can lead to urinary retention; many aminoglycosides can cause acute tubular necrosis. The commonly used drugs listed below often cause adverse reactions affecting the urinary system.

DRUG CLASS	DRUG	POSSIBLE ADVERSE REACTIONS
Aminoglycosides	amikacin sulfate, gentamicin sulfate, kanamycin sulfate, streptomycin sulfate, tobramycin sulfate	Nephrotoxicity, acute tubular necrosis
Antiarrhythmics	disopyramide phosphate	Urinary retention, urinary hesitancy
Anticholinergics	parasympatholytics	Urinary retention, urinary hesitancy
Antidepressants	All tricyclic antidepressants	Urinary retention, urinary hesitancy, nocturia, urinary tract dilatation
	trazodone hydrochloride	Hematuria, urinary frequency, urinary hesitancy
Antihypertensives	captopril	Proteinuria, nephrotic syndrome
	enalapril maleate	Decreased renal function
Anti-inflammatory agents	All nonsteroidal anti-inflammatory agents	Hematuria, glomerular and interstitial nephritis, renal papillary necrosis, proteinuria, nephrotic necrosis, nephrotic syndrome
Antineoplastics	carmustine	Decreased kidney size, renal failure (with large cumulative doses after prolonged therapy)
	cisplatin	Nephrotoxicity
	cyclophosphamide	Hemorrhagic cystitis, bladder fibrosis, tubular necrosis, nephrotoxicity
	methotrexate sodium	Severe nephropathy, hematuria, renal failure
	mitomycin	Nephrotoxicity
	streptozocin	Nephrotoxicity
Diuretics	acetazolamide	Renal calculi, crystalluria, renal colic, renal tubular acidosis
	amiloride hydrochloride	Transient increase in blood urea nitrogen (BUN) or serum creatinine concentration, bladder spasms
	furosemide	Asymptomatic uricosuria, allergic interstitial nephritis, transient increase in BUN
	mannitol	Urinary retention, uricosuria
	thiazides	Asymptomatic hyperuricemia

Adverse drug reactions continued

DRUG CLASS	DRUG	POSSIBLE ADVERSE REACTIONS
Narcotic analgesics	meperidine hydrochloride, morphine sulfate	Urinary retention
Psychotherapeutic agents	Aliphatic and piperidine phenothiazines (chlorpromazine, promazine, triflupromazine, thioridazine, mesoridazine)	Urinary retention, urine discoloration
	lithium carbonate	Glycosuria, polyuria
Uricosurics	probenecid	Urinary frequency, hematuria, renal colic
Vitamins	vitamin C (ascorbic acid)	Oxalate or urate renal stones (with long-term therapy at excessive doses)
	vitamin D (cholecalciferol or ergocalciferol)	With excessive doses: polyuria, albuminuria, hypercalciuria, nocturia, impaired renal function, renal calculi, proteinuria
Miscellaneous agents	acyclovir sodium	Transient increase in BUN and serum creatinine concentration, decreased renal function
	amphotericin B	Nephrotoxicity, renal calculi
	gold sodium thiomalate	Nephritis, acute tubular necrosis, nephrotic syndrome, glomerulonephritis with hematuria and transient proteinuria
	pentamidine isethionate	Nephrotoxicity
	vancomycin hydrochloride	Nephrotoxicity
	phenazopyridine	Urine color change to red or orange

Developmental considerations

If the client is young, pregnant, or elderly, be sure to investigate developmental status by exploring the areas described below.

Pediatric client. When assessing a pediatric client, try to involve the child and the parent or guardian in the interview. Of course, with an infant, pose your questions to the parent or guardian. However, let any client who can speak participate in the interview, using age-appropriate words. To help perform a thorough urinary assessment of a pediatric client, ask the following questions (directed to the parent or guardian):

Does the child have a persistent diaper rash or excessive thirst?
(RATIONALE: Persistent diaper rash suggests a urine composition change, which may result from renal dysfunction; excessive thirst typically indicates that urine output exceeds fluid intake.)

Has the child experienced recent urinary changes, such as difficulty urinating or a urine stream change?
(RATIONALE: Difficulty urinating or a urine stream change suggests urinary obstruction.)

Does the child cry when urinating?
(RATIONALE: Crying during urination may indicate pain or a burning sensation, suggesting a lower urinary tract infection.)

If the child has not been toilet trained, how many diapers does the child wet each day? Has this number changed recently?
(RATIONALE: A change in the number of diapers wet daily may indicate a urine volume change. For example, urine volume may decrease with a fever and increased perspiration.)

Has the child's bladder control deteriorated recently?
(RATIONALE: Stress may cause a child's bladder control to regress. Enuresis [bed-wetting] results from an emotional disturbance, small bladder capacity, or a urinary tract infection.)

Did the child learn to sit, stand, and talk at the expected time?
(RATIONALE: In a child who learned to sit, stand, and talk at the expected time, delayed toilet training may indicate a urinary system dysfunction.)

Does the child have a specific routine when urinating, for example, always urinating after a meal or before bed?
(RATIONALE: Determining the child's routine and attempting to maintain it can help prevent urine retention or loss of bladder control in a strange environment, such as a hospital.)

Pregnant client. When assessing a pregnant client, be aware that pregnancy normally increases urine volume and frequency and decreases urine specific gravity. Also, stay alert for signs and symptoms of urinary tract infection—the most common urinary problem during pregnancy. To assess a pregnant client, ask the following questions:

Do you ever have pain during urination or in the kidney area? (Point out this area to the client.) *Have you ever been diagnosed with a urinary tract infection?*
(RATIONALE: Painful urination or pain in the kidney area may indicate a urinary tract infection—a common problem in the pregnant client because of her increased risk of urine retention and infection.)

Elderly client. When assessing an elderly client, keep in mind that bladder muscles weaken with age, possibly leading to incomplete bladder emptying and chronic urine retention. Consequently, the elderly client has an increased risk of urinary tract infection, nocturia (excessive urination at night), and incontinence. To assess for these potential problems, ask the following questions:

How much and what types of liquid do you drink in the evening?
(RATIONALE: A high fluid intake in the evening can exacerbate nocturia or incontinence. Intake of natural diuretics, such as tea, coffee, and beer, are especially likely to cause these problems.)

Do you ever lose control of your bladder? If so, does this occur suddenly or do you feel a warning, such as intense pressure?
(RATIONALE: Bladder muscle weakening commonly impairs bladder control in the elderly client. This problem can lead to more serious urinary dysfunction.)

Health promotion and protection patterns

To continue the health history, determine the client's personal habits, sleep and wake patterns, and typical daily activities. Ask the following questions to identify potential urinary system problems:

Do you follow a special diet?
(RATIONALE: A diet that alters sodium intake or reduces fluid intake can affect urine output.)

Do you limit your salt intake?
(RATIONALE: Salt contains sodium, which increases fluid retention and can decrease urine output.)

Does the need to urinate awaken you at night? If so, how often? Does this happen only when you drink large amounts of liquid in the evening?
(RATIONALE: Pathologic nocturia can result from bladder cancer, lower urinary tract infection, or renal disease, such as polycystic kidney disease or chronic interstitial nephritis. Nonpathologic nocturia can result from a high intake of fluids—especially coffee, tea, or beer—in the evening.)

What is your occupation?
(RATIONALE: Assembly-line workers, nurses, and others with limited on-the-job access to lavatory facilities may develop urinary stasis and subsequent infection. Other workers also have a high risk of urinary dysfunction. For example, jackhammer operators may develop renal ptosis [kidney drop] from operating drills with a constant pounding movement.)

How many times do you urinate daily? Have you noticed any change in frequency?
(RATIONALE: Voiding pattern changes can result from a local urinary disorder, such as a bladder infection, or a systemic disorder, such as diabetes mellitus.)

Have you noticed any increase or decrease in the amount of urine you void each time?
(RATIONALE: A urine volume change may result from renal dysfunction, a fluid intake change, or a systemic disorder, such as diabetes insipidus or diabetes mellitus.)

How many glasses of liquid do you drink daily?
(RATIONALE: A low fluid intake usually leads to a low urine output; a high intake, to a high output).

Role and relationship patterns

Urinary system disorders can influence many role and relationship patterns. To discover the extent of this influence, ask the client the following questions:

Can you carry out toileting independently?
(RATIONALE: Determining whether a client needs assistance with toileting can help you plan interventions that take this need into account. Such planning can reduce the risk of incontinence or urine retention.)

If you have urinary frequency or nocturia, does it affect any family members?
(RATIONALE: Frequent trips to the bathroom can disturb the sleep of a spouse or other family members, straining family relationships.)

Have you noticed any local tenderness when you cleanse yourself after voiding? Do you ever have pain during sexual intercourse?
(RATIONALE: Bladder or urethral infection may cause perineal inflammation, leading to tenderness and dyspareunia [painful intercourse]. This, in turn, may impede the client's sexual behavior.)

Significance of weight and vital sign changes

When assessing a client's general physical status, the nurse should stay alert for changes in body weight and vital signs, which may indicate certain urinary problems. The table below summarizes the most common weight and vital sign changes, along with their possible implications.

SIGN	CHANGE	POSSIBLE URINARY IMPLICATION
Weight	Increase	Chronic renal failure
	Decrease	Polycystic kidney disease, chronic renal failure
Blood pressure	Increase	Acute glomerulonephritis, chronic renal failure, polycystic kidney disease
Pulse	Increase	Acute glomerulonephritis, chronic renal failure, pain caused by renal disorder (such as nephrolithiasis)
Temperature	Increase	Renal colic, urinary tract infection
Respiratory rate	Increase	Acute glomerulonephritis, pain caused by renal disorder (such as nephrolithiasis)
	Cheyne-Stokes respirations	Chronic renal failure

Physical assessment

Before assessing the client's urinary system, the nurse must do the following: Gather the necessary equipment and evaluate various factors that may reflect renal function, including body weight, vital signs, and body position. Also evaluate the status of related body structures. (For additional information, see *Significance of weight and vital sign changes.*)

Preparing for urinary system assessment

To perform a thorough physical assessment of the urinary system, gather the following equipment: a stethoscope, a sphygmomanometer with inflatable cuff, a scale, a gown and drapes to cover the client, and a specimen cup to collect a urine sample.

Physical assessment of the urinary system involves the basic techniques of inspection, palpation, percussion, and auscultation. However, perform these techniques in the following sequence: inspection, auscultation, percussion, and palpation. Note that palpating and percussing before ausculating may increase bowel motility, in turn interfering with sound transmission during renal artery auscultation.

Before beginning the physical assessment, ask the client to urinate into the specimen cup. The specimen can be assessed for color, odor, and clarity. Also have the client undress so that you can expose body parts, as appropriate. Provide a gown and drapes to prevent unnecessary exposure.

Because assessment of the urethral meatus requires exposure of the genitals, the client may be fearful or embarrassed. To help minimize such discomfort, explain each assessment step beforehand and reassure the client that drapes will be used appropriately throughout the assessment.

Body weight, vital signs, and body position

Begin the physical assessment by weighing the client and comparing the result with a baseline figure, if available. Stay alert for a gain or loss of 2 to 3 lb (1 to 1.4 kg) within 48 hours. This reflects a change in fluid status, not body mass, possibly resulting from chronic renal failure.

To assess the fluid status of a hospitalized client, measure weight at the same time daily, using the same scale, with the client wearing the same amount of clothing. If you cannot maintain these constants, document the differences for each weigh-in. (With a client who is at home, teach weight measurement using the same procedure.)

Measure and compare fluid intake and output daily. Because of insensible fluid losses from the skin and lungs, output should equal only about two thirds of intake over 24 hours. Hourly output for an adult normally ranges from 30 to 100 ml (1 to 3.3 oz); 24-hour output, 720 to 2,400 ml (25 to 80 oz). When measuring output, be sure to consider fluid loss from diarrhea, vomiting, fever, or wound drainage.

Validate daily weights and intake and output records by comparing them against each other: 1 ml of water weighs 1 g; therefore, if fluid intake exceeds urine output by 1,000 ml in 24 hours, weight should increase by about 2 lb (1 kg). If urine output exceeds fluid intake, the negative fluid balance should produce weight loss. Report any output decrease accompanying a weight gain of more than 6½ lb (3 kg) in 24 hours.

Next, obtain vital signs. Measure blood pressure in both arms for comparison. Also, take blood pressure readings with the client lying down and sitting up. Blood pressure that drops more than 40 mm Hg when the client sits up may indicate fluid volume depletion. Sustained severe hypotension (systolic pressure below 70 mm Hg) results in diminished renal blood flow and may cause acute renal failure. Hypertension, defined as several serial readings over 140/90 mm Hg at rest, can lead to renal insufficiency. Hypertension may result from vascular damage caused by a primary renal disorder.

Other abnormal vital sign findings may suggest additional problems. Fever, for instance, may mean an acute urinary tract infection. Tachycardia with normal or slightly elevated blood pressure suggests fluid overload. Other pulse abnormalities, such as bradycardia or dysrhythmia, may indicate potassium imbalance. A severe electrolyte imbalance may alter respiratory rate and character. For example, Kussmaul's respirations suggest severe acidosis or right-sided heart failure secondary to renal insufficiency.

Next, observe the client's body position, noting any abnormalities. Inability to lie flat in bed, for instance, may indicate severe respiratory distress, as in acute pulmonary edema; this disorder, in turn, may accompany primary renal failure. Such a client may sit with arms extended to the front, perhaps resting them on the overbed table. Constant position changes, on the other hand, may reflect an attempt to relieve severe stabbing flank pain from renal colic.

Assessing related body structures

Because the urinary system affects many body functions, chronic renal disease can cause the client to appear seriously ill. For example, the client may have dry skin with a grayish yellow cast, peripheral edema (swelling from excess fluid settling in the extremities), periorbital edema (swelling around the eyes), and ascites (peritoneal fluid). The client may seem fatigued, dyspneic (short of breath), and somewhat disoriented.

The nurse will begin by observing the client's general appearance and behavior, then by assessing orientation to person, place, and time as well as memory of the immediate past. Renal dysfunction may cause poor concentration and loss of recent memory. Chronic, progressive renal failure can lead to toxin accumulation and electrolyte imbalance, producing such neurologic signs as lethargy, confusion, disorientation, stupor, somnolence, coma, and convulsions. The following are guidelines for the remaining portions of the assessment.

Eyes. Using an ophthalmoscope, examine the internal eye—especially if the client has malignant hypertension. (For detailed information on how to examine the internal

Evaluating pitting edema

When assessing a client's urinary system, the nurse will check for and evaluate edema—buildup of excess sodium and water within interstitial spaces. Edema may be pitting or nonpitting. Pitting edema reflects a systemic cause—possibly renal disease. It occurs most commonly in dependent body parts, such as the legs, sacrum, and scrotum.

To assess for pitting edema, apply finger pressure to the client's skin, then release it. A small depression (pit) that remains after you release your finger indicates pitting edema. With severe pitting edema, the depression can take more than 30 seconds to rebound.

Next, assess the severity of pitting edema by pressing a finger against the swollen area for 5 seconds, then removing it quickly. Evaluate and document the pit with a scale approved by the health care facility. If the facility uses the widely accepted four-point scale, use the following guidelines:

+1: a barely perceptible pit accompanied by normal foot and leg contours
+2: a deeper pit accompanied by fairly normal contours
+3: a deep pit accompanied by foot and leg swelling
+4: an even deeper pit accompanied by severe foot and leg swelling.

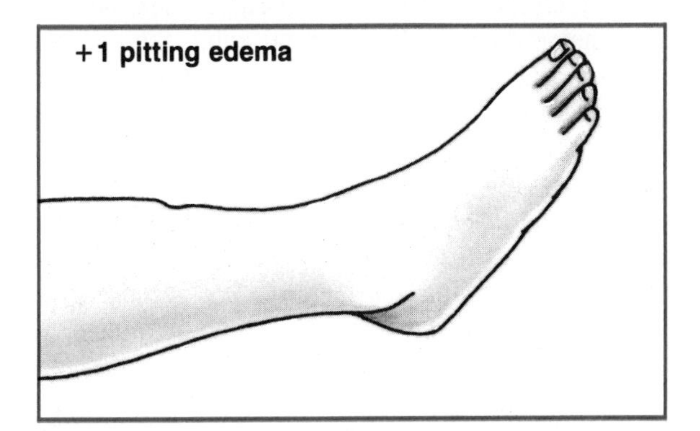
+1 pitting edema

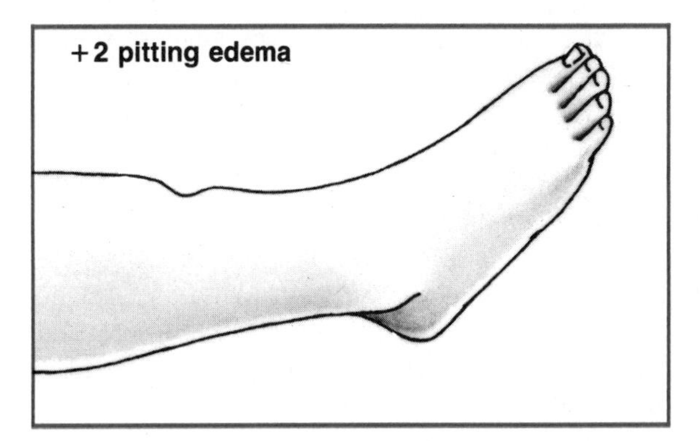
+2 pitting edema

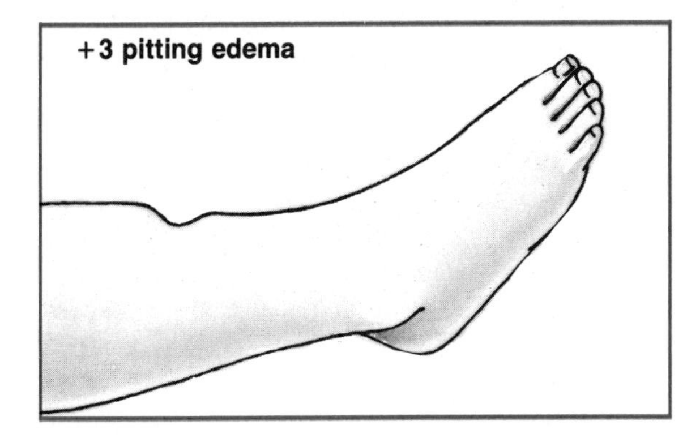
+3 pitting edema

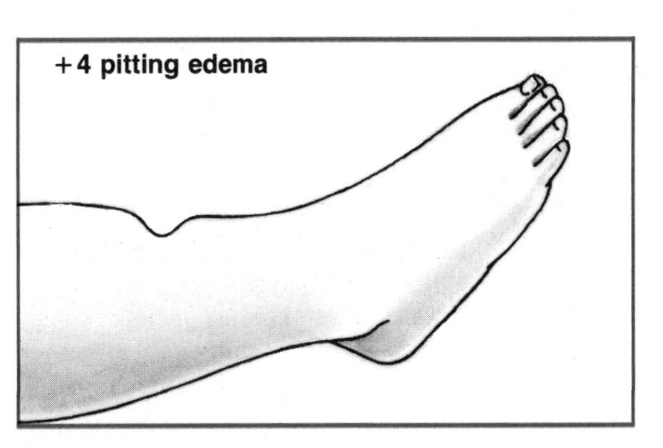
+4 pitting edema

eye, see Chapter 9, Eyes and Ears.) Various abnormal findings may indicate hypertension—a possible consequence or cause of renal disease. Check for thickened retinal arteriolar walls with small areas of infarction or hemorrhage, indicating damage to the intimal vascular layer of the retina; blurred disk margins, caused by papilledema (optic nerve head swelling); cotton-wool patches; and dilated, tortuous veins.

Skin, hair, and nails. Inspect the client's skin for a yellow-tan cast or pallor. Retention of urochrome pigment, which normally colors urine yellow, may cause a yellow-tan cast. Pallor typically stems from abnormally low hemoglobin concentration and hematocrit values, which gradually worsen as the kidneys fail. End-stage renal failure reduces erythropoietin production, leading to decreased RBC production. Also, uremic toxins shorten the RBC life span.

Inspect the client's skin for large ecchymoses (bruises) and petechiae (tiny purple or red spots)—characteristic signs of clotting abnormalities and decreased platelet adhesion that may reflect chronic renal failure. Observe for uremic frost—white or yellow urate crystals on the skin—indicating late-stage renal failure. Evaluate skin integrity by inspecting for cracks or tears. Because chronic renal disease impairs skin integrity and increases the risk of secondary infection, check for signs of secondary infection, such as reddened areas around cracks and tears or purulent drainage.

To assess the client's hydration status, inspect the mucous membranes in the mouth. Dryness reflects mild dehydration; parched, cracked lips with markedly dry mucous membranes and sunken eyes suggest severe dehydration. Inspect the skin for dryness and scratches; renal failure causes sweat and oil gland atrophy, resulting in subcutaneous calcium deposits. Chronic renal failure can lead to severe itching, which the client may try to ease by scratching hard.

Next, evaluate skin turgor by gently pinching the client's forearm skin with your thumb and index finger, then releasing it. (For details about this assessment technique, see Chapter 7, Skin, Hair, and Nails.) If the skin does not return to its normal position immediately, suspect advanced dehydration.

Inspect the client's neck veins for distention. (For a description of the technique, see Chapter 11, Cardiovascular System.) Also check for edema, abnormal buildup of excess sodium and water within the interstitial spaces. Sometimes accompanying renal disease, edema may be systemic or local; local edema may be pitting (an indentation that remains after pressing edematous skin with a finger) or nonpitting.

To check for signs of systemic nonpitting edema, inspect the eyelids for swelling or puffiness—signs of periorbital edema. Next, auscultate the lungs for bibasilar crackles, which may reflect pulmonary edema. Then inspect the abdomen for ascites (abnormal peritoneal fluid accumulation), and perform the fluid wave test. To assess for local edema, inspect the lowest (dependent) body portions (such as the ankles, sacrum, and scrotum) for swelling.

Determine if local edema is pitting or nonpitting by applying pressure with your fingertip. (For a description of this technique, see *Evaluating pitting edema,* page 399.) When accompanied by distended neck veins, pitting edema indicates fluid overload.

Inspection

Urinary system inspection includes examination of the abdomen and urethral meatus. Guidelines for this examination are described in the following paragraphs.

Abdomen

Help the client assume a supine position with arms relaxed at the sides. Make sure the client is comfortable and draped appropriately in this position. Then expose the abdomen from the xiphoid process to the symphysis pubis.

Inspect the abdomen for gross enlargements or fullness by comparing the left and right sides, noting any asymmetrical areas. In a normal adult, the abdomen is smooth, flat or scaphoid (concave), and symmetrical. Abdominal skin should be free of scars, lesions, bruises, and discolorations.

Abnormal abdominal inspection findings include gross enlargements or asymmetrical areas, suggesting a hernia, an enlarged liver, or an enlarged spleen. (For more on abdominal assessment findings, see Chapter 13, Gastrointestinal System.) Extremely prominent veins may accompany other vascular signs associated with renal dysfunction, for instance, elevated blood pressure and renal artery bruits. Such abnormalities as distention, skin tightness and glistening, and striae (streaks or linear scars caused by rapidly developing skin tension) may signal fluid retention. If ascites is suspected, perform the fluid wave test to confirm this condition. (For details on how to perform this test, see Chapter 13, Gastrointestinal System.) Ascites may suggest nephrotic syndrome, a condition characterized by increased urine protein levels, decreased serum albumin levels, and edema. Note and inquire about any surgical scars not mentioned in the client's history.

Urethral meatus

Help the client feel more at ease during your inspection by examining the urethral meatus last and by explaining beforehand how you will assess this area. Be sure to wear gloves. (For more information, see *Inspecting the urethral meatus.*)

Urethral meatus inspection may reveal several abnormalities. In a male client, a meatus deviating from the normal central location may represent a congenital defect. In any client, inflammation and discharge may signal urethral infection. Ulceration usually indicates a sexually transmitted disease.

Inspecting the urethral meatus

When inspecting the urethral meatus, the nurse will use the appropriate technique shown below.

Male urethral meatus
For a male client, drape him so that only the penis is exposed. Compress the tip of the glans penis with a gloved hand to open the urethral meatus, or ask the client to compress the glans himself. Normally, the meatus should be centrally located and show no discharge.

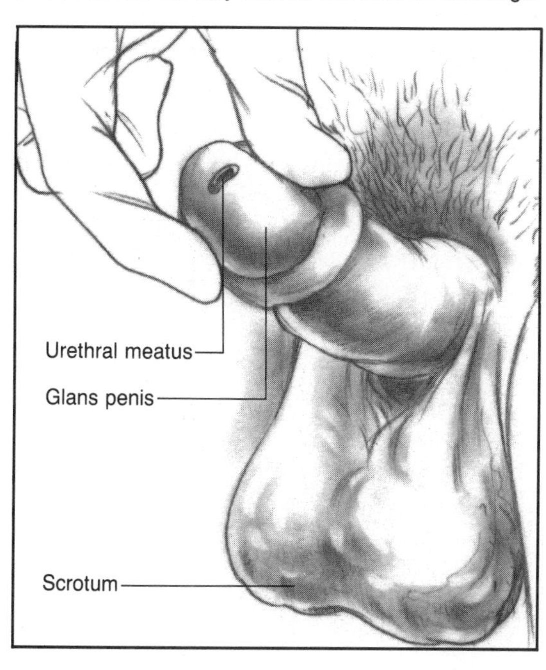

Female urethral meatus
For a female client, position her comfortably in the dorsal lithotomy position and drape her appropriately. Then spread her labia with a gloved hand and look for the urethral meatus, an irregular opening or slit normally located midline, superior to the vagina. Normally, the meatus is pink and free of swelling or discharge.

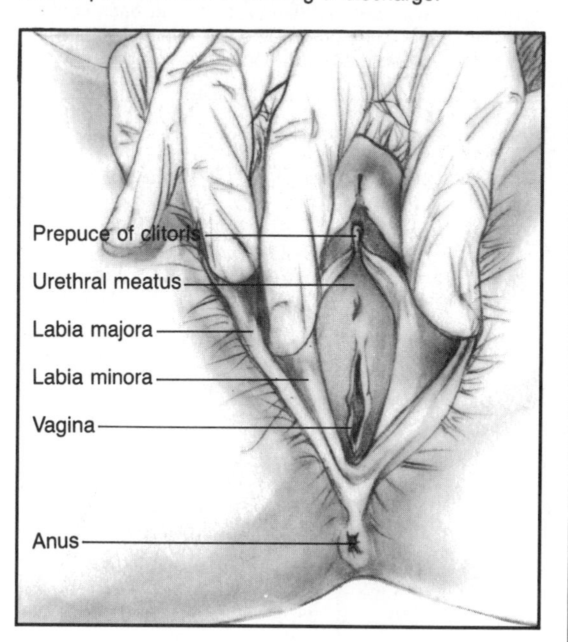

Auscultation

Auscultate the renal arteries in the left and right upper abdominal quadrants by pressing the stethoscope bell lightly against the abdomen and instructing the client to exhale deeply. Begin auscultating at the midline and work to the left. Then return to the midline and work to the right. Normally, systolic bruits (whooshing sounds) or other unusual sounds will not be heard. (For information about auscultating other abdominal areas, see Chapter 13, Gastrointestinal System.)

Abnormal auscultation findings include systolic bruits; in a client with hypertension, such bruits suggest renal artery stenosis.

Percussion

After auscultating the renal arteries, percuss the client's kidneys to detect any tenderness or pain, and percuss the bladder to evaluate its position and contents. (For more information, see *Percussing the urinary organs,* page 402.)

Abnormal kidney percussion findings include tenderness and pain, suggesting glomerulonephritis or glomerulonephrosis.

A dull sound heard on percussion in a client who has just urinated may indicate urine retention, reflecting bladder dysfunction or infection.

Percussing the urinary organs

In the urinary system, the nurse can percuss the kidneys and bladder using these techniques.

Kidney percussion
With the client sitting upright, percuss each costovertebral angle (the angle over each kidney whose borders are formed by the lateral and downward curve of the lowest rib and the spinal column). To perform mediate percussion, place your left palm over the costovertebral angle, and gently strike it with your right fist. To perform blunt percussion, gently strike your fist over each costovertebral angle. The normal client will feel a thudding sensation or pressure during percussion.

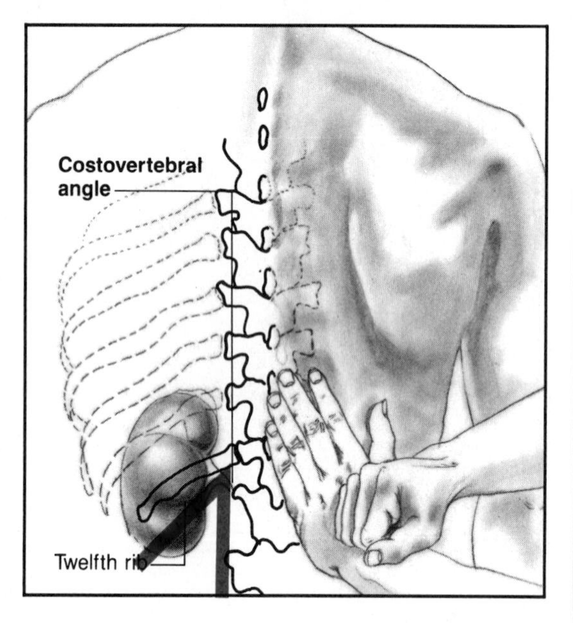

Bladder percussion
Next, using mediate percussion, percuss the area over the bladder, beginning 2" (5 cm) above the symphysis pubis. To detect differences in sound, percuss toward the base of the bladder. Percussion normally produces a tympanic sound. (Over a urine-filled bladder, it produces a dull sound.)

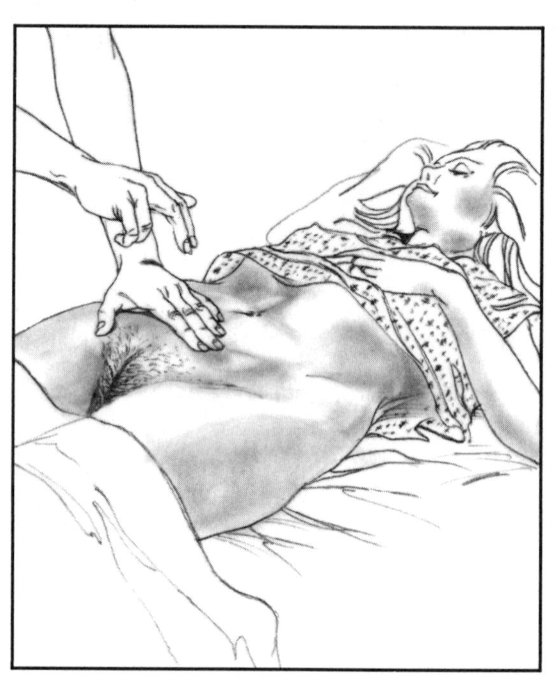

Palpation

Palpation of the kidneys and bladder is the next step in the physical assessment. Through palpation, the nurse can detect any lumps, masses, or tenderness. Optimum results are achieved by having the client relax the abdomen by taking deep breaths through the mouth. (For more information, see *Palpating the urinary organs.* For an advanced technique, see *Advanced assessment skills: Kidney palpation,* page 405.)

Abnormal kidney palpation findings may signify various problems. A lump, a mass, or tenderness may indicate a tumor or cyst. A soft kidney may reflect chronic renal disease; a tender kidney, acute infection. Unequal kidney size may reflect hydronephrosis, a cyst, a tumor, or another disorder. Bilateral enlargement suggests polycystic disease.

Abnormal bladder palpation findings include a lump or a mass, possibly signaling a tumor or a cyst, or tenderness, which may stem from infection. (For some common abnormal assessment findings associated with the urinary system, see *Integrating assessment findings,* page 404.)

Developmental considerations

Before physically assessing an infant or a child, note the ear position. In many cases, ears that are set low or at an unusual angle accompany urinary tract anomalies.

Palpating the urinary organs

In the normal adult, the kidneys usually cannot be palpated because of their location deep within the abdomen. However, they may be palpable in a thin client or in one with reduced abdominal muscle mass. (Because the right kidney is slightly lower than the left, it may be easier to palpate.) Keep in mind that both kidneys descend with deep inhalation.

If palpable, the bladder normally feels firm and relatively smooth. However, keep in mind that an adult's bladder may not be palpable.

Using bimanual palpation, the nurse should begin on the client's right side and proceed as follows:

Kidney palpation

Help the client to a supine position, and expose the abdomen from the xiphoid process to the symphysis pubis. Standing at the client's right side, place your left hand under the back, midway between the lower costal margin and the iliac crest. (See Step 1.)

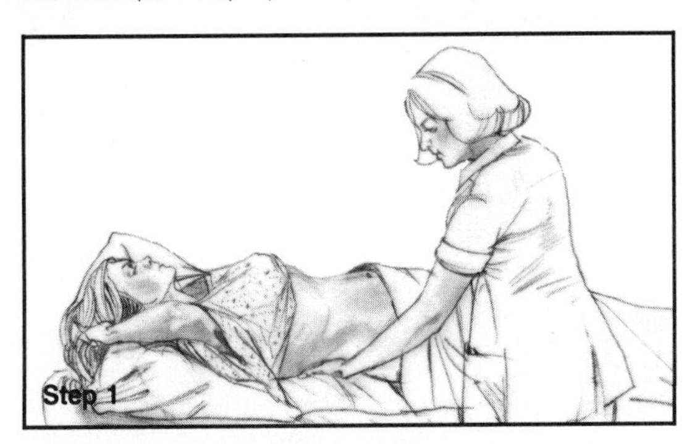
Step 1

Next, place your right hand on the client's abdomen, directly above your left hand. Angle this hand slightly toward the costal margin. To palpate the right lower edge of the right kidney, press your right fingertips about 1½″ (4 cm) above the right iliac crest at the midinguinal line; press your left fingertips upward into the right costovertebral angle. (See Step 2.)

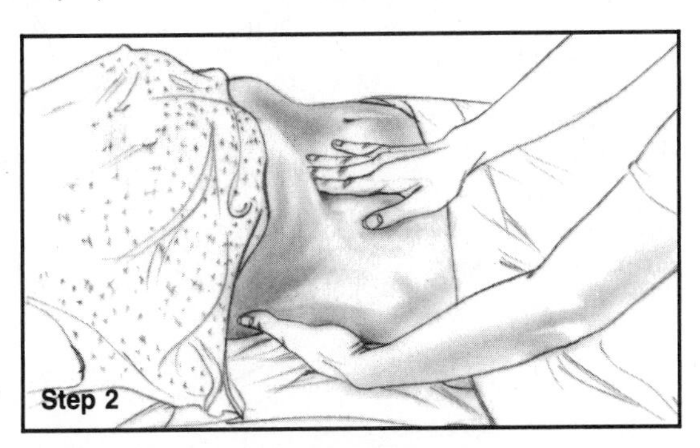
Step 2

Instruct the client to inhale deeply so that the lower portion of the right kidney can move down between your hands. (See Step 3.) If it does, note the shape and size of the kidney. Normally, it feels smooth, solid, and firm, yet elastic. Ask the client if palpation causes tenderness. (*Note:* Avoid using excessive pressure to palpate the kidney because this may cause intense pain.)

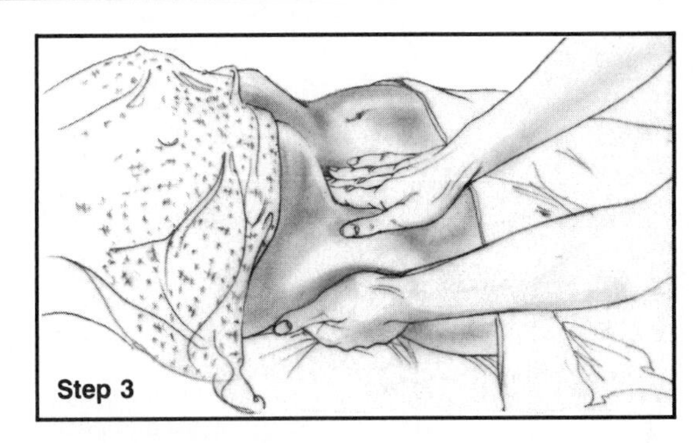
Step 3

To assess the left kidney, move to the client's left side and position hands as described above, but with this change: place your right hand 2″ (5 cm) above the left iliac crest. Then apply pressure with both hands as the client inhales. If the left kidney can be palpated, compare it to the right kidney; it should be the same size.

Bladder palpation

Before palpating the bladder, make sure the client has voided. Then locate the edge of the bladder by pressing deeply in the midline about 1″ to 2″ (2.5 to 5 cm) above the symphysis pubis. As the bladder is palpated, note its size and location and check for lumps, masses, and tenderness. The bladder normally feels firm and relatively smooth. (Keep in mind that an adult's bladder may not be palpable.) During deep palpation, the client may report the urge to urinate—a normal response.

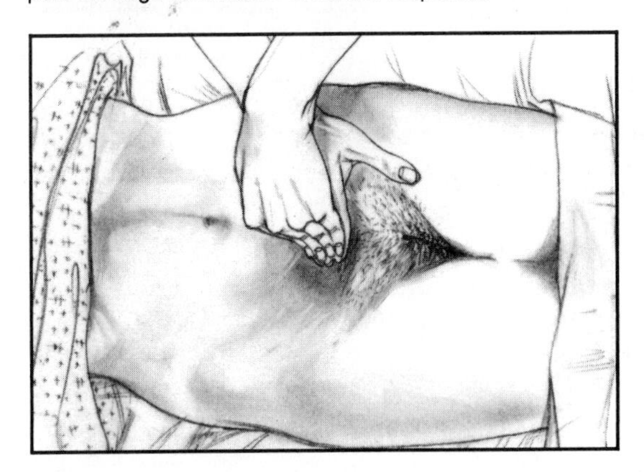

Integrating assessment findings

Sometimes, a cluster of assessment findings will strongly suggest a particular urinary system disorder. In the chart below, column one shows groups of presenting signs and symptoms—the ones that make the client seek medical attention. Column two shows related assessment findings that the nurse may discover during the health history and physical assessment. The client may exhibit one or more of these findings. Column three shows the possible disorder indicated by a cluster of these findings.

PRESENTING SIGNS AND SYMPTOMS	RELATED ASSESSMENT FINDINGS	POSSIBLE DISORDER
Oliguria possibly progressing to anuria; hematuria or smoky or coffee-colored urine	Poststreptococcal throat or skin infection Systemic lupus erythematosus Pregnancy Vasculitis Scleroderma Elevated blood pressure Periorbital edema progressing to dependent edema Ascites Pleural effusion	Acute glomerulonephritis
Oliguria; dark, smoky-colored urine; anorexia; vomiting	Crush injury or illness associated with shock (such as burn or trauma) Muscle necrosis Exposure to nephrotoxic agent (such as lead) I.V. pyelography using dye injection Recent aminoglycoside therapy Oliguria progressing to anuria Dyspnea Bibasilar crackles Dependent edema	Acute tubular necrosis
Proteinuria; hematuria; vomiting; pruritus (Client may be asymptomatic until advanced disease stage.)	Primary renal disorder (such as membranoproliferative glomerulonephritis or focal glomerulosclerosis) Elevated blood pressure Ascites Dyspnea Bibasilar crackles Dependent edema	Chronic glomerulonephritis
Urinary frequency; urinary urgency; burning sensation on urination; nocturia; cloudy hematuria; dysuria; low back or flank pain	Recurrent urinary tract infection Recent chemotherapy or systemic antibiotic therapy Recent vigorous sexual activity Female client Suprapubic pain on palpation Fever Inflamed perineal area	Cystitis
Severe radiating pain from costovertebral angle to flank, suprapubic region, and external genitalia; nausea and vomiting; hematuria	Strenuous physical activity in hot environment Previous renal calculi Recent kidney infection Fever and chills Poor skin turgor Concentrated urine Dry mucous membranes	Nephrolithiasis
Abdominal or flank pain; gross hematuria	Youth (especially under age 7) Congenital anomalies Firm, smooth, palpable abdominal mass in enlarged abdomen Fever Elevated blood pressure Urine retention	Wilms' tumor

ADVANCED ASSESSMENT SKILLS

Kidney palpation

The nurse can use the advanced palpation technique known as *capturing the kidney,* if the lower edge of the kidney cannot be palpated. This technique resembles—but usually proves more successful than—bimanual palpation.

1 To capture the right kidney, position your hands as for bimanual palpation. Place your left hand under the client, midway between the lower costal margin and the iliac crest. Then, place your right hand on the abdomen, directly above your left hand. Angle the right hand slightly toward the costal margin. Then instruct the client to inhale deeply. At the peak of inhalation, quickly press your hands together to capture the kidney. If the kidney can be palpated, note its contour and size and check for lumps, masses, and tenderness.

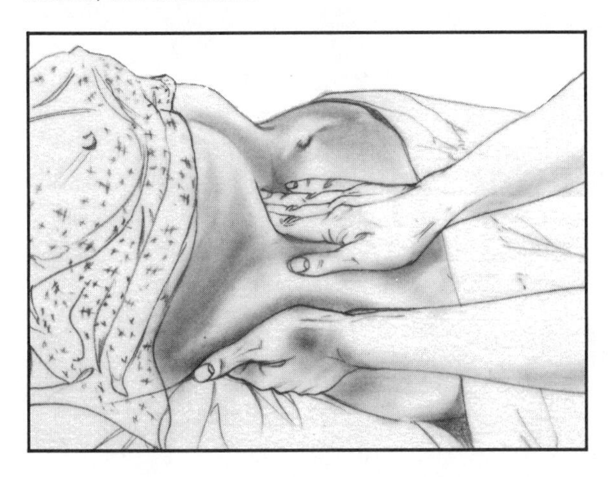

2 Now, ask the client to exhale slowly as you release your hands. If the kidney was captured, it will slide back into place. To capture the left kidney, repeat this technique on the client's left side.

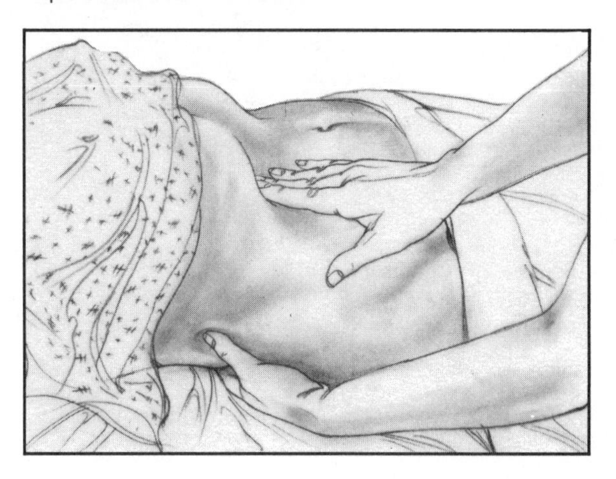

Throughout the abdominal assessment, the client's abdominal muscles must be relaxed. To promote relaxation, the parent can hold the child. If necessary, give an infant a bottle to prevent crying, which tenses the abdominal muscles.

After the child has been undressed to the diaper, ask the parent to help the child to a standing position so that you can observe the abdominal contour. The normal infant or child has a rounded or pot-bellied abdomen without masses. *Important:* If an upper abdominal mass is present, *do not* physically assess it further. If the mass is a nephroblastoma (Wilms' tumor), palpation could increase tumor cell spread.

The bladder of an infant or a child up to age 2 usually can be palpated and percussed to the umbilical level. (The superior margin of the bladder drops until adolescence, when it reaches the symphysis pubis level.)

In an elderly client, the kidneys are easier to palpate because of reduced abdominal muscle tone and mass. However, reduced muscle tone can prevent the bladder from emptying completely, resulting in up to 100 ml of residual urine. This client also may have little warning of the voiding urge. Along with residual urine, this can lead to incontinence during the assessment.

Documentation

Before beginning documentation, determine what the assessment findings may indicate; review and integrate the data collected about the client's urinary system, related body structures, weight, vital signs, and body position; and review the health history findings.

(Text continues on page 409.)

Common laboratory studies

For a client with urinary signs and symptoms, various laboratory studies can provide valuable clues to the possible cause, as shown in the chart below. (*Note:* Keep in mind that abnormal findings may stem from a problem unrelated to the urinary system.) Remember that values differ between laboratories, and check the normal value range for the specific laboratory.

TEST AND SIGNIFICANCE	NORMAL VALUES OR FINDINGS	ABNORMAL FINDINGS	POSSIBLE URINARY OR RELATED CAUSES OF ABNORMAL FINDINGS
Blood tests			
Albumin This protein normally remains in the plasma and does not pass through the glomerular membrane. With renal disease, however, it passes into the glomerular filtrate, leading to a below-normal blood level.	3.3 to 4.5 g/dl	Below-normal level	Nephrotic syndrome, nephritis, nephrosis, malnutrition, hypogammaglobulinemia
Total protein This test reflects the sum of albumin and globulin fractions in the serum.	6.6 to 7.9 g/dl	Above-normal level	Dehydration, vomiting, diarrhea, diabetic acidosis
		Below-normal level	Nephrosis
Blood urea nitrogen (BUN) This test reflects protein intake and renal excretory capacity and helps identify uremia (but less sensitively than the serum creatinine level).	8 to 20 mg/dl	Above-normal level	Renal disease, reduced renal blood flow, urinary tract obstruction
Creatinine This test provides a more sensitive measure of renal damage than BUN levels because renal impairment is usually the only cause of creatinine elevation.	*Males:* 0.8 to 1.2 mg/dl *Females:* 0.6 to 0.9 mg/dl	Above-normal level	Renal disease causing serious damage to at least half the nephrons in the kidneys
Electrolytes These tests provide a quantitive analysis of major extracellular electrolytes (sodium, calcium, chloride, and bicarbonate) and major intracellular electrolytes (potassium, magnesium, and phosphate).	*Sodium* 135 to 145 mEq/liter	Above-normal level	Inadequate water intake, water loss exceeding sodium loss (as in diabetes insipidus, impaired renal function, and prolonged hyperventilation), sodium retention (as in aldosteronism), excess sodium intake
	Potassium 3.8 to 5.5 mEq/liter	Above-normal level	Crush injury, reduced sodium excretion (possibly from renal failure)
		Below-normal level	Aldosteronism, body fluid loss, polyuria, diuretic therapy
	Chloride 100 to 108 mEq/liter	Above-normal level	Severe dehydration, acute tubular necrosis, renal failure, primary aldosteronism, metabolic acidosis
		Below-normal level	Chronic renal failure
	Calcium 4.5 to 5.5 mEq/liter	Above-normal level	Renal disease, parathyroid disorder
		Below-normal level	Renal failure, activated vitamin D insufficiency, parathyroid disorder
	Phosphate 1.8 to 2.6 mEq/liter	Above-normal level	Decreased tubular secretion

Common laboratory studies *continued*

TEST AND SIGNIFICANCE	NORMAL VALUES OR FINDINGS	ABNORMAL FINDINGS	POSSIBLE URINARY OR RELATED CAUSES OF ABNORMAL FINDINGS
Electrolytes (continued)	*Magnesium* 1.5 to 2.5 mEq/liter	Above-normal level	Renal failure, adrenal insufficiency
		Below-normal level	Primary aldosteronism, diuretic therapy
Osmolality Intracellular and extracellular osmolality are normally equal and reflect overall hydration and body fluid concentration.	280 to 295 mOsm/kg of water	Above-normal level	Dehydration, kidney dysfunction
		Below-normal level	Kidney dysfunction
Uric acid A purine metabolite, uric acid clears the body via glomerular filtration and tubular secretion.	*Males:* 4.3 to 8 mg/dl *Females:* 2.3 to 6 mg/dl	Above-normal level	Gout, impaired renal function
		Below-normal level	Defective tubular absorption
Urine tests			
Urinalysis This common screening test can indicate urinary or systemic disorders. Performed on a urine specimen of at least 5 ml, it may suggest absence of major disease (normal findings) or possible disease warranting further investigation (abnormal findings).	Straw color	Clear to black	Dietary changes; use of certain drugs; metabolic, inflammatory, or infectious disease
	Slightly aromatic odor	Fruity odor	Diabetes mellitus, starvation, dehydration
	Clear appearance	Turbid appearance	Renal infection
	Specific gravity between 1.005 and 1.020, with slight variations from one specimen to the next	Below-normal specific gravity	Diabetes insipidus, glomerulonephritis, pyelonephritis, acute renal failure, alkalosis
		Above-normal specific gravity	Dehydration, nephrosis
		Fixed specific gravity	Severe renal damage
	pH between 4.5 and 8.0	Alkaline pH (above 8.0)	Fanconi's syndrome (chronic renal disease), urinary tract infection, metabolic or respiratory alkalosis
		Acidic pH (below 4.5)	Renal tuberculosis, phenylketonuria, acidosis
	No protein	Proteinuria	Renal disease (such as glomerulosclerosis, acute or chronic glomerulonephritis, nephrolithiasis, polycystic kidney disease, acute or chronic renal failure)
	No ketones	Ketonuria	Diabetes mellitus, starvation, conditions causing acutely increased metabolic demands and decreased food intake (such as vomiting and diarrhea)
	No sugars	Glycosuria	Diabetes mellitus
		Fructosuria	Rare hereditary metabolic disorder, excess fructose ingestion
		Galactosuria	Rare hereditary metabolic disorder
		Pentosuria	Rare hereditary metabolic disorder, excess pentose ingestion

continued

Common laboratory studies *continued*

TEST AND SIGNIFICANCE	NORMAL VALUES OR FINDINGS	ABNORMAL FINDINGS	POSSIBLE URINARY OR RELATED CAUSES OF ABNORMAL FINDINGS
Urinalysis (continued)		Pentosuria	Rare hereditary metabolic disorder, excess pentose ingestion
	0 to 3 red blood cells (RBCs)/high-power field	Numerous RBCs	Urinary infection, obstruction, inflammation, trauma, or tumor; glomerulonephritis; renal hypertension; lupus nephritis; renal tuberculosis; renal vein thrombosis; hydronephrosis; pyelonephritis; parasitic bladder infection; polyarteritis nodosa; hemorrhagic disorder
	0 to 4 white blood cells (WBCs)/high-power field	Numerous WBCs	Urinary tract inflammation, especially cystitis or pyelonephritis
		Numerous WBCs and WBC casts	Renal infection (such as acute pyelonephritis and glomerulonephritis, nephrotic syndrome, pyogenic infection, and lupus nephritis)
	Few epithelial cells	Excessive epithelial cells	Renal tubular degeneration
	No casts (except occasional hyaline casts)	Excessive casts	Renal disease
		Excessive hyaline casts	Renal parenchymal disease, inflammation, glomerular capillary membrane trauma
		Epithelial casts	Renal tubular damage, nephrosis, eclampsia, chronic lead intoxication
		Fatty, waxy casts	Nephrotic syndrome, chronic renal disease, diabetes mellitus
		RBC casts	Renal parenchymal disease (especially glomerulonephritis), renal infarction, subacute bacterial endocarditis, vascular disorders, sickle cell anemia, scurvy, blood dyscrasias, malignant hypertension, collagen disease, acute inflammation
	Some crystals	Numerous calcium oxalate crystals	Hypercalcemia
		Cystine crystals (cystinuria)	Inborn metabolic error
	No yeast cells	Yeast cells in sediment	Genitourinary tract infection, external genitalia contamination, vaginitis, urethritis, prostatovesiculitis
	No parasites	Parasites in sediment	Genitourinary tract infection, external genitalia contamination

As the last step in the urinary system assessment, evaluate results of the client's diagnostic and laboratory studies. (For a summary of frequently used laboratory studies and their significance, see *Common laboratory studies.)* Reviewed along with history and physical findings, these results can provide a clear picture of the client's clinical status.

Considering assessment data is the first step in the nursing process. Based on these data, you should be able to formulate appropriate nursing diagnoses, and then plan, implement, and evaluate the client's nursing care. (For a case study that shows how to apply the nursing process to a client with a urinary disorder, see *Applying the nursing process,* pages 410 and 411.)

Documentation of data, including normal and abnormal findings, is the next step. The following example shows how to document some normal physical assessment findings:

> *Weight:* 157 lb
> *Vital signs:* Temperature 98.6° F., Pulse 72 and regular, Respirations 18 and regular, Blood pressure 130/70.
> Oriented to person, place, and time. Ophthalmoscopic examination normal. Skin color and integrity normal. No bruises, purpura, or uremic frost on skin. Abdomen flat with no visible hernias, prominent veins, pulsations, or lesions. Urethral meatus centrally located on glans penis and with no visible discharge. No bruits over renal arteries. Bladder percussion reveals tympanic sound. No costovertebral pain or tenderness. Left kidney not palpable; right kidney palpable, smooth, firm, and nontender.

The following example shows how to document some abnormal physical assessment findings:

> *Weight:* 270 lb
> *Vital signs:* Temperature 99.8° F., Pulse 96 and regular, Respirations 28 and regular, Blood pressure 184/106.
> Disoriented to person, place, and time. Ophthalmoscopic examination: disk margin blurred; retinal hemorrhages visible; arteries narrow and tortuous with vein compression. Skin color: pallor, multiple large bruises noted over extremities and trunk. Dry oral mucous membranes. Abdomen round with visible pulsations. Urethral meatus centrally located on glans penis with yellowish discharge present. Bruits auscultated over renal arteries. Bladder percussion reveals dull sound. Blunt percussion over kidneys elicits pain. Left costovertebral tenderness present. Bladder feels distended on palpation. Right kidney feels enlarged on palpation.

Be sure to document the other nursing process steps—nursing diagnosis, planning, implementation, and evaluation—as they are applied to the client with a urinary system disorder.

Chapter summary

To assess the client's urinary system effectively, the nurse must rely on health history data, physical assessment findings, and laboratory results. Chapter 14 describes how to gather and integrate this information. Here are the main points:

- Urinary system structures include the kidneys, ureters, bladder, and urethra.
- The nephron—the basic functional unit of the kidney—regulates fluid and electrolyte balance via glomerular filtration, tubular reabsorption, and tubular secretion. It also rids the body of waste products by excreting urine.
- Important urine characteristics include pH (which normally ranges from 4.5 to 8.0); specific gravity (which normally ranges from 1.008 to 1.030); and urine volume (which normally ranges from 720 to 2,400 ml per 24 hours).
- When obtaining the health history, establish a comfortable interview environment and use terms familiar to the client. Because urinary complaints may result from or cause problems in other body systems, the nurse should maintain a holistic approach by investigating complaints associated with related body structures.
- When obtaining the health history, explore the client's medication use. Such information may reveal whether the client is receiving treatment for a urinary dysfunction or suggest that an adverse drug reaction may have caused the dysfunction.
- When physically assessing the client's urinary system, measure weight and obtain vital signs besides using the standard techniques of inspection, palpation, percussion, and auscultation. Because signs of urinary dysfunction

Applying the nursing process

Assessment findings form the basis of the nursing process. Using them, the nurse formulates nursing diagnoses and develops appropriate planning, implementation, and evaluation of the client's care.

The table below shows how the nurse can use urinary system assessment data in the nursing process for the client described in the case history (shown at right). In the first column, history and physical assessment data are followed by a paragraph of mental notes. These notes help the nurse make important mental connections among assessment findings, aiding in development of the nursing diagnoses and planning.

The second column presents several appropriate nursing diagnoses; however, the information in the remaining three columns is based on the *first* nursing diagnosis. Although it is not part of the nursing process, documentation appears in the last column because of its importance. Documentation consists of an initial note using all components of the SOAPIE format and a follow-up note using the appropriate SOAPIE components.

ASSESSMENT	NURSING DIAGNOSES	PLANNING	IMPLEMENTATION
Subjective (history) data • Client states, "I have a burning sensation when I urinate. I go to the bathroom a lot and feel pressure each time." • Client reports that she had a urinary tract infection 2 weeks ago and has had five such infections in the past year. She asks why this keeps happening. • Client says she stopped taking the prescribed antibiotic because she felt better after several days. • Client states that she feels "cramping pain." **Objective (physical) data** • Vital signs: temperature 99° F. (37.2° C.), pulse 75 and regular, respirations 18 and regular, blood pressure 120/80. • Palpation causes abdominal and suprapubic pain. • Voided urine specimen appears cloudy and smells foul. • White blood cell (WBC) count 12,000/μl. • Urine culture is positive for *Escherichia coli.* **Mental notes** *Considered along with assessment and laboratory findings, the client's complaints suggest an inadequately treated urinary tract infection. Antibiotics usually prove effective against such infections; however, they must be taken for the prescribed period. Recurrent infection probably results from the client's lack of knowledge about personal hygiene and her subsequent noncompliance with the medication regimen. Improper personal hygiene easily can transfer normal intestinal flora, such as* E. coli, *to the urinary tract, where they cause infection.*	• Knowledge deficit related to lack of information about personal hygiene. • Alteration in urinary elimination patterns related to renal manifestations (urinary frequency and urgency). • Noncompliance with prescribed medication regimen for urinary tract infection related to a misunderstanding of the importance of completion of the regimen. • Alteration in comfort, pain related to infection and inflammation.	**Goals** Before leaving the clinic today, the client will: • verbalize the importance of proper personal hygiene • demonstrate proper personal hygiene technique on a doll. At the next followup visit, the client will: • state how improper hygiene can lead to a urinary tract infection • describe proper hygiene practices.	• Instruct the client to shower or bathe daily with an antibacterial soap to decrease the infection risk. • Instruct the client to avoid tub baths, especially bubble baths. Still water (as in tub baths) commonly serves as a bacterial medium; bubble baths can irritate the inflamed perineal area. • Using an anatomic model or doll, demonstrate how to clean the perineal area from front to back after bowel elimination to prevent bacterial transfer. • Advise the client to wear cotton underpants or underpants with a cotton crotch. Bacteria multiply best in a dark, moist environment; cotton underpants allow moisture to evaporate.

may manifest in other body systems, inspect related body structures (for example, the eyes, skin, hair, and nails).

• During inspection, examine the abdomen to detect any asymmetrical areas; hernias; veins; lesions; discolorations; bruises; scars; or signs of fluid retention, such as umbilical protrusion. Also inspect the client's urethral meatus for position, irritation, and discharge.

• Physical assessment should include auscultation of renal arteries in the upper abdominal quadrants, with particular attention to any systolic bruits.

• Percussion over the costovertebral angle may reveal kidney pain or tenderness; percussion over the bladder helps determine bladder size and fullness.

CASE HISTORY

Ms. Susan Hudson, age 24, is a single Caucasian female who works as a legal secretary. She visits the clinic for relief of a burning sensation during urination, urinary frequency, and urinary urgency.

EVALUATION	DOCUMENTATION BASED ON NURSING PROCESS DATA			
		Initial		**Follow-up**
At the next follow-up visit, the client: • correctly stated the relationship between personal hygiene and urinary tract infection. • accurately described the hygiene practices that she learned during the initial visit.	**S**	Client states, "I have a burning sensation when I urinate. I go to the bathroom a lot and feel pressure each time. I had a urinary tract infection 2 weeks ago with similar symptoms." Client states that she stopped taking the prescribed antibiotic after several days because she felt better. (She cannot remember the drug name or the dose but states that she took it four times a day.) She reports that this is the fifth time in the last year that the problem has occurred.	**S**	Client states, "I've finished all of the antibiotics the doctor prescribed, and I have not had any burning sensation when I urinate. I've been using the techniques you taught me." Client also reports no urinary frequency or urgency.
			O	No abdominal or suprapubic tenderness elicited on palpation. Urine appears clear.
			A	Repeat urine culture is negative. Repeat WBC count is 5,000/μl.
	O	Temperature 99° F., pulse 75 regular, respirations 18 regular, blood pressure 120/80. Abdominal and suprapubic tenderness elicited on palpation. Urine appears cloudy and smells foul. No hematuria noted.	**P**	Client complied with medication regimen and personal hygiene instructions. Physical assessment and laboratory data within normal limits.
			I	Discharge client to self-care.
	A	Knowledge deficit related to lack of information about personal hygiene.		
	P	Teach client about proper personal hygiene.		
	I	Instructed client about personal hygiene techniques that reduce the risk of urinary tract infection. Gave client a printed booklet to take home on proper feminine hygiene.		
	E	Demonstrated how to clean the perineal area on a doll, and client correctly returned the demonstration.		

• Try to palpate the client's kidneys and bladder, even though these organs usually cannot be palpated. When palpable, they normally feel smooth and firm with no lumps, masses, or tenderness.

• To complete the urinary system assessment, review the results of any laboratory studies ordered to assess renal function. Commonly ordered tests include routine urinalysis; creatinine clearance; serum electrolyte levels; and total protein, albumin, BUN, creatinine, and uric acid levels.

• Finally, document all assessment findings and use them in the nursing process to plan, implement, and evaluate the client's care.

Study questions

1. The nephron is the functional unit of the kidney. What are the structural components of the nephron and its three main activities?

2. Emily Augello, age 75, comes to the outpatient clinic complaining of pain and burning on urination, a fever of 100° F., and pain in the right kidney area. How would you document the following information related to your nursing assessment of Mrs. Augello?
- history (subjective) assessment data
- physical (objective) assessment data
- assessment techniques and special equipment used
- two appropriate nursing diagnoses
- documentation of your findings.

3. When Mrs. Augello leaves the outpatient clinic with a diagnosis of urinary tract infection, what instructions should you give her?

4. A client complains of nausea and sudden onset of severe abdominal pain and left-sided pain. The client states, "This pain is awful. My father always said the worst pain he suffered was when he passed a kidney stone." In your nursing assessment of this client, which critical areas should you focus on?

5. During your initial interview, a new client informs you that he has been taking furosemide (Lasix) for the past several months. Knowing this, what specific areas of the nursing assessment should you consider critical? What are the actions and possible adverse effects of furosemide?

Selected references

Alspach, J., and Williams, S. (1991). *Core Curriculum for Critical Care Nursing: AACN* (4th ed.). Philadelphia: Saunders.

Anthony, C., and Thibodeau, G. (1987). *Textbook of anatomy and physiology* (12th ed.). St. Louis: Mosby-Year Book.

Assessing Your Patients. (1984). Nursing Photobook Series. Springhouse, PA: Springhouse Corp.

Bowers, A., and Thompson, J. (1992). *Clinical manual of health assessment* (4th ed.). St. Louis: Mosby-Year Book.

Carnevali, D., and Patrick, M. (1986). *Nursing management for the elderly* (2nd ed.). Philadelphia: Lippincott.

Guyton, A. (1991). *Textbook of medical physiology* (8th ed.). Philadelphia: Saunders.

Henry, J. (1991). *Clinical diagnosis and management by laboratory methods* (18th ed.). Philadelphia: Saunders.

Holloway, N. (1988). *Nursing the critically ill patient* (3rd ed.). Redwood City, CA: Addison-Wesley.

McGuire, E. (1985). Clinical evaluation of the female lower urinary tract. *Urologic Clinics of North America,* 12(2), 225-229.

McEvoy, G. (Ed.). (1992). *American Hospital Formulary Service drug information.* Bethesda, MD: American Society of Hospital Pharmacists.

Richard, C. (1986). *Comprehensive nephrology nursing.* Boston: Little, Brown.

Tanago, E., and McAninch, J. (1991). *Smith's general urology* (13th ed.). East Norwalk, CT: Appleton & Lange.

Walsh, P., Stamey, T., and Vaughan, J. (1992). *Campbell's urology* (Vol. 1., 6th ed.). Philadelphia: Saunders.

Nursing research

Brown, S. (1990). Quantitative measurement of anxiety in patients undergoing surgery for renal calculus disease. *Journal of Advanced Nursing,* 15(8), 962-970.

Rose, M., Baigis-Smith, J., and Smith, D. (1990). Behavioral management of urinary incontinence in homebound older adults. *Home Healthcare Nurse,* 8(5), 10-15.

Simmons, R., and Abress, L. (1990). Quality-of-life issues for end-stage renal disease patients. *American Journal of Kidney Disease,* 15(3), 201-208.

Tuel, S., et al. (1990). Cost-effective screening by nursing staff for urinary tract infection in the spinal cord-injured patient. *American Journal of Physical Medicine and Rehabilitation,* 69(3), 128-131.

Voepel-Lewis, T., et al. (1990). Stress, coping, and quality of life in family members of kidney transplant recipients. *ANNA Journal,* 17(6), 427-431.

White, M., et al. (1990). Stress, coping, and quality of life in adult kidney transplant recipients. *ANNA Journal,* 17(6), 421-424, 431.

Skin, Hair, and Nails

Anatomy and physiology overview

■ Structures of the skin and nails

This photograph includes magnified views of the structures of the skin and nails.

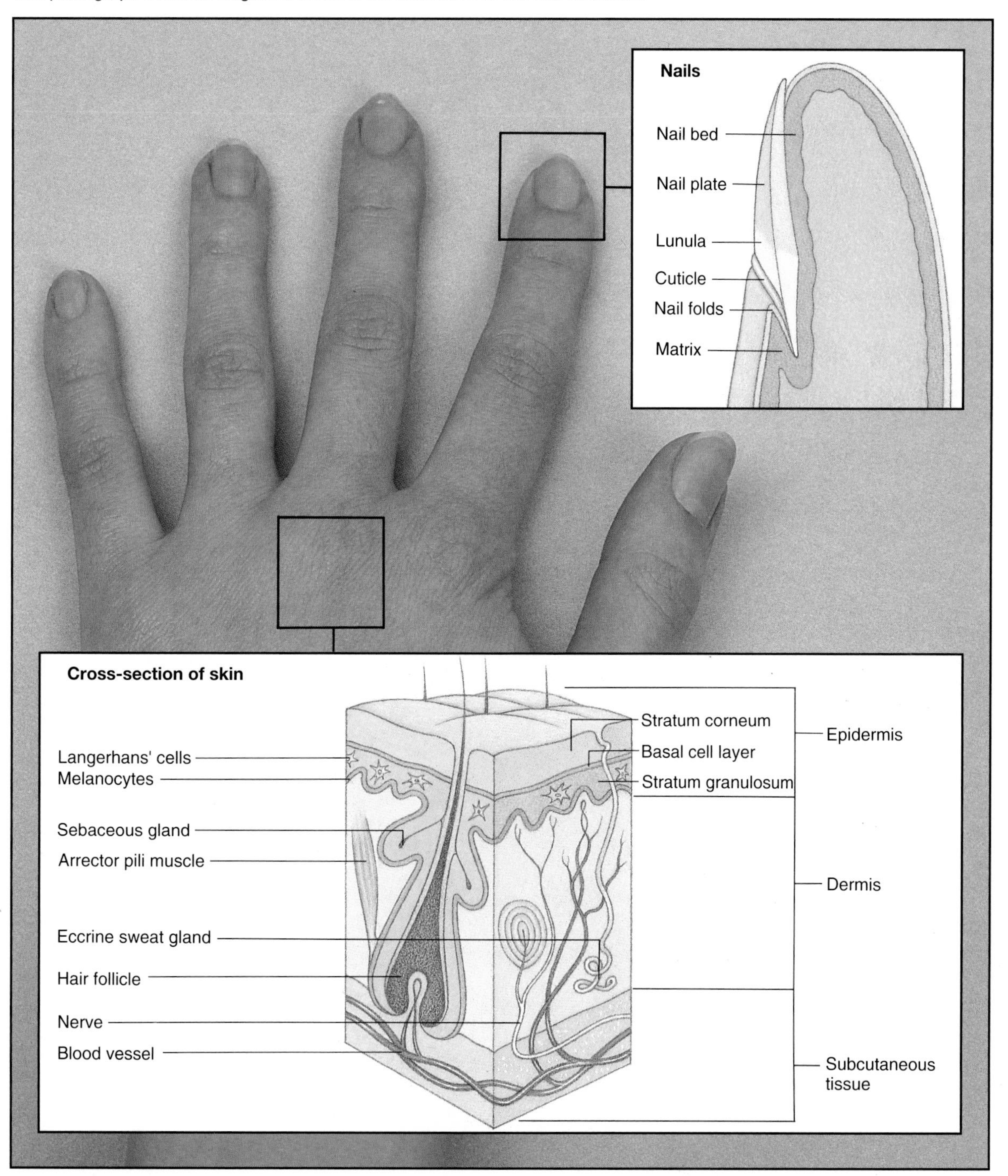

Assessment

■ Inspection

Inspect the skin from 3 to 6 feet to assess its color and condition. Freckles and birthmarks are normal variations.

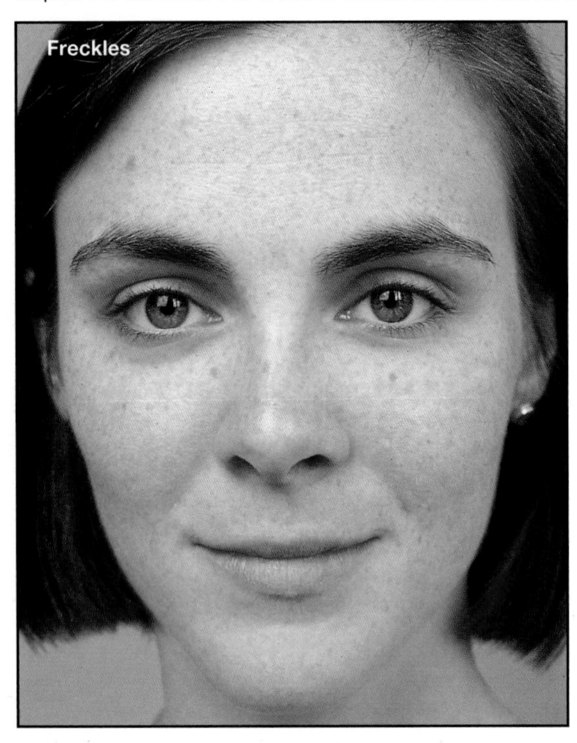
Freckles

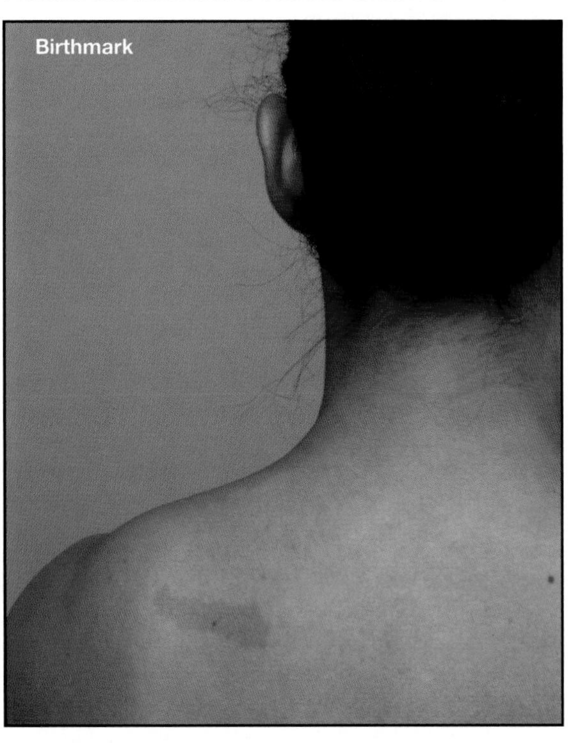
Birthmark

Inspect the hair to assess its quantity, texture, color, and distribution. Body hair distribution may be affected by race and ethnic origin.

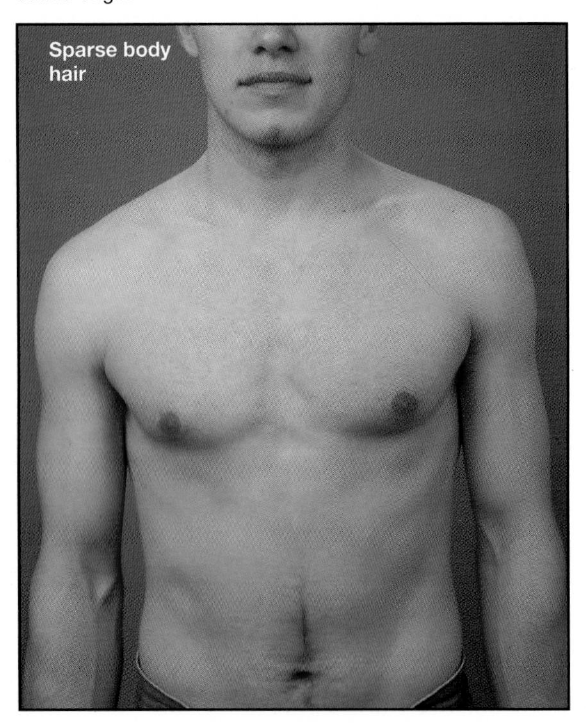
Sparse body hair

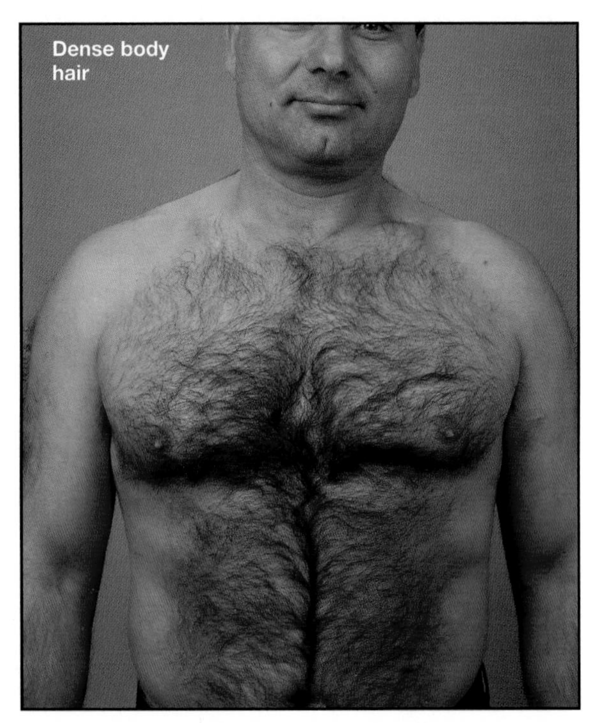
Dense body hair

Fingernail color and attachment

Inspect the fingernails, noting their color and angle of attachment, which normally is 160 degrees. The nail beds normally appear pink in Caucasian clients and may be brown in dark-skinned clients.

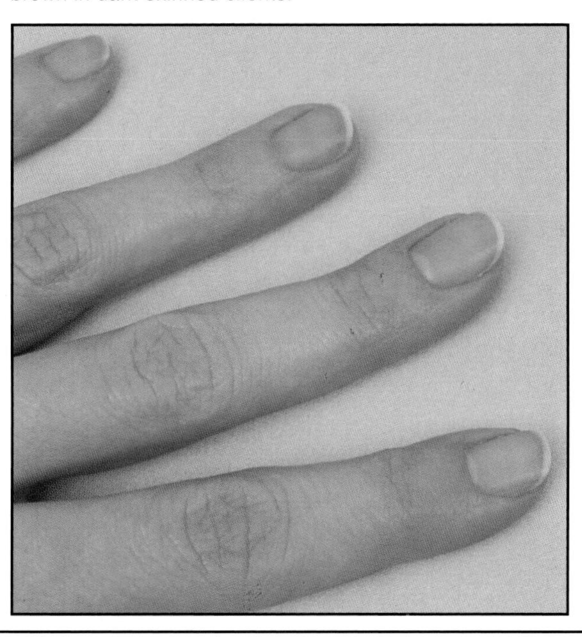

Fingernail consistency

Also inspect the fingernails for consistency, smoothness, and symmetry. Be aware that longitudinal ridges are a common normal variation.

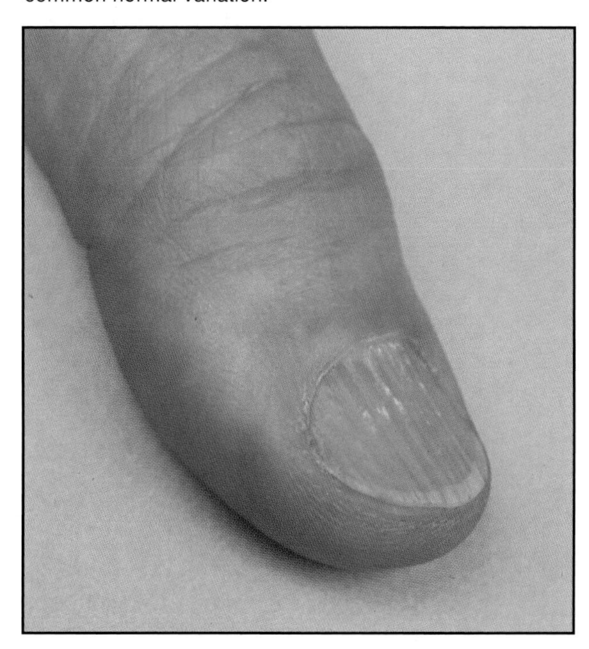

■ Palpation

Skin temperature

Assess the surface temperature of the skin with the dorsal aspect of the hand. The skin should feel warm to cool, and areas should feel the same bilaterally.

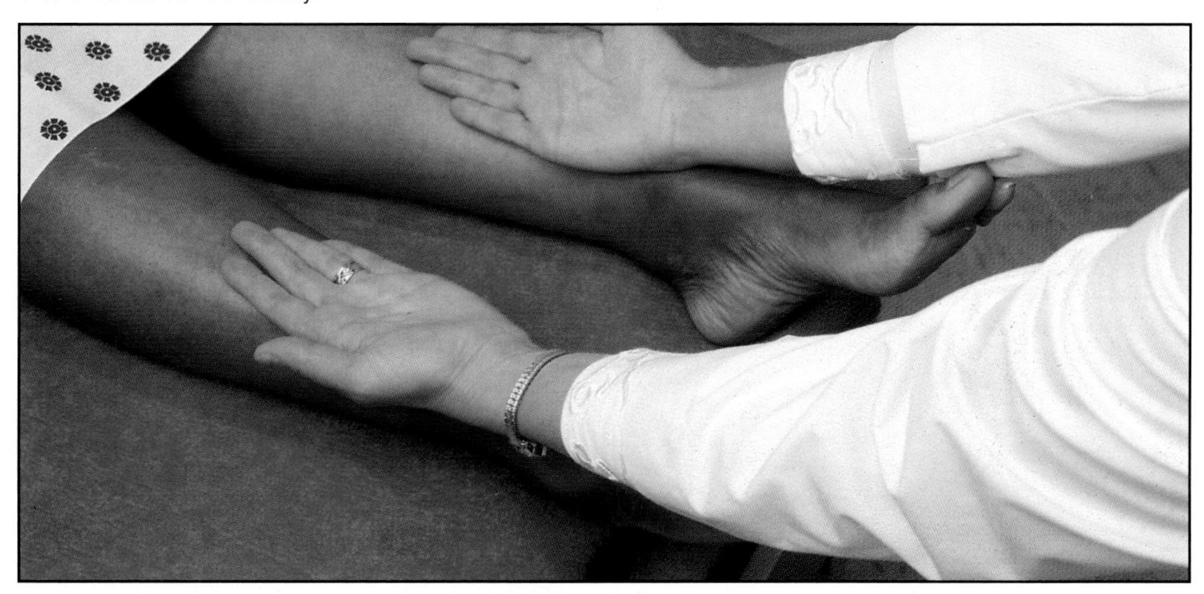

(continued)

ASSESSMENT

PALPATION (continued)

Skin turgor

Assess skin turgor (elasticity) by grasping and pulling up a fold of skin and then releasing it. Normally, the skin returns to its original shape immediately.

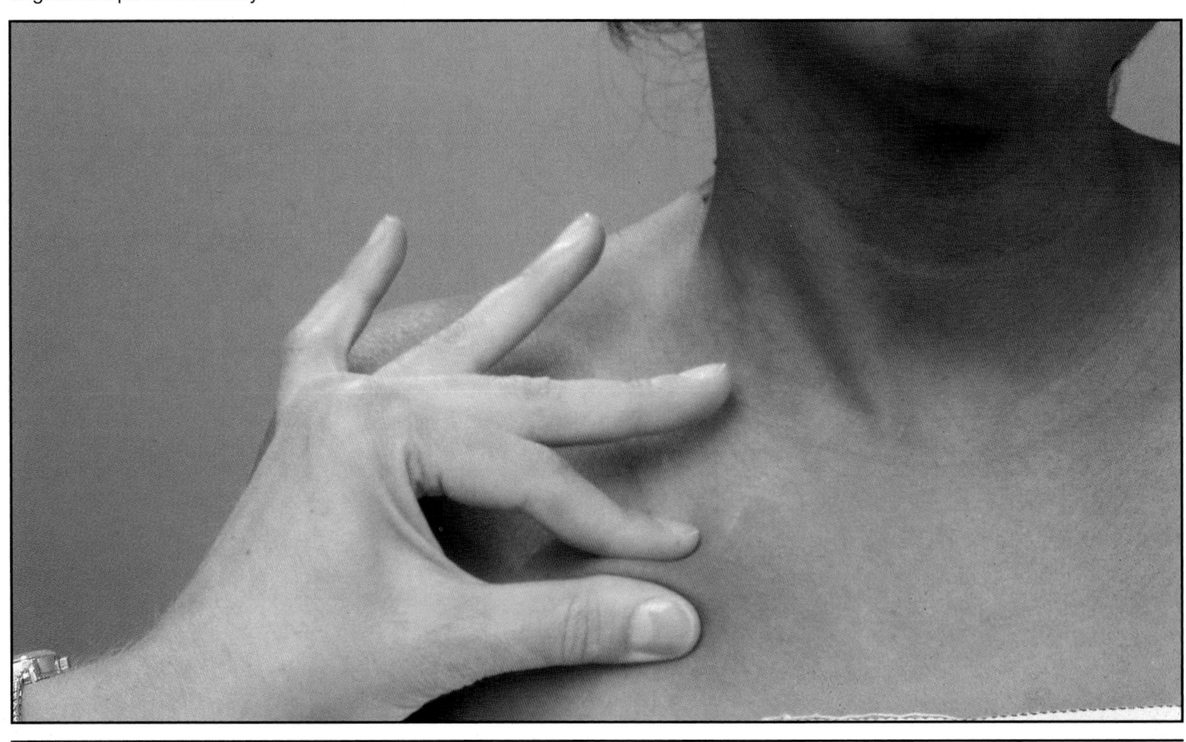

Capillary refill

Assess capillary refill by applying gentle pressure on the nail and inspecting the nail upon release of pressure. Normally, the nail blanches under pressure and returns to its original color rapidly when pressure is released.

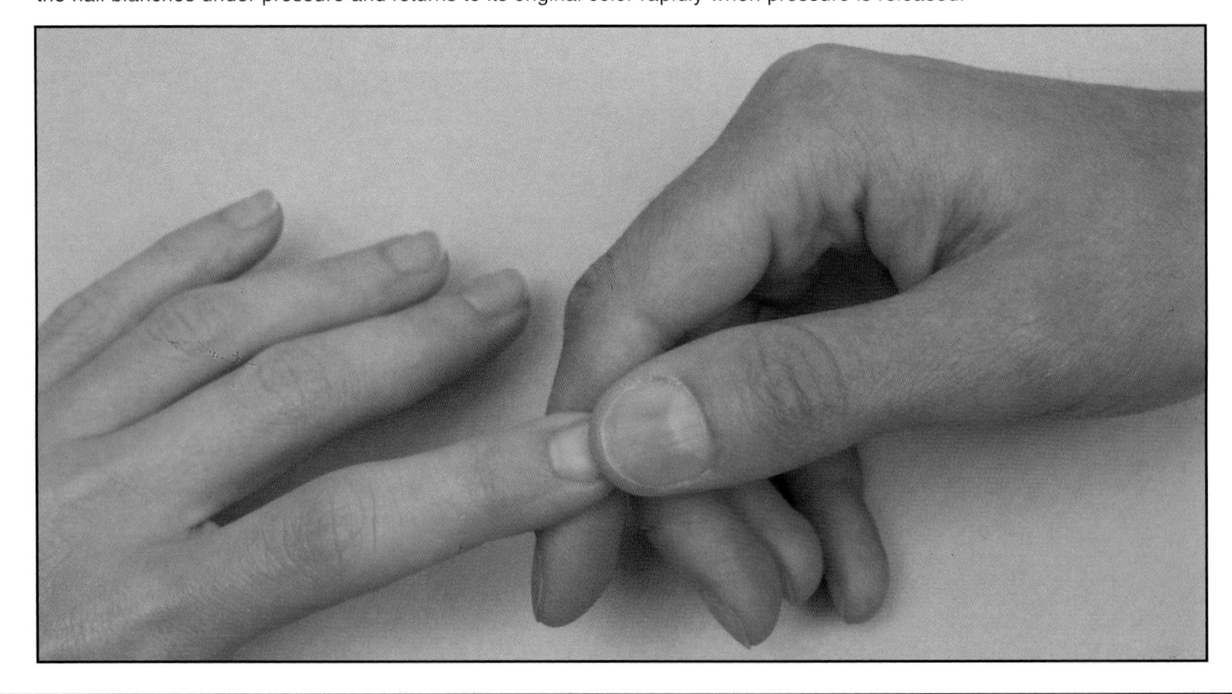

Ethnic considerations

■ Palm ridges

A dark-skinned client may have deeply pigmented ridges in the palms, which is a normal variation.

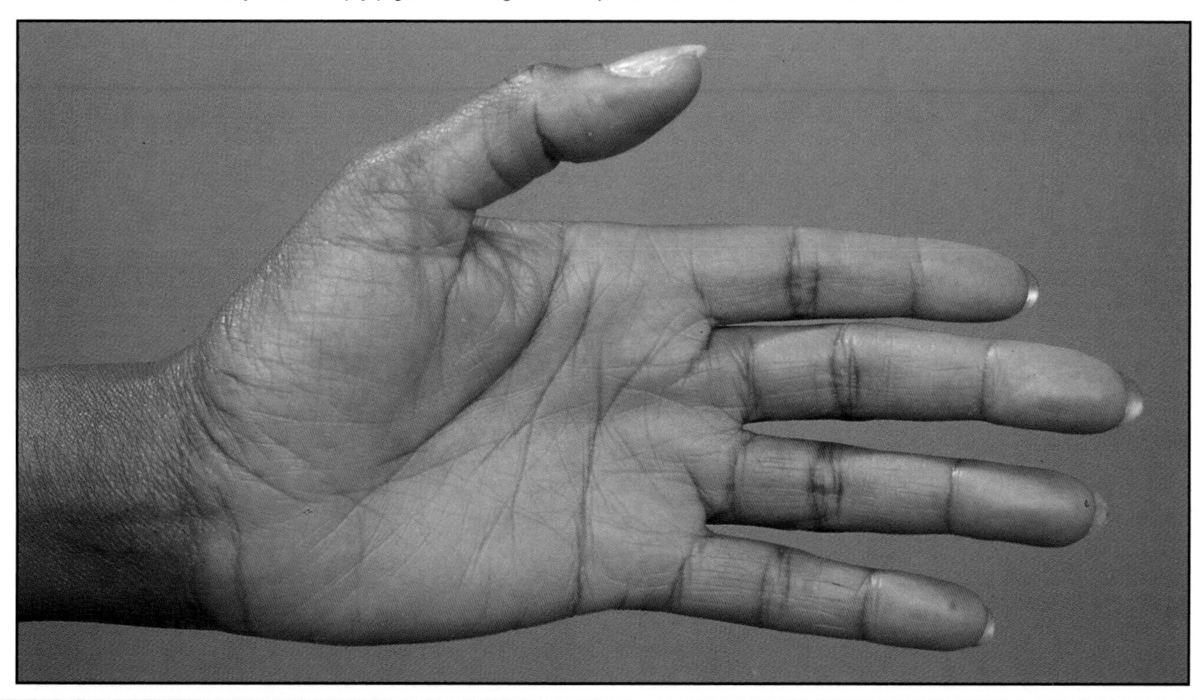

Developmental considerations

■ Pediatric client

Hemangioma simplex

Inspection may detect hemangioma simplex (strawberry mark) in a neonate. A normal variation, this soft, red, raised lesion results from vascular congestion.

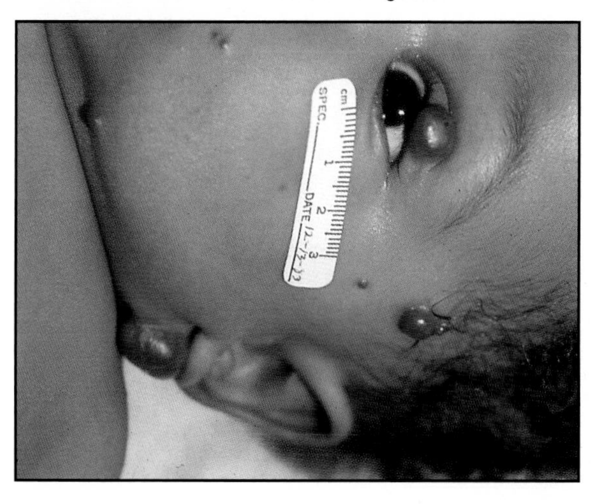

Mongolian spots

Inspection also may identify mongolian spots, normal neonatal skin lesions. Common in Blacks, Native Americans, and Asians, these flat, irregularly shaped lesions appear over the sacrum and buttocks; they typically resolve by about age 3.

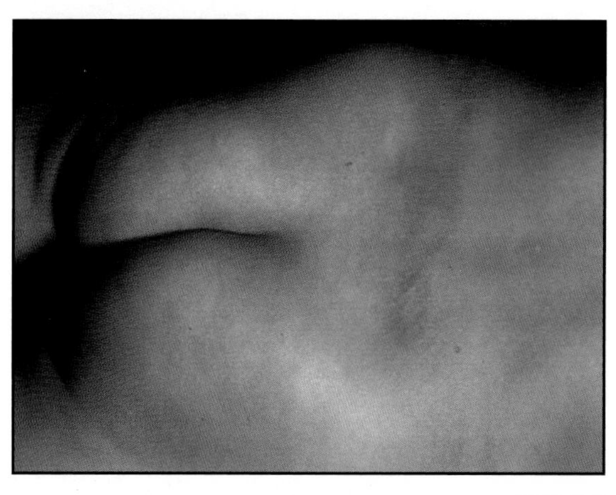

(continued)

DEVELOPMENTAL CONSIDERATIONS

PEDIATRIC CLIENT (continued)

Nevus flammeus

A neonate may display nevus flammeus (port-wine stain), which typically appears as a flat, irregular erythematous patch on the face or neck. This skin lesion may be normal or may accompany a neurologic disease.

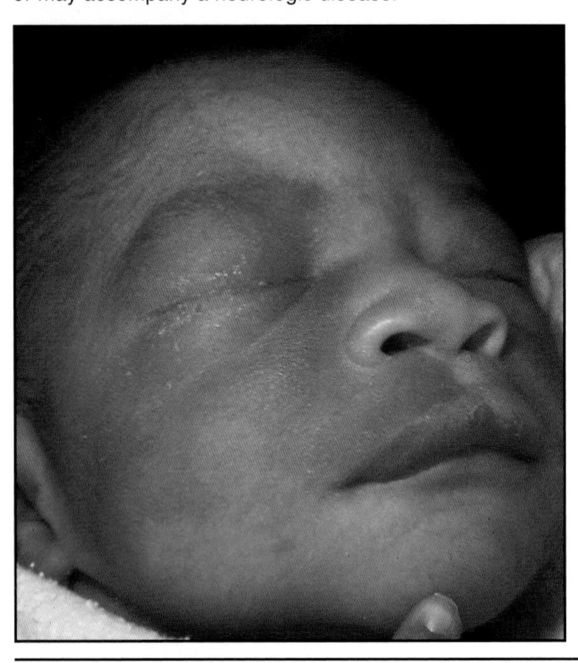

Acne

Acne lesions, which include comedones, papules, and pustules, commonly affect the face, back, and upper chest of adolescent clients.

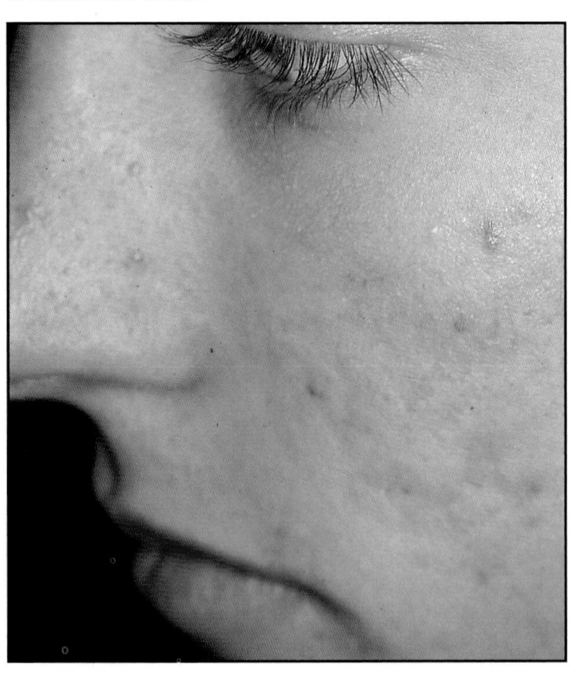

■ Elderly client

Thin, wrinkled skin

In an elderly client, the skin may become thin and may display wrinkles, which result from decreased skin elasticity.

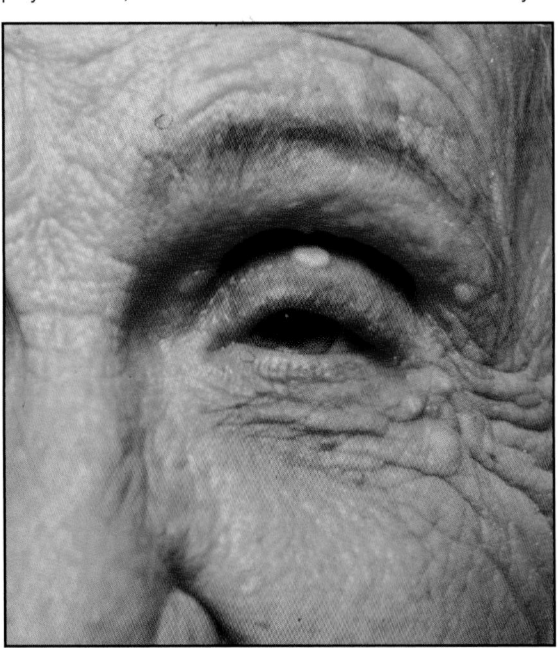

Senile lentigines

Also known as age spots or liver spots, senile lentigines are brown macules that may appear on sun-exposed areas in an elderly client.

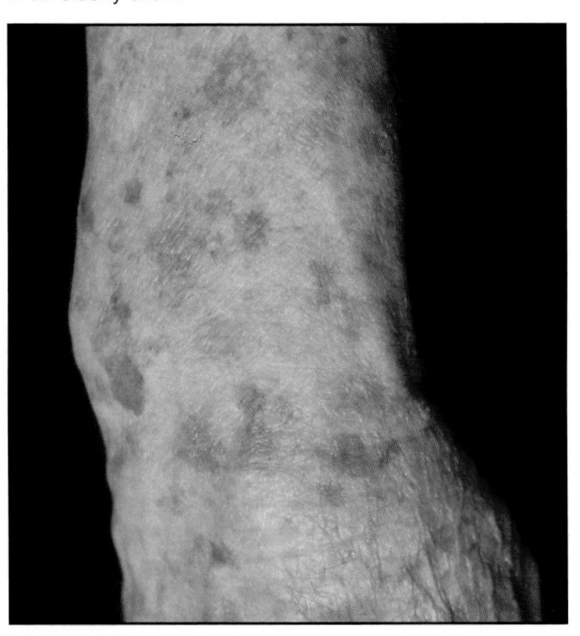

Common abnormalities

■ Skin color variations

Vitiligo

In vitiligo, an absence of melanocytes causes small, colorless, circumscribed areas.

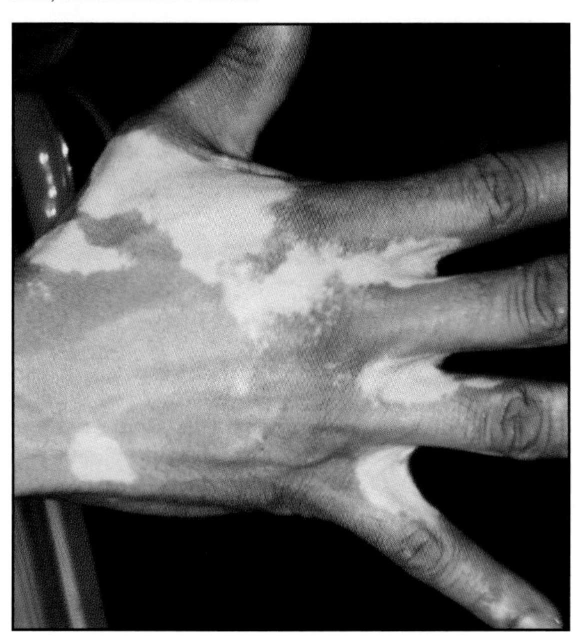

Jaundice

Liver dysfunction may result in jaundice, a yellow skin color that may be generalized or appear only in the sclera.

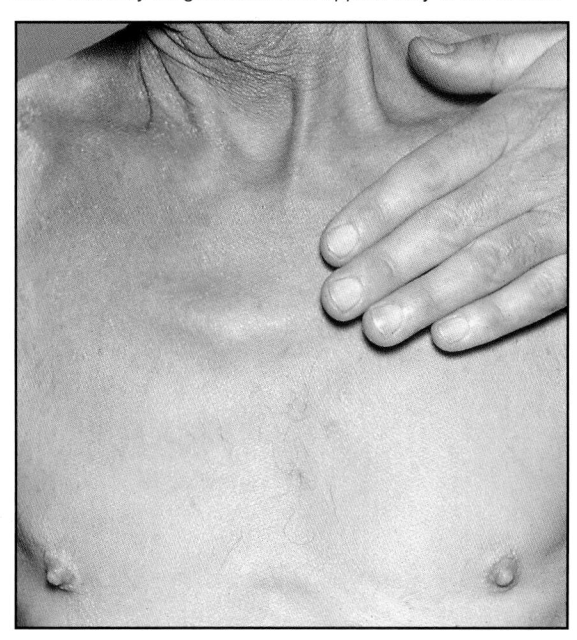

Albinism

A generalized absence of color, albinism is caused by an inherited defect in melanin metabolism of the skin and eyes.

Albinism in light-skinned client. A light-skinned client with albinism may have pale skin, hair color that ranges from white to yellow, and pupils that appear red because of translucent irides.

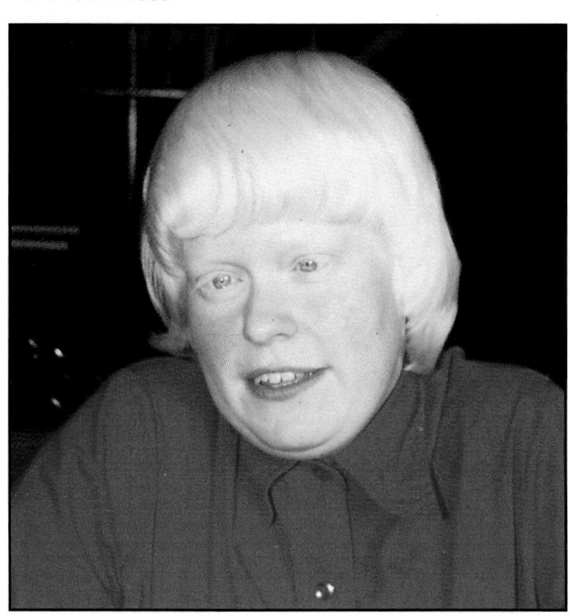

Albinism in dark-skinned client. A dark-skinned client with albinism may have white, yellow-tinged, or yellow-brown hair.

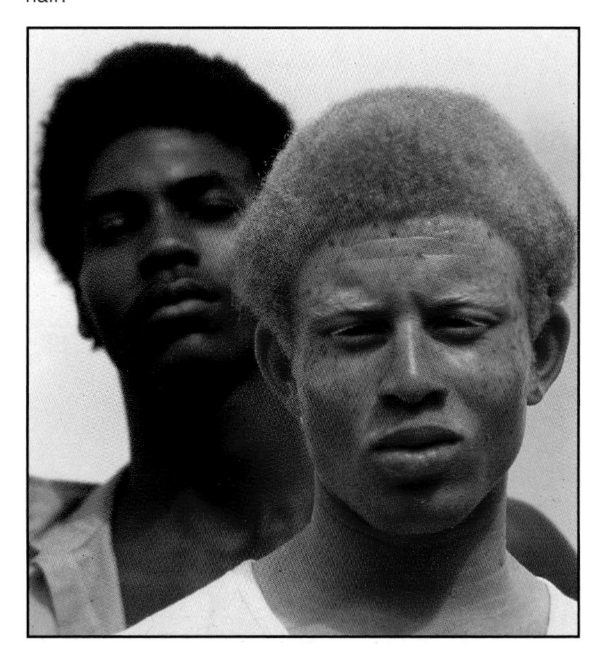

COMMON ABNORMALITIES

■ Skin lesions

Primary lesion

A primary lesion is any change in healthy skin in response to disease or external irritation. A type of primary lesion, a vesicle is a raised, circumscribed, fluid-filled lesion that is less than 0.5 cm (1/4") in diameter. Vesicles may result from varicella (chicken pox) as well as other causes.

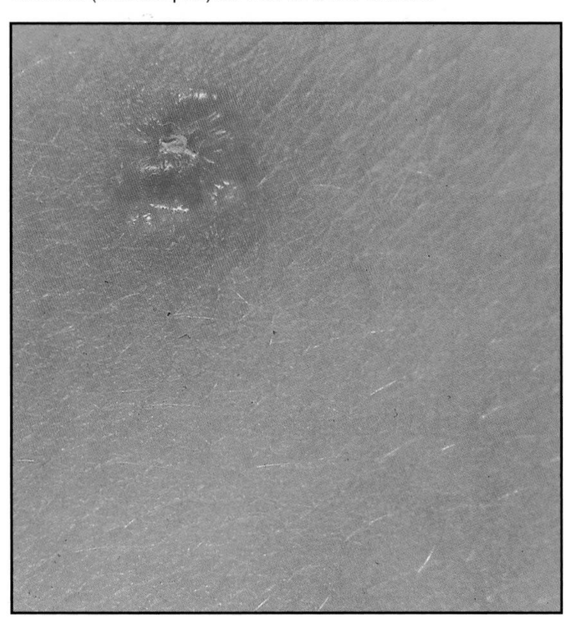

Secondary lesion

A secondary lesion results from a change in a primary lesion. A type of secondary lesion, a keloid is an overgrowth of collagenous scar tissue at the site of a skin wound. The new tissue is elevated, rounded, and firm with irregular margins.

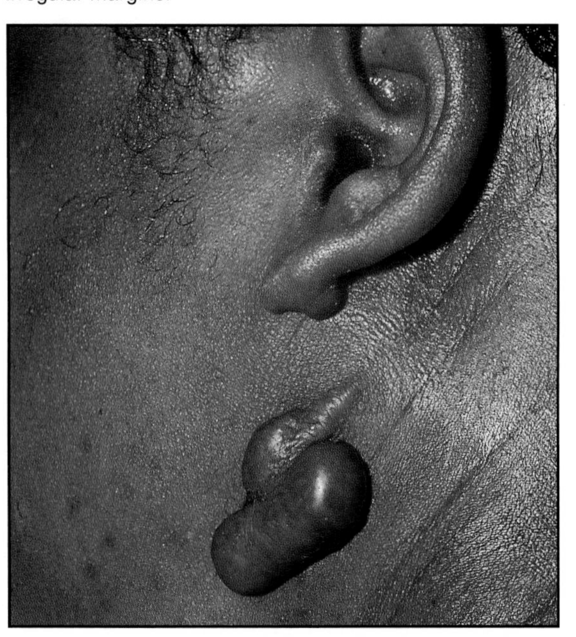

■ Skin lesion distribution

Localized

Skin lesions may be localized (distributed over a small area), as in contact dermatitis.

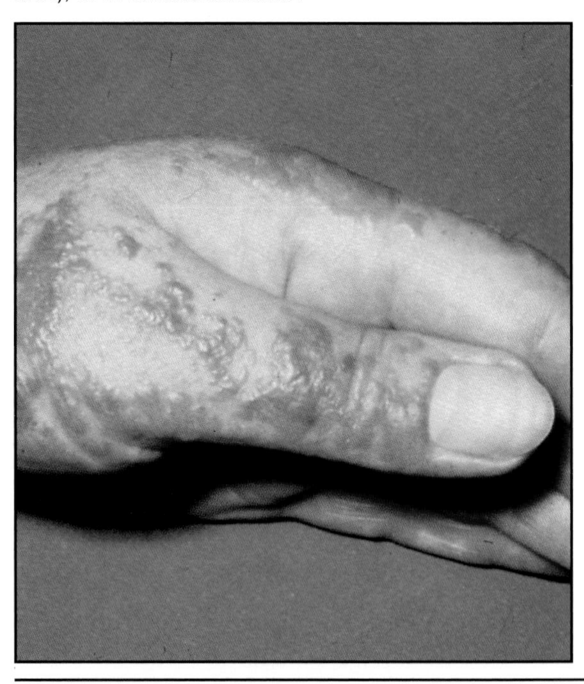

■ Skin lesion configuration

Annular

Annular configuration (arrangement of lesions in a circle) may occur in such disorders as tinea (ringworm).

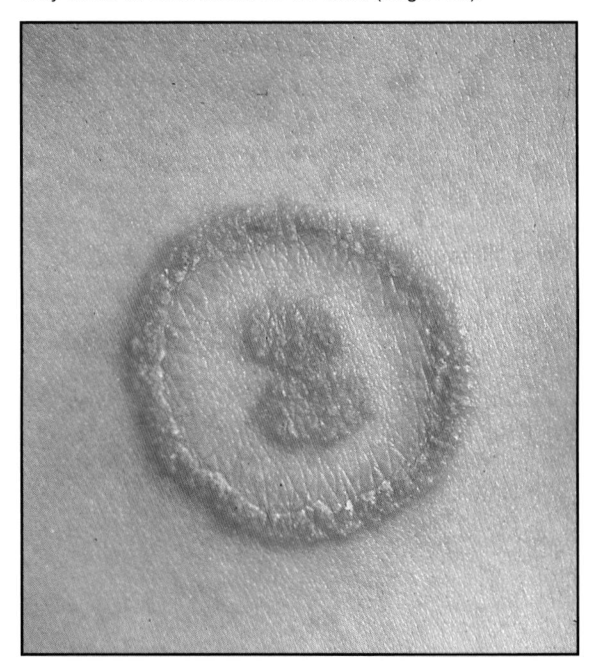

Regional

Skin lesions may display regional distribution (over a larger area), as in acne.

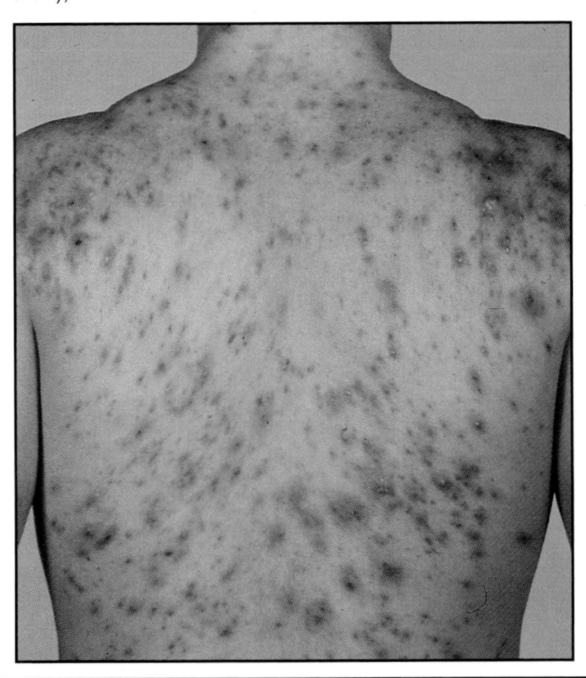

Generalized

Skin lesions also may display generalized distribution (over the entire body), as in rubeola (measles).

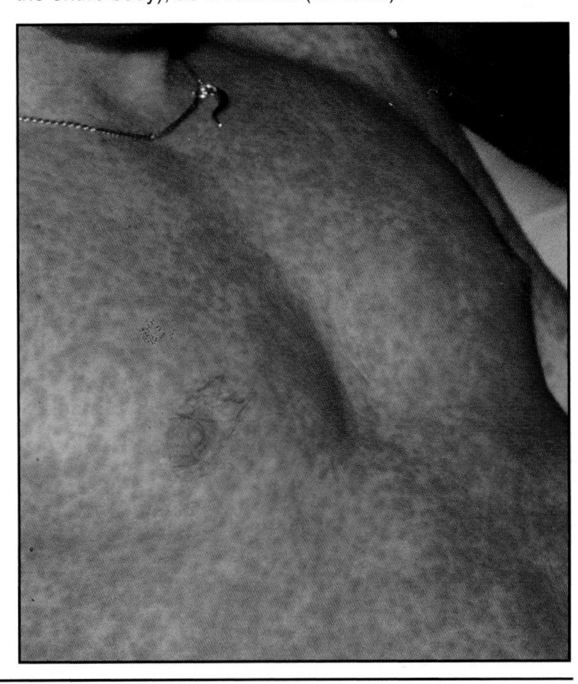

Linear

Linear configuration (arrangement of lesions in a line) may occur in such disorders as herpes zoster (shingles).

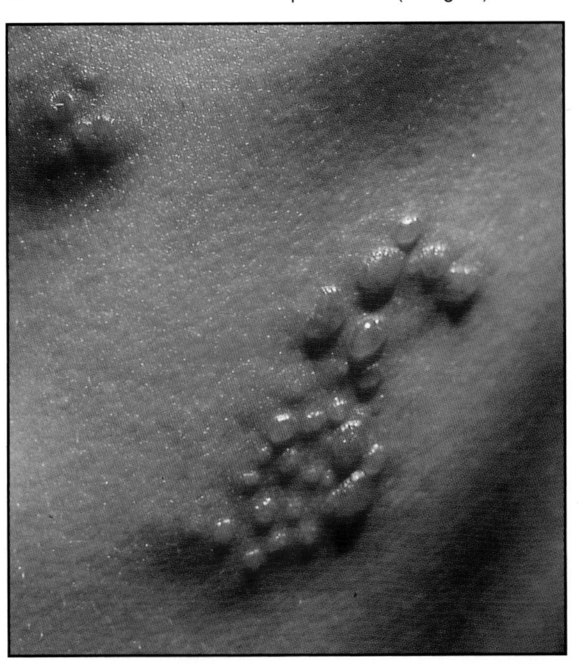

■ Nail abnormalities

Nail discoloration

Psoriasis may result in yellow discoloration of the nails and separation of the nail from the bed.

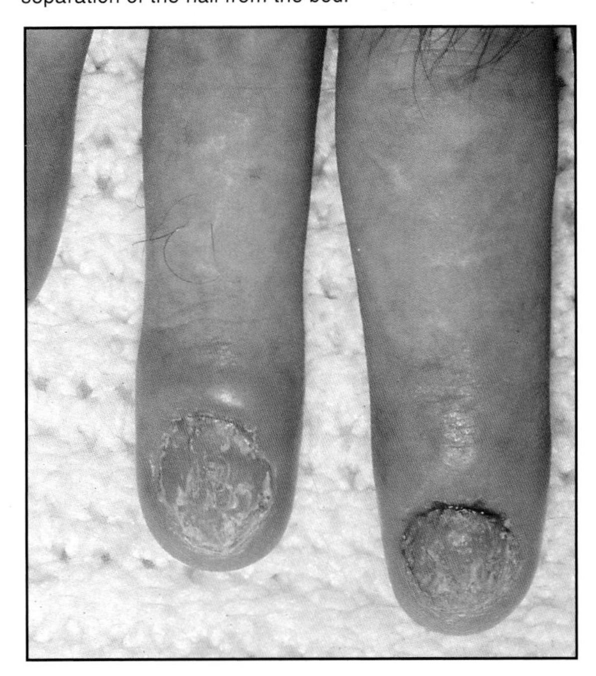

Head and Neck

Anatomy and physiology overview

■ Structures of the head and neck

This anterior view shows the structures of the head and neck.

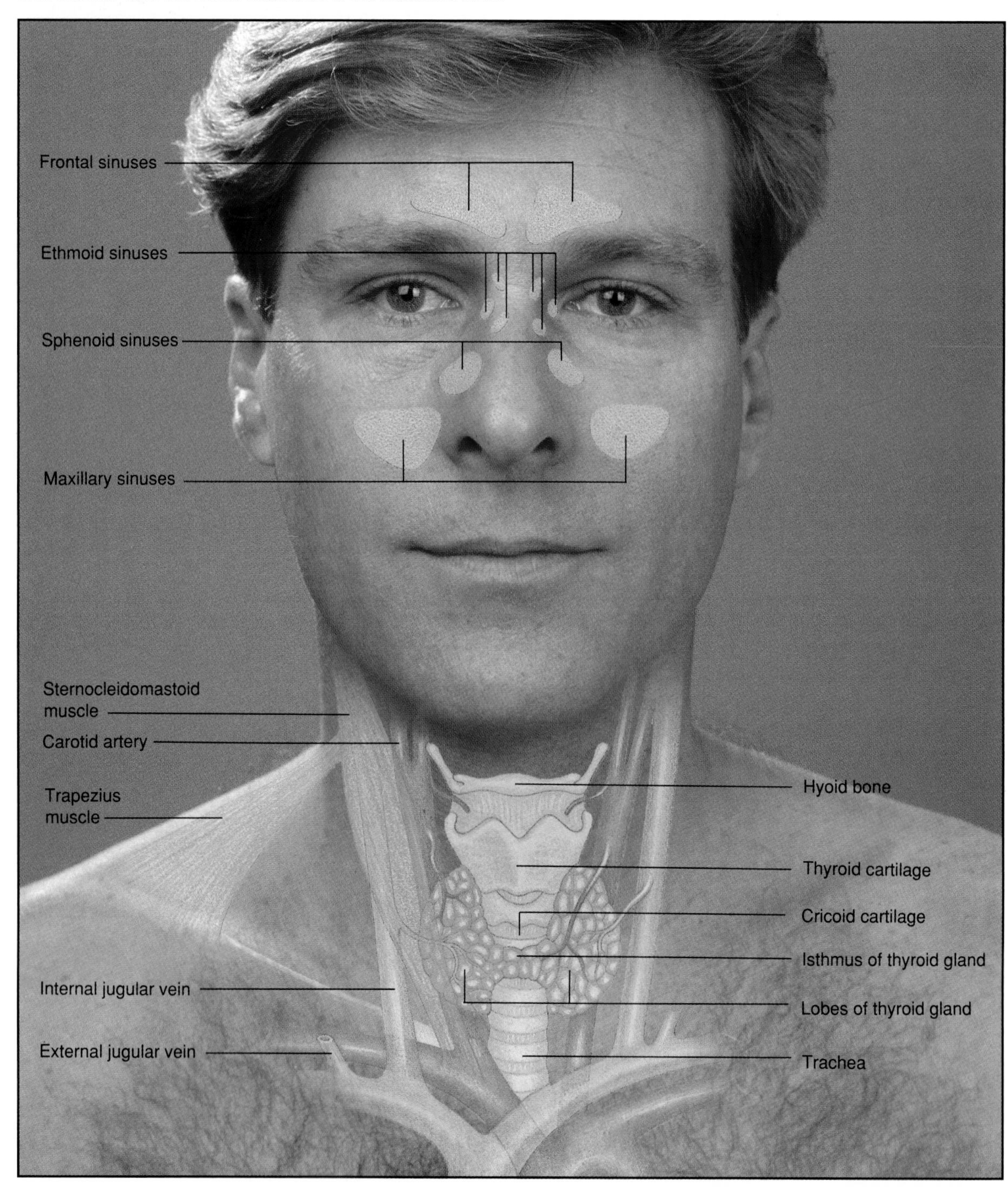

ANATOMY AND PHYSIOLOGY OVERVIEW

■ Structures of the mouth

This anterior view of the mouth shows its major structures. Underlying structures are illustrated in black.

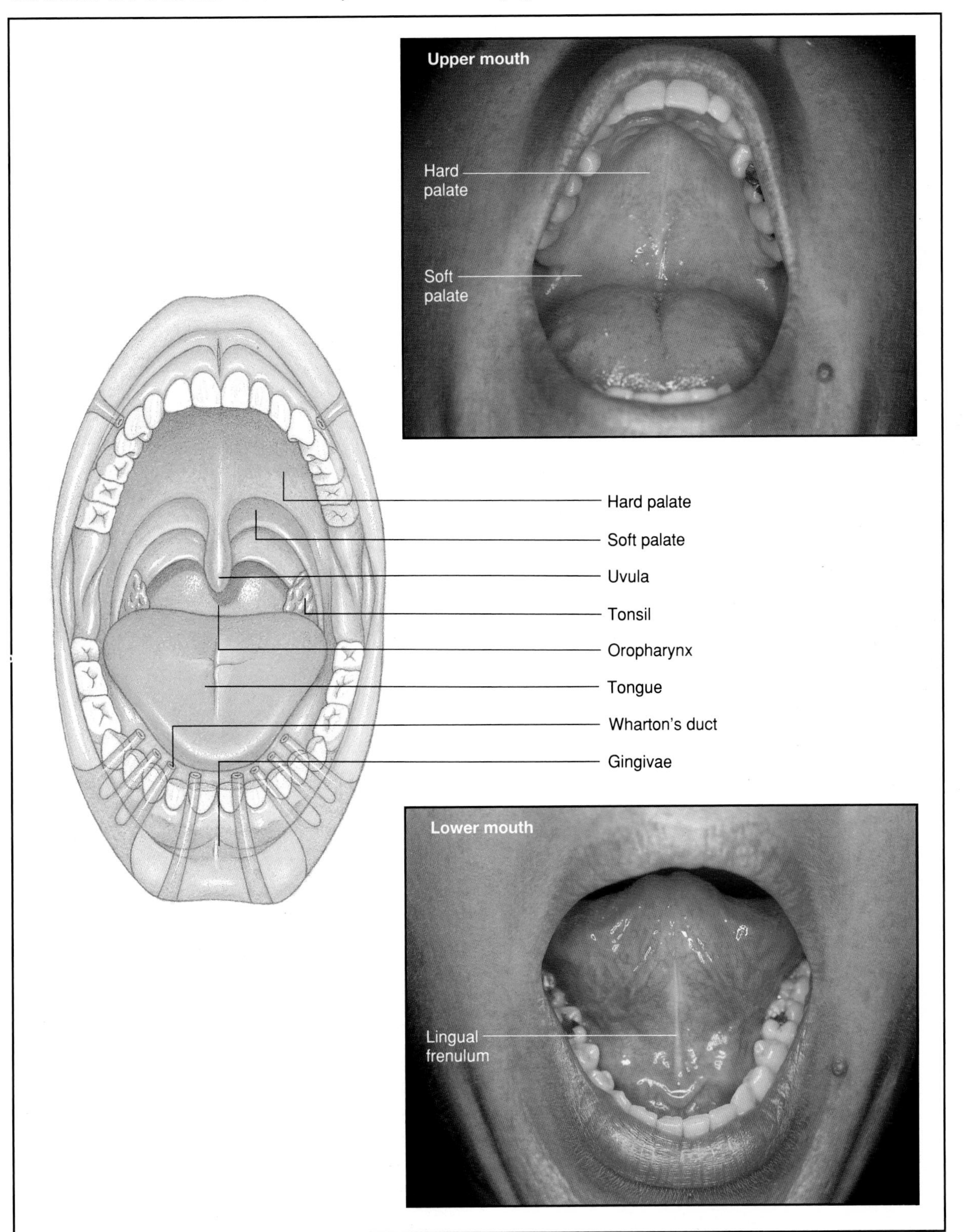

Assessment

■ Inspection

Head and face

Inspect the head and face for any abnormalities in size, shape, position, contour, or symmetry. When assessing for symmetry, particularly note the nasolabial folds and palpebral fissures. Normally, the head is normocephalic, erect, and midline, and the facial features are symmetrical.

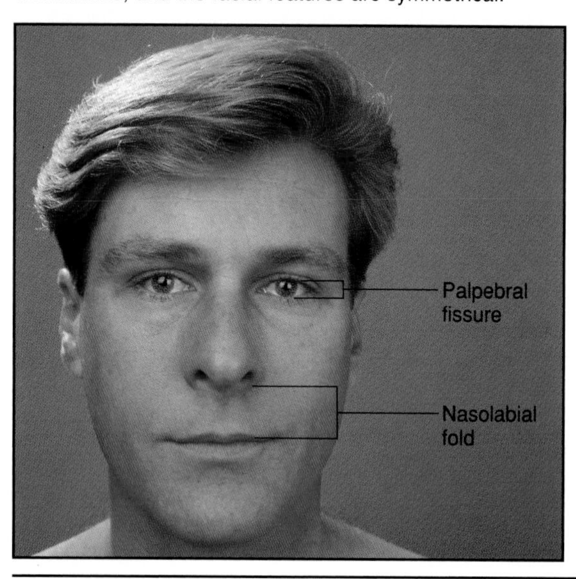

Internal nasal structures

Inspect the internal nasal structures with a nasoscope, nasal speculum and a small flashlight, or an ophthalmoscope handle with a nasal tip. The nasal mucosa and middle and inferior turbinates normally appear pink.

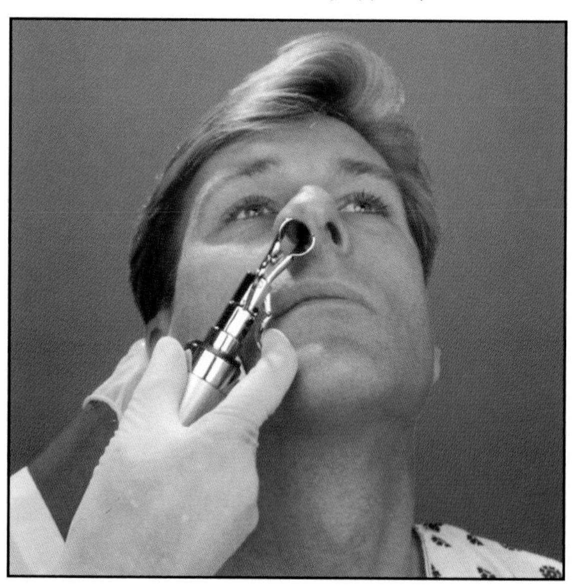

■ Palpation

Temporomandibular joints

Palpate the temporomandibular joints as the client opens and closes the mouth. Normally, the joints move smoothly and painlessly.

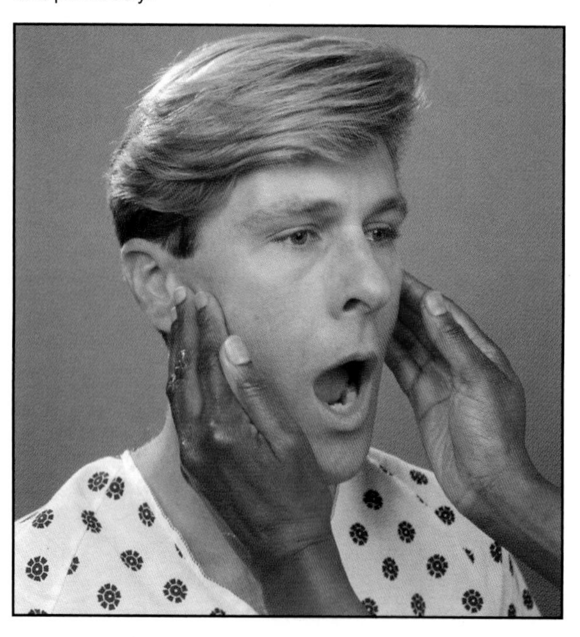

Tongue palpation

With a gloved hand, grasp the tongue with a 4" x 4" gauze pad and palpate it to assess consistency, mobility, and muscle tone. The tongue should be slightly rough, move freely, and have good muscle tone.

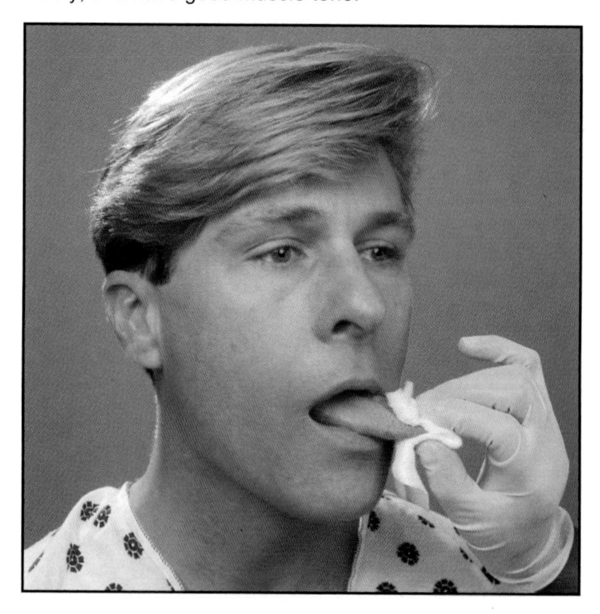

PALPATION (continued)

Palpation of the sinuses

Palpate the frontal sinuses by applying light pressure with the thumbs below the eyebrow. Normally, palpation detects no tenderness or swelling.

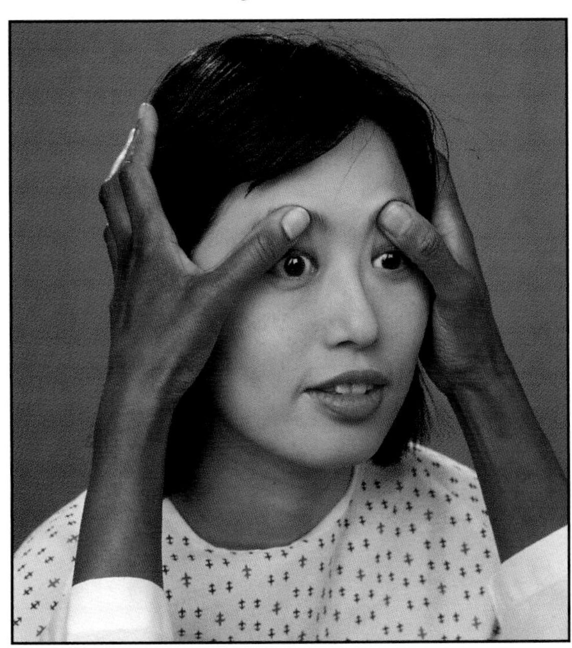

Palpate the maxillary sinuses by applying light pressure with the thumbs over the cheek bones. Normally, palpation detects no tenderness or swelling.

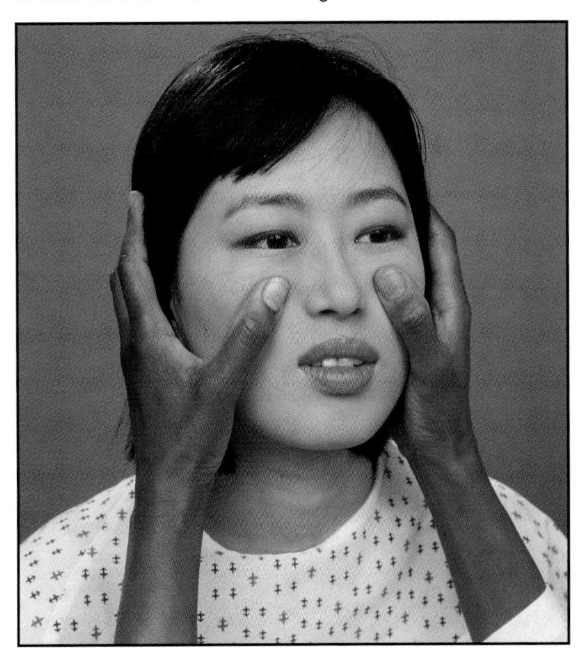

■ Percussion

Sinuses

Use direct percussion to assess the frontal sinuses. Light tapping above the eyebrow should elicit no tenderness.

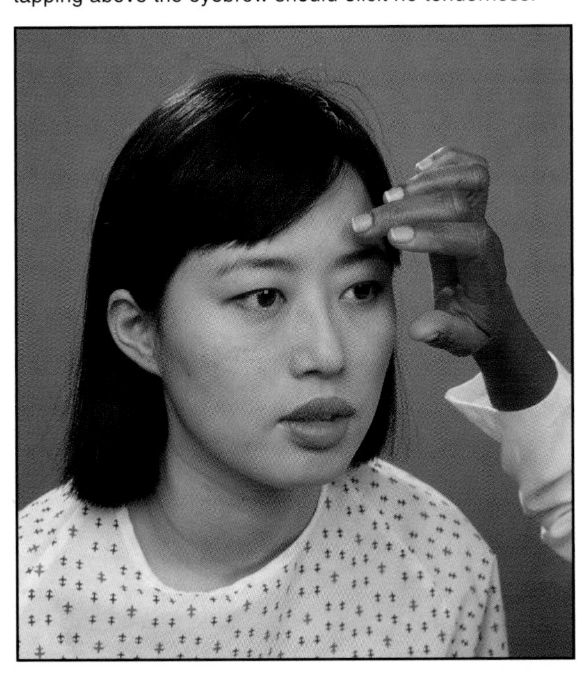

Use direct percussion to assess the maxillary sinuses. Light tapping below the eyes should elicit no tenderness.

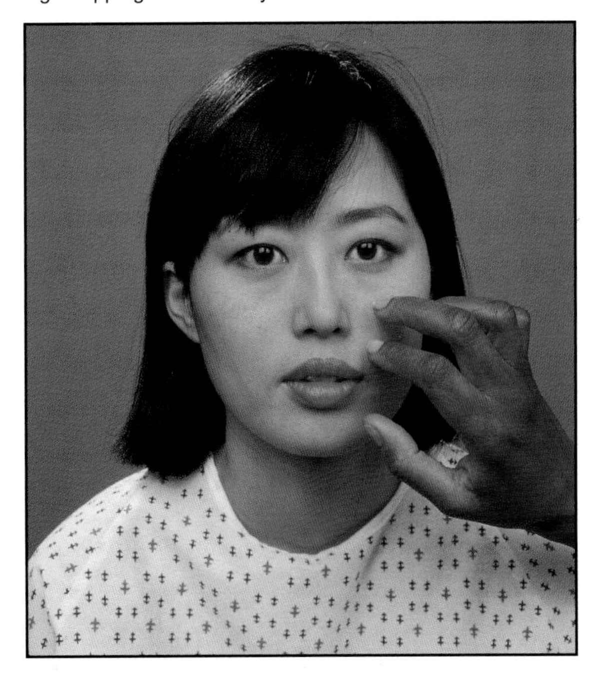

ASSESSMENT

■ Auscultation

Arteries

Auscultate the periorbital, temporal, and occipital arteries with the bell of the stethoscope, as shown in this photograph of temporal artery auscultation. Auscultation should not reveal any sounds in these arteries.

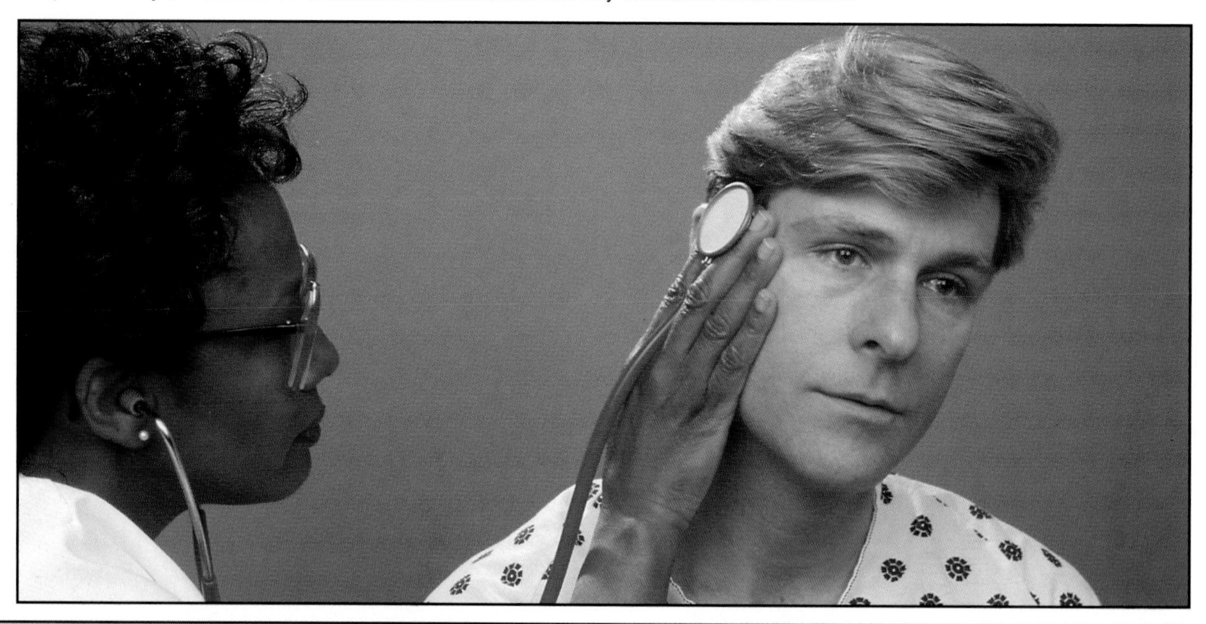

Developmental considerations

■ Pediatric client

Head circumference

For a child under age 2, assess head circumference by wrapping a tape measure around the head at its widest point.

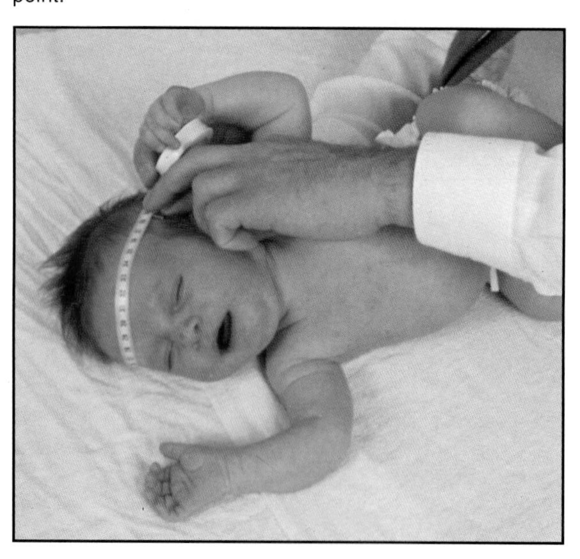

■ Elderly client

Gingival recession

An elderly client may display gingival recession, which may be accompanied by loose teeth.

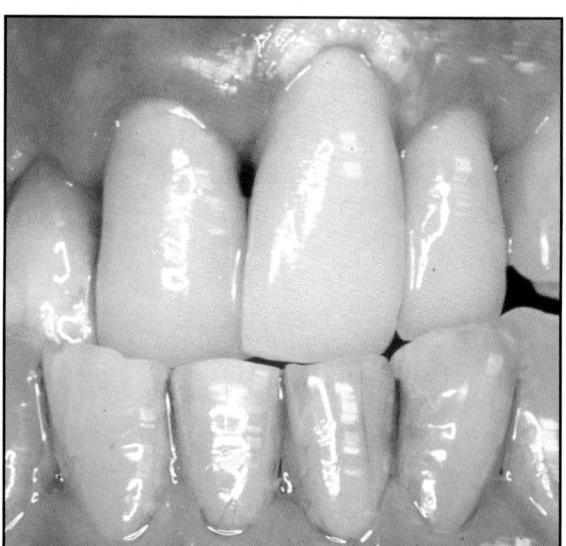

Common abnormalities

■ Nose

Nasal polyps

These benign, edematous growths result from continuous nasal pressure caused by chronic allergy, sinusitis, rhinitis, or recurrent nasal infections.

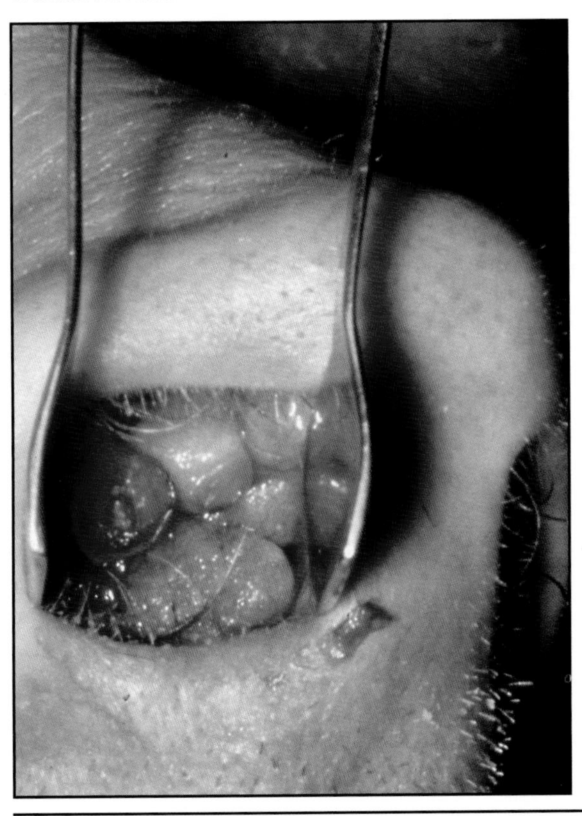

Inflamed tonsils

Red, enlarged tonsils may result from pharyngitis, which may be accompanied by exudate.

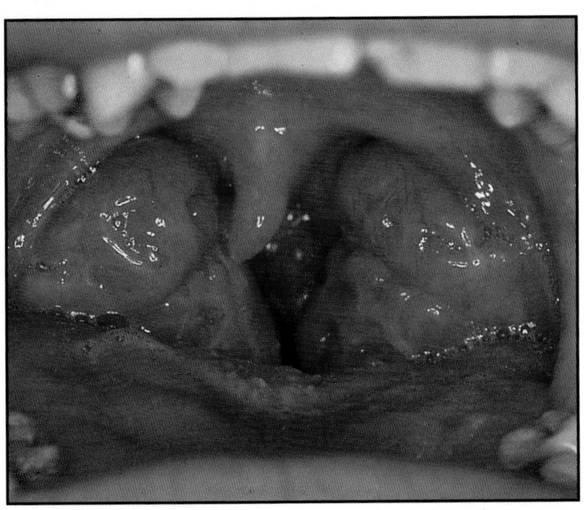

■ Mouth and oropharynx

Leukoplakia

This thickened white patch on the buccal membrane may be a precancerous lesion.

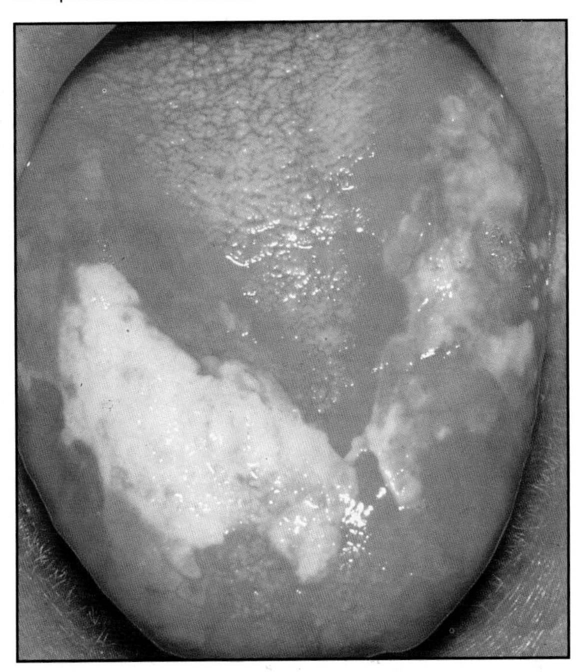

Glossitis

Tongue inflammation may be caused by pernicious anemia, streptococcal infection, or irritation from excessive smoking.

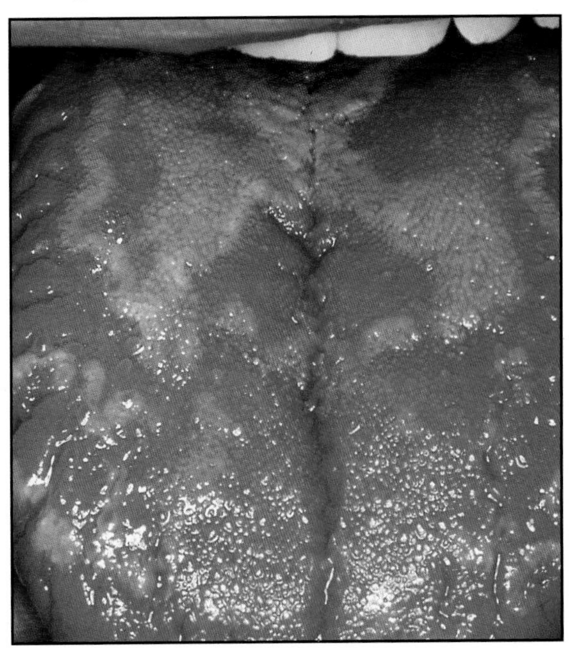

Eyes and Ears

Anatomy and physiology overview

■ Extraocular and intraocular structures

This close-up view of the face shows the extraocular and intraocular structures.

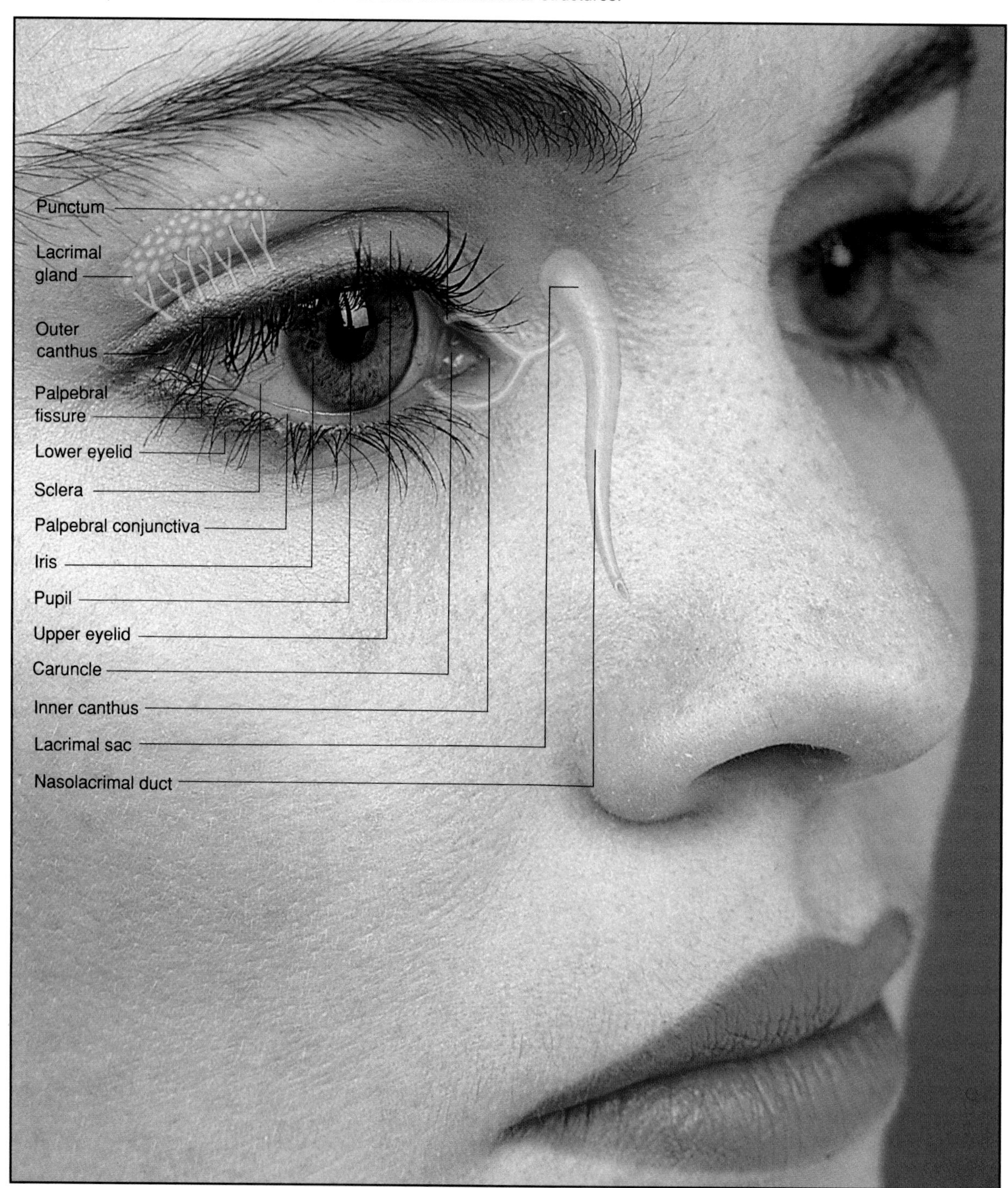

Assessment

■ Extraocular muscle function

Cover-uncover test

Use the cover-uncover test to assess extraocular muscle balance in each eye. At the moment of its uncovering, the eye should remain steady, without drifting.

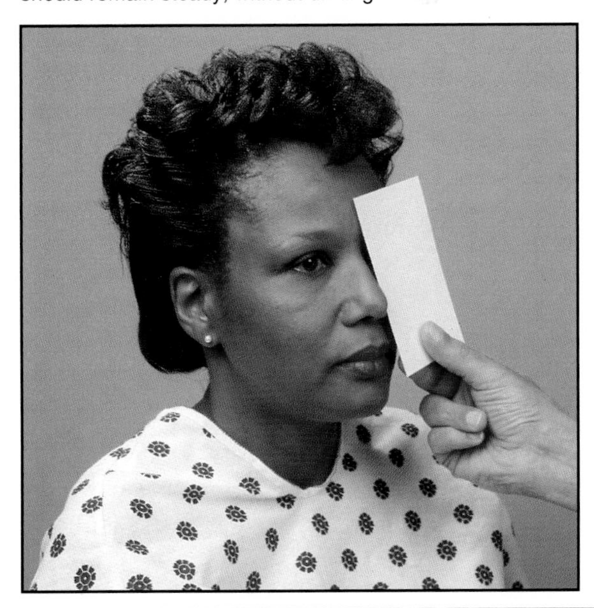

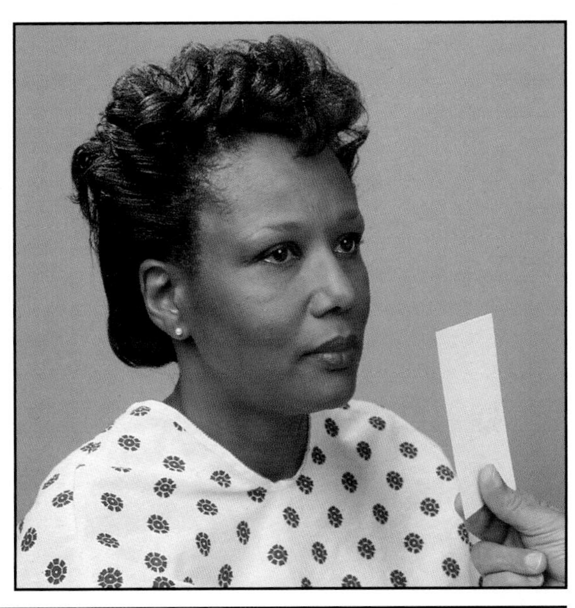

Corneal light reflex test

Perform the corneal light reflex by aiming a light at the bridge of the client's nose so that it falls on both corneas equally. Normally, the corneas reflect the light symmetrically.

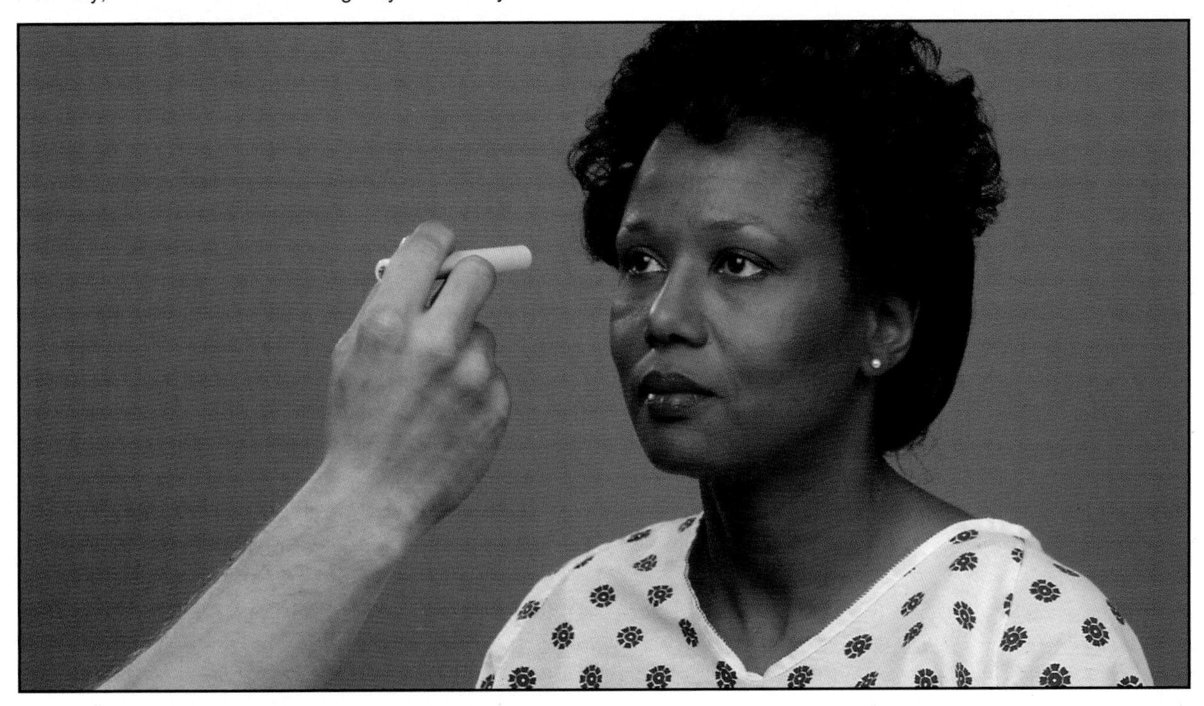

(continued)

ASSESSMENT

EXTRAOCULAR MUSCLE FUNCTION (continued)

Six cardinal positions of gaze test

To assess the function of the extraocular muscles and the cranial nerves responsible for their movement, perform the six cardinal positions of gaze test. The labels below explain which muscles and nerves are responsible for movements of each eye. Normally, the client's eyes remain parallel as they follow the moving object.

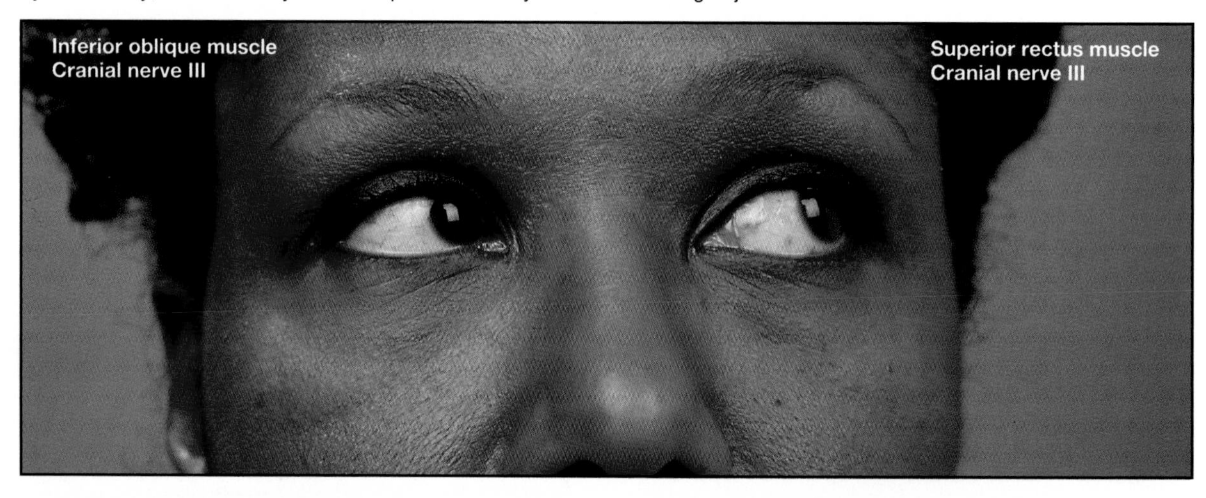

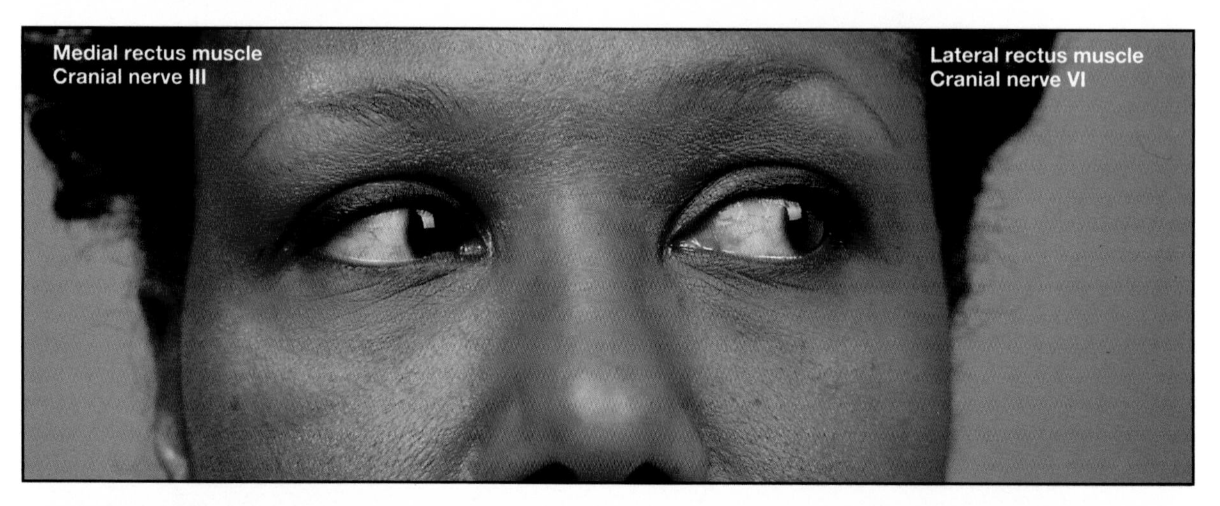

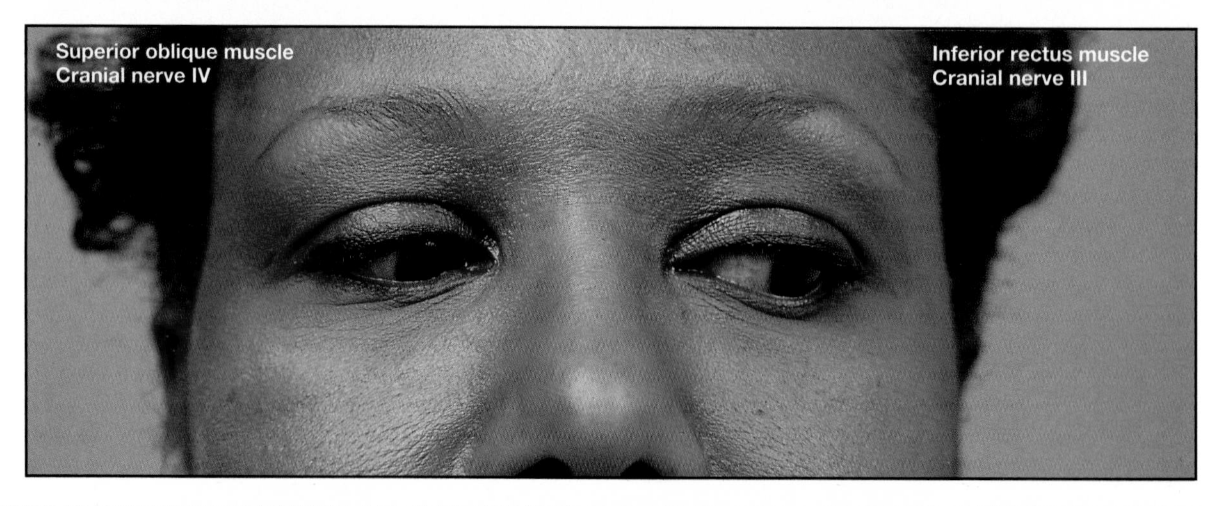

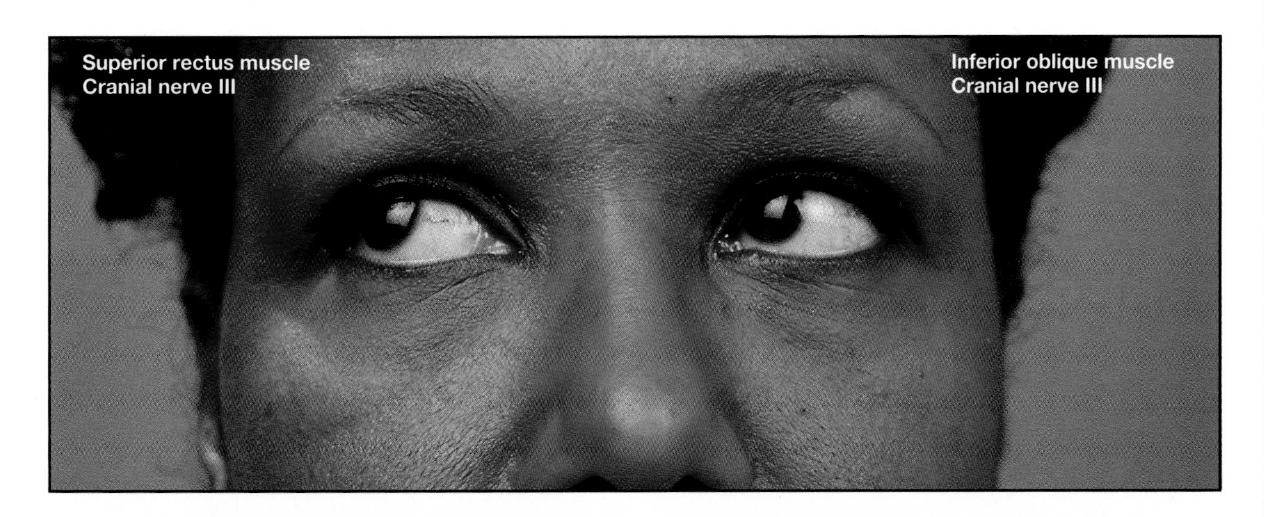
Superior rectus muscle
Cranial nerve III
Inferior oblique muscle
Cranial nerve III

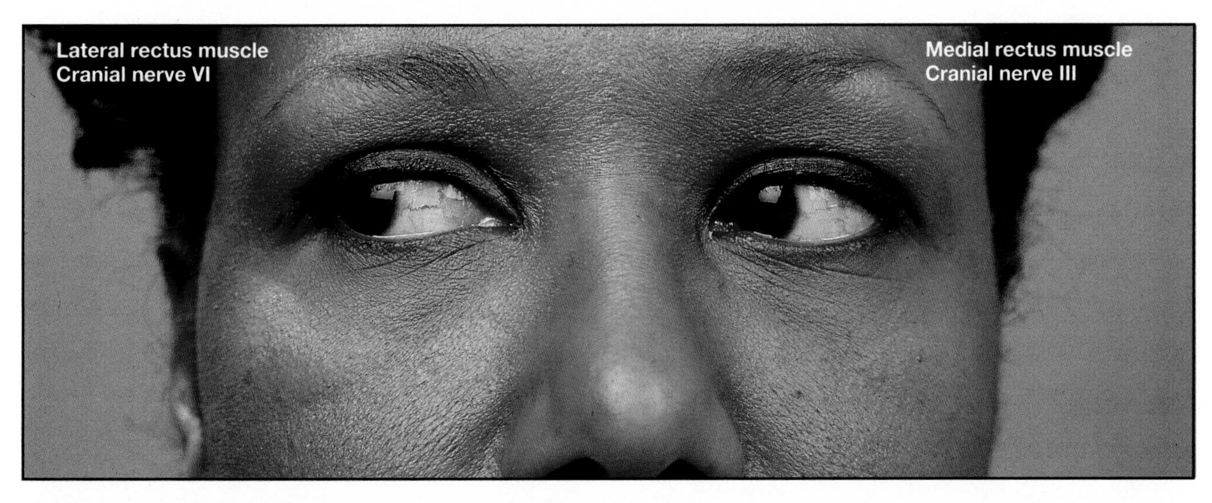
Lateral rectus muscle
Cranial nerve VI
Medial rectus muscle
Cranial nerve III

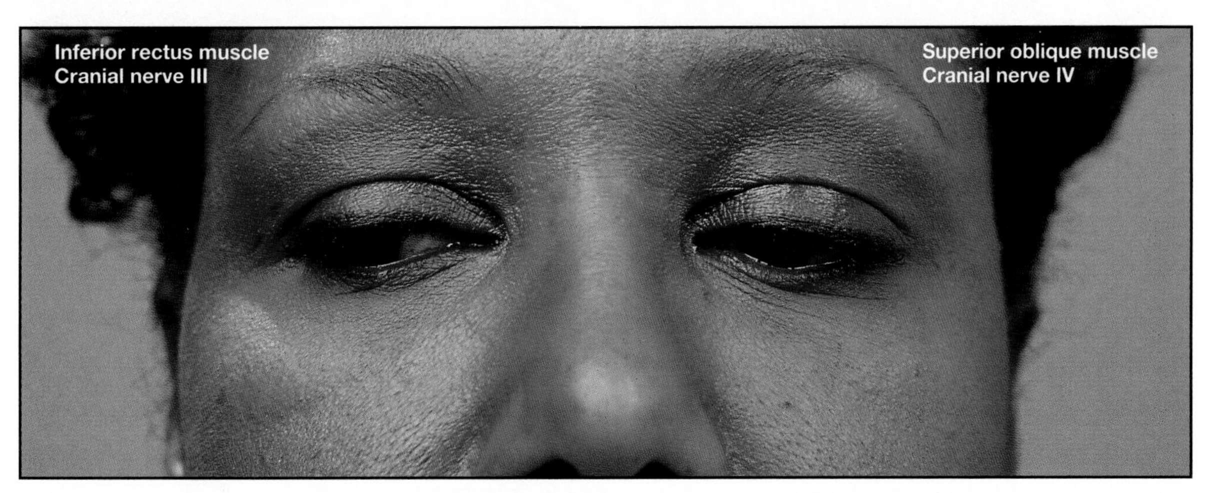
Inferior rectus muscle
Cranial nerve III
Superior oblique muscle
Cranial nerve IV

ASSESSMENT

■ Peripheral vision

Assess peripheral vision by testing the client's ability to identify an object moving in from the periphery of vision. Test each field as shown below. Each eye is tested separately, comparing the nurse's peripheral vision to the client's.

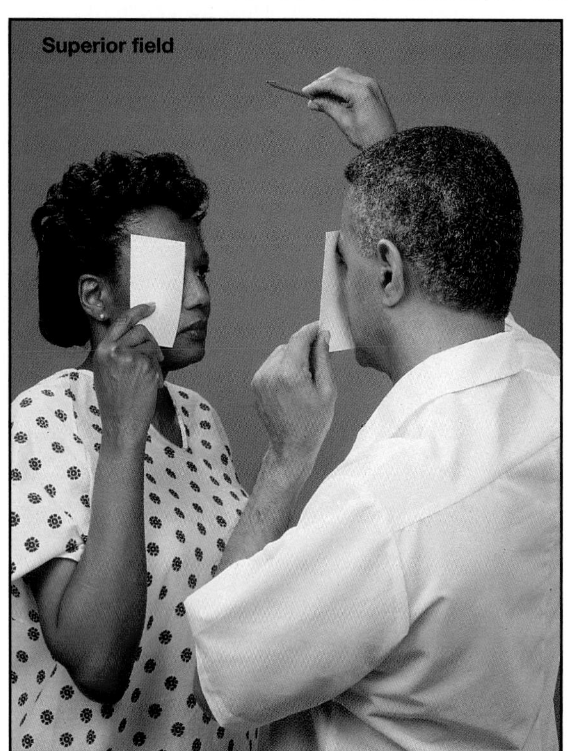
Superior field

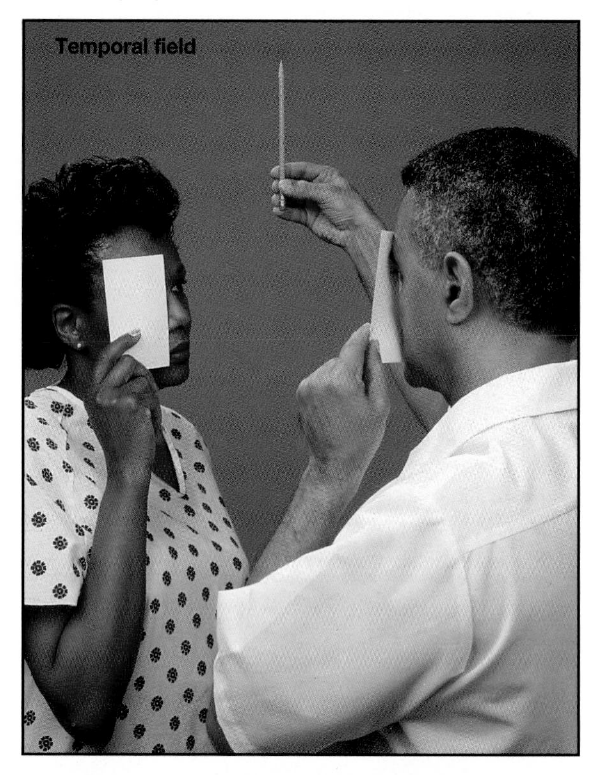
Temporal field

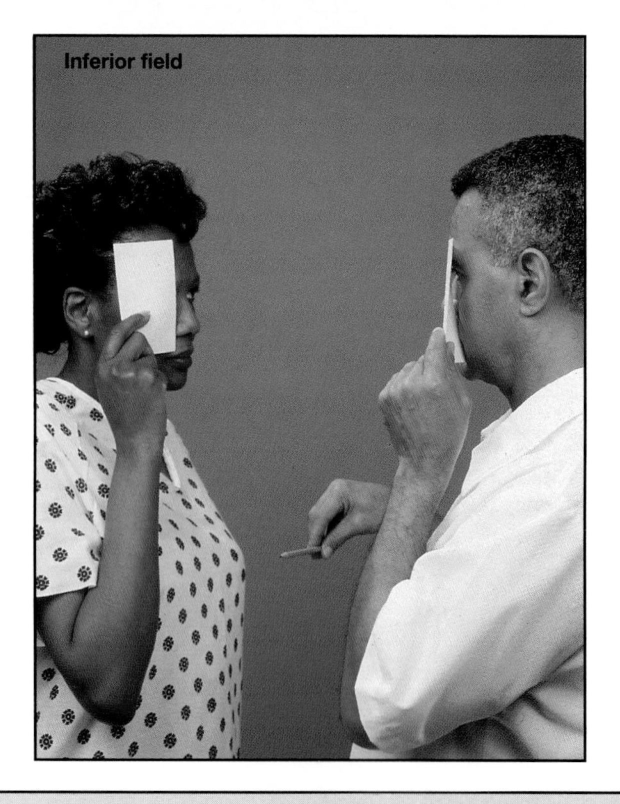
Inferior field

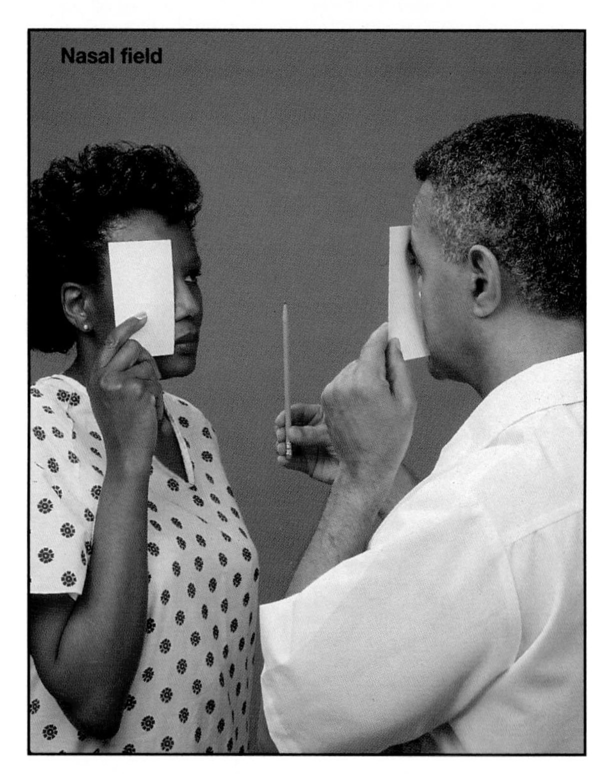
Nasal field

■ Inspection

Bulbar conjunctiva

To assess the bulbar conjunctiva, gently pull down the lower eyelid and examine it as the client looks up, down, left, and right. Normally, the bulbar conjunctiva appears clear and free from drainage.

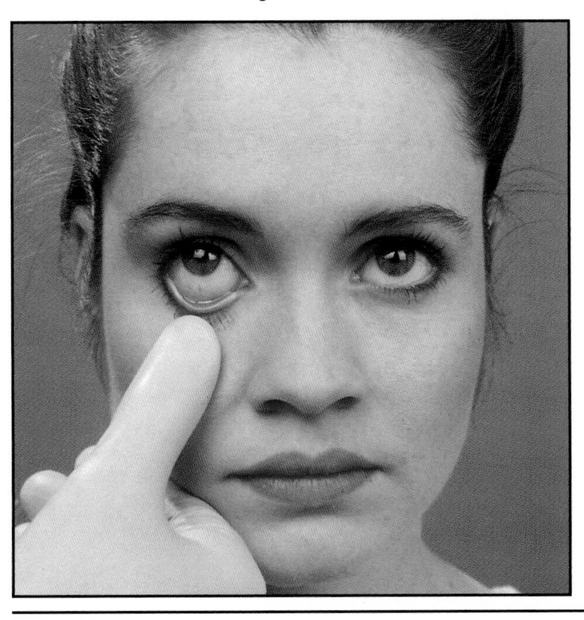

Palpebral conjunctiva

To assess the palpebral conjunctiva, gently evert the upper eyelid and inspect it as the client looks down. Normally, the palpebral conjunctiva appears pink and free from swelling.

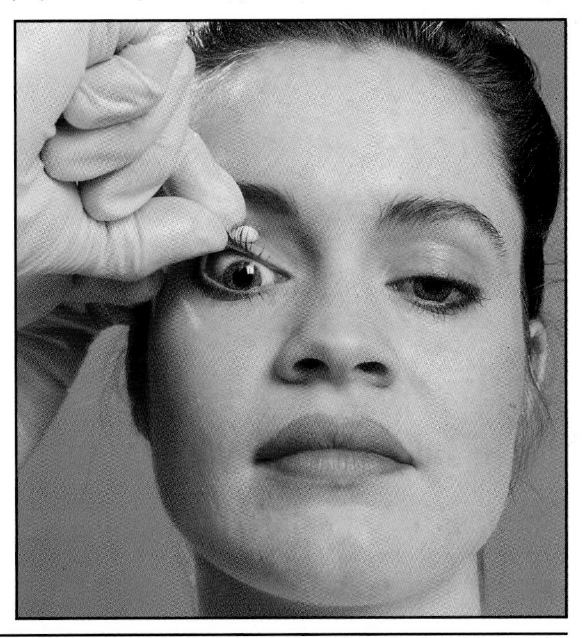

Cornea

Inspect the cornea by shining a light on it from several side angles. The cornea should be clear, transparent, and free from opacities or abrasions.

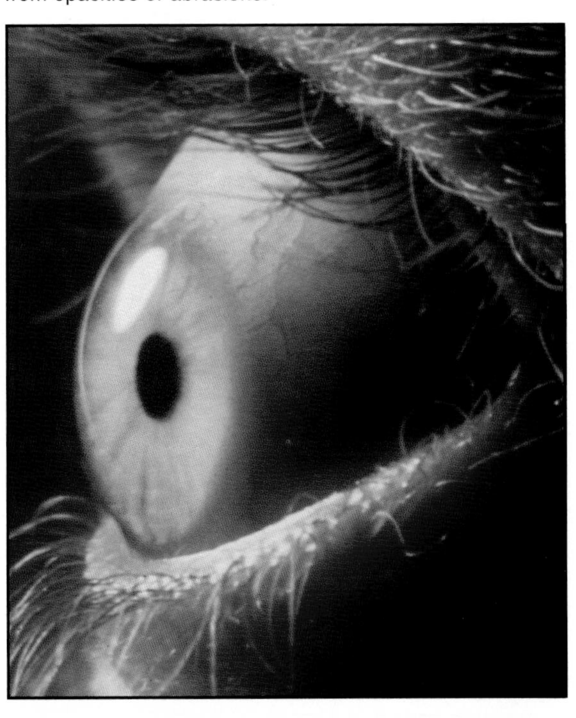

Corneal reflex

Test the corneal reflex by lightly stroking the cornea with a wisp of cotton. If cranial nerves V (the trigeminal nerve) and VII (the facial nerve) are intact, both eyes will close when either cornea is touched.

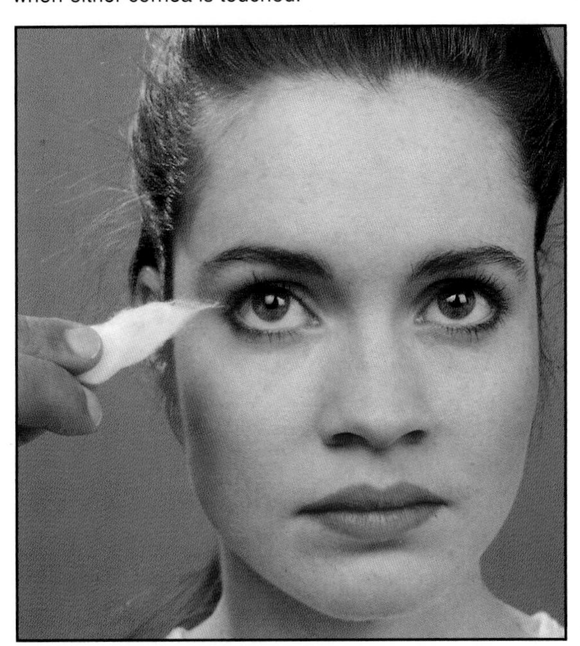

(continued)

ASSESSMENT

INSPECTION (continued)

Anterior chamber

With the client looking forward, inspect the anterior chamber by shining a light on the eyes from the side. The anterior chamber should be clear and transparent, and the iris should appear flat.

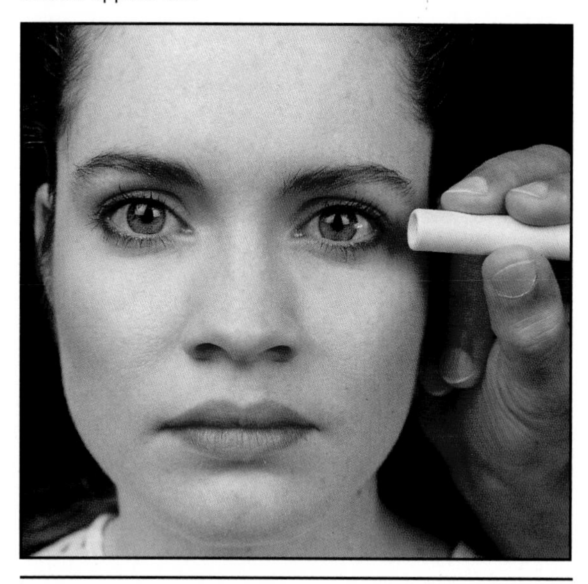

Pupillary accommodation

Assess accommodation by having the client stare at an object across the room. Normally, the pupils dilate. Then ask the client to focus on an object as you move it in from about 2' away. When the client changes focus, the pupils should converge and constrict equally on the object when it is 5 to 10 cm away.

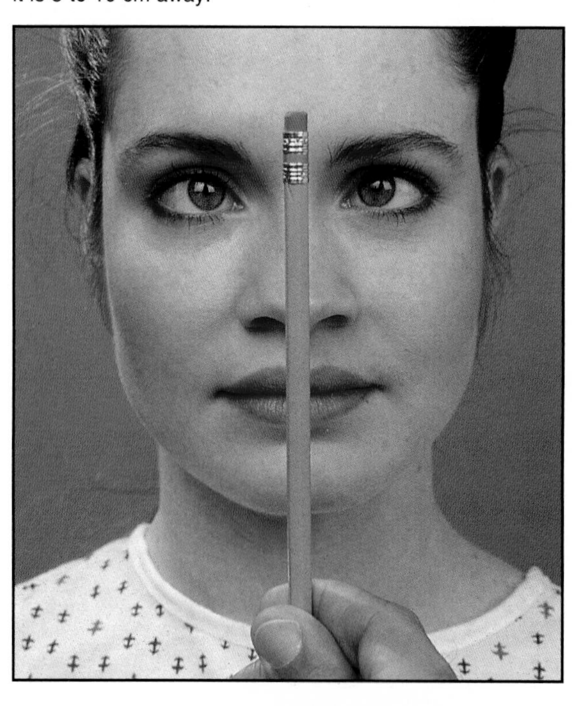

Pupillary reaction to light

First assess the client's pupils in normal room light (top photo). Then darken the room, and assess pupillary reaction by sweeping a light from the side of one eye to the center of its pupil (bottom photo). The pupils should react simultaneously, directly and consensually. Also note the size and equality of pupils, which should appear round and equal.

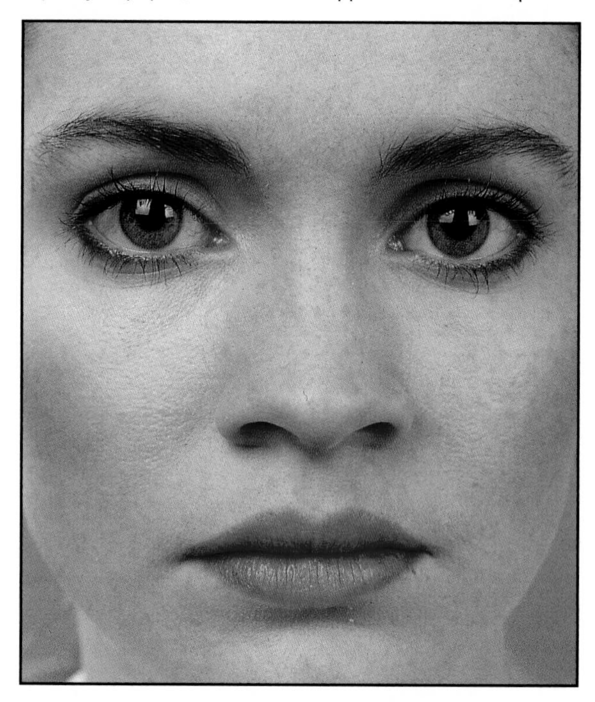

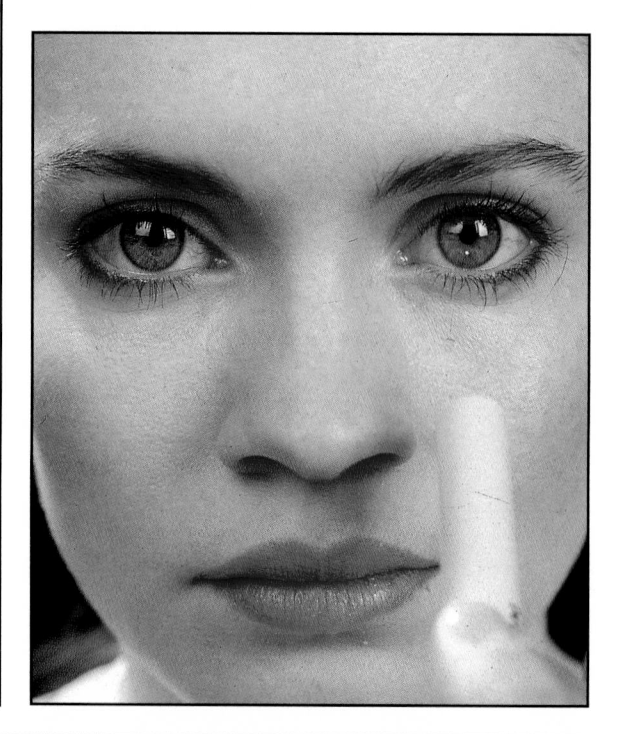

Palpation

Lacrimal gland

Assess the lacrimal gland by palpating the eyelid below the eyebrows with the index finger. Normally, palpation reveals no tenderness.

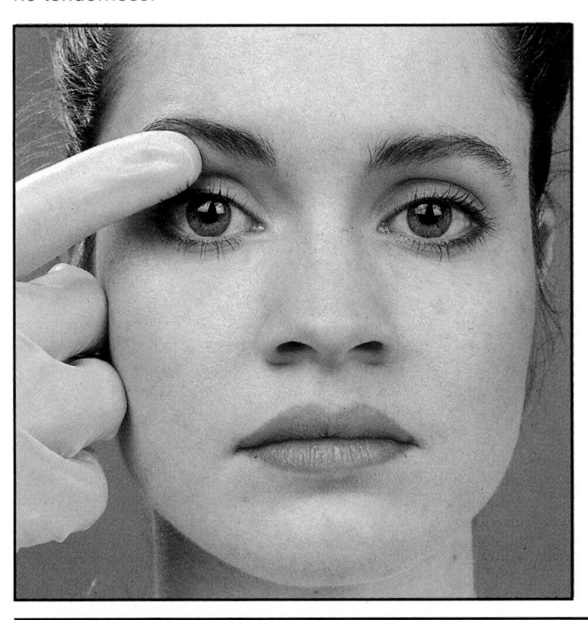

Lacrimal sac

To assess the lacrimal sac, palpate the lower orbital rim on the side closest to the nose and observe the punctum. Palpation should not elicit regurgitation of purulent material or excessive tearing.

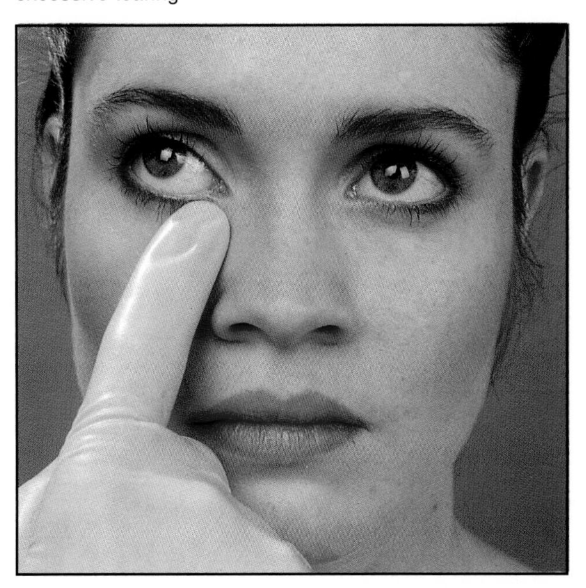

Ophthalmoscopic examination

Red reflex

In a darkened room, stand or sit about 1½" from the client. Using an ophthalmoscope, examine the client's eye while moving in at an oblique angle. When a small circle of light falls on the pupil, the red reflex should appear as a sharp, distinct orange-red glow through the pupil. Repeat this process for the other eye.

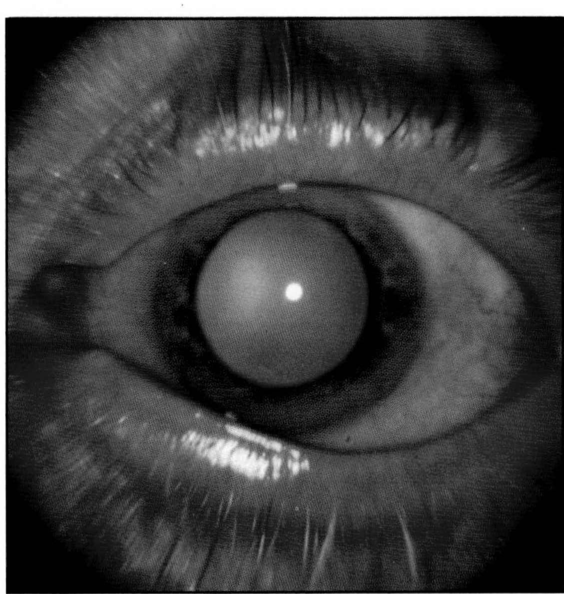

Retinal structures

Move closer to the client, adjusting the lens as needed to focus on retinal structures. The retinal vessels normally have an atriovenous ratio of 2:3 or 4:5. The optic disk should be orange-red with distinct margins. The physiologic cup is normally yellow-white and readily visible.

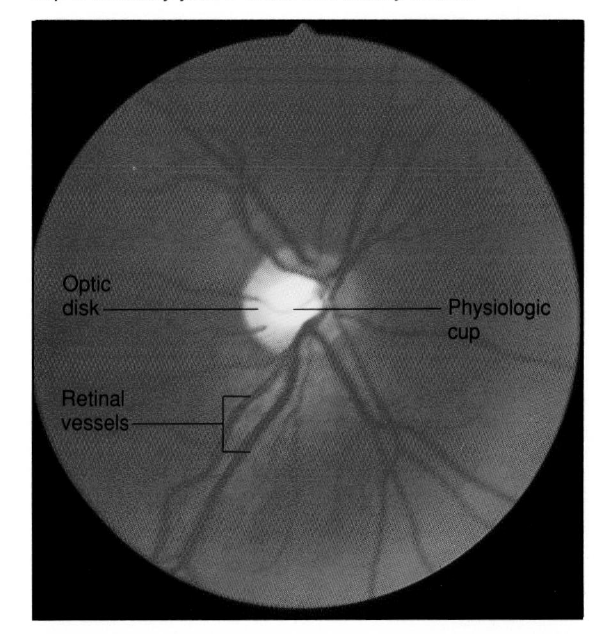

Ethnic considerations

Epicanthal folds

In Asian clients, skin folds that cover the inner canthus are a normal finding.

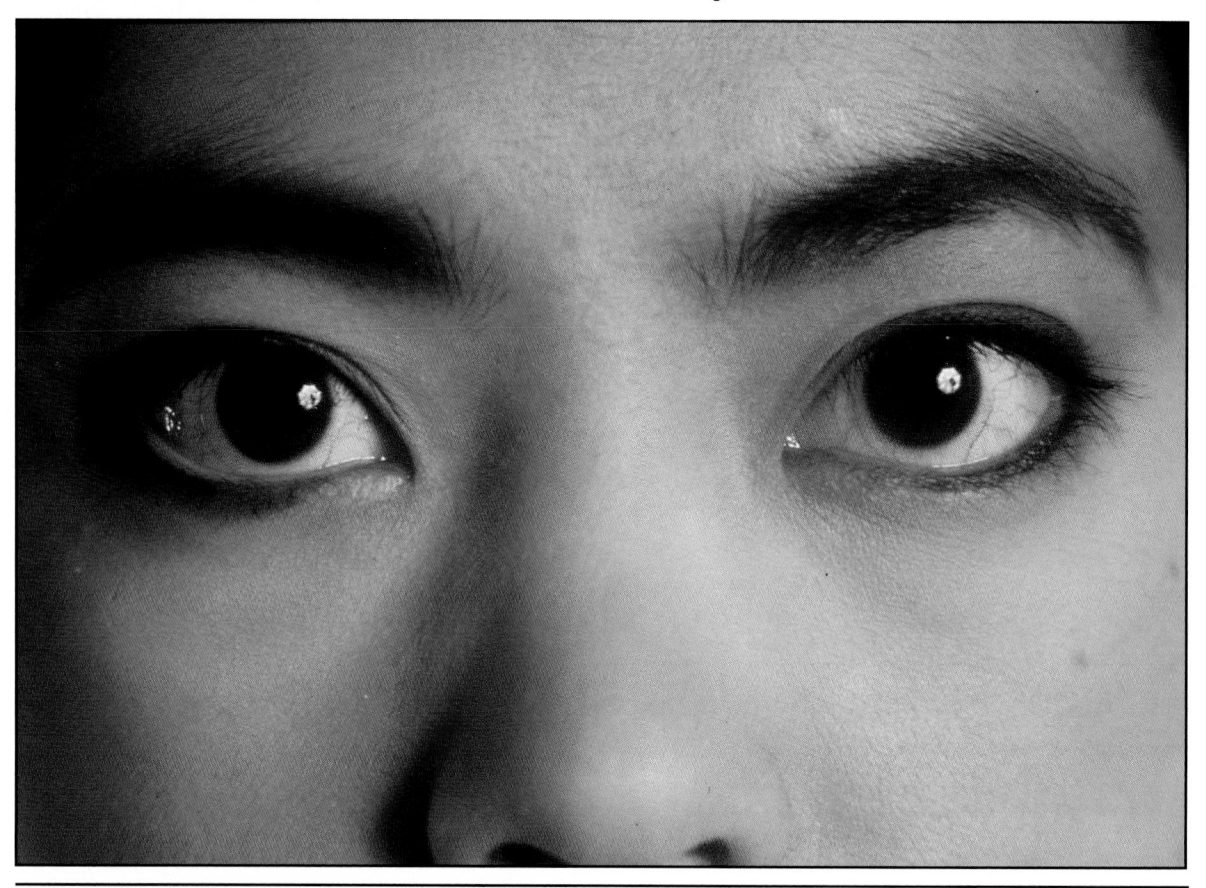

Optic disk and retina

The color of the optic disk and retina normally varies with the client's skin pigmentation. (Fair-skinned client, left photo; dark-skinned client, right photo).

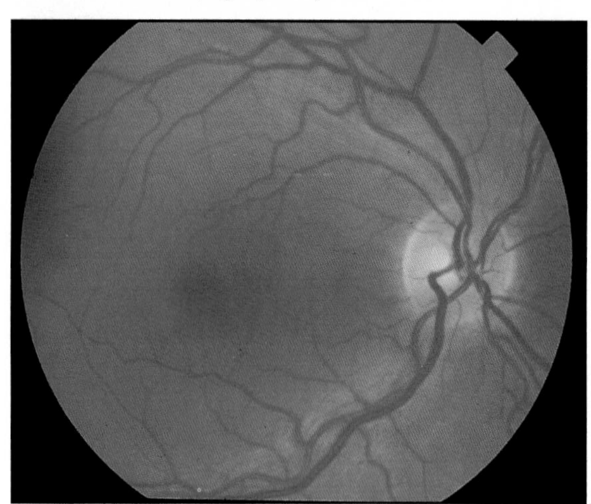

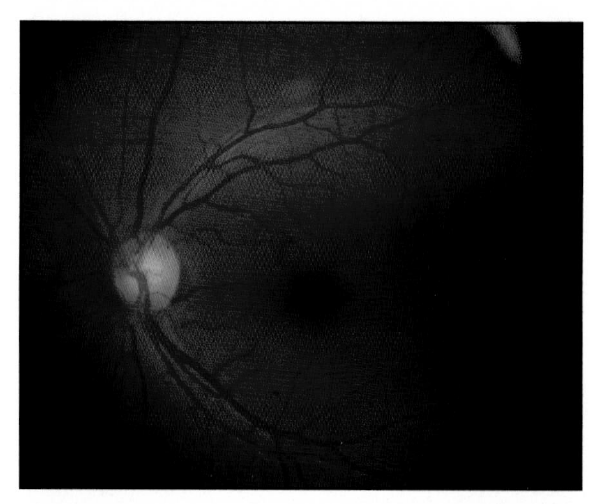

Developmental considerations

■ Pupil size variation

Pupil size depends on the client's age and normally ranges from 3 to 7 mm. Infants have small pupils that become larger during childhood and then progressively smaller throughout adulthood into old age.

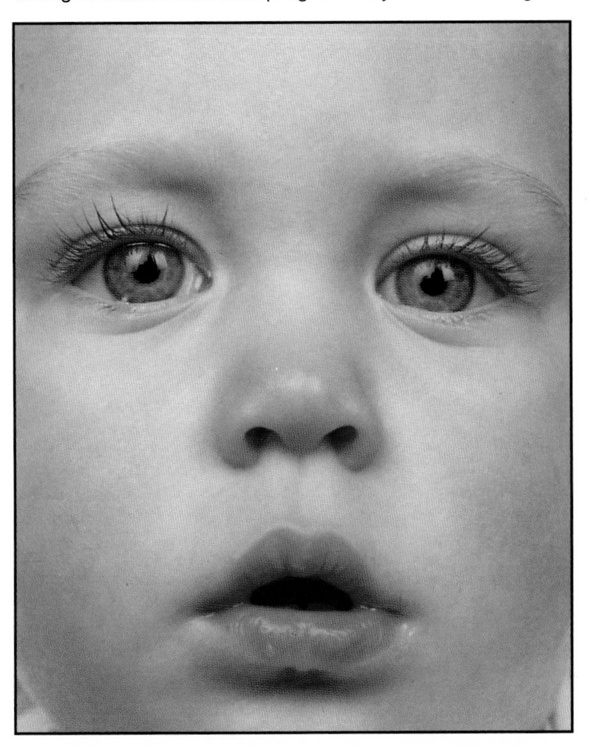

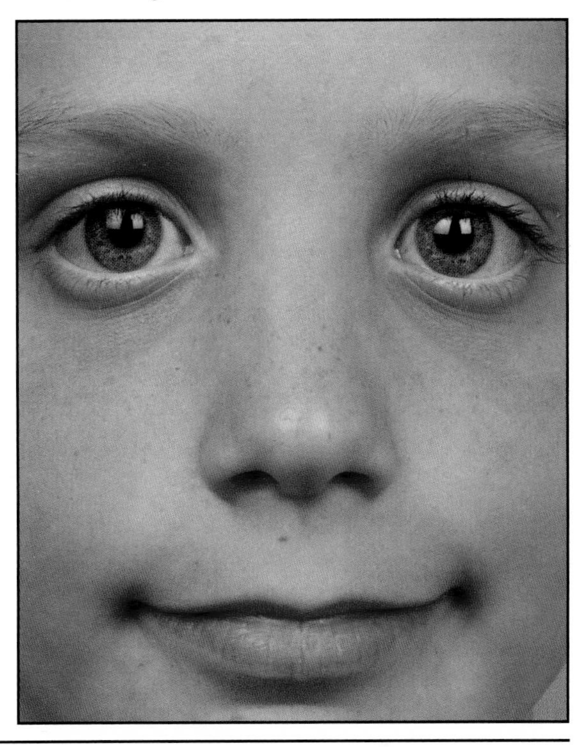

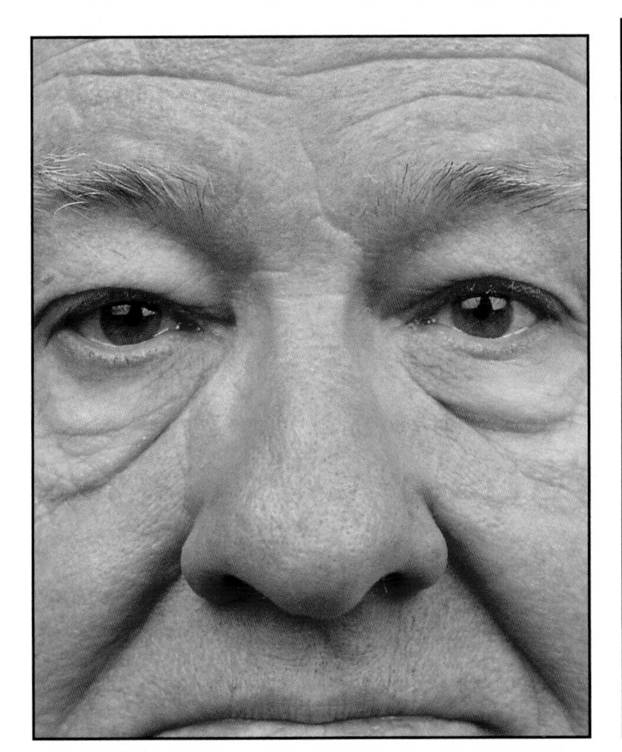

■ Arcus senilis

A thin, gray-white ring around the cornea results from lipid deposits and is normal in elderly clients.

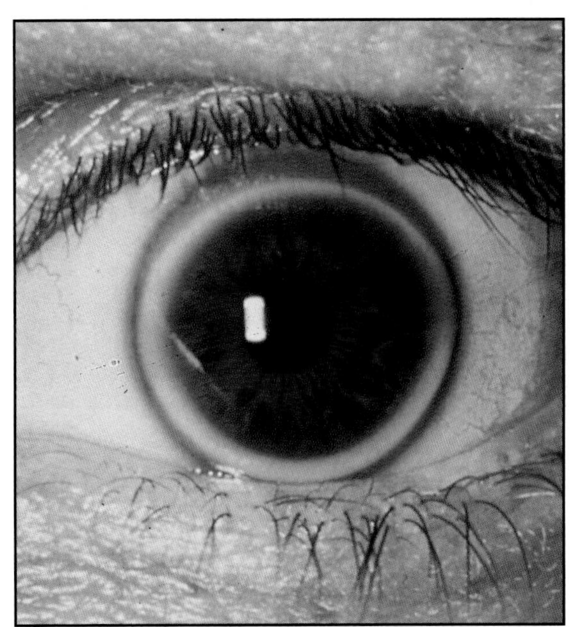

Common abnormalities

■ Esotropia

This condition may result from a disturbance in extraocular muscle function.

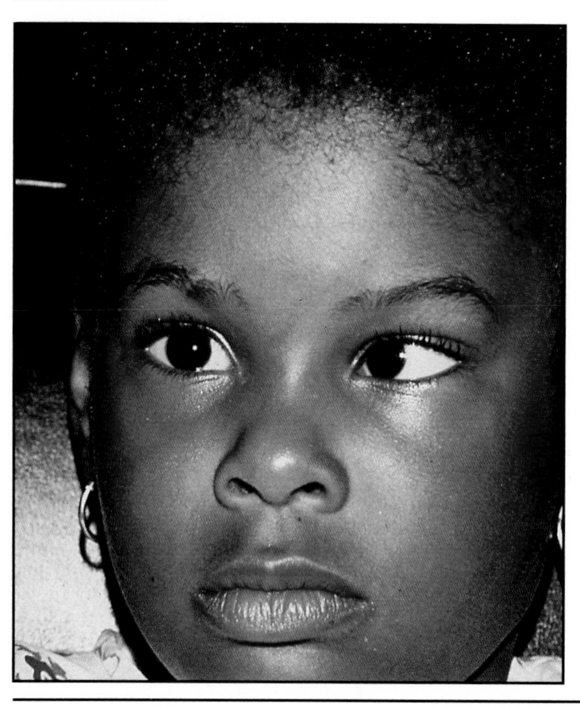

■ Ptosis

Drooping of the eyelid below the middle of the iris may be associated with abnormal extraocular muscle function, as in myasthenia gravis.

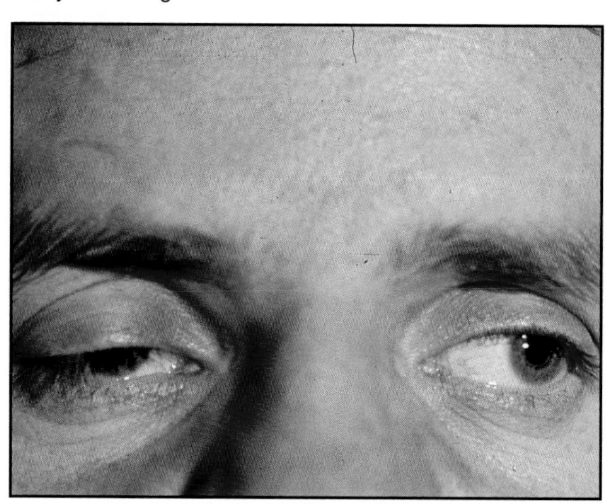

■ Ectropion

Eversion of the lower lid, which results from loss of muscle tone, displaces the punctum away from the inner canthus.

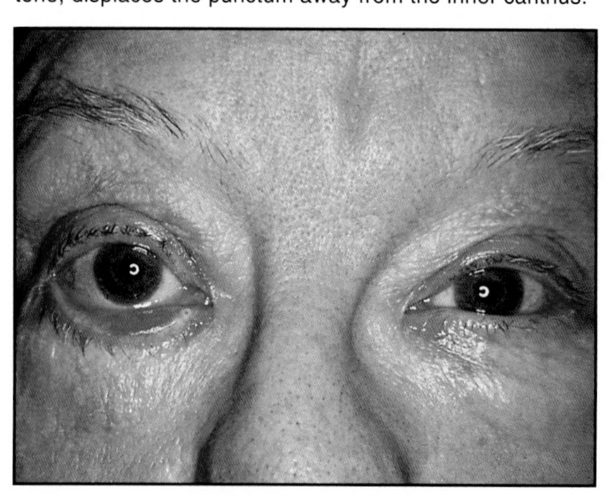

■ Entropion

Inversion of the lid and lashes, which can result from eyelid spasms or eyelid scars from styes, may damage the cornea.

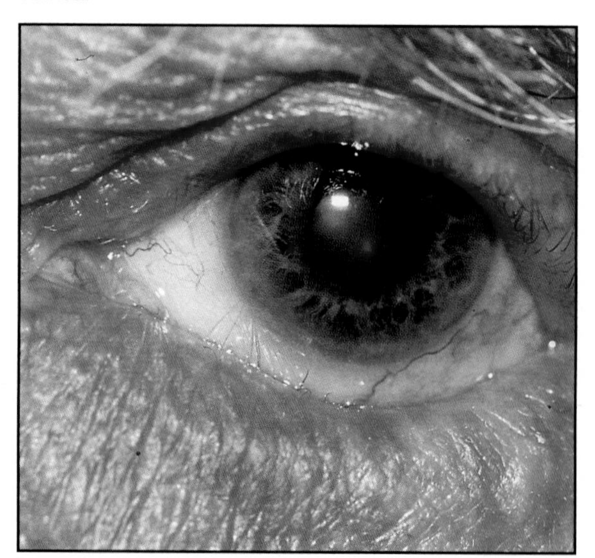

■ Xanthelasma

Soft, yellow spots on the eyelids result from elevated cholesterol deposits.

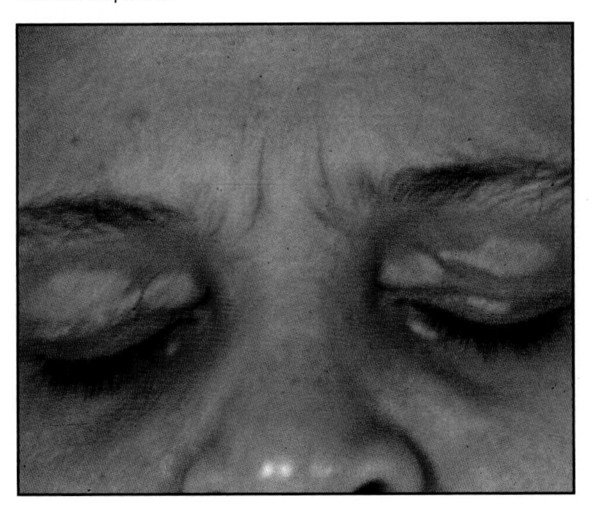

■ Inflamed conjunctiva

Red, engorged conjunctiva signals conjunctivitis, which may be caused by a bacterial or viral infection.

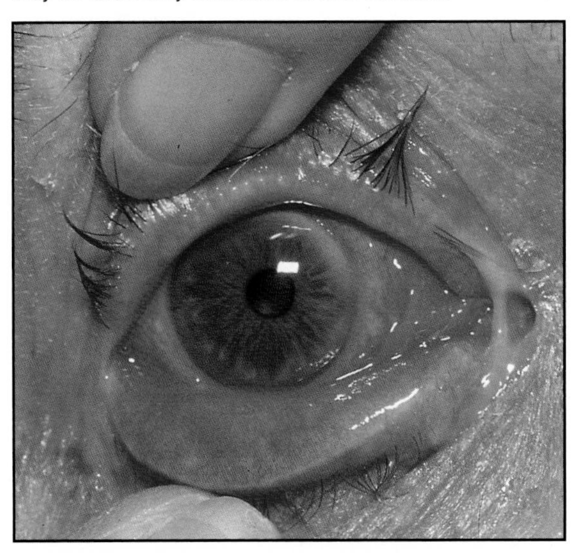

■ Red, swollen eyelid gland

A red, swollen sebaceous gland suggests a hordeolum (stye), which usually results from infection of an eyelash follicle.

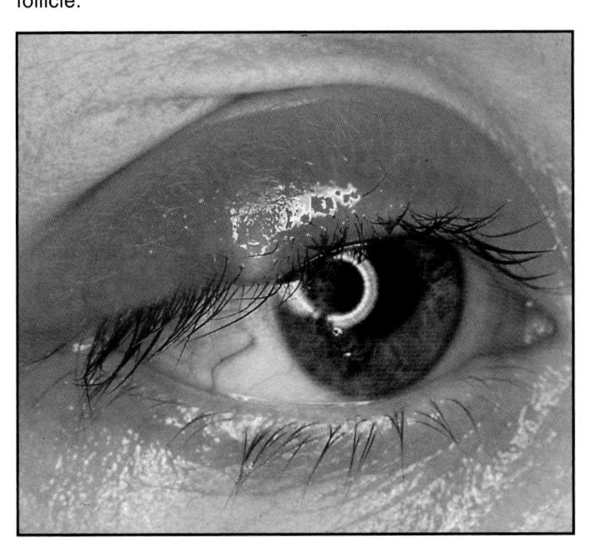

■ Eyelid nodule

A small, localized swelling of the eyelid indicates chalazion, an infection of the meibomian gland.

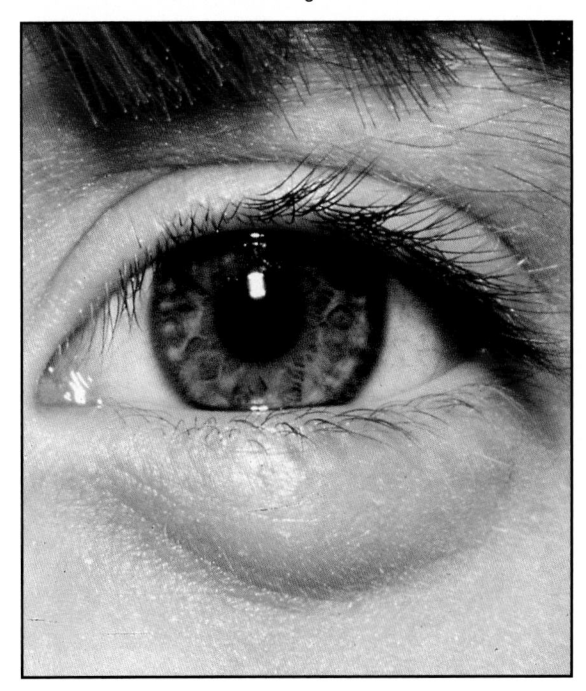

COMMON ABNORMALITIES

Corneal abrasions

These abrasions usually result from injury and may cause pain, inflammation, and photophobia.

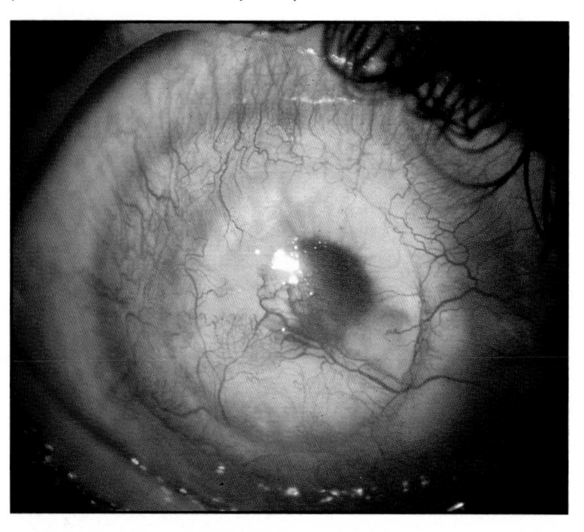

Papilledema

Characterized by blurred borders of the optic disk, this finding is associated with increased intracranial pressure.

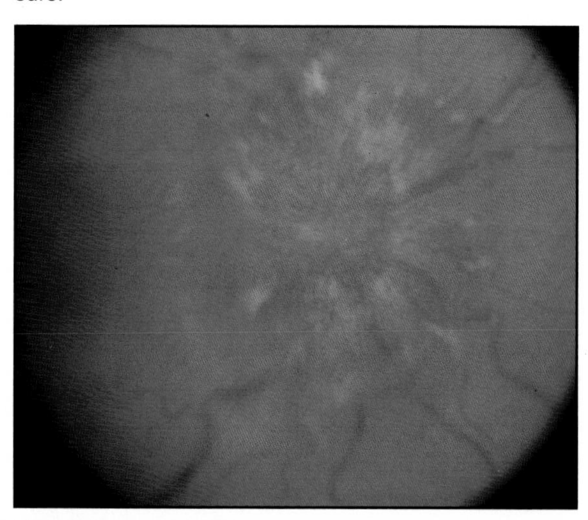

Optic disk atrophy

In this condition, the optic nerve fibers die and the tiny disk vessels begin to disappear. The atrophied disk appears whiter than normal. This abnormality is common in clients with multiple sclerosis or glaucoma.

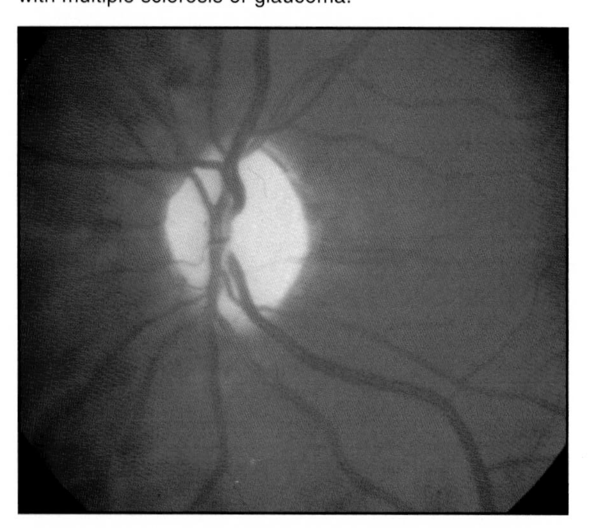

Cupped optic disk

The shape of the optic disk may change from round to cupped when the intraocular pressure increases, as in glaucoma.

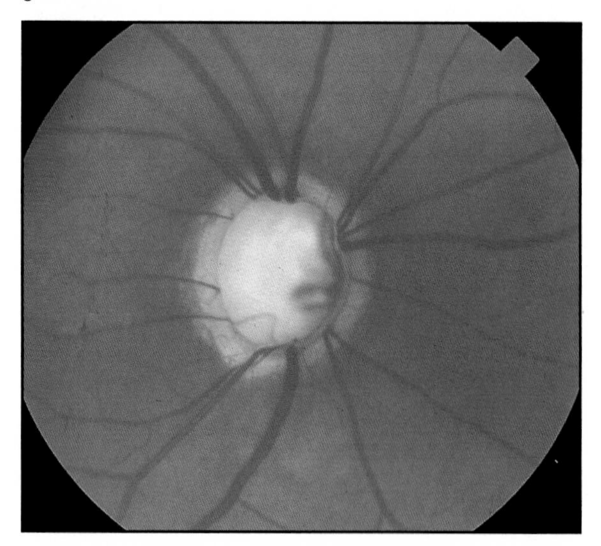

■ Superficial retinal hemorrhages

These hemorrhages appear as red, flame-shaped streaks in the fundus. They may be seen in clients with hypertension or papilledema.

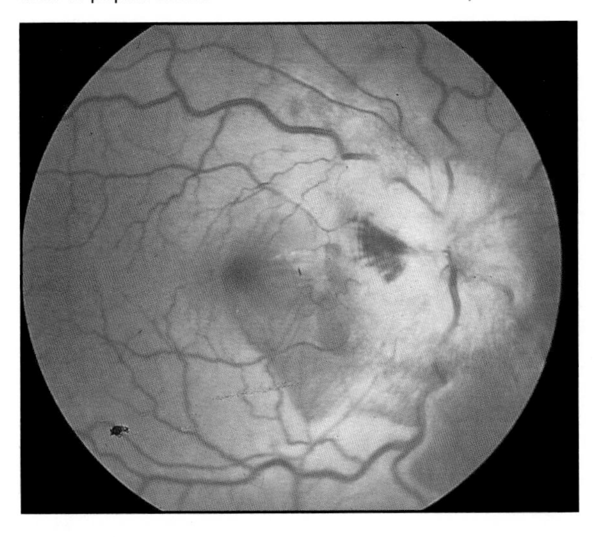

■ Soft exudates

Also known as cottonwool patches, these soft, yellow to gray exudates with irregular borders are retinal infiltrates that result from microinfarctions, which commonly occur in clients with hypertension

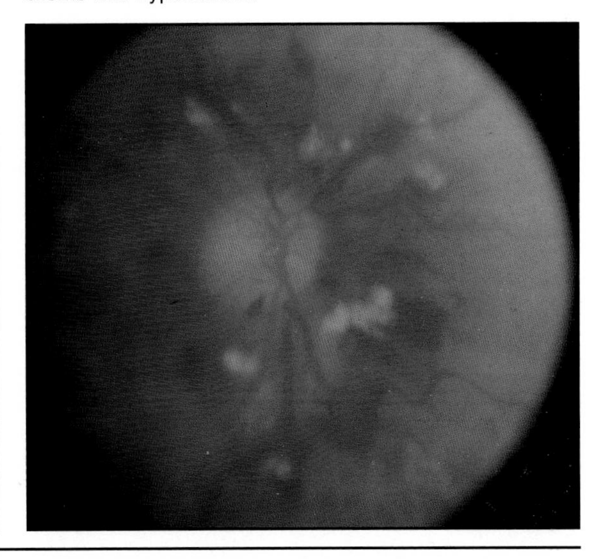

■ Hard exudates

Yellow exudates may be small and round with well-defined borders or may coalesce into larger irregular spots. These hard exudates are retinal infiltrates that may accompany diabetes or hypertension.

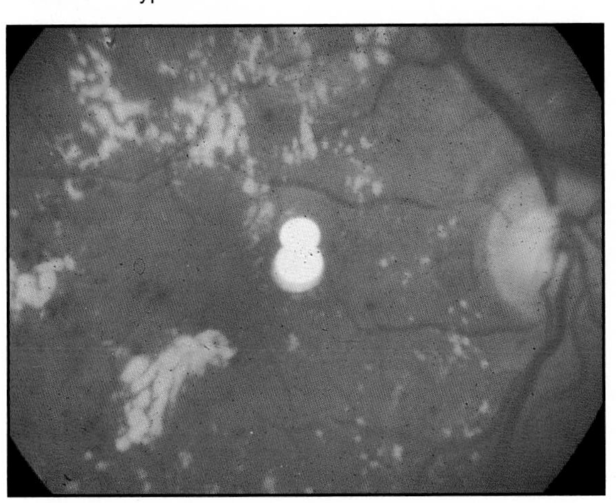

■ Lens opacities

Ophthalmic examination may uncover opacities of various shapes and colors. They may be caused by cataracts.

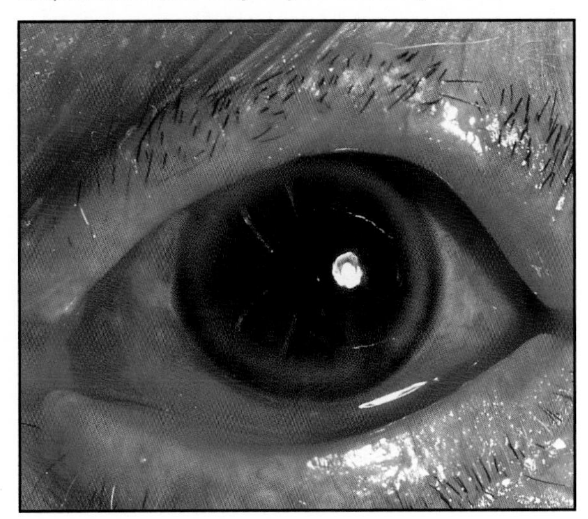

Anatomy and physiology overview

■ External ear structures and tympanic membrane

This photograph identifies the structures of the external ear, which serve as useful landmarks during assessment. The otoscopic view below shows the structural landmarks of the tympanic membrane.

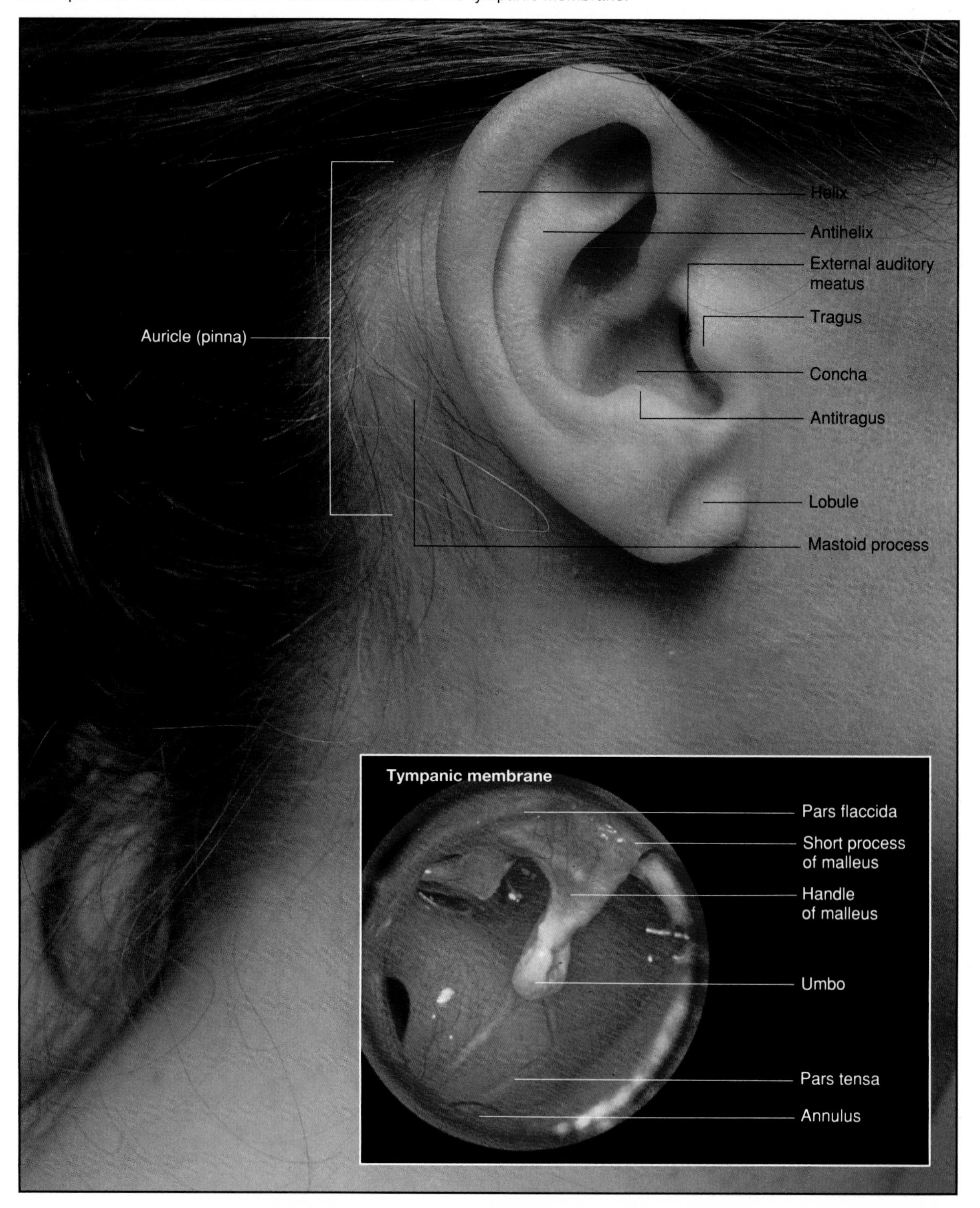

Assessment

■ Inspection

Ear position

Note the position of the auricle in relation to an imaginary line from the outer canthus of the eye to the protuberance of the occiput. The ear position should be almost vertical with no more than a 10-degree lateral-posterior slant.

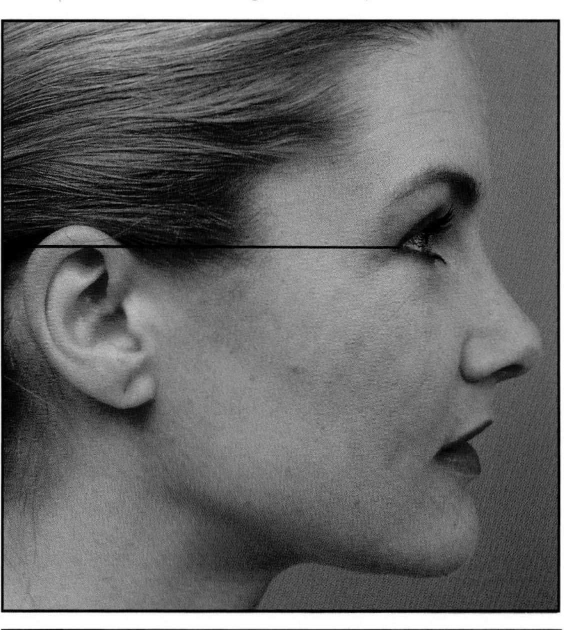

■ Palpation

Following the sequence shown, palpate the tragus, mastoid process, and helix. If tenderness is present, proceed carefully with the otoscopic examination.

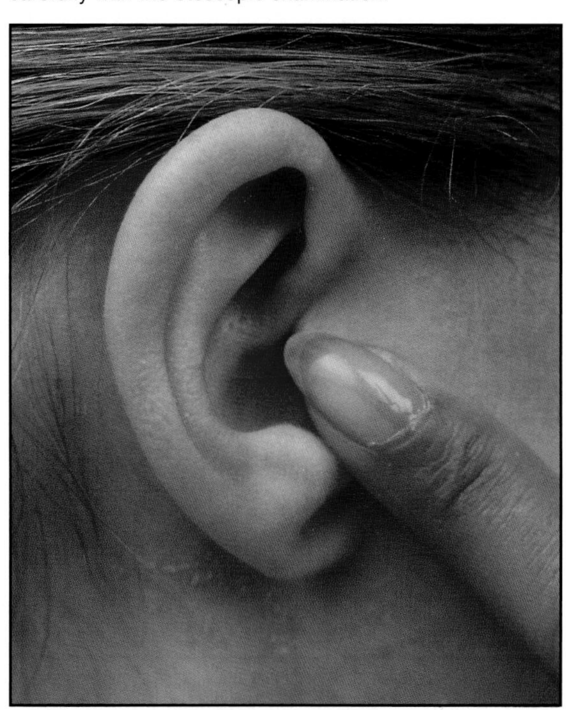

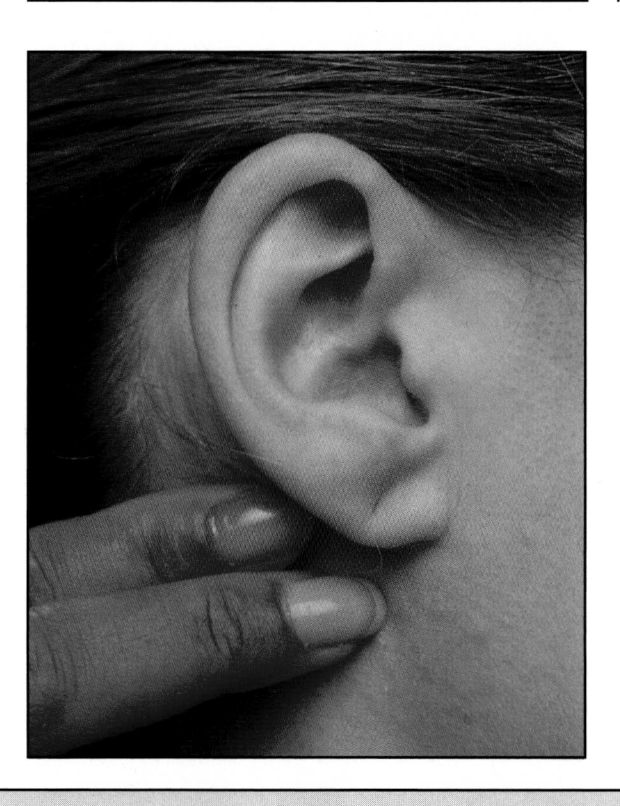

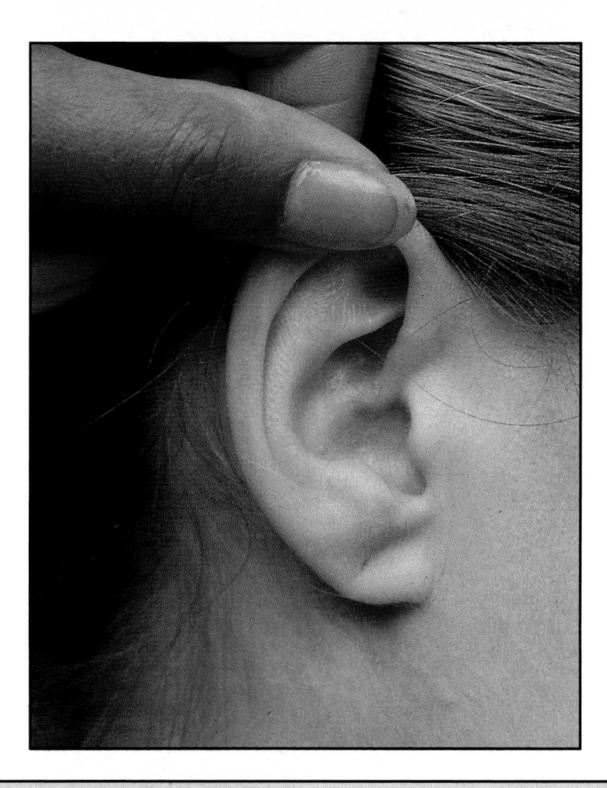

ASSESSMENT

■ Hearing screening

Rinne test

Perform the Rinne test for each ear to compare bone conduction to air conduction.

1 Assess bone conduction by placing the base of a vibrating tuning fork on the mastoid process. Note how many seconds pass before the client can no longer hear the tone.

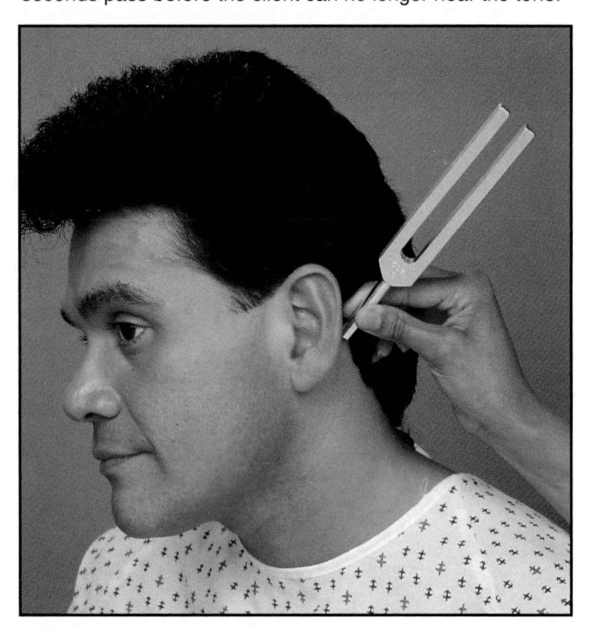

2 While the tuning fork is still vibrating, place the tines near the ear canal. Note how many seconds the client can hear the tone. This part of the test assesses air conduction. Normally, air conduction is twice as long as bone conduction (2:1) bilaterally.

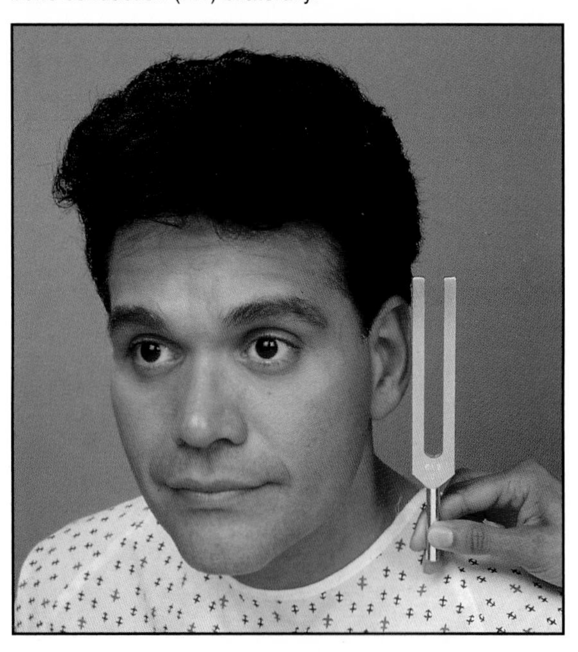

Weber's test

To evaluate bone conduction, perform Weber's test. Place a vibrating tuning fork midline at the top of the client's head or forehead. Normally, the client perceives the sound equally in both ears.

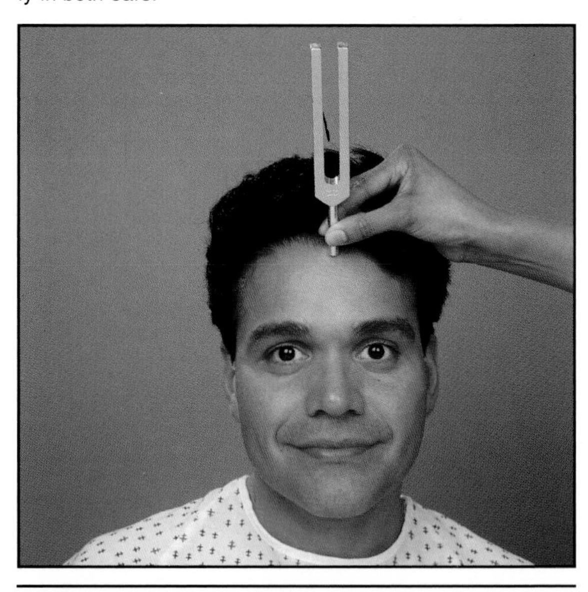

■ Otoscopic examination

To perform an otoscopic examination on an adult, tip the client's head to the side opposite from the ear being assessed. Straighten the ear canal by pulling the auricle up and back. Then gently insert the otoscope, and assess the external ear canal and the tympanic membrane. Normally, the external canal may have a small amount of cerumen, but has no inflammation or lesions. The tympanic membrane is pearl gray and intact with appropriately placed landmarks. The light reflex appears in the 7 o'clock position in the left ear and in the 5 o'clock position in the right ear.

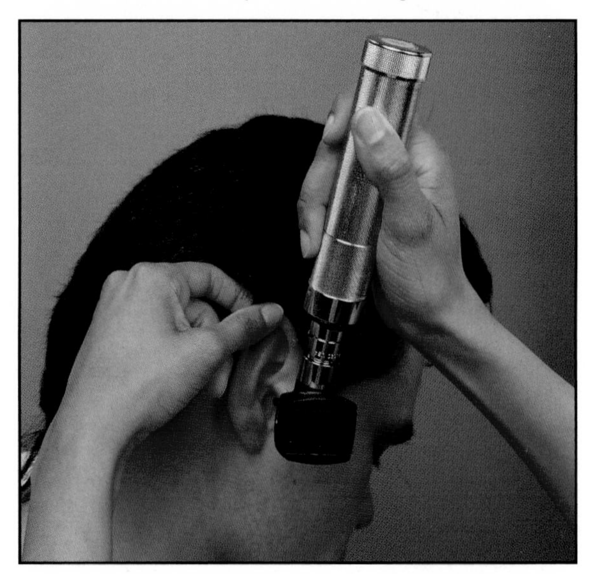

Developmental considerations

■ Pediatric otoscopic examination

When performing an otoscopic examination on an infant or young child, straighten the ear canal by pulling the auricle down and back.

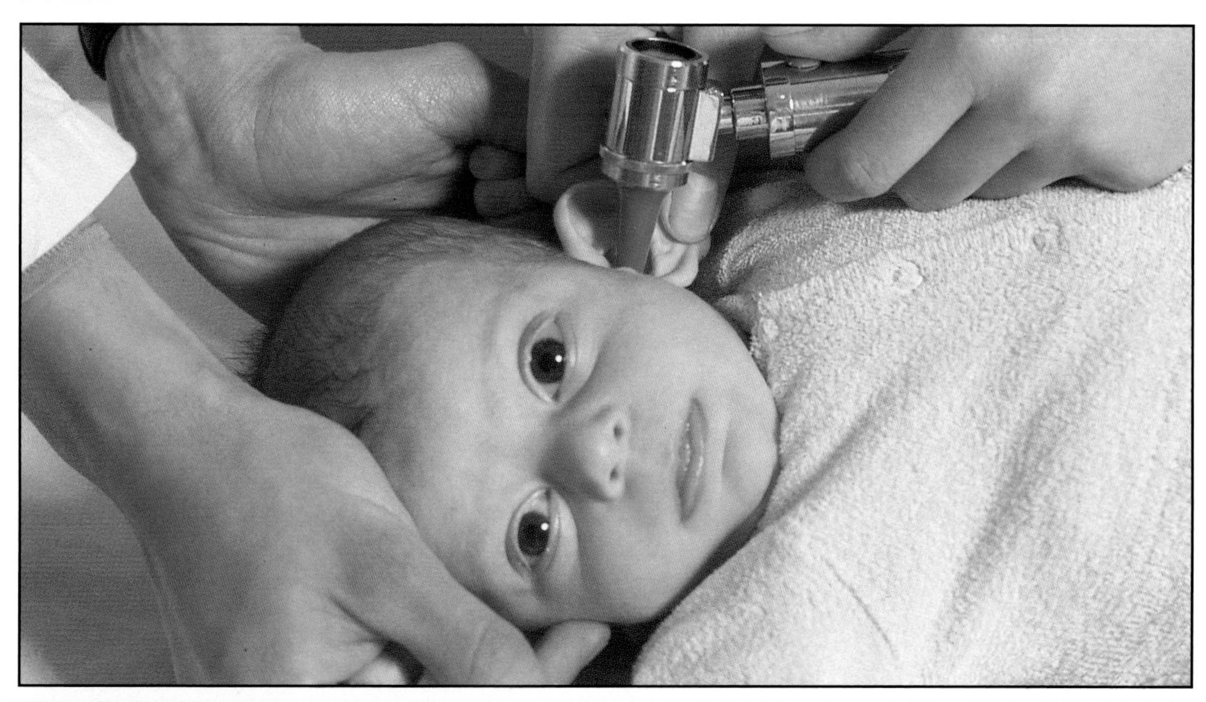

Common abnormalities

■ Red, bulging tympanic membrane

This otoscopic finding suggests inflammation caused by otitis media.

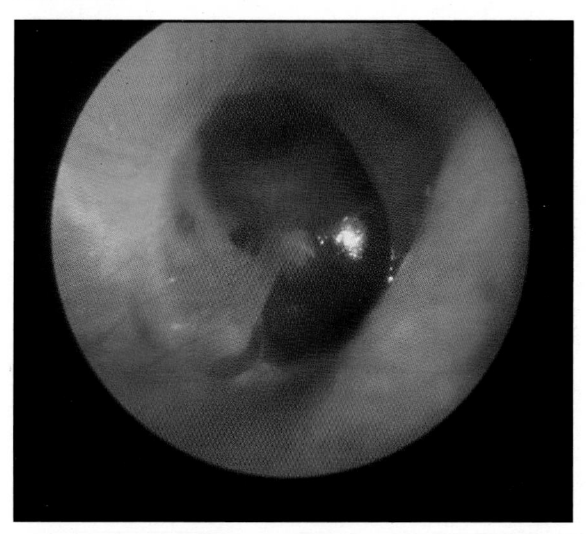

■ External ear canal drainage

Painless, purulent drainage from the external ear canal may indicate chronic suppurative otitis media, which can result from prolonged fluid accumulation in the middle ear.

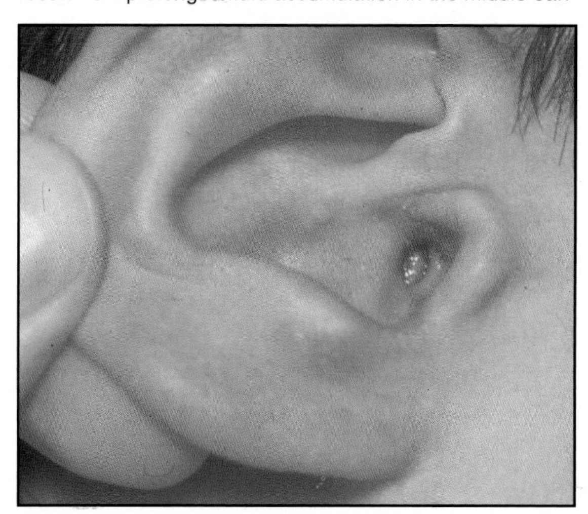

Respiratory System

Anatomy and physiology overview

■ Structures of the respiratory system

This anterior view of the thorax shows the structures of the respiratory system.

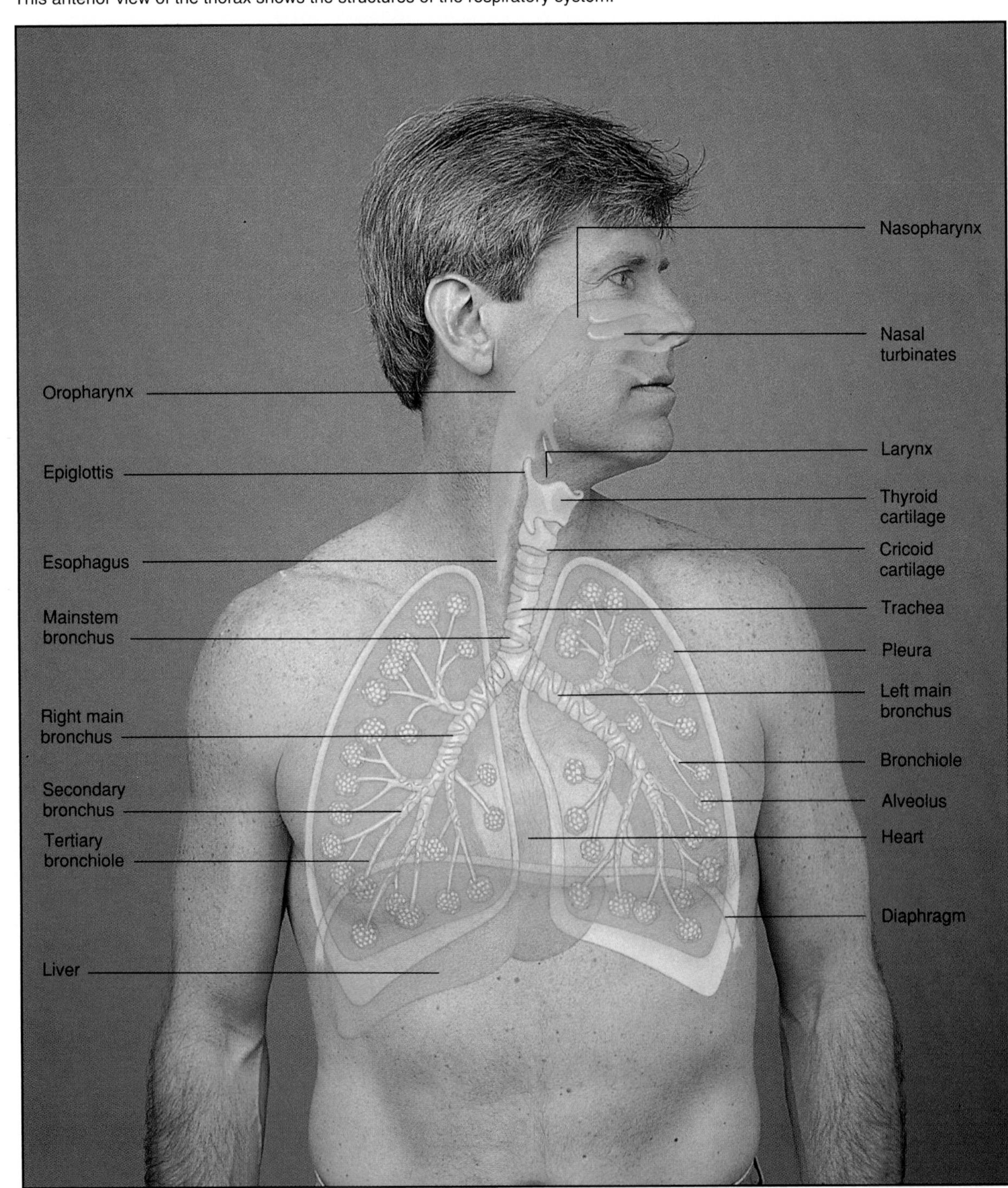

ANATOMY AND PHYSIOLOGY OVERVIEW

Thoracic landmarks

These anterior and posterior views of the thorax identify the thoracic landmarks.

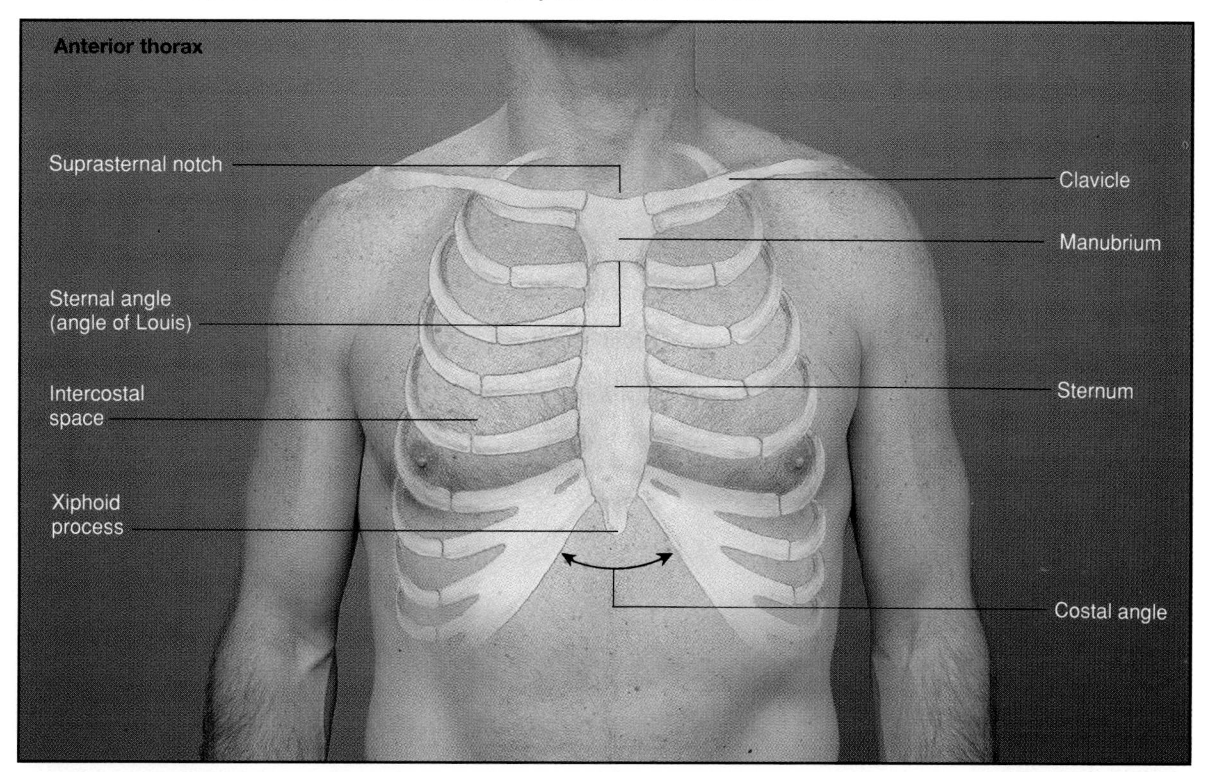

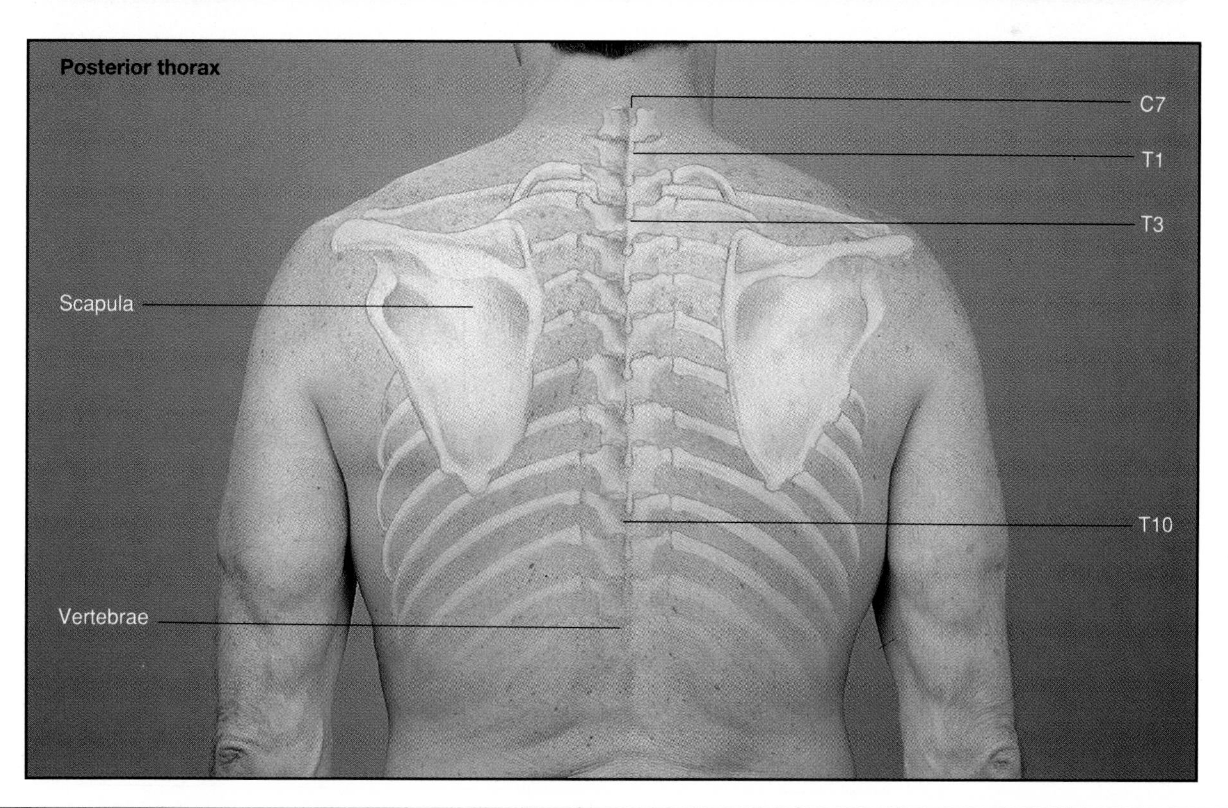

ANATOMY AND PHYSIOLOGY OVERVIEW

■ Lung lobes and anatomical lines

These anterior, posterior, and lateral views of the thorax show the relationship between the lung lobes and anatomical lines (imaginary lines that help the nurse identify underlying structures).

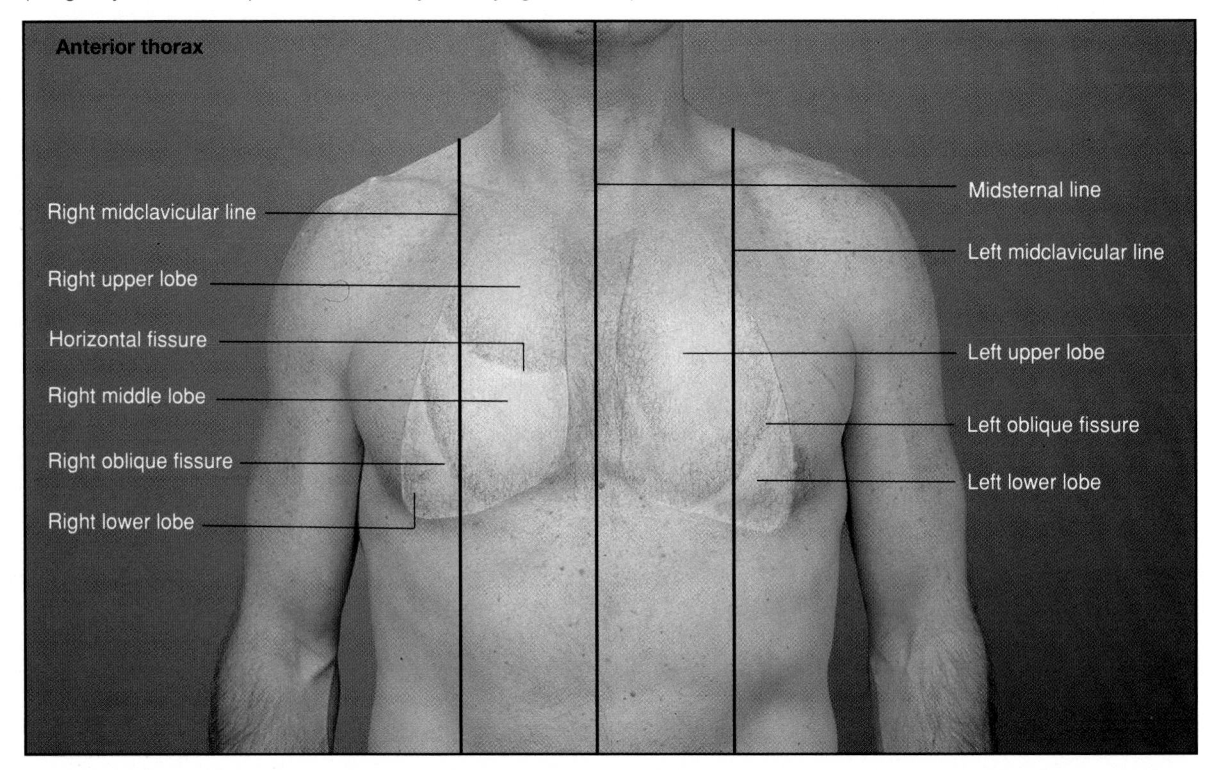

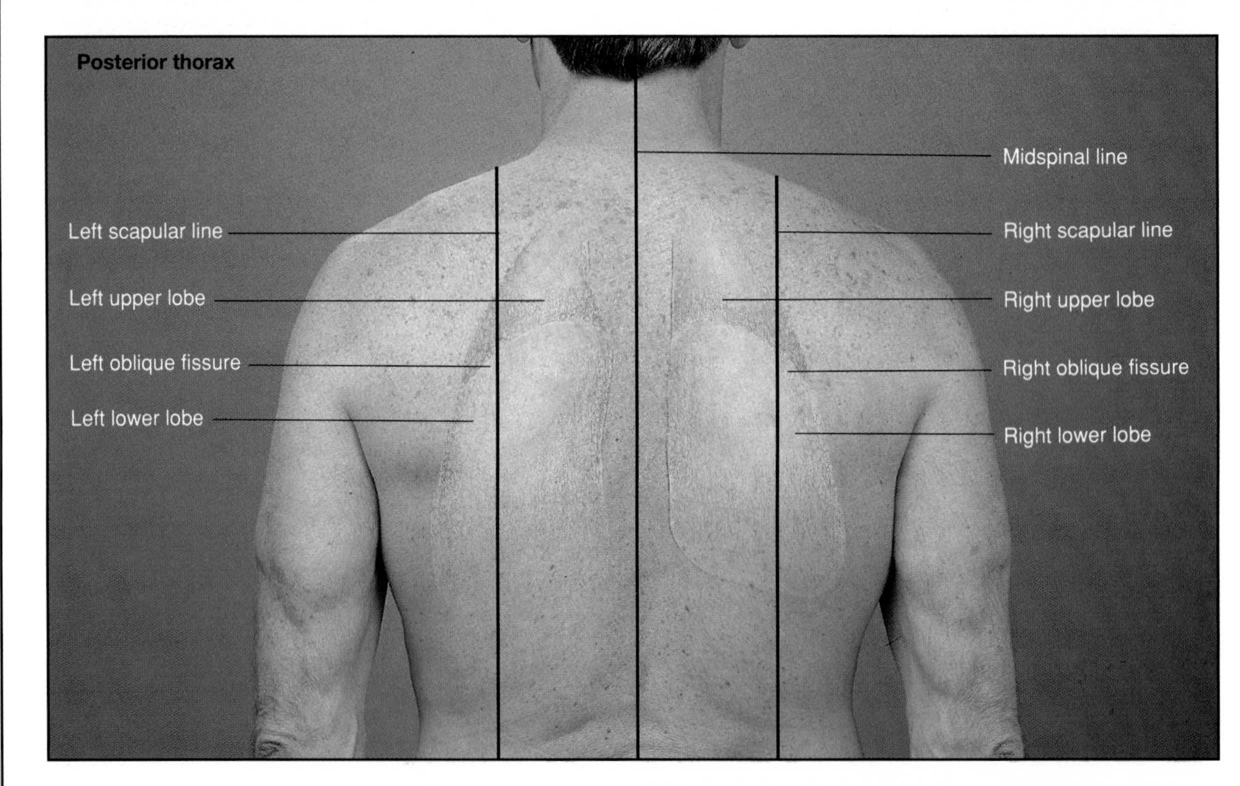

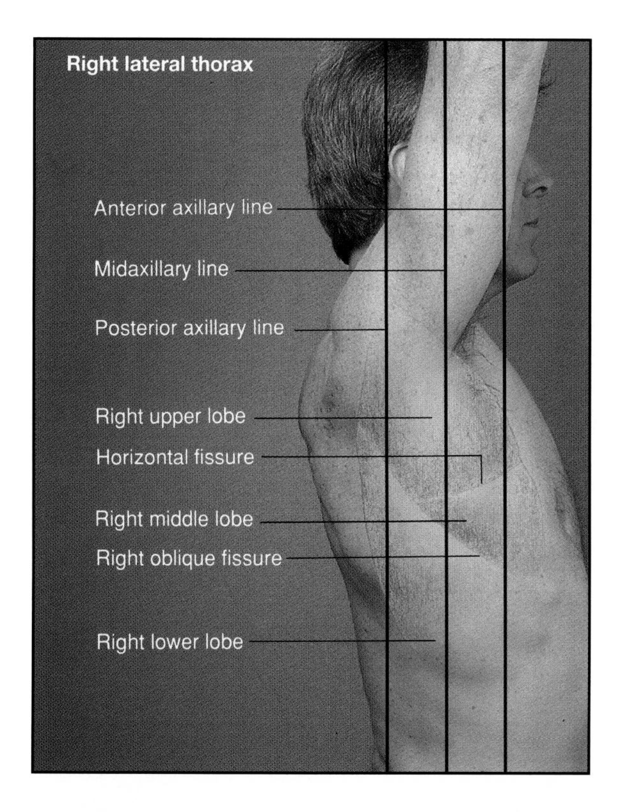

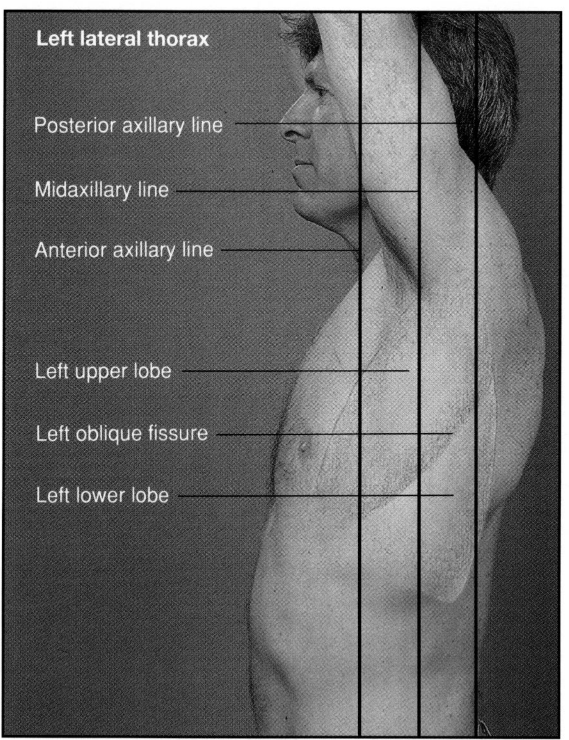

Assessment

■ Inspection

Mucous membranes

Inspect the mucous membranes, which normally appear pink, for color changes that suggest cyanosis. In dark-skinned clients, color changes are best detected by inspecting the oral mucosa and lips.

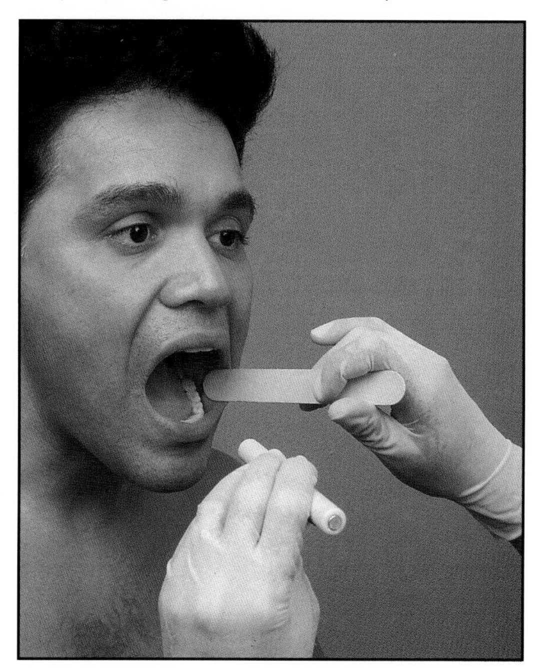

Fingernails

Inspect the fingertips for clubbing. The angle between the fingernail and the point where it enters the skin normally is about 160 degrees.

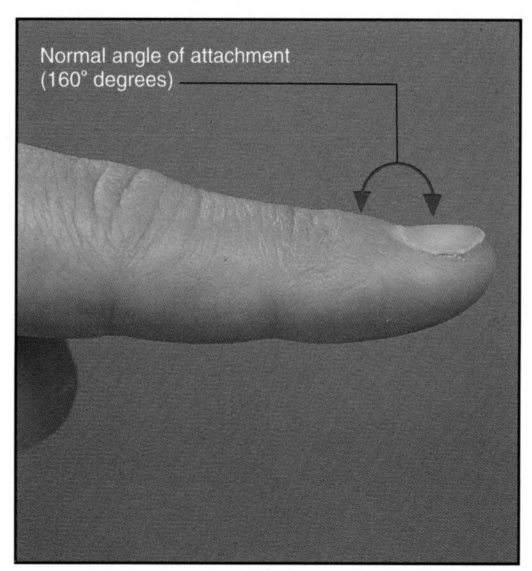

(continued)

ASSESSMENT

INSPECTION (continued)

Chest

Inspect the chest from the front and side to assess the lateral and anteroposterior diameters. In an adult, these diameters have a 1:2 ratio.

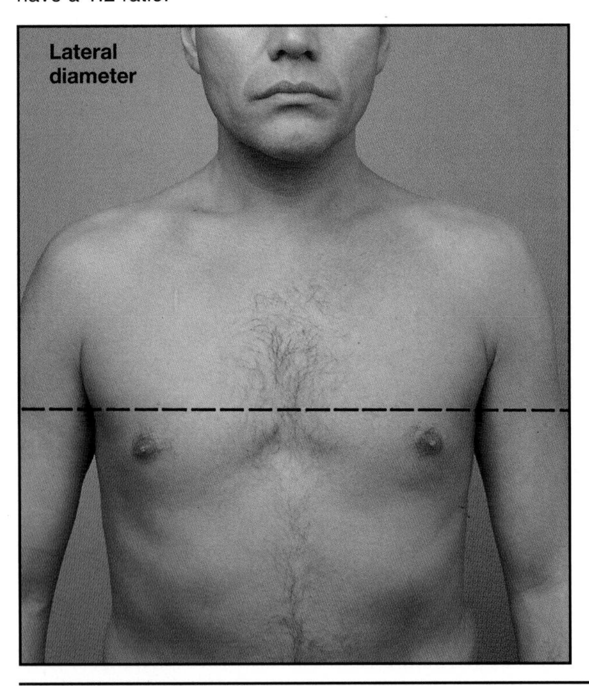

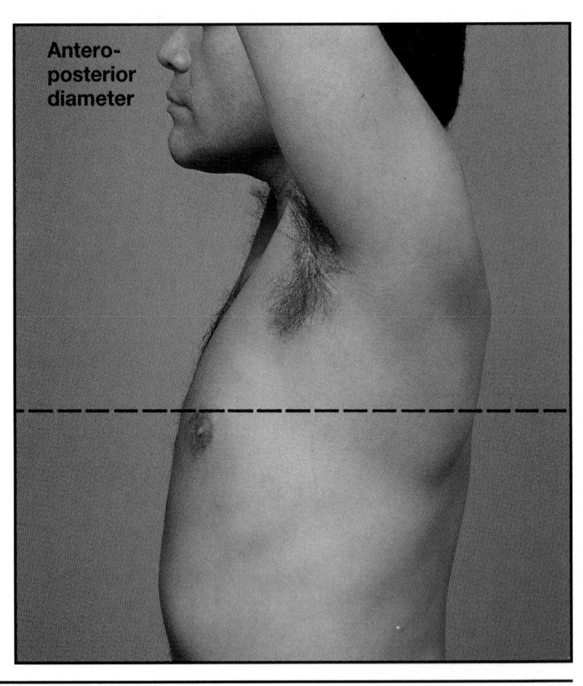

■ Palpation

Tracheal position

Palpate the trachea by placing one thumb on either side of the trachea above the suprasternal notch. The trachea normally is midline.

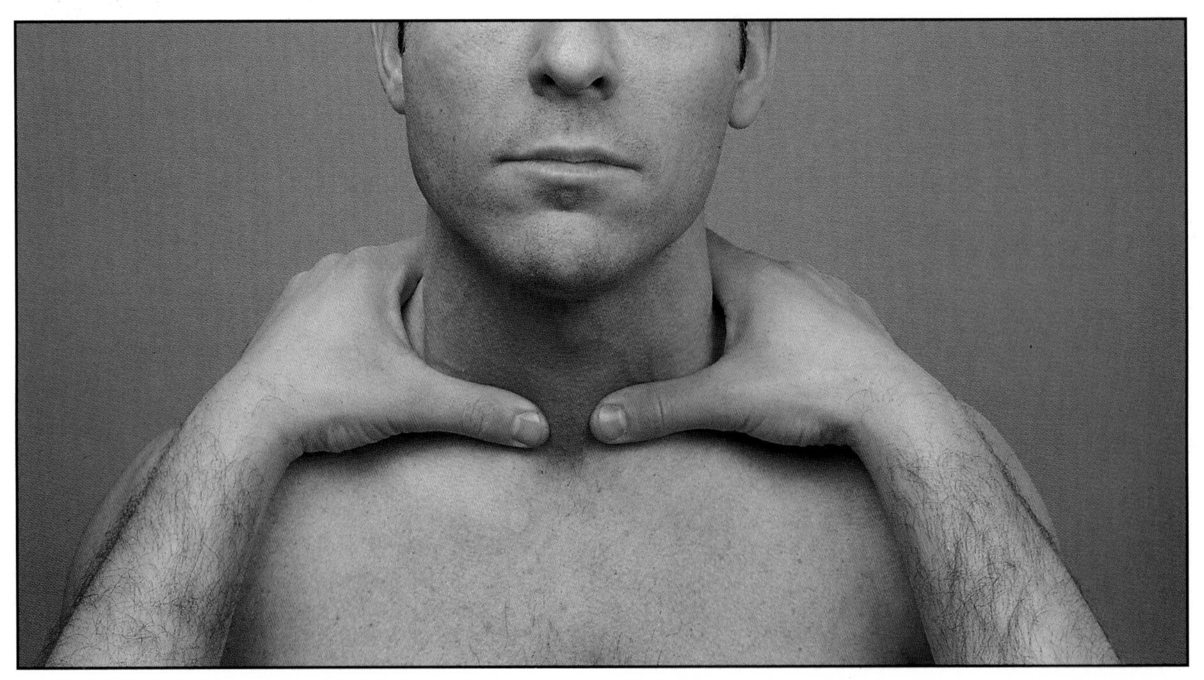

PALPATION (continued)

Respiratory excursion

Palpate the anterior and posterior thorax to assess respiratory excursion.

1 Place the hands at the second intercostal space. During inspiration, assess for simultaneous separation of the thumbs, indicating symmetrical expansion of the chest.

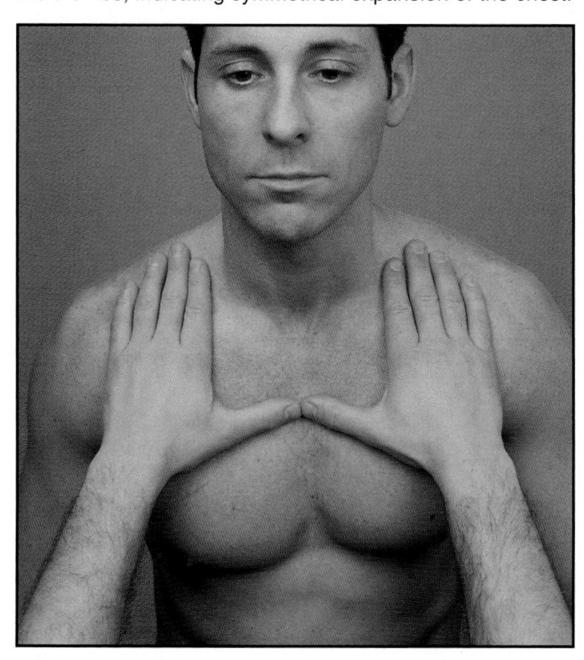

2 Place the hands at the fifth intercostal space. During inspiration, assess for simultaneous separation of the thumbs, indicating symmetrical expansion of the chest.

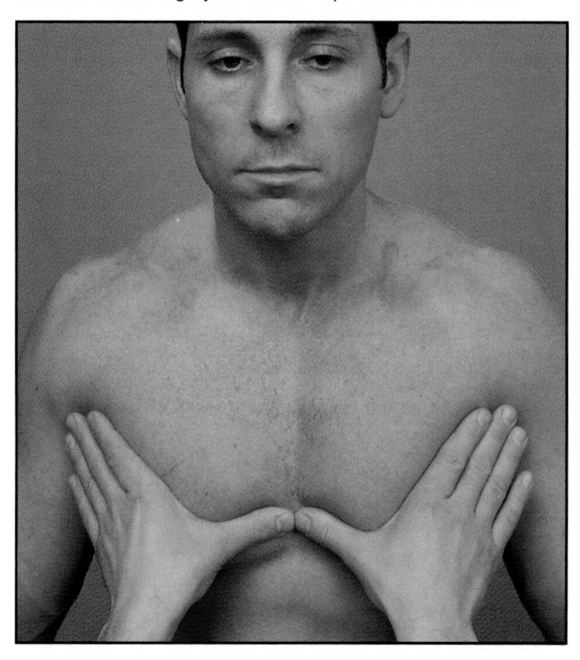

3 Place the hands at the infrascapular area (tenth rib). During inspiration, assess for simultaneous separation of the thumbs, indicating symmetrical expansion of the chest.

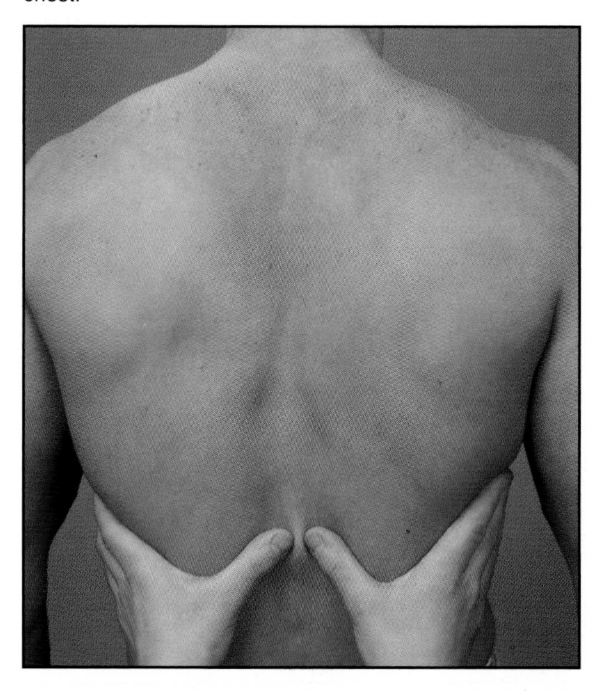

4 Place the hands at the interscapular area. During inspiration, assess for simultaneous separation of the thumbs, indicating symmetrical expansion of the chest.

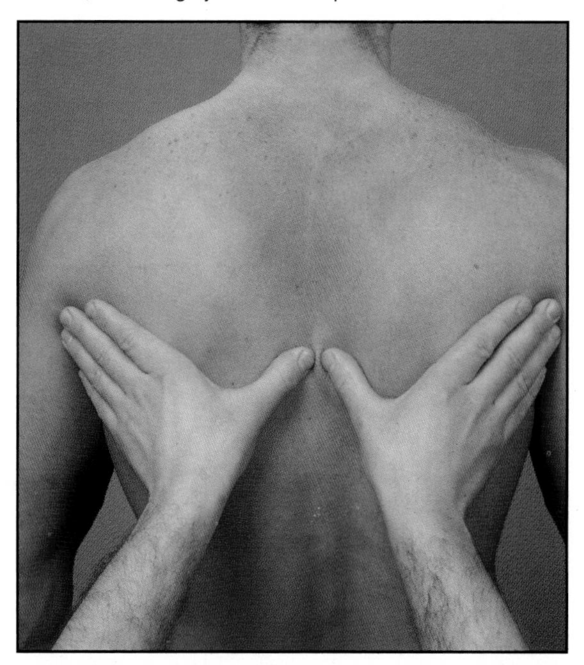

(continued)

ASSESSMENT

PALPATION (continued)

Palpation sequence

Follow this sequence to palpate the anterior thorax.

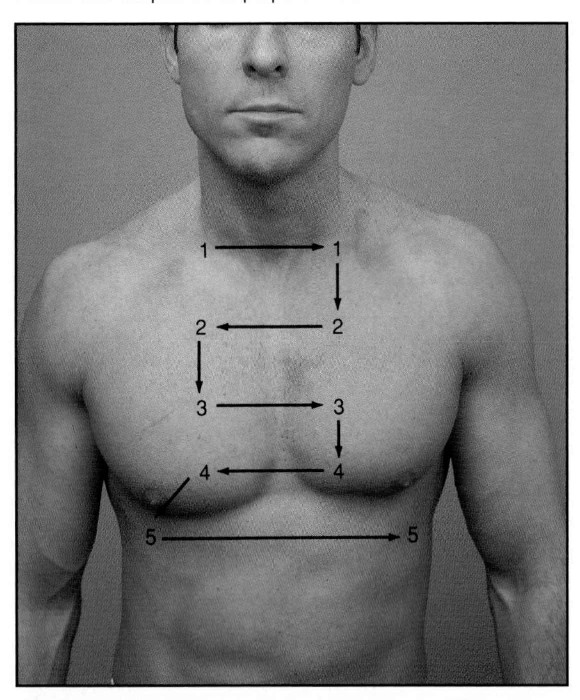

Follow this sequence to palpate the posterior thorax.

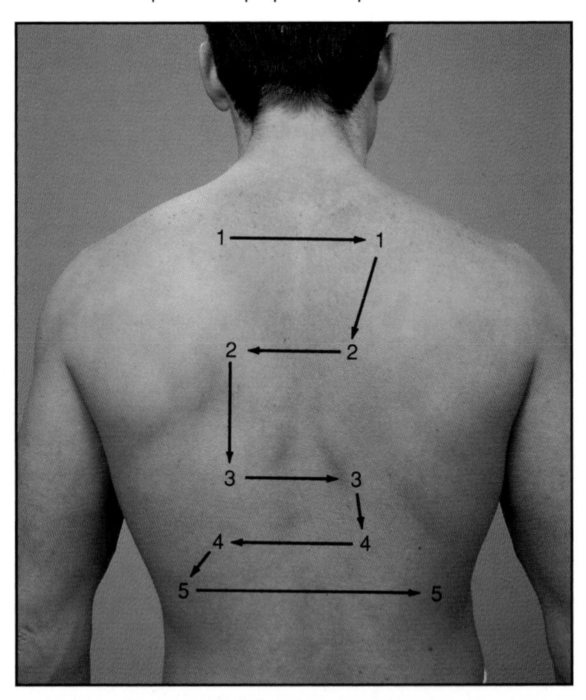

Tactile fremitus

Palpate for tactile fremitus by placing the palms of the hands in various areas of the client's anterior thorax. Fremitus normally occurs in equal intensity on both sides of the chest.

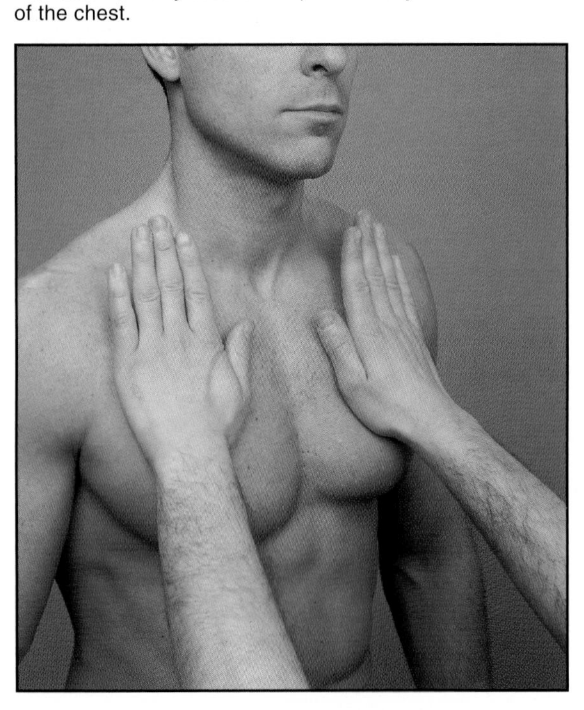

Palpate for tactile fremitus by placing the palms of the hands in various areas on the client's posterior thorax. Fremitus normally is greater close to the bronchi and decreases toward the periphery of the lungs.

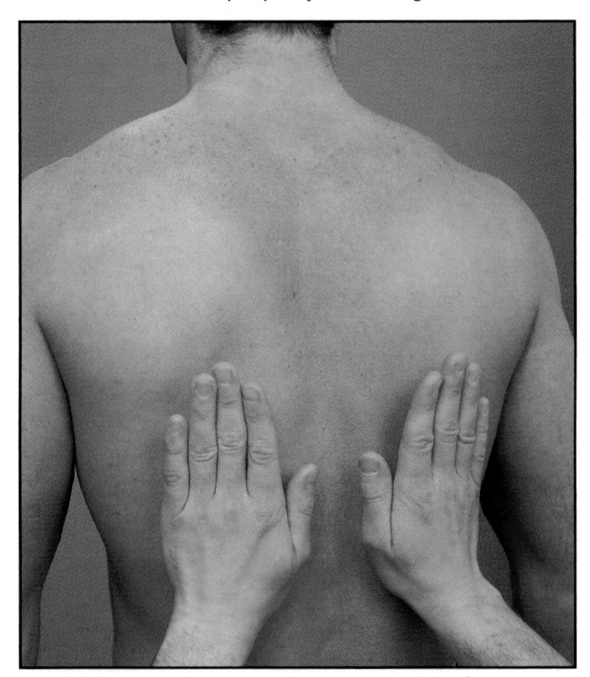

■ Percussion

Percussion and auscultation sequence

Follow this sequence to percuss and auscultate the anterior thorax.

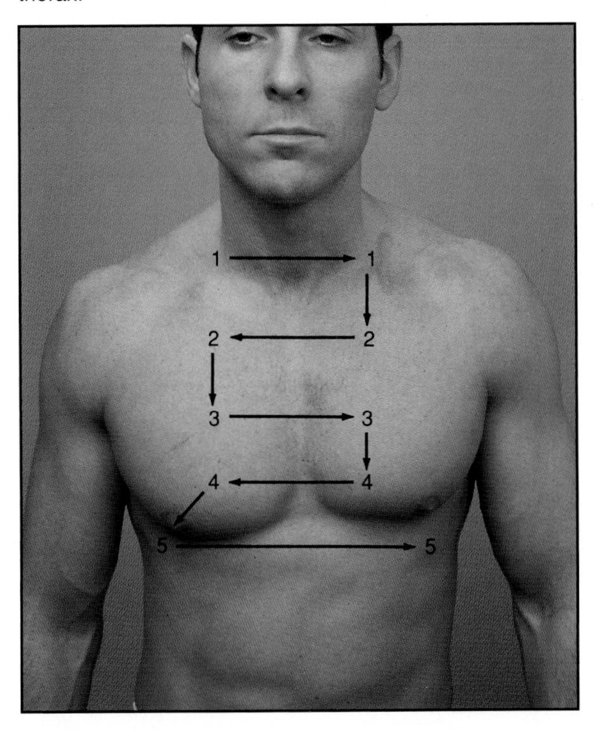

Follow this sequence to percuss and auscultate the posterior thorax.

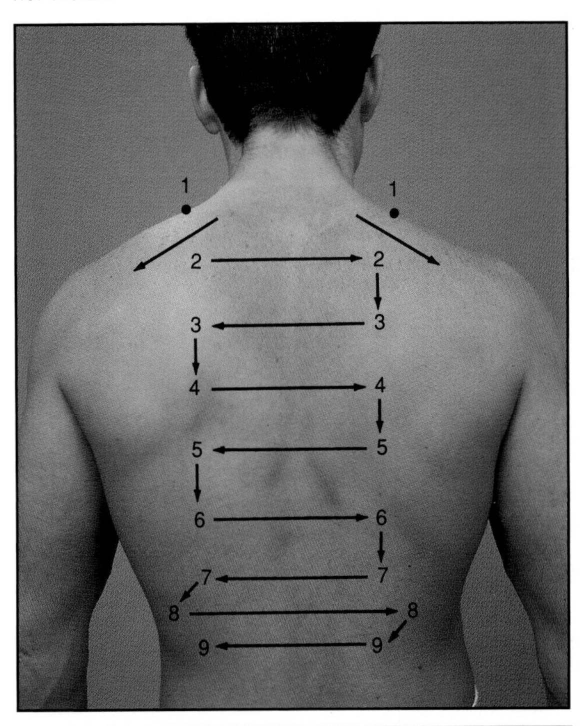

Follow this sequence to percuss and auscultate the lateral thorax.

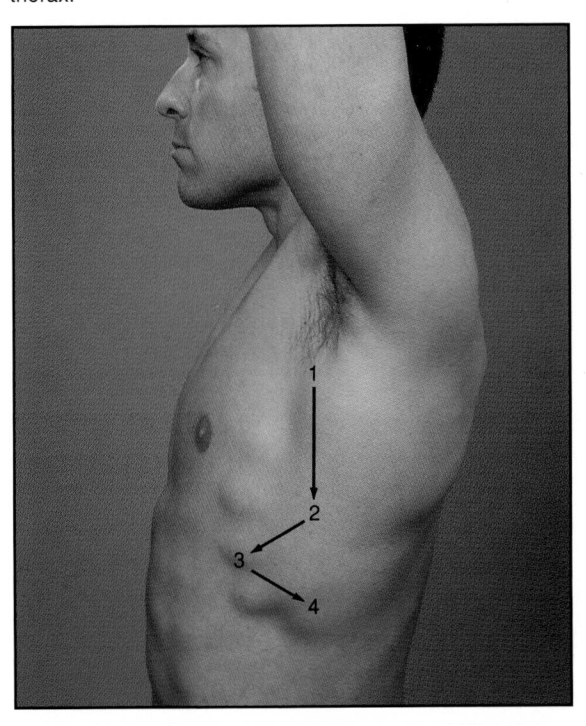

Diaphragmatic excursion

Percuss and mark the posterior thorax during full inspiration and expiration to assess diaphragmatic excursion, which normally measures 1¼" to 2¼" (3 to 6 cm).

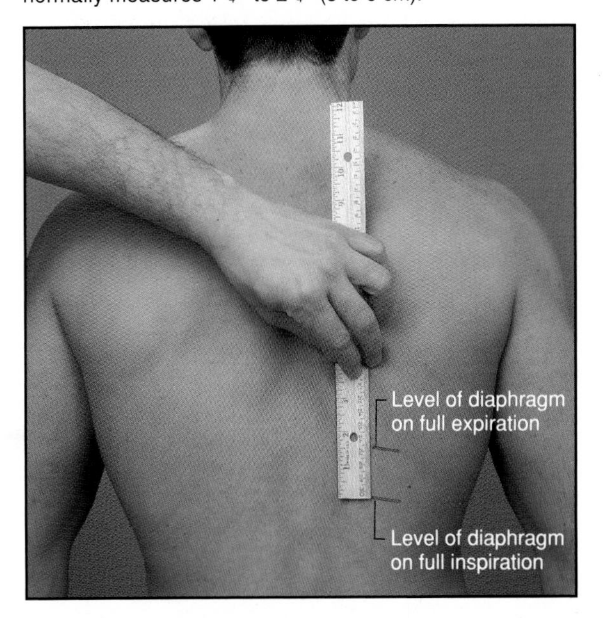

(continued)

ASSESSMENT

PERCUSSION (continued)

Indirect percussion

Use mediate (indirect) percussion to assess the thorax. Percussion detects resonance over healthy lung tissue.

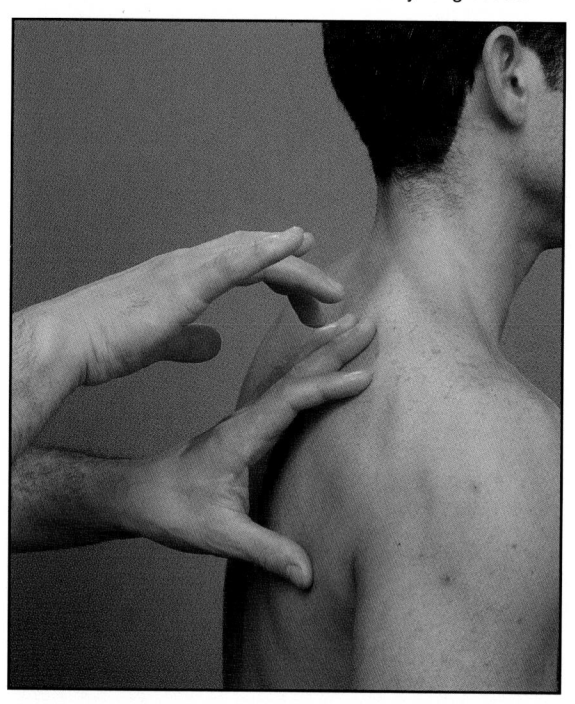

Direct percussion

As an alternative, use direct percussion to assess the thorax.

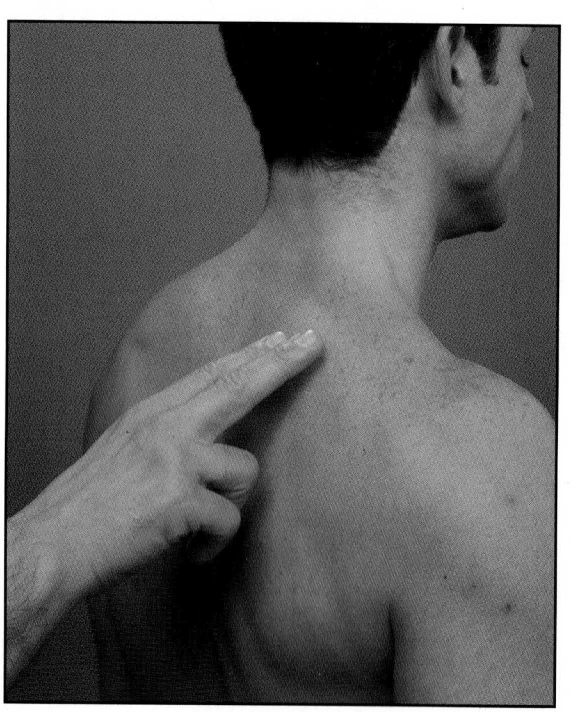

■ Auscultation

Breath sound locations

Auscultate over the anterior thorax. Auscultation normally detects bronchial (tracheal) sounds (loud, high-pitched sounds) over the trachea, bronchovesicular sounds (soft, breezy sounds) over the mainstem bronchi, and vesicular sounds (soft, swishy, breezy sounds) in the periphery of the lungs. The ratio of inspiration to expiration is 1:2 for bronchial sounds, 1:1 for bronchovesicular sounds, and 3:1 for vesicular sounds.

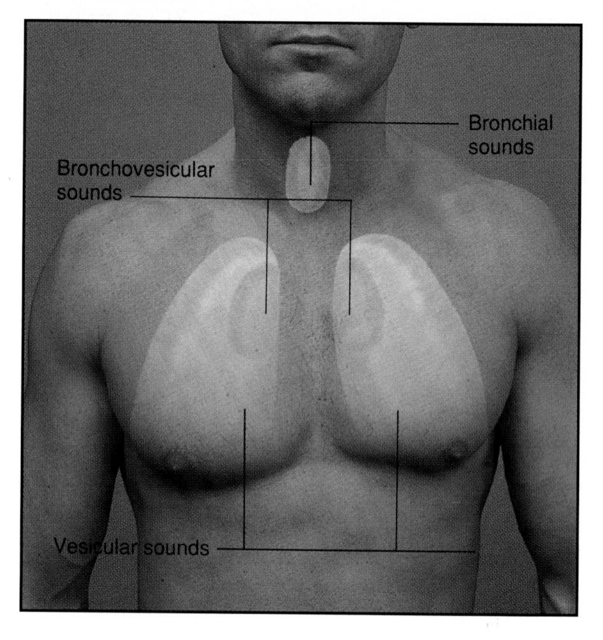

Auscultate the posterior thorax. Auscultation normally detects bronchovesicular breath sounds between the scapulae and vesicular breath sounds in the periphery of the lungs.

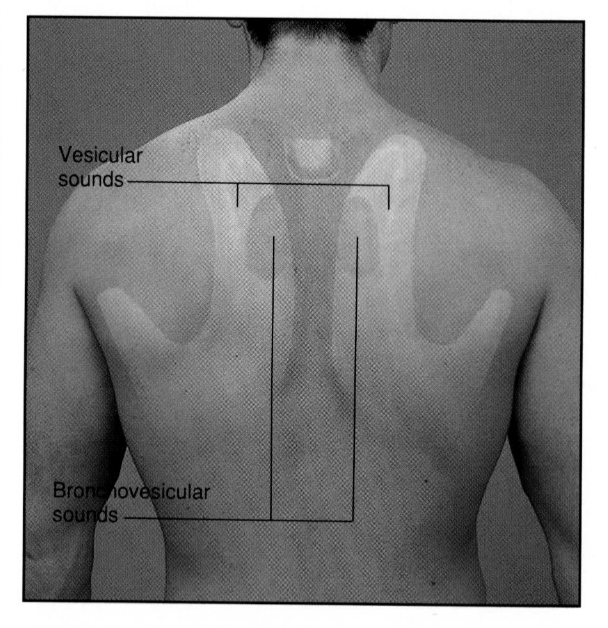

Breath sound auscultation

Auscultate for tracheal sounds over the trachea.

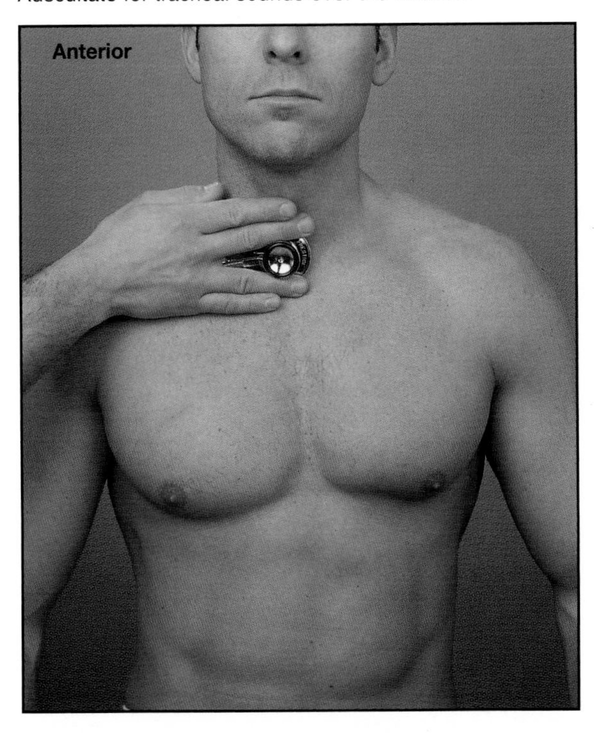

Auscultate for bronchial sounds over the manubrium.

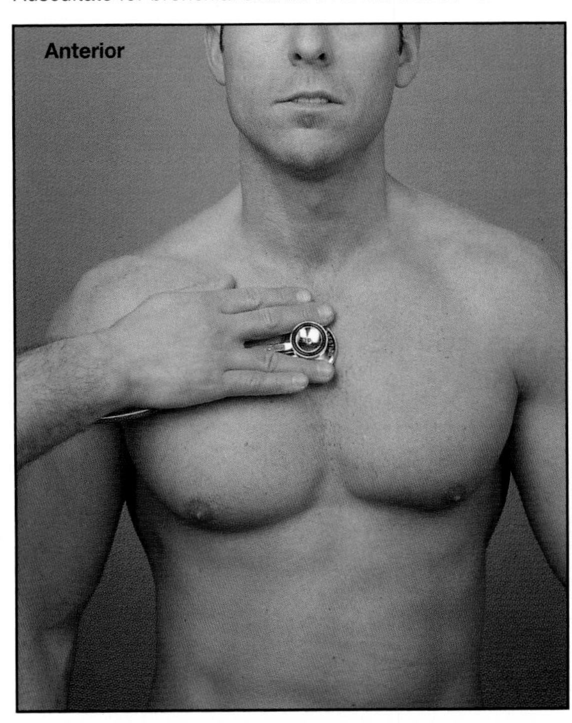

Auscultate for bronchovesicular sounds over the mainstem bronchi on the anterior thorax and between the scapulae on the posterior thorax.

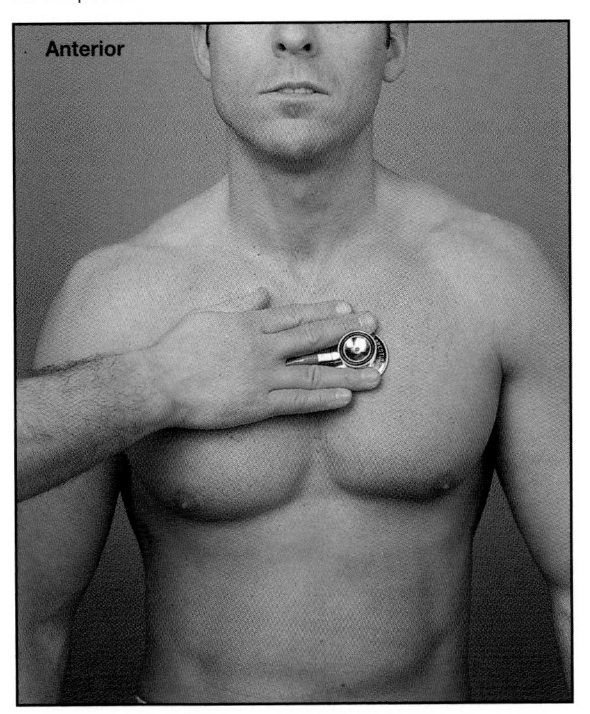

Auscultate for vesicular sounds in the periphery of the lungs on the anterior, posterior, and lateral thorax.

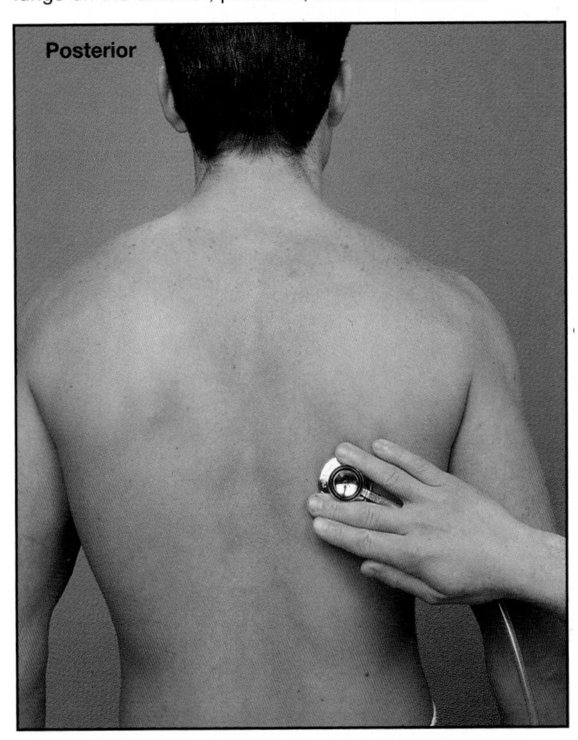

Cardiovascular System

Anatomy and physiology overview

■ Cardiovascular structures

This anterior view of the thorax and neck shows the cardiovascular structures.

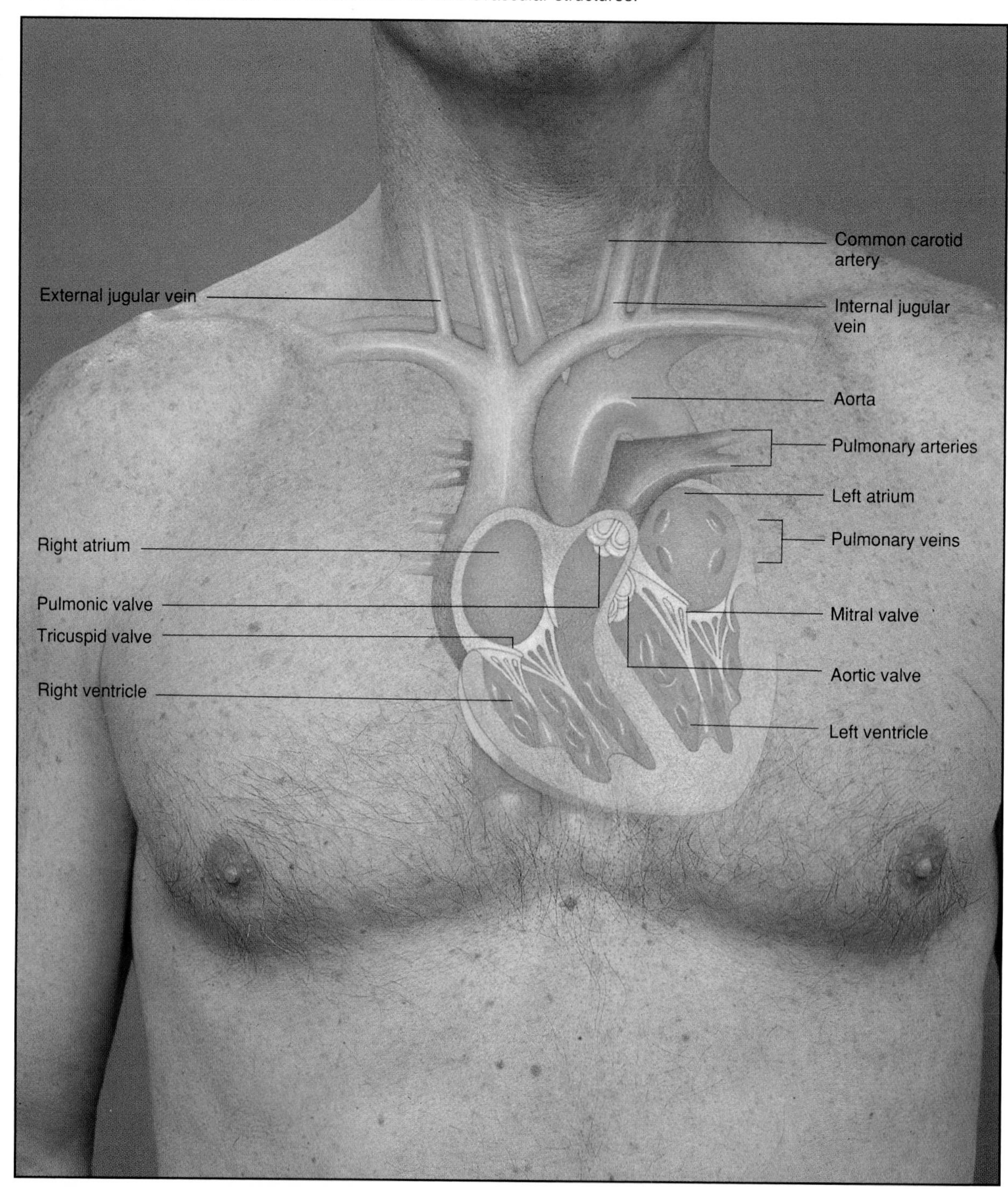

ANATOMY AND PHYSIOLOGY OVERVIEW

■ Cardiac landmarks

This anterior view of the thorax shows the anatomic landmarks used for cardiac assessment.

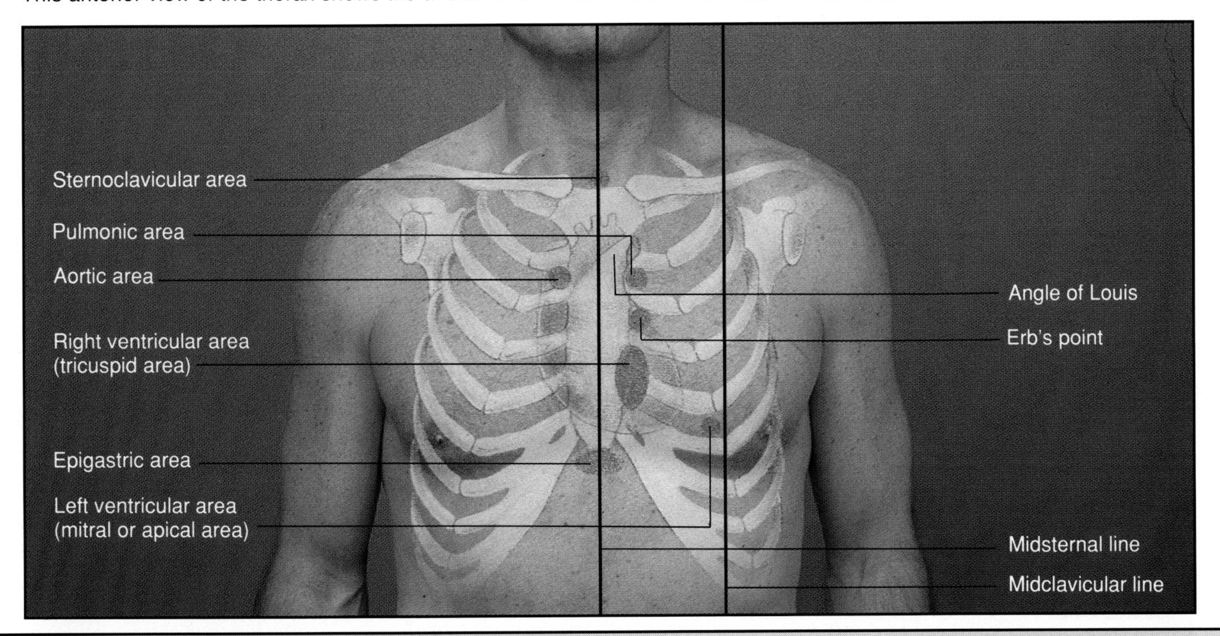

Assessment

■ Inspection

Neck veins

Inspect the neck veins with the client sitting at a 45-degree angle with the head turned slightly away from the side being examined. Use tangential lighting to cast small shadows along the neck, which allow you to see pulse wave movements more clearly. The jugular veins should not appear distended, unless the client has right-side heart dysfunction.

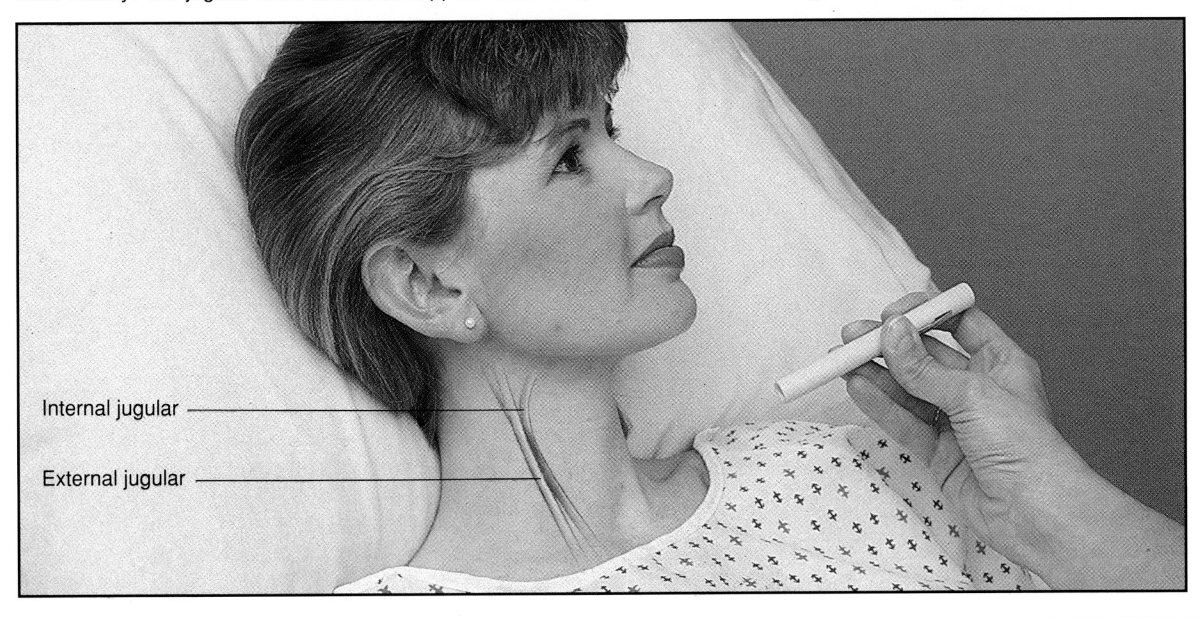

ASSESSMENT

■ Palpation

Central and peripheral pulses

Through palpation, assess the pulse rate, rhythm, symmetry, contour, and strength at each central and peripheral pulse site. Pulse rates usually range from 60 to 100 beats/minute in adults. Pulses normally feel regular in rhythm and equal in strength bilaterally. Their contour typically has a smooth upstroke and downstroke. Pulses with a normal amplitude can be palpated easily and can be obliterated only with strong finger pressure.

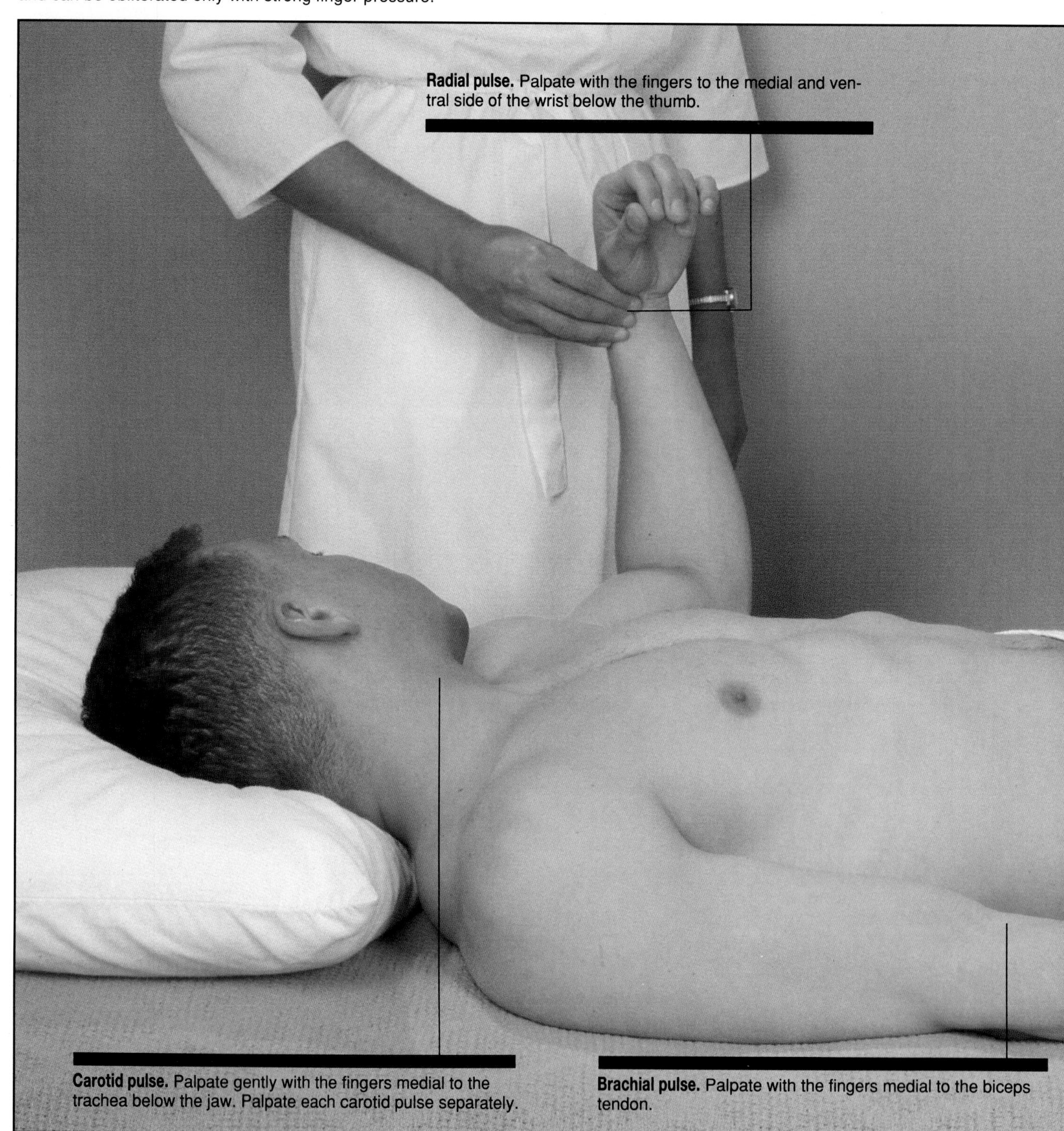

Radial pulse. Palpate with the fingers to the medial and ventral side of the wrist below the thumb.

Carotid pulse. Palpate gently with the fingers medial to the trachea below the jaw. Palpate each carotid pulse separately.

Brachial pulse. Palpate with the fingers medial to the biceps tendon.

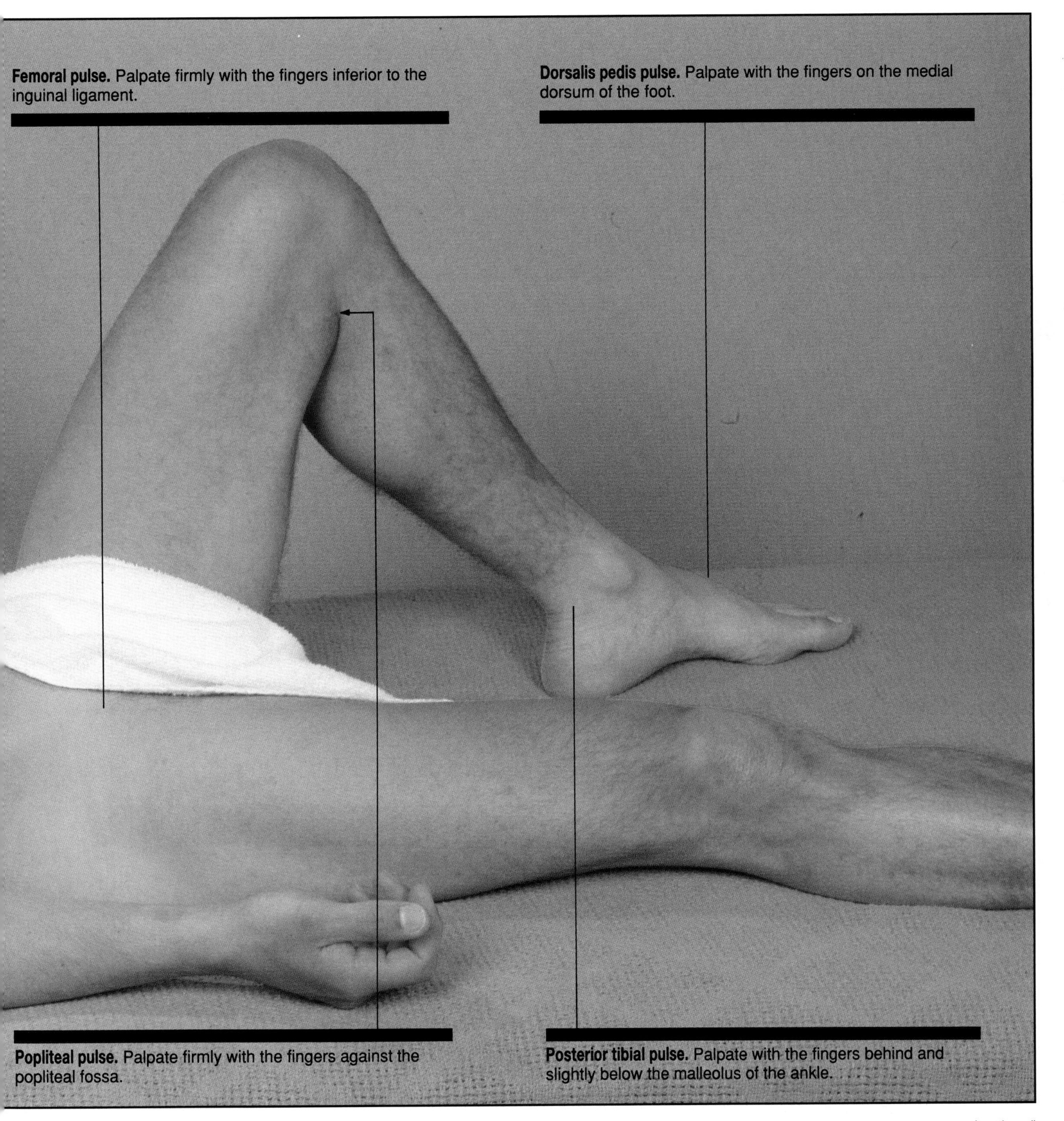
Femoral pulse. Palpate firmly with the fingers inferior to the inguinal ligament.
Dorsalis pedis pulse. Palpate with the fingers on the medial dorsum of the foot.
Popliteal pulse. Palpate firmly with the fingers against the popliteal fossa.
Posterior tibial pulse. Palpate with the fingers behind and slightly below the malleolus of the ankle.

(continued)

ASSESSMENT

PALPATION (continued)

Precordium

Using the pads of the fingers, palpate the precordium in six specific areas. Particularly note the size of any pulsations and any abnormal thrills, lifts, or heaves.

Sternoclavicular area. Assess by palpating at the sternal notch. A slight pulsation may be palpable.

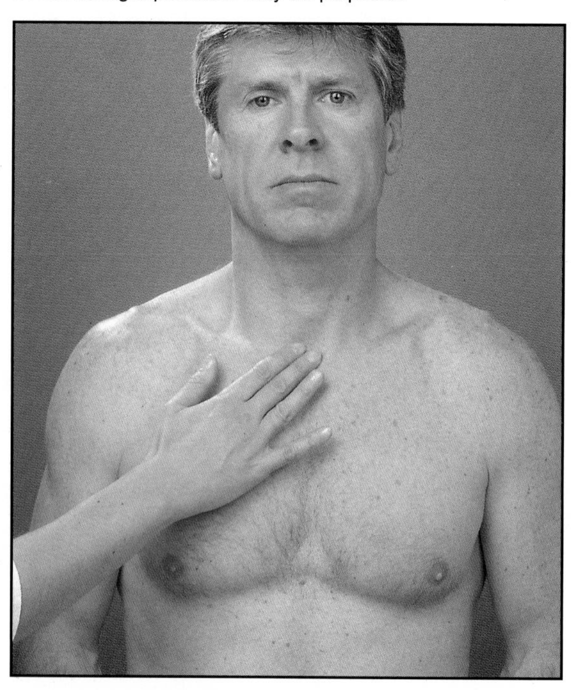

Aortic area. Assess by palpating at the second intercostal space on the right sternal border. Normally, pulsations are not palpable here.

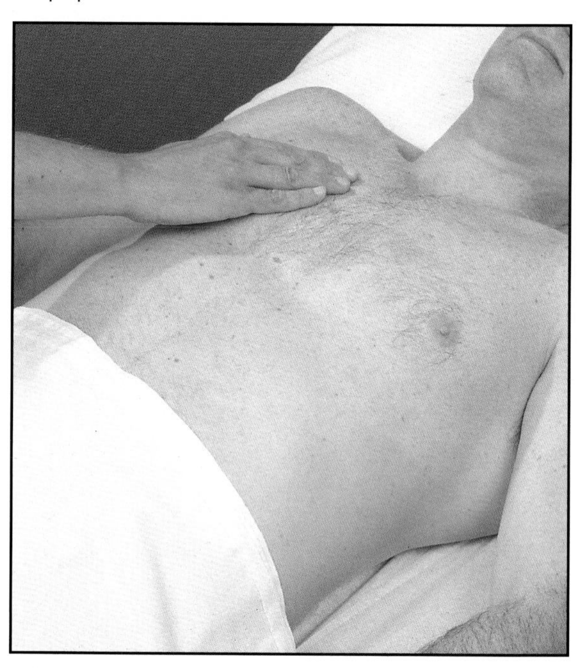

Left ventricular area. Assess by palpating at the fifth intercostal space at the midclavicular line. For most clients, this is the point of maximum impulse (PMI).

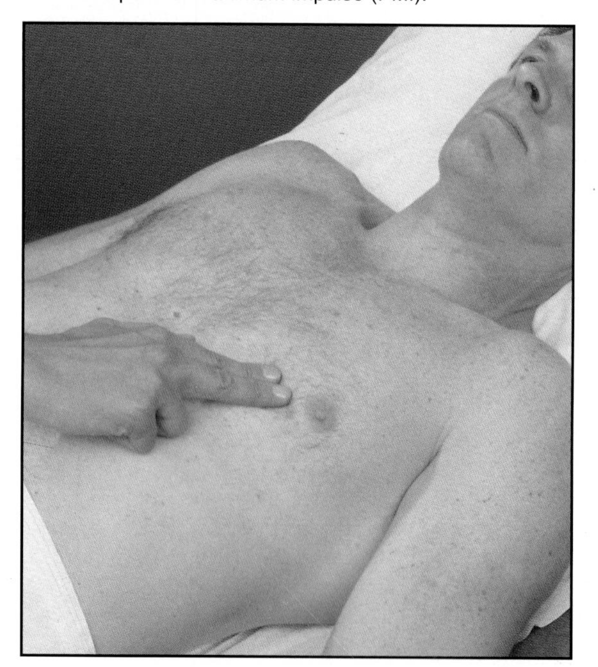

Epigastric area. Assess by palpating below the xiphoid process in the costal angle. An abdominal aortic pulsation may be palpable, especially in a thin client.

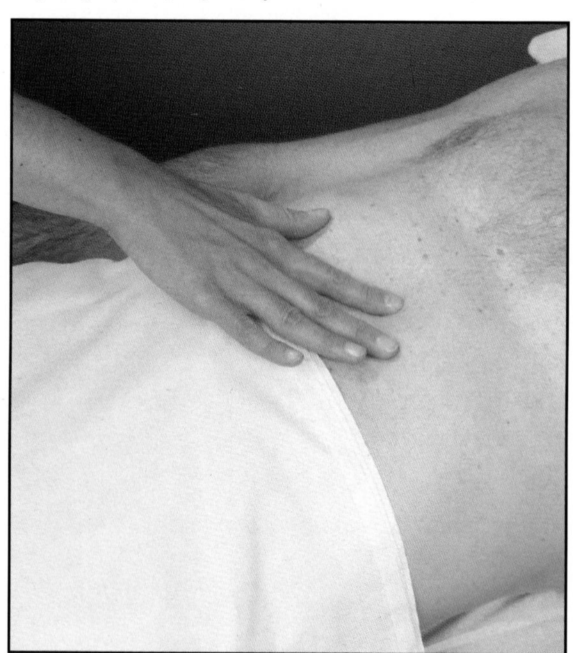

Pulmonic area. Assess by palpating at the second intercostal space on the left sternal border. Pulsations normally are not palpable here.

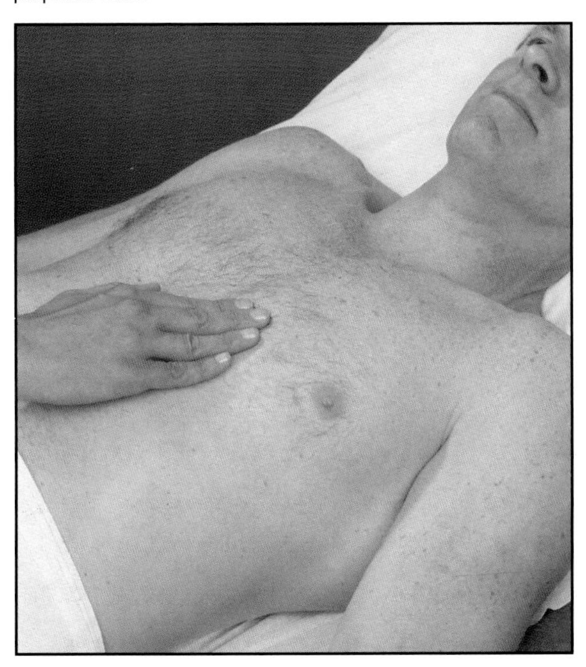

Right ventricular area. Assess by palpating at the fifth intercostal space on the left sternal border. Pulsations normally are not palpable here.

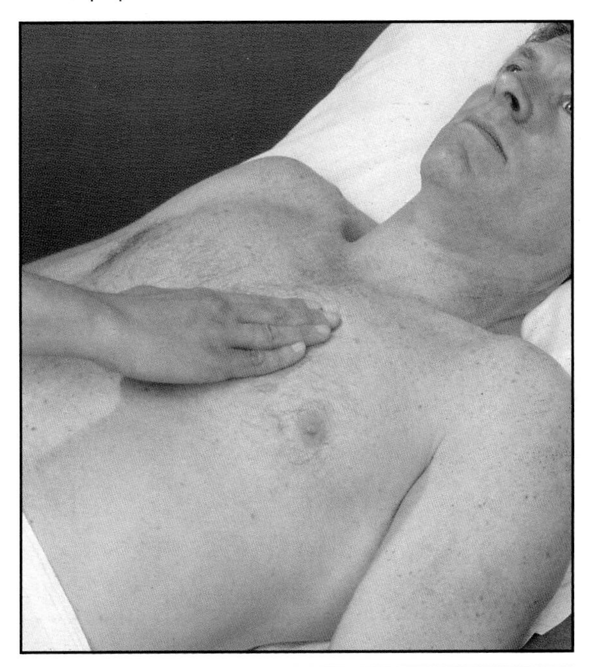

■ Percussion

Heart

Use mediate (indirect) percussion to assess heart size. From the anterior left axillary line, percuss toward the sternum along the fifth intercostal space. The percussion note should change from resonance to dullness at the midclavicular line, indicating the left border of the heart.

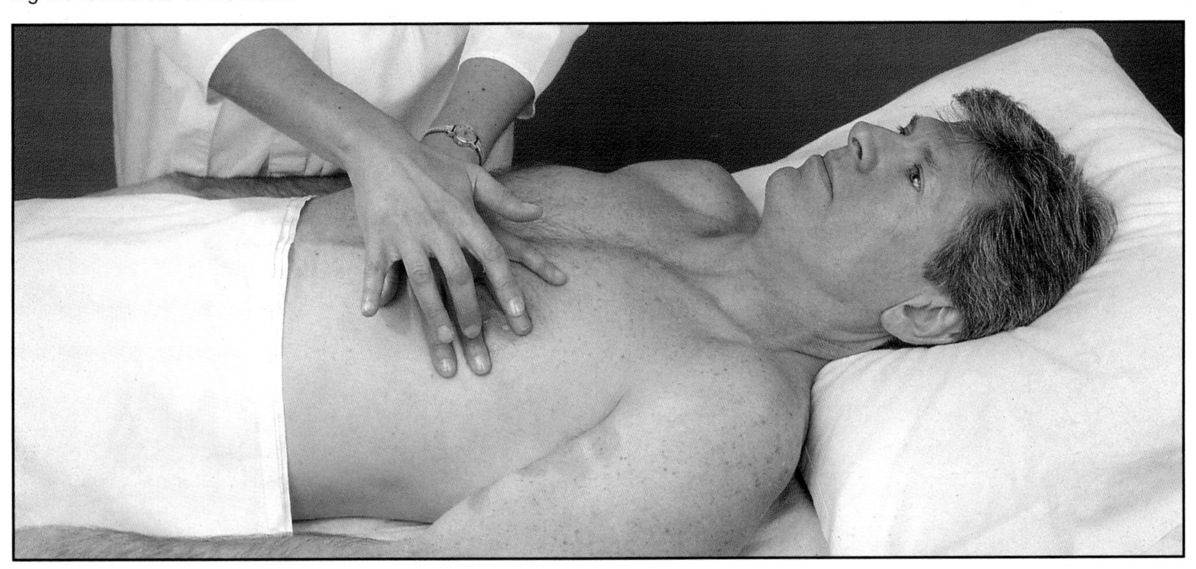

ASSESSMENT

■ Auscultation

Positions for cardiac auscultation

Various client positions may be used for cardiac auscultation, as shown below.

Supine position. This is the most commonly used position. The nurse usually stands to the right of the client.

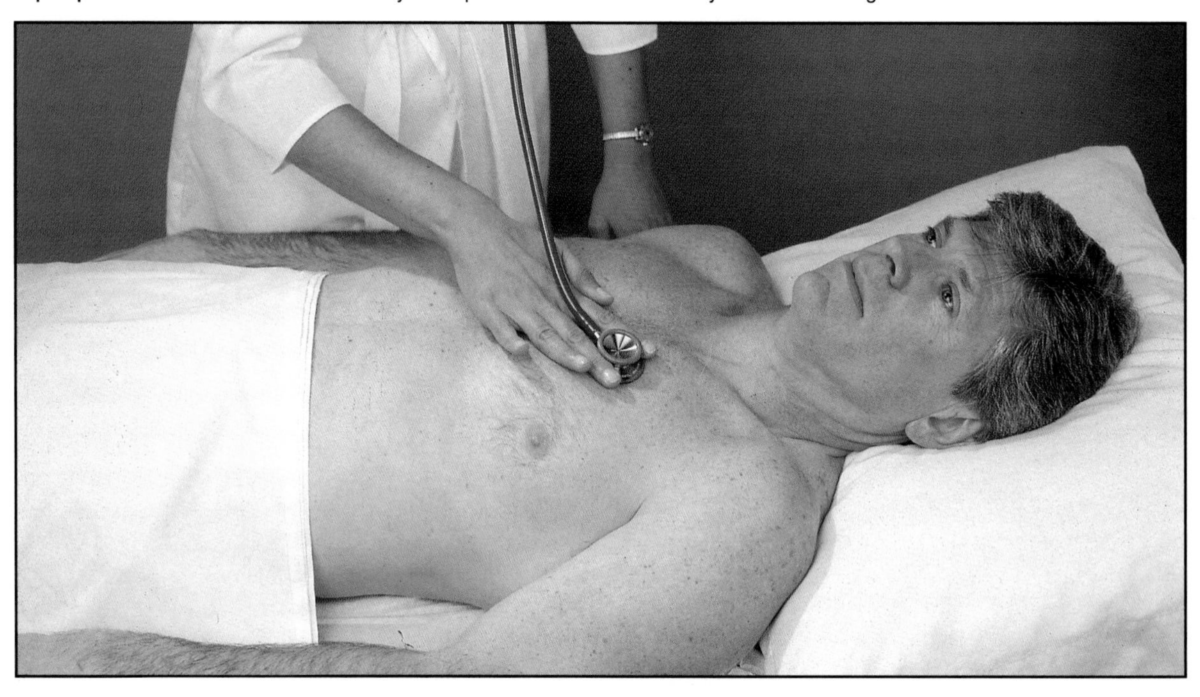

Left-lateral recumbent position. This position is best for hearing low-pitched sounds, such as third and fourth heart sounds and sounds related to atrioventricular valve problems.

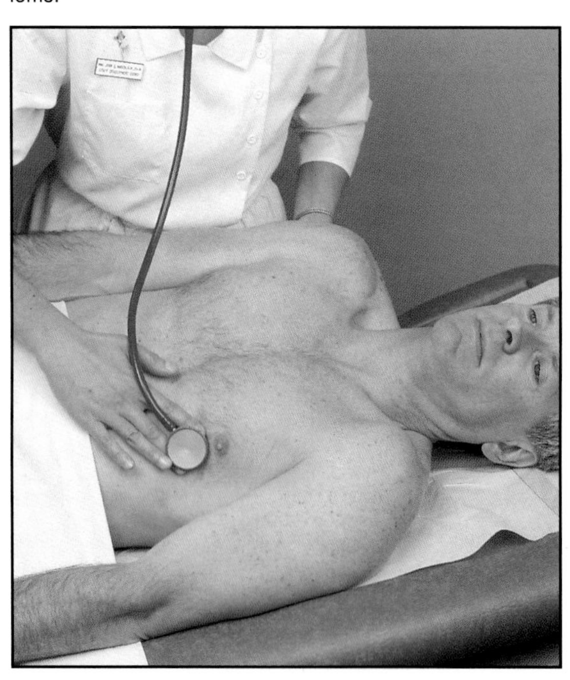

Forward-leaning position. This position is best for hearing high-pitched sounds related to semilunar valve problems, such as aortic and pulmonic valve murmurs.

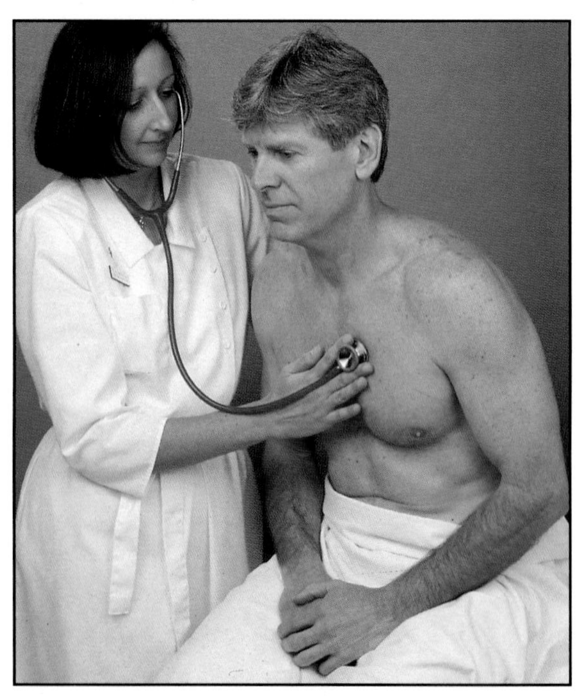

Heart sounds

In four different areas, auscultate heart sounds, assessing their pitch, intensity, duration, timing in the cardiac cycle, quality, location, and radiation. Normal heart sounds are relatively high pitched. S_1 and S_2 vary in intensity with the auscultation area. They last for a fraction of a second and are followed by slightly longer periods of silence. Use the diaphragm of the stethoscope at all four areas to detect high-pitched sounds, such as S_1, S_2, ejection clicks, opening snaps, and some murmurs and rubs. Then use the bell of the stethoscope at all four areas to detect low-pitched sounds, such as S_3, S_4, and some murmurs. Ventricular filling sounds, S_3, and S_4 should be heard best at the mitral or tricuspid areas.

Aortic area. Auscultate at the aortic area, which lies in the second intercostal space along the right sternal border. Normally, S_1 is quieter than S_2.

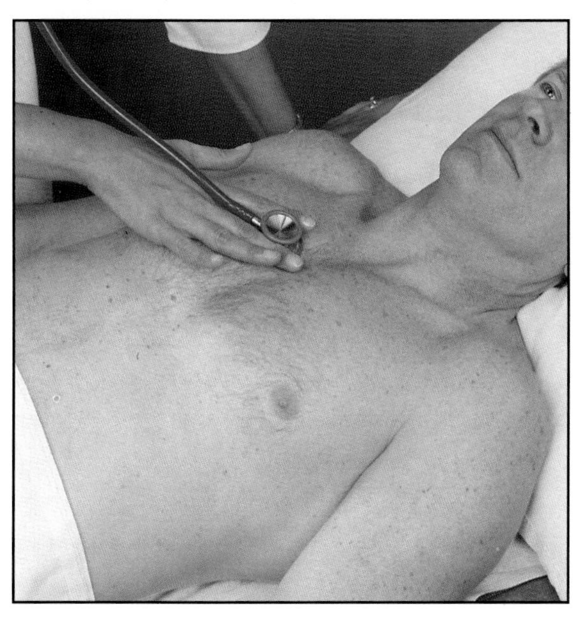

Pulmonic area. Auscultate at the pulmonic area, which lies in the second intercostal space along the left sternal border. Here, S_1 normally is quieter than S_2, and a split S_2 may be heard during inspiration.

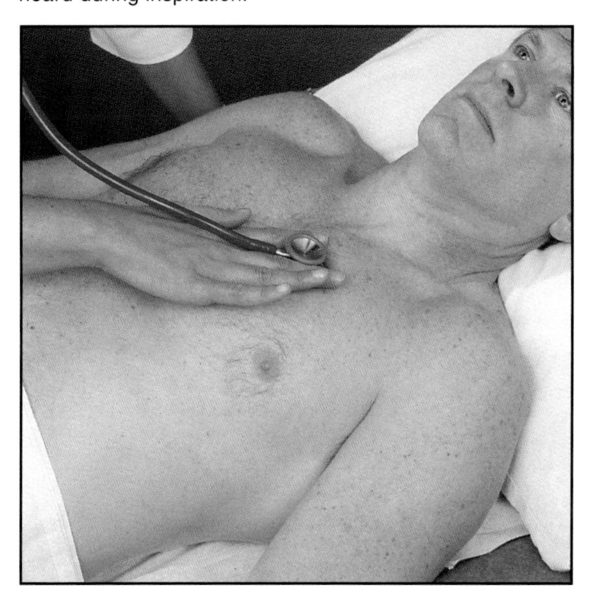

Tricuspid area. Auscultate at the tricuspid (right ventricular) area, which lies in the fourth intercostal space along the left sternal border. In this location, S_1 normally is louder than S_2, and a split S_1 may be heard.

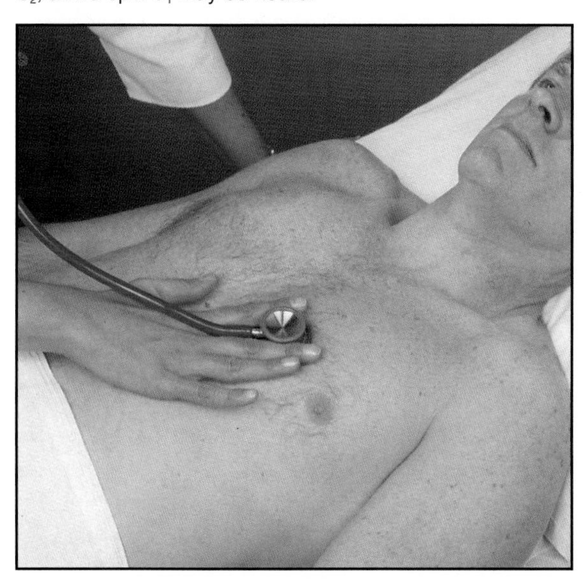

Mitral area. Auscultate at the mitral area (apex), which lies in the fifth intercostal space near the midclavicular line. Normally, S_1 is louder than S_2 here.

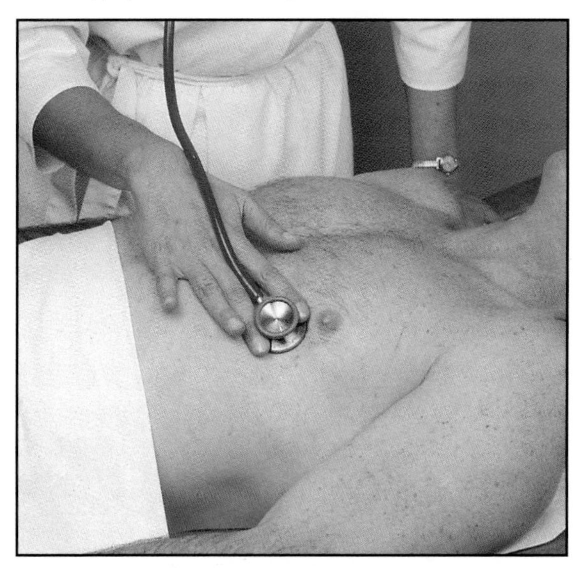

(continued)

ASSESSMENT

AUSCULTATION (continued)

Heart sound timing

While auscultating heart sounds, palpate the carotid pulse to determine the timing of the sound in the cardiac cycle. The first heart sound (S_1) should occur simultaneously with the carotid pulsation.

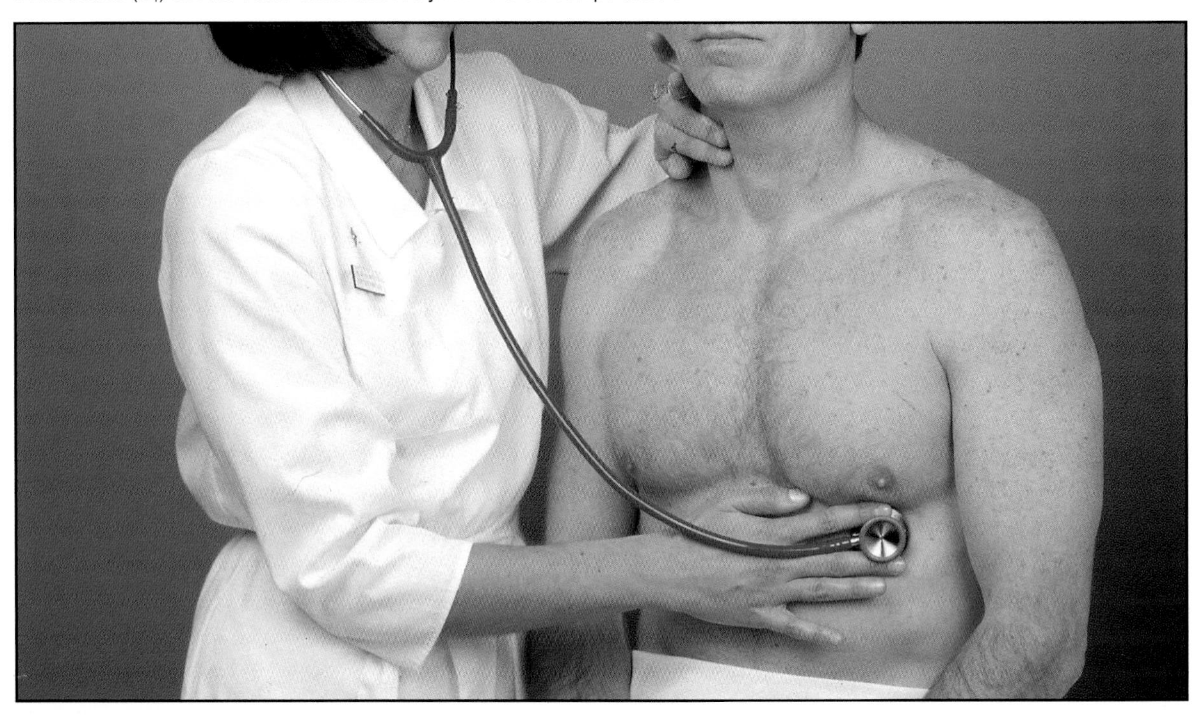

Carotid arteries

While the client holds the breath, auscultate each carotid artery with the bell of the stethoscope. Normally, auscultation detects no vascular sounds.

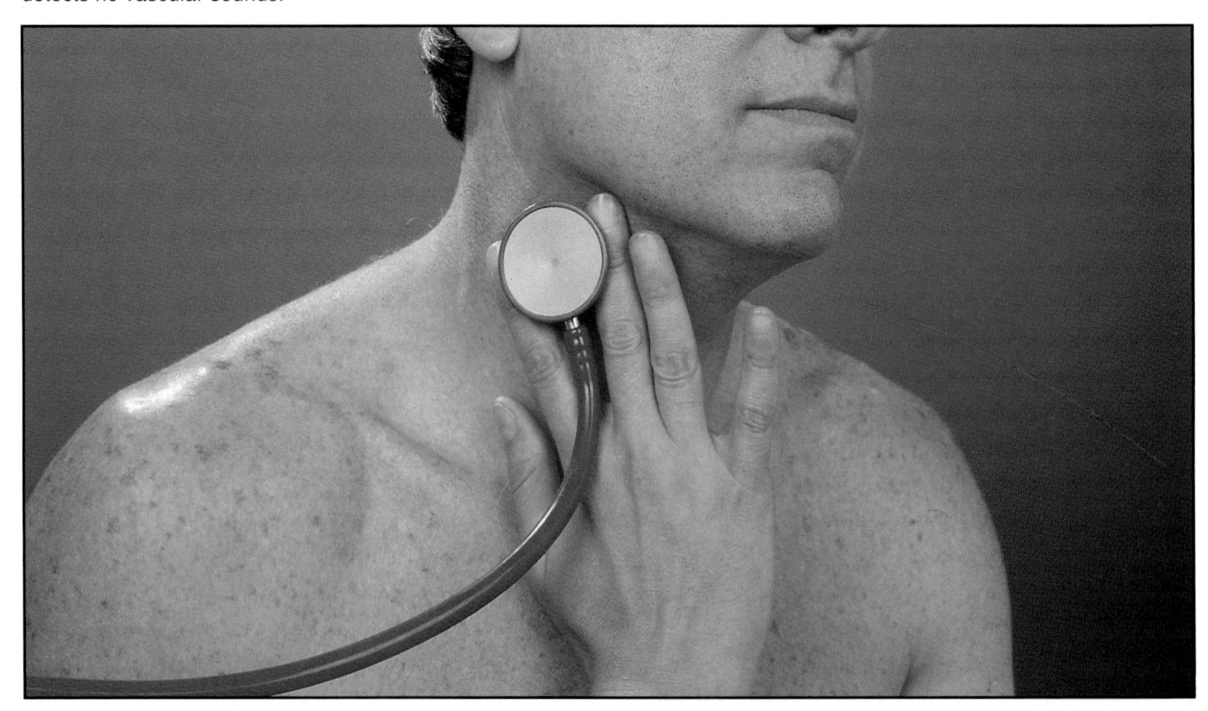

Common abnormalities

■ Leg abnormalities

Venous insufficiency

Venous insufficiency can produce any of these abnormalities in the legs: wet, open lesions with red or purplish edges (as shown), cyanosis when the legs are dangling, brown discoloration, and marked edema.

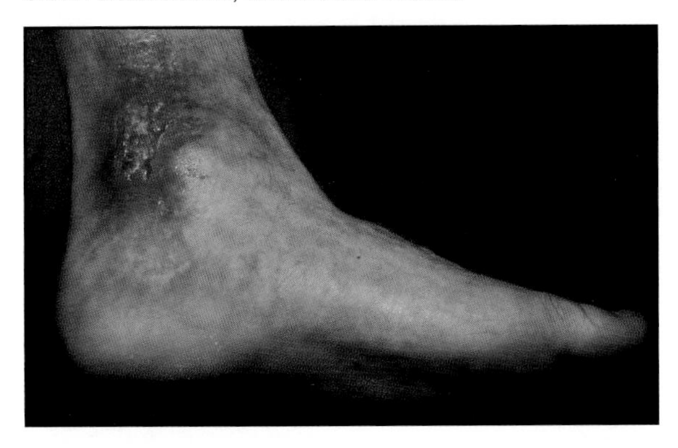

Varicose veins

These dilated, tortuous veins usually affect the legs. They can result from congenital weakness of the valves or venous wall, deep vein thrombophlebitis, and conditions that promote prolonged venostasis.

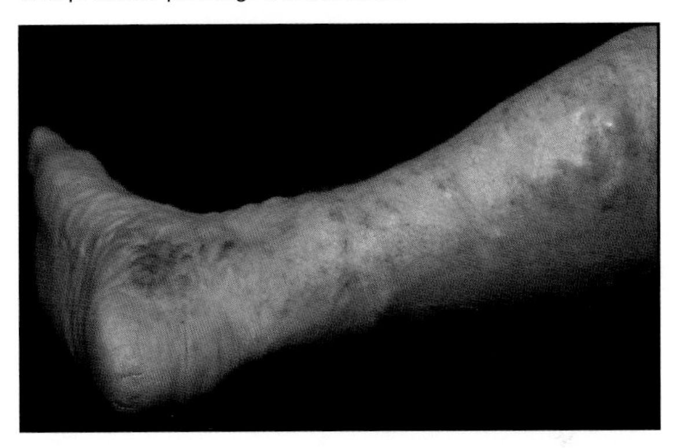

Arterial obstruction

Acute arterial obstruction can produce any of these abnormalities in the legs: decreased or absent pulses, pallor upon elevation, skin mottling (as shown), and coolness to the touch.

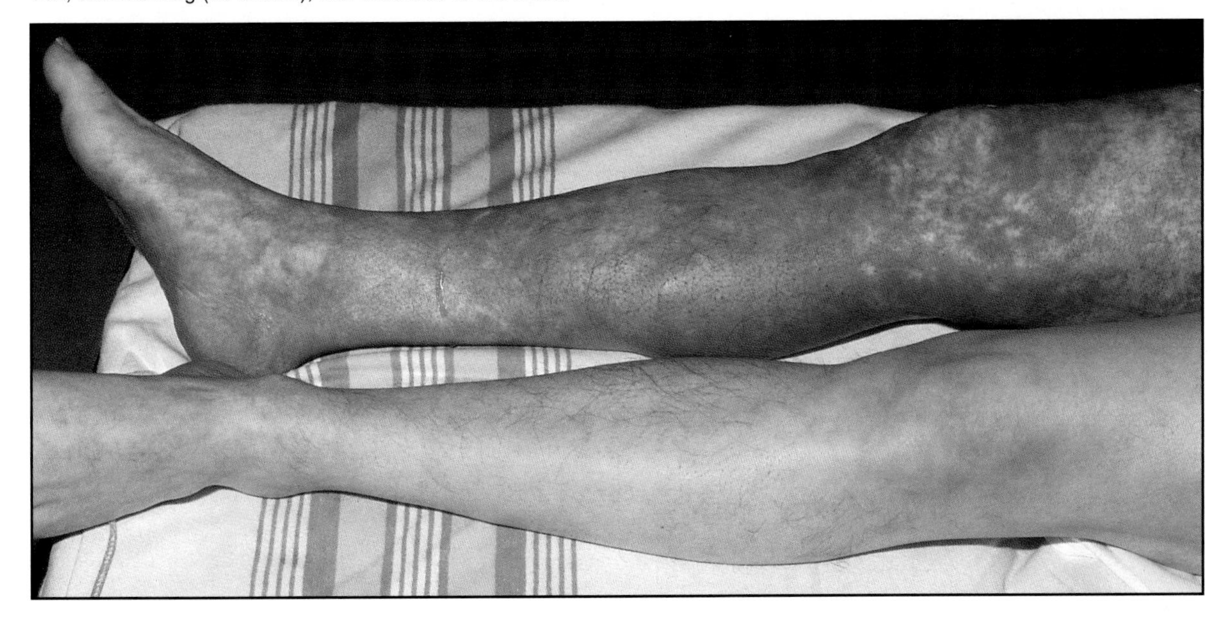

COMMON ABNORMALITIES

■ Peripheral cyanosis and clubbing

Cyanosis that appears only on the fingers, feet, nose, or ears may result from such disorders as peripheral arterial occlusion, shock, or right-side heart failure. Finger clubbing is associated with chronic cyanosis of congenital heart disease and chronic fibrotic changes in the lungs.

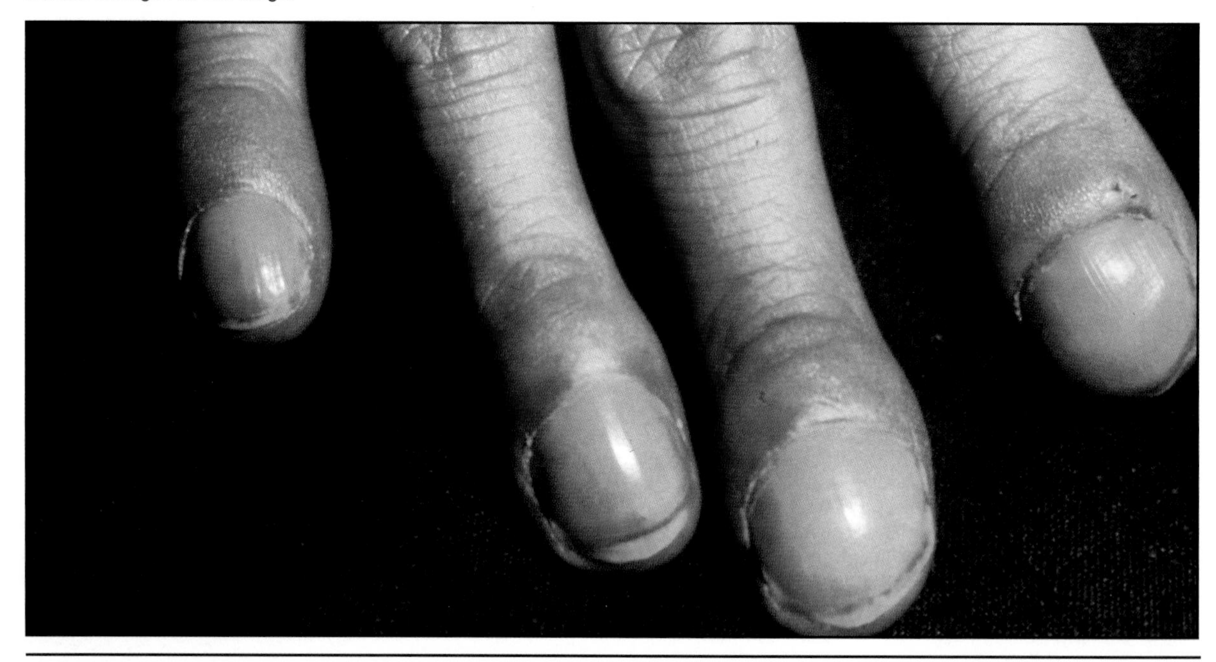

■ Pitting edema

When finger pressure produces a small depression (pit) that does not rebound immediately, the client has pitting edema, which typically reflects congestive heart failure or venous insufficiency.

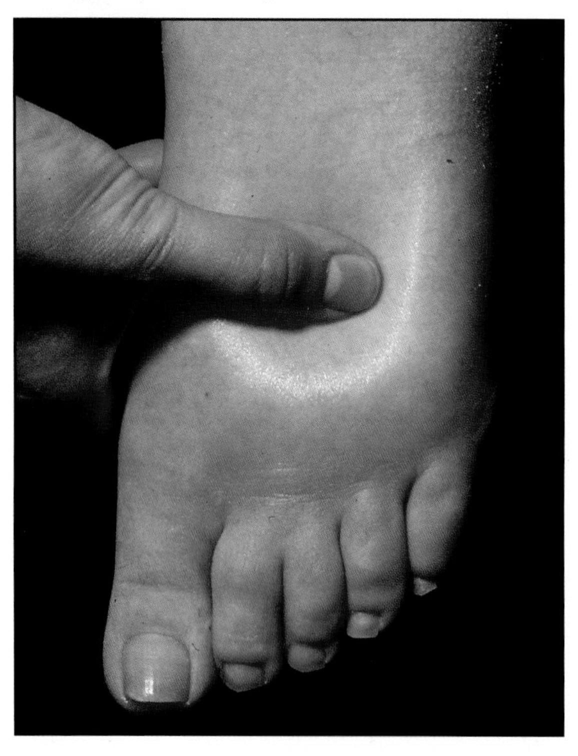

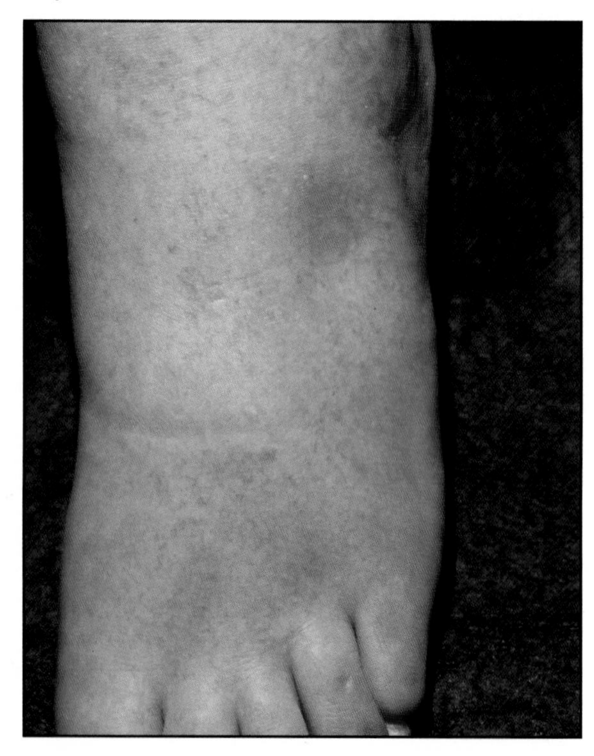

Female and Male Breasts

Anatomy and physiology overview

■ Structures of the breast

This lateral view of the female breast shows its structures.

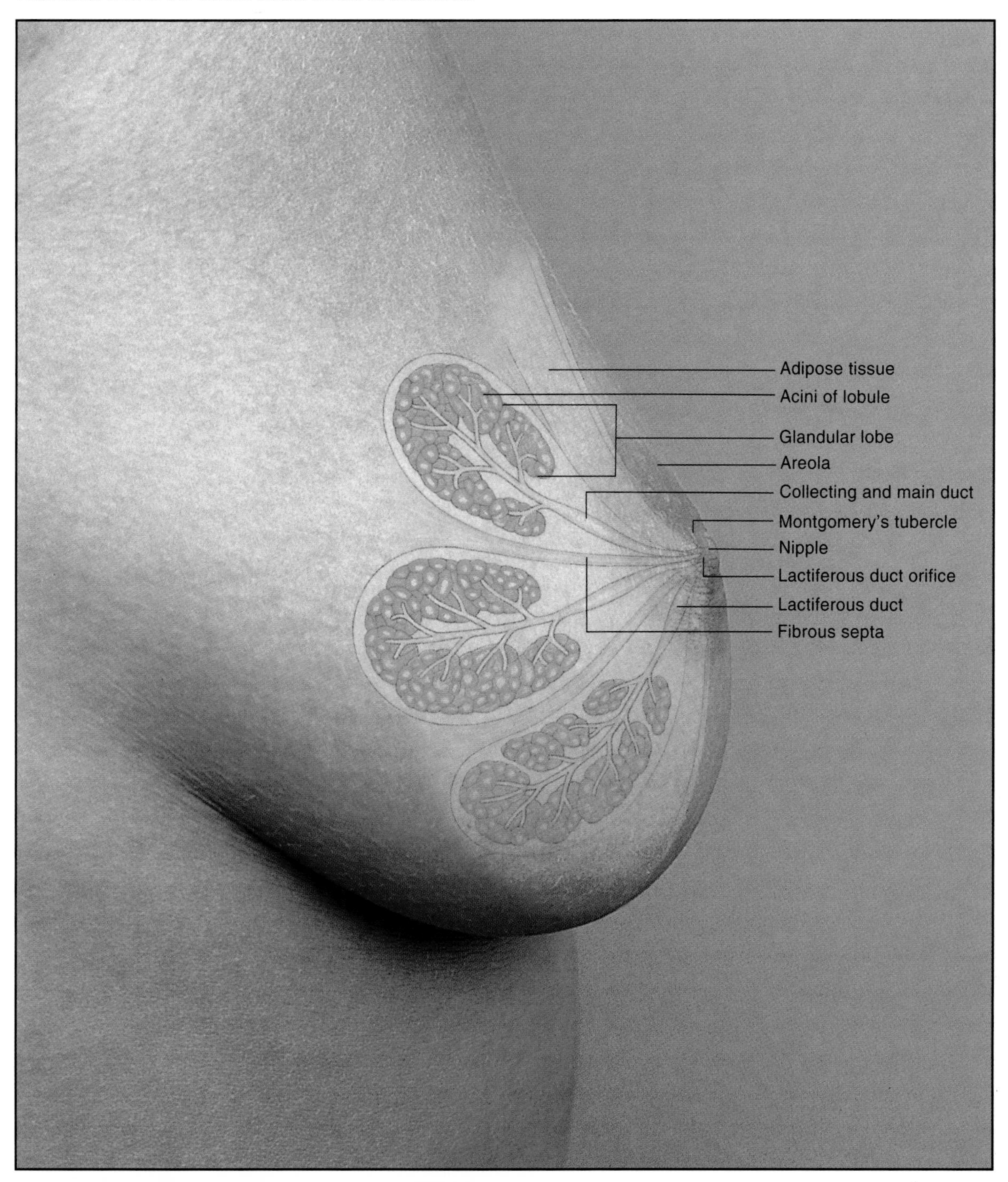

ANATOMY AND PHYSIOLOGY OVERVIEW

■ Lymph drainage and quadrants of the breast

This anterior view shows the quadrants of the breast and the location of the lymph nodes.

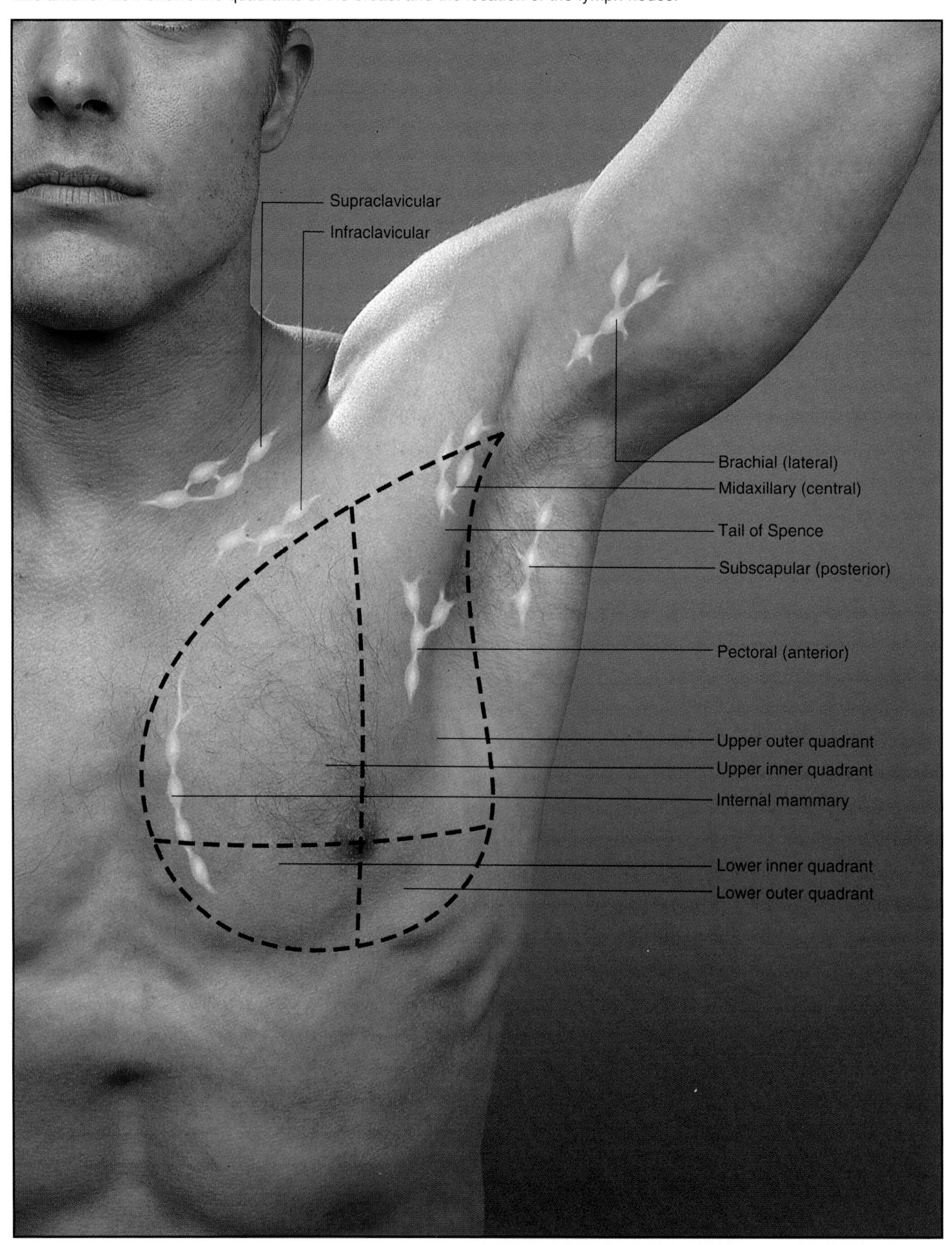

Assessment

■ Inspection

Breasts

With the client in at least three of the four positions shown, note the size, shape, symmetry, and color of the breasts. Normally, the breasts are similar in size, convex in shape (except in normal-weight men), fairly symmetrical, and consistent in color with the rest of the body. Also, inspect the nipples and areolae for size, shape, color, lesions, and symmetry. The nipples and areolae should be similarly round or oval, of equal size, similar in color, and free of lesions. Both nipples should point outward and slightly upward.

Sitting with arms at sides. Begin inspecting the breasts with the client seated and with her arms resting at each side.

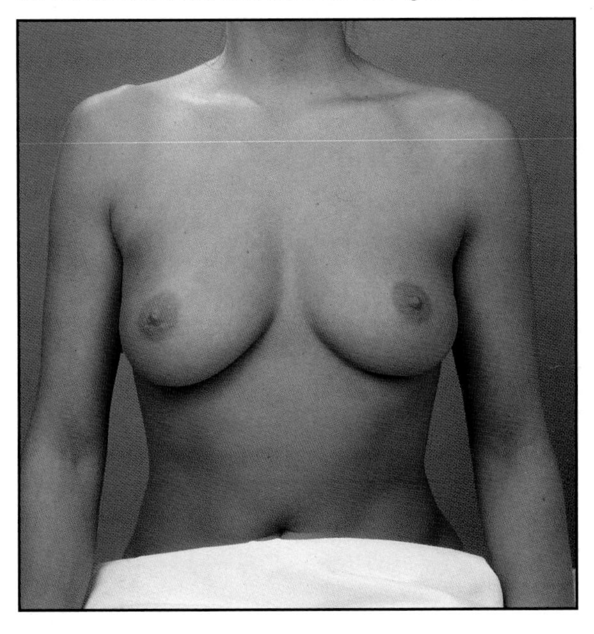

Sitting with hands on hips. Inspect the breasts as the client places her hands against her hips. This position reveals any hidden retraction or dimpling.

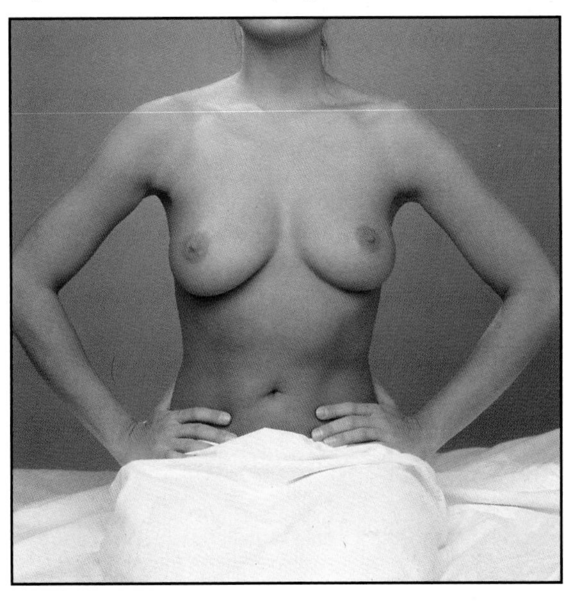

Sitting with arms overhead. Inspect the breasts as the client raises her arms over her head. This position also helps reveal any hidden retraction or dimpling.

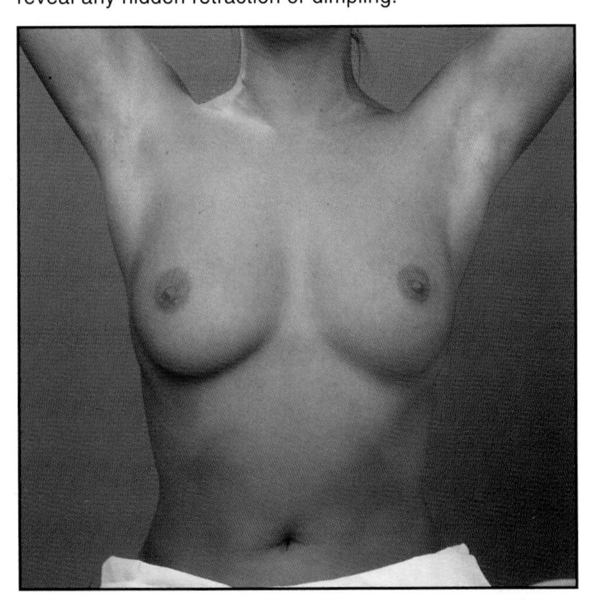

Standing and leaning forward. Inspect the breasts as the client leans forward from the waist. This position is best for inspecting large breasts.

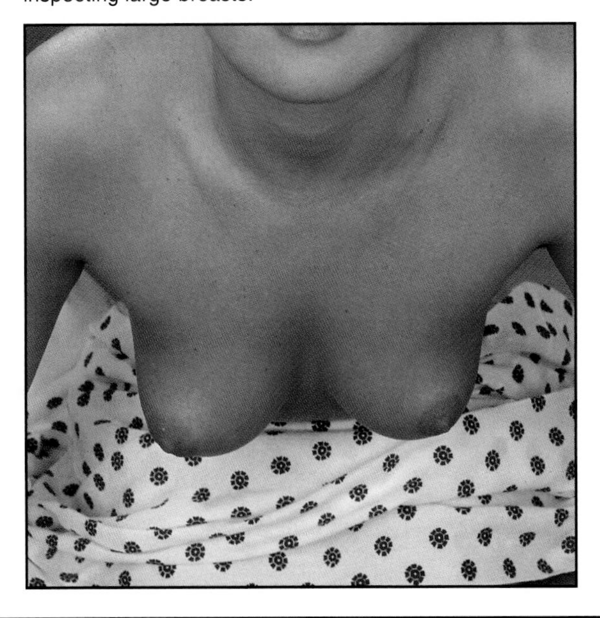

ASSESSMENT

Palpation

Axillae

With the client seated, palpate the axillae. Palpating one or two small, nontender, freely movable, central lymph nodes is normal.

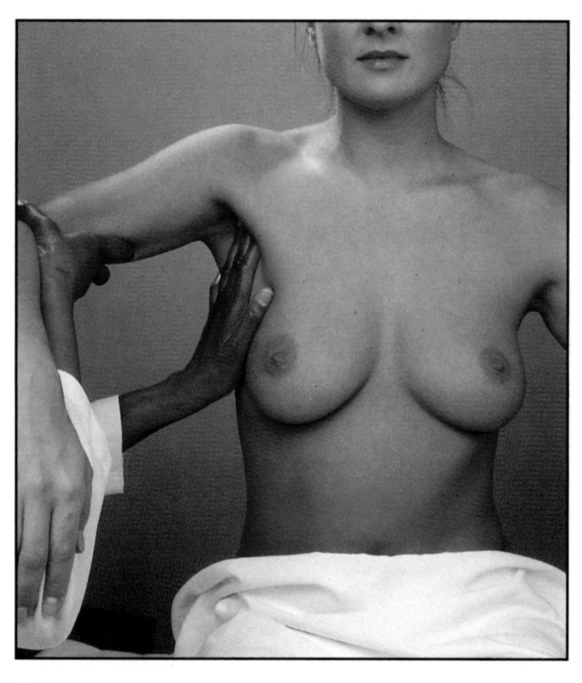

Breasts

With the client supine and her arm above her head, place a small pillow under the shoulder of the breast being examined. Using the fingertips, palpate the breast circularly from the center to the periphery, including the tail of Spence. In a young client, the breasts should feel firmly elastic; in an older client, they may feel more granular or stringy. In a premenopausal client, the breasts normally may be tender one week before the menstrual period. However, they should not have masses, induration, or inflammation.

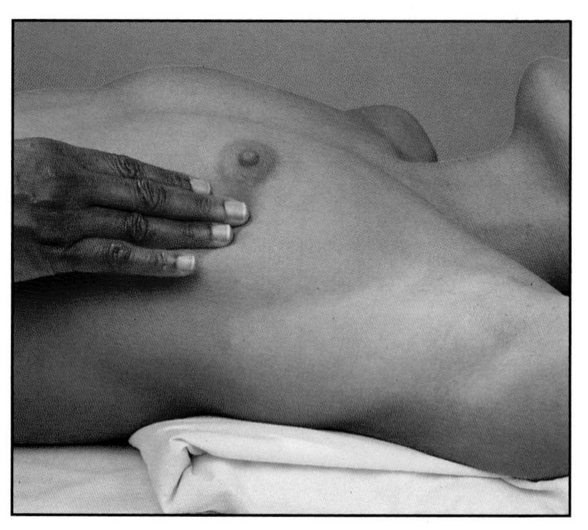

Breast mass

If a mass is suspected, gently move or compress the breast tissue to look for dimpling. Normally, this technique produces no dimpling.

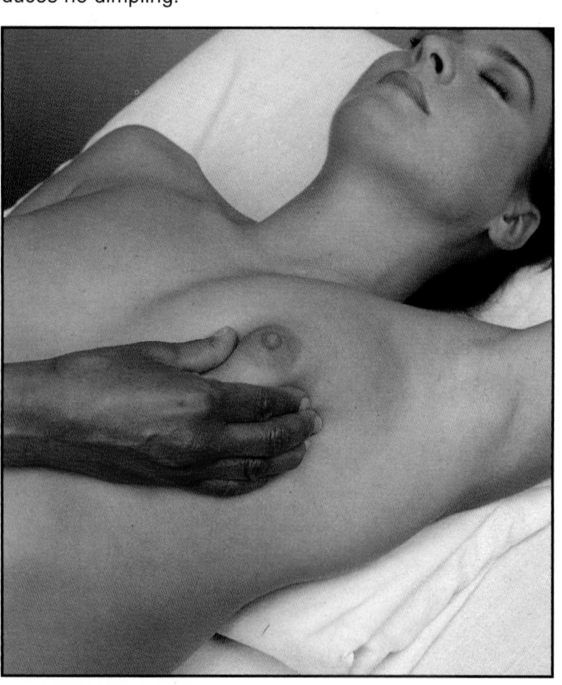

Areola and nipple

Palpate the areola and nipple, and compress the nipple between the thumb and index finger. This normally produces nipple erection and puckering of the areola.

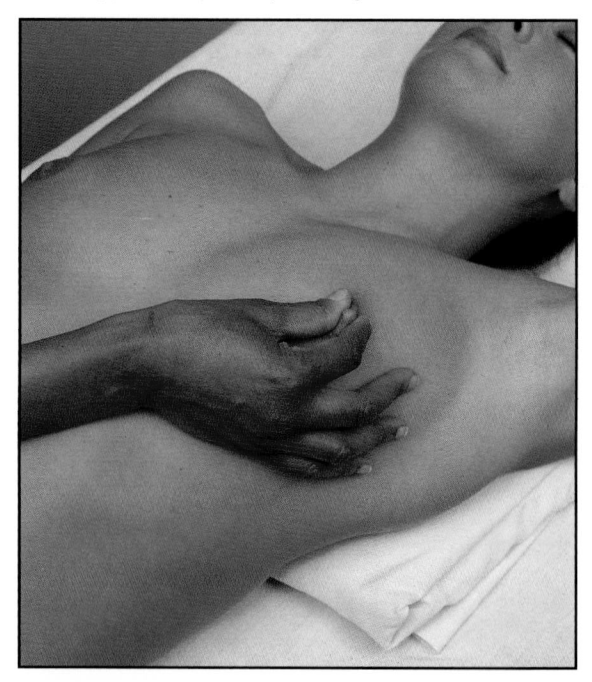

Common abnormalities

■ Nipple retraction

Retraction of the nipple may result from breast cancer.

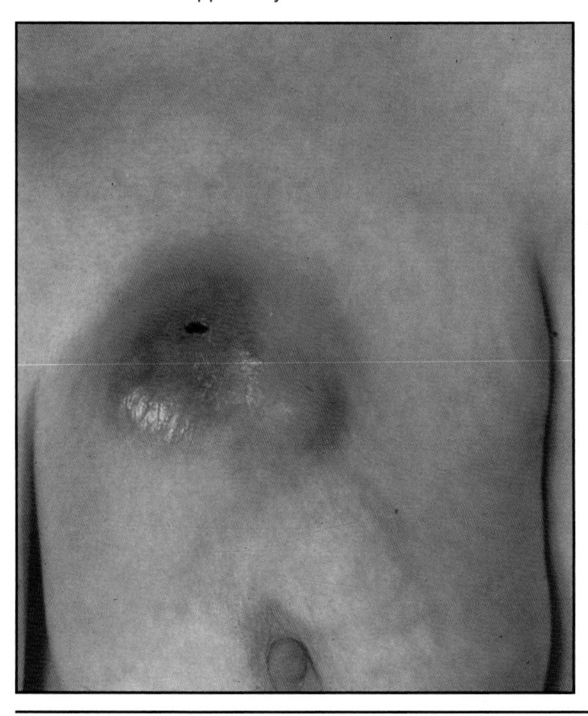

■ Asymmetrical breasts

Asymmetrical breasts may indicate a breast disorder or may be normal, especially during adolescence.

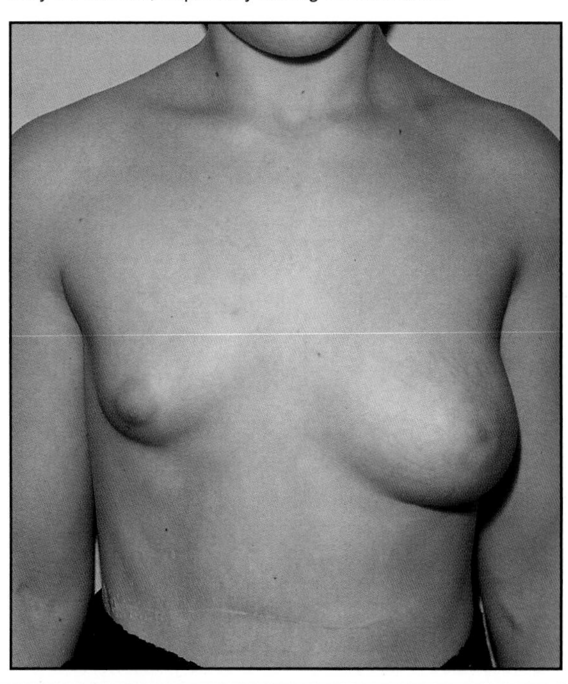

■ Gynecomastia

Unilateral or bilateral breast enlargement in an adult male may be caused by an estrogen-secreting tumor, liver disease, or use of certain drugs. In an adolescent male, it may result from normal hormonal changes.

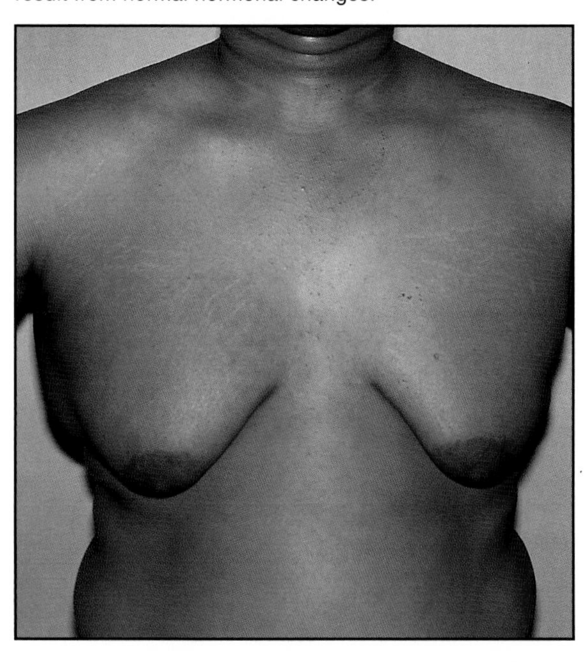

■ Eczema-like nipple changes

A red, scaly, eczema-like area over one nipple and areola may be a sign of Paget's disease.

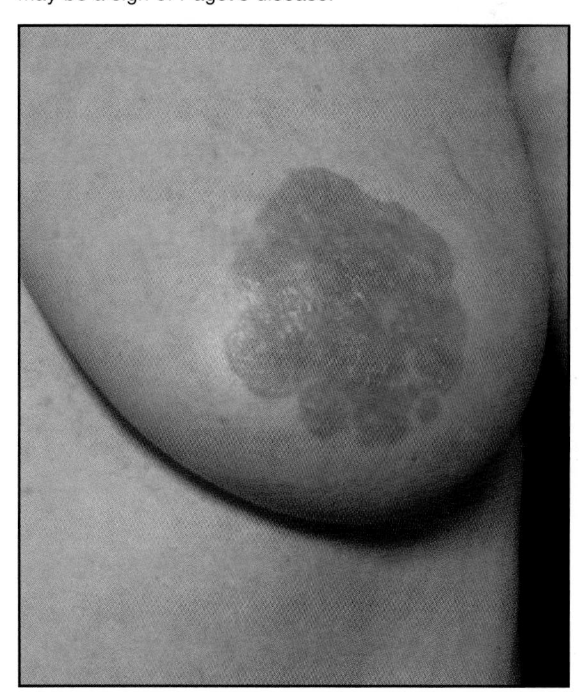

Gastrointestinal System

Anatomy and physiology overview

■ Structures of the gastrointestinal system

This anterior view shows the structures of the gastrointestinal (GI) system.

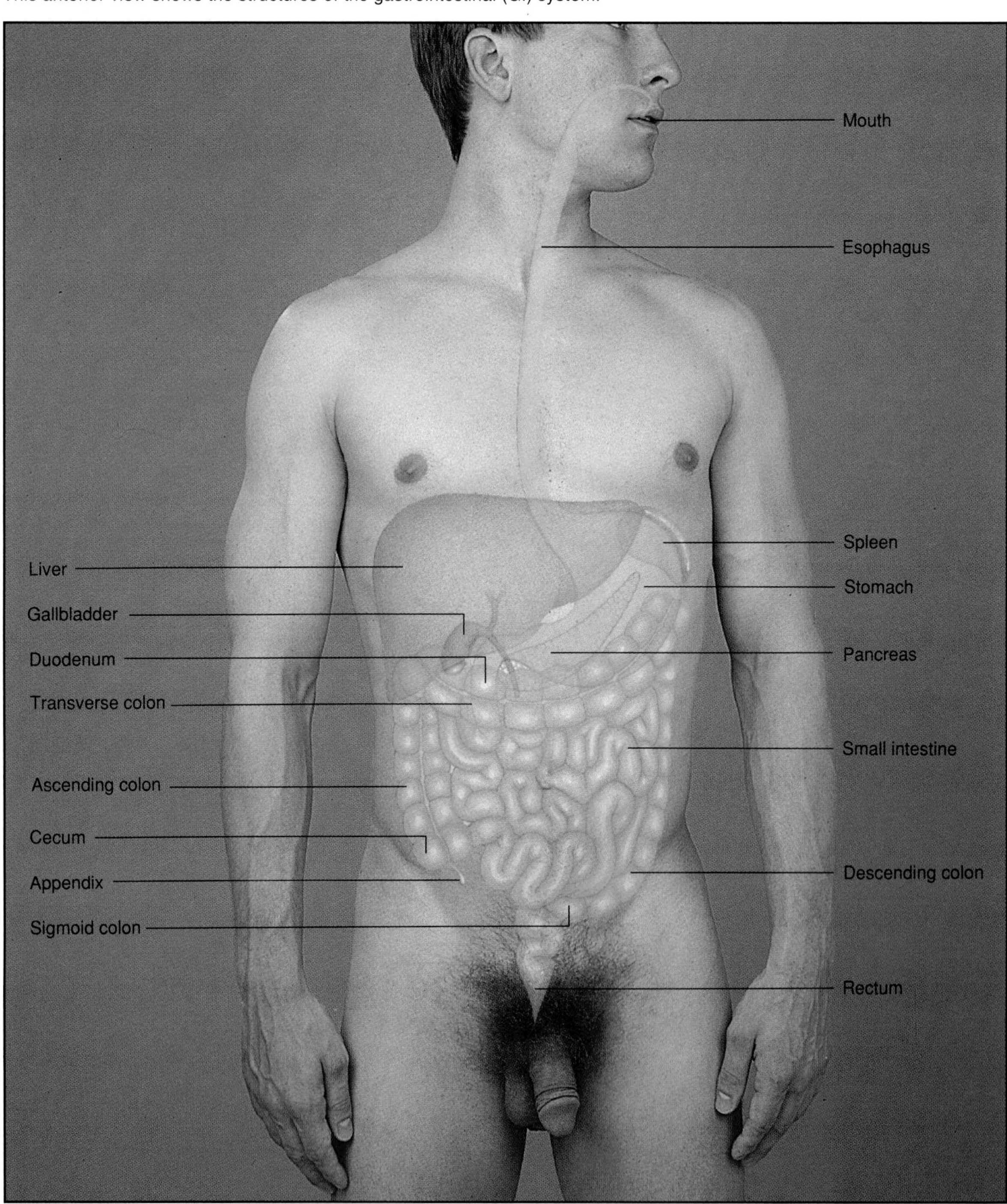

■ Abdominal landmarks

These anterior views divide the abdomen into sections using the quadrant and nine region methods. These sections serve as anatomical landmarks during assessment.

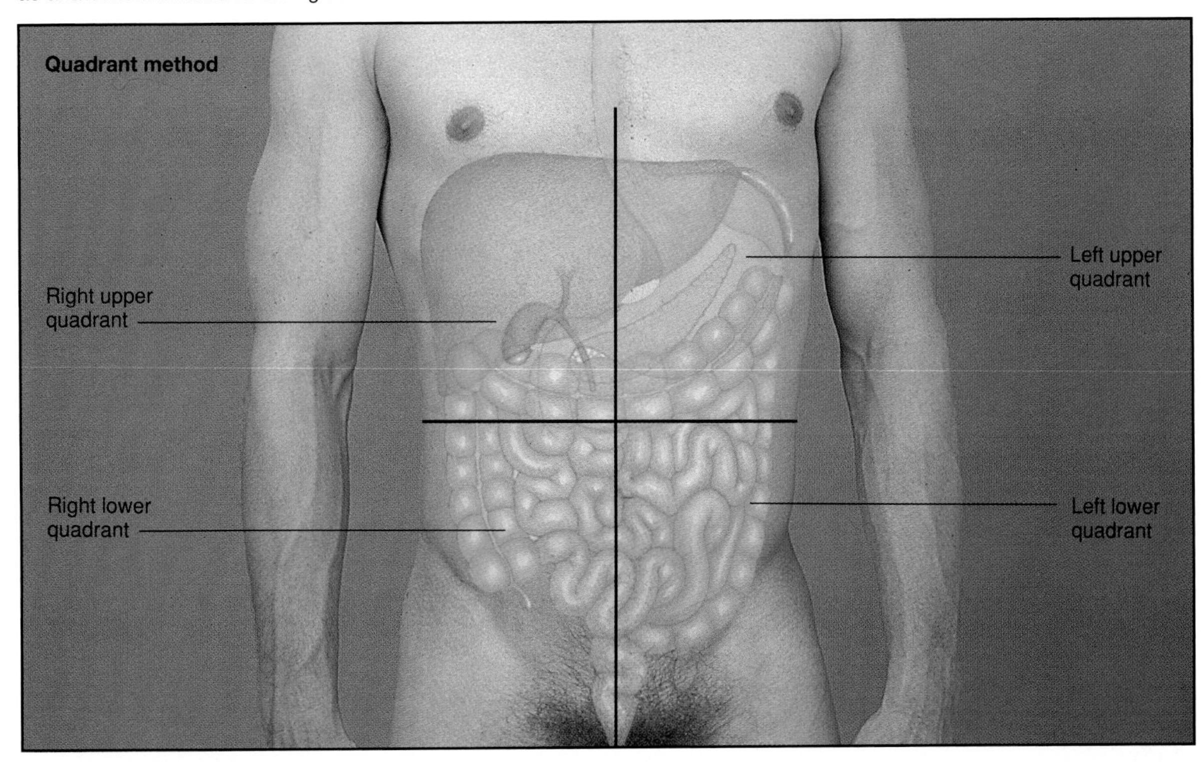

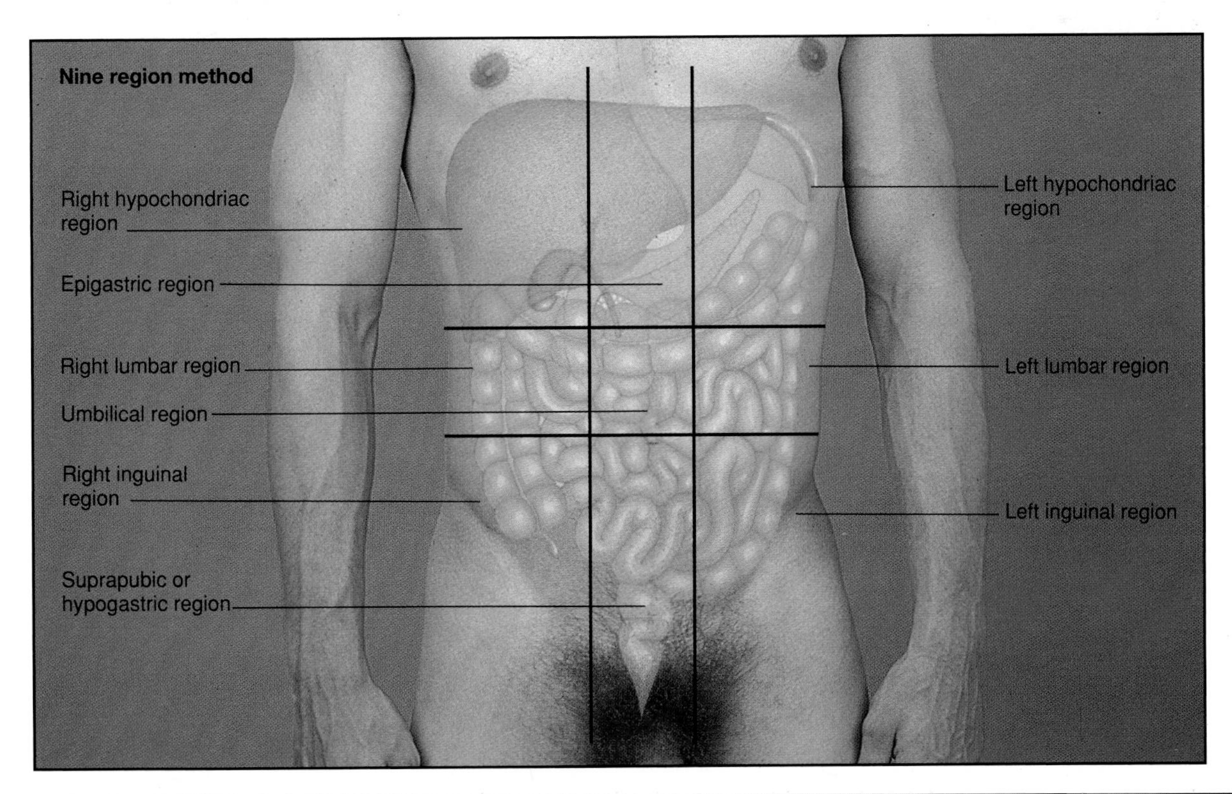

Assessment

■ Auscultation

Bowel sounds and vascular sounds

Using the diaphragm of the stethoscope, auscultate for bowel sounds in all abdominal quadrants. These soft, bubbling sounds normally occur every 5 to 15 seconds. Using the bell of the stethoscope, assess for abdominal vascular sounds in these auscultatory sites. Here, auscultation normally detects no vascular sounds.

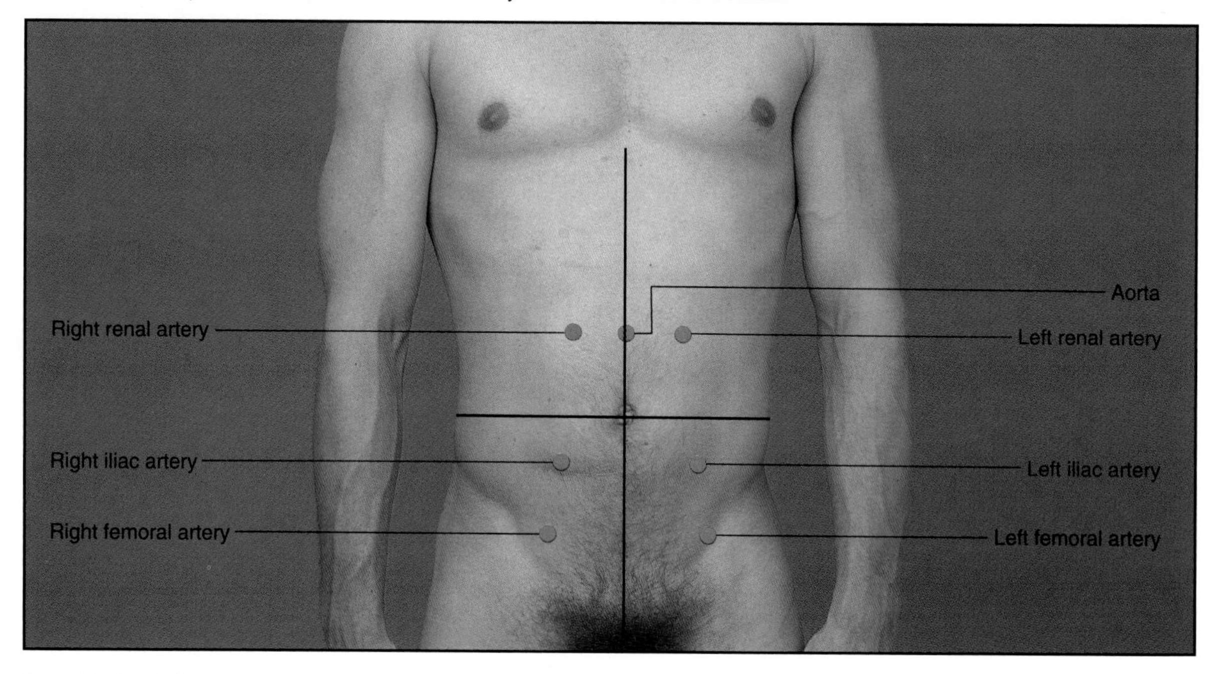

Scratch technique

Perform the scratch technique to identify the lower border of the liver. To do this, place the diaphragm of the stethoscope over the approximate location of the lower border. Auscultate while lightly scratching at the midclavicular line from the right iliac crest and upward. The scratching noise should become louder over the liver.

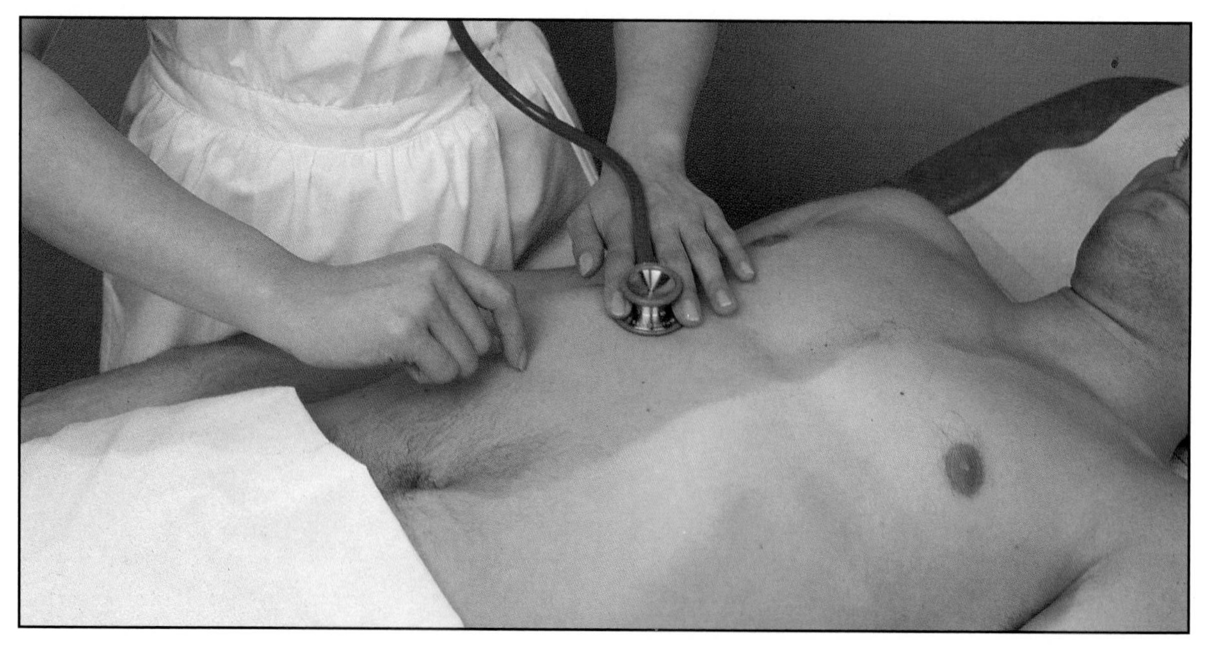

■ Percussion

Abdomen

Use mediate (indirect) percussion to assess the abdominal quadrants. Normal percussion notes range from tympany to dullness, depending on intestinal contents.

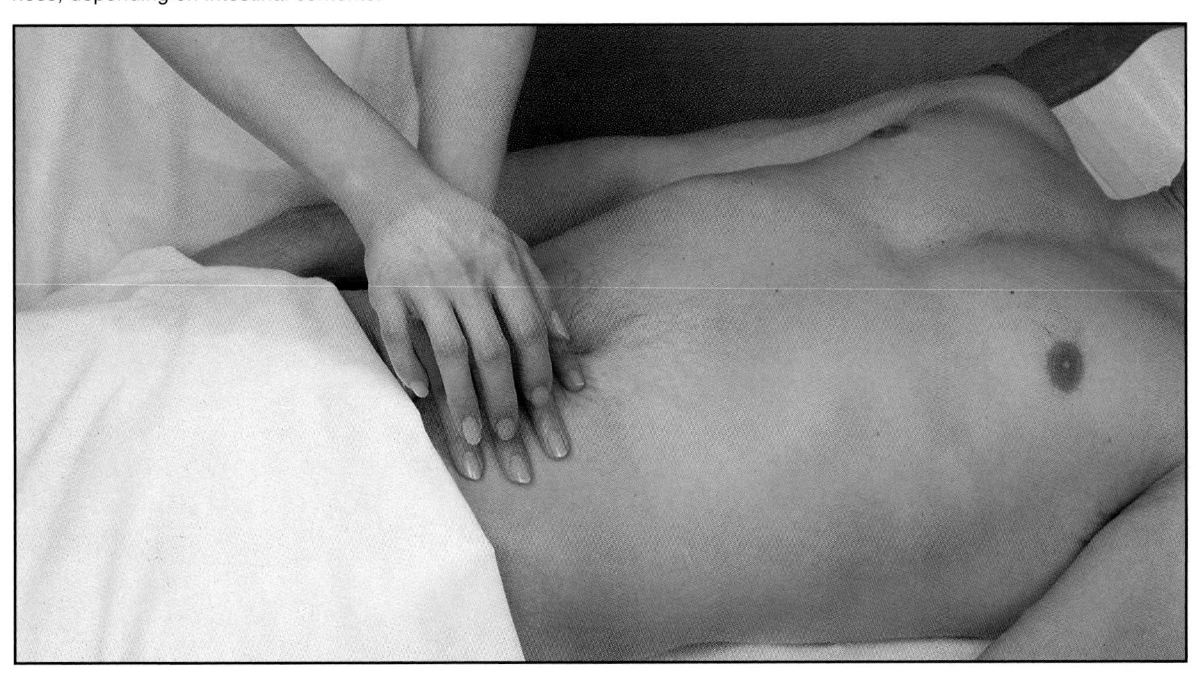

Liver size

Use mediate percussion along the right midclavicular line to estimate the size of the liver, which usually ranges from 6 to 12 cm.

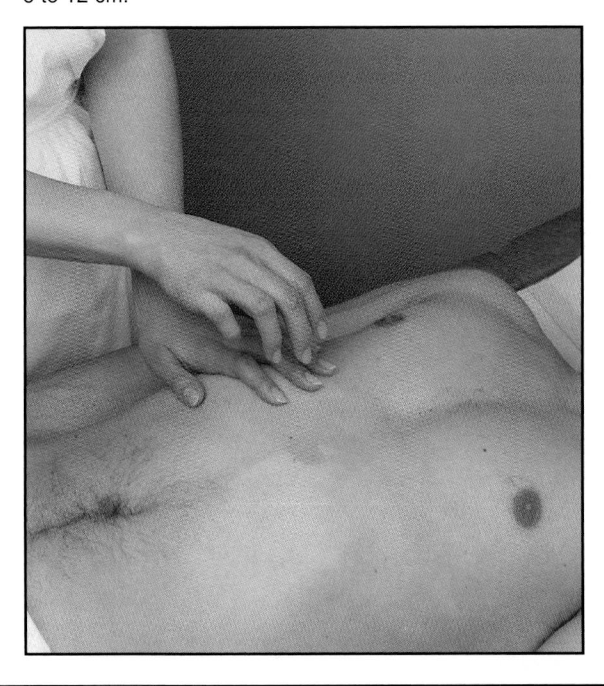

Liver tenderness

Use fist percussion to detect tenderness over the liver or gallbladder. To do this, place one hand flat over the client's lower right rib cage along the midclavicular line. Then strike the back of this hand with the other hand clenched in a fist. Fist percussion normally elicits no tenderness.

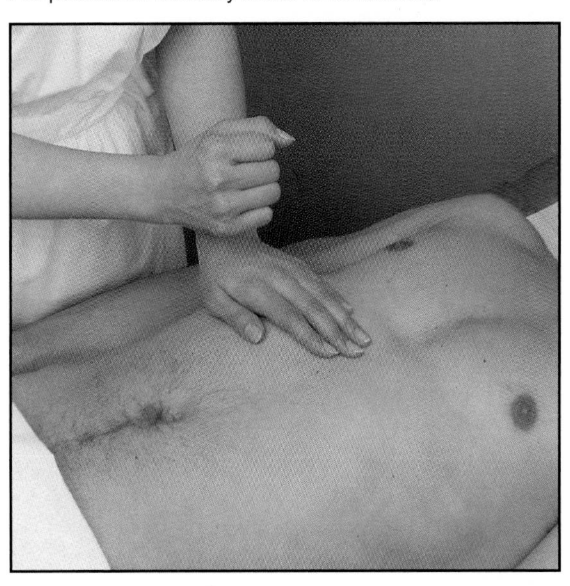

(continued)

ASSESSMENT

PERCUSSION (continued)

Test for shifting dullness

With the client supine, percuss the abdomen and note where tympany changes to dullness (below left). Then repeat this procedure with the client lying on one side (right). Normally, the border between tympany and dullness remains the same when the client changes position.

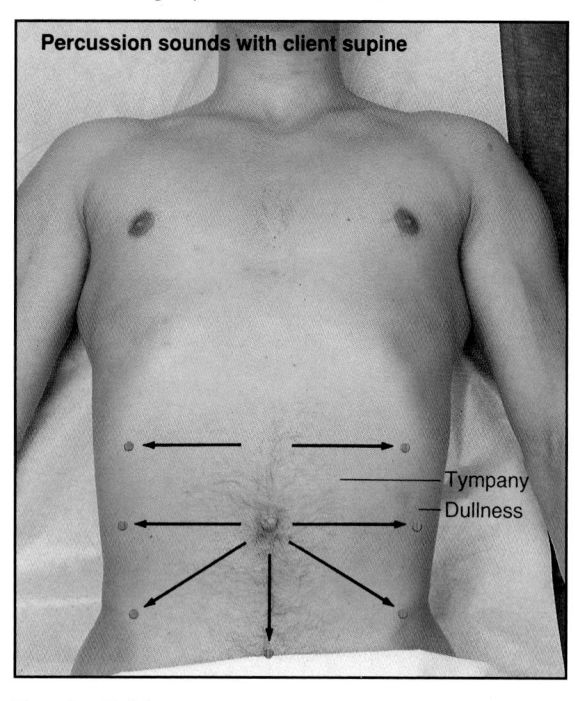

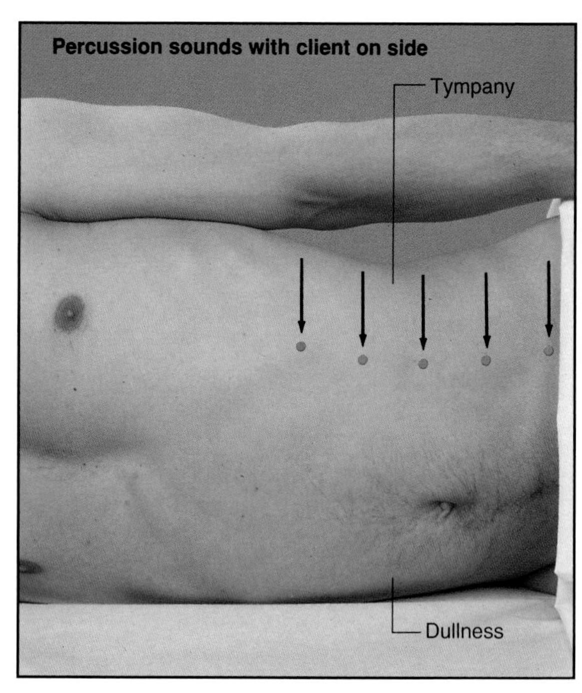

Test for fluid wave

With the client supine, have an assistant place the hand and forearm firmly on the client's abdomen at the midline. This minimizes wave transmission through adipose tissue. Place your hand firmly against one side of the client's abdomen. With the opposite hand, tap on the opposite side of the abdomen. Normally, a fluid wave cannot be felt.

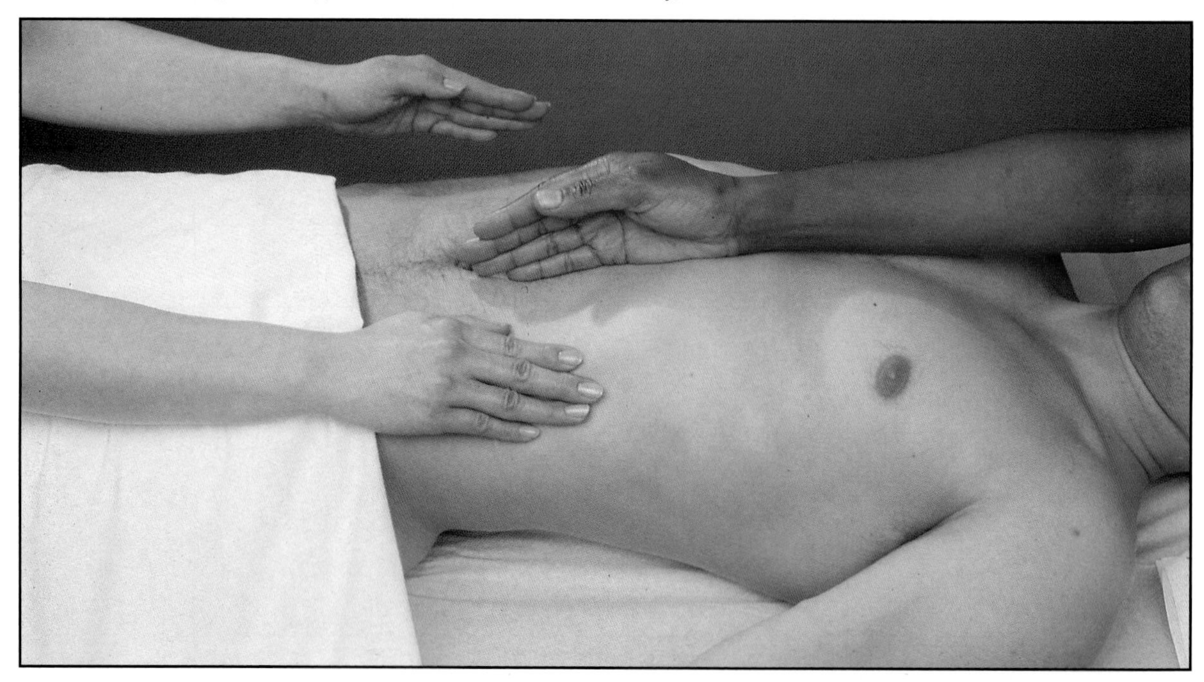

■ Palpation

Light abdominal palpation

Lightly palpate all quadrants to assess consistency and areas of tenderness. Normally, the abdomen is soft and nontender.

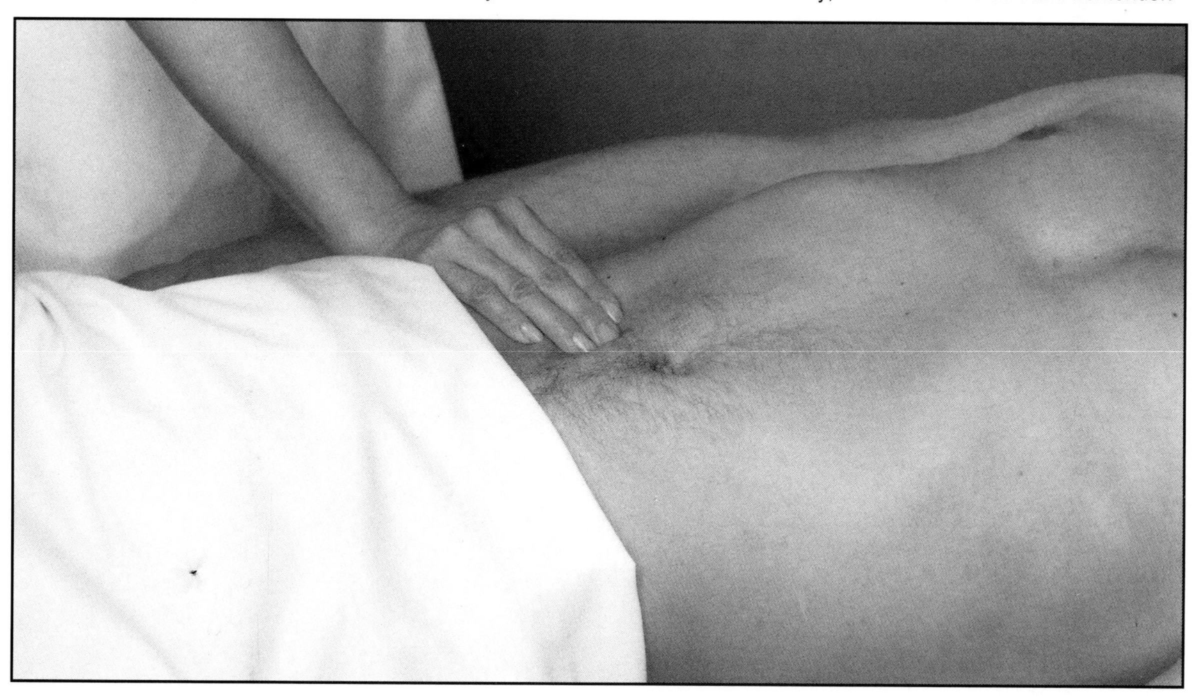

Deep abdominal palpation

Deeply palpate all four quadrants with one hand or, if the client is obese, with two hands. Abdominal organs should feel normal in size and consistency. Deep palpation should not detect any masses, tenderness, or muscle resistance.

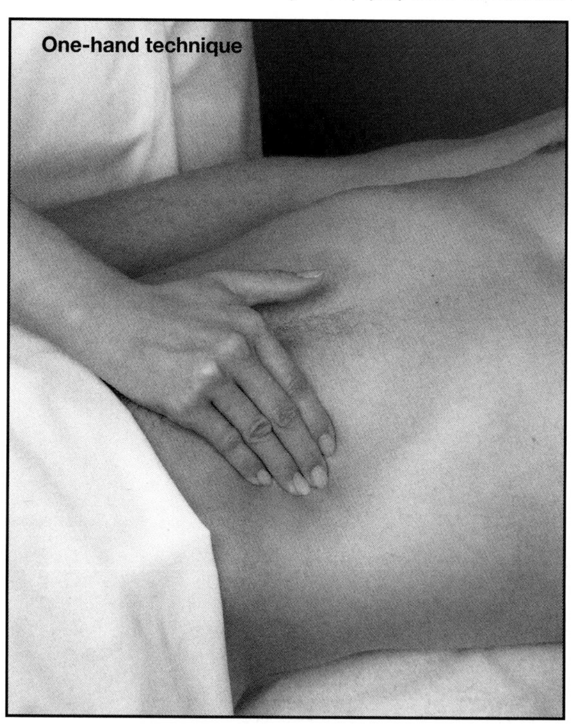

One-hand technique

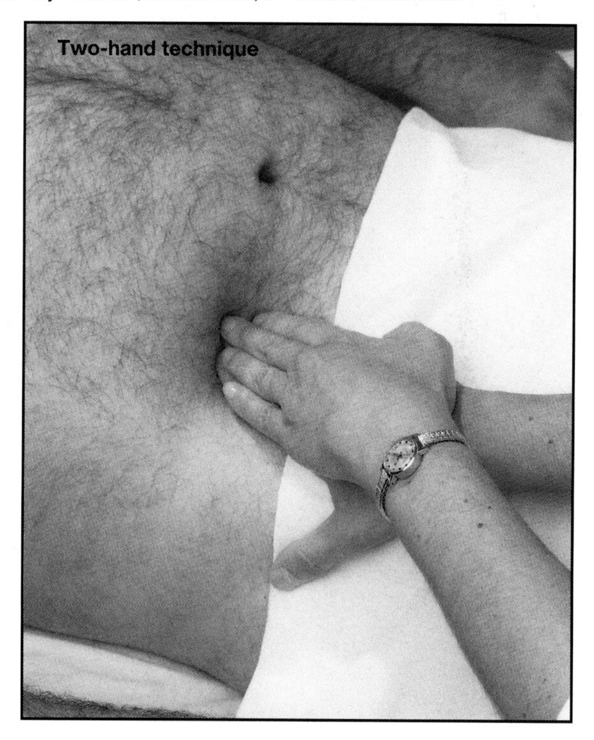

Two-hand technique

Common abnormalities

■ Symmetrical abdominal distention

This assessment finding may result from excessive fluid, gas, or severe malnutrition.

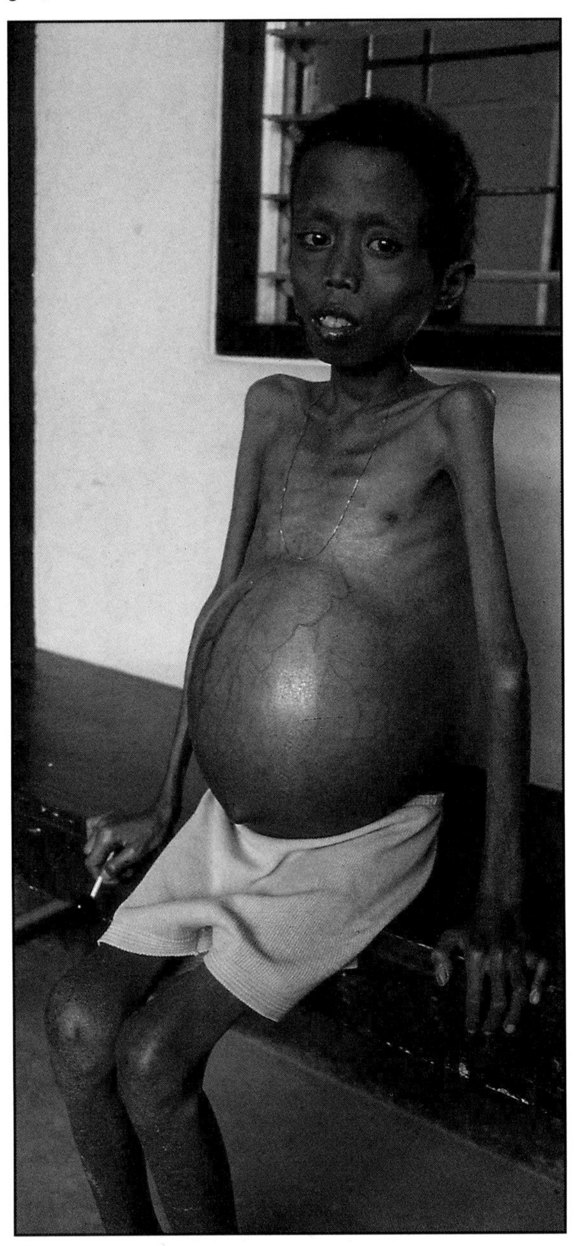

■ Striae

Abdominal lines may be caused by rapid, prolonged skin stretching. They initially appear pink or blue, then turn white or silver. Cushing's syndrome may cause them to turn purplish.

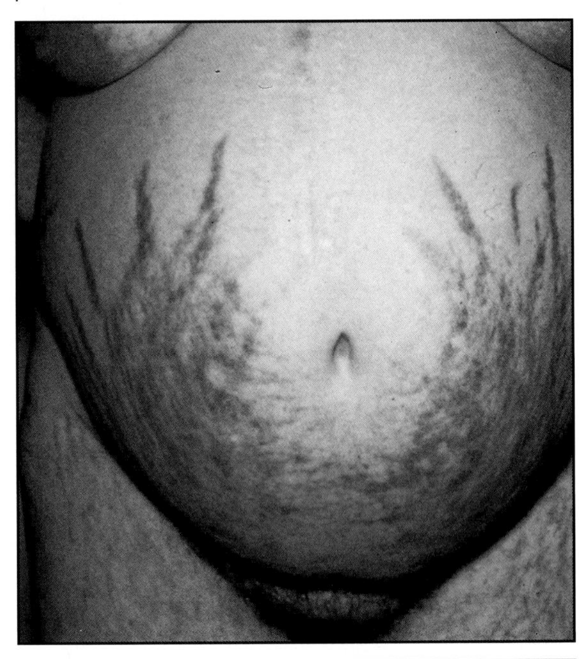

■ Incisional hernia

After surgery, a patient may display an incisional hernia, which is the protrusion of an organ through the opening made by an abdominal incision.

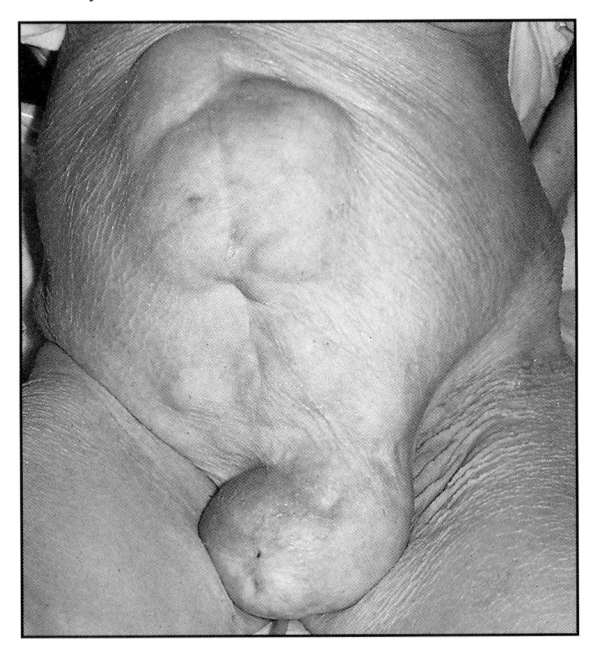

Urinary System

Anatomy and physiology overview

■ Structures of the urinary system

This anterior view of the torso shows the structures of the urinary system.

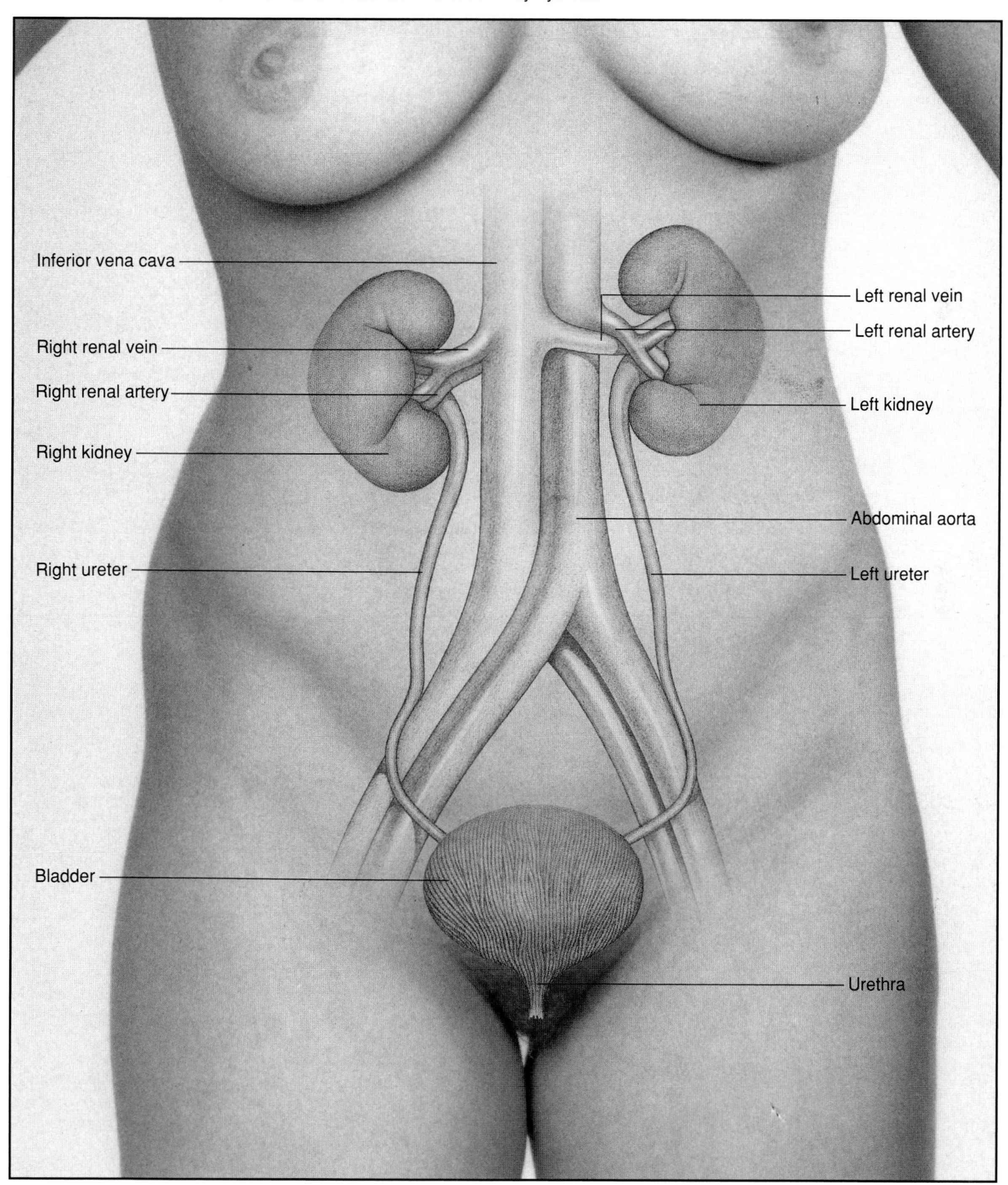

Assessment

■ Inspection

Urethral meatus

Male client. Inspect the urethral meatus while compressing the tip of the glans penis with a gloved hand. (If the client is uncircumsized, first retract the foreskin.) Normally, the meatus is centrally located and free of discharge.

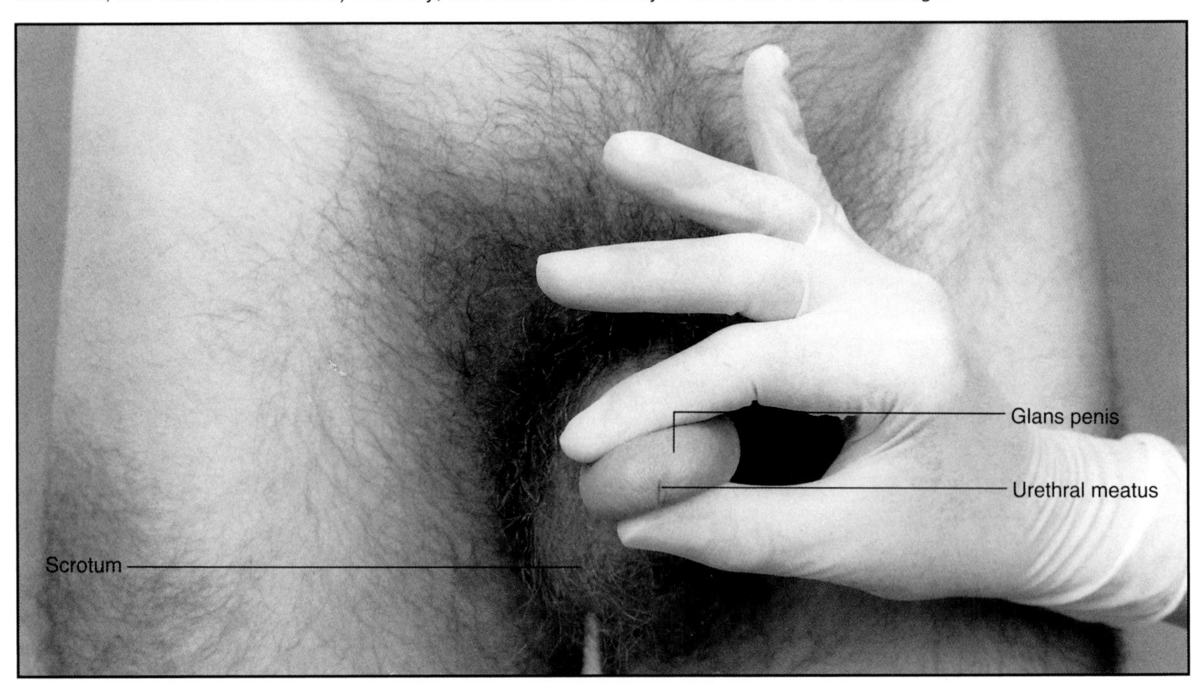

Female client. After placing the client in the lithotomy position, inspect her urinary meatus while separating the labia with a gloved hand. Normally, the meatus is pink and shows no swelling or discharge.

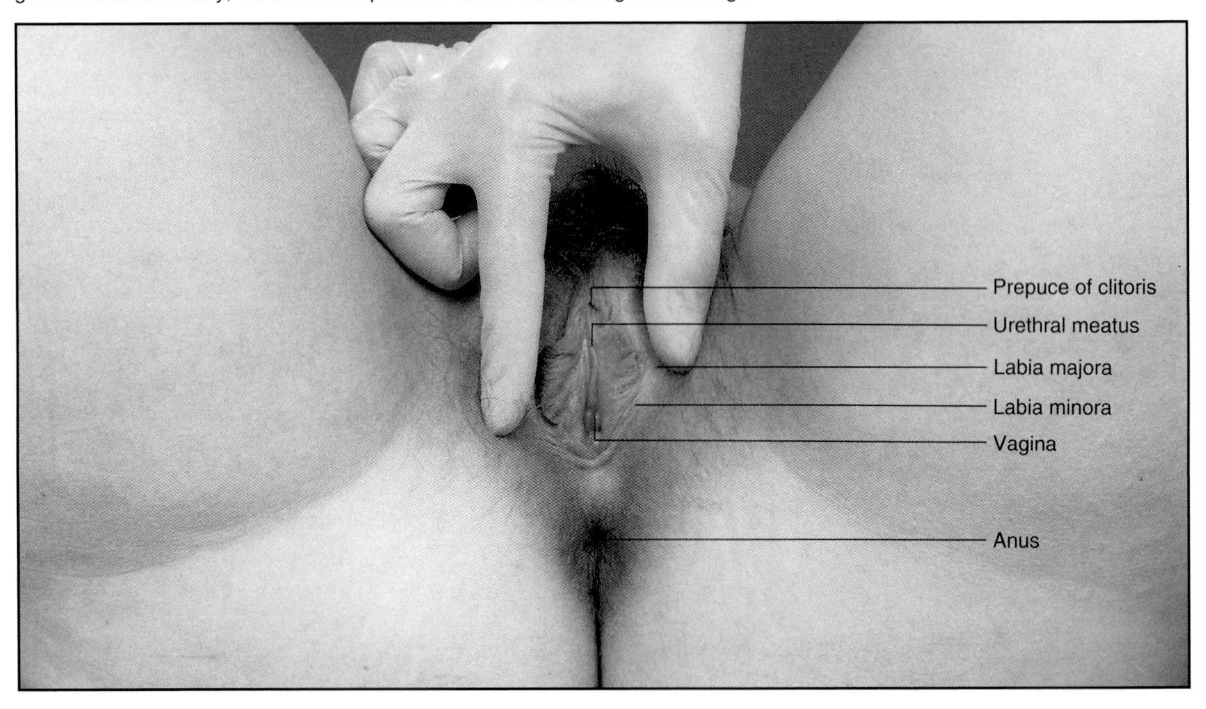

■ Percussion

Kidneys

To percuss the kidneys, place the left palm over the client's costovertebral angle and strike it with the right fist. Repeat this procedure over the opposite costovertebral angle. The client may report feeling a thudding sensation, but normally will feel no tenderness or pain.

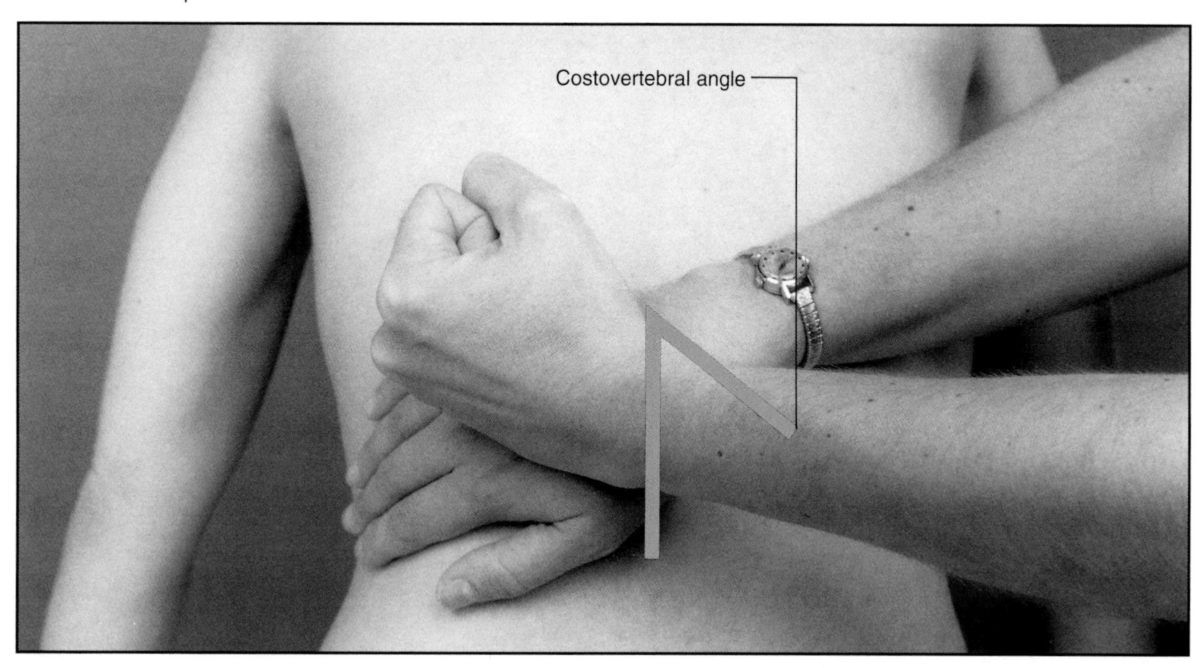

Bladder

To assess the bladder, use mediate (indirect) percussion beginning 2" (5 cm) above the symphysis pubis. To detect differences in sound, percuss toward the base of the bladder. Percussion normally produces tympany or, over a urine-filled bladder, dullness.

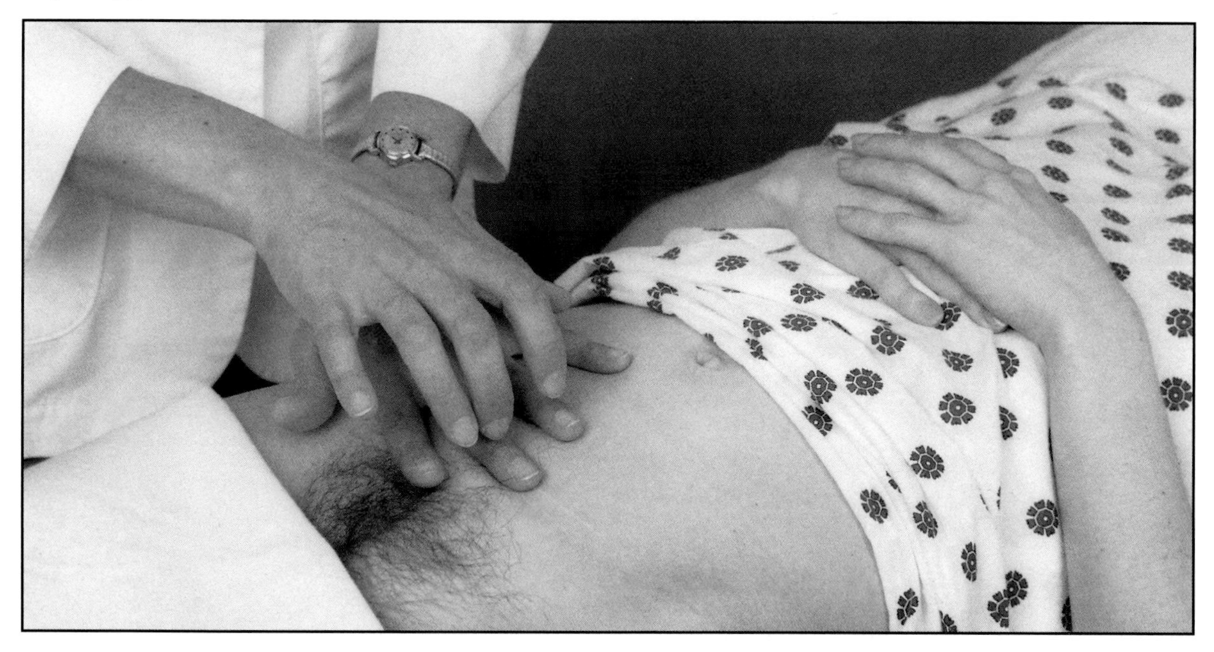

ASSESSMENT

■ Palpation

Kidneys

1 Place the left hand midway between the lower costal margin and the iliac crest, and the right hand on the abdomen above the left hand. While the client inhales deeply, quickly press the hands together to attempt to capture the kidney.

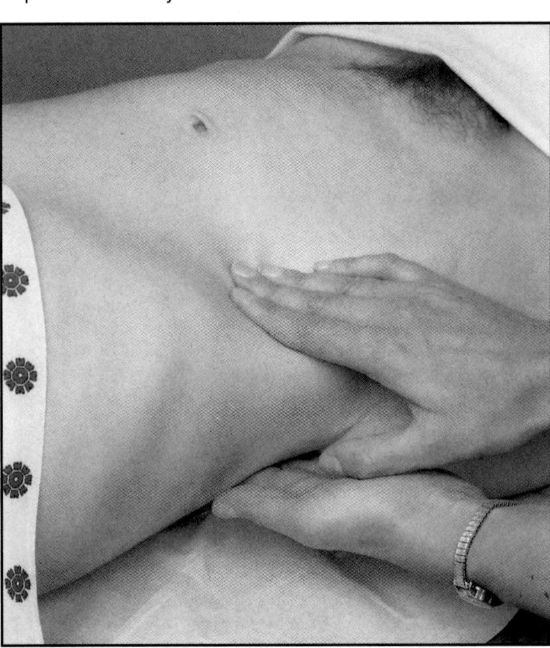

2 While the client exhales, slowly release your hands. If the kidney was captured, it will slide back into place. Usually, the kidneys are not palpable in an adult. If palpable, the kidneys should be smooth, solid, firm, and nontender. The kidneys should be equal in size bilaterally.

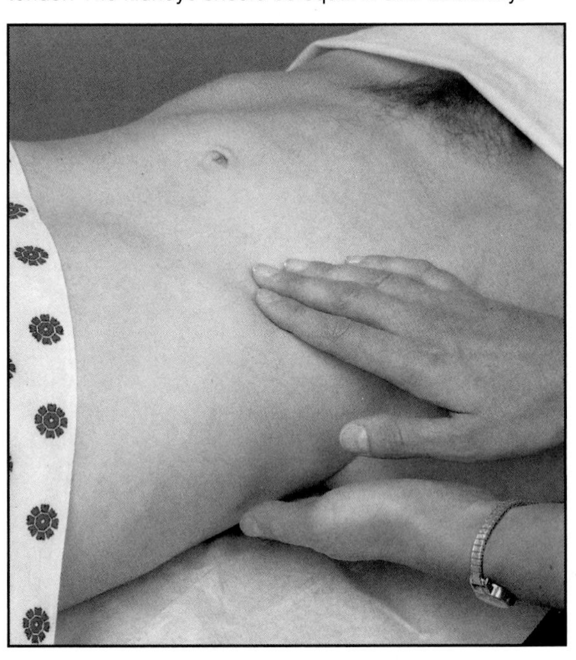

Bladder

Before palpating the bladder, have the client void. Palpate 1" to 2" (2.5 to 5 cm) above the symphysis pubis. If palpable, the bladder should feel firm and relatively smooth. (The empty bladder normally is not palpable.)

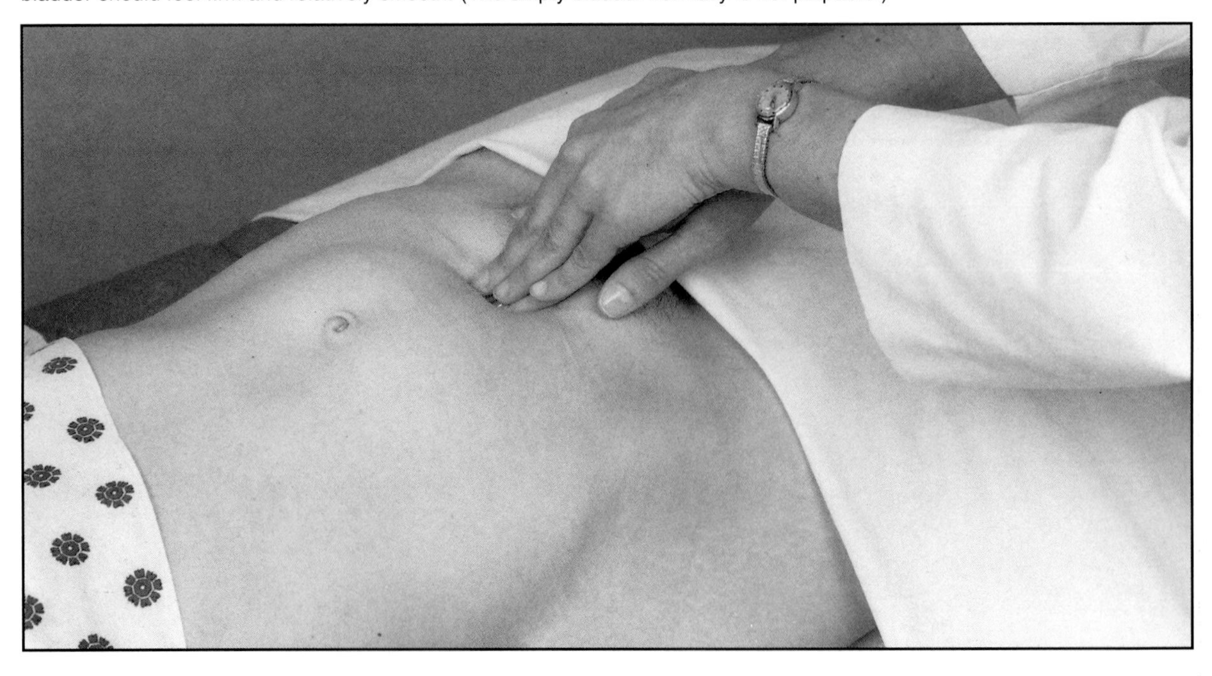

Female Reproductive System

Anatomy and physiology overview

■ Structures of the female reproductive system

This frontal view identifies the internal structures of the female reproductive system. The lithotomy view below shows the external structures and landmarks.

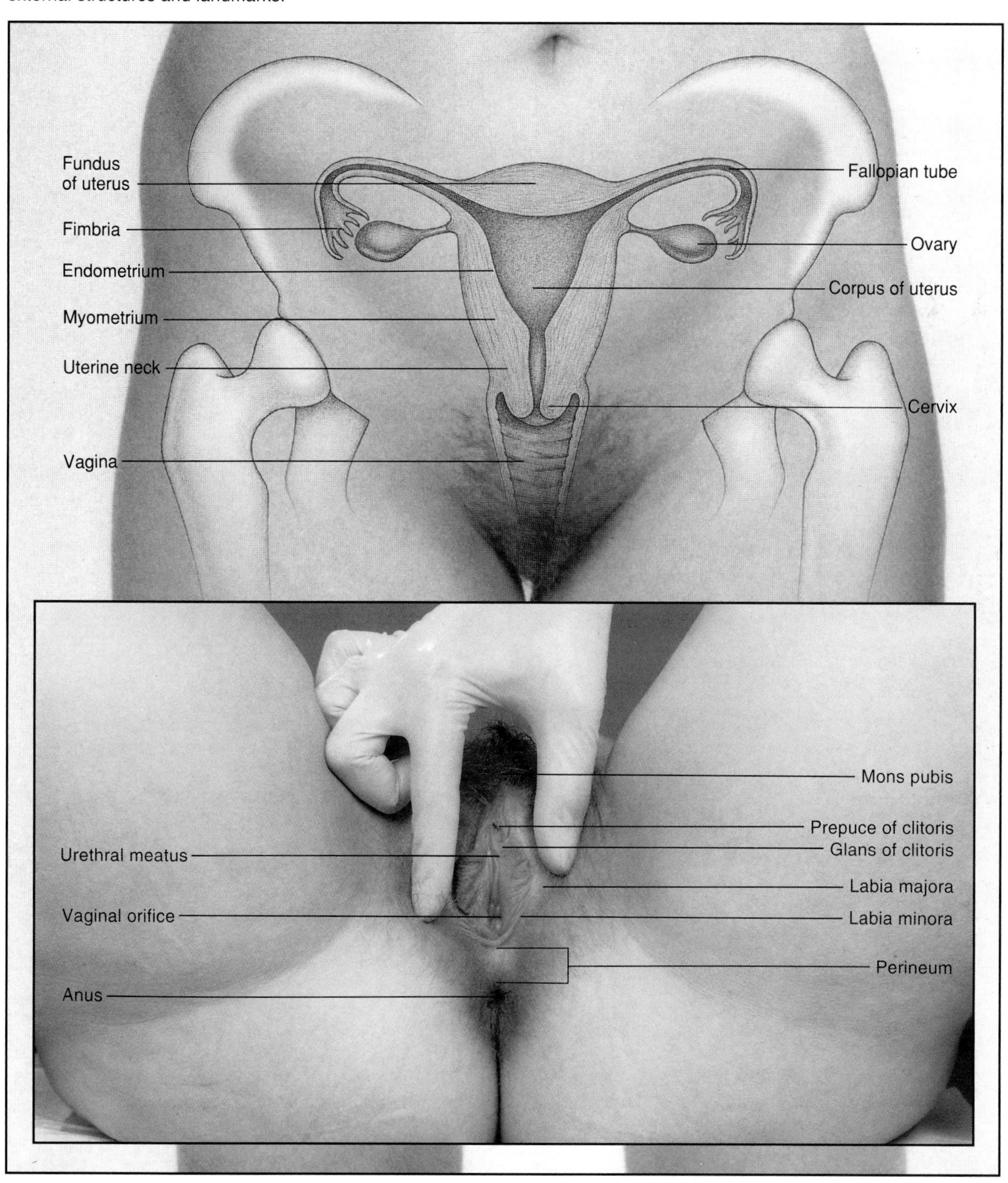

Common abnormalities

■ Cervical polyps

These bright-red, fragile, soft protrusions into the cervical canal may arise from endometrial or endocervical tissue. They usually result from localized inflammation. The photograph below shows cervical polyps with cervical prolapse.

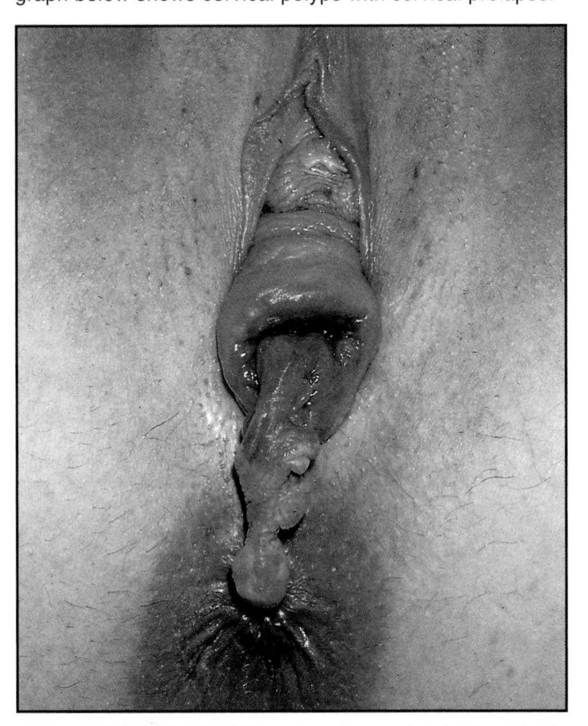

■ Venereal warts

Dark pink to pale, cauliflower-like lesions indicate venereal warts (condylomata acuminata), which are caused by a virus.

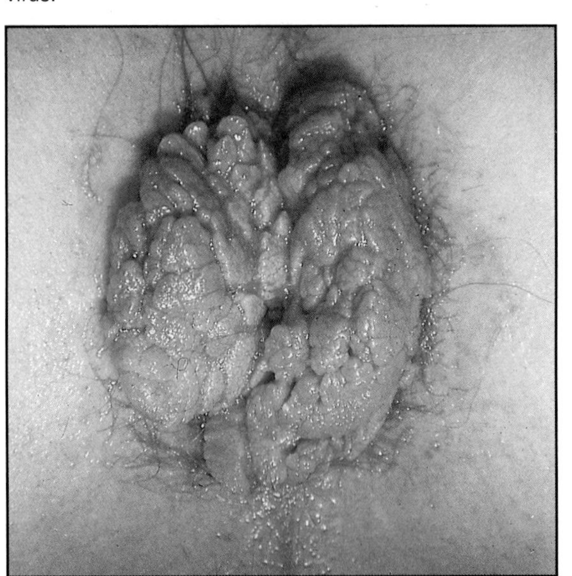

■ Uterine prolapse

Displacement of the uterus into the vagina may be caused by weak pelvic muscles or ligaments.

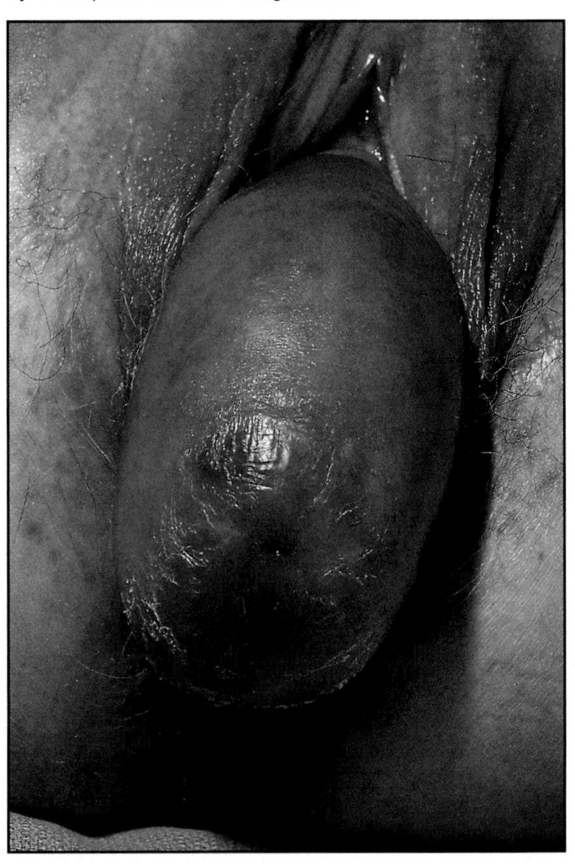

■ Inguinal mass

Bulging in the inguinal area suggests an inguinal hernia, which may be congenital or may result from obesity, muscular weakness, surgery, or illness.

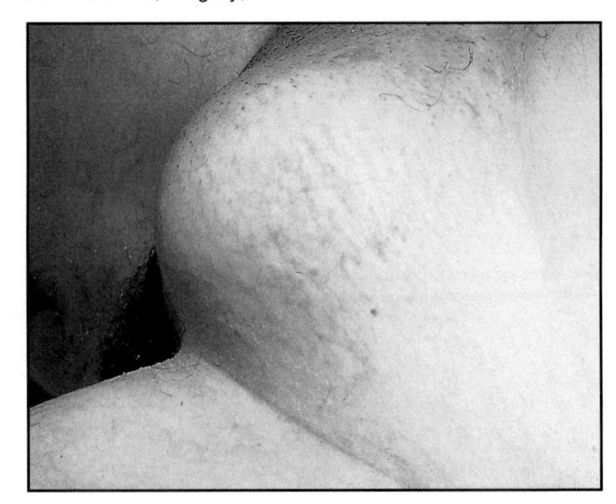

Male Reproductive System

Anatomy and physiology overview

■ Structures of the male reproductive system

This lateral view of the pelvis shows the structures of the male reproductive system and associated landmarks.

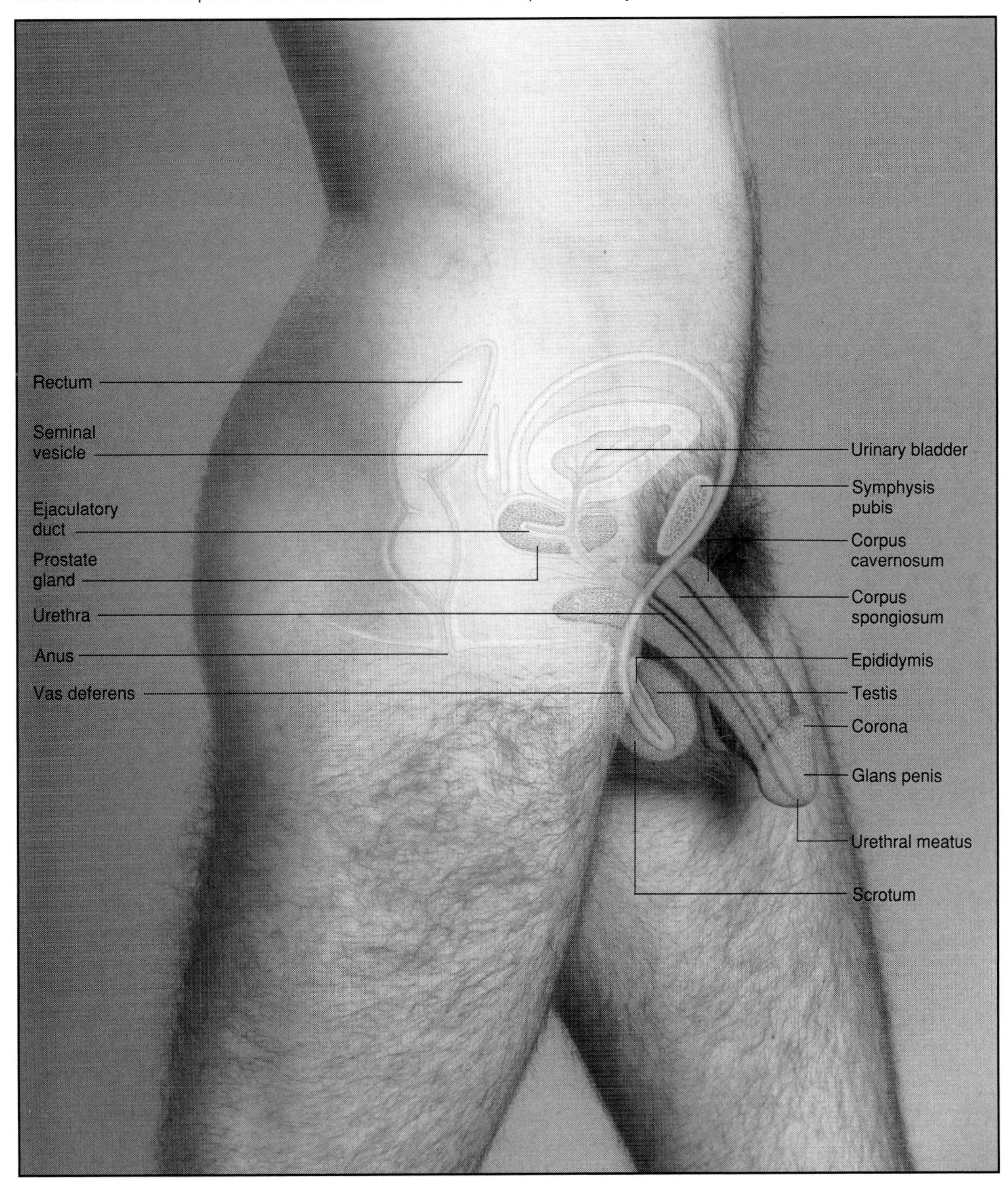

Assessment

■ Inspection

Penis and scrotum

Inspect the penis and scrotum. Normally, the organs are of appropriate size, the skin is intact with no lesions, and the pubic hair is distributed evenly. The left testicle usually hangs slightly lower than the right, but both should hang freely in the scrotum.

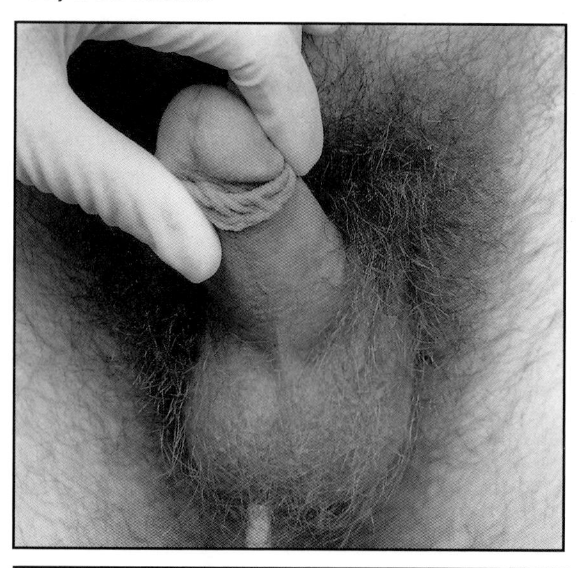

Scrotum and testes

While wearing gloves, palpate the scrotum between the thumb and first two fingers. Normally, the scrotal skin is rough without nodules or lesions, and the testes are small, smooth, oval, and freely movable.

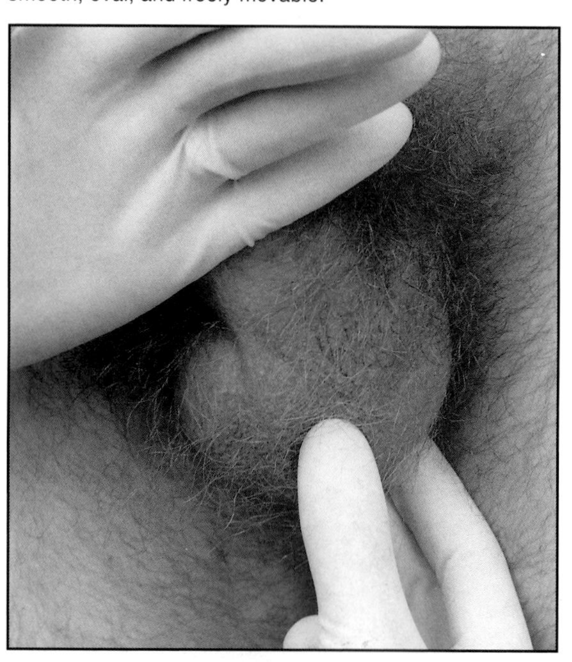

■ Palpation

Penis

While wearing gloves, palpate along the length of the penis, using the thumb and first two fingers. The nonerect penis should feel soft, nontender, and free of nodules.

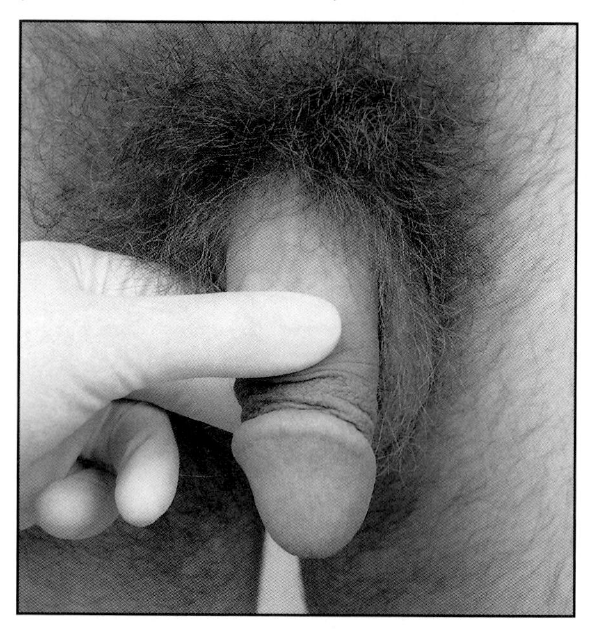

Epididymis and vas deferens

Continue the assessment by palpating the epididymis and vas deferens on the posterolateral scrotal surface. The epididymis should feel like a firm ridge of tissue lying vertically on the testicular surface. The vas deferens should feel like a smooth cord and be freely movable.

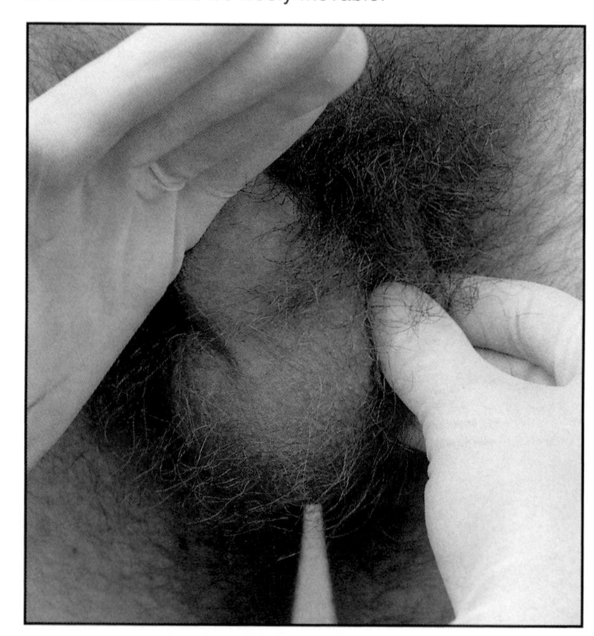

Common abnormalities

■ Venereal warts

Dark pink to pale, cauliflower-like lesions indicate veneral warts (condylomata acuminata), which are caused by a virus.

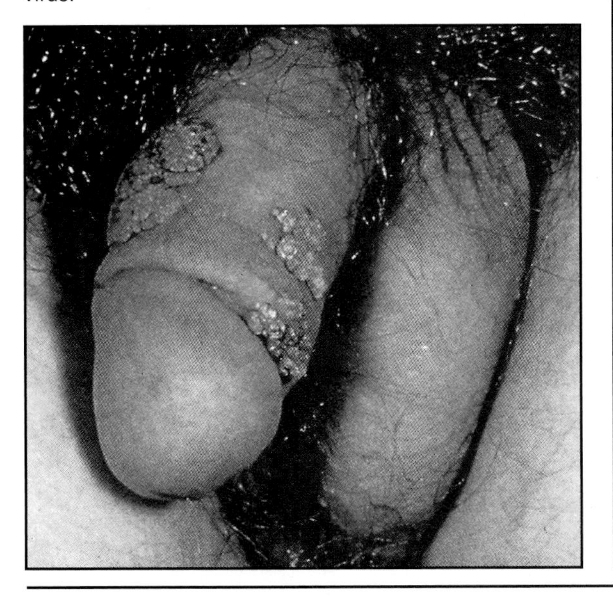

■ Ulcerative lesions

Painful, recurring genital lesions may result from genital herpes.

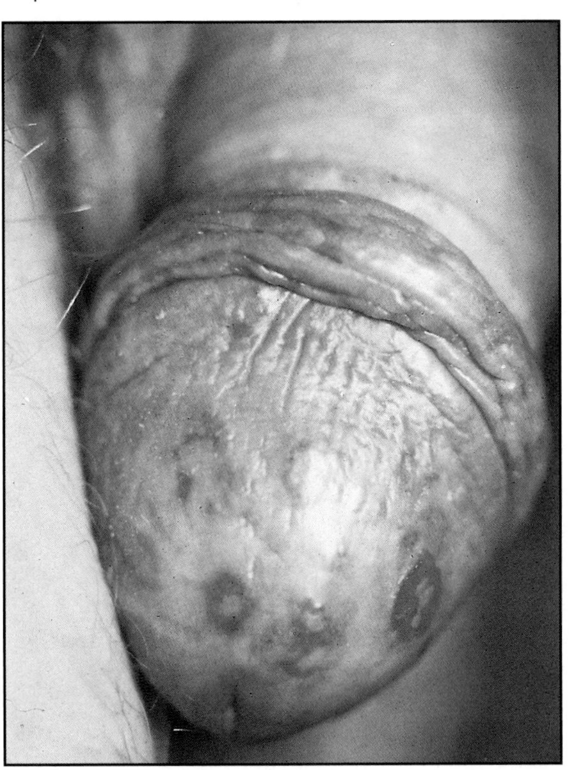

■ Chancres

Red, painless, indurated lesions (as in the circled areas) are characteristic of primary syphilis.

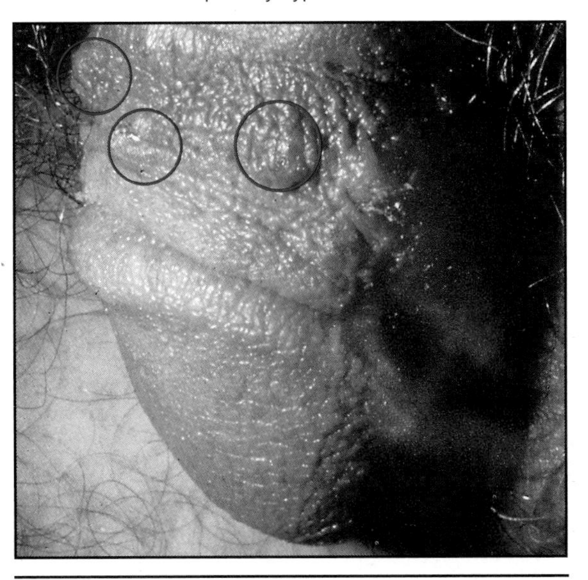

■ Inguinal mass

Bulging in the inguinal area suggests an inguinal hernia, which may be congenital or may result from obesity, muscular weakness, surgery, or illness.

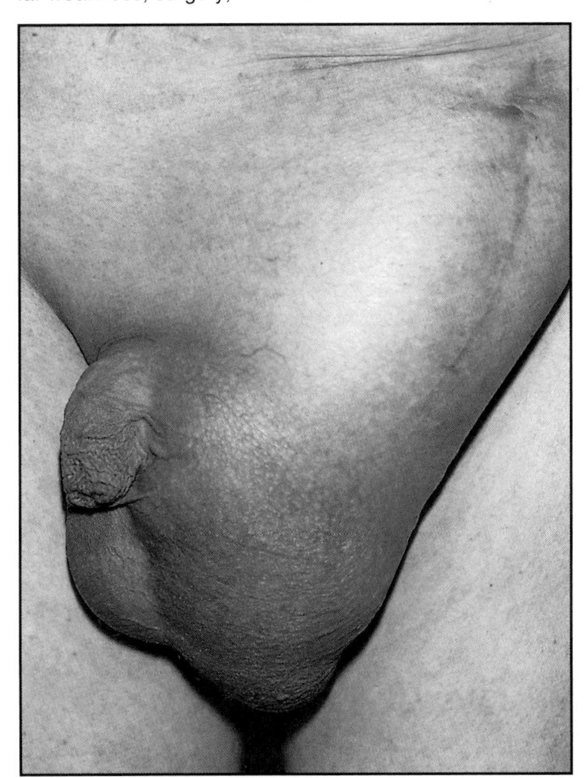

Nervous System

Anatomy and physiology overview

■ Structures of the central nervous system

This view of the head and neck shows the structures of the central nervous system (CNS).

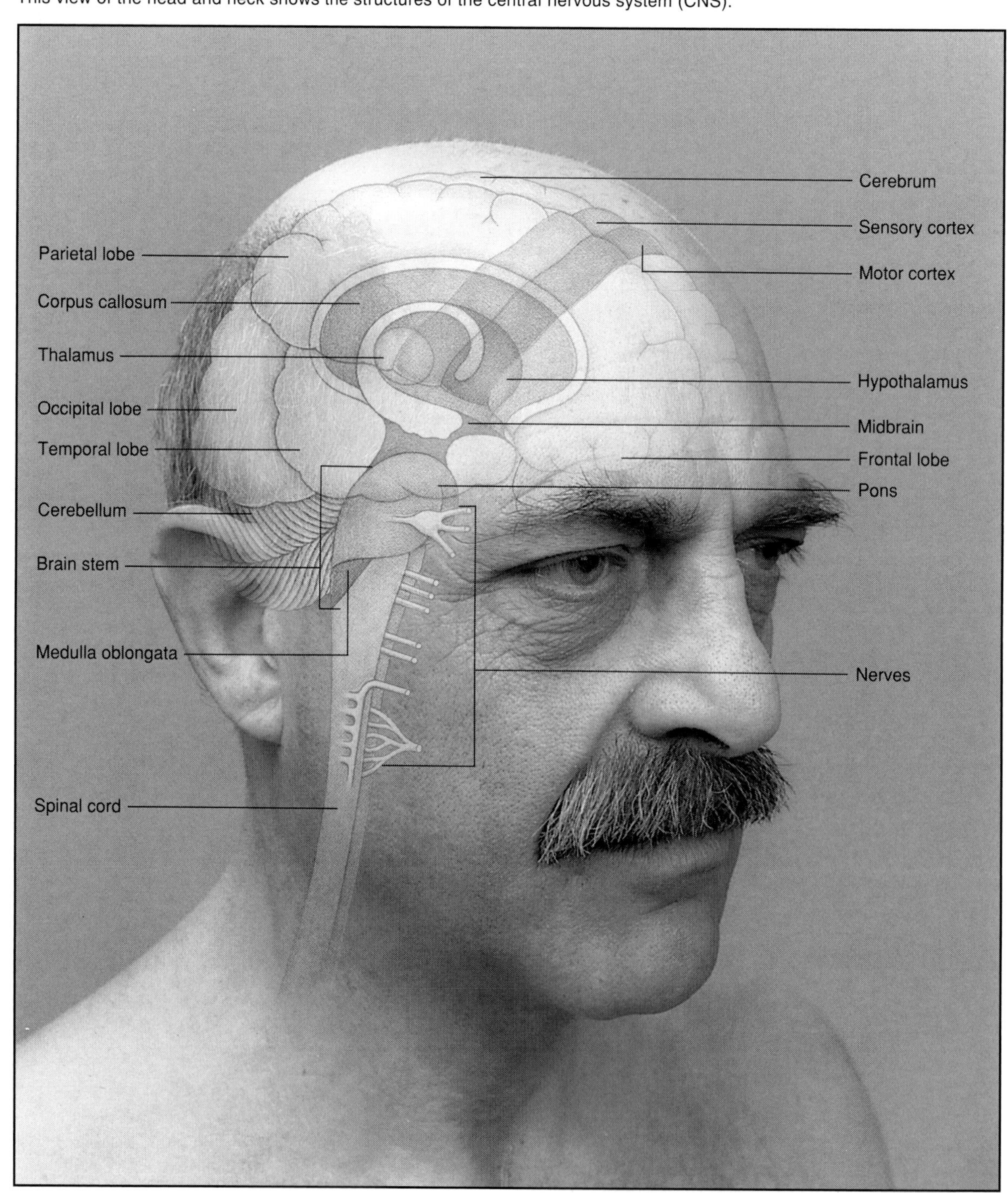

Assessment

■ Cranial nerves

Olfactory nerve (CN I)

After assessing the patency of each nostril, have the client close both eyes. Then occlude one nostril, hold an aromatic substance under the nose, and ask the client to identify it. Repeat for the other nostril. Normally, the client should be able to identify the odor in both nostrils.

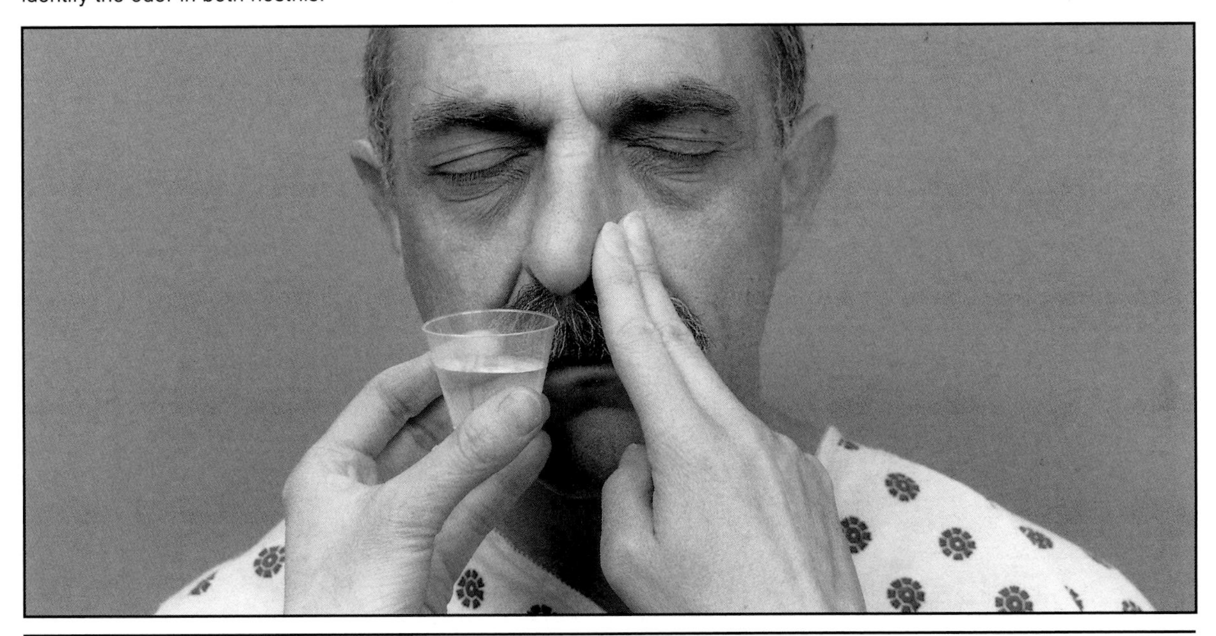

Trigeminal nerve (CN V)

Motor portion. To assess the motor portion of CN V, palpate the temporal and masseter muscles with the client's jaws clenched. Then try to open the client's clenched jaws. The jaws should clench symmetrically and remain closed against resistance.

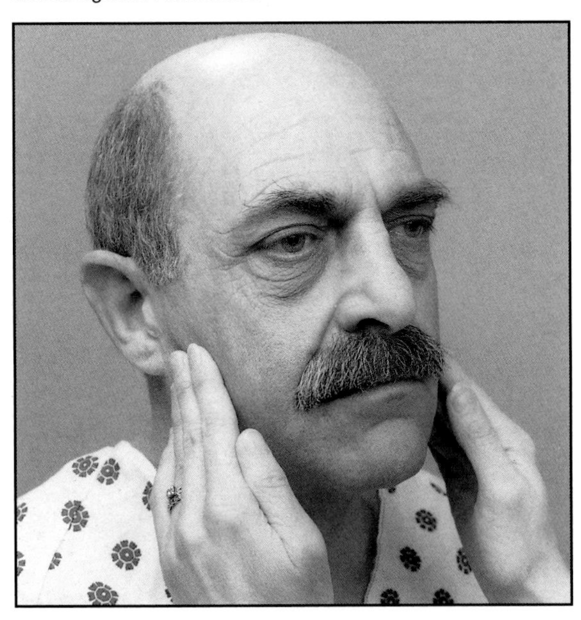

Sensory portion. While the client's eyes are closed, assess the sensory portion of CN V by testing the client's response to light touch and sharp stimuli on the forehead, cheek, and jaw. Normally, the client reports feeling light touch and sharp stimuli in all three areas bilaterally.

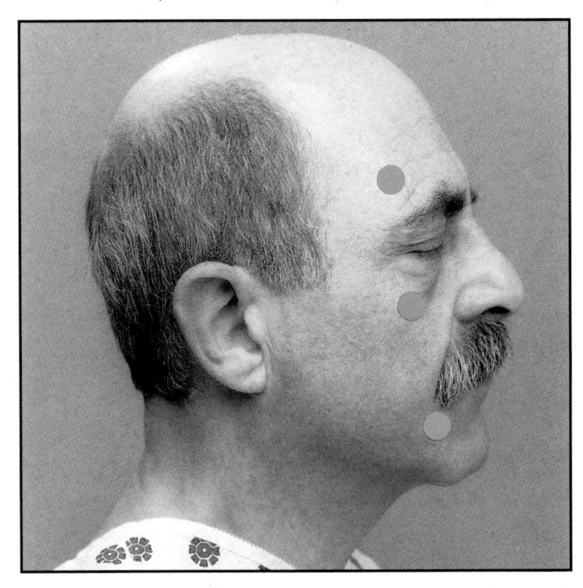

(continued)

ASSESSMENT

CRANIAL NERVES (continued)

Facial nerve (CN VII)

Motor portion. Ask the client to wrinkle the forehead, raise and lower the eyebrows, smile to show teeth, puff out the cheeks, and squeeze the eyes shut. Normally, facial movements are symmetrical.

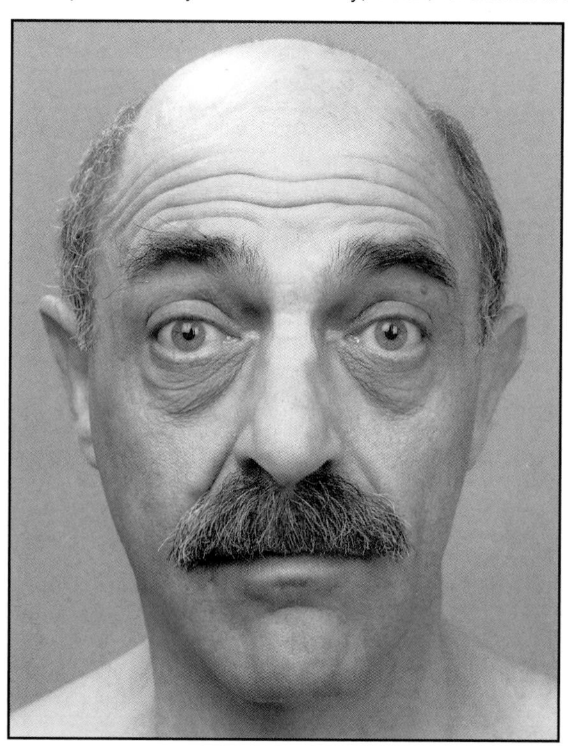

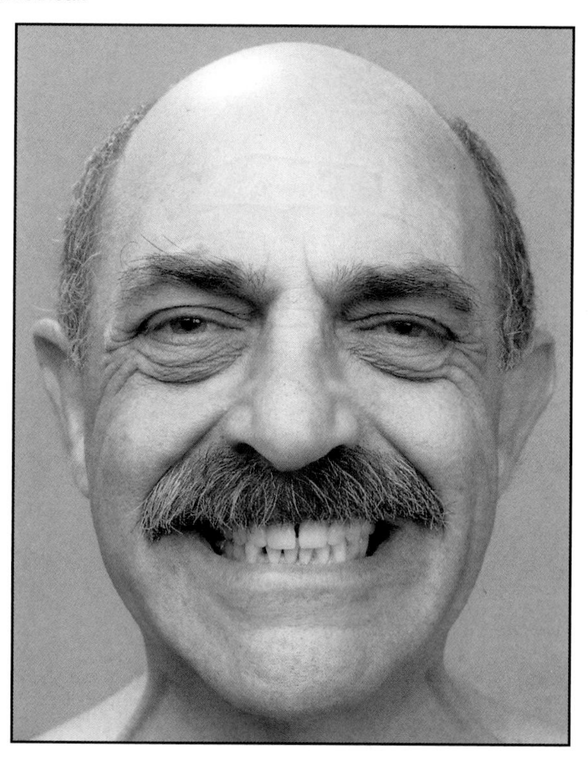

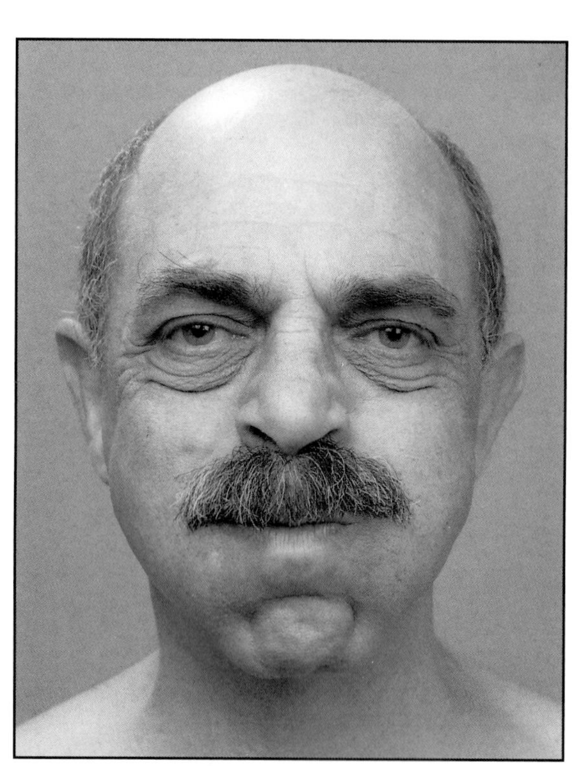

Sensory portion. While the client's eyes are closed, test the taste sensation to sweet, salt, sour, and bitter flavors bilaterally on the anterior two-thirds of the tongue. A client with an intact CN VII reports symmetrical taste sensations.

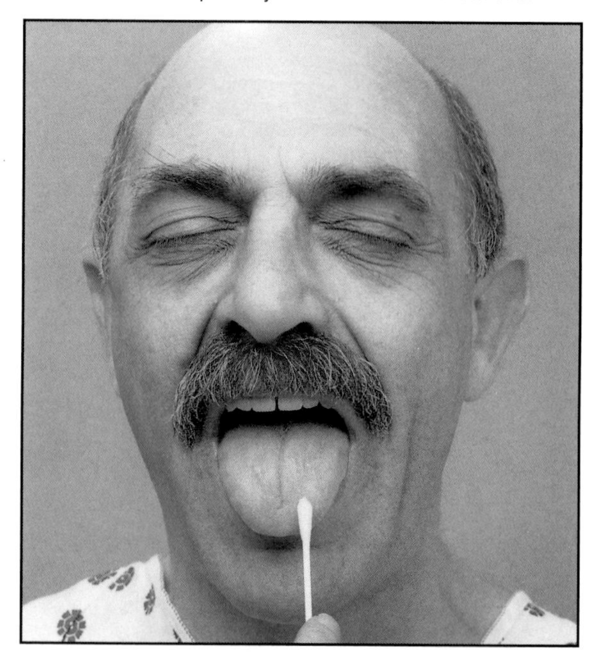

Glossopharyngeal and vagus nerves (CN IX and X)

Motor portion. Because CN IX and X have overlapping functions, they are tested together. Observe the client's soft palate and uvula as the client says "ah." The soft palate and uvula should rise symmetrically, and the uvula should remain midline.

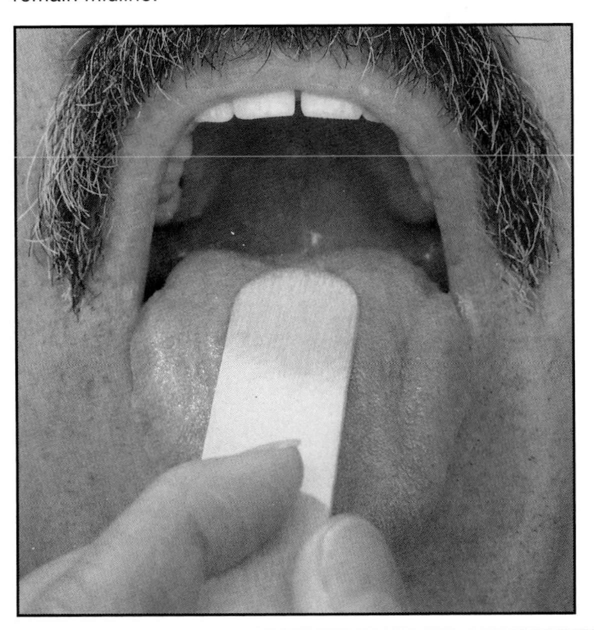

Sensory portion. While the client's eyes are closed, test the taste sensation to sweet, salt, sour, and bitter flavors bilaterally on the posterior third of the tongue. Normally, the client reports symmetrical taste sensations.

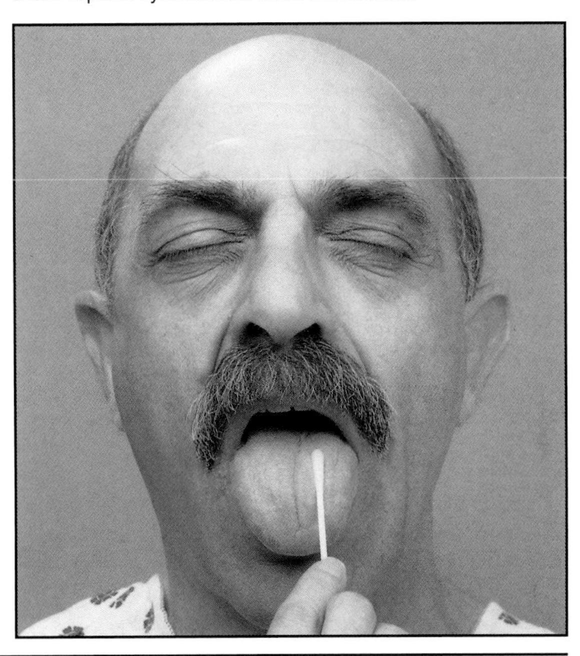

Spinal accessory nerve (CN XI)

1 Press down on the shoulders while the client shrugs them. Note shoulder strength and symmetry while inspecting and palpating the trapezius muscle. Normally, both shoulders should be able to overcome the resistance equally well.

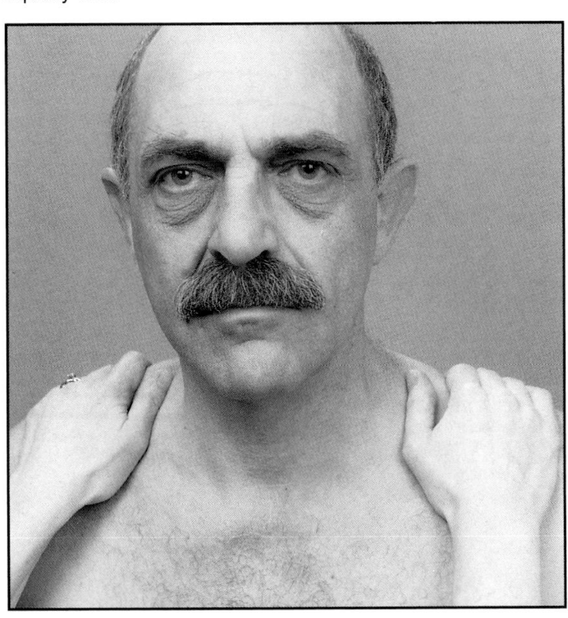

2 Then have the client attempt to turn the head against hand resistance. Repeat on the opposite side. The neck should overcome resistance equally in both directions.

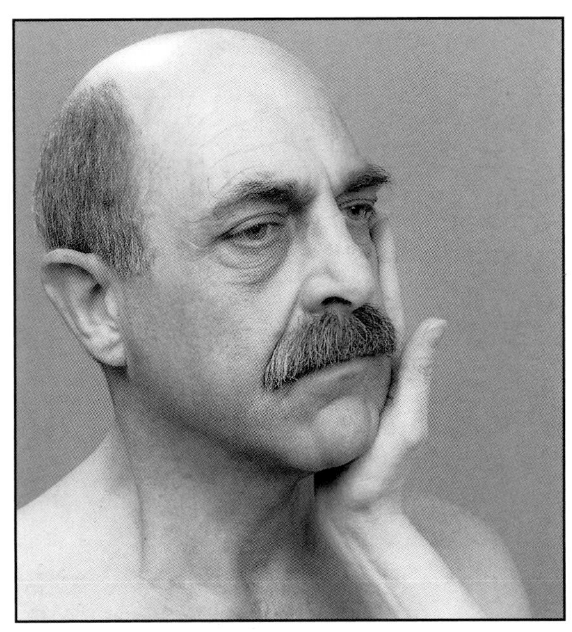

(continued)

ASSESSMENT

CRANIAL NERVES (continued)

Hypoglossal nerve (CN XII)

While the client sticks out the tongue, note its position and mobility. Normally, the tongue is midline and displays a full range of motion. Also with the tongue in a normal position, the client's speech should be clear.

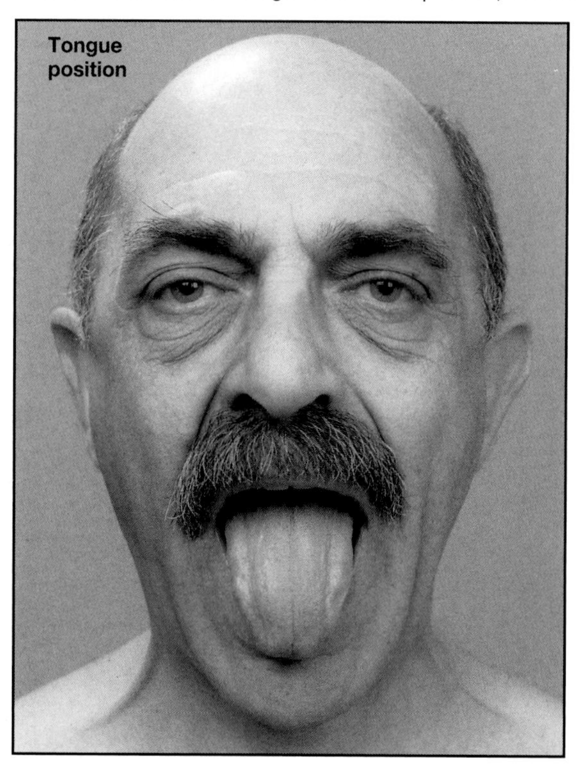

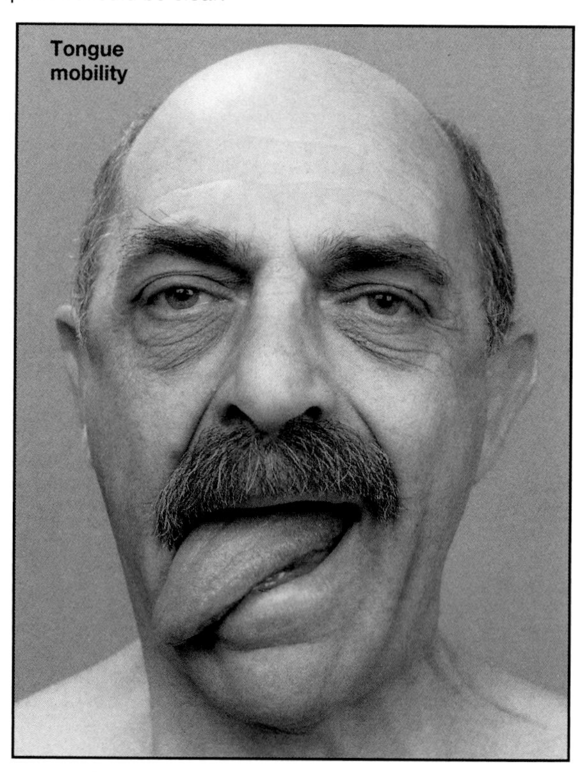

■ Cerebellar function

Coordination

Leg coordination. Have the client lie supine and slide one heel down the shin of the opposite leg. Repeat with the other leg, noting the ease, speed, and accuracy of this maneuver. Normally, leg movements are coordinated.

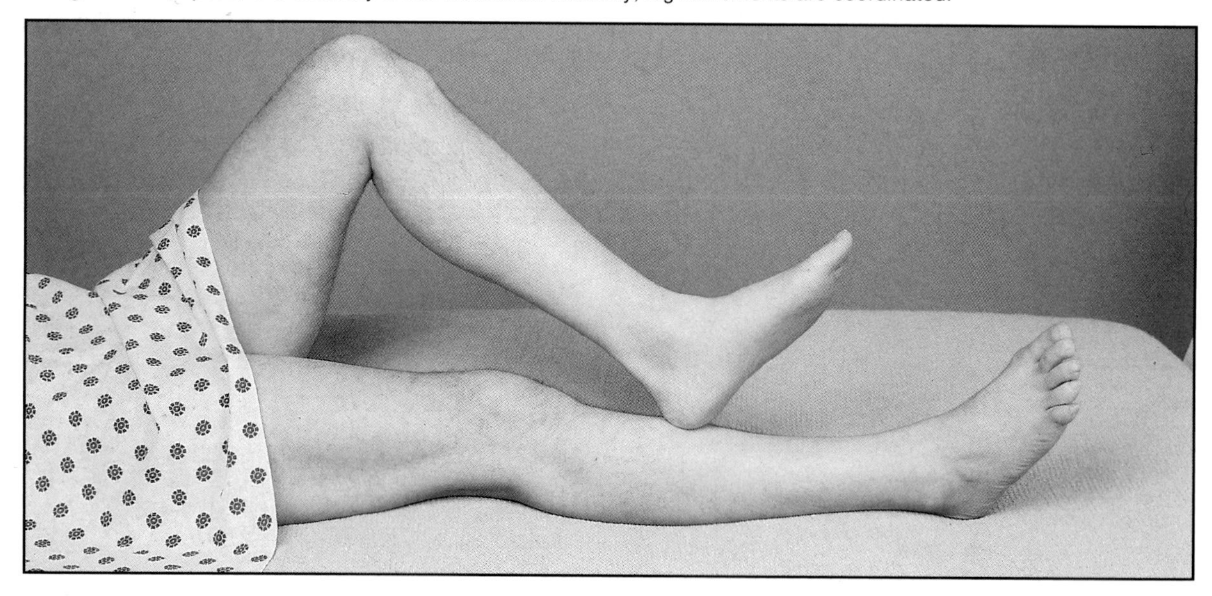

CEREBELLAR FUNCTION (continued)

Balance

Romberg test. Have the unsupported client stand with feet together and arms at side. Observe the client's ability to maintain balance with both eyes open and then with them closed. A client with normal cerebellar function demonstrates minimal swaying with eyes closed (a negative Romberg test).

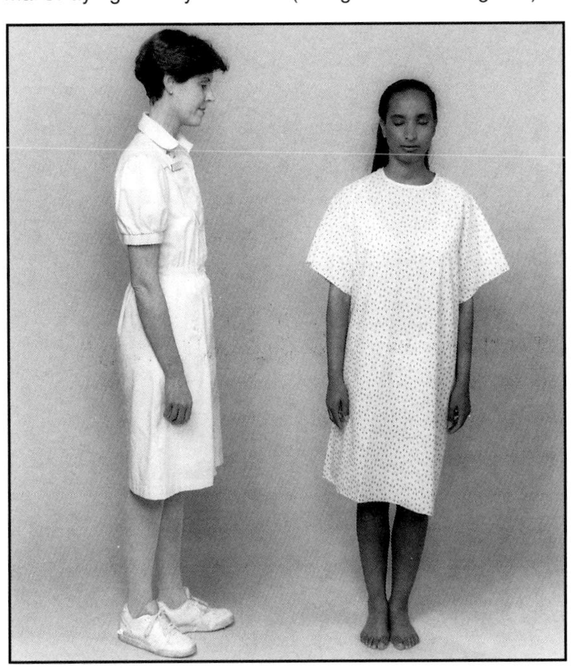

Tandem-gait walking. Ask the client to walk heel-to-toe in a straight line. Normally, the client's tandem gait is balanced and coordinated.

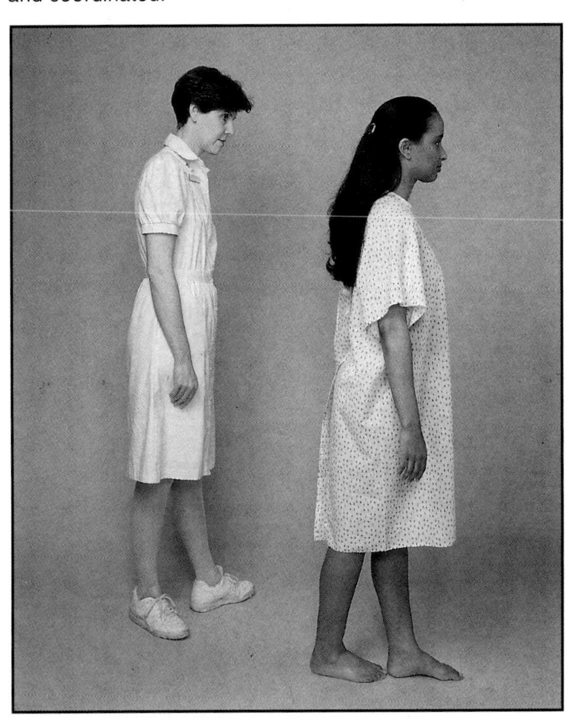

Heel and toe walking. Have the client walk on the heels and then walk on the toes. The client's heel and toe walking should be balanced and coordinated.

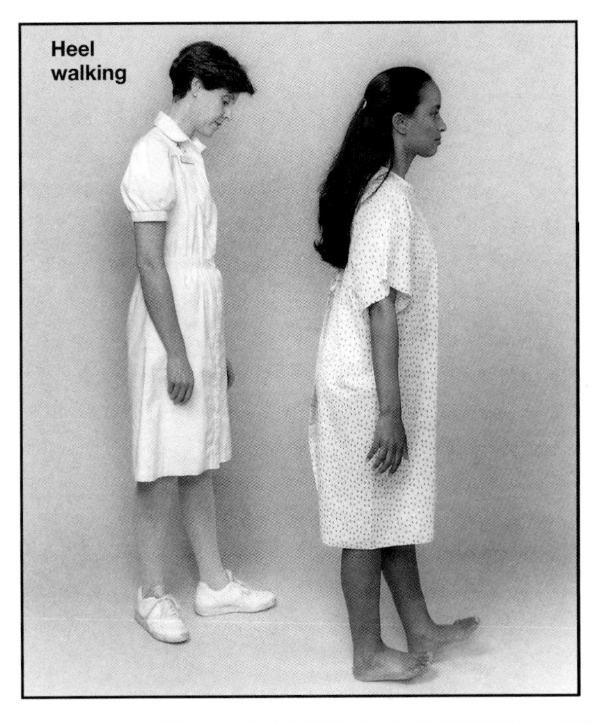

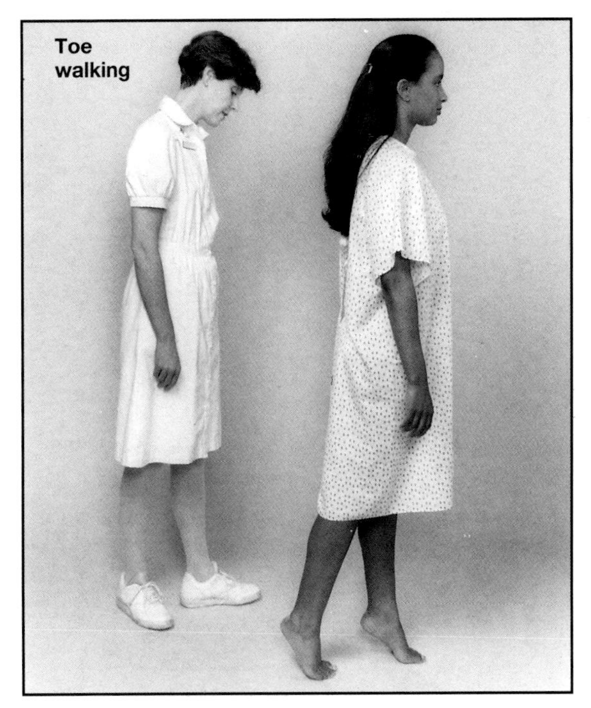

ASSESSMENT

■ Sensory system

Light touch

While the client's eyes are closed, use a wisp of cotton to test light-touch sensation in all extremities. The client should feel a similar light-touch sensation bilaterally.

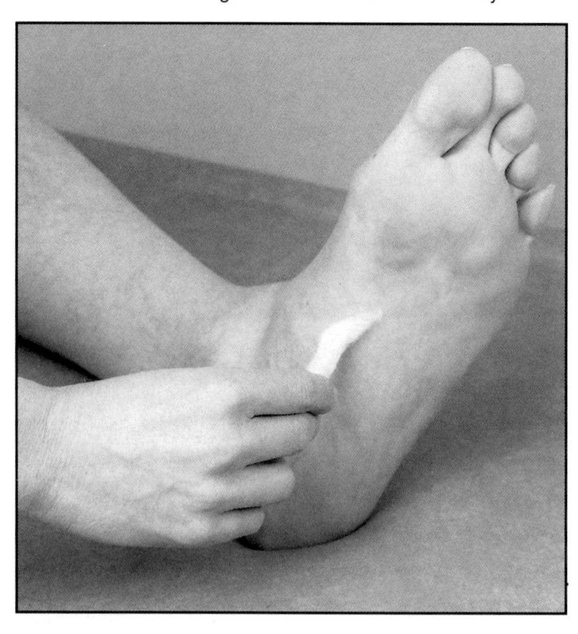

Superficial pain

While the client's eyes are closed, use a sharp object to evaluate superficial pain sensations in all extremities, taking care not to puncture the skin. The client should feel a similar superficial pain bilaterally.

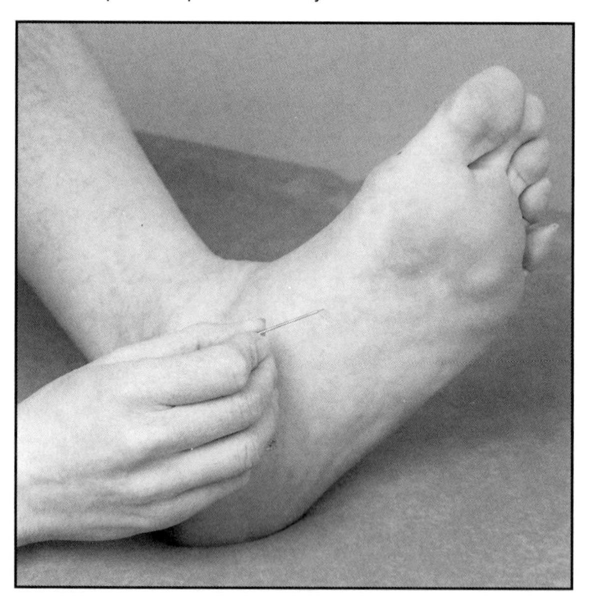

Temperature

If the client displays abnormal pain sensations, assess temperature sensation while the client's eyes are closed. Using test tubes that contain hot and cold water, test temperature sensation in the extremities. The client should feel a similar temperature sensation bilaterally.

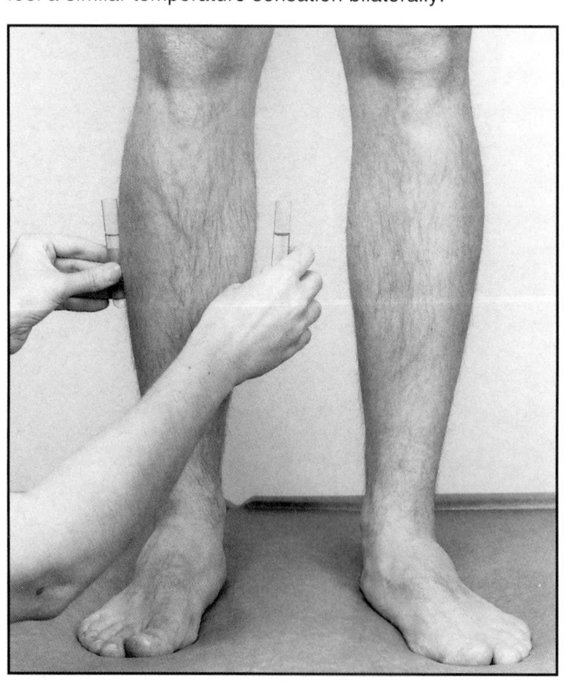

Vibration

While the client's eyes are closed, place the base of a vibrating tuning fork on a bony prominence, proceeding from distal to proximal areas. Have the client describe the sensation and state when the sensation stops. The client should feel a similar vibration bilaterally in all areas. If the response to vibration is normal distally, further testing is unnecessary.

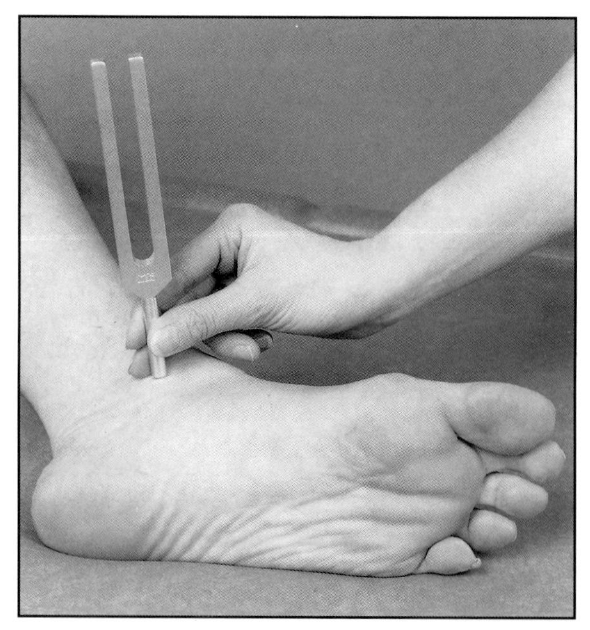

Position

While the client's eyes are closed, move a toe or finger up or down and ask the client to describe the position. Repeat on the other side of the body. The client normally can identify the position correctly.

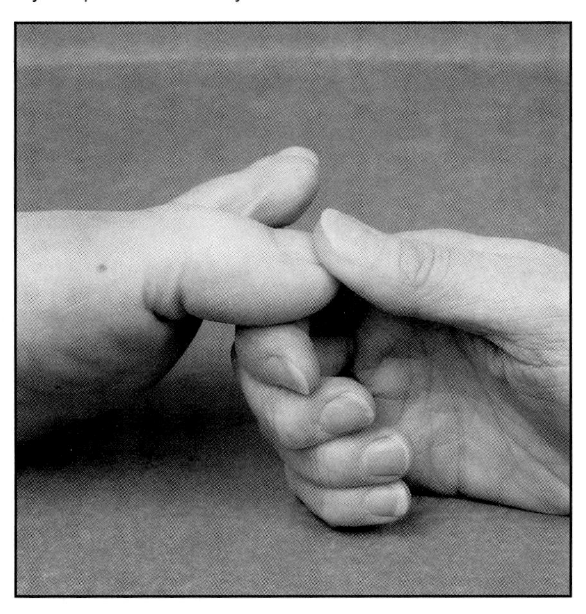

Number identification

While the client's eyes are closed, trace a large number on the client's palm, using a blunt object. Number identification should be correct when traced in either palm.

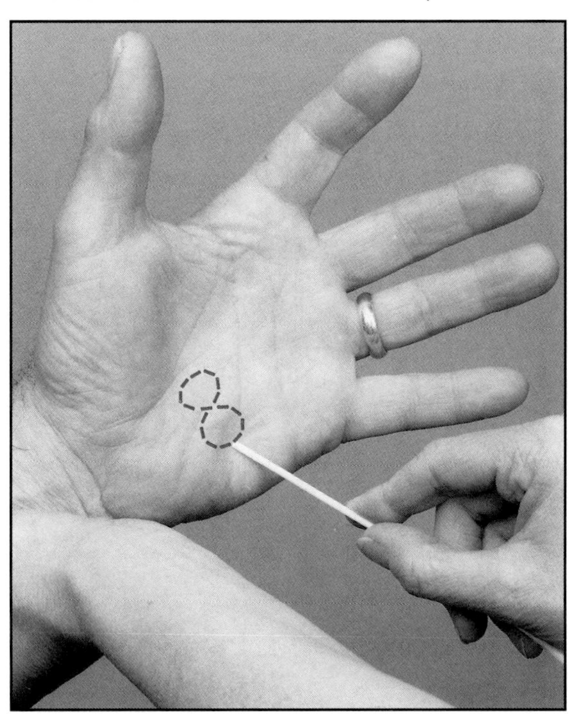

Stereognosis

Have the client keep the eyes closed and attempt to identify a familiar object by feel. Object identification should be correct with either hand.

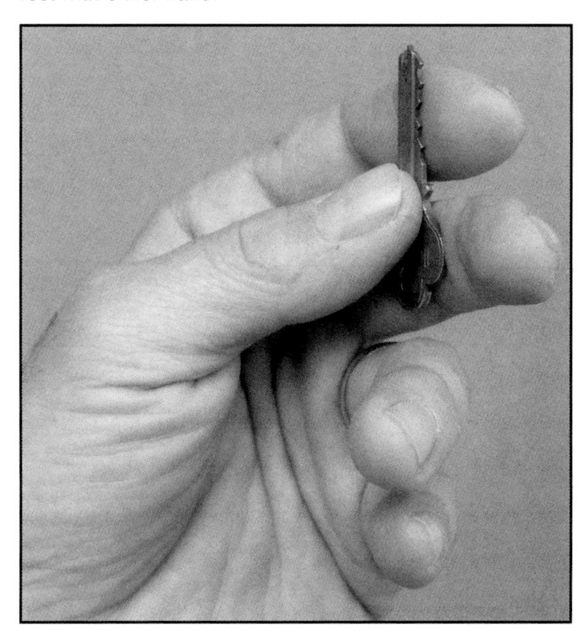

Two-point discrimination

While the client's eyes are closed, touch one or two sharp objects to the client's skin. After assessing whether the client can feel one or two points, note the smallest distance between the two points at which the client can still discriminate between them. Be aware that acuity typically varies in different parts of the body. On the finger pads, for example, the distance may be less than 5 mm; on the back, much greater.

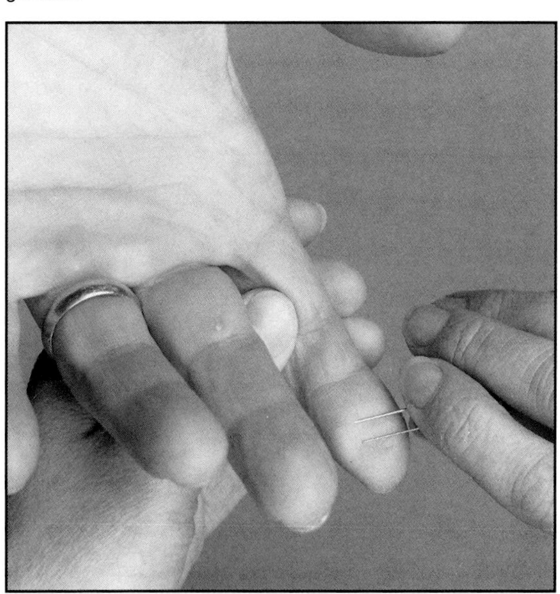

ASSESSMENT

■ Reflexes

Deep tendon reflexes

Biceps. Place your thumb or finger over the biceps tendon and tap it lightly with the reflex hammer. Repeat on the other arm. The normal response is brisk elbow flexion (++ bilaterally).

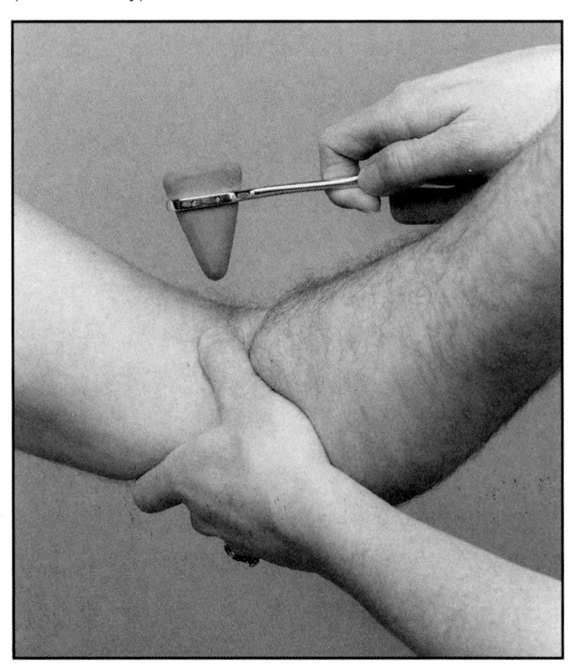

Triceps. Tap the reflex hammer directly over the triceps tendon at its insertion point. Repeat on the other arm. The normal response is brisk elbow extension and triceps muscle contraction (++ bilaterally).

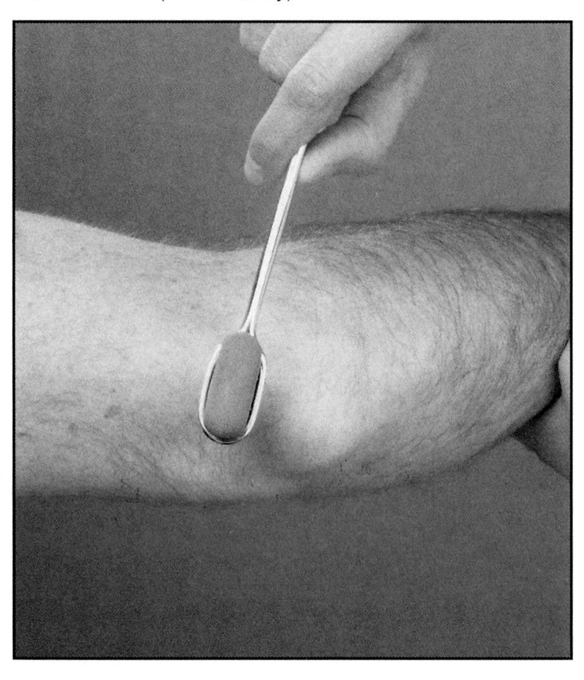

Quadriceps (knee-jerk). Tap the patellar tendon with the reflex hammer. Repeat on the other leg. The normal response is knee extension and quadricep contraction (++ bilaterally).

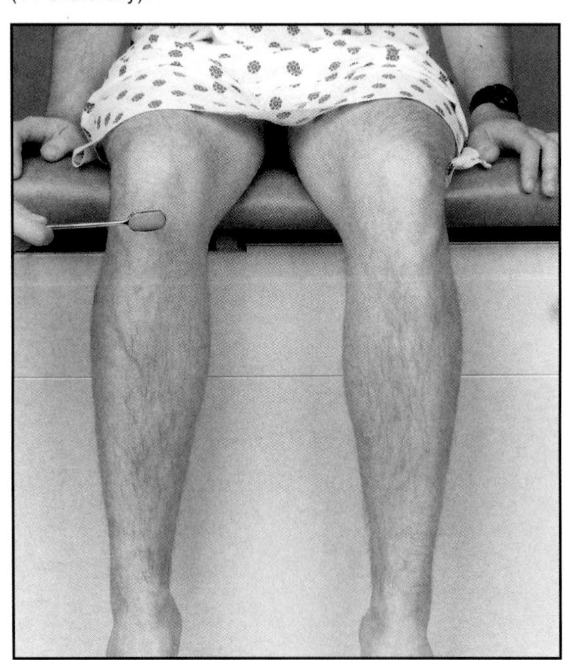

Achilles (ankle jerk). Tap the achilles tendon with the reflex hammer. Repeat on the other leg. The normal response is plantar flexion followed by muscle relaxation (++ bilaterally).

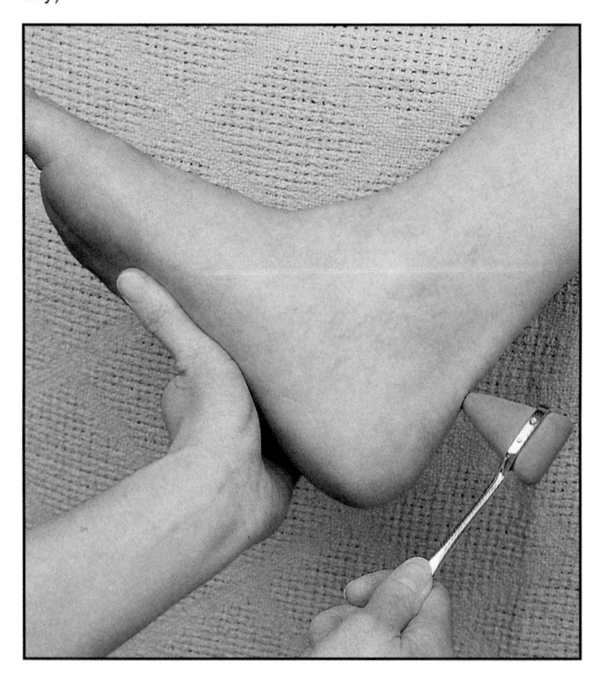

Brachioradialis (supinator). Tap the reflex hammer on the styloid process of the radius, about 1" to 2" above the wrist. Repeat on the other arm. The normal response is elbow flexion, forearm supination, and finger and hand flexion (++ bilaterally).

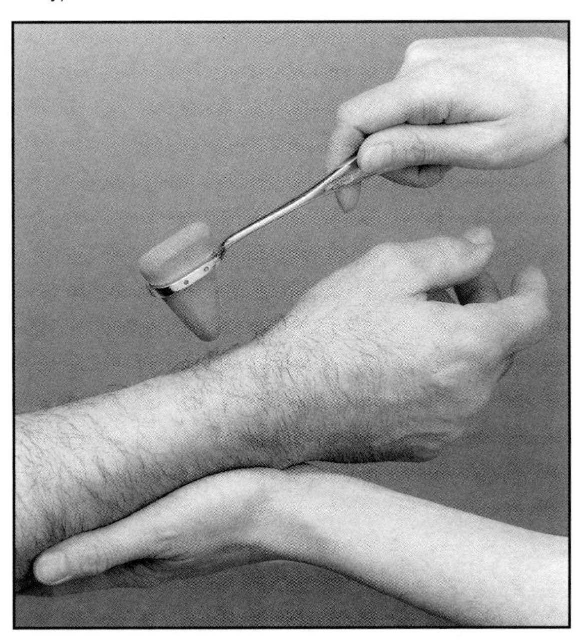

Grasp. Stimulate the palm of the client's hand with your index and middle fingers. The normal response is no grasping on stimulation (++ bilaterally).

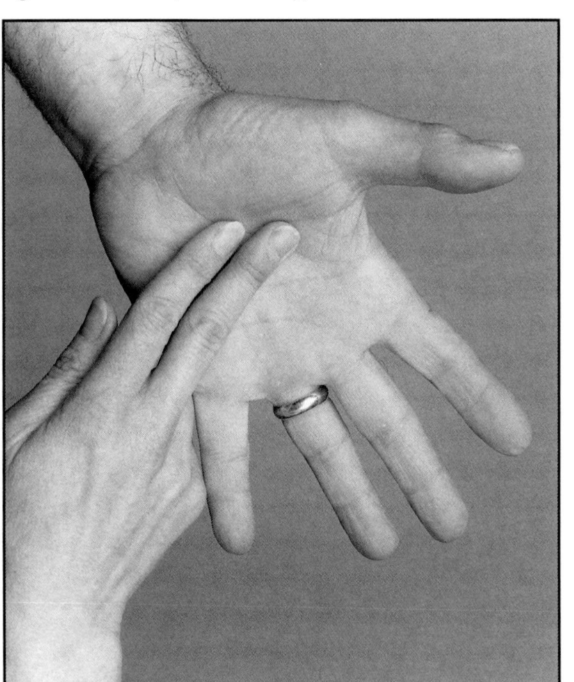

Superficial reflexes

Abdominal. Using the handle of the reflex hammer, stroke each side of the client's upper and lower abdomen. Normally, the abdominal muscles contract and the umbilicus deviates towards the stimulated side.

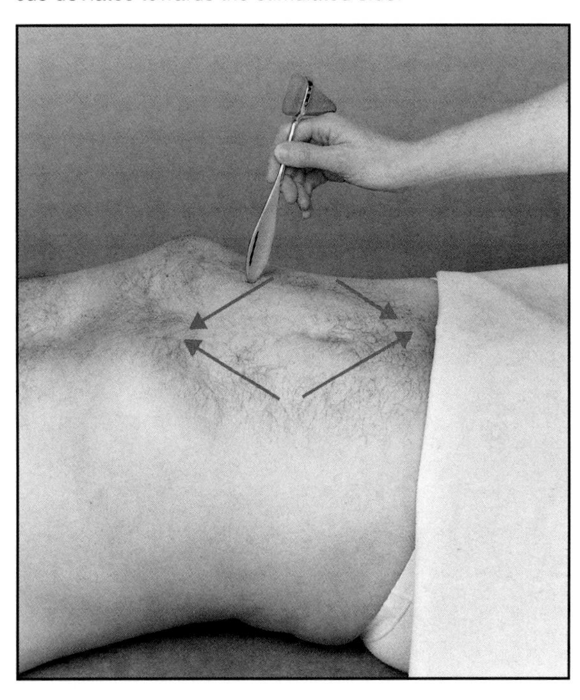

Plantar. Using the handle of the reflex hammer, stroke the lateral aspect of the sole of the client's foot. The normal response is toe flexion.

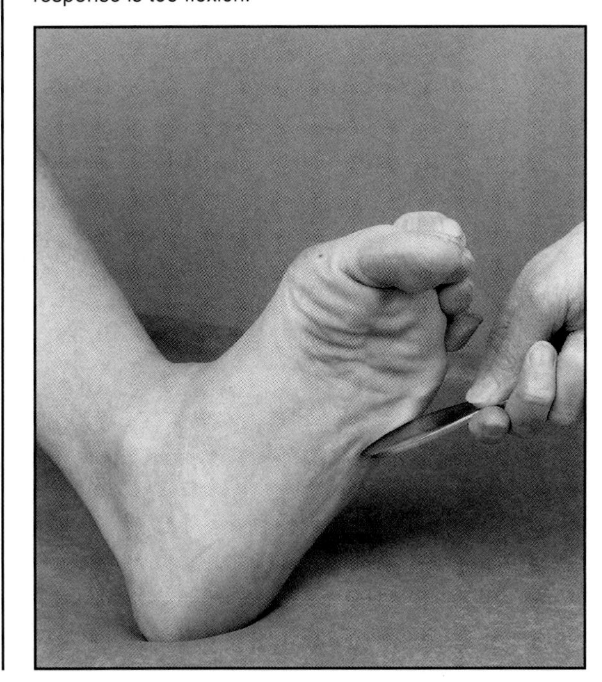

Musculoskeletal System

Anatomy and physiology overview

■ Structures of the musculoskeletal system

This anterior view of the body shows the structures of the musculoskeletal system.

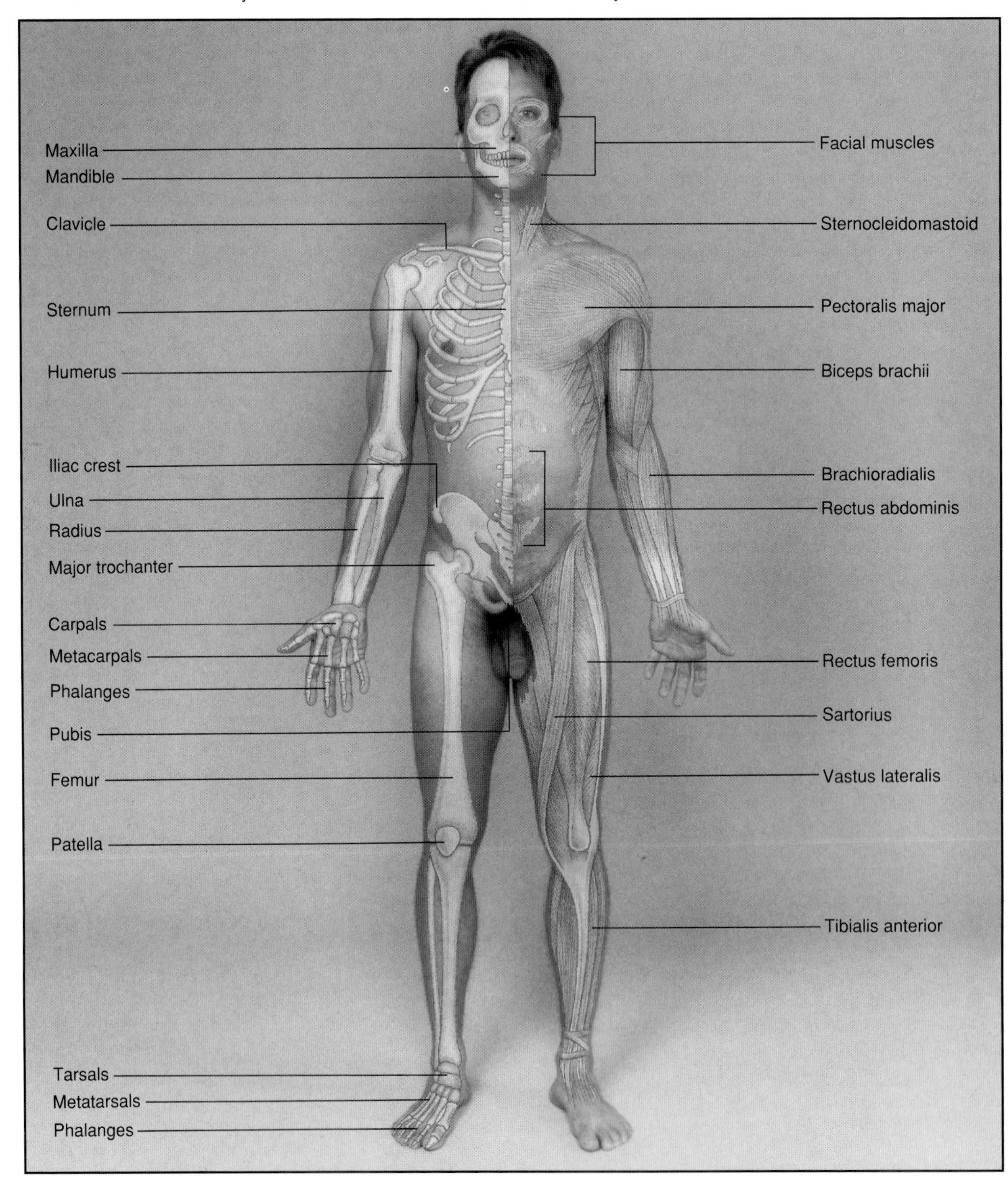

ANATOMY AND PHYSIOLOGY OVERVIEW

STRUCTURES OF THE MUSCULOSKELETAL SYSTEM (continued)

This posterior view of the body shows the structures of the musculoskeletal system.

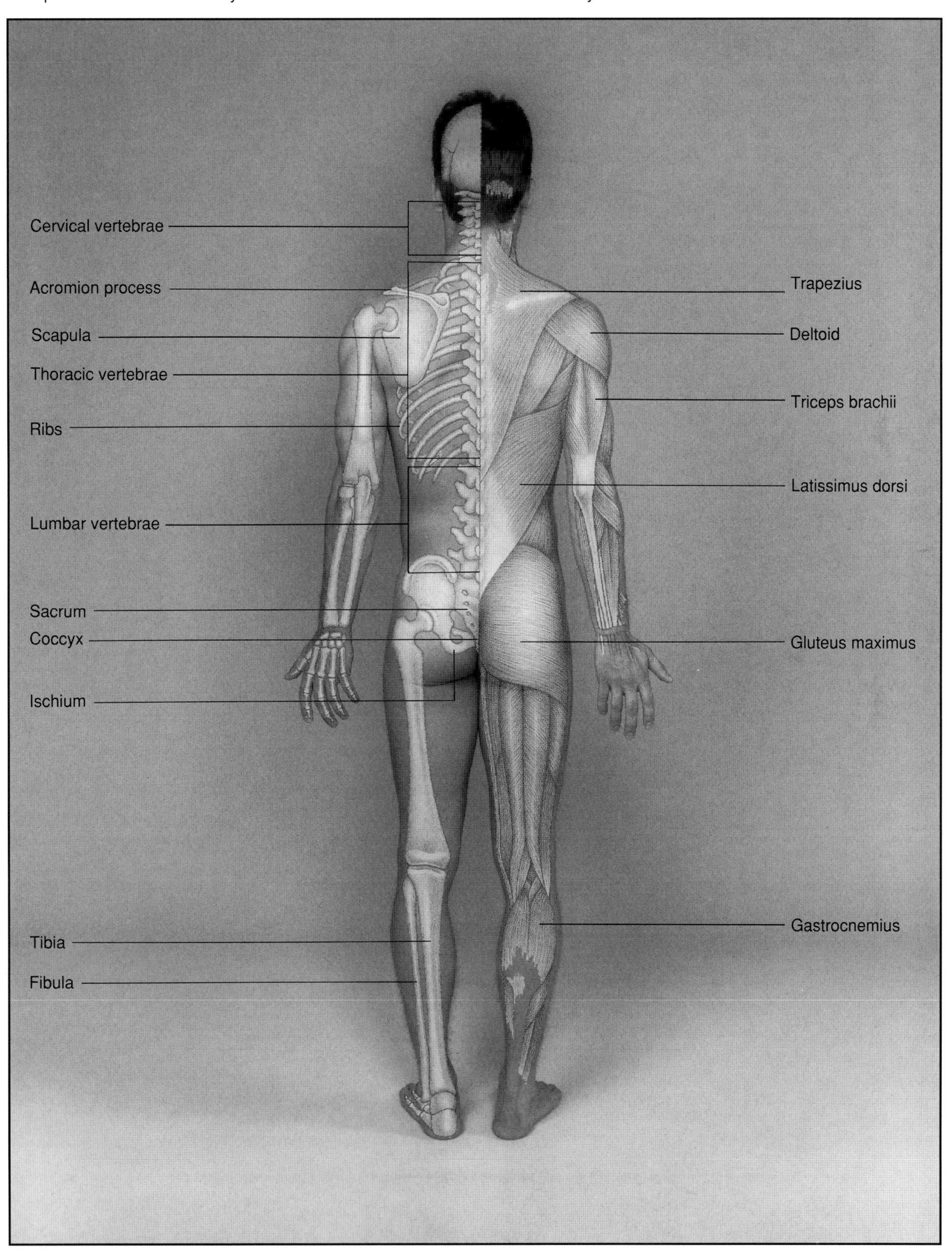

Assessment

■ Inspection

Spinal curvature

With the client standing straight, assess body symmetry, posture, and spinal alignment. Repeat the inspection with the client bending forward from the waist. The posture should be erect and symmetrical, and the spine should be midline with normal curvature but no lateral deviation.

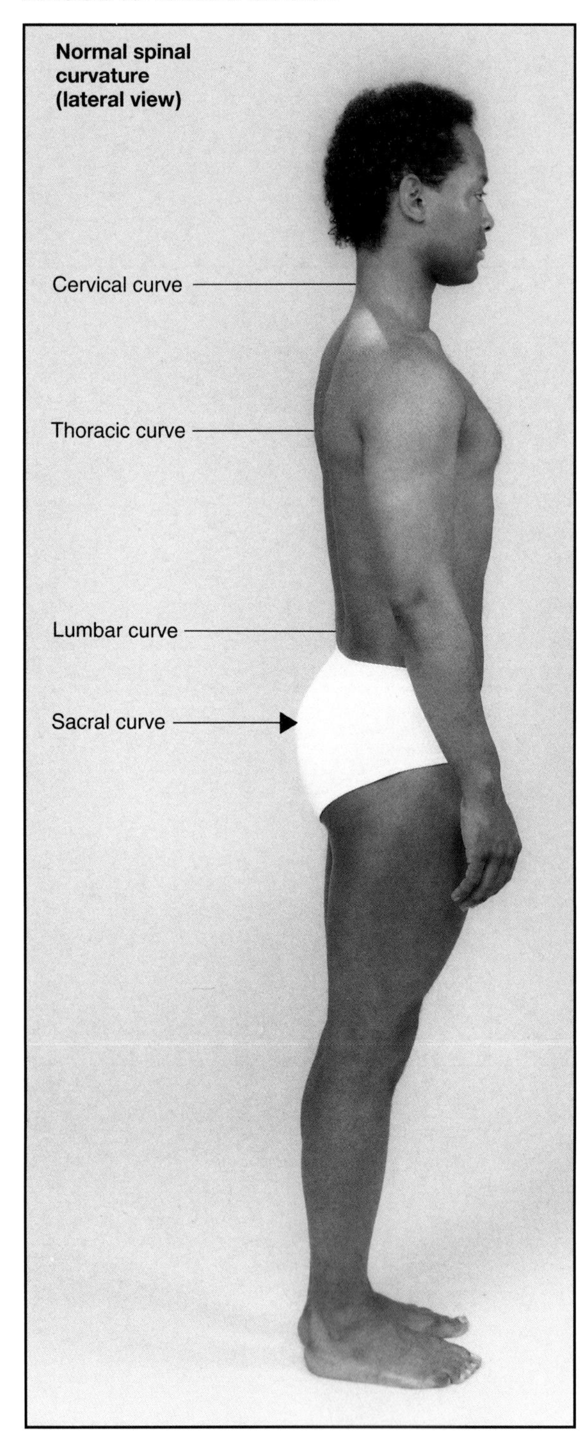

Normal spinal curvature (lateral view)

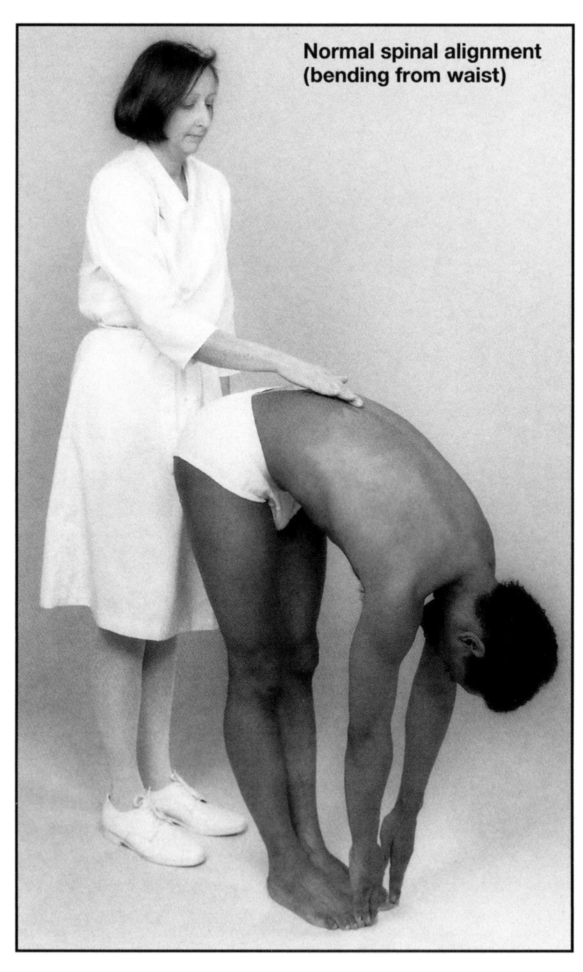

Normal spinal alignment (bending from waist)

Gait

Inspect the client's gait to assess phases, cadence, stride length, base of support, and posture. Normally, the stride length is symmetrical, and the gait is smooth, rhythmic, and coordinated with conformity of phases. Also note the movement of the arms, which should swing in opposition.

Stance phase. The components of the stance phase include heel strike, flat foot, midstance, and push off.

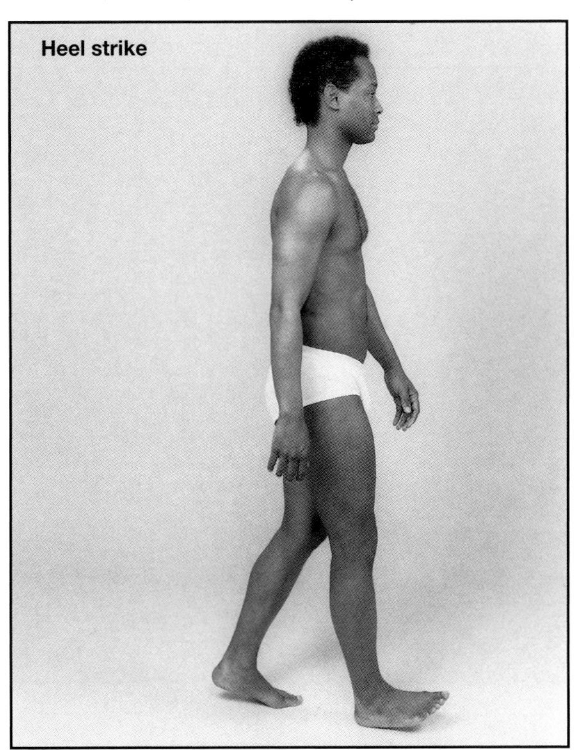

Stance phase. The components of the stance phase include heel strike, flat foot, midstance, and push off.

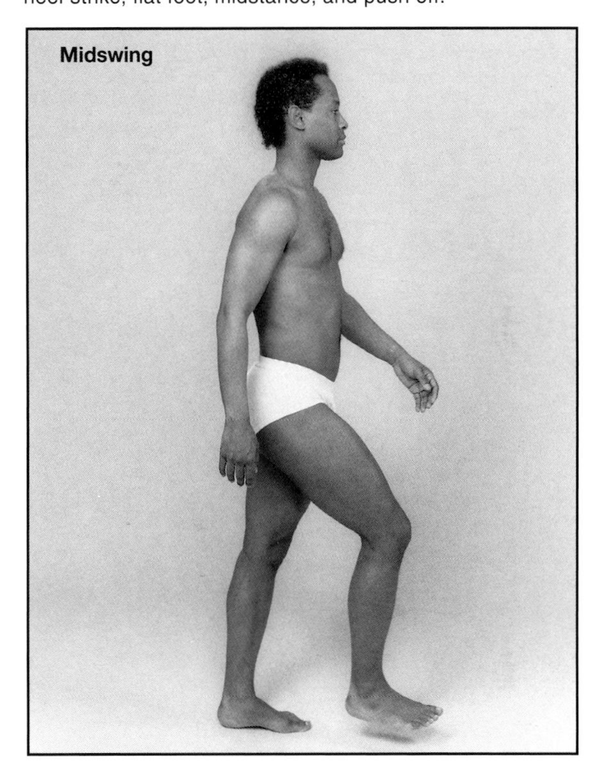

Extremity lengths

Arm length. Measure each arm from the acromion process to the tip of the middle finger. Normally, arm length should not differ by more than $^3/_8$" (1 cm).

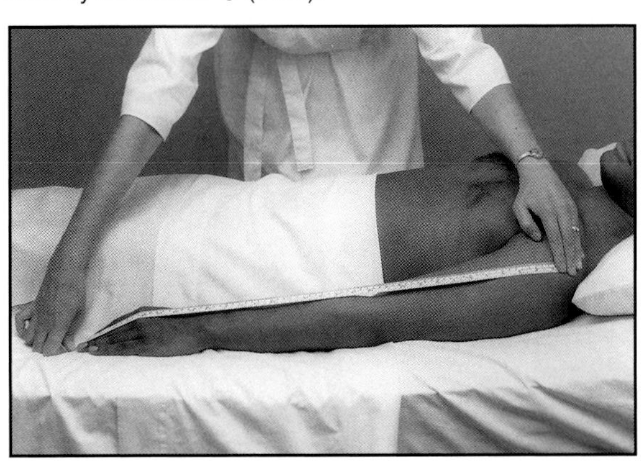

Leg length. Measure each leg from the anterior superior iliac spine to the medial malleolus. Normally, leg length should not differ by more than $^3/_8$" (1 cm).

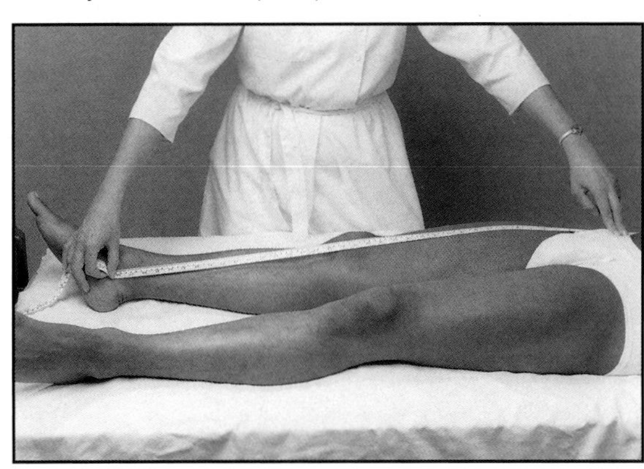

ASSESSMENT

■ Muscle strength and joint range of motion

Muscle strength is tested against resistance. Joint range of motion (ROM) is tested by measuring joint movement. After testing the cervical spine and neck as shown, assess the other major muscle groups and joints.

Cervical spine and neck muscle strength

To assess the muscle strength of the sternocleidomastoid and trapezius, have the client perform ROM against hand resistance. Normally, the cervical spine and neck have active ROM with grade 5 muscle strength on a scale of 0 to 5.

To assess cervical spine flexion and neck muscle strength, ask the client to touch the chin to the chest as you apply hand resistance to the client's forehead.

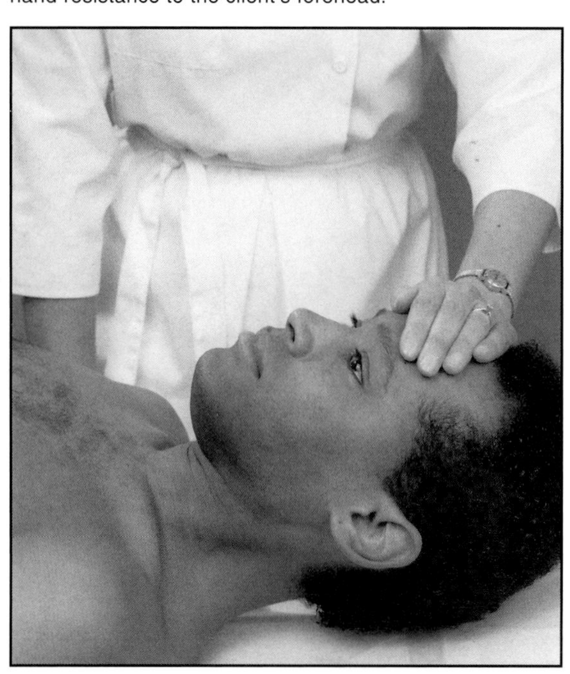

To assess cervical spine rotation and neck muscle strength, ask the client to push against your left hand positioned at the side of the face as you palpate the sternocleidomastoid on the opposite side.

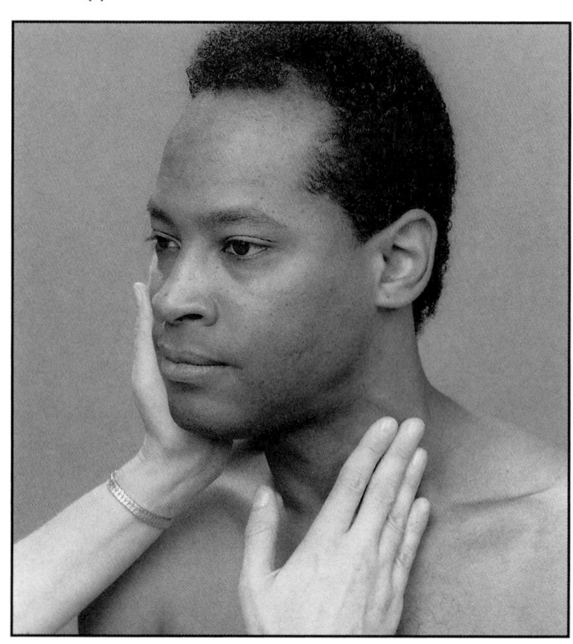

Cervical spine and neck range of motion

Have the client move the head and neck through the full range of motion. Normal ROM of the neck includes 45-degree flexion, 55-degree hyperextension, 70-degree rotation, and 40-degree lateral bending.

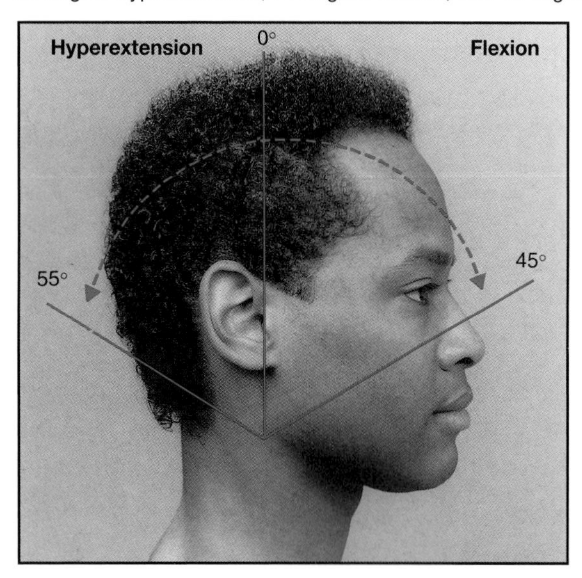

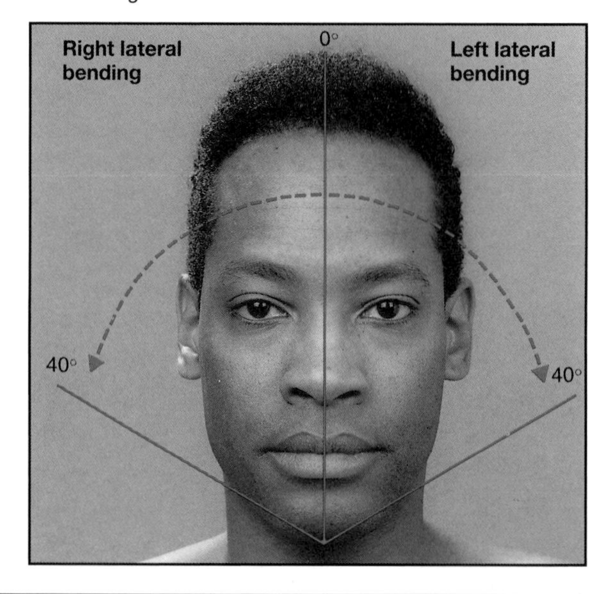

Developmental considerations

■ Pediatric client

Spinal convexity

The neonate normally displays a generalized convexity (C-shape) of the spine.

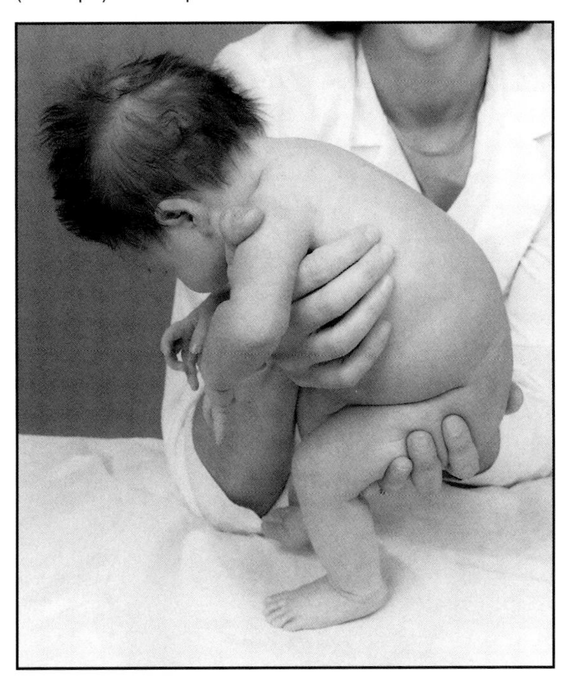

Lumbar concavity

The toddler normally may have a lumbar concavity (lordosis). By school age, the spine should assume the normal adult spinal curvature.

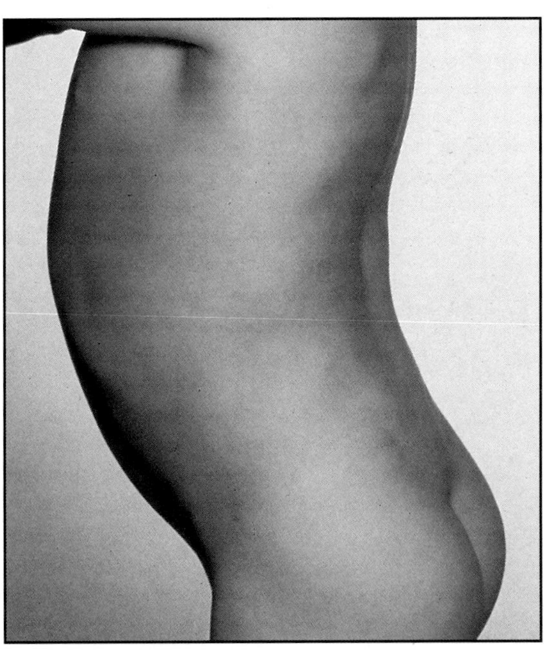

Common abnormalities

■ Scoliosis

This lateral deviation of the spine may result from congenital spinal malformation, poliomyelitis, or skeletal dysplasias.

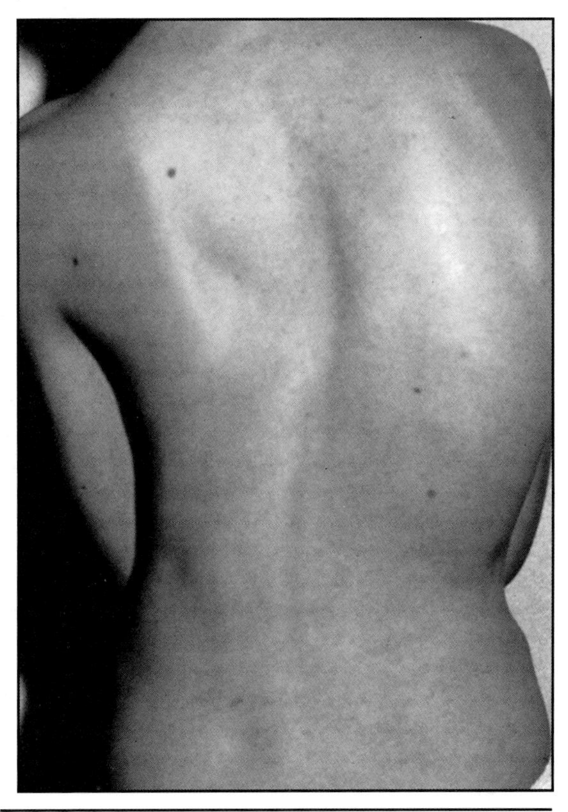

■ Nodular abnormalities

Heberden's nodes

These bony overgrowths of the distal interphalangeal joints may result from osteoarthritis.

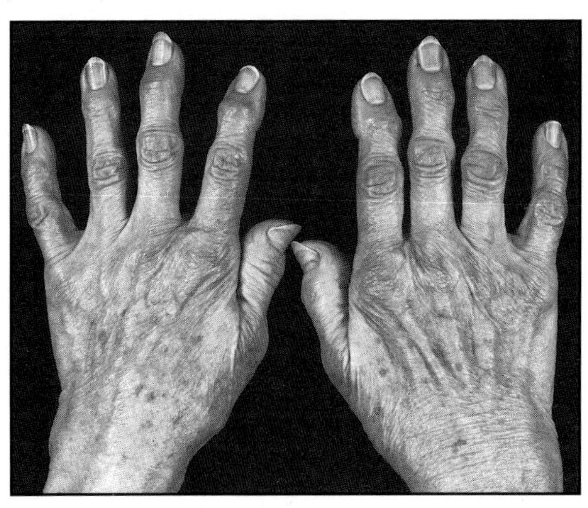

(continued)

COMMON ABNORMALITIES

NODULAR ABNORMALITIES (continued)

Rheumatoid nodules

These nodules commonly are accompanied by ulnar deviation and swan neck deformity of the fingers in rheumatoid arthritis.

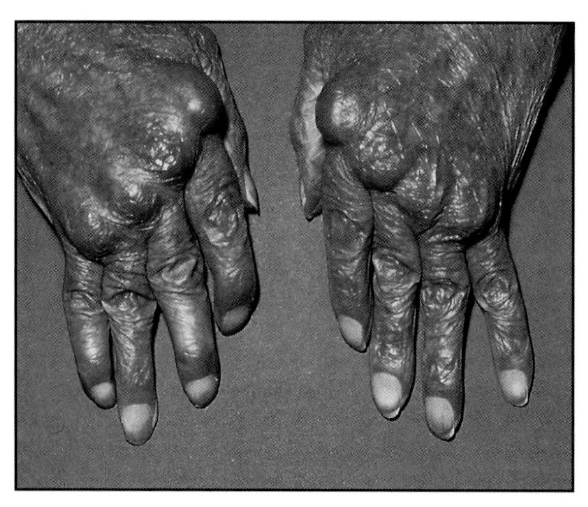

Gouty deformities

Joint deformities can result from gouty arthritis when uric acid is deposited in the joints.

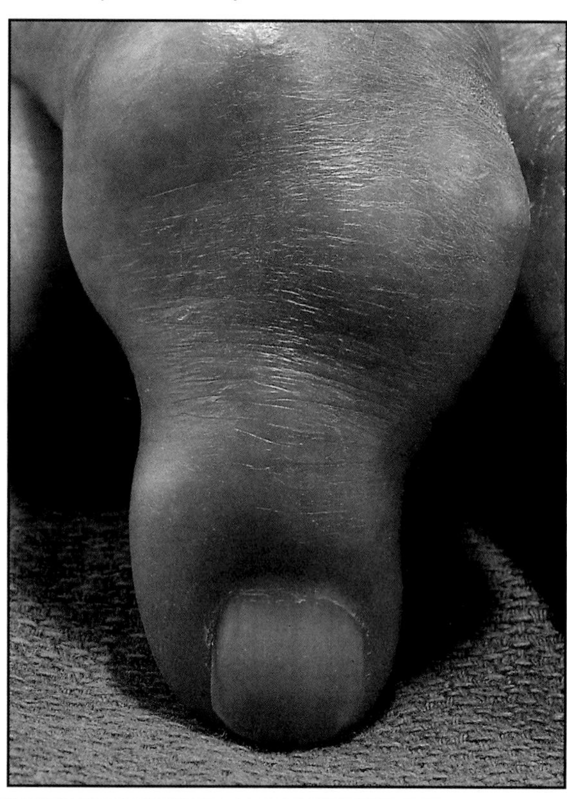

■ Foot abnormalities

Hallux malleous

Sometimes called hammer toe, this hyperextension of the metatarsophalangeal joint with flexion of the proximal toe joint commonly is associated with ill-fitting shoes.

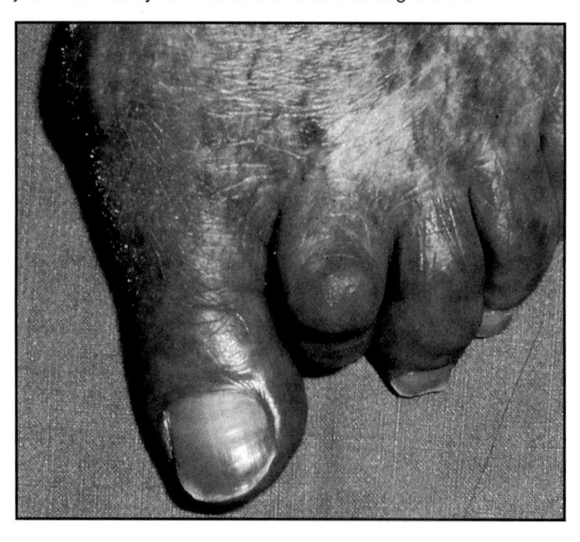

Hallux valgus

Lateral deviation of the great toe may cause the great toe to underlap the second toe. This abnormality may result from heredity, arthritis, or ill-fitting shoes.

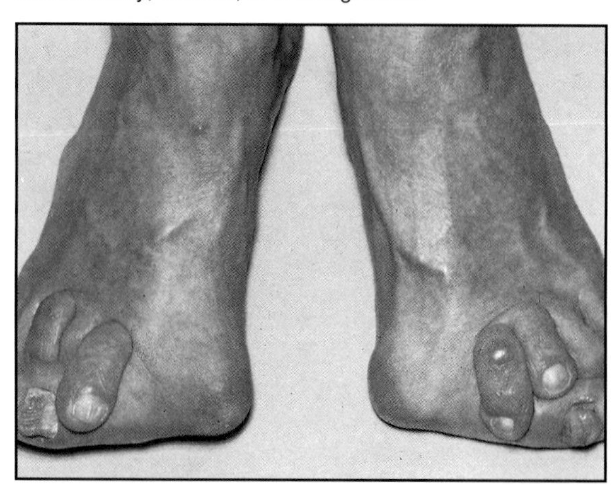

Immune System and Blood

Anatomy and physiology overview

■ Structures of the immune system

This anterior view of the body shows the structures of the immune system.

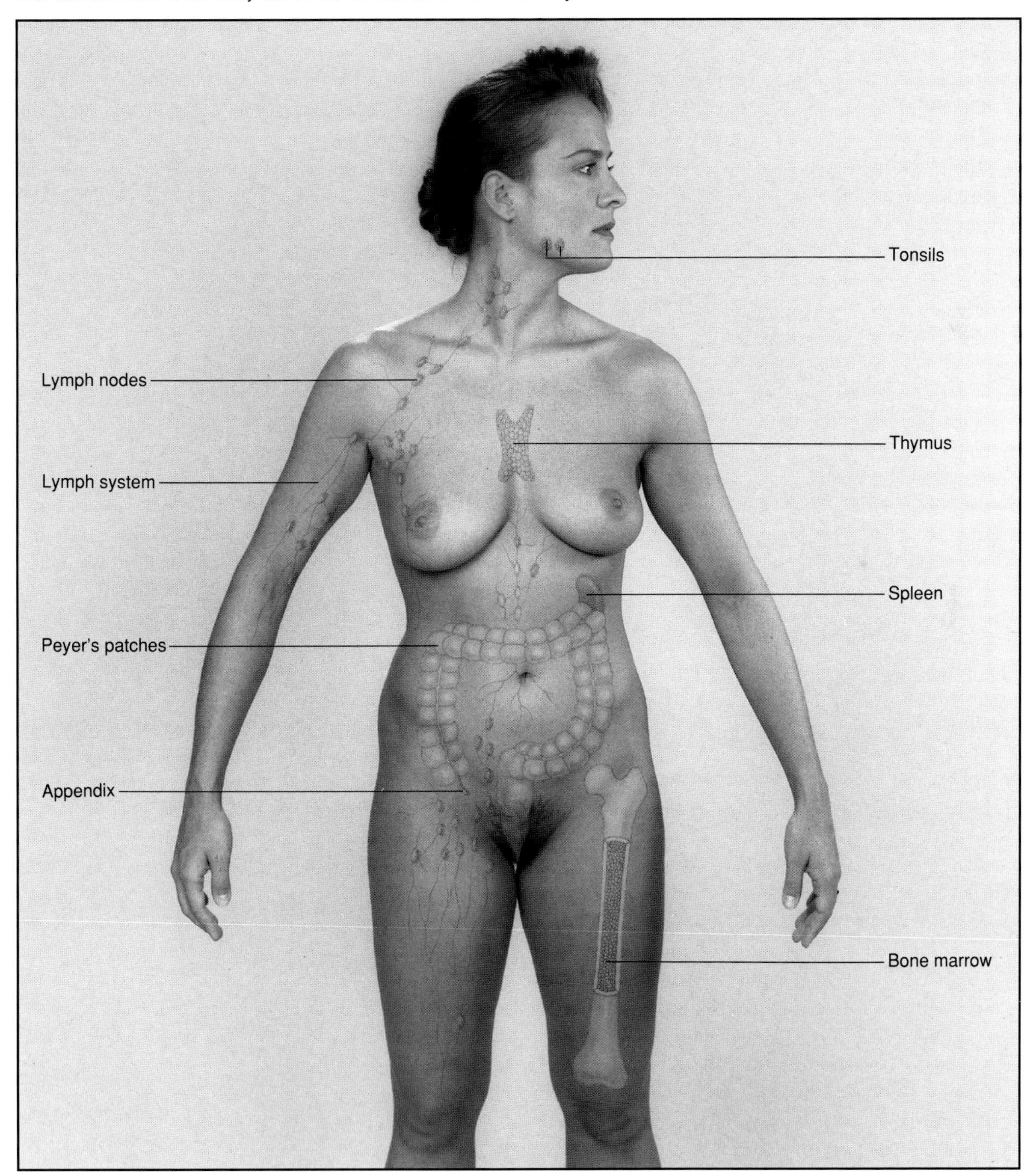

(continued)

ANATOMY AND PHYSIOLOGY OVERVIEW

STRUCTURES OF THE IMMUNE SYSTEM (continued)

Head and neck lymph nodes

This view of the head and neck shows the superficial lymph nodes in these areas.

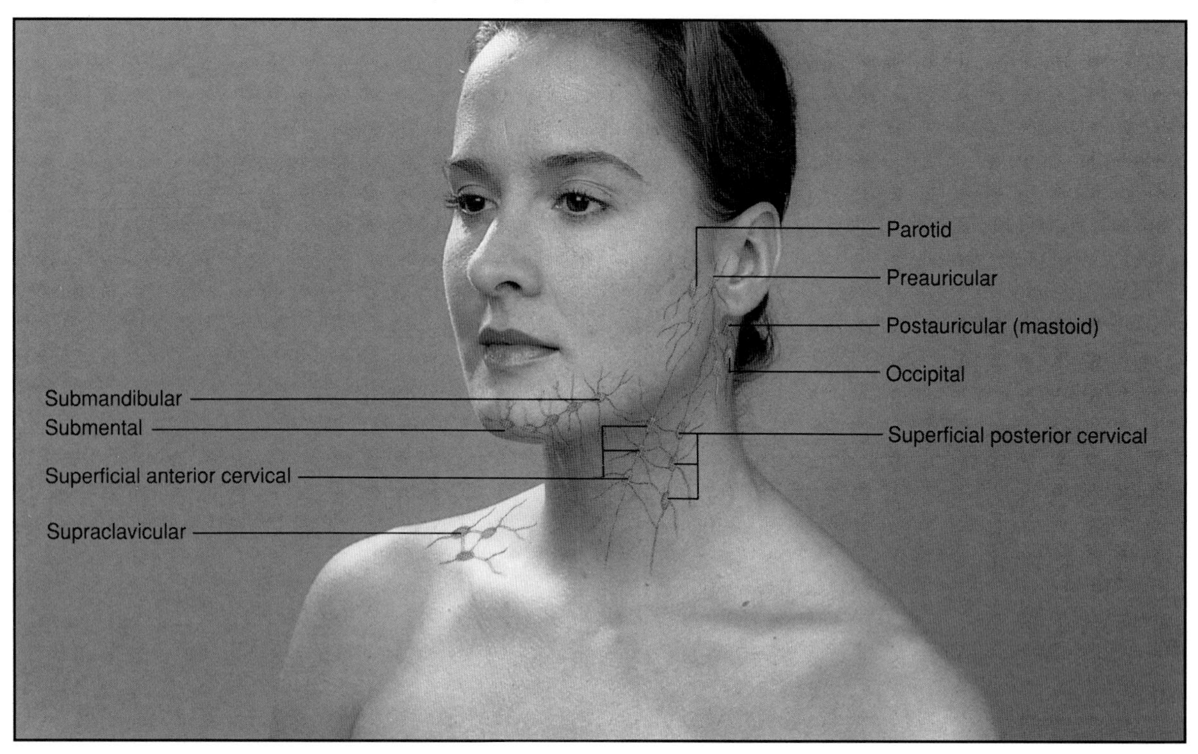

Axillary and epitrochlear lymph nodes

This anterior view of a portion of the chest and right arm shows the axillary and epitrochlear lymph nodes.

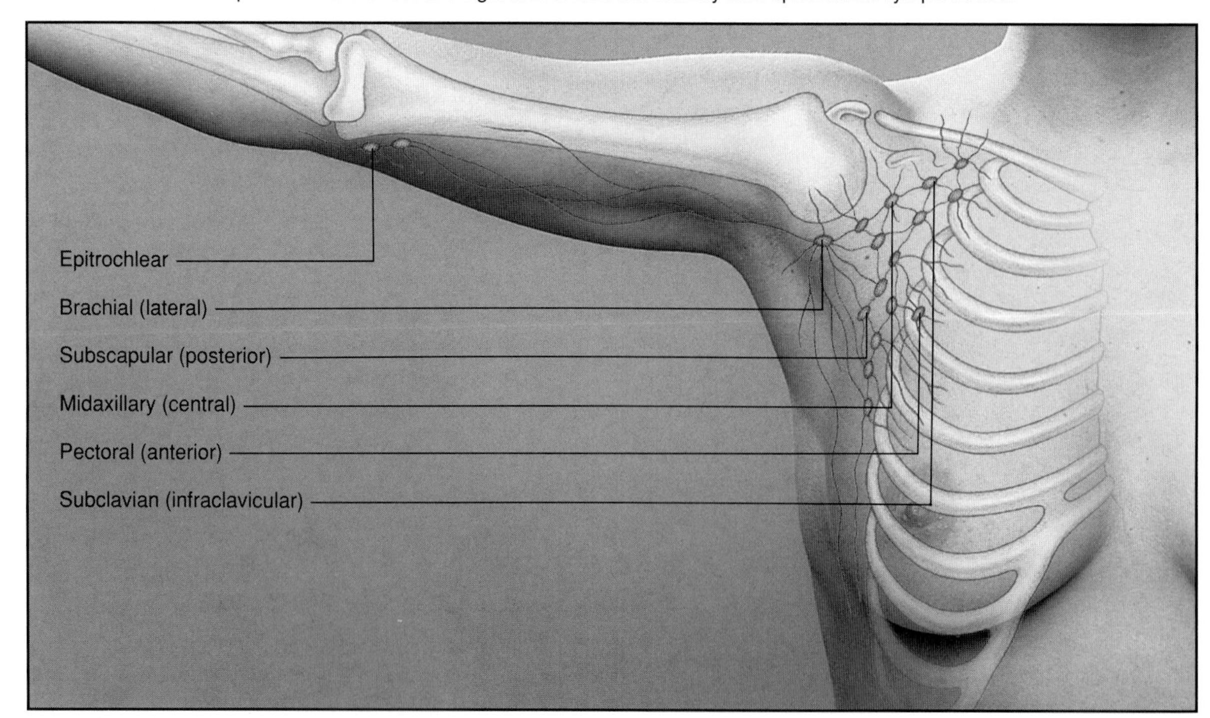

Inguinal nodes

This anterior view of the legs shows the inguinal lymph nodes.

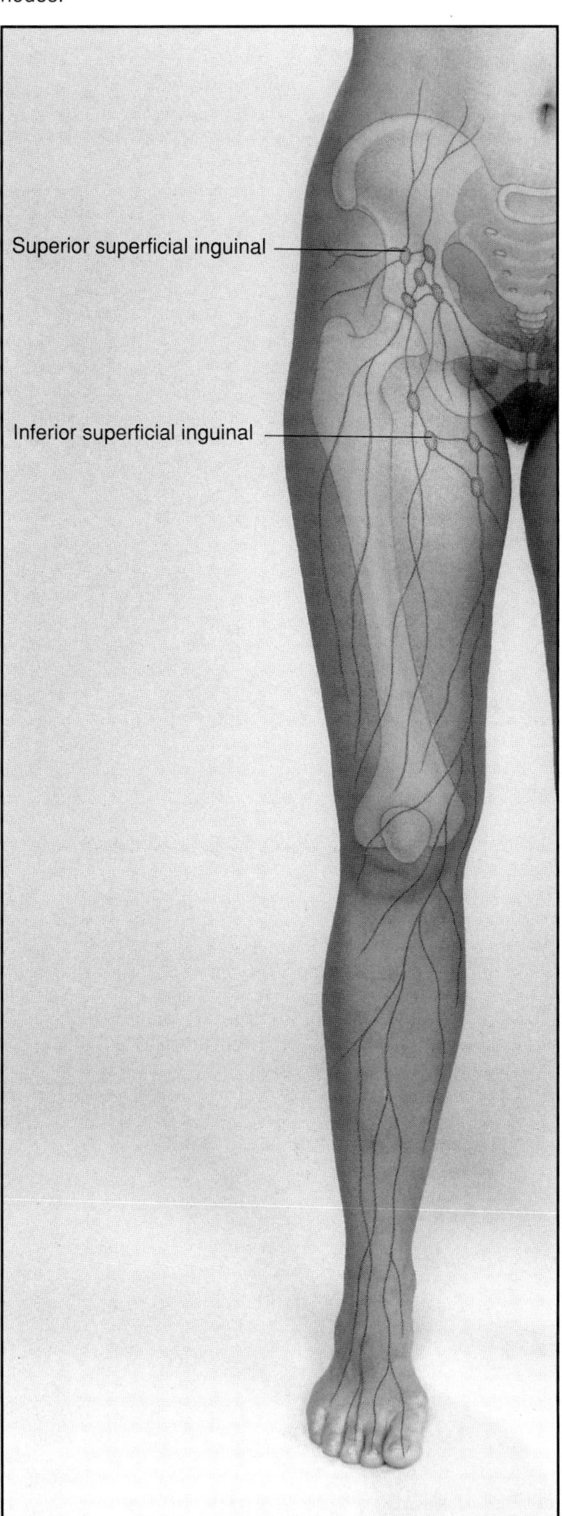

Popliteal lymph nodes

This posterior view of the legs shows the popliteal lymph nodes.

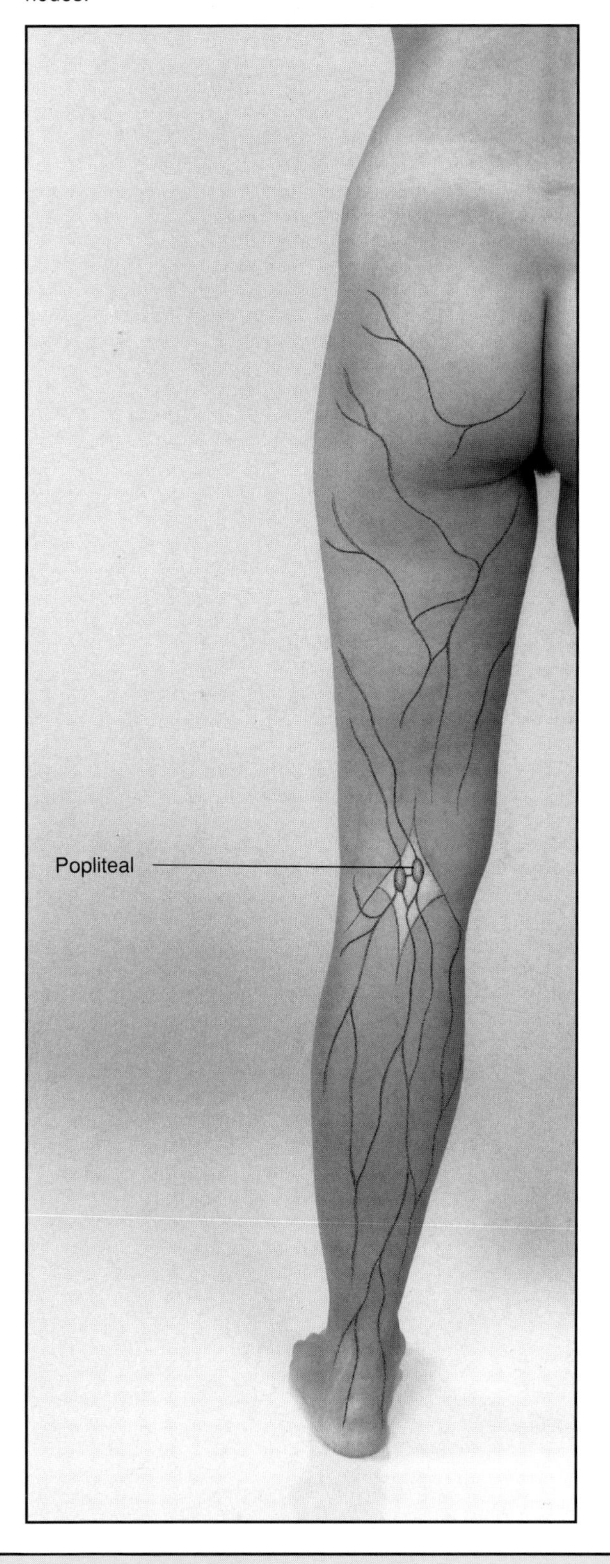

Assessment

■ Inspection and palpation

Inspect and gently palpate the head and neck, axillary, epitrochlear, inguinal, and popliteal areas with the pads of the index and middle fingers. Normally, lymph nodes are not palpable, tender, or hot to the touch. If palpable, however, superficial lymph nodes should be less than 3 cm, firm, oval or round, well-defined, mobile, nontender, symmetrical, and nonpulsating.

Head and neck lymph nodes

Parotid and preauricular. To assess the parotid and preauricular lymph nodes, palpate in front of the ear.

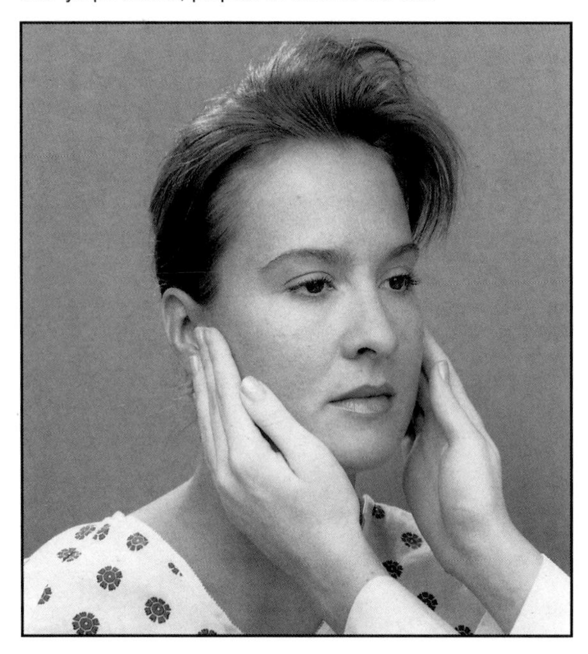

Postauricular. To assess the postauricular lymph nodes, palpate behind the ear over the mastoid process.

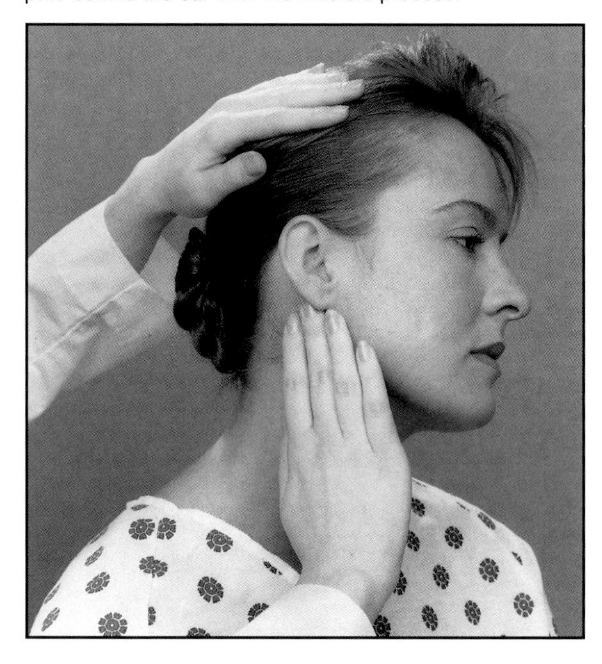

Occipital. To assess the occipital lymph nodes, palpate behind the ear at the occiput (base of the skull).

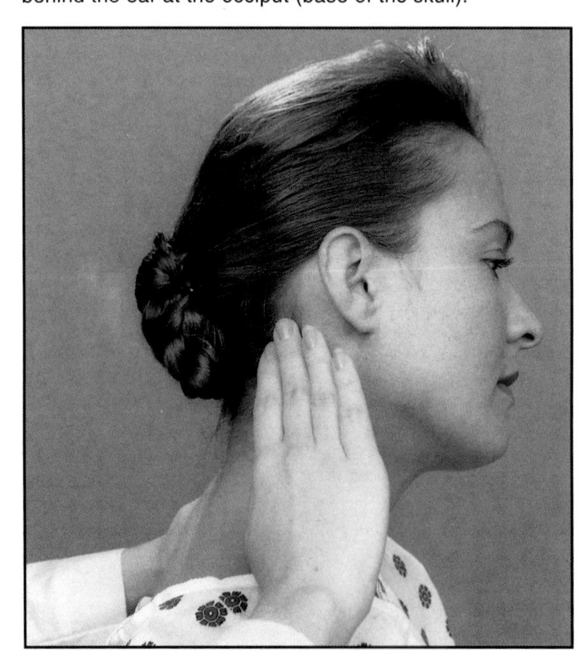

Submandibular. To assess the submandibular lymph nodes, palpate over the edge of the mandible.

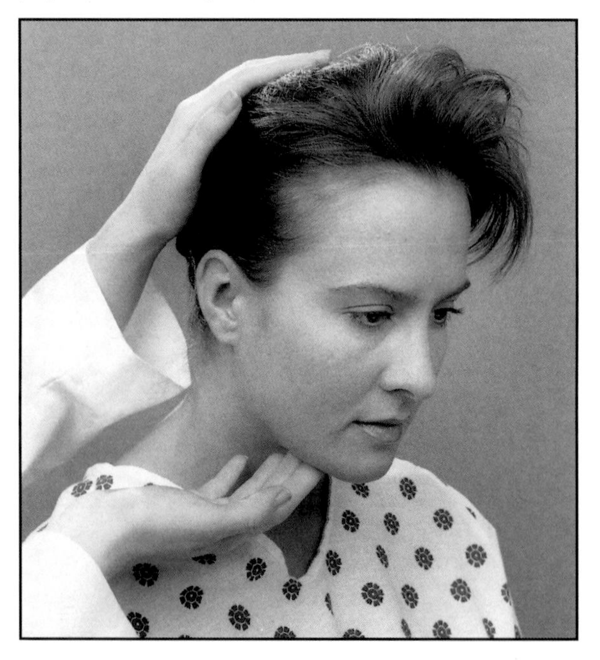

Submental. To assess the submental lymph nodes, palpate under the chin.

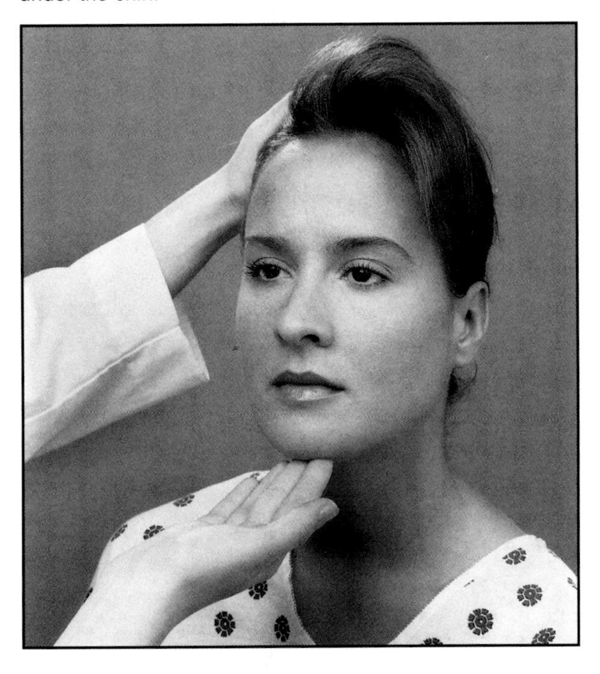

Superficial cervical. To assess the superficial cervical lymph nodes, palpate over the sternocleidomastoid muscle.

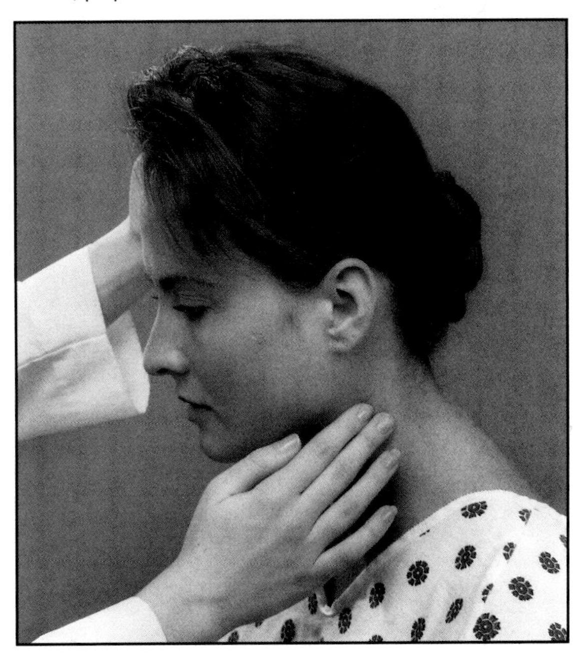

Superficial posterior cervical. To assess the superficial posterior cervical lymph nodes, palpate over the anterior surface of the trapezius muscle.

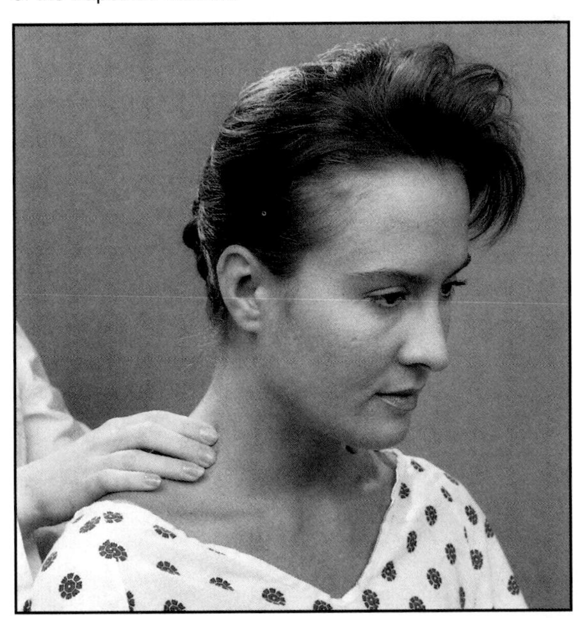

Supraclavicular. To assess the supraclavicular lymph nodes, palpate the supraclavicular area by hooking the index finger over the clavicle lateral to the sternocleidomastoid muscle.

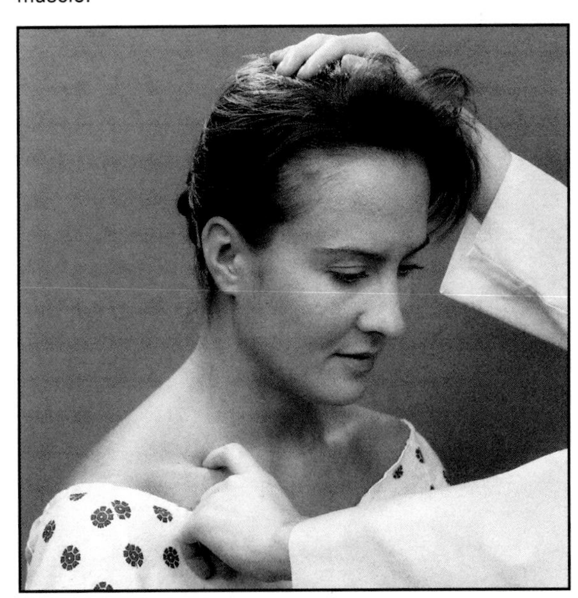

ASSESSMENT

INSPECTION AND PALPATION (continued)

Axillary and epitrochlear lymph nodes

Central, lateral, and subscapular. To assess the central, lateral, and subscapular nodes, place the hand as high in the axilla as possible. Then palpate the axillary nodes.

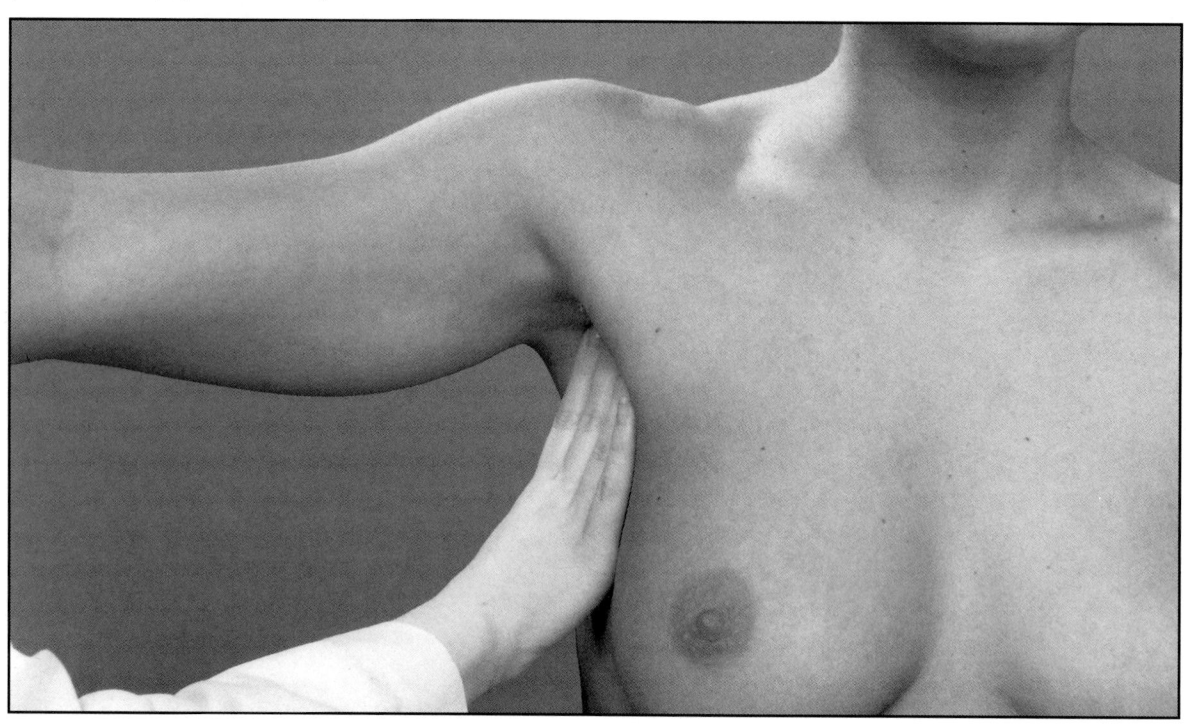

Infraclavicular. To assess the infraclavicular lymph nodes, palpate below the clavicle.

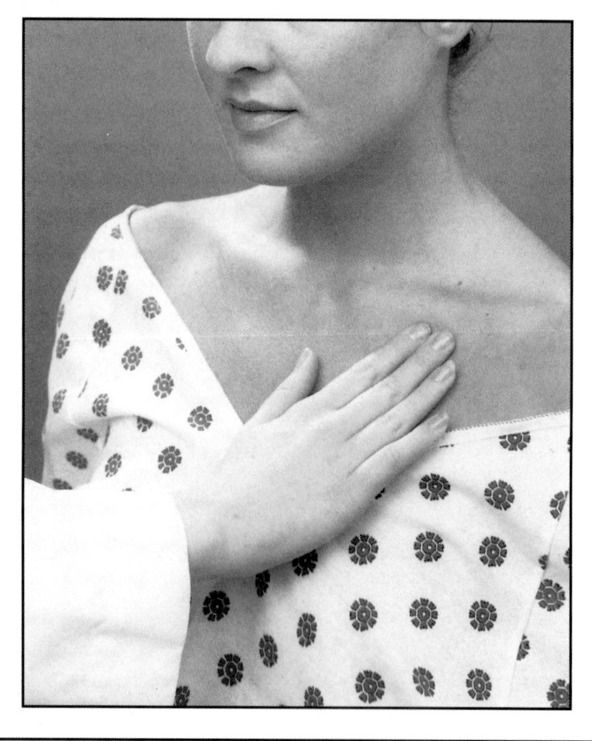

Epitrochlear. To assess the epitrochlear lymph nodes, palpate in the depression above and posterior to the medial area of the elbow.

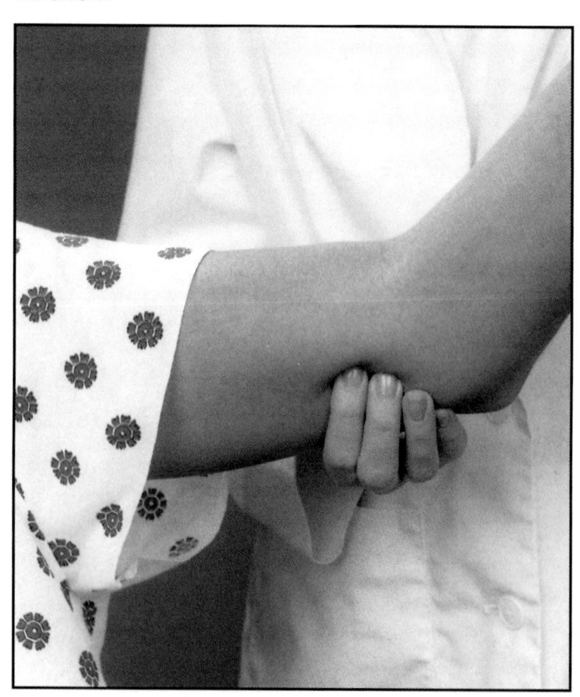

Inguinal and popliteal lymph nodes

Inferior superficial inguinal. To assess the inferior superficial inguinal lymph nodes, palpate below the junction of the saphenous and femoral veins.

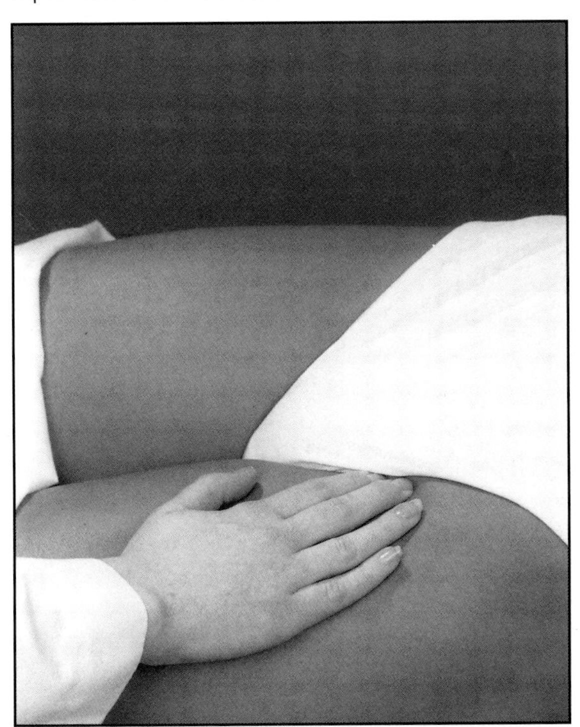

Superior superficial inguinal. To assess the superior superficial inguinal lymph nodes, palpate along the saphenous veins from the inguinal area to the abdomen.

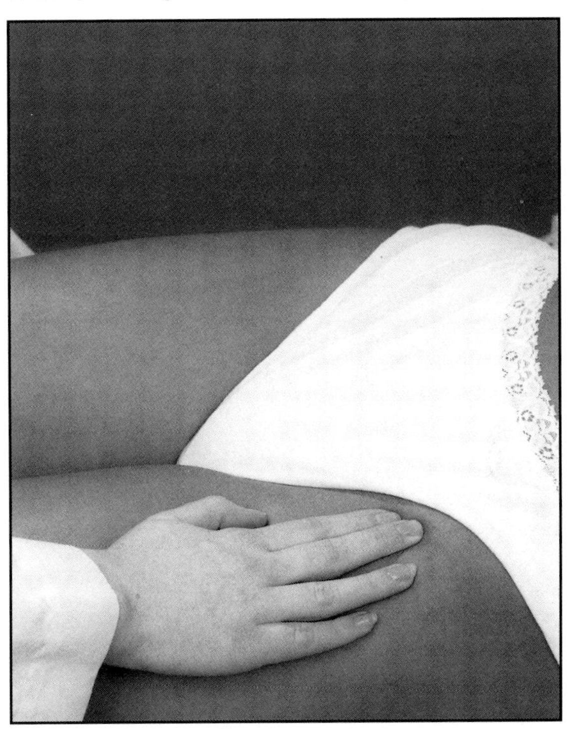

Popliteal. To assess the popliteal lymph nodes, palpate along the posterior muscles at the back of the knee.

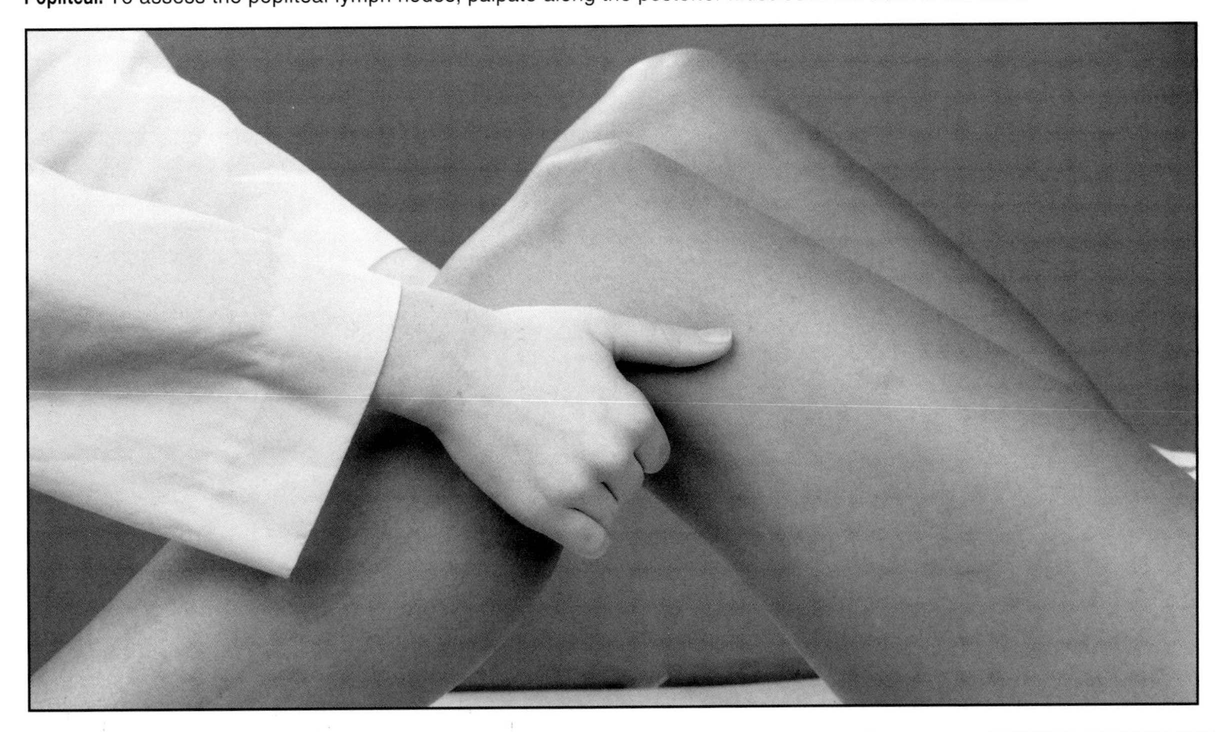

Common abnormalities

■ Kaposi's sarcoma

This rare vascular tumor is characterized by widespread purple or blue patches, plaques, or nodular skin lesions. Until recently, Kaposi's sarcoma was found primarily in elderly men of Mediterranean descent (classical form) and in young men of African descent (endemic form). More recently, the epidemic form has been found in men with acquired immunodeficiency syndrome (AIDS).

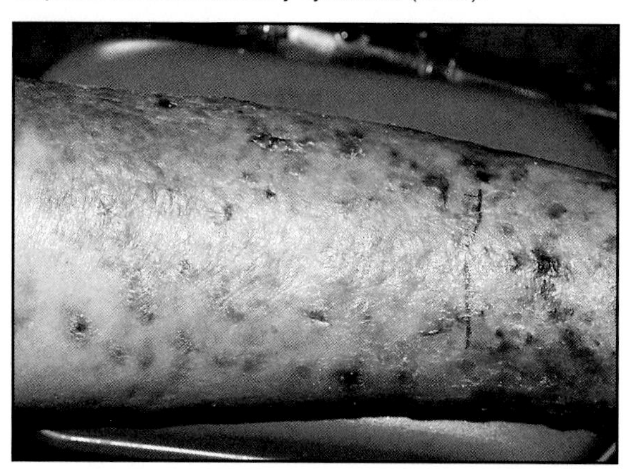

■ Wasting syndrome

This syndrome is characterized by weight loss of more than 10%, chronic diarrhea, and chronic weakness. It commonly is associated with AIDS.

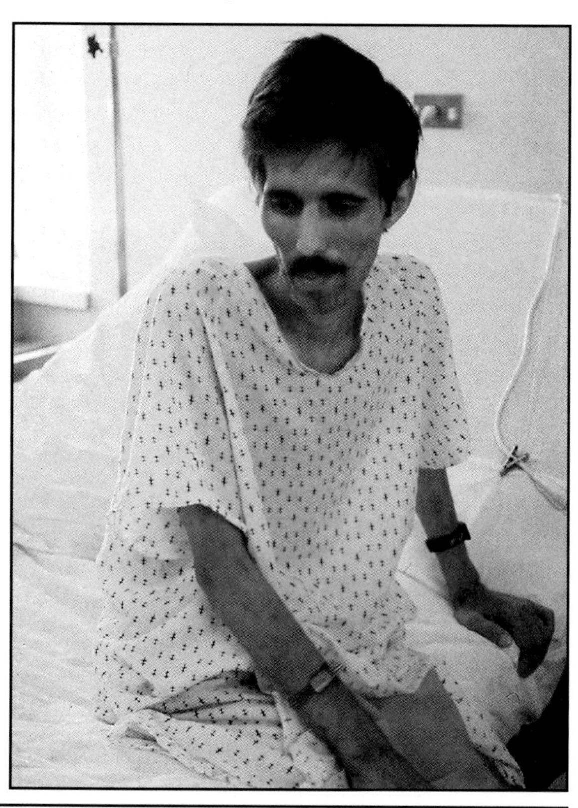

■ Discoid lesions

These raised, red, scaling plaques with central atrophy usually erupt on the face, scalp, ears, neck, arms, and other sunlight-exposed areas of the body. They may result from discoid lupus erythematosus, which is an immune disorder that affects only the skin.

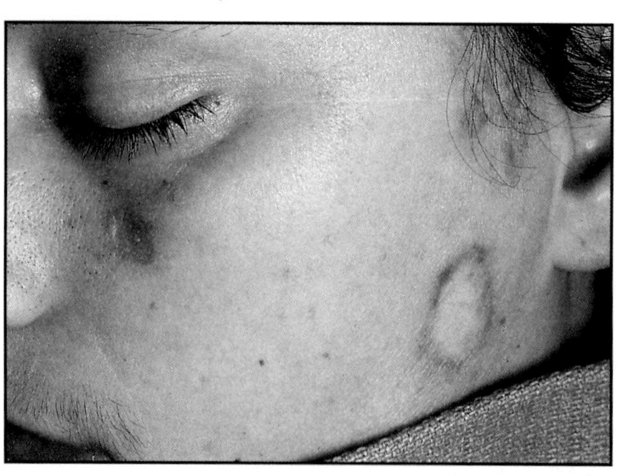

■ Raynaud's phenomenon

This condition is characterized by intermittent bilateral attacks of ischemia of the fingers, toes, and sometimes ears and nose. It is associated with systemic lupus erythematosus, which is an immune disorder that affects various body systems and may produce such signs as sclerodactyly (finger deformity), ulcerations, and chronic paronychia (skin infection at nail margin).

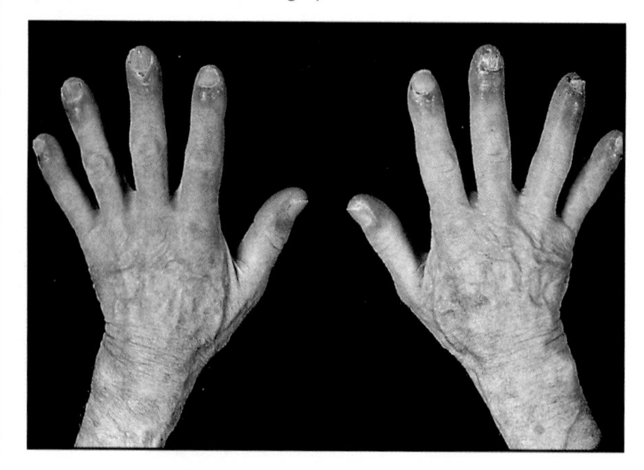

Endocrine System

Anatomy and physiology overview

■ Structures of the endocrine system

These anterior views show the structures of the endocrine system.

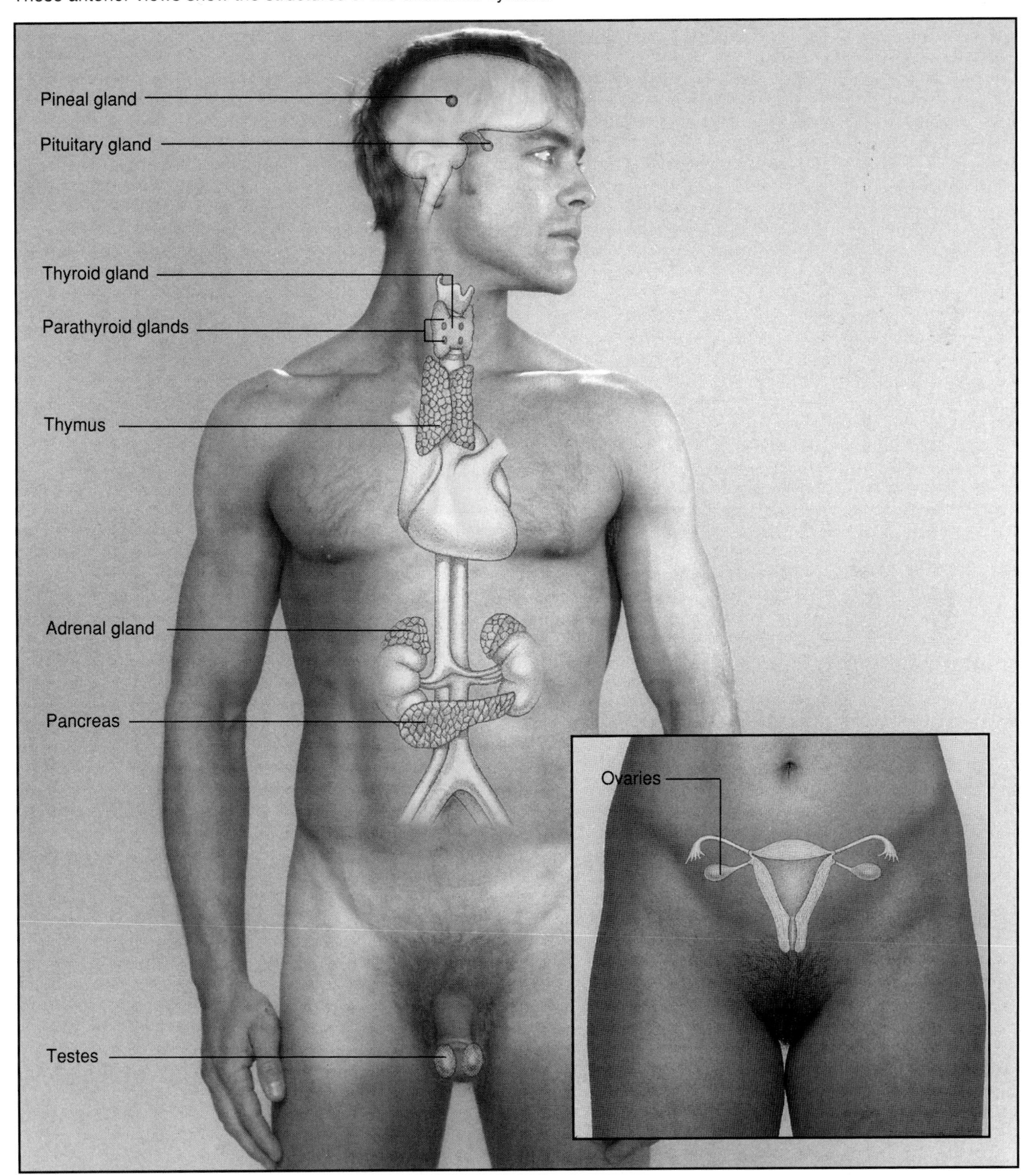

(continued)

ANATOMY AND PHYSIOLOGY OVERVIEW

STRUCTURES OF THE ENDOCRINE SYSTEM (continued)

Thyroid gland and related structures

This anterior view of the neck shows the thyroid gland and related anatomical structures.

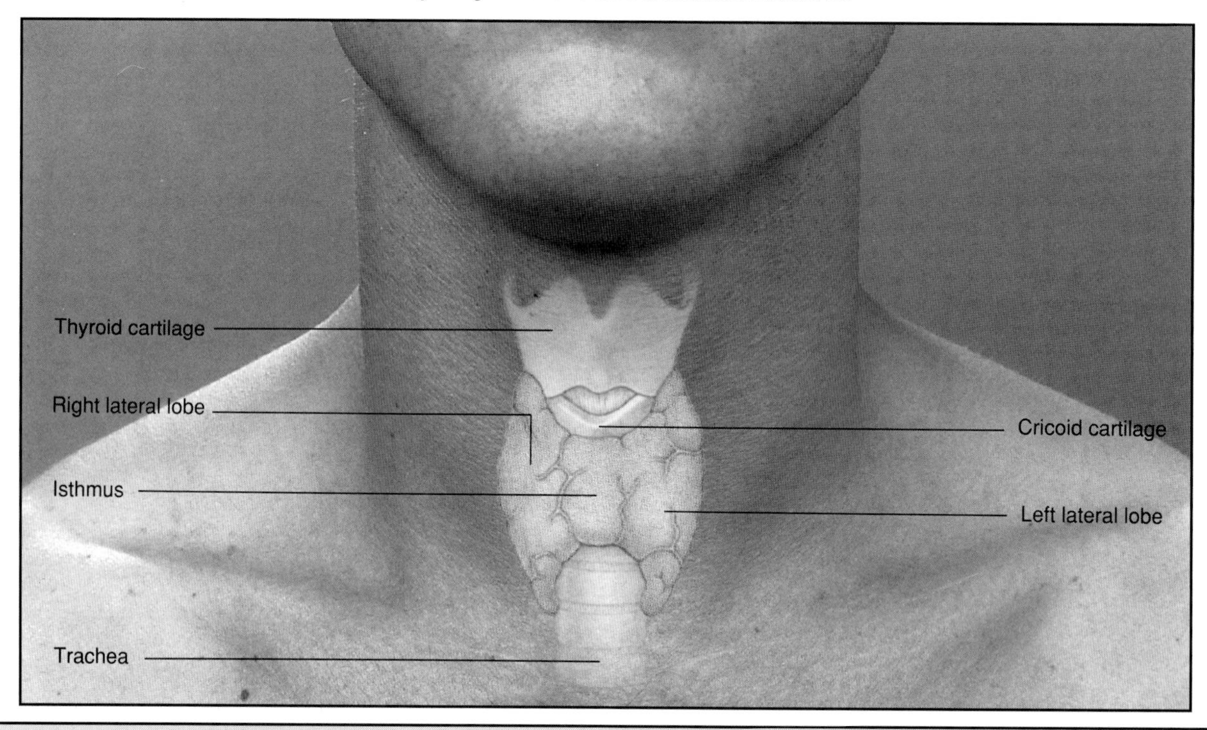

Assessment

■ Inspection

Neck

Inspect the neck first with it held straight, then slightly extended, and finally while the client swallows water (not shown). Normally, the neck and trachea are symmetrical, and the larynx, trachea, and thyroid move up and down as the client swallows.

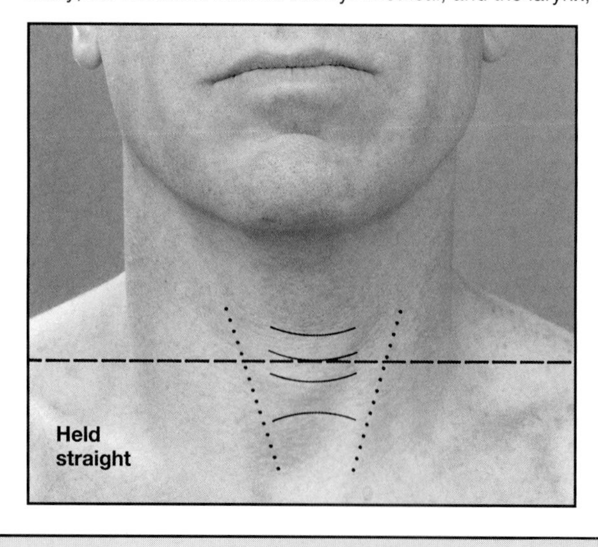

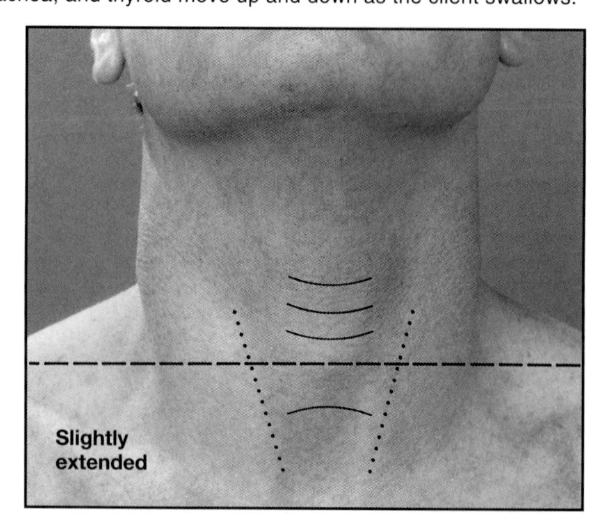

ASSESSMENT

■ Palpation

Thyroid

Palpate the thyroid from in front of or behind the client as shown below. Normally, the thyroid gland is not tender.

1 Stand behind the client and gently place the fingers on either side of the trachea, just below the cricoid cartilage. Palpate the thyroid isthmus as the client swallows.

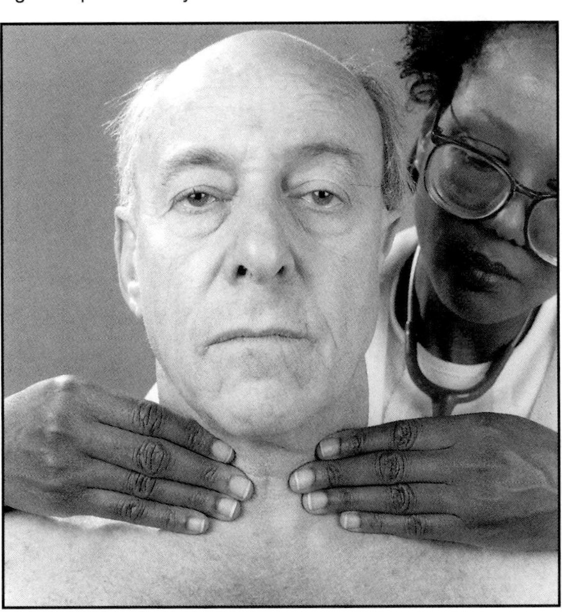

2 Palpate one lobe of the thyroid at a time. To palpate the right lobe, have the client tilt the head to the right. Move the thyroid cartilage to the right, have the client swallow, and palpate the main body of the thyroid.

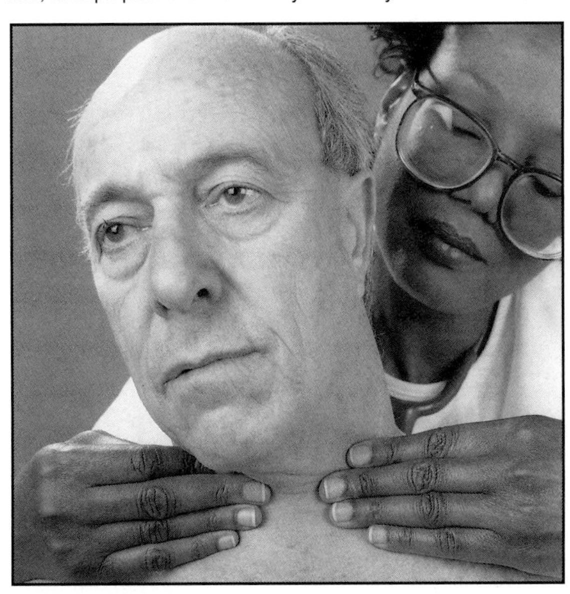

3 To palpate the right lateral border, move the fingers of your left hand between the trachea and the right sternocleidomastoid. Place the fingers of your right hand behind the right sternocleidomastoid, press your hands together, and palpate the right lobe as the patient swallows. Using the opposite hands, repeat steps 2 and 3 on the other side of the neck to palpate the left lobe.

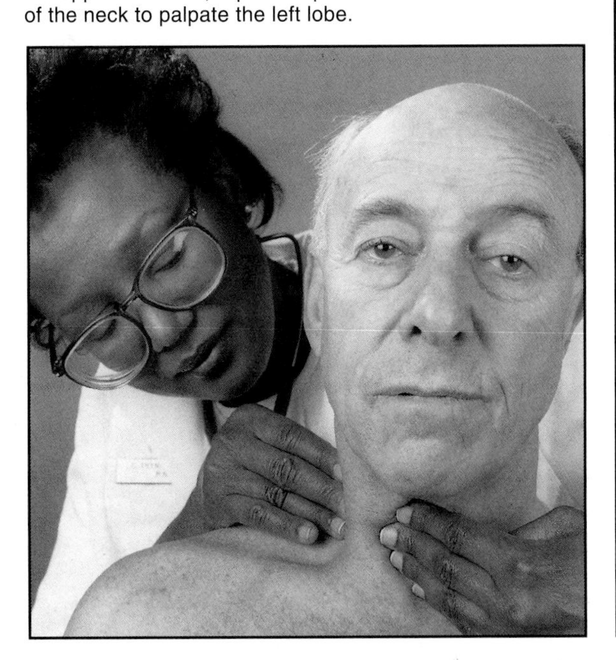

■ Auscultation

Thyroid

If palpation reveals an enlarged thyroid gland, auscultate it for bruits with the bell of the stethoscope while the client holds his or her breath. Normally, auscultation detects no bruits.

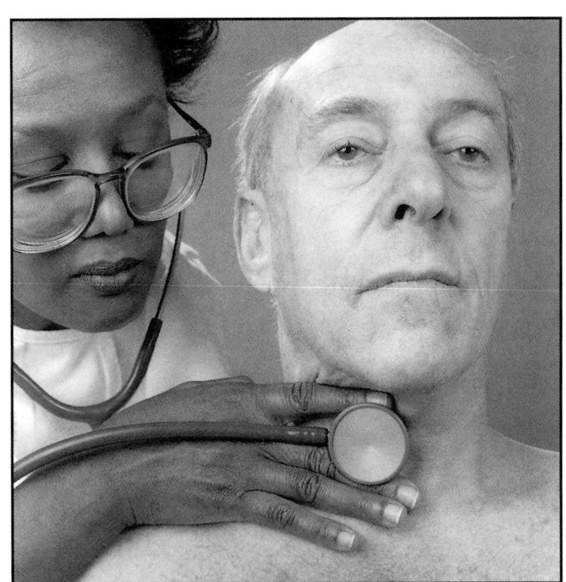

Common abnormalities

■ Exophthalmos

Eyeball protrusion accompanied by lid lag is a common sign of hyperthyroidism.

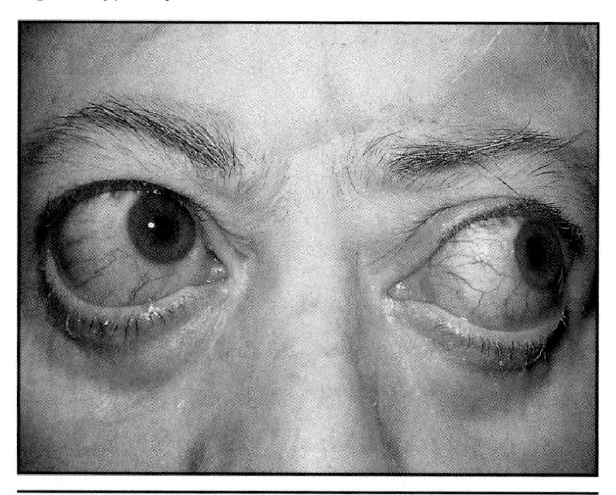

■ Acromegaly

This condition may produce an enlarged supraorbital ridge and thickened nose and ears. It is caused by excess production of the growth hormone somatotropin, which may result from an anterior pituitary tumor.

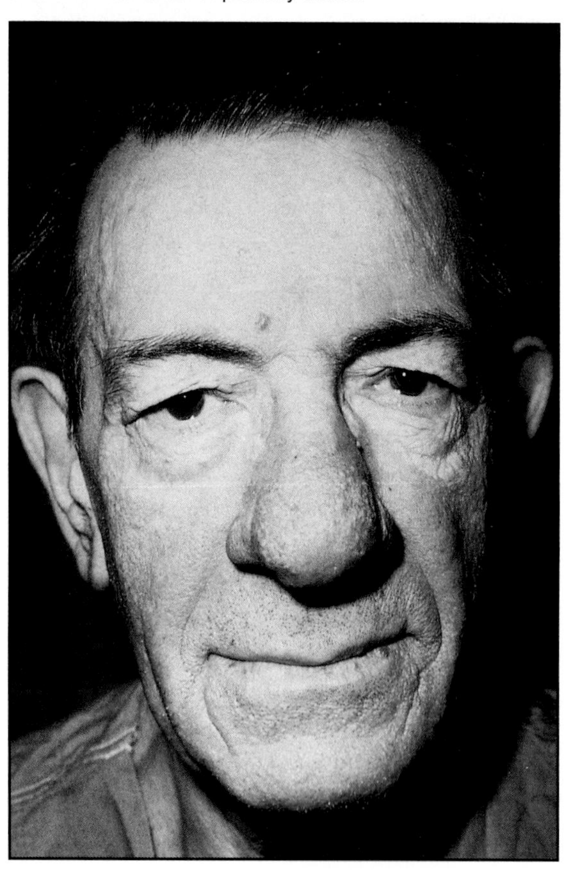

■ Goiter

A diffusely enlarged goiter may be caused by Graves' disease, Hashimoto's thyroiditis, or iodine deficiency (endemic goiter). A nodular goiter may be benign or malignant.

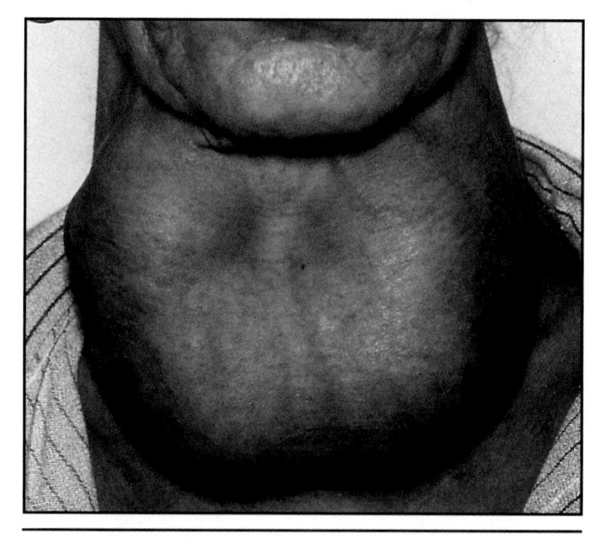

■ Buffalo hump

Fat deposits that concentrate around the interscapular area are characteristic of Cushing's syndrome.

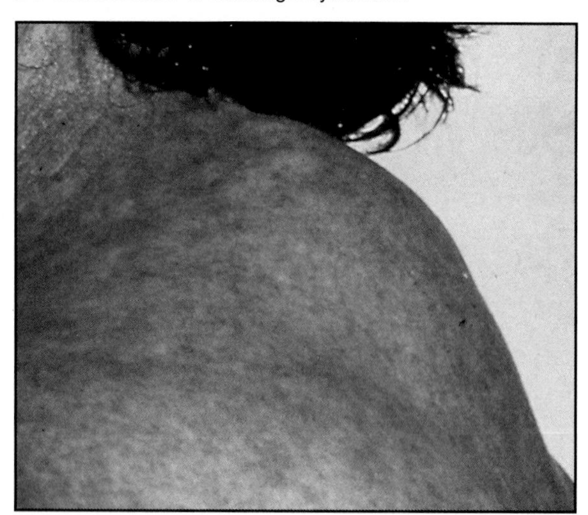

Perinatal and Neonatal Assessment

Prenatal assessment

■ Inspection

Skin

Melanotropin normally increases during pregnancy, causing brownish hyperpigmentation of facial skin, also known as chloasma, melasma, or the mask of pregnancy.

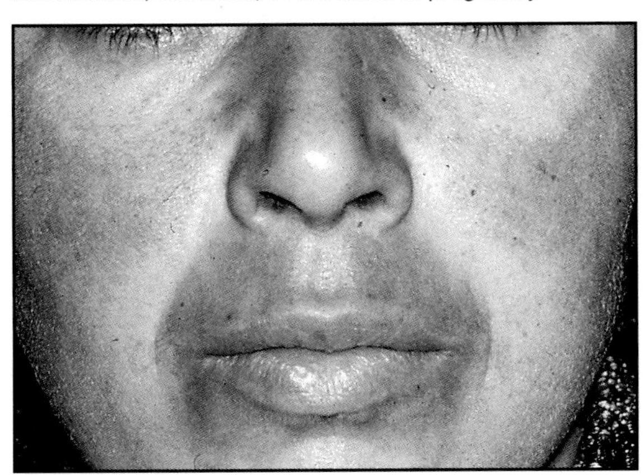

Breasts

In a pregnant client, the areolae and nipples darken, and the breasts may display striae (stretch marks) and an increased venous pattern.

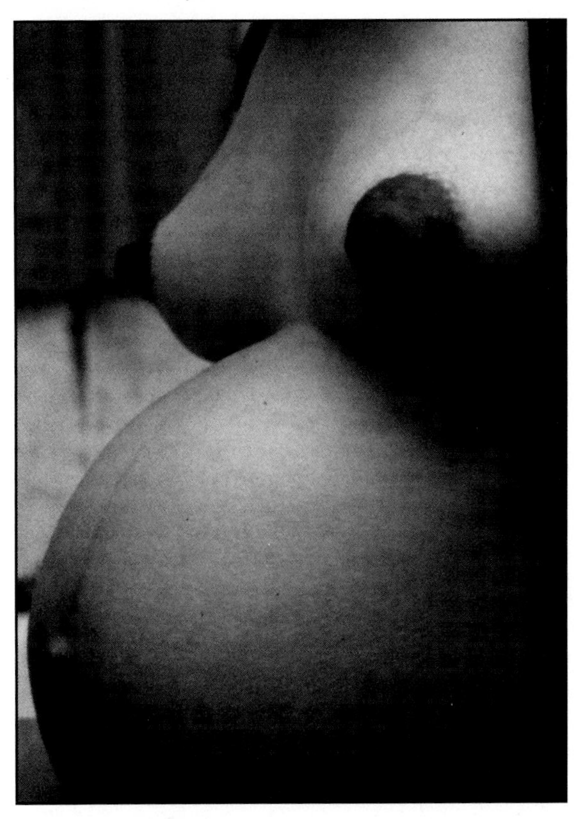

Abdomen

Linea nigra (a brownish-black pigmented line at midline) and striae may appear on the pregnant client's abdomen.

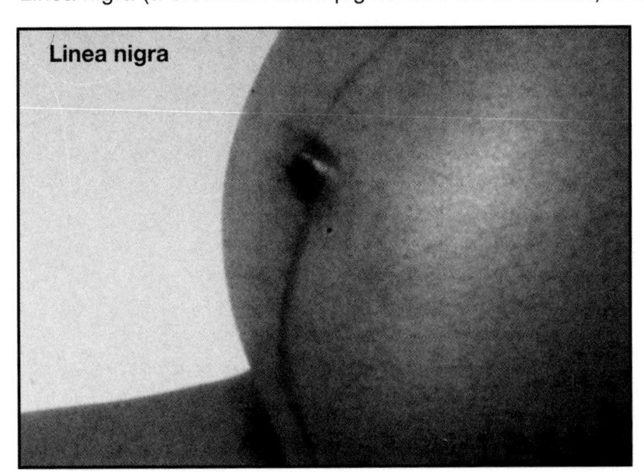

Linea nigra

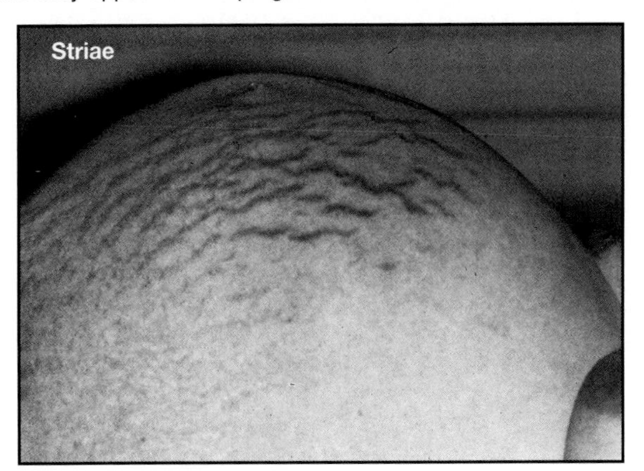

Striae

PRENATAL ASSESSMENT

■ Palpation

Fundus

To assess fundal height, begin palpating above the normal location of the uterus for this stage of pregnancy. Then palpate down toward the symphysis pubis to the point where the soft abdomen ends and the firm fundal edge begins. Along the anterior abdominal wall, measure the distance from the top of the fundus to the notch at the inferior edge of the symphysis pubis. At 12 to 13 weeks, the fundus can be felt just above the symphysis pubis; at 16 weeks, the fundus is about midway between the symphysis pubis and the umbilicus; at 20 weeks, it can be felt at the umbilical level.

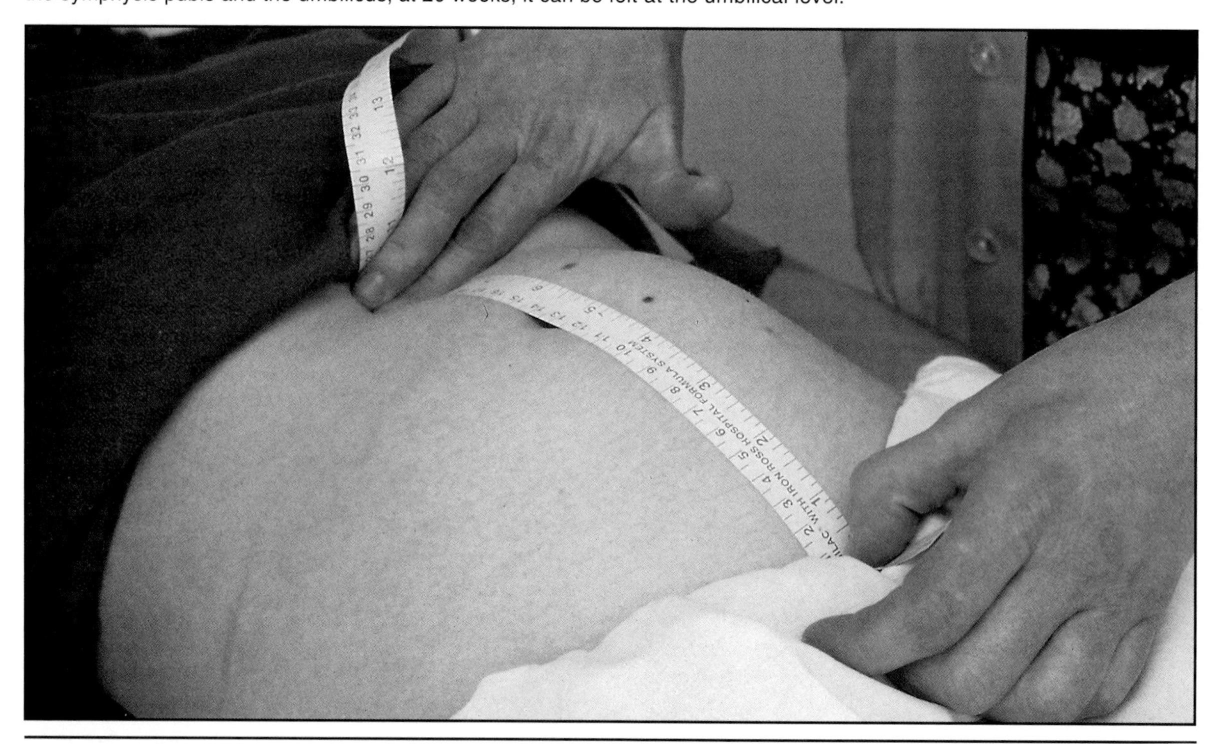

■ Auscultation

Using an ultrasound stethoscope (left below) or fetoscope (right), auscultate fetal heart sounds beginning at the midline about midway between the umbilicus and the symphysis pubis. Move the stethoscope or fetoscope from side to side, if needed, to the point where the heart sounds are loudest.

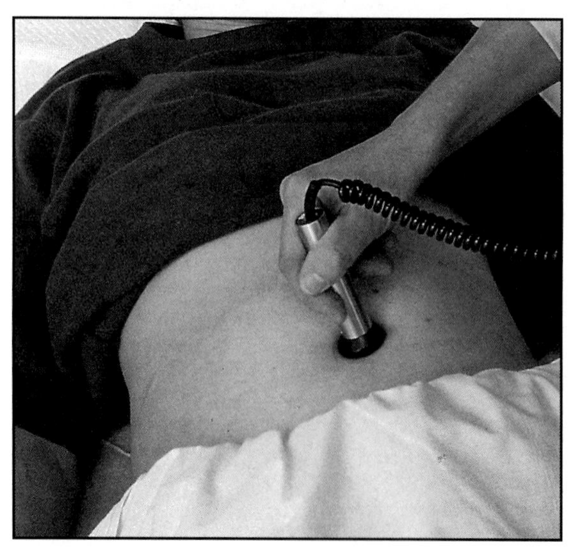

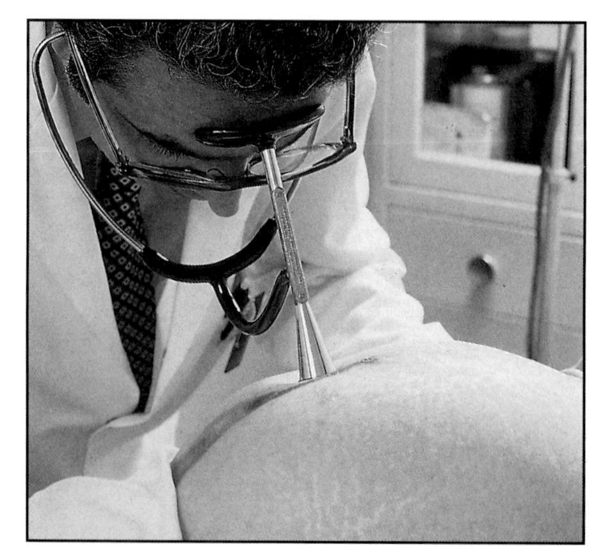

Neonatal assessment

■ Inspection

Skin and hair

Vernix caseosa. A gray-white, cheeselike, protective skin covering is normal immediately after birth. It typically diminishes after several days.

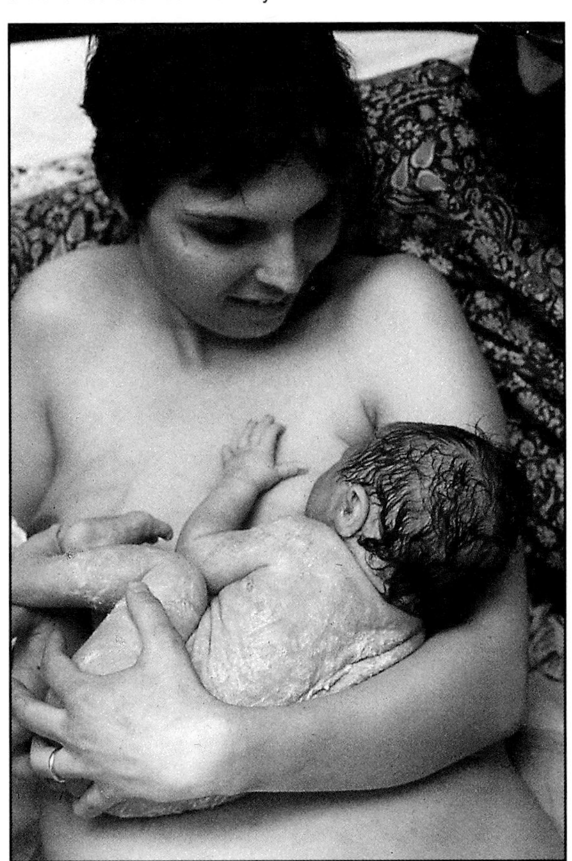

Capillary hemangioma. These small reddened areas on the upper eyelids, bridge of the nose, and nape of the neck normally disappear as the skin thickens.

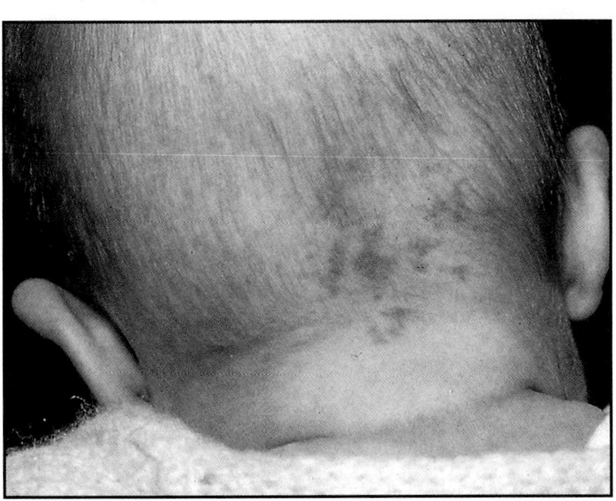

Milia. White papules, caused by accumulated sebum in the sebaceous glands, commonly affect the nose, cheeks, and chin and disappear in 2 to 3 weeks.

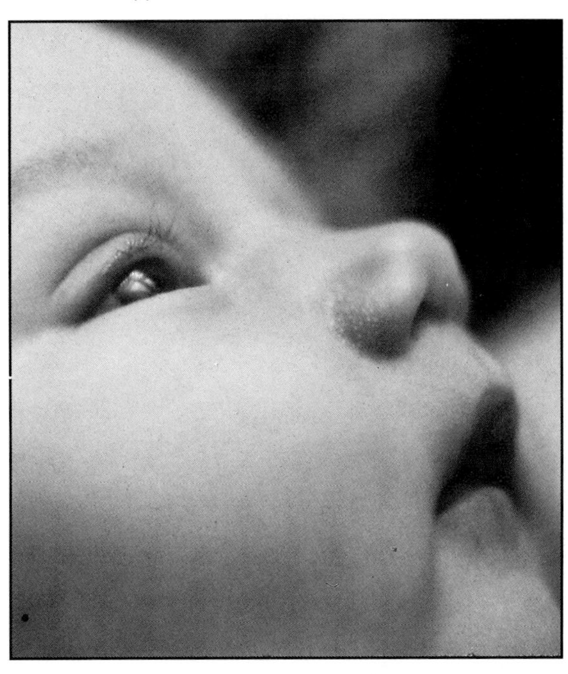

Head

Head molding results from an overlap of cranial bones. This normal finding commonly occurs with vaginal delivery.

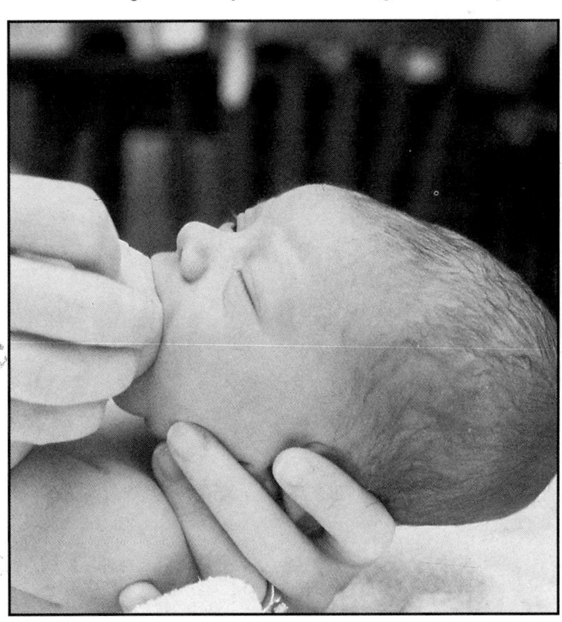

(continued)

NEONATAL ASSESSMENT

INSPECTION (continued)

Chest

Circumference. Measure the chest at the nipple line. The normal chest circumference ranges from 12" to 13" (30 to 33 cm) or 3/4" to 1 1/2" less than the head circumference.

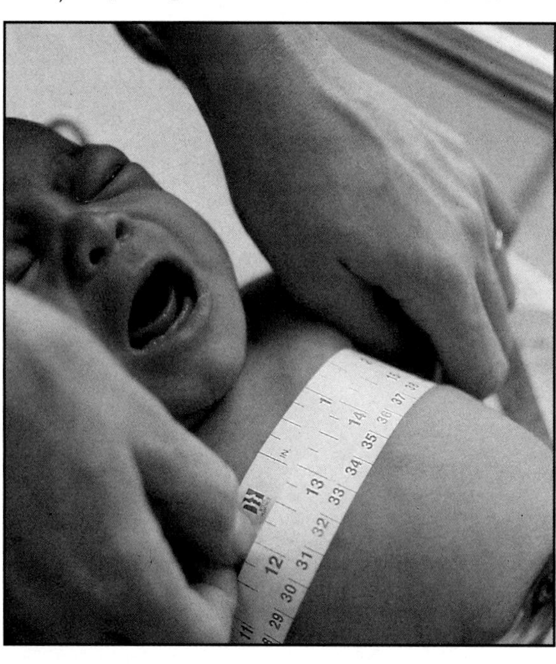

Back

Inspect the back, noting spinal position and alignment of shoulders, scapulae, and iliac crests. Normally, the spine is straight and shows no dimpling, and the shoulders, scapulae, and iliac crests are in planar alignment.

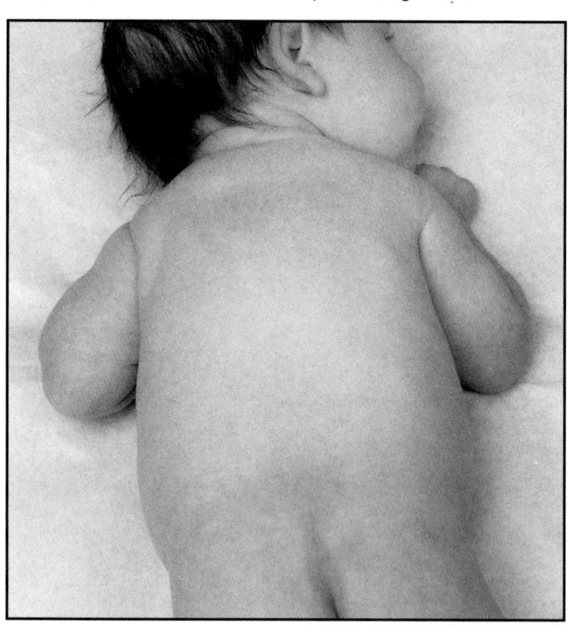

Abdomen

Inspect the abdomen, noting its size, shape, and condition. Normally, the abdomen is round and dome-shaped, and has no visible masses. The umbilical stump normally falls midline and is soft, moist, and white at birth.

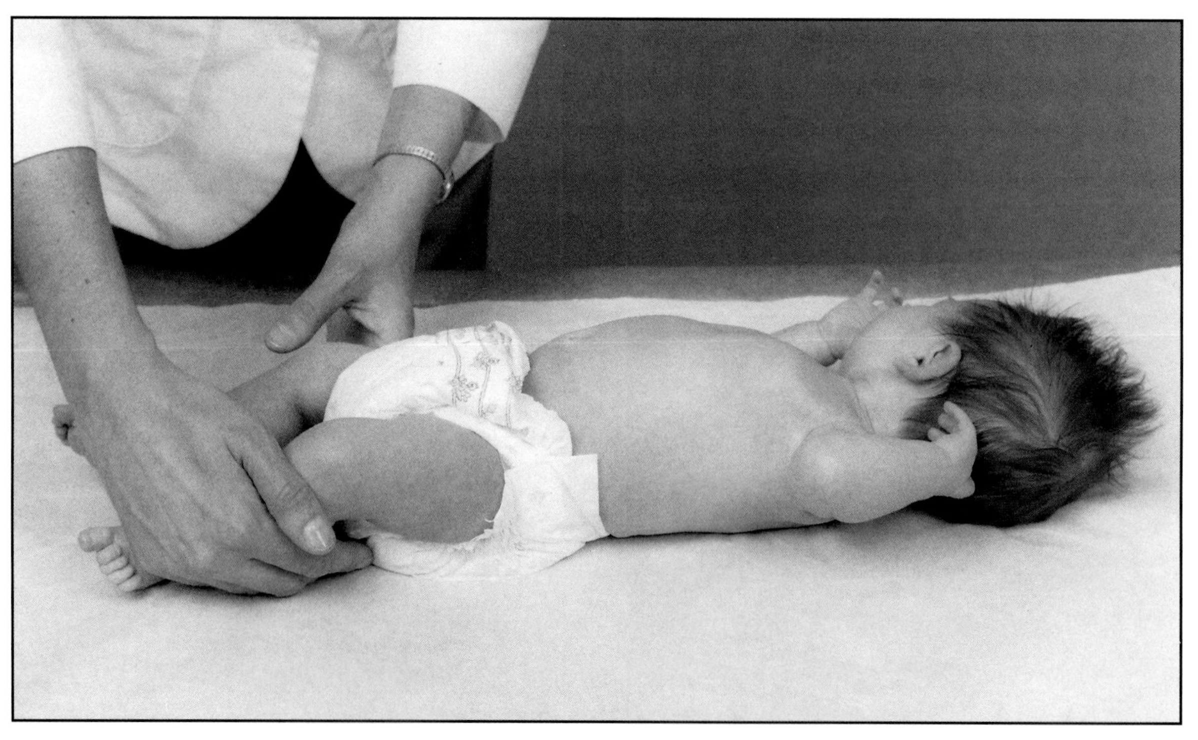

Extremities

To assess hip joint stability, perform Ortolani's maneuver. With the neonate supine, grasp the legs by placing your thumb on the inner aspect of the thigh and your fingers on the greater trochanter. Adduct the neonate's legs with the hips and knees flexed at a 90-degree angle. Then abduct the legs until the lateral aspects of the knees touch the table. An audible or palpable click indicates an unstable joint.

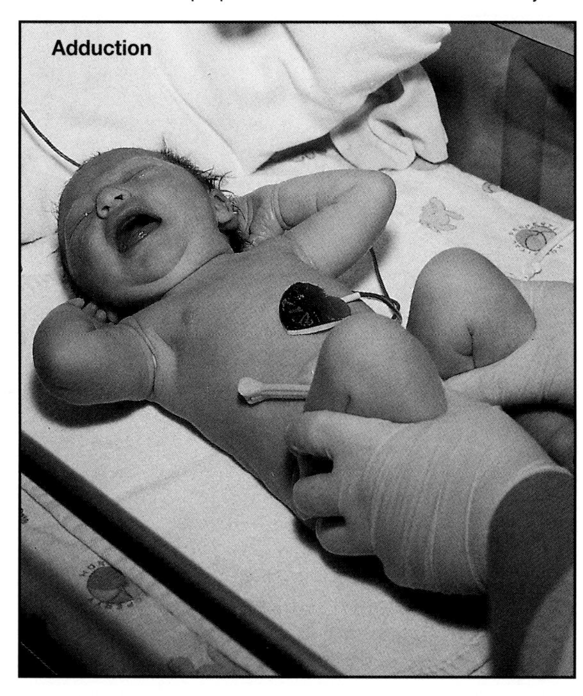
Adduction

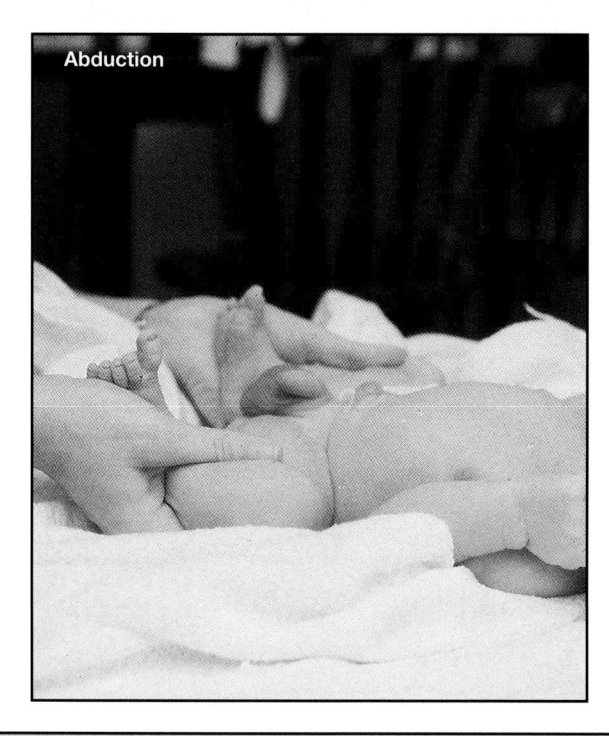
Abduction

Gluteal folds

Inspect the gluteal folds, which normally are symmetrical. Asymmetrical gluteal folds may indicate hip dislocation.

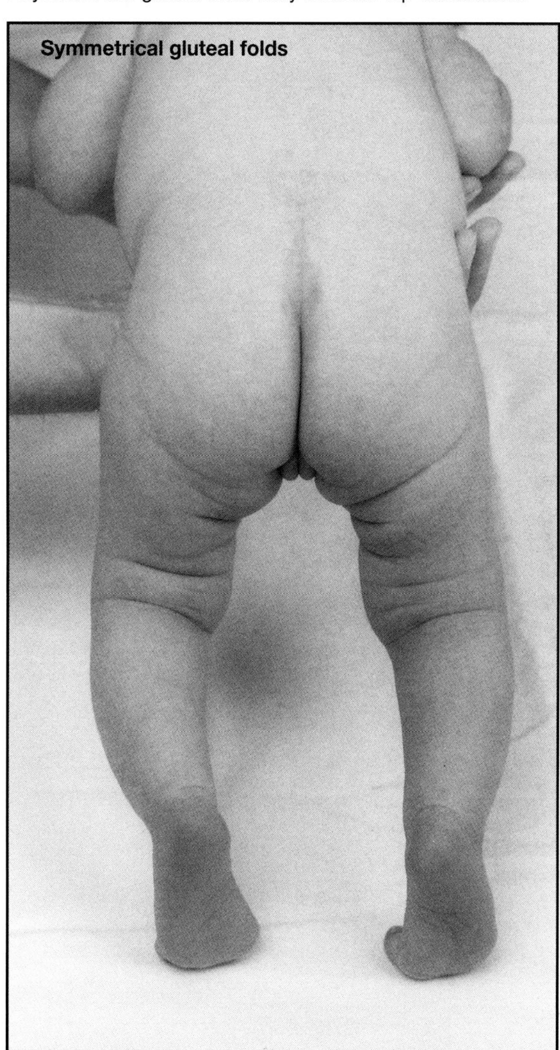
Symmetrical gluteal folds

(continued)

NEONATAL ASSESSMENT

INSPECTION (continued)

Anus and genitalia

After assessing the anus of a male neonate, inspect the scrotal sacs and testes. Also note the condition of the foreskin and the location of the urinary meatus. Normally, the anus is patent, the testes descended, the foreskin difficult to retract, and the urinary meatus at the penile tip.

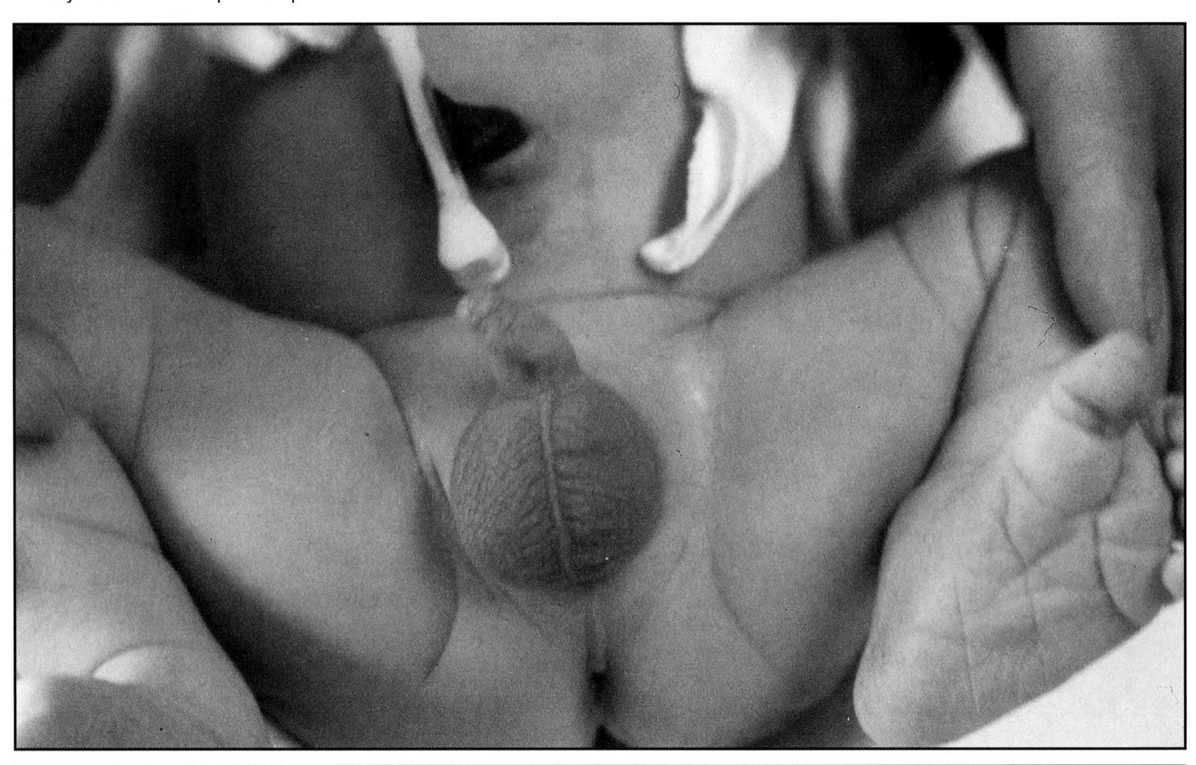

■ Palpation

Fontanels

Gently palpate the anterior and posterior fontanels. Normally, the fontanels are soft and slightly concave. The anterior closes about 18 months after birth; the posterior closes by 3 months.

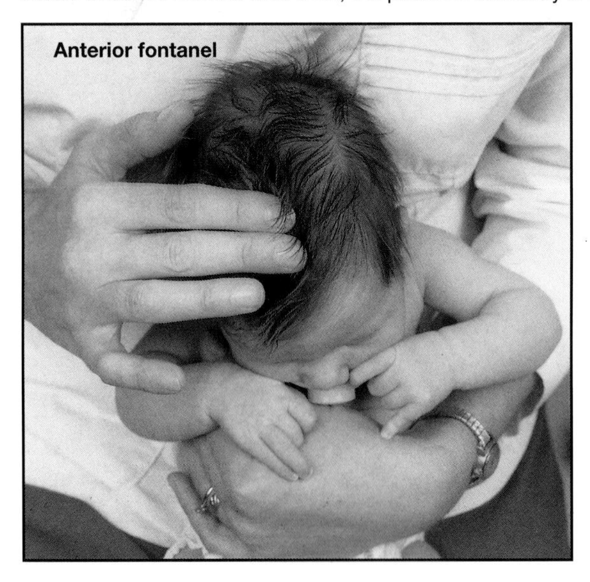
Anterior fontanel

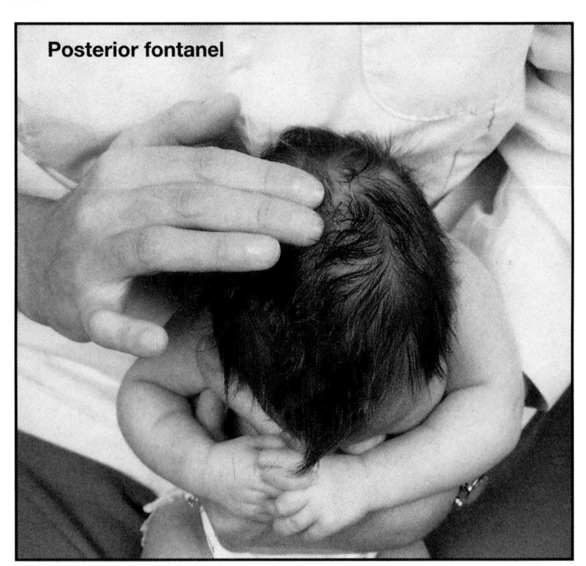
Posterior fontanel

PALPATION (continued)

Spine

Palpate the spine with the neonate in a prone position. Normally, the spinal processes are thin and well-formed.

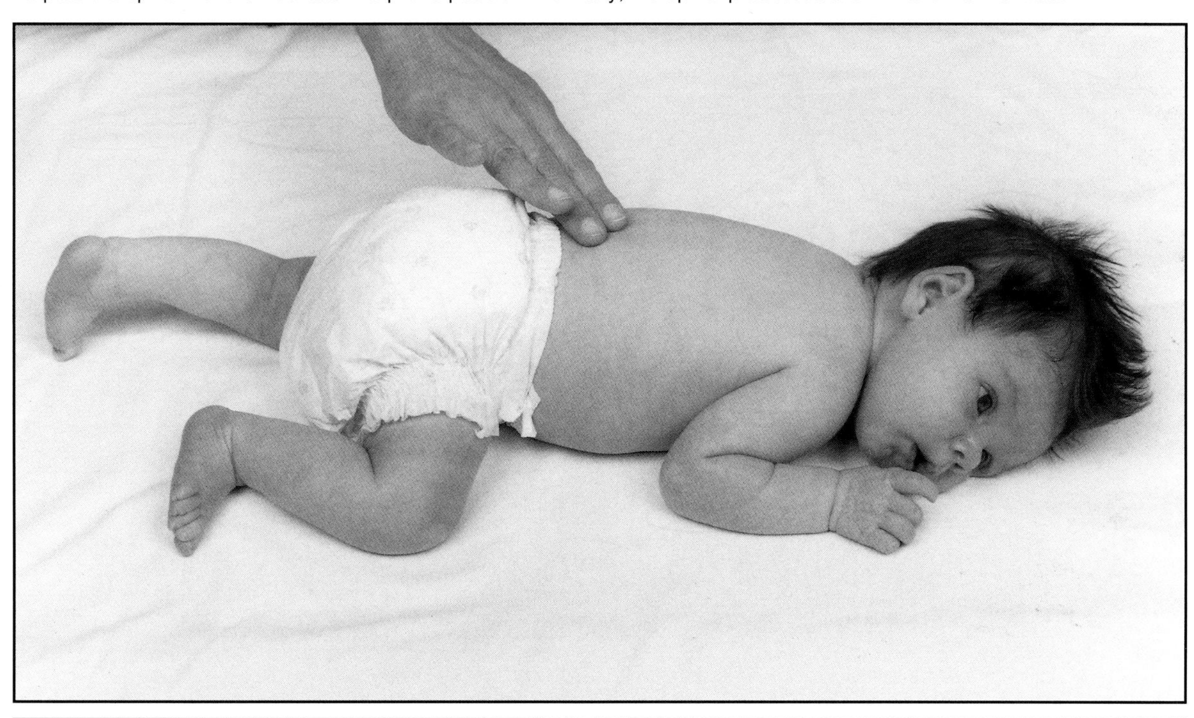

■ Reflex tests

Sucking or rooting

Touch the neonate's lip, cheek, or corner of the mouth. Normally, the neonate will turn the head toward the stimulus and open the mouth.

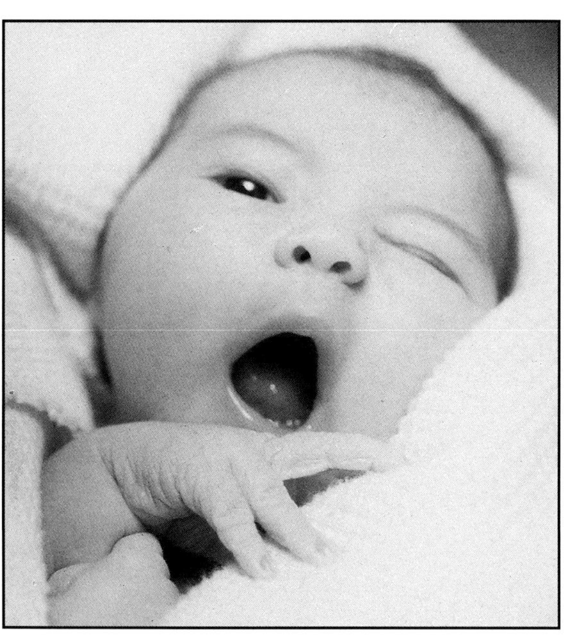

Extrusion

Touch or depress the neonate's tongue. Normally, the neonate will force the tongue outward.

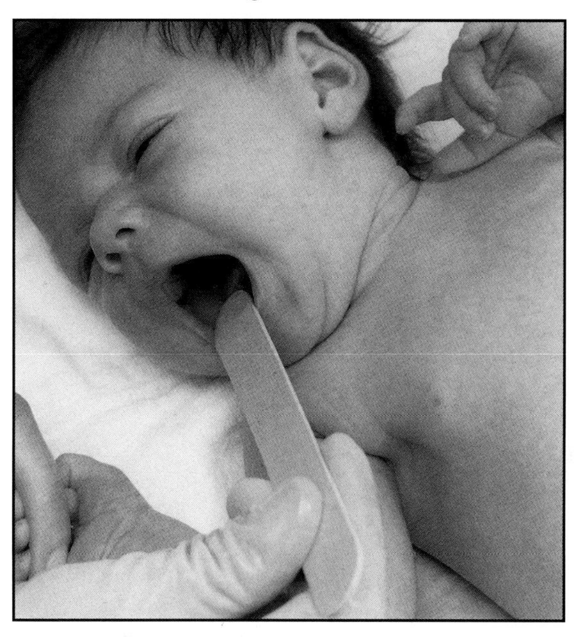

(continued)

NEONATAL ASSESSMENT

REFLEX TESTS (continued)

Babinski's reflex

Stroke the side of the neonate's foot from the heel to the toes and across the ball of the foot. Normally, the neonate hyperextends and fans out the toes and dorsiflexes the great toe.

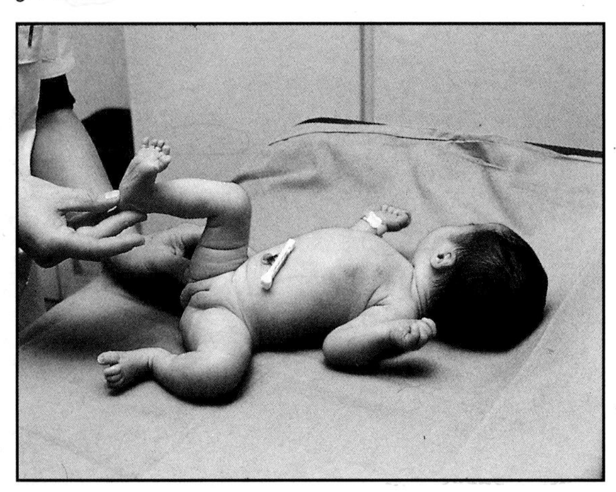

Palmar grasp

Apply pressure to the palm of the neonate's hand. Normally, the neonate's fingers will curl around the examiner's finger.

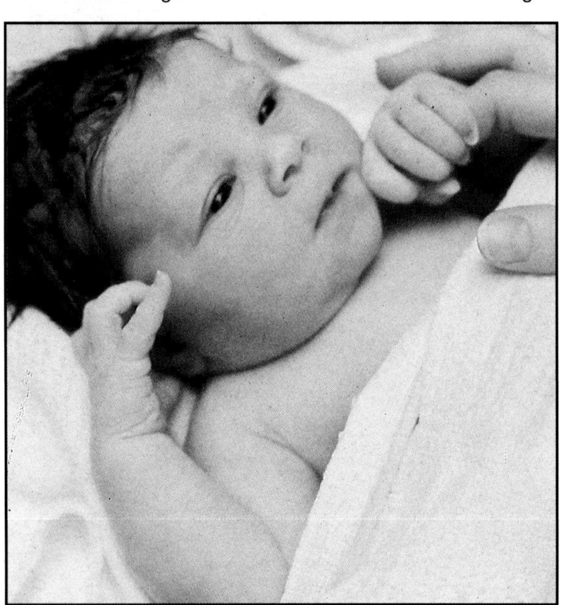

Moro or "startle"

While the neonate is lying quietly, provide a sudden stimulus, such as a hand clap. Normally, the neonate will flex the arms and legs symmetrically in an embracing motion.

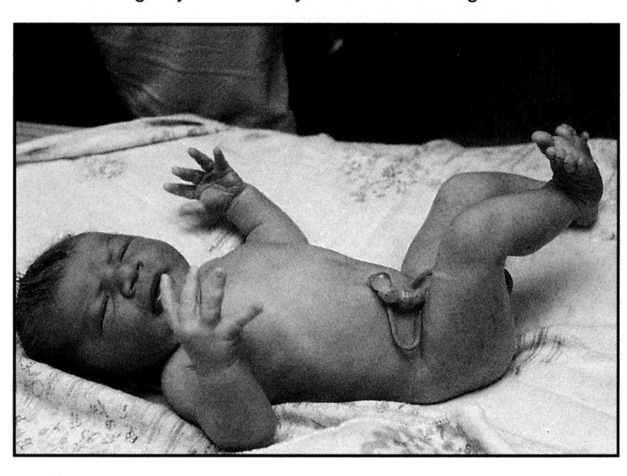

Tonic neck or "fencing"

With the neonate supine, turn the head from midline to one side. Normally, the extremities will extend on the side toward which the neonate is turned, and the opposite extremities will flex.

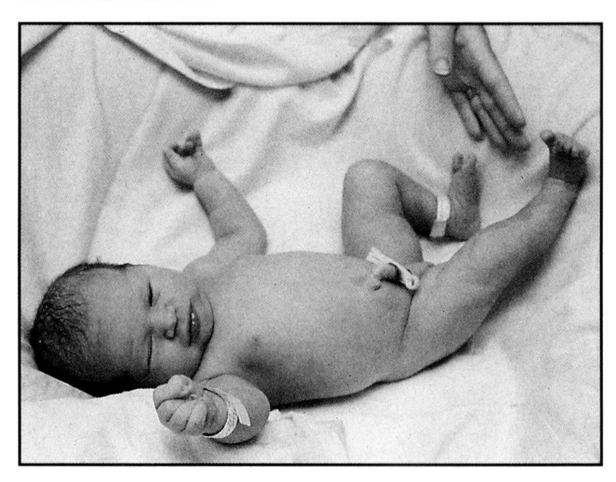

15

Female Reproductive System

Objectives

After reading and studying this chapter, you should be able to:

1. Identify the location of the female reproductive organs.
2. Compare the variations in estrogen and progesterone levels and actions.
3. Develop interview questions that will elicit information about the female client's reproductive system status.
4. Define the normal physical characteristics of premenarchal, adolescent, mature, and postmenopausal women.
5. Describe, step-by-step, a physical assessment of the female reproductive organs and external genitalia.
6. Differentiate normal from abnormal findings during physical assessment of the female reproductive system.
7. Describe two different clusters of abnormal assessment findings that indicate possible female reproductive system disorders.
8. Explain specimen collection techniques for selected diagnostic tests, including the Papanicolaou (Pap) test.
9. Identify representative adverse reactions to drugs that affect the female reproductive system.
10. Document the assessment findings for a female client with a reproductive system disorder.

Introduction

In the past, women were discouraged from discussing reproductive system problems, privately or publicly. Recently, however, women's health care issues have emerged as important discussion topics. Reproductive concerns such as contraception, infertility, and premenstrual syndrome (PMS) are commonly discussed in clinics and women's support groups. Because of their knowledge, nurses are particularly qualified to provide health care services and instruction related to these concerns.

Most nurses will encounter clients with reproductive health problems in hospitals; others will meet them in clinics or physicians' offices. Reproductive health education includes various teaching opportunities. For example, a premenarchal girl may have questions about menstruation; a young woman about to become sexually active may have questions about contraception; a married couple may have questions about contraception, conception, and pregnancy; and a woman past the childbearing years may have questions about menopause. This chapter provides information to assist the nurse in handling these and related health assessment and teaching activities.

Chapter 15 reviews female reproductive anatomy and physiology (including the hormonal cycle and its relationship to menstruation) as well as developmental and maturational changes. Then it discusses use of the health history for gathering subjective data about the client. The health history questions relate to menstruation, procreation, sexually transmitted diseases, contraception, reproductive tract infections and abnormalities, sexuality, and development and maturity. The questions suggest individualized approaches for the premenarchal girl, the adolescent, and the older woman.

Also described in this chapter is the basic physical assessment, including special client preparation and relaxation techniques, external reproductive organ inspection, and guidelines for assisting with an internal pelvic assessment. The chapter also discusses advanced internal pelvic assessment techniques, describes how to collect specimens for diagnostic tests, and explains some

Glossary

Abortion: spontaneous or induced termination of pregnancy before the fetus becomes viable (about 20 weeks).
Anovulation: lack of ovulation.
Anteflexed uterus: normal position in which the uterine corpus flexes forward at an acute angle.
Anteverted uterus: normal position in which the uterine corpus flexes forward, but less acutely than if anteflexed.
Breakthrough bleeding: vaginal spotting or bleeding that occurs between periods and is caused by the failure of progestin (usually taken in combination with estrogen as an oral contraceptive) to support the endometrium adequately.
Cervical ectropion: eversion of the epithelium onto the cervix.
Climacteric: period from onset to end of hormonal and related changes that ceases reproductive function.
Cystocele: herniation of the bladder through the anterior vaginal wall.
Dysmenorrhea: menstrual discomfort or pain.
Dyspareunia: painful or difficult sexual intercourse.
Enterocele: herniation of intestine through the vaginal wall.
Gravida: number of pregnancies, regardless of their outcomes.
Menarche: onset of menstrual periods, usually occurring between age 9 and 17.
Menopause: cessation of menstrual periods with the decline of cyclic hormonal production and function usually between the ages of 45 and 60 but may stop earlier in life, for example, as a result of illness or the surgical removal of the uterus or both ovaries.
Multigravida: woman who has been pregnant several times.
Multiparity: condition of having two or more pregnancies that resulted in viable fetuses.
Nulliparity: condition of never having delivered a viable infant.
Osteoporosis: loss of bone density, occurring most frequently in menopausal women.
Papanicolaou test (or smear): cytologic study of cervical tissue sample, performed most frequently to detect cervical cancer.
Parity: condition of having delivered an infant or infants, alive or dead, during the viability period (fetus weighing 500 g or more or having an estimated 20-week gestation); multiple birth is a single parity.
Premenstrual syndrome (PMS): a cyclic cluster of signs and symptoms, such as breast tenderness, fluid retention, and mood swings, usually occurring after ovulation and before or during menses; characterized by at least 7 symptom-free days, usually in the first half of the menstrual cycle.
Puberty: period when secondary sexual characteristics begin to appear and sexual reproductive ability occurs.
Rectocele: herniation of the rectum through the posterior vaginal wall.
Retroflexed uterus: normal position in which the uterine corpus flexes toward the rectum at an acute angle.
Retroverted uterus: normal position in which the uterine corpus flexes toward the rectum, but at a less acute angle than if retroflexed.
Vaginitis: inflammation of the vaginal mucosa.

normal and abnormal assessment findings. The chapter includes a case study, showing how to integrate the female reproductive system assessment into the nursing process.

Anatomy and physiology review

The female reproductive system consists of external and internal genitalia, which develop and function according to the hormonal influences that also affect fertility, childbearing, and the ability to experience sexual pleasure. External genitalia include the mons pubis, clitoris, labia majora, labia minora, and the adjacent structures (Bartholin's glands, Skene's glands, and the urethral meatus). Internal genitalia include the vagina, uterus, ovaries, and fallopian tubes. (For information about these structures, see *Female genitalia,* pages 416 and 417.)

In the years before menarche (initial onset of menstrual periods) and after childbearing, the uterus changes in size and shape. (For a comparison of these changes, see *Developmental changes in the uterus and cervix,* page 418.)

Hormonal function and the menstrual cycle

The hypothalamus, ovaries, and pituitary gland secrete hormones that affect the buildup and shedding of the uterine lining during the menstrual cycle. Through a network of positive and negative feedback loops from the hypothalamus to the pituitary and to the ovaries and back to the hypothalamus and pituitary, ovulation

Menstrual cycle

The average menstrual cycle usually occurs over 28 days, although the normal cycle may range from 22 to 34 days. The cycle is regulated by fluctuating hormone levels that, in turn, are regulated by negative and positive feedback mechanisms. The flow chart represents the menstrual cycle.

Menstrual (preovulatory) phase
The cycle starts with menstruation (cycle day 1), which usually lasts 5 days. As the cycle begins, low estrogen and progesterone levels in the bloodstream stimulate the hypothalamus to secrete gonadotropin-releasing hormone (GnRH). In turn, this substance stimulates the anterior pituitary to secrete follicle-stimulating hormone (FSH) and luteinizing hormone (LH). When the FSH level rises, LH output increases.

Proliferative (follicular) phase and ovulation
The proliferative phase lasts from cycle day 6 to day 14. During this phase, LH and FSH act on the ovarian follicle (mature ovarian cyst containing the ovum), causing estrogen secretion, which in turn stimulates the buildup of the endometrium. Late in the proliferative phase, estrogen levels peak, FSH secretion declines, and LH secretion increases, surging at midcycle (around day 14). Then, estrogen production decreases, the follicle matures, and ovulation occurs. Normally, one follicle matures during the ovulatory process and is released from the ovary during each cycle.

Luteal (secretory) phase
During the luteal phase, which lasts about 14 days, FSH and LH levels drop. Estrogen levels decline initially, then increase along with progesterone levels as the corpus luteum (progesterone-producing yellow structure that develops after the follicle ruptures) begins functioning. During this phase, the endometrium responds to progesterone stimulation by becoming thick and secretory in preparation for implantation of a fertilized ovum.

About 10 to 12 days after ovulation, the corpus luteum begins to diminish as do estrogen and progesterone levels, until the hormone levels are insufficient to sustain the endometrium in a fully developed secretory state. Then the endometrial lining is shed (menses).

Decreasing estrogen and progesterone levels stimulate the hypothalamus to produce GnRH, and the cycle begins again.

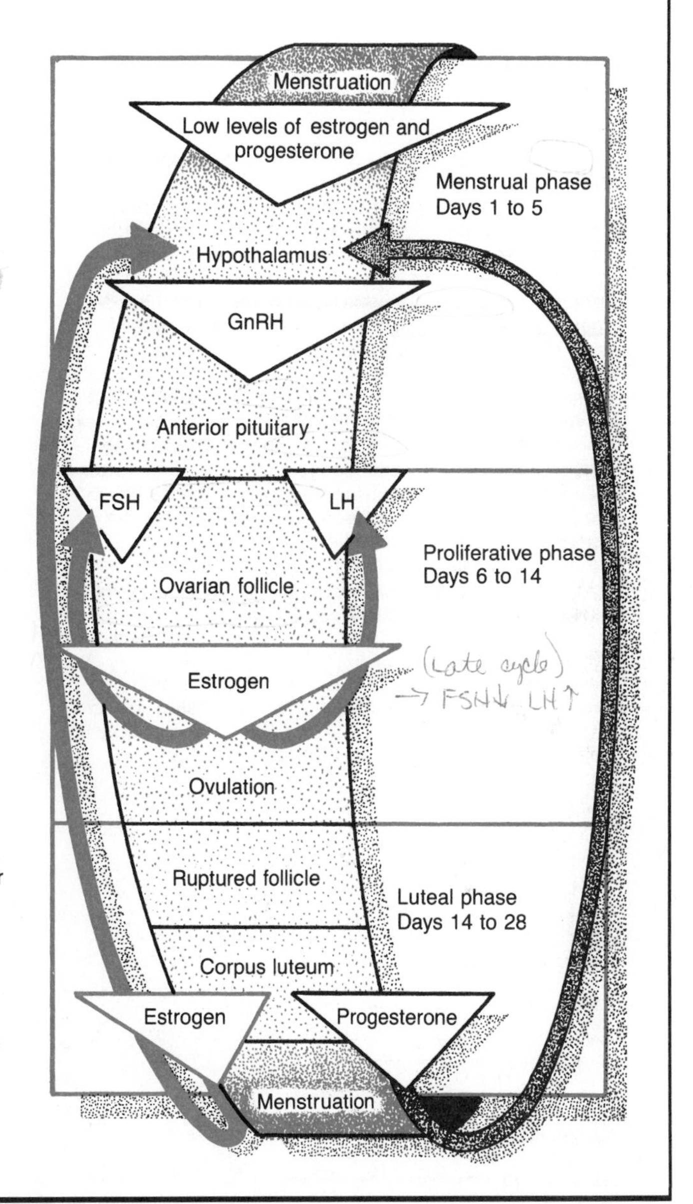

occurs. (For a description of this process, see *Menstrual cycle.*)

Physiology of menopause

Menopause (cessation of menses) varies in onset, usually occurring between age 40 and 55, with the average about age 51. Menstrual periods cease from an exhaustion of ovarian follicles capable of responding to follicle-stimulating hormone (FSH) and luteinizing hormone (LH) released by the pituitary gland. The term *menopause* is used after menses are absent for 1 year. *Climacteric* is a broader word for the transitional years from reproductive fertility to infertility, when several physiologic and psychosocial changes occur, including menopause.

The hormonal changes include decreased estrogen and progesterone levels and increased testosterone secretion. However, the woman is not totally estrogen-deficient because a weaker form of estrogen, estrone, is produced in the peripheral tissues by a weak androgen, androstenedione. Uninhibited by ovarian estrogen and progesterone, the pituitary increases FSH and LH production.

The predominant physiologic and anatomic reproductive system changes that occur from estrogen decline

(Text continues on page 418.)

Female genitalia

External and internal structures comprise the female genitalia.

External genitalia

The vulva contains the external female genitalia that are visible on inspection. The mons pubis is the cushion of adipose and connective tissue covered by skin and coarse, curly hair in a triangular pattern over the symphysis pubis (the joint formed by union of the pubic bones anteriorly). The labia majora border the vulva laterally from the mons pubis to the perineum (muscle, fascia, and ligaments between the anus and vulva). The labia minora, two moist lesser mucosal folds, darker pink to red, lie within and alongside the labia majora.

When the labia are spread, the introitus (vaginal orifice) and the urethral meatus are visible. Less easily visible are the multiple orifices of Skene's glands, mucus-producing glands located on both sides of the urethral opening. Openings of the two mucus-producing Bartholin's glands are located laterally and posteriorly on either side of the inner vaginal orifice. The hymen, a tissue membrane varying in size and thickness, may completely or partially cover the vaginal orifice. A disrupted hymen appears as remnants of uneven mucosal tissue tags, called myrtiform caruncles.

→ disrupted hymen

Internal genitalia

The vagina, a highly elastic muscular tube, is located between the urethra and the rectum. Approximately 6 to 7 cm (2½" to 2¾") long anteriorly and 9 cm (3½") long posteriorly, the vagina lies at a 45-degree angle to the long axis of the body.

The uterus, a small, firm, pear-shaped, muscular organ, rests between the bladder and the rectum and usually lies at almost a 90-degree angle to the vagina. However, other locations may be normal. The mucous membrane lining the uterus is called the endometrium; the muscular layer, the myometrium. In pregnancy, the elastic, upper uterine portion (the fundus) accommodates most of the growing fetus until term. The uterine neck (isthmus) joins the fundus to the cervix, the uterine part extending into the vagina. The fundus and the isthmus make up the corpus, the main uterine body.

Although anteflexed or anteverted above and over the empty bladder in most women, the uterus can be midplane (its long axis parallel to the long axis of the body), retroverted, or retroflexed.

Two fallopian tubes attach to the uterus at the upper angles of the fundus. Usually nonpalpable, these 7- to 14-cm (2¾" to 5½") long, narrow tubes of muscle fibers have fingerlike projections, called fimbriae, on the free ends that partially surround the ovaries. Fertilization of the ovum usually occurs in the outer third of the fallopian tube.

Palpable, oval, almond-shaped organs approximately 3 to 3.5 cm (1¼" to 1½") long, 2 cm (¾") wide, and 1 to 1.5 cm (¼" to ½") thick, the ovaries usually lie near the lateral pelvic walls, a little below the anterosuperior iliac spine.

View of external genitalia in lithotomy position

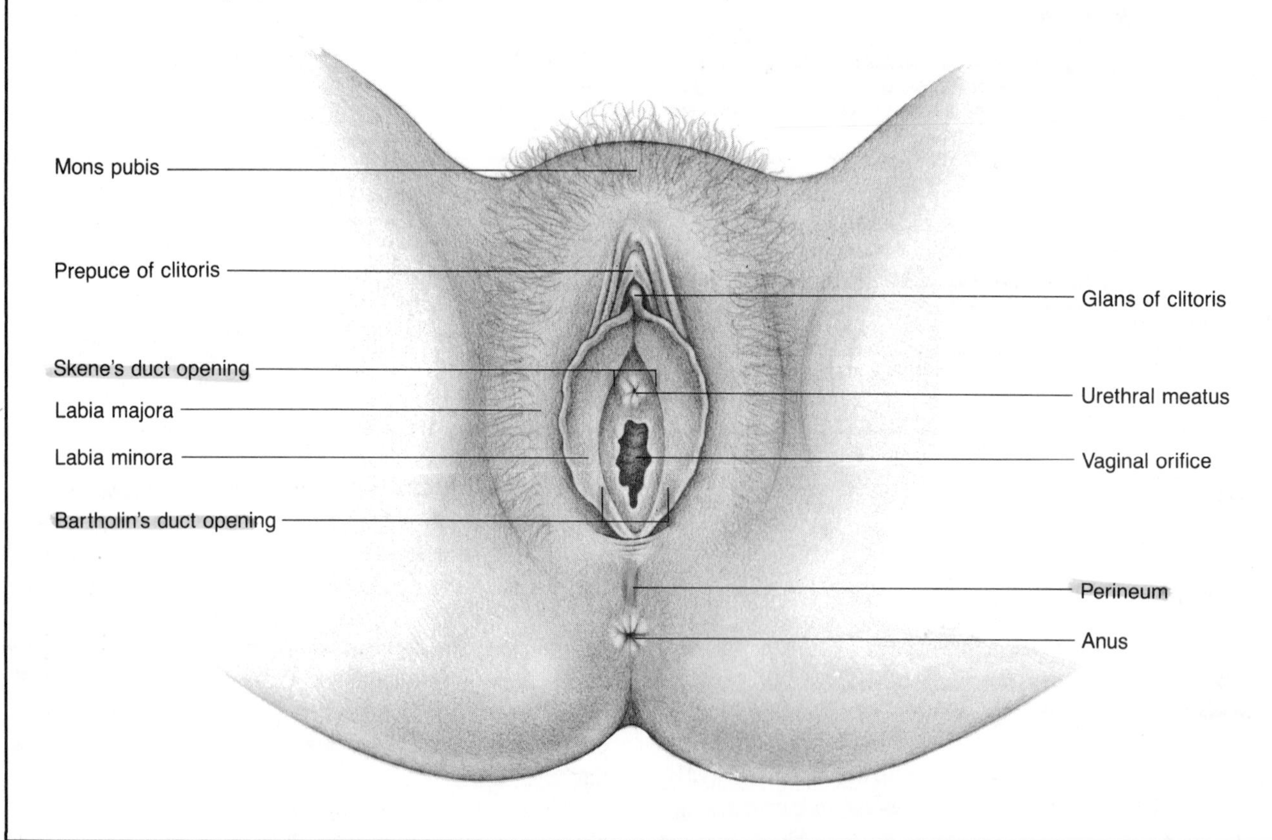

Lateral view of internal genitalia

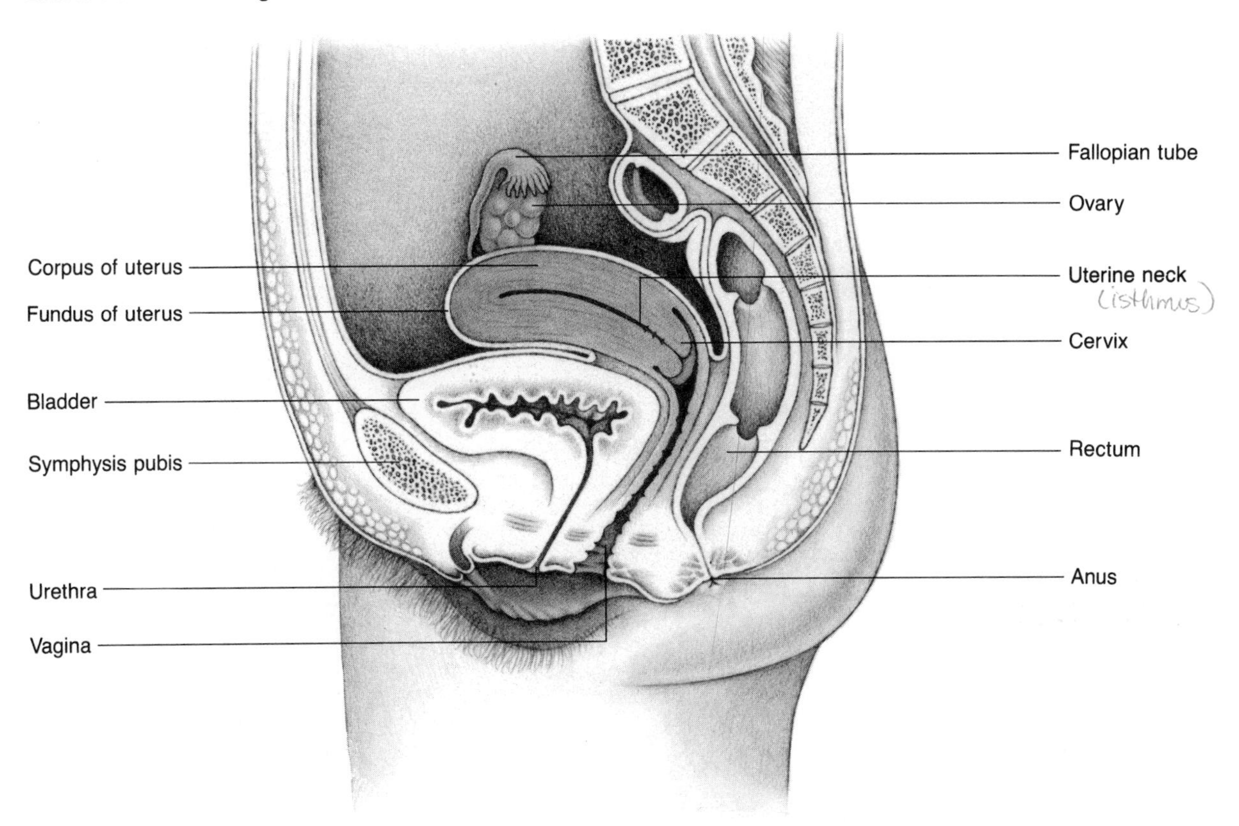

Anterior cross-sectional view of internal genitalia

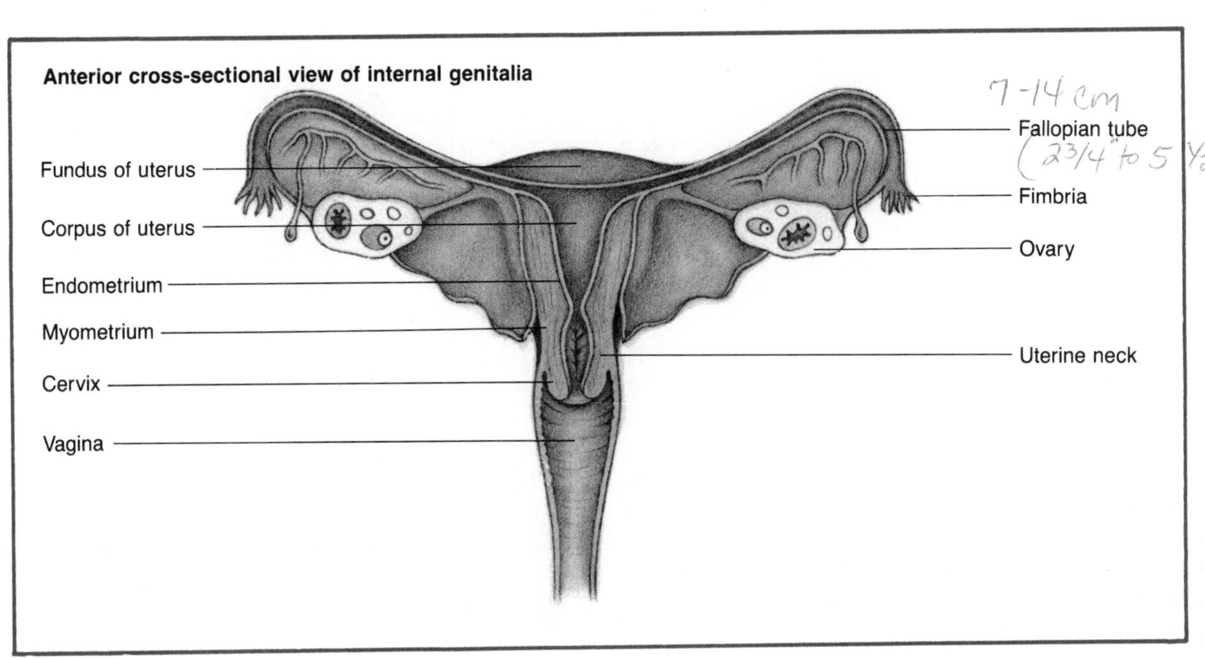

Developmental changes in the uterus and cervix

Over a woman's lifetime, the size of the uterine corpus and cervix changes as does the percentage of space these parts occupy. For example, of the space filled by the whole uterus in a premenarchal female, one third may be uterine corpus, and two thirds may be cervix. In the adult multiparous female, the uterine corpus may occupy two thirds of the space available, whereas the cervix may fill a third. The illustrations below show the changes for a premenarchal, adult nulliparous, and adult multiparous woman.

The central opening of the cervix (the external os), visible by speculum, is round and closed in a nulliparous woman. In a parous women, the opening is an irregularly shaped slit.

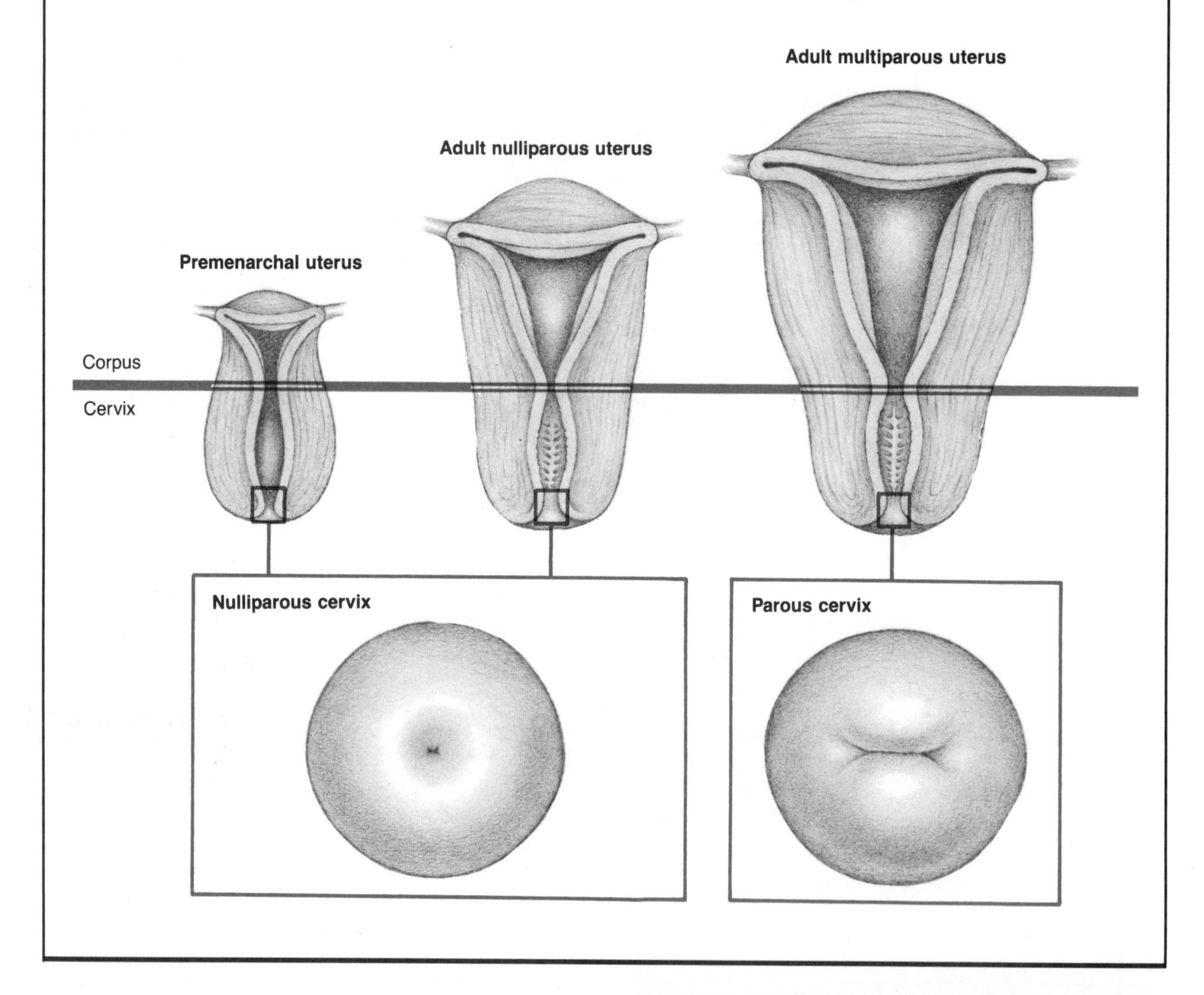

include vasomotor symptoms, such as hot flushes or flashes, and urogenital tissue atrophy, causing decreased elasticity and thinning of the vaginal walls and urinary frequency. Other systems affected by estrogen loss include the integumentary system, as evidenced by sparse, gray pubic hair; the cardiovascular system, as evidenced by an increased risk of heart disease; and the musculoskeletal system, as evidenced by osteoporosis.

Health history

Adequate and accurate data are the keys to a successful health history interview. In some cultures, discussing female physiologic function or problems is taboo. For example, some cultures do not permit women to be examined by a man or discuss sexual topics. Often sheltered, these women sometimes do not understand their bodies. Recognizing cultural taboos helps the nurse anticipate client responses and behavior. The nurse faced with obtaining an accurate health history from such a client learns to ease difficult interview situations by providing the client with detailed information and explanations. Sometimes a phrase like "I realize how uncomfortable this is for you, but to help you, I need to know . . . " encourages the client's candor and assures her that such confidential information is essential.

Terminology and language pose further barriers to obtaining accurate data. The nurse must be certain of what a client's statements mean. An easy way to avoid erroneous conclusions while clarifying information is to interpret and repeat the client's statements for verification. The client can then correct any misunderstandings. For example, a client may complain of itching "down there." The nurse can determine what "down there" means by saying to the client, "Down there in your private parts?" or by using pictures or by asking the client to point to the area.

If language presents a barrier, attempt to find an objective interpreter. Because health history data is confidential, using a family member or friend as an interpreter may be undesirable. Translations should not be condensed by the interpreter, because valuable information may be lost.

During the reproductive health history interview, follow these guidelines:

- Obtain health history data in a comfortable environment that protects the client's privacy. Conduct the interview at an unhurried pace; otherwise the client may overlook important details. Ideally, the client should remain seated and dressed until the physical assessment. This ensures client comfort and confidence.
- Use terms that the client understands. Explain technical language.
- Focus questions on the reproductive system, but maintain a holistic approach by inquiring about the status of other body systems and psychosocial concerns. Reproductive system problems may cause the client other problems, such as self-image, sexual functioning, and overall wellness. When choosing health history questions, consider their relevance and practicality for the client. For example, asking an 80-year-old woman the date of her first menstrual period is pointless. Conversely, asking her about menopause, irregular bleeding, and estrogen replacement therapy would be appropriate.
- Always ask the health history questions before the client is in the lithotomy position. In many busy medical practices or health clinics, the client is asked to undress, get on the examination table, and wait for the physician to come in and begin the examination and interview. Some women find this practice demeaning as well as anxiety-producing.

The following questions are designed to help the nurse assess the female client's reproductive system. They include rationales describing the significance of the answers and, where appropriate, nursing interventions to incorporate into the client's care plan.

Health and illness patterns

To assess health and illness patterns, the nurse should ask about the client's current, past, and family health status as well as developmental considerations.

Current health status

Because current health status is foremost in the client's mind, begin the interview by exploring this topic. Then, carefully document the client's own words, using the *PQRST* method to help the client completely describe the main complaint and any others. (For a detailed explanation of this method, see *Symptom analysis* in Chapter 3.) The following questions about reproductive function cover the menstrual, procreative, and contraceptive history.

When was the first day of your last menstrual period (LMP)?
(RATIONALE: Knowing when the last true menses occurred is necessary to evaluate such conditions as pregnancy or abnormal bleeding episodes.)

Was that period normal compared with your previous periods?
(RATIONALE: Determine what is usual for the client and how the menstrual period has changed. Some pregnant women continue to have what appear to be menses, but with different characteristics. The client could interpret a change, such as spotting [small amounts of bloody discharge from the vagina], as a period; spotting could indicate an ectopic pregnancy, a cervical infection, or a problem with hormonal support of the endometrium.)

When was the first day of your previous menstrual period (PMP)?
(RATIONALE: The answer to this question may reveal a pattern of irregularity. A change in menstrual flow from PMP to LMP may signal pregnancy or another condition, such as anovulation.)

How often do your periods occur?
(RATIONALE: The cycle length, from day 1 of one menses to day 1 of the next, should be more than 21 and fewer than 35 days. Deviations could indicate ovulatory problems, fibroid tumors, or a malignant process.)

How long do your periods normally last?
(RATIONALE: The usual flow duration is 3 to 7 days, varying for each woman from cycle to cycle. Extremely long or short periods may signal an abnormality, such as anovulation or anorexia nervosa.)

How would you describe your menstrual flow? How many pads or tampons do you use on each day of your period?
(RATIONALE: How many heavy flow days, the heaviest flow day, and whether blood clots are expelled are important factors that help supply an idea of the client's normal pattern. Heavy flow and clots that constitute a new pattern could indicate uterine fibroids. Women who use oral contraceptives or an intrauterine device [IUD] report wide variations in the menstrual flow. [The usual flow is between 30 and 80 ml per cycle.])

Are you currently using an oral contraceptive? If so, what do you use? How long have you used it?
(RATIONALE: Many oral contraceptives can cause adverse reactions, such as headaches, chest pain, or breast tenderness. An elderly client need not be questioned about current contraceptive use. However, a climacteric client may be questioned because conception is possible until the client completes menopause.)

If you do not use oral contraceptives, what method of contraception do you use? How long have you used it? If it is a device, is it in good condition?
(RATIONALE: Discussion of contraceptive methods and proper usage could reveal a knowledge deficit. Troublesome adverse reactions to any method should be queried. For example, a diaphragm may cause urinary discomfort, spermicides may cause vaginal irritation, and an IUD may increase the risk of pelvic inflammatory disease [PID]. Besides, various anatomic changes, wear, and improper care may cause a diaphragm to fit improperly, compromising its effectiveness. Instruct the client that annual checks for fit and periodic checks for deterioration of the diaphragm are needed.)

Do you currently take any prescription or over-the-counter medications? If so, what are they? How often do you take them?
(RATIONALE: Some medications interfere with oral contraceptive action. For example, barbiturates may reduce oral contraceptive effectiveness. Other medications, such as phenothiazines, for example, can cause a false-positive result on a urine pregnancy test. For additional information, see *Adverse drug reactions.*)

Are you using any recreational drugs or alcohol? If so, what do you use? How much do you use? How long have you used it?
(RATIONALE: Illicit drug or alcohol use can be hazardous. For example, acquired immunodeficiency syndrome can be passed by shared, contaminated needles. Marijuana use can produce a false-positive result on a urine pregnancy test. Taken during pregnancy, such drugs as cocaine can cause severe drug withdrawal symptoms, as well as possible long-term adverse neurologic effects in newborns. Alcohol abuse can cause fetal alcohol syndrome, a condition in which the infant has low birth weight and possible congenital anomalies).

Do you smoke? If so, how much do you smoke? How long have you smoked?
(RATIONALE: Smoking is a health hazard for pregnant and nonpregnant women. Smoking increases the risk of cardiovascular disease and thrombi [blood clots] in women using oral contraceptives. Smoking during pregnancy is associated with fetal growth retardation and fetal and infant morbidity and mortality.)

Do you have any unusual signs or symptoms of infection, such as discharge, itching, painful intercourse, sores or lesions, fever, chills, or swelling?
(RATIONALE: Such signs and symptoms could result from a sexually transmitted disease [STD], candidiasis (*Monilia* infection), vaginitis, or toxic shock syndrome. Commonly, women try to treat infections themselves by douching, frequently washing away the "evidence" of the infectious organism. Urge a client seeking a reproductive system health assessment not to douche or use creams or jellies for at least 72 hours before the assessment. Douching, unless medically indicated, is not recommended as a routine activity because it may wash away normal vaginal flora, upsetting the pH balance and predisposing the client to infection. Remember especially to tell this to an elderly client, who may douche regularly because she was told when young that it was the proper way to keep clean and to prevent infection.)

Does your sexual partner have any signs or symptoms of infection, such as genital sores or penile discharge?
(RATIONALE: Such symptoms may result from STD. If the client's sexual partner has infection symptoms and is untreated, instruct the client to insist her partner undergo diagnostic testing [to prevent spreading STD].)

Adverse drug reactions

When obtaining a health history to assess a female client's reproductive system, the nurse must ask about current drug use. Many drugs can affect the menstrual cycle or sexual desire. For example, certain antipsychotics can cause menstrual irregularities; many antihypertensives can decrease the libido. The commonly used drugs listed below may produce adverse reactions in the female reproductive system and in other body systems as well.

DRUG CLASS	DRUG	POSSIBLE ADVERSE REACTIONS
Androgens	danazol	Vaginitis with itching, dryness, burning, or bleeding; amenorrhea
	fluoxymesterone, methyltestosterone, testosterone	Amenorrhea and other menstrual irregularities; virilization, including clitoral enlargement
Antidepressants	amitriptyline hydrochloride, desipramine hydrochloride, doxepin hydrochloride, imipramine hydrochloride, nortriptyline hydrochloride, trazodone hydrochloride, trimipramine maleate	Changed libido, menstrual irregularity
Antihypertensives	clonidine hydrochloride, reserpine	Decreased libido
	methyldopa	Decreased libido, amenorrhea
Antipsychotics	chlorpromazine hydrochloride, perphenazine, prochlorperazine, promazine hydrochloride, thioridazine hydrochloride, trifluoperazine hydrochloride, haloperidol	Inhibition of ovulation (chlorpromazine only), menstrual irregularities, amenorrhea, changed libido, false-positive result on pregnancy test
Beta-blockers	atenolol, labetalol hydrochloride, nadolol, propranolol hydrochloride, metoprolol	Decreased libido
Cardiac glycosides	digoxin, digitoxin	Changes in cellular layer of vaginal walls in postmenopausal women
Cytotoxics	busulfan	Amenorrhea with menopausal symptoms in premenopausal women, ovarian suppression, ovarian fibrosis and atrophy
	chlorambucil	Amenorrhea
	cyclophosphamide	Gonadal suppression (possibly irreversible), amenorrhea, ovarian fibrosis
	methotrexate	Menstrual dysfunction, infertility
	tamoxifen	Vaginal discharge or bleeding, menstrual irregularities, pruritus vulvae (intense itching of the female external genitalia)
	thiotepa	Amenorrhea
Estrogens	chlorotrianisene; conjugated estrogens, esterified estrogens, estradiol, estrone, ethinyl estradiol	Altered menstrual flow, dysmenorrhea, amenorrhea, cervical erosion or abnormal secretions, enlargement of uterine fibromas, vaginal candidiasis
	dienestrol	Vaginal discharge, uterine bleeding with excessive use

continued

Adverse drug reactions continued

DRUG CLASS	DRUG	POSSIBLE ADVERSE REACTIONS
	diethylstilbestrol	Breakthrough bleeding, altered menstrual flow, dysmenorrhea, amenorrhea, cervical erosion, altered cervical secretions, enlargement of uterine fibromas, vaginal candidiasis, change in libido, increased risk of vaginal cancer in female offspring
Thyroid hormones	levothyroxine sodium, thyroid USP, thyrotropin, and others	Menstrual irregularities with excessive doses
Progestins	hydroxyprogesterone caproate, medroxyprogesterone acetate, norethindrone, norethindrone acetate, norgestrel, progesterone	Breakthrough bleeding, dysmenorrhea, amenorrhea, cervical erosion and abnormal secretions
Steroids	dexamethasone, hydrocortisone, prednisone	Amenorrhea and menstrual irregularities
Miscellaneous	lithium carbonate, L-tryptophan	Decreased libido
	spironolactone	Menstrual irregularities, amenorrhea, postmenopausal bleeding

Are you sexually active? If so, when was the last time you had intercourse?
(RATIONALE: Answers to these questions help assess some reproductive system disorders, such as infections, and provide clues for the physical assessment as well. Knowing that a client has never had intercourse is important because the examiner then should be prepared to begin the physical assessment with a small speculum.)

Are you satisfied with communication between you and your partner about your sexual needs? Are your needs for affection and intimacy being met?
(RATIONALE: If the client shows dissatisfaction with her sexuality or sexual relations, some simple self-help educational materials, such as a book, may be helpful. If the client wants help with problems related to sexual dysfunction, refer her to a specialist.)

Past health status

To collect data about the client's past health history, ask the following questions related to the female reproductive system:

Do you ever bleed between periods? If so, how much and for how long?
(RATIONALE: Bleeding between menstrual periods can indicate problems, such as hormonal imbalance or cancer.)

Do you ever have vaginal bleeding after intercourse?
(RATIONALE: Postcoital bleeding can indicate a vaginal infection with *Trichomonas* or other organism.)

Have you had any uncomfortable signs and symptoms before or during your periods?
(RATIONALE: Uncomfortable signs and symptoms before the period, such as irritability, headache, abdominal bloating, breast tenderness, and constipation, can indicate PMS. Dysmenorrhea [discomfort or pain during menstruation] is common for some women. A change in pattern may be significant. For example, a woman with minimal menstrual discomfort who develops dysmenorrhea could have also developed uterine fibroids. For severe problems, suggest that the client keep a menstrual-cycle calendar so that she can identify her signs and symptoms as they appear during the menstrual cycle. This provides a sense of control, which may help the client feel better. Other help includes instruction about stress-reducing techniques and avoidance of salty foods, chocolate, and caffeine.)

Has anyone ever told you that something is wrong with your womb or other female organs?
(RATIONALE: The answer to this question provides information about previous problems as well as the client's readiness or reluctance to discuss them.)

Have you ever had a sexually transmitted disease (STD) or other genital or reproductive system infection?

(RATIONALE: Repetitive infections may indicate several problems. For example, a woman who continues to have candidal infections may have diabetes mellitus. Constant STD reinfections may mean an untreated partner or multiple partners. PID from such organisms as *Chlamydia trachomatis* and *Neisseria gonorrhoeae* can cause sterility.)

Have you had surgery for a reproductive system problem?
(RATIONALE: Tubal ligation, dilatation and curettage, and hysterectomy are common gynecologic surgical procedures.)

Have you ever been pregnant?
(RATIONALE: Specific data about the prenatal, labor, delivery, and postpartum periods; complications; neonatal weight; outcome; problems; treatments; and sequelae, if any, are important particularly in women in the childbearing years.)

Have you ever had problems conceiving?
(RATIONALE: Lack of pregnancy after more than 1 year of regular coitus without contraception may indicate a fertility problem and the need for referral to a gynecologist or a fertility specialist if the couple desires. The couple trying unsuccessfully to conceive may be experiencing stress and anxiety and may welcome a counseling referral.)

Family health status

The nurse asks about family reproductive history because several reproductive problems tend to appear from generation to generation. The following questions relate to family health status of the reproductive system:

Has anyone in your family ever had any reproductive problems?
(RATIONALE: Spontaneous abortion, menstrual difficulties, multiple births, congenital anomalies, or difficult pregnancies can have a familial tendency.)

Has anyone in the family had hypertension, diabetes mellitus, gestational diabetes (diabetes occurring only during pregnancy), obesity, or heart disease?
(RATIONALE: Such conditions tend to be familial and could affect the health of the pregnant client and her fetus. For example, eclampsia or diabetes may develop during the pregnancy.)

Has any immediate member of your family had gynecologic surgery?
(RATIONALE: The client's answer could indicate a familial history of endometriosis, fibroid tumors, or ovarian or cervical cancer.)

Developmental considerations

Young or elderly clients require special assessment of the reproductive system, using the following questions. (For pregnant clients, see Chapter 22, Perinatal and Neonatal Assessment.)

Pediatric client. Although the nurse may obtain reproductive history data from a parent or guardian, the child can best describe her own perceptions. Usually a parent or guardian accompanies the child seeking reproductive system health care, perhaps for a vaginal discharge or related problem. Attempt to interview the parent alone and then the child alone, especially if sexual abuse is suspected. Besides establishing a basis for trust, singular interviews permit the child freedom to express concerns. The following questions are addressed specifically to a child:

What name would you like me to call you?
(RATIONALE: If the client appears upset and fearful, help her feel safe and less apprehensive by using a nickname.)

What problem brings you here? How can I help you?
(RATIONALE: The premenarchal girl, age 7 or older, can express her understanding of situations and her feelings and ideas about specific problems.)

Adolescent client. Bodily changes occurring as sexual maturity approaches may precipitate fears and questions in the adolescent girl, who may be reluctant to express them. Anticipating these concerns, offer opportunities for questions and explanations to help the girl understand her body and its functions.

Adolescents need simple explanations. Open-ended questions with prefaces, such as "A lot of girls have questions about their bodies and their development. Maybe you have similar questions about . . . (your periods, birth control, and so forth)" are ways to introduce a topic and provide concise explanations.

At what age did you first notice hair on your pubic area? When did you first notice your breasts growing?
(RATIONALE: In females, the appearance of secondary sex characteristics is the most accurate physical maturity indicator. Pubic hair growth usually begins between ages 8 and 14. For information about breast development, see Chapter 12, Female and Male Breasts.)

How do you feel you are developing compared with your friends?
(RATIONALE: Adolescent girls need assurance that they are normal when their development seems to lag behind

that of their peers. Unless no maturational changes occur by age 14, most girls can be reassured that they will menstruate normally when their bodies are ready.)

Have you noticed any moistness on your underpants?
(RATIONALE: Infection as well as increasing estrogen and androgen production from the ovaries result in increased vaginal secretions. To deal with body changes, the adolescent client must understand them. Any signs of infection should be evaluated and frank, open explanations provided. Sometimes, clear visual aids further teaching and data collection.)

Have you experienced any new feelings or emotions? If so, would you like to talk about them?
(RATIONALE: During this time of rapid change in the body and the emotions, confusion and misinformation proliferate. Routine physical assessments for school or camp, during which evolving sexual changes can be evaluated, present ideal opportunities for the client to ask questions and for you to provide supportive information. Sexuality knowledge and understanding should be assessed and anticipatory preventive health information provided. If the client expresses negative or unhealthy feelings, offer appropriate assessment and counseling referrals.)

Have you noticed any blood on your underpants?
(RATIONALE: Although ovarian estrogen production may be potent enough to trigger the first menstrual flow, ovulation may not occur for some time. Adolescent girls commonly complain of irregular menses, which are caused by anovulation. Usually, no medical therapy is indicated unless heavy bleeding, which may cause anemia, occurs. The hypothalamic-pituitary-ovarian axis takes time to begin the coordinated functioning that stimulates ovulation. The young adolescent needs reassurance that these changes are normal.)

When did you begin having menstrual periods?
(RATIONALE: The mean onset of menarche is age 12.8; the normal age range, 9.1 to 17.7. By age 14, if no menses occur and no secondary sex characteristics appear, the adolescent should be evaluated medically; no menses occurring by age 16, regardless of secondary sex characteristics, also warrants medical evaluation.)

How old were you when you first had sex? Do you ever have pain with sex?
(RATIONALE: Many adolescents are sexually active. Asking the questions in this manner assumes sexual activity and is nonthreatening.)

Climacteric client. During the climacteric, some women have various discomforting signs and symptoms. (The most common symptom is hot flashes.) Lasting as long as 10 years, the climacteric, a period of hormonal changes resulting in the end of reproductive capability, includes menopause. In some women, the hormonal and physical changes relate to changes in self-concept. Explain to a climacteric client that while her body is changing, until menopause occurs she should continue previous contraceptive and reproductive health practices. During the reproductive history interview, the following questions are appropriate for a climacteric client:

Do you experience hot flushes or flashes? If so, how bothersome are they?
(RATIONALE: Menopausal experiences are subjective. Hot flashes or flushes may bother one woman and not another.)

Do you experience vaginal dryness, pain, or itching during sexual intercourse?
(RATIONALE: Such symptoms are caused by decreased estrogen levels that lead to decreased vaginal secretions. When teaching the client, you may wish to include information on appropriate lubricants.)

Are you experiencing menstrual irregularities?
(RATIONALE: Reassure the client that climacteric menstrual irregularities are common, but refer a client with excessive or frequent bleeding to a physician.)

Do you practice contraception?
(RATIONALE: The woman may become pregnant during the climacteric if she does not practice contraception because she thinks that she can no longer conceive.)

Are you having any problems or changes you attribute to menopause? What are they? Could anything else be causing these problems or changes?
(RATIONALE: Help the client differentiate between the signs and symptoms related to menopause and those related to stress caused by other life changes.)

How do you feel about approaching menopause (or menopause if it has occurred)?
(RATIONALE: This question allows the client to vent feelings about menopause and life changes occurring during that time. Listen actively.)

Are you receiving hormone therapy for menopause?
(RATIONALE: Some women need medical assistance during menopause—for example, estrogen replacement therapy, which can decrease symptoms but increases the

risk of uterine cancer. Studies indicate that even a woman without bothersome symptoms may need hormone replacement therapy to prevent osteoporosis. Smoking, a slight frame, low weight, and a maternal family history of osteoporosis are factors increasing osteoporosis risk.)

If you have completed menopause, have you had any bleeding?
(RATIONALE: Any bleeding in a postmenopausal woman, except that associated with estrogen-progesterone replacement therapy, is abnormal and a possible sign of endometrial carcinoma.)

Health promotion and protection patterns

The health history continues with assessment of the client's nutrition, sleep and wake patterns, and health behaviors. The following questions help obtain this information:

Do you eat a well-balanced diet?
(RATIONALE: Eating patterns can affect the reproductive system at any age. For example, anorexia nervosa can cause menstrual irregularities.)

Do you have urinary problems that interfere with your sleep?
(RATIONALE: Voiding-pattern changes caused by infections and reproductive structure changes, such as cystocele [herniation of the urinary bladder into the vaginal wall] can interfere with the client's sleep.)

Do you have regular health checkups, including gynecologic examinations?
(RATIONALE: A client's health practices can indicate how active she is in her own health care.)

When was your last Pap test?
(RATIONALE: A Pap test can detect precancerous and cancerous cell changes in the cervix. It may also detect human papillomavirus [which causes venereal warts], *Chlamydia trachomatis,* and herpes simplex, which may not produce symptoms but may cause abnormal cellular changes. Regular Pap tests help detect such problems. Remind the client that she needs a Pap test even if the uterus has been removed surgically.)

Have you any questions about your reproductive organs or sexual activity?
(RATIONALE: The client's questions may be significant to her health. The elderly client, for example, may want to discuss her sexual activity. The adolescent client may have questions that she is reluctant to ask.)

Are you currently having any problems that you feel are related to your reproductive system or any other problems that we have not talked about?
(RATIONALE: These questions offer the client a chance to air any concerns. For instance, pelvic pain, one of the most common complaints in women, could be discussed, if relevant and unaddressed previously.)

Role and relationship patterns

Reproductive system disorders can affect many role and relationship patterns. Ask the following questions to assess the extent of this effect:

Have you noticed any changes in your sexual interest, frequency of intercourse, or sexual functioning?
(RATIONALE: Changes in libido [psychic energy or instinctual drive associated with sexual desire or pleasure] or sexual function could indicate pain, infection, hormonal changes, disease [for example, diabetes mellitus], changes in mental status [for example, depression], or altered role and relationship patterns.)

Are you experiencing any sexual problems?
(RATIONALE: Physical problems in the reproductive system can alter sexual relationships. The client's answer may lead not only to exploring possible changes in client sexual relations, but also to assessing whether a physical problem is contributing to the changes.)

Physical assessment

In most health care facilities, a nurse assists a physician or nurse practitioner with a gynecologic assessment. In some health care facilities, the nurse performs the assessment. The first part of this section describes how to prepare for a female reproductive system assessment and how to inspect the external genitalia. The second portion explains how to perform a complete gynecologic assessment—an advanced assessment skill.

Preparing for the assessment

Before beginning the assessment, gather the necessary equipment and supplies. (For detailed information, see *Gynecologic assessment equipment*, page 426.)

Gynecologic assessment equipment

When assisting with a gynecologic assessment, the nurse assembles the equipment needed before helping the client into position and draping her. Below is a description of necessary equipment and guidelines for use.

Gloves
Proper-fitting and medically clean examination gloves protect the examiner and the client from infection. If the examiner works alone, one hand must be reserved for handling specimen containers, slides, and equipment.

Specula
Several sizes and types of sterilized specula should be available. The two most commonly used vaginal specula are the Graves and the Pederson. The Graves speculum is available in 3½" to 5½" lengths by ¾" to 1½" widths. It has a spoon-shaped flare at the distal blade ends, which helps in visualizing the cervix and in examining multiparous clients. The Pederson speculum is narrow, flat, and appropriate for children, females who have not been sexually active, as well as nulliparous and some postmenopausal women.

Plastic specula are available in several sizes. Some make loud clicking noises when the blades are opened. Warn the client about this before the assessment begins. Because of surface tension factors and possible rough edges found on some low-cost brands, plastic specula can be difficult to introduce into the vagina. Furthermore, forcing such a speculum can tear the mucous membrane lining.

Lubricant
The examiner applies a water-soluble lubricant to the fingers for the bimanual assessment. Because the lubricant is bacteriostatic, it may change the cells obtained for the Papancolaou (Pap) test, making accurate cell analysis difficult. It should not be used during the speculum assessment. The lubricant is available in tubes or individual packets.

Spatula, swabs, and endocervical brush
A spatula is used to obtain cells from the endocervix (internal cervix) and ectocervix (external cervix) for the Pap test. A cotton-tipped swab may be used to obtain specimens from the cervical os and the vaginal pool. The examiner also can use an endocervical brush. Controversy exists over which is the better implement. Each health care facility may prefer using a different technique.

Large and small swabs are used to clean the cervix or vaginal wall before certain procedures, to apply medication, or to obtain specimens for culture.

Glass slides and cover slides
Glass slides are used for wet mounts to diagnose several vaginal infections, such as *Trichomonas vaginalis* or *Candida albicans.* Normal saline solution or potassium hydroxide may be added to the specimen on the slide to create a wet mount. Both solutions are available in dropper bottles. The cover slide is placed on top of the specimen to protect it.

For Pap tests, use glass slides. Note the client's name, date, and origin of smear sample on the frosted portion of the glass before the assessment begins. Usually one slide is used for the endocervical specimen, one for the ectocervical specimen, and, occasionally, one for the vaginal wall. Some health care facilities place endocervical and ectocervical smears on the same slide.

Cytologic fixative
Have a spray can or bottle of cytologic fixative available for immediate fixation of the Pap smear samples. The fixative preserves the tissue cells to allow for accurate interpretation.

Culture bottles or plates
Many examiners routinely use bottles or plates to test culture for *Neisseria gonorrhoeae*, the microorganism causing gonorrhea. If bottles of culture medium are used, keep them upright to hold the carbon dioxide (CO_2) in the bottle. The medium is a modified Thayer-Martin (MTM) combination of hemoglobin, gonococcal growth-enhancing chemicals, and antimicrobial agents. The CO_2 is heavier than air, so the lid of the MTM container may be removed with the container bottle upright to apply the specimen to the medium. If a round culture plate is used, add a CO_2 tablet after the specimen is applied and keep the plate warm to allow incubation.

Sponge forceps
Sponge forceps are used for such procedures as applying pressure or medication with a gauze sponge or for cleansing. Keep at least one pair in a sterilizing solution.

Mirror
A hand mirror is useful for clients who want to watch the assessment. Because this provides an opportunity to teach the client about her body, offer her the mirror.

Light source
Good lighting is essential. If a goose-necked lamp is used, the examiner must remember not to touch the lamp with the contaminated gloved hand.

Keep in mind that many women feel significant anxiety when undergoing a gynecologic assessment. Some are modest and uncomfortable exposing their genitalia. Others are fearful because of lack of knowledge, past painful examinations, or accounts of painful experiences. Some women express reluctance to have a gynecolgic assessment because of negative feelings about their own sexuality or fear of what may be found.

Thoroughly and accurately assessing an extremely tense woman is almost impossible. The assessment takes longer and is more uncomfortable for the tense client than for the relaxed one. Merely telling the client to relax is ineffective. The guidelines that follow will help you (whether assisting or performing the assessment) relieve the client's anxiety and help her to relax.

Ask if this is the client's first gynecologic assessment. If it is, explain the procedure so that the client knows what to expect. If it is not, ask the client about previous assessment experiences, which may help her express feelings. Stand beside the examination table, hold the client's hand, talk to her during the assessment, explain what is occurring and what will occur next, and avoid using such words as hurt or pain. Every client needs supportive assurances.

Using pictures and the equipment, explain the assessment procedure, even if the client has had gynecologic assessments. Showing how the speculum works and advising that although the instrument may look menacing, it should not cause undue discomfort can reduce the client's apprehension.

Because a full bladder produces discomfort and interferes with accurate palpation, tell the client to empty her bladder before the assessment begins.

No one other than the assessment participants should be in the room during the assessment. The room should be environmentally comfortable; a cold room increases tension and discomfort.

In most instances, the client should be in the lithotomy position for the assessment. (For a review, see *Client positioning and draping guidelines*, Chapter 4.) The client's heels should be secure in the stirrups or the knees comfortably placed in the knee supports if they are used. Adjust the foot or knee supports so that the legs are equally and comfortably separated and symmetrically balanced. With unpadded stirrups, the client's shoes or socks remain on. If the client chooses to be barefoot, use paper towels as padding.

The buttocks must extend about ½" over the table end. Because the position is precarious, the client may need help, direction, and ample time to assume it. The hips and knees will be flexed and thighs abducted. The client places her feet (or knees) in the stirrups and "inches" down to the proper position. A pillow placed beneath her head may help her to relax the abdominal muscles. Her arms should be at her side or over her chest. This also reduces abdominal muscle tension. The examiner sits on a movable swivel stool an arm's length away from and between the client's abducted legs. In this way, equipment can be reached readily and the genitalia can be seen and palpated easily.

An alternative position for the client who cannot assume the lithotomy position because of age, arthritis, back pain, or other reasons is Sims' (left lateral) position. To assume this position, the client lies on her left side almost prone with her buttocks close to the edge of the table, her left leg straight, and her right leg slightly bent in front of her left leg.

Privacy and adequate draping give the client a sense of security. If the client prefers no draping, that is her prerogative. If she wishes to watch the assessment, supply a hand mirror for her to hold.

To help the client relax as the assessment begins (or immediately before), describe what she will feel. For example, she will feel her inner thigh being touched, then her labia, then a finger slightly in the vaginal opening pressing on the muscle (the bulbocavernous muscle) in the lower vaginal wall. Explain that tightening this muscle when tense is normal and show the client how to relax by inhaling slowly and deeply through the nose, exhaling through the mouth, and concentrating on breathing regularly to relax the muscle. If the client begins to tense up and hold her breath, remind her to breathe and relax. A ceiling poster or mobile may help distract her.

Assure the client that the assessment will take little time and that before each new step, she will be told what to expect. Positioning the drape low on the client's abdomen allows her to see the examiner. The examiner and client must be able to give and take visual cues. Remember, gentle words and actions soothe; jerky movements alarm. Also, idle conversation may make the client more tense.

If the client has never had intercourse or is extremely nervous, more than one appointment may be necessary to complete the assessment. The examiner decides, based on the urgency of the chief complaint and the client's anxiety, whether to perform the assessment over two or three visits. Coaching a nervous client in how to relax may help in a difficult assessment; however, if relaxation fails, administering a tranquilizer or even general anesthesia may be necessary. The latter is especially true with young children.

Male examiners should be attended by a female assistant for the client's emotional comfort and the examiner's legal protection.

Inspection

In many cases, a complete gynecologic assessment is not required but inspection of the client's external genitalia is, especially if the client complains of sores or itching. Routine bathing is an excellent time to inspect the client's external genitalia. Wash your hands, then take the following steps during the inspection.

Position the client supine with the pubic area uncovered, and begin the assessment by determining sexual maturity. Inspect pubic hair for amount and pattern. Normally, pubic hair is thick and appears on the mons pubis as well as the inner aspects of the upper thighs. Then, using a gloved index finger and thumb, gently spread the labia majora and look for the following: labia majora and labia minora, which should be pink and moist with no lesions, and normal cervical discharge, which varies in color and consistency, being clear and stretchy before ovulation, white and opaque after ovulation, and usually odorless and nonirritating to the mucosa. No other discharge should be present.

Abnormal findings

If a male pubic hair distribution pattern exists, note clitoral size as well as any other masculinization signs, such as a deepened voice. The client may need referral to an endocrinologist. Other readily apparent abnormalities include varicosities (distended superficial vessels on the labia), which can indicate increased pressure in the pelvic region seen in pregnancy and uterine tumor; lesions, such as an ulceration or a wartlike growth (condyloma acuminatum); organisms, such as *Pediculus pubis* (lice) or nits (minute white louse eggs attached to the pubic hair shaft); and edema of the mons pubis, labia majora, labia minora, urethral orifice, vaginal introitus, or the surrounding skin.

Frothy, malodorous, green or gray watery discharge may indicate infection with *Trichomonas* or *Hemophilus* organisms. Purulent, green-yellow urethral or vaginal discharge may indicate gonorrhea; a heavy gray-white discharge, *Chlamydia trachomatis;* and an inflamed vulva with a cheeselike discharge, candidiasis (a yeastlike infection). Specimens of all discharges should be cultured and examined microscopically in the laboratory. (For a description of some common abnormal assessment findings, see *Integrating assessment findings.)*

Developmental considerations

The labia majora on an infant or young child are soft and somewhat resilient compared with the firmer labia of a mature woman. Labial agglutination (adhesion of the labia minora) may be seen in some infants or toddlers. Extensive adhesion makes voiding difficult. The consequent urinary retention may invite urinary tract infections.

In a child of any age, an inflamed vulva with open irritated areas could indicate sexual abuse. If sexual abuse is suspected, follow the health care facility protocol for reporting such cases.

Pubic hair growth begins in early puberty and is sparse, long, and fine and found along the labia. In adolescents, the hair texture is similar to an adult's but not as thick and is limited to the mons pubis. The hair quantity increases, thickens, and extends to the inner aspects of the thighs as the adolescent becomes an adult.

On inspection, the elderly client's external genitalia show thinning and atrophy of the labia majora. The clitoris also appears smaller than in a younger woman. The pubic hair becomes sparse, thin, brittle, gray, and straight.

Advanced assessment skills

With experience, some nurses choose to practice in facilities specializing in women's health care, where after appropriate preparation, they may perform complete gynecologic assessments. (For information on how to perform this assessment, see *Advanced assessment skills: Using the speculum,* pages 430 to 432, and *Advanced assessment skills: Bimanual palpation,* pages 433 to 436.)

As part of the complete gynecologic assessment, obtain a Pap smear, a routine cancer-screening test, after examining the cervix. Also obtain other specimens if an abnormal cervical or vaginal discharge indicates infection. (For guidelines on obtaining specimens for culture, see *Obtaining specimens for culture,* page 437.)

Abnormal findings

If the client is estrogen deficient, as after menopause, the vaginal mucosa may be pale with rugae loss. A shorter depth, dry or shiny appearance, less elastic quality, and easily cracked surface indicate a need for estrogen therapy.

Swelling or tenderness of Bartholin's glands could indicate infection; any discharge from the gland should be cultured.

Pregnancy enlarges the cervix; cancer hardens it. Women with PID may experience severe pain when the cervix is manipulated.

A blue-colored (cyanotic) cervix can indicate pelvic congestion from a tumor or pregnancy. Infection may give the cervix a bright red or spotted red appearance (erythema). A cervix projecting low into the vagina can indicate uterine prolapse (displacement of the uterus from its normal position) caused by weak pelvic muscles or ligaments. A less severe prolapse may occur when the client bears down. Urinary leakage when the client bears down indicates stress incontinence.

A cystocele (protrusion of the bladder into the vagina) or a rectocele (protrusion of the rectum into the vagina) may be observed in a woman with weak pelvic muscles. A laterally placed cervix can indicate a uterine tumor or uterine adhesion to the peritoneum.

Any cervical surface abnormalities, such as ulcerations, masses, nodules, or surface irregularities should be assessed carefully and considered malignant until proven otherwise. Sometimes the endocervical lining, outward on the cervical surface, gives the area around the external os a velvety red appearance. Called a cervical ectropion or eversion, this tissue is friable (bleeds

Integrating assessment findings

Sometimes, a cluster of abnormal assessment findings will strongly suggest a particular female reproductive disorder. In the chart below, column one shows groups of presenting signs and symptoms—the ones that make the client seek medical attention. Column two shows related assessment findings that the nurse may discover during the health history and physical assessment. The client may exhibit one or more of these findings. Column three shows the possible disorder indicated by a cluster of these findings.

PRESENTING SIGNS AND SYMPTOMS	RELATED ASSESSMENT FINDINGS	POSSIBLE DISORDER
Heavy discharge with yeasty, sweet odor or no odor for 3 to 4 days; dysuria; pruritus; dyspareunia (painful or difficult sexual intercourse)	Increased emotional stress Oral contraceptive use Previous pregnancy Diabetes mellitus Antibiotic use Steroid use White, curdlike, thick discharge on cervix and vagina Vulvovaginal edema	Candidiasis
Mild pelvic discomfort, low back pain, or deep dyspareunia possible; localized pain and tenderness possible; abnormal uterine bleeding, occasional menstrual irregularities; delayed menstruation, followed by persistent bleeding, possible	Age 20 to 40 Cysts detected on bimanual palpation	Functional ovarian cysts (follicle cysts, corpus luteum cysts)
Watery discharge with lesions or sores and blisters on external genitalia; mild itching and pain	Teens to early 30s Recent urinary tract or gynecologic examination Frequent intercourse without male use of condom Fever Enlarged inguinal lymph nodes Yellow-gray film on cervix	Genital herpes (herpes simplex virus, type I or II)
Excessive, prolonged uterine bleeding; menstrual pain referred to rectum and lower sacrum; pain on defecation; dysuria; constipation	Age 25 to 45 History of menstrual disturbances Multiple tender nodules palpable along the uterosacral ligaments or in the rectovaginal septum Pain on palpation of uterus	Endometriosis
Abdominal pain (in the later stage of disease); lower abdominal mass; ascites possible; irregular postmenopausal bleeding possible but infrequent	History of urinary frequency and constipation Early-stage menopause, postmenopause, nulliparity Displaced cervix Solid, bilateral ovarian mass on bimanual palpation	Ovarian carcinoma
Pain in later invasive stage of disease; abnormal uterine bleeding; spotting for days to months	History of previous estrogen therapy, nulliparity, obesity, and possible diabetes, hypertension Previous curettage, sterility, or poor fertility Menopause Red or brown vaginal discharge Uterine or adnexal mass, usually nontender, detected on palpation Cervical lesion	Endometrial cancer

easily) when the Pap test sample is obtained. Because an early carcinoma may resemble an ectropion, evaluation is indicated.

Polyps—bright-red, fragile, soft protrusions into the cervical canal—may be visible when they protrude from the external os. They may arise from the endometrium or the endocervical tissue, and may bleed easily when the Pap test sample is obtained. Areas where the mucosa has eroded bleed easily when touched.

Small, smooth, round, raised yellow cysts (Nabothian cysts) appear with or after chronic cervicitis or with cervical gland duct obstructions. They are harmless, but may indicate an underlying problem.

(Text continues on page 432.)

ADVANCED ASSESSMENT SKILLS

Using the speculum

The following guidelines describe how the nurse performs an assessment using a speculum. Put on gloves before beginning. After touching the genitalia, touch no equipment that will be handled by others: this examination requires medically aseptic technique. (To prevent spreading fecal matter to the vagina and urethra, do not palpate areas close to the anus until assessment completion, if at all.) Then proceed as follows.

1 To avoid startling the client, touch her thigh before touching her genitalia, and explain the next procedures. Then gently spread the labia majora with the left hand, insert the right index finger into the vagina about 4 to 5 cm (1½" to 2"), turn the finger pad upward, and milk the urethra and Skene's glands very gently by exerting upward pressure on either side of the urethra and then directly over it.

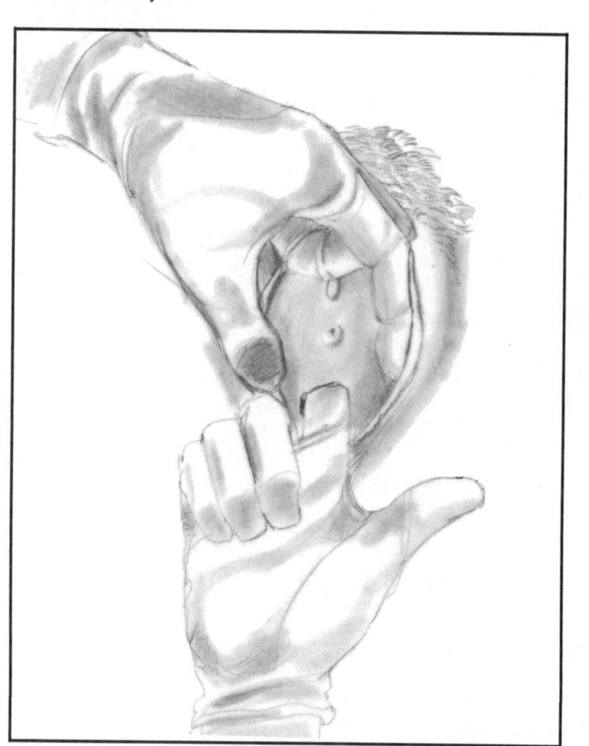

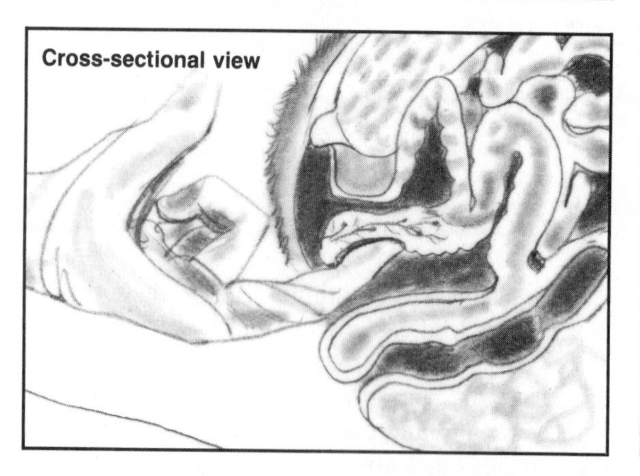

2 Rotate the index finger downward and, using the thumb and index finger, palpate the areas of Bartholin's glands (at the 5 and 7 o'clock positions) in the vaginal walls at the introitus. The areas should feel smooth with no swelling, masses, or tenderness.

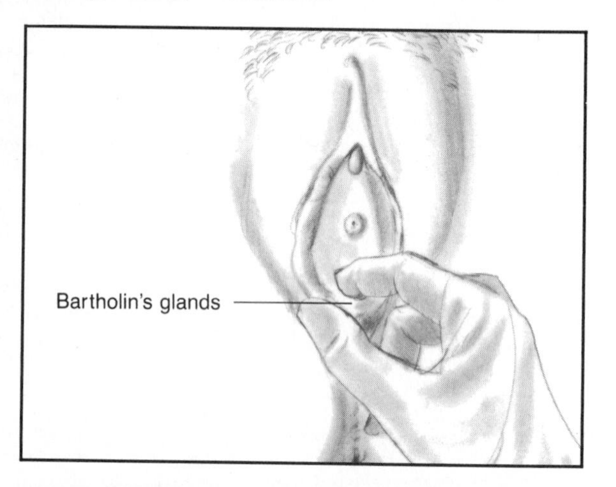

3 Place the index and middle fingers on either side of the vaginal opening and spread the fingers to separate the opening. To check pelvic support, ask the client to bear down. Some slight muscle bulging is normal. Assess vaginal tone by having the client tighten her vaginal muscles around your two fingers. Tone should be greater in women who have not borne children vaginally. Next palpate the perineum between the index finger and thumb. The tissue should feel smooth and thick in nulliparous women and thicker and rigid in multiparous women.

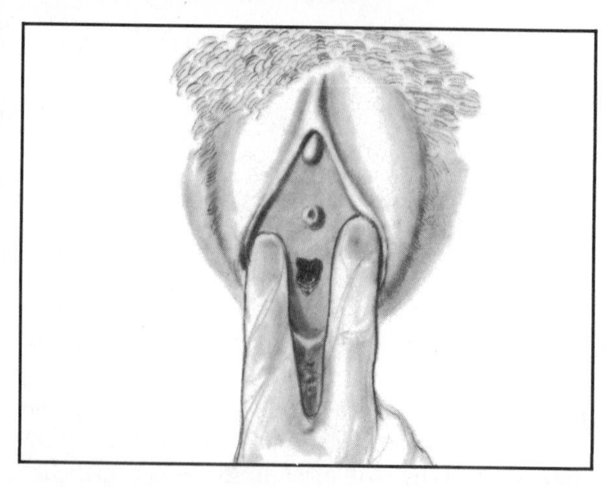

4 After evaluating vaginal outlet tone, prepare to use the speculum, which should be placed in a clean warming drawer or in clear warm water, for warmth and lubrication. (A cold speculum increases muscle tenseness.)

First, place the index and middle fingers of one hand inside the vaginal orifice to spread it apart about 2.5 cm (1″). Exert downward pressure with the fingers while introducing the closed speculum with the opposite hand over the spread fingers at about a 45-degree angle. This maneuver bypasses the sensitive urethra adjacent to the anterior vaginal wall. Hold the blades closed with the index and middle fingers of the introducing hand, and insert the speculum at about a 45-degree angle. Make sure not to pinch or pull skin or hair.

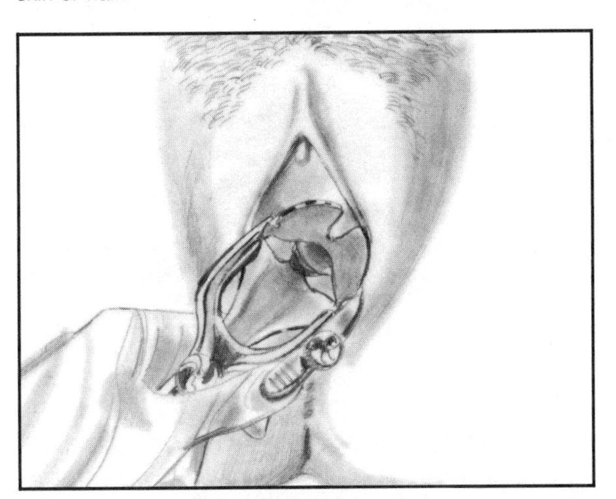

5 Once the blades pass the introitus, rotate the speculum to a horizontal plane and remove the fingers, exerting downward pressure. Maintain pressure in a downward and posterior manner on the blades until the instrument is completely inserted.

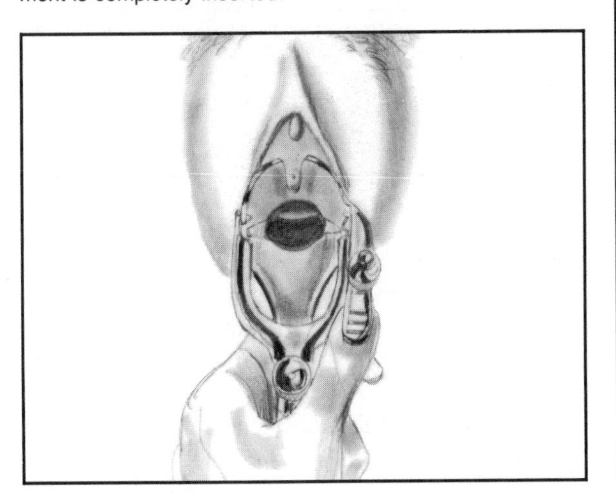

6 Open the speculum blades and look for the cervix. If you cannot see it, reposition the speculum more anteriorly, posteriorly, or laterally until the complete cervix appears. The speculum may have to be removed, the cervix located digitally, and the speculum reinserted. Tell the client when the speculum will be moved or reinserted.

To fix the blade of the metal speculum in open position, tighten the thumbscrew. During speculum repositioning maneuvers, remind the client to relax. The cervix will be more posterior with the anteverted or anteflexed uterus and more anterior with the retroverted or retroflexed uterus.

The cervix should be shiny pink. However, it may be pale if the client is anemic or menopausal. Pregnancy gives it a bluish purple cast (Chadwick's sign). The cervix, with a diameter of about 2 to 3 cm (¾″ to 1¼″), projects about 1 to 3 cm (¼″ to 1¼″) into the vagina. The cervix position correlates with the position of the uterus; it should be midline.

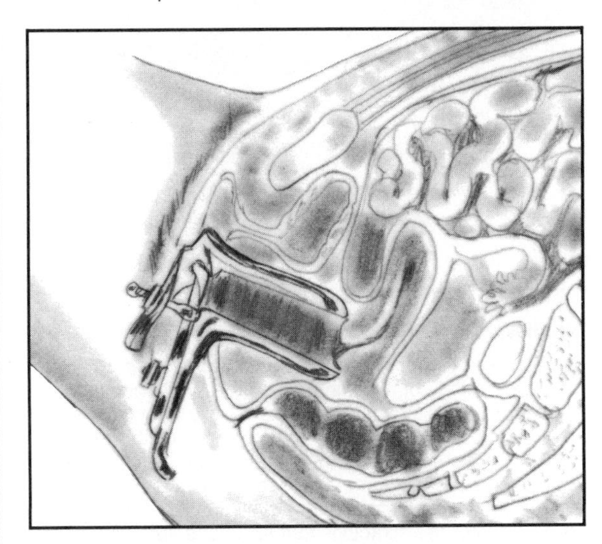

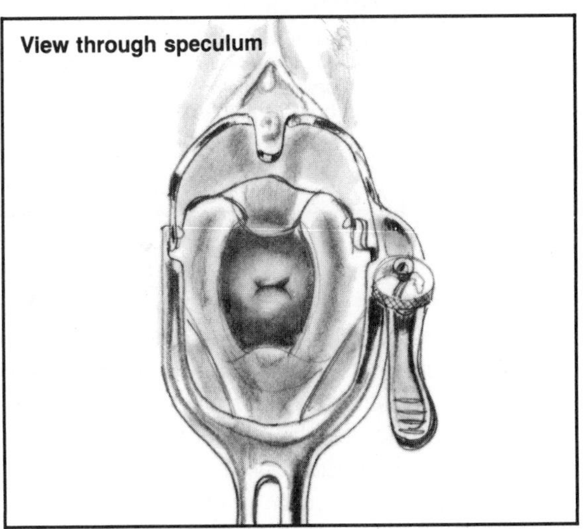
View through speculum

continued

ADVANCED ASSESSMENT SKILLS continued

Using the speculum continued

7 After inspecting the cervix, obtain an endocervical specimen by inserting a cotton-tipped swab, an endocervical brush, or the longer serrated end of a spatula about 0.5 cm into the cervical os and rotating the instrument 360 degrees clockwise. Then smear the specimen onto a glass slide with a smooth, painting motion; too much pressure can destroy the cells. Then spray the slide with cytologic fixative.

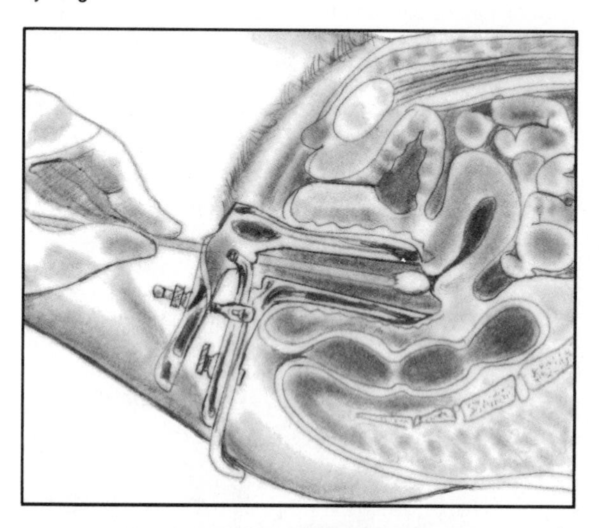

8 Retrieve a specimen from the ectocervix (the outer layer of the cervix) with the softly curved end of the spatula. Some health care facility protocols permit collecting both the ectocervical and endocervical smears simultaneously on the same slide (one on each end). Regardless, the procedure is the same: Place the curved end of the spatula in the os, apply pressure while turning it 360 degrees, transfer the scrapings to a slide, and spray the slide with fixative.

If the client has no cervix, as after a complete hysterectomy, scrape the vaginal cuff and obtain a vaginal pool specimen with a cotton-tipped applicator from the posterior vaginal area. If the client has dry mucosa, the applicator tip can be moistened with normal saline solution. Prepare the slide specimen as described previously; label the slide to indicate where the specimen came from.

A vaginal wall specimen may be needed to evaluate the maturation index (estrogen and progesterone influence on the cells). Take this specimen by scraping the blunt end of a spatula along the lateral middle third of the vagina wall.

Transfer specimens from all cervical areas to the slide and spray with cytologic fixative. (Note: If the specimen is too thick, it may be inadequate for microscopic examination.)

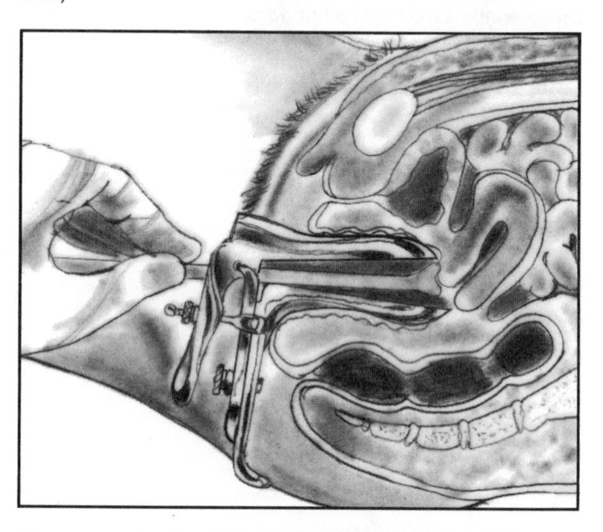

9 After collecting all the specimens, unlock the speculum thumbscrew and begin to withdraw the speculum. Slowly rotating the blades in a moderately open fashion, inspect the vaginal wall for abnormalities, such as lesions, discharge, swelling, abnormal color, and the presence or absence of rugae. Women with adequate estrogen levels have pink, moist, rugose vaginal walls.

Finally, close the speculum blades just before the distal ends reach the area adjacent to the urethral meatus and the introitus (to avoid trauma to the area), making sure that no mucosa, skin, or hair remains between the closed blades before withdrawing them. Place the speculum into a soaking solution or container or discard it if it is disposable.

Cervical carcinoma, if visible, appears as hard, granular, friable lesions usually beginning near the os and growing outward irregularly.

Venereal warts (condylomata acuminata) are dark pink to pale, cauliflowerlike lesions on the mucosal surface. They may or may not be visible and resemble irregular, small bumps on the cervix.

Ulcerations may indicate trauma or infection. Herpes simplex, type I or II, causes ulcerative lesions, whereas trichomonal infection usually produces strawberry spots (punctate hemorrhages).

Bleeding from the os may occur with menses or signal another problem. Purulent or malodorous discharge indicates an infection requiring culture or cytologic evaluation.

With hyperplasia and increasing blood supply, the pregnant uterus softens; however, the tumorous uterus

(Text continues on page 436.)

ADVANCED ASSESSMENT SKILLS

Bimanual palpation

After inspecting the cervix and obtaining a Papancolaou smear and any other specimens, the examiner bimanually palpates the internal genitalia as follows. Use your dominant hand internally for the most comfortable approach, but try your other hand if this seems awkward.

1 Put on clean gloves and apply lubricant. Lubricant comes in a tube or foil packet and may be squeezed onto a disposable gauze or paper square for easy use. Never touch the tube end with your gloved fingers; instead, allow the lubricant to drop freely onto the fingers. Discard the packet after one use.

After lubricating the index and middle fingers of your gloved hand, introduce them into the vagina using downward and posterior pressure. With your thumb abducted and your other two fingers flexed, palpate every aspect of the vaginal wall with the palmar surfaces of your fingers, rotating them as necessary. Rugae, a normal finding, feel like small ridges running concentrically around the vaginal wall. Note any nodules, tenderness, or other abnormalities. Women with small vaginal openings may need to be examined with one finger.

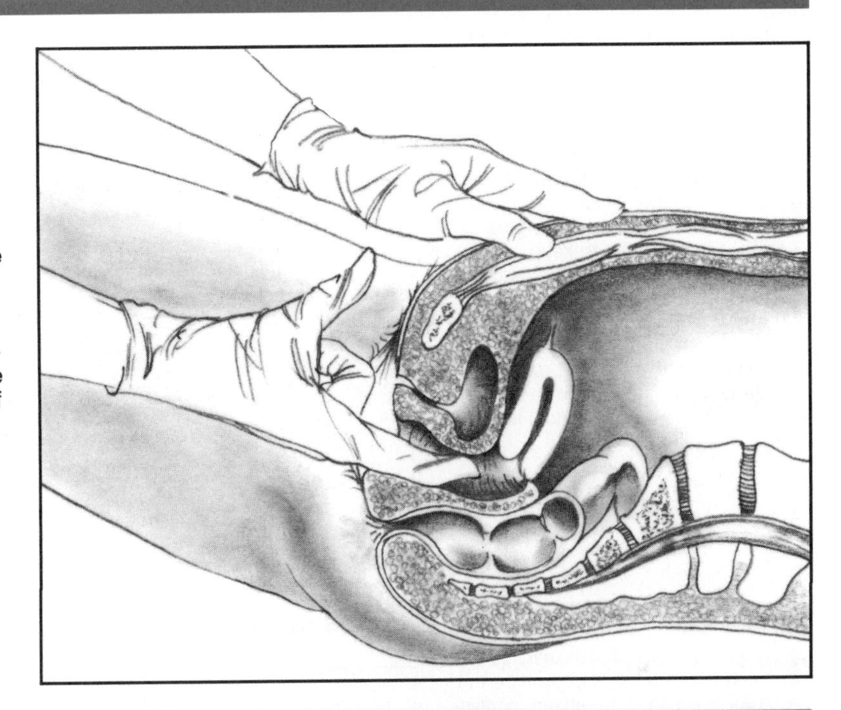

2 Insert your fingers deeper until the cervix is located with the palmar surface of the fingers. Grasp the cervix gently between your fingers and feel the surface. Also run your fingers around the circumference. Gently moving the cervix from side to side 1 to 2 cm (½" to ¾"; this should not hurt the client), assess the size, shape, position, consistency, regularity of contour, mobility, and sensitivity of the cervical surface. It should feel firm, smooth, mobile, and nontender when moved and touched. The cervix of an older woman is smaller and is usually recessed, as in a prepubertal girl; a pregnant woman's cervix is usually softened and enlarged. The os should admit your index finger about 1 cm (¼") or less, unless the woman is pregnant. The cervix, usually in the midline, should point posteriorly, anteriorly, or midplane.

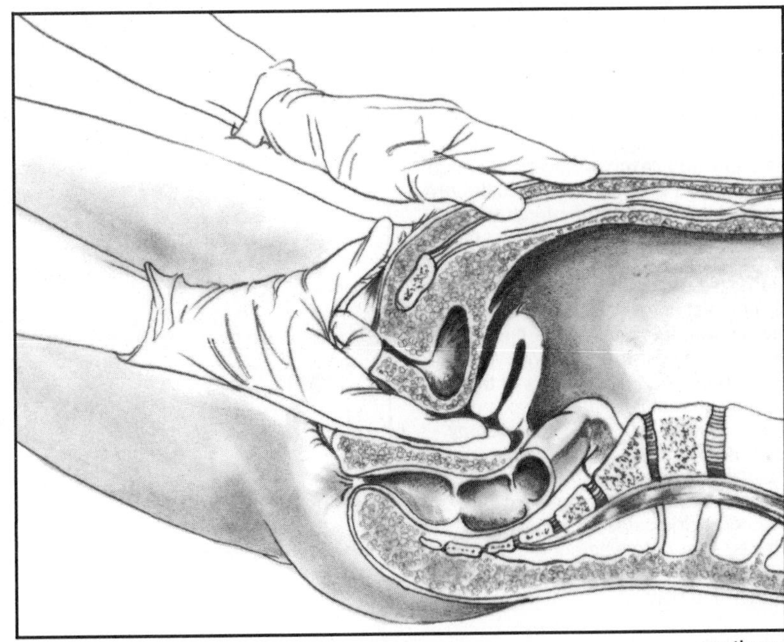

continued

ADVANCED ASSESSMENT SKILLS continued

Bimanual palpation continued

3 Position your hands for examination of the uterus. Place your external hand on the abdomen between the umbilicus and symphysis pubis. Then, inserting the first and second fingers of your examining hand into the vagina and pressing the bent digits of the fingers remaining outside the vagina against the perineum, reach under and behind the cervix and lift the uterus toward the abdomen and toward your external hand, which is applying pressure toward the internal fingers. Keep the wrist straight to keep your internal hand and forearm in a straight line. Most examination tables have a step at the examiner's end, allowing the examiner to step up and elevate one knee. Then, stabilize the elbow of the examining hand on the elevated knee, or on the hip if no step or stool is available.

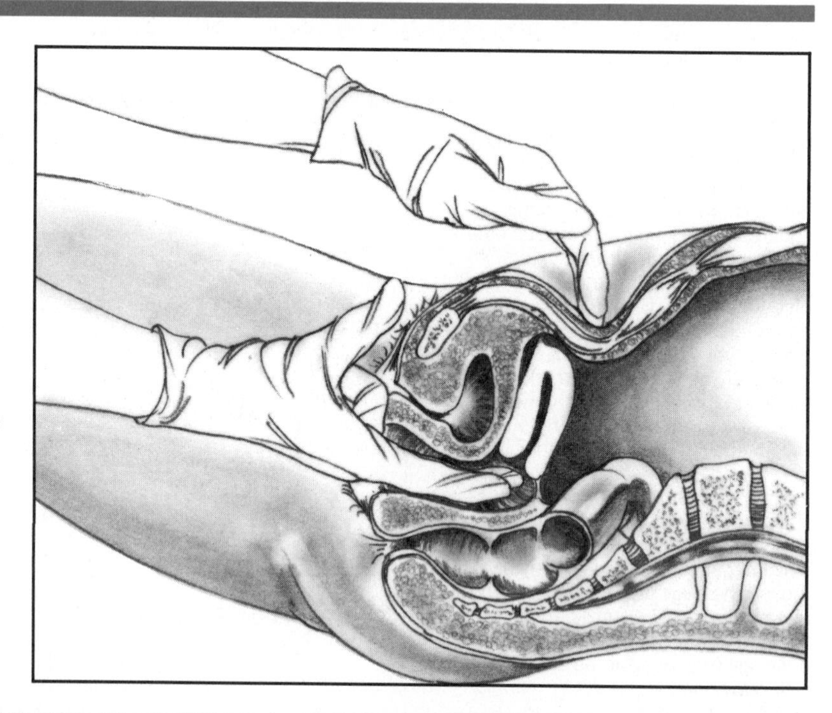

4 After inserting your examining hand into the vagina, examine the uterus for position, size, shape, consistency, tenderness, mobility, and surface regularity. If your internal fingers can move underneath and behind the cervix without encountering an obstacle in the cul-de-sac (a deep recess formed by the peritoneum as it covers the lower posterior wall of the uterus and upper portion of the vagina), the uterus is probably anteflexed, anteverted, or midplane. If you encounter an obstacle (the body of the uterus), the uterus is posteriorly positioned, either retroflexed or retroverted. (Flexion indicates that the uterus is bent upon itself; version refers to a deflection of the long axis of the uterus from the long axis of the body, either anteriorly or posteriorly. Midplane position means the long axis of the uterus is parallel to the long axis of the body.) The position of the cervix may be a clue to the uterine position. A cervix pointing anteriorly indicates a retroverted uterus; a cervix pointing posteriorly indicates an anteverted uterus. Also note whether the uterus lies midline or deviates to the left or right of the pelvis.

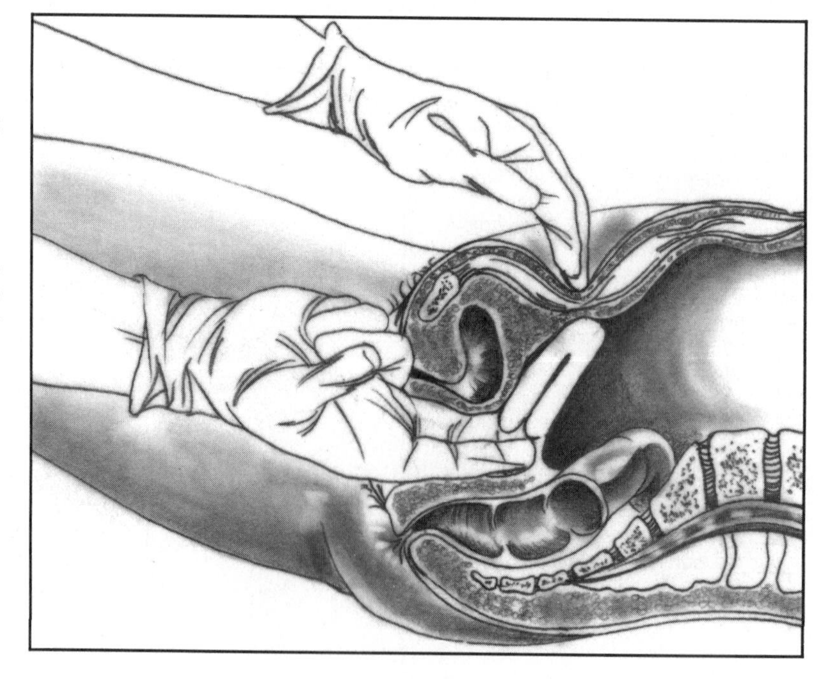

5 Determine whether the uterus is normal size, enlarged, or immature. If it is enlarged, the size is estimated in weeks of gestation. For example, the size of a uterus enlarged by a tumor might be 12 weeks. The normal nonpregnant uterus is small and fits comfortably beneath the symphysis pubis in the pelvis; it is not palpable by abdominal examination. The uterus of a postmenopausal woman is usually smaller than before menopause.

Unless an abnormality or pregnancy changes the shape of the uterus, it is pear-shaped and symmetrical. Note any deviations; for example, a protruding mass on the fundal surface.

Normally, the muscular composition of the uterus makes it feel firm. Although the uterus is not particularly tender on palpation (unless the woman is menstruating), some tenderness normally may occur. The ligaments suspending the uterus in the pelvis allow the uterus to be slightly mobile on the anterior to posterior plane. Limited mobility may indicate a pathologic condition, such as carcinoma, infection, or scarring.

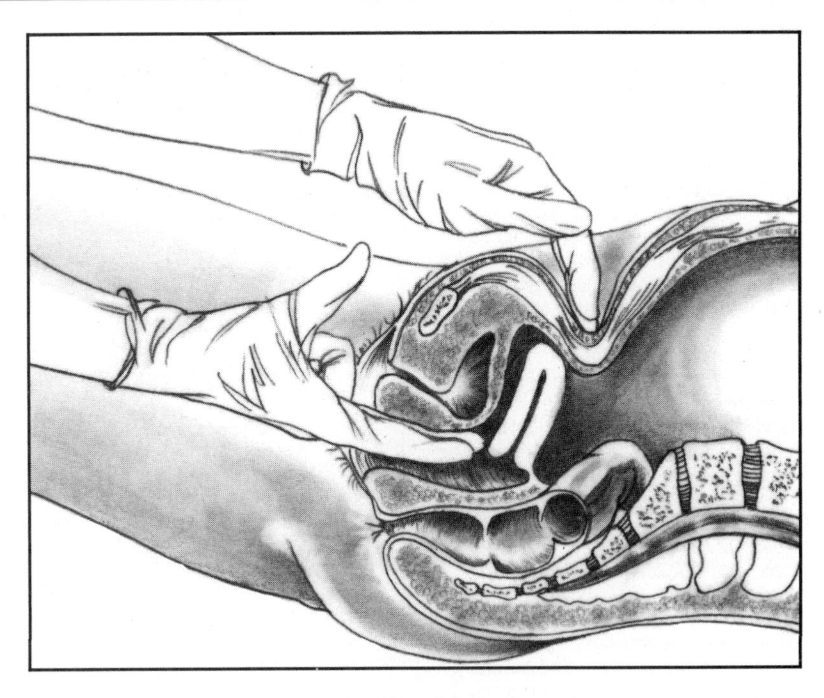

6 Assess the right and left adnexal areas (ovaries and fallopian tubes). Place your internal fingers deeply inward and upward toward the external hand on the right lower abdominal quadrant and lift your internal fingers as the external hand is swept down and inward toward the symphysis pubis. This maneuver allows the ovary and any masses to slip between the fingers of your two hands; it should be repeated on the left side.

If palpable, the ovaries are mobile, oval, somewhat flattened, firm, smooth, almond-shaped organs approximately 3 × 2 × 1 cm (1¼″ × ¾″ × ¼″). They may be sensitive to palpation. The ovaries of a postmenopausal woman or prepubertal girl should not be palpable. Normal fallopian tubes are usually not palpable or sensitive. The round ligaments may be palpable as cordlike apparatuses in the adnexa.

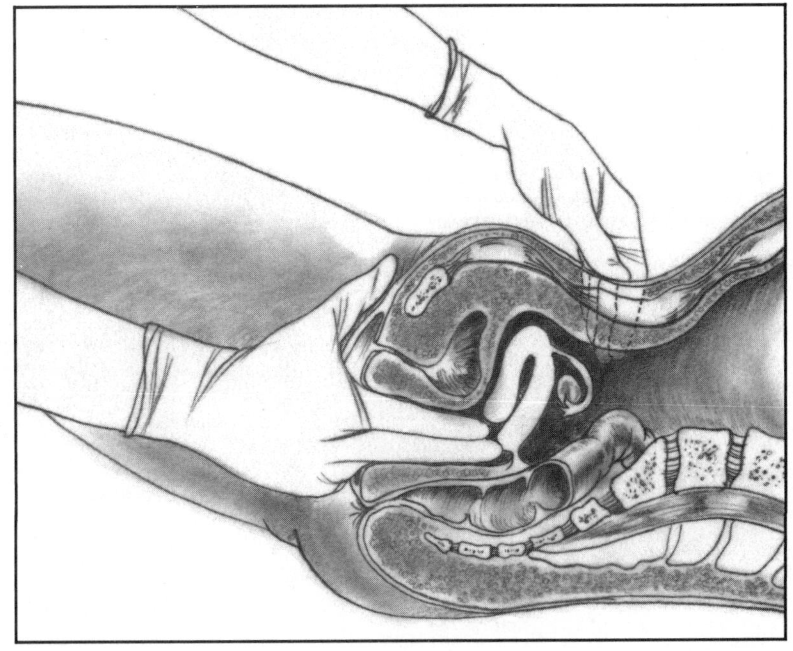

continued

ADVANCED ASSESSMENT SKILLS continued

Bimanual palpation continued

7 After completing the bimanual assessment, prepare for rectovaginal palpation. Change the glove of your internal hand to prevent transfer of vaginal organisms into the rectum. Be careful not to touch the anal area with the index finger that will be introduced into the vagina. Changing gloves also prevents a positive occult blood test result of rectal contents (caused by introducing vaginal or cervical blood into the rectum with a contaminated glove). An inadvertently contaminated index finger must be newly gloved before the assessment proceeds.

The rectovaginal assessment is useful for examining women with small vaginal openings that permit only one finger to be introduced. The finger used rectally can lift organs anteriorly that cannot be reached by the finger used vaginally.

Explain the procedure to the client. Then, after lubricating the index and middle fingers of your gloved examining hand, ask the client to bear down, as if to have a bowel movement (she should be assured she will not), and carefully insert your middle finger into the rectum. Inspect for hemorrhoids or other painful areas and avoid these lesions when inserting your finger. Next, as you insert your index finger into the vagina, tell the client to stop bearing down and to relax using the techniques taught earlier. Use the finger in the vagina to find the cervix and keep it from being confused with a mass by the finger in the rectum.

Sweep the rectum within the reach of your examining finger. No masses or nodules should be felt. A high percentage of rectal growths can be felt by the examining hand. The rectovaginal assessment provides a more complete evaluation of the posterior side of the uterus.

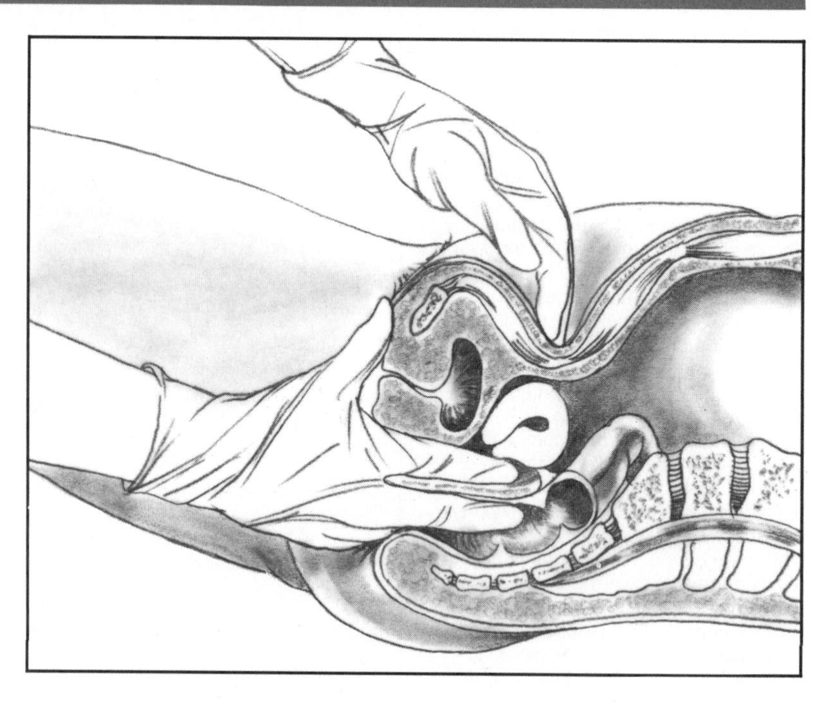

The posteriorly positioned uterus must be examined rectally to examine its surface characteristics. The anteriorly positioned or midplane uterus is also assessed posteriorly when the rectovaginal assessment is performed. Reevaluation of the adnexa and the cul-de-sac may reveal masses or nodules not palpated during the bimanual assessment.

After withdrawing your gloved finger from the client's rectum, check it for stool color and note any blood. When the examination is complete, clean the client with tissue in a front-to-back motion to remove excess lubricant. Help her to a sitting position. Wash your hands and advise the client to wash her hands if she has touched her genitals.

may feel hard, especially if cancerous. Excessive tenderness usually indicates disease, especially infection. The pregnant uterus is normally somewhat tender.

A palpable ovary in a postmenopausal woman or prepubescent girl is abnormal. Any abnormal ovarian enlargement in any age client should be evaluated medically. Although common and usually benign in young fertile women, ovarian cysts should also be evaluated.

Documentation

Before documenting, the nurse evaluates the reproductive system assessment findings by reviewing all the data, especially from the health history interview and the physical assessment. The nurse also evaluates the results of diagnostic studies (such as cultures) or other laboratory tests (such as the Pap test and the human

Obtaining specimens for culture

This chart describes the equipment and techniques used to obtain specimens for culture studies that may accompany assessment of the female reproductive system.

ORGANISMS	SPECIMEN SITE	EQUIPMENT	PROCEDURE
Neisseria gonorrhoeae	Endocervix	• Cotton-tipped swab • Thayer-Martin medium culture plate or bottle	• Insert a sterile cotton-tipped swab 0.5 cm into the cervical os, then rotate 360 degrees. Leave applicator in the os 10 to 30 seconds to absorb secretions. • Inoculate culture medium with specimen by simultaneously rotating the swab and patterning a Z on a culture plate or in the bottle. • Place tightly capped bottle on its side or culture plate face up in a warm environment within 15 minutes of obtaining the specimen.
	Anus	• Cotton-tipped swab • Thayer-Martin medium culture plate or bottle	• Insert sterile cotton-tipped swab into the rectal canal 2.5 cm (1″), then rotate the swab 360 degrees, move it from side to side, and leave it in place for 10 to 30 seconds. • Apply specimen to culture medium as described above.
	Oropharynx	• Cotton-tipped swab • Thayer-Martin medium culture plate or bottle	• Swab oropharynx with a sterile cotton-tipped swab. • Apply specimen to culture medium as described above.
Chlamydia trachomatis	Endocervix	• Special swab (provided with test medium) • Special medium slide • Acetone	• Enzyme immunoassay: Collect specimen on a special swab, place in a provided medium, and send for analysis by spectrophotometer. • Monoclonal antibody test: Apply specimen collected with endocervical brush on a slide, allow to dry, and apply acetone.
Candida albicans *Trichomonas vaginalis* *Hemophilus vaginalis*	Vaginal secretions from posterior vaginal pool	• Cotton-tipped applicator • Normal saline solution • Potassium hydroxide (KOH) • Glass slides and coverslips	• Dip the wooden end of a cotton-tipped applicator into the vaginal secretion pool without touching the mucosa, then into a drop of solution placed on a slide. If both normal saline solution and KOH slides are needed, place the tip in the saline drop first, then the KOH. • Apply glass coverslips and send to laboratory for microscopic examination as soon as possible.

chorionic gonadotropin test) that may have been done. Normal findings for the Pap test, which is used to detect cervical cancer, are Class I and indicate the absence of abnormal cells. Abnormal findings may be Class II (atypical, but nonmalignant cells present), Class III (dysplasia, a cell abnormality), Class IV (suggestive of, but inconclusive for, malignancy), or Class V (conclusive for malignancy).

The human chorionic gonadotropin test, commonly known as the pregnancy test, measures the level of hormones produced by the placenta. Normal values vary with the trimester of pregnancy from 500,000 IU/24 hours (first trimester); to 10,000 to 25,000 IU/24 hours (second trimester); to 5,000 to 15,000 IU/24 hours (third trimester). In a pregnant client, above-normal values may indicate multiple pregnancy or erythroblastosis fetalis; below-normal values, threatened abortion or ectopic (out-

(Text continues on page 440.)

Applying the nursing process

Assessment findings form the basis of the nursing process. Using them, the nurse formulates the nursing diagnoses and develops appropriate planning, implementation, and evaluation of the client's care.

The table below shows how the nurse can use female reproductive system assessment data in the nursing process for the client described in the case history (shown at right). In the first column, history and physical assessment data appear, followed by a paragraph of mental notes. These notes help the nurse make important mental connections among assessment findings, aiding in development of the nursing diagnoses and planning.

The second column presents several appropriate nursing diagnoses; however, the information in the remaining columns is based on the *first* nursing diagnosis. Although it is not part of the nursing process, documentation appears in the last column because of its importance. Documentation consists of an initial note using all components of the SOAPIE format and a follow-up note using the appropriate SOAPIE components.

ASSESSMENT	NURSING DIAGNOSES	PLANNING	IMPLEMENTATION
Subjective (history) data • Client states, "My periods aren't regular. They come every 12 to 36 days and last from 1 to 10 days." • Client reports a heavy menstrual flow (six to seven extra-absorbent pads a day) during the 10-day periods and light flow (one pad a day) during the shorter periods. • Client states, "I've been feeling really tired lately; I have no energy. I've missed a lot of school since this problem started. I'm scared; I don't know what's happening." • Client reports cramps during heavy-flow periods. • A 24-hour dietary recall reveals dietary intake low in iron and vitamin C. **Objective (physical) data** • Client crying and clinging to her mother. • Conjunctiva slightly pale. • Hematocrit (HCT) 32%; hemoglobin (Hb) 10.8 g. • Red blood cell (RBC) indices and laboratory test results indicate iron-deficiency anemia. • Breast budding and pubic hair growth appropriate for age. • Assessment by gynecologist reveals no abnormal masses on inspection with a Pederson speculum and bimanual palpation. Hymen intact. Cervix pink with no lesions or abnormal discharge. **Mental notes** *Because this client is so young, she probably has not had a gynecologic assessment before. I will need to allay her anxiety by letting her express her feelings and by explaining procedures carefully to her. She may be unfamiliar with the anatomy of the reproductive system and the reason for the maturational changes she is experiencing. Fatigue may be related to stress, caused by fear and anxiety, and to a low hemoglobin from heavy menstrual flow. Client may not be getting sufficient iron in her diet to compensate for blood loss; she probably needs to improve nutrition and take an iron supplement.*	• Altered nutrition: less than body requirements, related to poor dietary habits. • Knowledge deficit related to body functions, maturational changes, and nutrition. • Cardiac output: potential for alteration, related to low hemoglobin. • Ineffective individual coping related to physical alteration in body.	**Goals** Before leaving the clinic today, the client will: • list foods high in iron and vitamin C and explain the importance of improved dietary intake of foods containing these substances. • discuss basic anatomy of female reproductive system and explain the maturational changes she is experiencing. At the follow-up visit, the client will: • discuss potential adverse reactions to iron preparations. • bring in a menstrual-cycle calendar kept during the previous month.	• Give the client a list of foods high in iron and vitamin C and explain why she should include them in her diet. • Explain the importance of iron supplements to the client. Advise her to take the supplement ½ hour after meals for optimal absorption and to expect black stools and constipation. Advise increasing fluid and fiber intake to prevent constipation. • Using clear illustrations and language appropriate to the client's educational level, teach her about reproductive system anatomy, the menstrual cycle, and the maturational changes she is experiencing. • Teach the client to keep a menstrual-cycle calendar that includes menstrual period dates, flow characteristics, and signs and symptoms she notices before, during, and after her menstrual period. • Ask the client to keep a 7-day diet history and bring it to the next visit.

CASE HISTORY

Shelly Jordan is a 13-year-old Black female eighth grader. Her mother brought her to the clinic. She complains of "funny periods" since the onset of menses 6 months ago and reports extreme fatigue.

DOCUMENTATION BASED ON NURSING PROCESS DATA

Initial

S Client states, "My periods have not been regular since they started 6 months ago. They come every 12 to 36 days and last from 1 to 10 days. I'm really tired, have missed a lot of school, and I'm afraid something is wrong with me."

O Bimanual palpation of internal pelvic organs reveals no tenderness, pain, or masses. Inspection with speculum reveals pink cervix with no abnormal discharge. Pale conjunctiva. Dietary recall reveals diet low in iron and vitamin C. Crying and clinging to mother. HCT 32%; Hb 10.8 g; RBC indices indicate iron-deficiency anemia.

A Altered nutrition: less than body requirements, related to poor dietary habits.

Client very fearful, needs mother's support. Menses irregular with heavy flow.

P Instruct the client about nutritional needs and supplemental iron use, including potential adverse reactions.Using anatomic models and a booklet for the client to take home and read, teach client about female reproductive system and menstrual cycle. Show client how to keep menstrual-cycle calendar.

I Client taught that iron supplements should be taken ½ hour after meals and also taught potential adverse reactions. Client taught about anatomy of female reproductive system, including the menstrual cycle and normal maturational changes.

E Client discussed supplemental iron use and explained importance of eating properly. She discussed female reproductive organs and menstrual cycle in quiet, embarrassed manner.

Follow-up

S Client states, "I feel a lot better. I read the booklet you gave me and showed it to my girlfriend, Sonia, so that she would know these things too. I've been taking my iron like you told me, ½ hour after I eat. I've been trying to eat better, but still go out with my friends on Friday nights for fast food."

O Client appears more relaxed and discusses menstrual problems more freely. Conjunctiva pink. Repeat HCT is 37%; Hb 12 g.

A Client's fears reduced with increased understanding of her body. Physical assessment and laboratory data within normal limits. Dietary habits improved; client complied with medication regimen.

P Follow-up visit in 6 months. Continue to gain client's trust and allow her to discuss concerns and questions she may have about her developing body and feelings of sexuality.

EVALUATION

At the next follow-up visit, the client:

- brought in a 7-day diet history that shows she has eaten dark-green leafy vegetables, liver, and fresh fruits.
- explained the female reproductive anatomy and the maturational changes she is experiencing.
- shared her previous month's menstrual-cycle calendar.
- reported taking iron supplement ½ hour after meals, drinking more fluids, and eating foods high in fiber; she is not constipated.

side the uterus) pregnancy. In a nonpregnant client, measurable levels of human chorionic gonadotropin suggest ovarian tumor, melanoma, multiple myeloma, or gastric, hepatic, pancreatic, or breast cancer.

The assessment data become the first step in the nursing process. From these data the appropriate nursing diagnoses are formed, allowing the nurse to plan, implement, and evaluate the client's nursing care. (For a case study that shows how to apply the nursing process to female reproductive dysfunction, see *Applying the nursing process,* pages 438 and 439.)

The documented physical assessment findings clearly, accurately, and concisely describe the collected data, including normal and abnormal findings. The following example shows how to document normal findings related to the female reproductive system:

> External genitalia: no lesions, inflammation, edema, varicosities, or other abnormalities visible. Labia majora, labia minora, clitoris intact. Hair pattern of mature female. Vagina: pink, without lesions or inflammation. Cervix: pink, no lesions, small ectropion area around external os. Clear mucus discharge from os. No odor. Uterus: midline, retroverted, pear-shaped, about 6 cm long, mobile, nontender, symmetrical, firm. Adnexa: no masses palpated; ovaries firm, about 3 x 2 cm, small, smooth, mobile, slightly tender. Rectovaginal area: no masses, nodules, or bleeding. Hard stool felt on palpation of rectum.

The following example shows how to document abnormal findings:

> External genitalia: Three tender ulcerations each less than 1 mm on right labia minora. Clear fluid from lesions. No other external abnormalities. Vagina: 1 x 1 cm pale, irregular, firm, nontender papular lesion on the midleft vaginal wall. Cervix: small (less than 1 mm), round, velvety red lesion projecting from external os—nontender, movable. Bleeds easily when touched with spatula. Uterus: anteflexed, pregnant 12-week size, hard, irregular shape, nontender, somewhat fixed, deviated to left. Adnexa: right ovary 5 x 6 cm, with several nodular masses about 0.5 to 1 cm, tender, mobile, ovoid. Rectovaginal area: 2-cm irregular hard mass, nontender, fixed, anterior rectal wall.

Chapter summary

To assess the female client's reproductive system effectively, the nurse relies on health history data, physical assessment findings, and laboratory results. Chapter 15 describes how to gather and integrate this information. Here are the major points discussed in this chapter:

- The female reproductive system includes the external genitalia (labia minora, labia majora, and clitoris) adjacent structures (Bartholin's glands, Skene's glands, and the urethral meatus), and the internal genitalia (vagina, uterus, fallopian tubes, ovaries, and supporting structures).
- The menstrual cycle functions by a complex network of hormonal substances produced by the hypothalamus, the pituitary, and the ovaries. The positive and negative feedback responses from these structures influence the normal menstrual cycle and ovulation. Decline of ovarian hormones eventually results in cessation of reproductive function at menopause.
- The health history should be obtained before the physical assessment. During the health history interview, the client remains seated and dressed. Depending on the reason for the evaluation, questioning should cover menstruation, procreation, contraception, STDs, other pathology or reproductive system abnormalities, sexuality, and developmental and cultural concerns.
- The questions for females of specific age-groups, such as the premenarchal girl and the elderly woman, should be formulated with sensitivity and specially focused to obtain accurate data.
- When obtaining the health history, the nurse must explore the client's use of medications, including oral contraceptives. Subsequent information may reveal whether the client receives hormone therapy for reproductive system dysfunction or whether an adverse drug reaction caused a dysfunction.
- A gynecologic assessment requires careful client preparation, psychologically and physically. Equipment for the assessment and related diagnostic studies should be ready before the examiner approaches the client. Inspection with the speculum and bimanual palpation are performed using medically aseptic technique.
- During the assessment, the labia minora and labia majora, the vagina, and the cervix are inspected. All external and internal structures are palpated, including the rectovaginal area.

• To complete the female reproductive system assessment, the nurse reviews the results of any laboratory tests (cultures or smears). The specimens most commonly obtained for laboratory study include cervical tissue for the Pap test; exudate samples for culture and identification of *Neisseria gonorrhoeae, Chlamydia trachomatis,* and other sexually transmitted microorganisms; and wet mounts.
• Finally, the nurse documents all assessment findings and uses them in the nursing process to plan, implement, and evaluate the client's care.

Study questions

1. Maryellen Crowder, age 15, comes to the school clinic for information about contraception. Upon questioning her, you learn that she has little knowledge about the normal menstrual cycle and none about contraception. What basic facts about the menstrual cycle would you teach her?

2. Having her first gynecologic assessment today, Maryellen is frightened and anxious. What steps can you take to help her relax during the assessment?

3. How would you explain the actions of estrogen and progesterone during the menstrual cycle to a client?

4. What questions would you ask to obtain information about the female reproductive system of an adolescent and a menopausal client?

5. Florence Devon, age 35 and married, complains of a white, thick vaginal discharge of 2 weeks' duration. Mrs. Devon reports that the discharge has no foul odor and that she has pain with intercourse and painful vaginal itching most of the time. She has tried a nonprescription cream but has had no relief. Physical assessment reveals erythematous (inflamed) and edematous (swollen) external genitalia, especially the labia. The vagina and cervix are also inflamed, swollen, and tender to the touch. A white, curdlike discharge appears on the internal surfaces. A 10% potassium hydroxide wet smear shows many hyphae and spores, indicative of *Candida albicans.*

How would you document the following information related to your nursing assessment of Mrs. Devon?
• history (subjective) assessment data
• physical (objective) assessment data
• assessment techniques and special equipment
• nursing diagnoses
• documentation.

Selected references

Cancer statistics. (1991). New York: American Cancer Society.

Edelman, C., and Mandle, C. (1990). *Health promotion throughout the lifespan* (2nd ed.). St. Louis: Mosby-Year Book.

Funch, D. (1986). Socioeconomic status and survival for breast and cervical cancer. *Women's Health,* 11(3-4), 37-54.

Key, T., and Resnik, R. (1990). Maternal changes in pregnancy. In D. Danforth and J. Scott (Eds.), *Danforth's obstetrics and gynecology* (6th ed.). Philadelphia: Lippincott.

Kim, M., McFarland, G., and McLane, A. (1991). *Pocket guide to nursing diagnoses* (4th ed.). St. Louis: Mosby-Year Book.

Morrison-Beedy, D., and Robbins, L. (1989). Sexual assessment and the aging female. *Nurse Practitioner,* 14(12), 35, 38-39, 42, 45.

Muscari, M. (1987). Obtaining the adolescent sexual history. *Pediatric Nursing,* 13(5), 307-310.

Sloane, E. (1985). *Biology of women* (2nd ed.). New York: Wiley & Sons.

Tanner, J. (1962). *Growth and adolescence* (2nd ed.). Oxford: Blackwell Scientific.*

Nursing research

Smith, K., Turner, J., and Jacobsen, R. (1987). Health concerns of adolescents. *Pediatric Nursing,* 13(5), 311-315.

Heitkemper, M., et al. (1991). GI symptoms, function, and psychophysiological arousal in dysmenorrheic women. *Nursing Research,* 40(1), 20-26.

Walton, J., and Youngkin, E. (1987). The effect of a support group on self-esteem of women with premenstrual syndrome. *JOGNN,* 16(3), 174-178.

*Landmark publication

16

Male Reproductive System

Objectives

After reading and studying this chapter, you should be able to:
1. Identify and locate the normal male reproductive organs and structures.
2. Explain normal physiologic function of the male reproductive system, including the sexual act, spermatogenesis, and hormonal control.
3. Discuss health history questions designed to elicit information about a male client's reproductive system.
4. Identify the important classes of drugs that affect the male reproductive system.
5. Conduct a physical assessment of the penis and scrotum, including inspection and palpation.
6. Examine the inguinal area for hernias.
7. Explain how to palpate the prostate gland.
8. Describe normal and abnormal findings detected during physical assessment of the penis, scrotum, inguinal area, and prostate gland.
9. Discuss the most important laboratory tests used to evaluate sexual and reproductive function and detect sexually transmitted diseases or other disorders.
10. Document male reproductive system assessment findings using the nursing process.

Introduction

Assessing the male reproductive system, although potentially uncomfortable for the nurse and client, is an essential part of a complete health assessment. Careful assessment may uncover actual or potential problems or concerns that the client usually would not volunteer willingly. Such information may be crucial. Many common disorders of the male reproductive system carry potentially serious physiologic or psychological consequences. For example, sexual or reproductive dysfunction, such as impotence or infertility, can dramatically affect the client's quality of life. Also, sexually transmitted diseases—the most common communicable diseases in the United States—can produce devastating complications unless detected and treated early.

This chapter begins with a review of male reproductive system anatomy and physiology, including normal sexual and reproductive function and hormonal control. It then discusses the steps involved in assessing a male client's reproductive system, covering health history and physical assessment. It presents normal and abnormal assessment findings, including information about relevant laboratory tests. It also demonstrates how to document such assessment findings using the nursing process.

Anatomy and physiology review

The male reproductive system consists of two major organs—the penis and testicles—and associated structures, including transport ducts, the prostate gland, and inguinal structures. (For detailed information about these organs and structures, see *The male reproductive system*, pages 444 and 445.) This system serves three

Glossary

Androgens: male sex hormones, primarily testosterone.
Circumcision: surgical removal of the prepuce (foreskin) of the penis.
Cryptorchidism: developmental abnormality in which the testes fail to descend into the scrotum.
Ejaculation: forceful emission of semen from the urethral meatus at sexual climax.
Epispadias: congenital opening of the urethral meatus on the dorsal surface of the penis.
Erection: state of penile swelling and rigidity usually associated with sexual arousal.
Hernia, inguinal: protrusion of the bowel through the abdominal wall into the inguinal canal.
Hydrocele: abnormal collection of spermatic fluid in the tunica vaginalis of the scrotum.
Hypospadias: congenital opening of the urethral meatus on the ventral surface of the penis.
Paraphimosis: abnormal condition in which a retracted prepuce cannot move back over the glans penis.
Phimosis: abnormal tightness of the prepuce preventing its retraction from the glans penis.
Puberty: developmental stage during which the secondary sex characteristics appear and the ability to reproduce is attained.
Semen: viscous secretion discharged during ejaculation, containing sperm and fluids produced by the prostate, bulbourethral, and other glands.
Sperm: spermatozoa, the mature male sex or germ cells contained in semen.
Spermatogenesis: process of sperm formation.

basic functions: sexual reproduction, male sex hormone secretion, and urine elimination. (For information on urine elimination, see Chapter 14, Urinary System.)

Male sexual function

The male sexual act occurs in three stages: erection, lubrication, and emission and ejaculation. Erection, a neurovascular reflex controlled by the autonomic nervous system, can result from physical or psychological stimulation. It begins with the transmission of parasympathetic impulses via the spinal sacral nerves to the penile vasculature, producing increased arterial dilation and decreased venous outflow. As these changes occur, blood fills the erectile tissue and causes the penis to become elongated and rigid. The same parasympathetic impulses stimulate the bulbourethral glands to secrete mucus, which flows through the urethra to aid lubrication for intercourse. As sexual stimulation increases, the scrotal skin thickens and the testes increase in size, rotate anteriorly, and elevate.

When sexual stimulation reaches a critical point, the spinal cord reflex mechanisms emit rhythmic sympathetic impulses from the first and second lumbar vertebrae to the genitals. Emission begins as contractions in the epididymis, the vas deferens, and the ampulla expel sperm into the internal urethra. Contractions in the seminal vesicles then expel a mucoid fluid containing fructose, fibrinogen, prostaglandin, and other substances that nourish and protect sperm and provide energy for motility after ejaculation. The contractions propel the fluid-sperm mixture—now known as seminal fluid or semen—along the internal urethra to the prostate gland, which secretes a thin, milky, alkaline fluid (prostatic fluid) that helps protect the sperm in the acidic vaginal environment, and then to the bulbourethral glands, which secrete more mucus.

In response to filling of the internal urethra, more rhythmic impulses are sent, this time to the muscles that encase the base of the erectile tissue. Eventually, these impulses cause peristaltic pressure changes that forcefully expel the semen from the urethral meatus—a process known as ejaculation—and produce the accompanying pleasurable sensations of orgasm.

After orgasm and ejaculation, the penile vessels gradually constrict, causing blood flow back out of the erectile tissue and the return of the penis to its normal, flaccid state.

Spermatogenesis

Spermatogenesis—sperm formation—is a continuous process that begins when a male reaches puberty, usually during early adolescence. Spermatogenesis normally continues throughout life.

Triggered by the action of male sex hormones, spermatogenesis begins in the seminiferous tubules with epithelial cells called spermatogonia. (For more information, see *Understanding spermatogenesis*, page 446.)

After formation is complete, sperm pass from the seminiferous tubules through the vasa recta into the epididymis, where they mature. Only a small number of sperm can be stored in the epididymis; most of them move into the vas deferens, where they are stored until sexual stimulation triggers emission. Length of storage

The male reproductive system

As shown in these illustrations, the male reproductive system consists of the penis, the scrotum and its contents, the prostate gland, and the inguinal structures.

Penis

Internally, the cylindrical penile shaft consists of three columns of erectile tissue bound together by heavy fibrous tissue. Two corpora cavernosa form the major part of the penis; on the underside, the corpus spongiosum encases the urethra. The penile shaft terminates distally in the glans penis, a cone-shaped expansion of the corpus spongiosum that is highly sensitive to sexual stimulus. The expanded

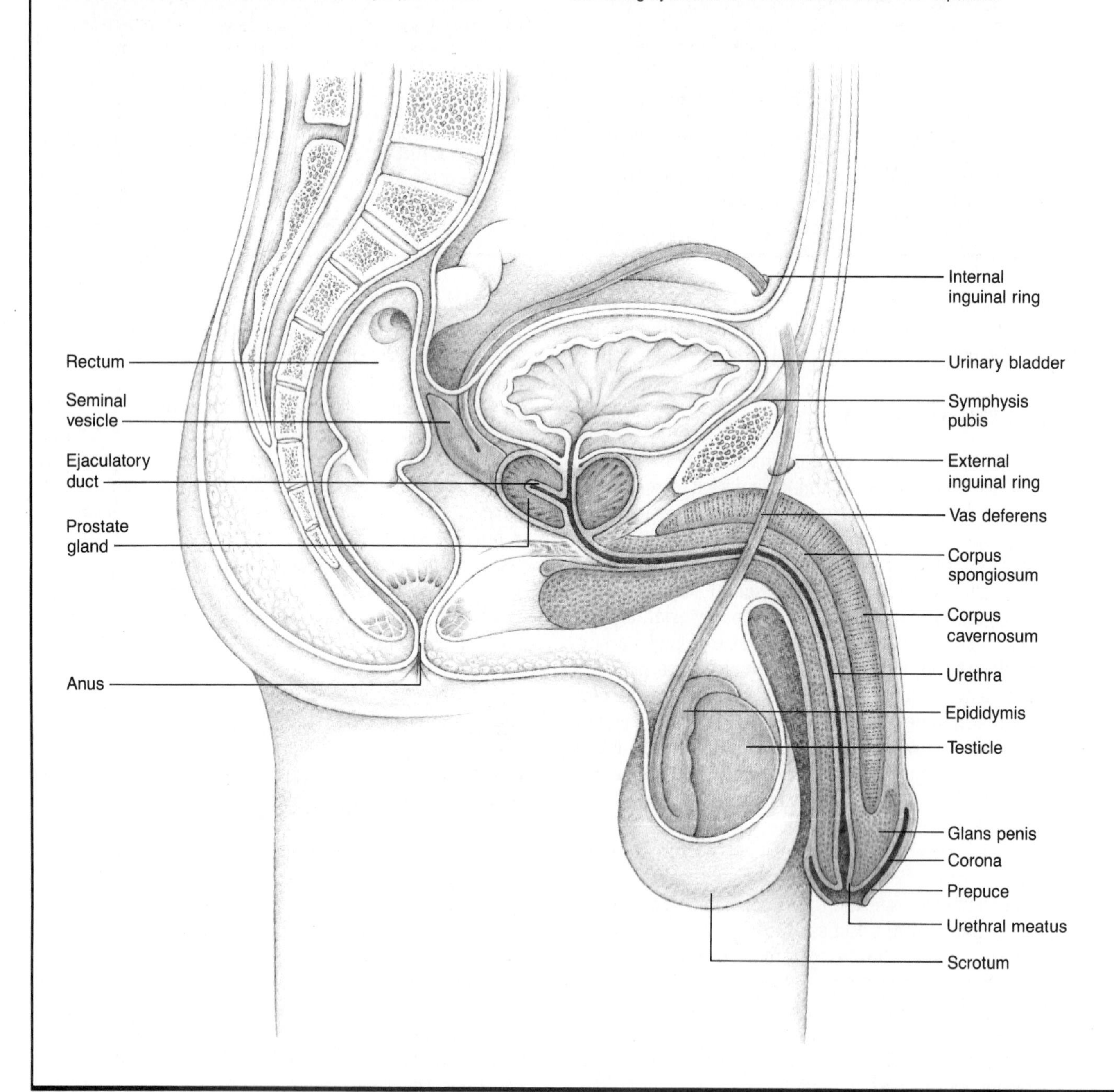

lateral margin of the glans forms a ridge of tissue known as the corona. Thin, loose skin covers the penile shaft. In an uncircumcised male, a skin flap—the foreskin, or prepuce—covers the corona and much of the glans. The urethral meatus opens through the glans to allow urination and ejaculation.

Scrotum

The penis meets the scrotum, or scrotal sac, at the penoscrotal junction. The scrotum itself consists of a thin layer of skin overlying a tighter, muscle-like layer, which in turn overlies the tunica vaginalis, a serous membrane covering the internal scrotal cavity. Externally, the median raphe (seam of union of the two halves) continues from the penis to superficially bisect the scrotal skin. Internally, a septum divides the scrotum into two sacs, each containing a testis, an epididymis, and spermatic cord. Each testis measures about 2″ (5 cm) long by 1″ (2.5 cm) wide and weighs about ½ oz (15 g). The testes contain the seminiferous tubules, where spermatogenesis takes place.

A complex duct system conveys sperm from the testes to the ejaculatory ducts near the bladder. From the seminiferous tubules, newly formed sperm travel to the epididymis—a tubular reservoir for sperm storage and maturation that curves over the posterolateral surface and upper end of the testes. Mature sperm then move from the epididymis to the vas deferens. This duct begins at the end of the epididymis, passes up through the external inguinal canal, and descends near the bladder fundus, where it enters the ejaculatory duct inside the prostate gland. The vas deferens is enclosed within the spermatic cord, a compact bundle of vessels, nerves, and muscle fibers.

Prostate gland

Lying under the bladder and surrounding the urethra, the walnut-sized (approximately 1½″ [4 cm] in diameter) prostate gland consists of three lobes—the left and right lateral lobes and the median lobe. The prostate continuously secretes prostatic fluid—a thin, milky alkaline fluid. During sexual activity, prostatic fluid adds volume to the semen and enhances sperm motility and possibly fertility by neutralizing the acidity of the urethra and of the woman's vagina.

Inguinal structures

The spermatic cord travels from the testis through the inguinal canal, exiting the scrotum through the external inguinal ring and entering the abdominal cavity through the internal inguinal ring. The external inguinal ring is located just above and lateral to the pubic tubercle; the internal ring, about ½″ (1 cm) above the midpoint of the inguinal ligament, between the pubic tubercle of the symphysis pubis and the anterior superior iliac spine. Between the two rings lies the inguinal canal. Lymph nodes from the penis, scrotal surface, and anus drain into the inguinal lymph nodes. Lymph nodes from the testes drain into the perivenacaval nodes in the abdomen.

time may depend on how often the male ejaculates, but sperm can be stored and remain fertile for many weeks. After ejaculation, the life span of sperm is 24 to 72 hours at body temperature.

The number and motility of sperm affect fertility. A sperm count (the number of sperm in ejaculated semen) below 20 million per ml or poor motility of ejaculated sperm may cause infertility.

Hormonal control and sexual development

The male sex hormones, also known as androgens, are produced in the testes and the adrenal glands. The most significant male sex hormone—testosterone—is secreted by Leydig's cells, located in the testes between the seminiferous tubules. These cells become numerous during puberty, and remain in large numbers throughout life. Testosterone, which is responsible for the development and maintenance of male sex organs and secondary sex characteristics, is required for spermatogenesis.

Male sexuality also is affected by other hormones. Two of these—luteinizing hormone (LH), also known as interstitial cell-stimulating hormone, and follicle-stimulating hormone (FSH)—directly affect testosterone secretion. (For an explanation of this process, see *Regulation of male sex hormones*, page 447.)

Testosterone secretion begins in utero. Starting at approximately the second month of gestation, release of chorionic gonadotropins from the placenta stimulates Leydig's cells in the male fetus to secrete testosterone. Absence or presence of fetal testosterone directly affects sexual differentiation of the fetus. With testosterone, fetal genitalia will develop into a penis, scrotum, and other male organs; without testosterone, fetal genitalia will develop into a clitoris, vagina, and other female organs.

During the last 2 months of fetal life in utero, testosterone normally causes the testes to descend into the scrotum. If the testes are undescended after birth, administration of exogenous testosterone may correct the problem.

During early childhood, a boy does not secrete gonadotropins and consequently has little circulating testosterone. Pituitary secretion of gonadotropins—which usually occurs between ages 11 and 14—produces an increase in testicular function and testosterone secretion and marks the onset of puberty. During puberty, the penis and testes enlarge and the male reaches full adult sexual and reproductive capability. Puberty also marks the onset of male secondary sexual characteristics: distinct body hair distribution; skin changes, such as increased secretion by sweat and sebaceous glands; deepening of the voice from laryngeal enlargement; increased musculoskeletal development; and other intracellular and extracellular changes.

Understanding spermatogenesis

Spermatogenesis––the formation of mature sperm within the seminiferous tubules—occurs in several stages:

- Spermatogonia, the primary germinal epithelial cells, grow and develop into primary spermatocytes. Both spermatogonia and primary spermatocytes contain 46 chromosomes, consisting of 44 autosomes and the two sex chromosomes, X and Y.
- Primary spermatocytes divide to form secondary spermatocytes. No new chromosomes are formed in this stage—the pairs only divide. Each secondary spermatocyte contains half the number of autosomes, 22—one secondary spermatocyte contains an X chromosome; the other, a Y chromosome.
- Each secondary spermatocyte then divides again to form spermatids.
- Finally, the spermatids undergo a series of structural changes that transform them into mature spermatozoa, or sperm. Each spermatozoan is composed of a head, neck, body, and tail. The head contains the nucleus; the tail, a large amount of adenosine triphosphate (ATP), which provides energy for sperm motility.

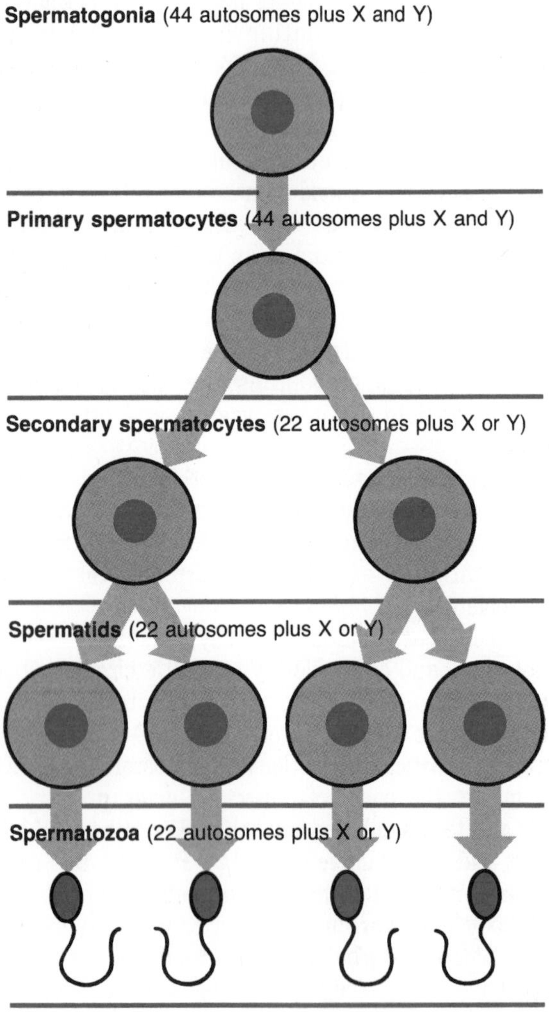

Spermatogonia (44 autosomes plus X and Y)

Primary spermatocytes (44 autosomes plus X and Y)

Secondary spermatocytes (22 autosomes plus X or Y)

Spermatids (22 autosomes plus X or Y)

Spermatozoa (22 autosomes plus X or Y)

After full physical maturity is reached—usually by age 20—sexual and reproductive function remain fairly consistent throughout the rest of life. Although a man normally should never lose the ability to reproduce, he may experience subtle changes in sexual function with aging. For example, an elderly man may require more time to achieve an erection, may experience less firm erections, may have reduced ejaculatory volume, and, after ejaculation, may take longer to regain an erection.

Health history

Interviewing a male client about his reproductive system requires sensitivity and tact, tempered with a professional approach. The initial goal should be to establish a rapport with the client so that he will relax and confide. An uncomfortable client may withhold valuable information.

One particularly sensitive area of questioning involves sexual performance. Many men tend to equate their sexual and reproductive functioning with their identities as men, and may view sexual problems as signs of diminished masculinity. Older men may view a decrease in sexual ability as a sign of lost youth and declining health.

A client having a problem with sexual function may be uncomfortable discussing it. Although further questioning is indicated to obtain an accurate picture of the problem, the nurse should remember to ask such questions in a sensitive manner and assure the client that his replies will be kept strictly confidential. To put such a client at ease, begin the interview with general questions regarding his health as it relates to the male reproductive system, then proceed to the more sensitive areas, reserving questions about sexual function until the end of the health history.

During the interview, keep in mind that each client has his own individual views on sexuality and reproduction, many of which may reflect cultural and religious background. To ensure accurate and useful history data, take these views into account and remain nonjudgmental and supportive.

While assessing the client's health and illness patterns, health promotion and protection patterns, and role and relationship patterns, use terminology that the client can understand. Medical terminology may be confusing, especially to a younger client, and may lead to misun-

Regulation of male sex hormones

In males, a negative feedback mechanism controls the release of sex hormones by stimulating the hypothalamus. In this system, the hypothalamus secretes substances—gonadotropin-releasing hormones (GnRH)—that stimulate the anterior pituitary. Once stimulated, the anterior pituitary releases luteinizing hormone (LH) and follicle-stimulating hormone (FSH). Both LH and FSH are found in plasma and urine as gonadotropins.

FSH acts on the germinal epithelial cells of the seminiferous tubules to promote complete spermatogenesis. LH acts on the Leydig's cells in the testes, causing these cells to mature and secrete testosterone—the hormone necessary for normal growth and development of male sex organs. Normal testosterone production develops and maintains the male secondary sex characteristics, such as thickened skin and increased growth of muscles and body hair.

Unlike the female hormonal cycle, male hormonal function is continuous and constant. When testosterone concentrations rise, the body sends negative feedback messages to the hypothalamus to keep testosterone levels stable.

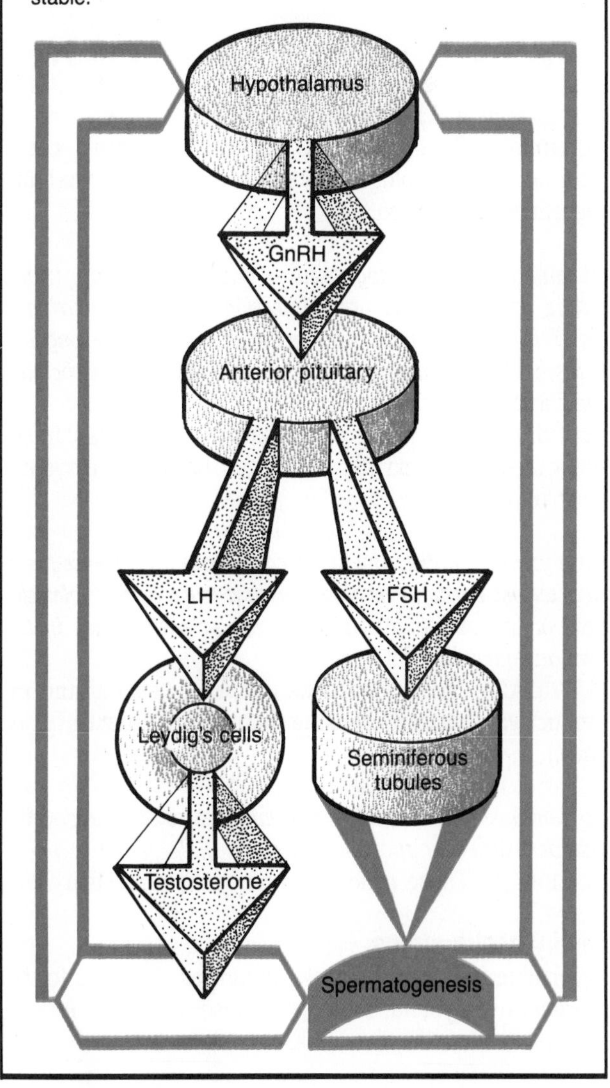

derstandings and inaccurate assessment findings. On the other hand, slang terms may project an undesirable image of informality and intimacy.

Health and illness patterns

Begin the health assessment by obtaining information about the client's health and illness patterns. To do so, explore the client's current, past, and family health status as well as developmental considerations.

Current health status

Because current health status is the client's most pressing concern, begin the health history by exploring this area. Using the *PQRST* method, ask the client to describe his chief complaint and any others. (For a detailed explanation of this method, see *Symptom analysis* in Chapter 3.) Be sure to document the client's description in his own words. To investigate the client's current health status further, ask the following questions about the male reproductive system:

Have you noticed any changes in the color of the skin on your penis or scrotum?
(RATIONALE: Reddened penile skin may indicate an inflammation; reddened scrotal skin could result from orchitis—inflammation of the testes. Dark blue to black discoloration may point to gangrene. Altered skin integrity may occur in sexually transmitted diseases, inflammatory disorders, and cancer. Small skin lumps on the scrotum may be sebaceous cysts.)

If you are uncircumcised, can you retract and replace the foreskin easily?
(RATIONALE: Inability to retract the prepuce [foreskin] from the glans penis [phimosis] sometimes occurs in uncircumcised men. Inability of the retracted prepuce to return to its normal position over the glans penis [paraphimosis] could, if untreated, impair local circulation and lead to edema and even gangrene of the glans penis.)

Have you noticed the appearance of a sore, lump, or ulcer on your penis?
(RATIONALE: Such findings may point to a sexually transmitted disease, an inflammatory disorder, or cancer.)

Have you noticed any discharge or bleeding from the opening where urine comes out?
(RATIONALE: Copious amounts of thick, yellowish discharge may indicate gonorrhea. Thin, watery discharge may point to nonspecific urethritis or prostatitis. Bloody discharge may indicate infection or cancer in the urinary or reproductive tract.)

Have you noticed any swelling in your scrotum?
(RATIONALE: Scrotal swelling may point to inguinal hernia, hematocele, epididymitis, or testicular tumor.)

Are you experiencing any pain in the penis, testes, or scrotal sac? If so, where? Does the pain radiate? If so, to where? What measures aggravate or relieve the pain? When does it occur?
(RATIONALE: Dull, aching pain in the scrotal sac may indicate inguinal hernia. Sudden onset of extremely sharp pain may point to testicular torsion. Sharp pain of more gradual onset usually indicates infection, such as orchitis or epididymitis.)

Have you felt a lump, painful sore, or tenderness in the groin?
(RATIONALE: These findings may point to a tumor or an infection.)

Do you get up during the night to urinate? Do you have urinary frequency, hesistancy, or dribbling; or pain in the area between your rectum and penis, hips, or lower back?
(RATIONALE: These signs and symptoms are especially significant in men over age 50; they may point to a prostate problem, such as benign prostatic hypertrophy or prostatic cancer.)

Do you have any difficulty achieving and maintaining an erection during sexual activity? If so, do you have erections at other times, such as on awakening?
(RATIONALE: The ability to achieve an erection is an important diagnostic clue in evaluating the cause of impotence.)

Do you have any difficulty with ejaculation?
(RATIONALE: Problems with ejaculation—such as premature, retarded [delayed], or retrograde [backward] ejaculation—may provide clues to the underlying cause of impotence or other sexual problems.)

Do you ever experience pain from erection or ejaculation?
(RATIONALE: Painful erection or ejaculation may point to inflammation in the genitourinary tract.)

What medications (prescribed, over-the-counter, and street drugs) do you take? At what dosage and for what reason?
(RATIONALE: Certain medications can interfere with reproductive system function. For more information, see *Adverse drug reactions.*)

Past health status

Continue data collection by questioning the client about any past health problems. This information is important because other body system dysfunction or past reproductive system problems may affect the present condition of the reproductive system. Important questions to include in this part of the assessment are:

Have you fathered any children? If so, how many and what are their ages? Have you ever had a problem with infertility? Is it a current concern?
(RATIONALE: If infertility is a problem, further exploration will be required. This is best done by a professional who specializes in this field.)

Have you ever had surgery on the genitourinary tract or for a hernia? If so, where, when, and why? Did you experience any complications after surgery?
(RATIONALE: Surgery may predispose the client to adhesions or may alter reproductive structure and function.)

Have you ever experienced trauma to the genitourinary tract? If so, what happened, when did it occur, and what if any symptoms have developed as a result?
(RATIONALE: Trauma to the genitourinary tract could alter normal physiologic processes and affect sexual and reproductive function.)

Have you ever been diagnosed as having a sexually transmitted disease or any other infection in the genitourinary tract? If so, what was the specific problem? How long did it last? What treatment was provided? Did any associated complications develop?
(RATIONALE: Depending on its nature and course, infection can cause infertility and other reproductive system abnormalities.)

Have you had diabetes mellitus, cardiovascular disease (such as arteriosclerosis), neurologic disease (such as multiple sclerosis or amyotropic lateral sclerosis), or malignancy in the genitourinary tract?
(RATIONALE: These conditions can affect sexual and reproductive function, causing impotence, infertility, or both.)

Do you have a history of undescended testes or an endocrine disorder, such as hypogonadism?
(RATIONALE: These conditions may cause infertility.)

Family health status

Determine the client's family history as it relates to the reproductive system, looking for disorders with known familial tendencies. Questions to ask include:

Adverse drug reactions

When obtaining a health history to assess a male client's reproductive system, the nurse should ask about current drug use. Several drugs affect male reproductive system function, producing erectile difficulties and associated adverse reactions.

DRUG CLASS	DRUG	POSSIBLE ADVERSE REACTIONS
Anticonvulsants	carbamazepine, primidone	Impotence
Antidepressants	amitriptyline hydrochloride, amoxapine, desipramine hydrochloride, doxepin hydrochloride, imipramine hydrochloride, maprotiline hydrochloride, nortriptyline	Increased or decreased libido, impotence, testicular swelling
	trazadone	Priapism, impotence, decreased or increased libido, retrograde ejaculation
	isocarboxazid, phenelzine, tranylcypromine sulfate	Transient impotence
Antihypertensives	clonidine hydrochloride, methyldopa, nadolol, reserpine	Decreased libido, impotence; ejaculatory failure (methyldopa only)
	guanabenz	Impotence
	prazosin hydrochloride	Impotence, priapism
Beta blockers	atenolol, propranolol hydrochloride, labetolol, timolol maleate, nadolol, pindolol, metoprolol	Decreased libido, ejaculatory failure, impotence; priapism (labetolol only)
Antipsychotics	chlorpromazine hydrochloride, fluphenazine, perphenazine, prochlorperazine, thioridazine hydrochloride, thiothixene, haloperidol	Priapism, impotence, change in libido
Benzodiazepines	alprazolam, clonazepam, chlordiazepoxide, diazepam, flurazepam hydrochloride, lozazepam	Increased or decreased libido
Anticholinergics	atropine sulfate, belladonna alkaloids, glycopyrrolate, hyoscyamine, propantheline bromide	Impotence
Androgenic steroids	fluoxymesterone, methyltestosterone, testosterone	Increased or decreased libido, oligospermia, decreased ejaculatory volume, priapism or excessive sexual stimulation, testicular atrophy, impotence
	danazol	Testicular atrophy
Corticosteroids	beclomethasone, betamethosone, cortisone, dexamethasone, flunisolide, hydrocortisone, meprednisone, methylprednisolone, paramethasone, prednisolone, prednisone, triamcinolone	Possibly increased or decreased motility and number of sperm when administered over a prolonged period
Miscellaneous agents	spinonolactone	Decreased libido, impotence

Has anyone in your family had infertility problems?
(RATIONALE: Infertility often has a familial tendency.)

Has anyone in your family had a hernia?
(RATIONALE: Hernias also tend to occur in families.)

Developmental considerations

If the client is young or elderly, be sure to investigate developmental status by exploring the areas described below.

Pediatric client. When assessing a male child, try to involve both the child and the parent or guardian in the interview. Obviously, the parent or guardian will answer for an infant or very young child. Questions to ask include:

Did the mother use any hormones during pregnancy?
(RATIONALE: Some hormones taken during pregnancy can have an adverse effect on the development of a male child's reproductive system.)

If the child is uncircumcised, what hygienic measures do you use?
(RATIONALE: Poor hygiene increases the risk of infection under the prepuce.)

Do you notice any scrotal swelling when the child cries or has a bowel movement?
(RATIONALE: This finding may point to an inguinal hernia.)

Did the child exhibit any genitourinary abnormalities at birth? If so, what if any treatment was received?
(RATIONALE: If uncorrected, congenital defects such as hypospadias and epispadias can lead to further problems.)

Adolescent client. When interviewing an adolescent, determine his knowledge of sexual and reproductive function and his level of sexual development by asking the following questions:

Do you have pubic hair? If so, at what age did it appear?
(RATIONALE: Normally, pubic hair appears between ages 12 and 14, usually indicating normal sexual development.)

How would you describe your sexual activity?
(RATIONALE: This question gives the adolescent client the opportunity to ask questions and express concerns about sexual function. It also allows the nurse to share information and clear up any misconceptions the client may have.)

If you are sexually active, do you use condoms for intercourse?
(RATIONALE: This question elicits information on the adolescent client's knowledge of contraception and prevention of sexually transmitted diseases. It also gives the nurse a chance to teach the client about the proper use of prophylactics for these purposes.)

Elderly client.
When interviewing an elderly client, ask questions that elicit information about changes in sexual patterns.

Have you experienced any change in your frequency of or desire for sex?
(RATIONALE: Depression, loss of partner, or physical illness may cause these changes.)

Have you noticed any changes in your sexual performance?
(RATIONALE: Such physiologic changes as slower and less-firm erections, longer time required to reach orgasm, and decreased ejaculatory volume normally occur with age or may result from use of certain drugs or from physical illness.)

Health promotion and protection patterns

Continue the health history by eliciting information about the client's life-style to determine his risk of trauma or disease to the reproductive system.

Do you examine your testes periodically? Have you been taught the proper procedure?
(RATIONALE: Testicular cancer, the most common form of cancer in males between ages 15 and 30, is treated most successfully after early detection. For more information, see *Testicular self-examination*.)

If you are sexually active, do you have more than one partner?
(RATIONALE: Having multiple sex partners increases the risk of acquiring sexually transmitted disease.)

Do you take any precautions to prevent contracting sexually transmitted disease or acquired immunodeficiency syndrome (AIDS)? If so, what do you do?
(RATIONALE: Take this opportunity to discuss measures for preventing these disorders, such as use of condoms during intercourse and avoiding exchange of body fluids during any sexual activity.)

What is your job?
(RATIONALE: Certain occupations—for example, construction or assembly-line work with heavy machinery—put a client at increased risk for genital injury.)

Testicular self-examination

To help detect abnormalities early, every male should examine his testes once a month. Instruct the client to follow this procedure:

1 If possible, take a warm bath or shower before beginning; the scrotum, which tends to contract when cold, will be relaxed, making the testes easier to examine.

2 With one hand, lift the penis and check the scrotum (the sac containing the testes) for any change in shape, size, or color. The left side of the scrotum normally hangs slightly lower than the right.

3 Next, check the testes for lumps and masses. Locate the crescent-shaped structure at the back of each testis. This is the epididymis, which should feel soft.

4 Use the thumb and first two fingers of your left hand to squeeze the spermatic cord gently; it extends upward from the epididymis, above the left testis. Then repeat on the right side, using your right hand. Check for lumps and masses by palpating along the entire length of the cord.

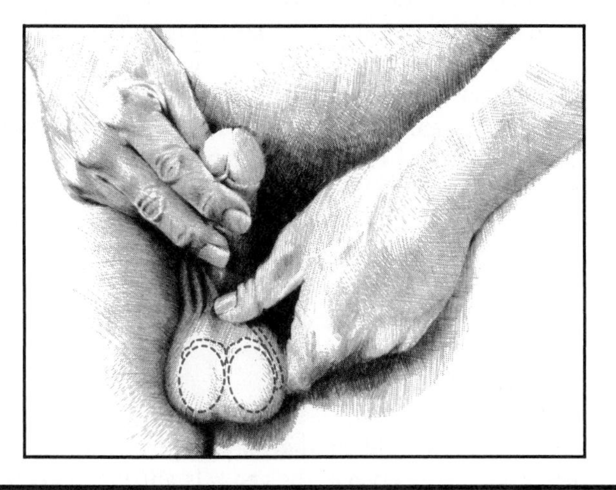

5 Next, examine each testis. To do so, place the index and middle fingers on its underside and the thumb on top, then gently roll the testis between the thumb and fingers. A normal testis is egg-shaped, rubbery-firm, and movable within the scrotum; it should feel smooth, with no lumps. Both testes should be the same size.

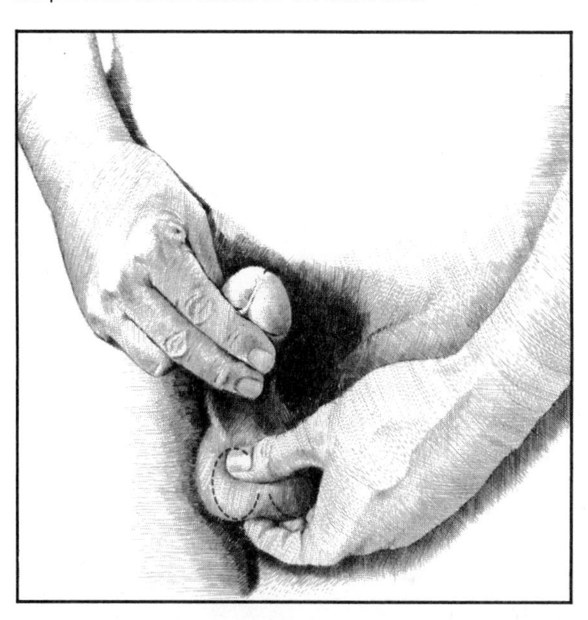

6 Promptly report any lumps, masses, or changes to the physician.

Are you now or have you been exposed to radiation or toxic chemicals?
(RATIONALE: Such exposure may increase the client's risk of developing infertility or testicular cancer.)

Do you engage in sports or in any activity that requires heavy lifting or straining? If so, do you wear any protective or supportive devices such as a jock strap, protective cup, or truss?
(RATIONALE: Any activity involving heavy lifting or abdominal straining can increase the risk of hernia formation. Certain sports activities—for example, playing the catcher's position in a baseball or softball game—can predispose the client to genital trauma.)

Would you describe yourself as being under a lot of stress?
(RATIONALE: Stress can adversely affect sexual and reproductive function.)

Role and relationship patterns

Conclude the data collection by obtaining information about the client's role and relationship patterns.

What is your self-image? Do you consider yourself attractive to others?
(RATIONALE: A poor self-image and lack of self-confidence can predispose a client to sexual dysfunction.)

What is your cultural and religious background? Do any cultural or religious factors affect your beliefs or practices regarding sexuality and reproduction?
(RATIONALE: Knowledge of the client's cultural and religious beliefs may help explain normal variants and identify potential risk factors; for example, an increased risk of contracting AIDS or a sexually transmitted disease if use of condoms is prohibited for cultural or religious reasons.)

Do you have a supportive relationship with another person?
(RATIONALE: Problems with family or other relationships can produce stress, which in turn can cause sexual dysfunction.)

Are your sexual practices heterosexual, homosexual, or bisexual?
(RATIONALE: The answer to this question provides information about the client's possible risk level for certain sexually transmitted diseases and forewarns of certain sexual practices that can injure the anal sphincter, which may be noted during the physical assessment.)

If you are experiencing sexual difficulty, is it affecting your emotional and social relationships?
(RATIONALE: Feelings of emotional or social isolation can increase stress, which in turn can exacerbate sexual dysfunction.)

Physical assessment

After the health history, the nurse should perform a complete physical assessment of the client's reproductive system. This assessment should cover four major areas: a general inspection of the groin; inspection and palpation of the penis and scrotum; inspection and palpation of the groin to detect any hernias; and palpation of the prostate gland in men over age 50 and in other men with probable prostate problems.

Preparing for physical assessment

Before beginning the physical assessment, wash your hands and gather the following equipment: gloves, water-soluble lubricant, and a flashlight.

Instruct the client to urinate before assessment begins (to reduce discomfort from a full bladder) and to undress to expose the groin area. (If the client wishes, he may wear a gown to prevent unnecessary exposure.)

Because reproductive system assessment involves exposure and handling of the genitals, the client may feel anxious and embarrassed. To help minimize such discomfort, explain each assessment step before performing it and expose only the necessary areas. Remember that for any client to feel comfortable during physical assessment, the nurse also must feel at ease and project a calm, professional demeanor. If the client detects that the nurse is uncomfortable, he will tend to feel the same.

Some men may object to being examined by a female. If the client is uncomfortable in such a situation, a female nurse might defer to a male nurse or physician.

In some instances, a client may attempt to relieve his embarrassment by using language that a female nurse may find offensive. If this occurs, the nurse should continue the assessment in a professional manner. If the situation should escalate to the point that the female nurse feels threatened, the assessment should then be deferred to a male nurse or physician.

A sexually related disease of great concern to all health care professionals is AIDS. Homosexual men and intravenous drug users, two high-risk groups, are entitled to the same assessment and nursing care as other persons. Many of these clients live in almost constant fear of acquiring AIDS. They are aware that many health care professionals do not feel comfortable touching them, particularly their genitals. When assessing such a client, make an extra effort to maintain a professional, nonjudgmental attitude and demeanor.

Inspection

Physical assessment of the male reproductive system begins with inspection of the genitals and inguinal area. Be sure to put on gloves before starting.

Penis

Inspection of the penis should start with an evaluation of the color and integrity of the penile skin. Over the shaft, the skin should appear loose and wrinkled; over the glans penis, taut and smooth. The skin should be pink to light brown in Caucasians and light to dark brown in Blacks, and free of scars, lesions, ulcers, or breaks of any kind.

If the client is uncircumcised, ask him to retract his prepuce to allow inspection of the glans penis. Normally, the client should be able to retract the prepuce with ease, revealing a glans with no ulcers or lesions, and then easily replace it over the glans after inspection. A white substance (smegma) may be present.

The urethral meatus, a slit-like opening, should be located at the tip of the glans. Inspection of the urethral meatus should reveal no discharge.

Scrotum

Inspection of the scrotum should begin with evaluation of the amount, distribution, color, and texture of pubic hair. Pubic hair should cover the symphysis pubis and scrotum.

Next, inspect the scrotal skin for obvious lesions, ulcerations, induration, or reddened areas, and evaluate the sac for size and symmetry. The scrotal skin should be coarse and more deeply pigmented than the body skin. The left testicle usually hangs slightly lower than the right; both should hang freely in the scrotum.

Inguinal area

Inspect the inguinal area for obvious bulges—a sign of hernias. Then ask the client to bear down as if passing a stool as you inspect again. (Bearing down increases intra-abdominal pressure, which pushes any herniation downward and makes it more easily visible.)

Abnormal findings

Inspection of the penis may reveal lesions or similar problems. If so, document the location, size, and color of any lesions as well as the presence of any exudate. Lesions may indicate a sexually transmitted disease. Inspection of the prepuce of an uncircumcized client may reveal phimosis (abnormal tightness of the prepuce that prevents its retraction from the glans penis) or paraphimosis (strangulation of the glans penis caused by a prepuce that will not return over the glans).

Inspection of the urethral meatus may detect epispadias (a congenital defect involving opening of the urethral meatus on the dorsal surface of the penis), hypospadias (a congenital defect involving opening of the urethral meatus on the ventral surface of the penis), or a discharge. If discharge is present, obtain a smear to send for culture and sensitivity testing. Discharge indicates infection and possibly a sexually transmitted disease, such as gonorrhea.

On inspection of the scrotum, note absence of pubic hair or presence of bald spots; these are abnormal. So are lesions, ulcers, induration, or reddened areas, which may indicate an infection or inflammation. Absence of pubic hair may indicate a vascular or hormonal problem.

Inspection of the inguinal area may reveal obvious bulging, which may indicate a hernia.

Palpation

After inspection, palpate the penis and scrotum for structural abnormalities; then palpate the inguinal area for hernias.

Penis

To palpate the penis, gently grasp the shaft between the thumb and first two fingers and palpate along its entire length, noting any indurated, tender, or lumpy areas. The nonerect penis should feel soft and free of nodules.

Scrotum

Like the penis, the scrotum can be palpated using the thumb and first two fingers. Palpation begins with examination of the scrotal skin by feeling its rough, wrinkled surface for nodules, lesions, or ulcers.

Normally, the right and left halves of the scrotal sac are identical in content and feel the same. The testes are felt as separate, freely movable oval masses low in the scrotal sac. Their surface should feel smooth and even in contour. Slight compression of the testes should elicit a dull, aching sensation that radiates to the client's lower abdomen. This pressure-pain sensation should not occur when the other structures are compressed. No other pain or tenderness should be present.

Absence of a testis may result from temporary migration. The cremasteric muscle surrounding the testicles contracts in response to certain stimuli, such as cold air, cold water, or touching the inner thigh. This contraction raises the contents of the scrotum toward the inguinal canal. When the muscle relaxes, the scrotal contents resume their normal position. This temporary migration is normal, and may occur throughout the course of the assessment.

The epididymis is palpated on the posterolateral surface by grasping each testicle between the thumb and forefinger and palpating up from the epididymis to the spermatic cord or vas deferens up to the inguinal ring. The epididymis should palpate as a ridge of tissue lying vertically on the testicular surface. The vas deferens should feel like a smooth cord and be freely movable. The arteries, veins, lymph vessels, and nerves, which are located next to the vas deferens, may be felt as indefinite threads.

Any lumps, nodular areas, or areas of swelling should be transilluminated. To perform this technique, darken the room, then hold a flashlight behind the scrotum and direct its beam through the mass. If the swollen area contains serous fluid, it will transilluminate, marked by an orange-red glow; if the area contains blood

Applying the nursing process

Assessment findings form the basis of the nursing process. Using them, the nurse formulates nursing diagnoses and develops appropriate planning, implementation, and evaluation of the client's care.

The table shows how the nurse can use male reproductive system assessment data in the nursing process for the client described in the case history (shown at right). In the first column, history and physical assessment data appear, followed by a paragraph of mental notes. These notes help the nurse make important mental connections among assessment findings, aiding in development of the nursing diagnoses and planning.

The second column presents several appropriate nursing diagnoses; however, the information in the remaining three columns is based on the *first* nursing diagnosis. Although it is not part of the nursing process, documentation appears in the last column because of its importance. Documentation consists of an initial note using all components of the SOAPIE format and a follow-up note using the appropriate SOAPIE components.

ASSESSMENT	NURSING DIAGNOSES	PLANNING	IMPLEMENTATION
Subjective (history) data • Client states, "I have a sore on my penis, I can't believe it! About a month ago, I was at a party where I had sex with a woman named Sheila. After the party was over, the guys told me they thought Sheila was dirty." • Client states, "I don't have any trouble urinating, but I'm afraid the sore is a sign of syphilis." • Client reports no sexual contacts since the fraternity party. **Objective (physical) data** • Vital signs: Blood pressure 138/88, temperature 99° F. (37.2° C.), pulse 100 and regular, respirations 24 and regular. • Young, anxious male—wringing hands and pacing. • Inspection reveals an oval indurated ulcer, with raised edges and clear exudate. • Palpation reveals firm, enlarged inguinal lymph nodes bilaterally about 1 cm in diameter, freely movable. • Laboratory culture of ulcer exudate is positive for syphilis. **Mental notes** *Penile sore is typical of syphilitic chancre. Will need to ask Sheila and others who have had contact with her to come to the health clinic for evaluation and treatment, if necessary.*	• Anxiety related to penile ulcer. • Fear related to infectious process in reproductive system. • Disturbance in self-concept and body image related to penile ulcer. • Impaired tissue integrity related to penile ulcer.	**Goals** By the time of the first follow-up visit, the client will: • describe the basics of the transmission of and treatment for syphilis. • verbalize fears and anxieties about being infected with syphilis. • explain the importance of using condoms during intercourse. • provide the names of other individuals who may be infected.	• Client given written pamphlets describing syphilis. • Client shown videotape about syphilis. • Explained to client the importance of examinations for Shelia and others who had sexual contact with her.

or tissue, it will not. A lump or mass anywhere in the scrotal sac should be described according to its placement, size, shape, consistency, tenderness, and response to transillumination.

Inguinal area

After assessing the penis and scrotum, palpate the client's inguinal area for hernias—protrusion of the bowel through the abdominal wall into the inguinal or femoral canal or, in some cases, into the scrotum. (For more information, see *Palpating for hernias in the inguinal area,* page 456.)

Abnormal findings

On palpation, the penis may have indurated, tender, or lumpy areas, which may indicate Peyronie's disease—characterized by a fibrous band in the corpus cavernosum.

The scrotum may have surface nodules, which may be sebaceous cysts. Abnormal pain or tenderness may be caused by an inflammation, such as orchitis or epididymitis.

CASE HISTORY

Mr. Tom Sloan, age 20, is a single college student who has come to the university health care clinic because of a sore on his penis.

EVALUATION	DOCUMENTATION BASED ON NURSING PROCESS DATA			
		Initial		**Follow-up**
At the first follow-up visit: • the client described the transmission of and treatment for syphilis. • the client was less anxious about ulcer on penis. • the client verbalized the importance of using condoms. • the client said he would encourage Shelia and his friends to come to the clinic for evaluation and treatment, if needed.	**S**	Client states, "I have a sore on my penis. I don't have any trouble urinating, but I'm afraid the sore is a sign of syphilis."	**S**	Client states, "I spoke to my friends who were at this party and they're scared and worried. Does this information go to our parents?"
	O	Anxious client with oval ulcer on top of penile shaft. Ulcer is indurated with raised edges; clear exudate. Enlarged inguinal lymph nodes bilaterally on palpation, 1 cm in diameter, firm, freely movable. Laboratory report is positive for syphilis.	**O**	Client anxious. Ulcer healing. Inguinal lymph nodes not palpable.
	A	Anxiety related to penile ulcer. Client is upset with himself and worried about what others will think.	**A**	Encourage client to assure his friends that test results are confidential, and encourage them to come to the clinic for treatment.
	P	Teach client about disease to reduce anxiety. Teach the importance of condom use. Ascertain which other students were involved.	**P**	Teach general student body about venereal diseases and assist those who wish to be tested. Provide information about sexually transmitted diseases that client can post on dormitory bulletin boards.
	I	Client provided with film and written literature on syphilis and use of condoms. Discussed with client the need to treat other involved parties.		
	E	Client verbalizes correct information concerning syphilis and use of condoms. Reluctant to provide information on other participants.		

Absence of a testis may be from congenital maldescent, or cryptorchidism. In this condition, one or both testes fail to descend from the abdomen into the scrotal sac. Fixed or tender areas in the scrotum may indicate a testicular tumor.

In males of any age-group, palpation of the inguinal area may reveal three major types of hernias. An *indirect inguinal hernia* occurs when the herniation enters the internal inguinal canal, possibly descending into the scrotum. A *direct inguinal hernia* develops when the herniation penetrates the inguinal canal through an abnormal opening in the abdominal wall. A *femoral hernia* occurs in the femoral canal, a potential space located below the inguinal ligament lateral to the pubic tubercle. (For some common abnormal assessment findings associated with the male reproductive system, see *Integrating assessment findings,* page 457.)

Developmental considerations

While assessing a client's reproductive system, keep in mind important developmental considerations. Although

Palpating for hernias in the inguinal area

The nurse should palpate the inguinal area for inguinal and femoral hernias during assessment of the male reproductive system.

Palpating for inguinal hernias

To palpate a client's inguinal area for hernias, the nurse first should place the index and middle finger of each hand over each external inguinal ring and ask the client to bear down or cough to increase intra-abdominal pressure momentarily. Then, with the client relaxed, proceed as follows: Gently insert the middle or index finger (if the client is an adult) or the little finger (if the client is a young child) into the scrotal sac and follow the spermatic cord upward to the external inguinal ring, to an opening just above and lateral to the pubic tubercle known as Hesselbach's triangle. Holding the finger at this spot, ask the client to bear down or cough again. A hernia will palpate as a mass or bulge.

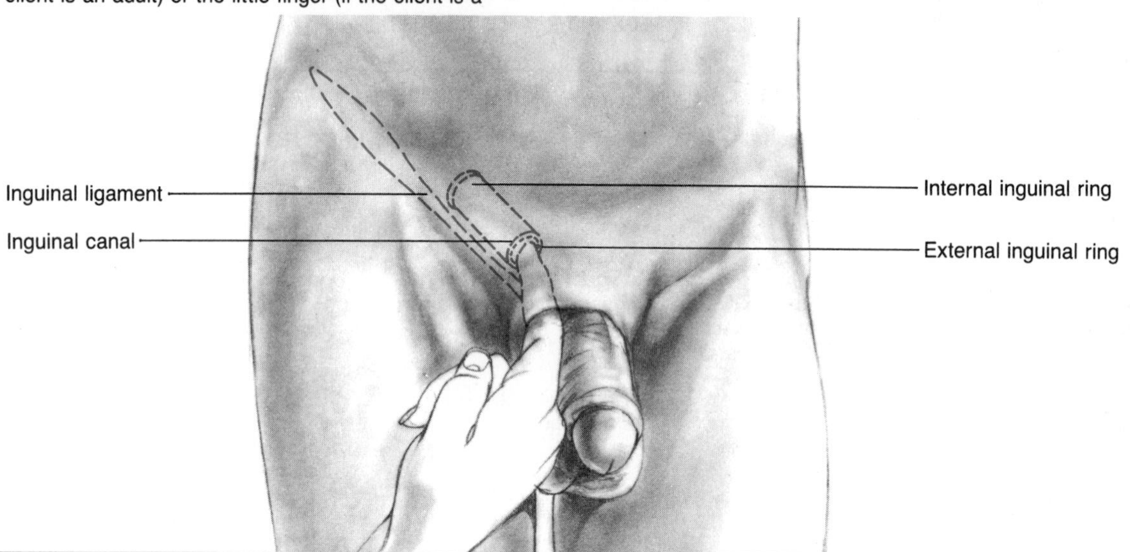

Palpating for femoral hernias

To palpate for a femoral hernia, place the right hand on the client's thigh with the index finger over the femoral artery. The femoral canal is then under the ring finger in an adult client and between the index and ring finger in a child. A hernia here will palpate as a soft bulge or mass.

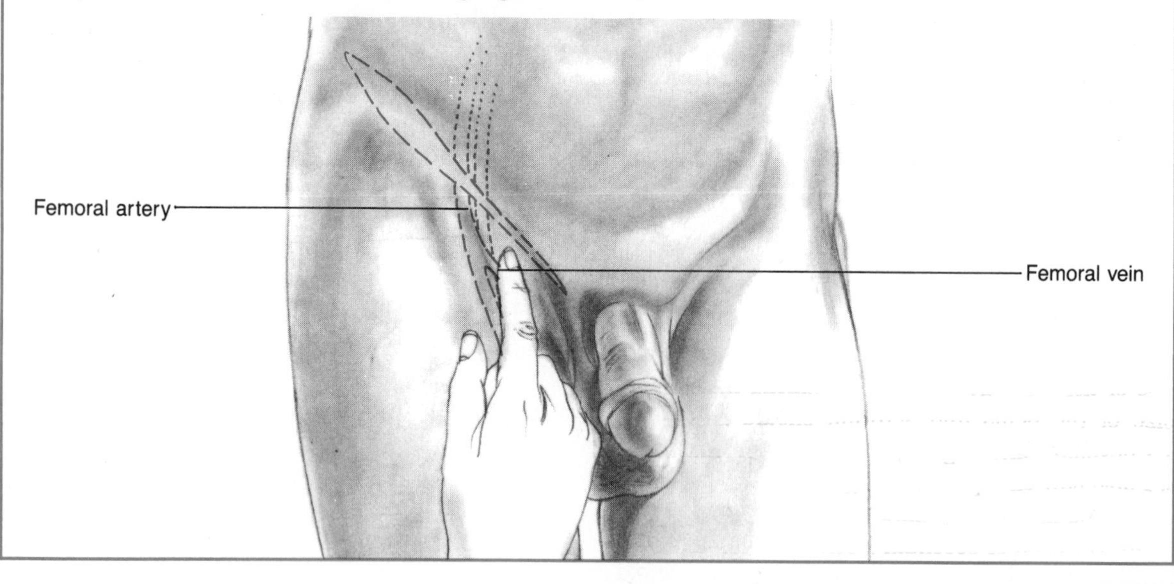

Integrating assessment findings

Sometimes, a cluster of assessment findings will strongly suggest a particular male reproductive system disorder. In the chart below, column one shows groups of presenting signs and symptoms—the ones that make the client seek medical attention. Column two shows related assessment findings that the nurse may discover during the health history and physical assessment. The client may have one or more of these related findings. Column three shows the possible disorder indicated by a cluster of these findings.

PRESENTING SIGNS AND SYMPTOMS	RELATED ASSESSMENT FINDINGS	POSSIBLE DISORDER
Changes in urination pattern, such as hesitancy, incontinence with dribbling, reduced caliber and force of urine stream, and possibly retention	Enlarged, firm, slightly elastic, smooth, possible tender prostate Client over age 50 Burning on urination if accompanied by urinary tract infection	Benign prostatic hypertrophy
Painful genital lesions that recur	Fever Painful, tender scrotal or inguinal mass Tender, enlarged inguinal lymph nodes Possible dysuria Sexual contact with an infected partner	Genital herpes
Large scrotal or inguinal mass, possibly painful and tender, that appears translucent on transillumination	Recent scrotal infection, particularly epididymitis Infant or adult client	Hydrocele
Scrotal or inguinal mass; unilateral or bilateral scrotal swelling, with pain and tenderness	Fever Possible nausea and vomiting Recent infection, especially epididymitis or mumps Impotence Possible infertility	Orchitis
Changes in urination pattern, such as frequency, urgency, hesitancy and nocturia; dysuria and lower back pain; penile discharge and thin, watery, possibly blood-tinged semen	Enlarged, tender, boggy prostate (firm in chronic cases) Fever and chills Diminished libido and impotence Recent urinary tract infection Possible infertility	Prostatitis
Sore on penis, sore on or near anal canal	Single or multiple eroded papules Palpated lesion feels cartilagenous Bisexual or homosexual activity with someone who has anal lesion Bilateral inguinal node enlargement	Primary syphilis
Painful, constant erection without sexual desire	Erect penis History of sickle cell anemia History of spinal cord lesion	Priapism
Dysuria (painful urination), urinary frequency, dripping from tip of penis	Swollen urethral meatus White or yellow discharge from urethral meatus Thrombophlebitis of the dorsal penile vein Culture of discharge positive for *Neisseria gonorrhoeae*	Gonorrhea

the size of the male genitals varies among individuals, the size of the penis and scrotum should match the client's developmental age, as should other characteristics. Pubic hair on a preschool-aged child or extremely small genitals in an adult male should be recognized as abnormal. Absence of secondary sex characteristics after puberty is abnormal, as are secondary sex characteristics before puberty.

The genitals change in appearance throughout the life span. In an infant, the scrotum is pink, small, and wrinkled, with a well-defined median raphe (seam of union of the two halves). Both testes should be easily palpated in the scrotal sac at birth. The penis should appear pink and smooth. In neonates, small white cysts

ADVANCED ASSESSMENT SKILLS

Palpating the prostate gland

Because palpation of the prostate usually is uncomfortable and may embarrass the client, the nurse should begin by explaining the procedure and reassuring the client that the procedure should not be painful.

To palpate the prostate, follow these steps:

1 Have the client urinate to empty the bladder and reduce discomfort during the examination.

2 Ask the client to stand at the end of the examination table, with his elbows flexed and his upper body resting on the table. If the client cannot assume this position because he is unable to stand, have him lie on his left side with his right knee and hip flexed or with both knees drawn up toward his chest.

3 Wear a sterile glove on your examining hand and apply water-soluble lubricant to the gloved index finger.

4 Inspect the skin of the perineal, anal, and posterior scrotal surfaces. The skin should appear smooth and unbroken, with no protruding masses.

5 Introduce the gloved, lubricated index finger into the rectum, pad down. Instruct the client to relax to ease passage of the finger through the anal sphincter.

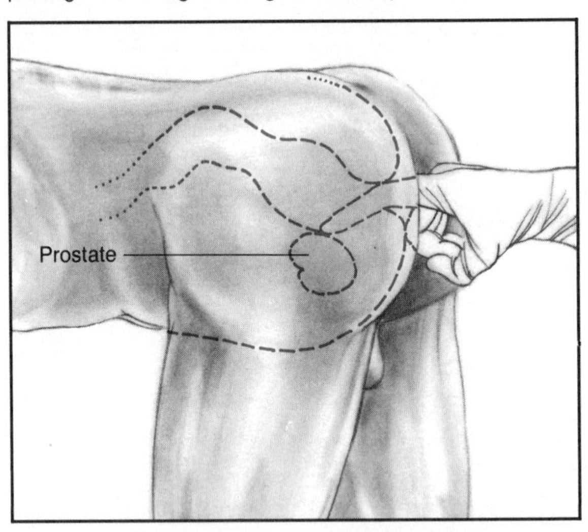

6 Using the pad of the index finger, palpate the prostate on the anterior rectal wall, located just past the anorectal ring. The prostate should feel smooth and rubbery. Normal size varies, but usually is about the size of a walnut. The prostate should not protrude into the rectal lumen. The proximal portions of the seminal vesicles sometimes may be palpated above the superolateral to midpoint section of the gland as corrugated structures.

on the distal prepuce are considered a normal finding. In an uncircumcised infant, the prepuce usually is tight for 2 to 3 months after birth. It does not retract easily but should retract enough to allow urine to flow freely from the urinary meatus. When assessing an uncircumcised infant, retract the prepuce only enough to expose the urethral meatus. Forced retraction may cause tearing of the prepuce from the glans. (By age 3 or 4, the child's prepuce should be completely retractable.) If an infant has been circumcised, the penis may appear reddened.

During infancy, any congenital malformations, such as epispadias (urethral opening on dorsal side of penis), hypospadias (urethral opening on ventral side of penis), or cryptorchidism (undescended testes), should be detected.

Throughout childhood, the scrotum and penis remain hairless and pink. The genitals grow in proportion to the child, but usually remain rather small.

During puberty, the genitals enlarge and develop and the secondary sex characteristics appear, including pubic hair and typical male facial and body hair distribution.

By the end of puberty, the male reaches full adult sexual appearance and functional capability.

After full maturity is reached, the genitals do not change much in appearance until the male reaches about age 50. At this point, several changes may start to develop: the pubic hair turns grey or white, and the scrotal skin becomes less taut over the testes, giving the scrotum a more pendulous appearance.

Advanced assessment

Prostate palpation usually is done by a physician as part of a rectal assessment. However, if the client has not scheduled a separate rectal assessment, the nurse may

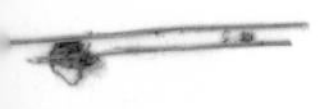

palpate the prostate during the reproductive system assessment. (For a detailed explanation, see *Advanced assessment skills: Palpating the prostate gland.*)

Tenderness, asymmetry, enlargement, bogginess, rough or nodular surface, and protrusion of the gland into the rectum represent significant abnormal findings of prostate palpation. When enlargement is present, determine the degree and classify according to the following categories:

- Grade I—less than 1 cm protrusion into the rectum
- Grade II—1 to 2 cm protrusion into the rectum
- Grade III—2 to 3 cm protrusion into the rectum
- Grade IV—greater than 3 cm protrusion into the rectum

In benign prostatic hypertrophy, a relatively common disorder in men age 50 and older, the prostate is enlarged, protrudes into the rectum, and feels soft, boggy (nonfirm, mushy), and nontender.

In prostatic cancer, also common in men over age 50, palpation typically reveals a hard, fixed, firm prostate or a fixed lesion on the prostate.

Common laboratory studies

For a male client with signs and symptoms of a reproductive system problem, various laboratory studies can provide valuable clues to the possible cause, as shown in the chart below. (*Note*: Keep in mind that abnormal findings may stem from a problem unrelated to the male reproductive system.) Remember that values differ between laboratories, and check the normal value range for the specific laboratory.

TEST AND SIGNIFICANCE	NORMAL VALUES OF FINDINGS	ABNORMAL FINDINGS	POSSIBLE CAUSES OF ABNORMAL FINDINGS
Semen tests			
Semen analysis This test quantifies the number of sperm in a semen sample to evaluate fertility.	60 to 150 million/ml	Below-normal level	Male infertility
Blood tests			
Serum alpha-fetoprotein By measuring the glycoprotein produced by tumors, this test helps detect testicular cancer and monitors the effectiveness of cancer treatment.	<30 ng/ml	Above-normal level	Testicular cancer, ineffective treatment
Venereal disease research laboratory (VDRL) test This test screens for or confirms diagnosis of syphilis.	Nonreactive	Reactive	Syphilis
Serum acid phosphatase By measuring the phosphatase enzymes produced by prostatic tumors, this test helps detect prostatic cancer.	0 to 1.1 Bodansky unit/ml; 1 to 4 king Am strong units/ml; 0.13 to 0.63 Bessey-Lowery-Brock units/ml	Above-normal levels	Prostatic cancer
Urine tests			
Divided urine test This test detects bacteria in prostatic fluid or a urine sample.	Absence of bacteria	Presence of bacteria	Prostatitis
Culture and sensitivity Using a common culture medium, this test detects infectious microorganisms in exudate, urine, or lesions.	Absence of infectious microorganisms	Presence of infectious microorganisms	Infection of kidney, bladder, or urethra

Documentation

Before documenting assessment findings, the nurse should use the following guidelines to review and integrate the data collected from the health history and physical assessment. The review of data should include any laboratory and diagnostic studies ordered by the physician. (For a summary of typical laboratory studies, see *Common laboratory studies,* page 459.) Along with history and physical findings, these results can provide a clear picture of the client's clinical status.

Gathering assessment data may be considered the first step in the nursing process. Based on these data, formulate appropriate nursing diagnoses—the basis for planning, implementing, and evaluating the client's nursing care. (For a case study that shows how to apply the nursing process to a male client with a reproductive system disorder, see *Applying the nursing process,* pages 454 and 455.)

After completing the assessment, document the findings in a clear, concise, and comprehensive manner. The following example shows how to document some normal physical assessment findings:

> Normal male pubic hair distribution. Penis circumcised; no lesions, inflammation, or structural alterations; urethral opening patent. Testes descended and symmetrical without redness, masses, or tenderness. Prostate small and nontender.

The following example shows how to document some abnormal physical assessment findings:

> Normal male pubic hair distribution. Testes descended; no scrotal masses. Circumcised penis with two small raised vesicles on lip of circumcised fold; no penile discharge. Rectal assessment elicits pain and reveals firm, enlarged, tender, boggy prostate gland.

Be sure to document the other nursing process steps—nursing diagnoses, planning, implementation, and evaluation—as they are applied for a client with a reproductive system disorder.

Chapter summary

Effective assessment of the male reproductive system requires a complete health history and physical assessment, and, in some cases, analysis of pertinent laboratory test results. Chapter 16 discusses how to gather and integrate this information. Here are the chapter highlights:

- Male reproductive system structures include the penis, scrotum, prostate gland, and inguinal structures.
- The penis functions to eliminate urine and, when erect, as the male sex organ.
- The scrotum and its contents, including the testes, produce sperm and male sex hormones (primarily testosterone).
- Testosterone affects sperm production, sexual function, and the development of male secondary sexual characteristics, such as growth of facial and body hair, increased muscle mass, and deepened voice.
- To ensure accurate and complete assessment findings, the client and the nurse must be comfortable with discussing sexual and reproductive function and assessing the genitalia and other structures.
- Drugs from the following classes can affect the male reproductive system: anticonvulsants, antidepressants, antihypertensives, antineoplastics, antipsychotics, phenothiazines, benzodiazepines, anticholinergics, and androgenic steroids.
- Assessing the male reproductive system begins with a comprehensive health history that focuses primarily on sexual and reproductive function.
- Physical assessment of the male genitalia includes inspecting and palpating the penis and scrotum for structural abnormalities.
- Inspection and palpation of the inguinal area can detect a direct inguinal hernia, an indirect inguinal hernia, or a femoral hernia.
- Palpation of the prostate gland and seminal vesicles is performed through a rectal examination.
- To complete the assessment, the nurse should review the results of any laboratory tests ordered to evaluate reproductive system dysfunction, such as semen analysis or serum alpha-fetoprotein levels.
- Findings obtained from assessment of the male reproductive system are used to identify nursing diagnoses and plan nursing care appropriate to the client's specific problem or dysfunction.

Study questions

1. How would you describe the regulation of male sex hormones?

2. The nurse is assessing Mr. Yin, age 26, to rule out the presence of hernias. How would you proceed to inspect and palpate the inguinal area? What typical physical assessment findings for three types of hernias—inguinal, scrotal, and femoral—might you find?

3. How would you integrate a client's cultural and developmental background into the health history and physical assessment of the male reproductive system?

4. Mr. Johnson, age 24, comes to the clinic complaining of a left testicular mass. How would you proceed with a complete assessment?

5. Mr. Donovan, age 24, arrives in the emergency department complaining of a penile discharge and urethral redness. How would you document the following information related to your nursing assessment of Mr. Donovan?
- history (subjective) assessment data
- physical (objective) assessment data
- assessment techniques and any special equipment
- two appropriate nursing diagnoses
- documentation of your findings.

Selected references

Brown, M., and Hudak, C. (1984). *Student manual of physical examination* (2nd ed.). Philadelphia: Lippincott.

Guyton, A. (1992). *Human physiology and mechanisms of disease* (5th ed.). Philadelphia: Saunders.

Henry, J. (1991). *Clinical diagnosis and management by laboratory methods* (18th ed.). Philadelphia: Saunders.

McEvoy, G. (Ed.). (1992). *American Hospital Formulary Service drug information.* Bethesda, MD: American Society of Hospital Pharmacists.

Rudy, E., and Gray, V. (1986). *Handbook of health assessment* (2nd ed.). East Norwalk, CT: Appleton & Lange.

Tanagho, E., and McAninch, J. (1991). *Smith's general urology* (13th ed.). East Norwalk, CT: Appleton & Lange.

Walsh, P., Retik, A., Stamey, T., and Vaughan, E. (1992). *Campbell's urology* (6th ed.). Philadelphia: Saunders.

Nursing research

Danielson, R., et al. (1990). Reproductive health counseling for young men: What does it do? *Family Planning Perspectives,* 22(3), 115-121.

Ganong, L., and Markovitz, J. (1987). Young men's knowledge of testicular cancer and behavioral intentions toward testicular self-exam. *Patient Education and Counseling,* 9(3), 251-261.

17

Nervous System

Objectives

After reading and studying this chapter, you should be able to:

1. Identify the major components of the two anatomical divisions of the nervous system.
2. Describe the neuron and explain how it conducts an impulse.
3. Identify the function of each of the 12 cranial nerves and describe one assessment technique for each.
4. Formulate interviewing questions that provide information about the status of the client's nervous system.
5. Describe representative neurologic adverse reactions to commonly used drugs.
6. Explain the differences between a neurologic screening assessment, a complete neurologic assessment, and a neuro check.
7. Describe how to assess a client's level of consciousness.
8. List the cognitive skills evaluated in a complete mental status examination.
9. Describe three tests of cerebellar function.
10. Identify the five sensations evaluated in a complete sensory examination, and describe a test for each.
11. Differentiate between normal and abnormal neurologic findings in pediatric, adult, and elderly clients.
12. Document a neurologic assessment accurately and comprehensively.

Introduction

The nurse may encounter signs and symptoms of nervous system disorders in clients of any age. Cerebrovascular accidents (CVAs, or strokes)—the third most common cause of death in the United States—produce varying degrees of neurologic dysfunction, mostly in elderly clients. Young adults are more likely to suffer traumatic injuries to the nervous system, especially the spinal cord and brain. Degenerative neurologic disorders, such as Huntington's chorea or multiple sclerosis, cause a progressive deterioration of the nervous system and can occur at any age. Nervous system infections (meningitis, encephalitis, brain abscess) and cancer (brain and spinal cord tumors) also affect clients in different age groups.

Nervous system disorders can affect the functioning of other body systems, and disorders in other systems can affect the nervous system. Signs of neurologic dysfunction accompany various non-neurologic disorders, such as renal failure, respiratory insufficiency, vitamin deficiencies, toxin exposure, and diabetes. As a result, expect to encounter neurologic signs and symptoms in clients with various primary disorders.

Some common signs and symptoms of neurologic dysfunction include changes in level of consciousness, disorientation, inability to understand or use language, slurred speech, paralysis or paresis (weakness), unstable gait, dizziness or vertigo, numbness or tingling, blurred or double vision, and headache. Any of these warning signs warrants a nervous system assessment.

This chapter prepares you to perform nervous system assessment. It begins with a review of nervous system anatomy and physiology and explains how the nervous system detects, transmits, interprets, and responds to sensory stimuli. Next, it presents questions to ask during the neurologic health history, including rationales and, when appropriate, nursing interventions.

Glossary

Anosmia: loss of sense of smell, indicating malfunction of cranial nerve I (olfactory).
Aphasia: inability to understand or use language (or both) secondary to damage to the language control centers in the frontal and temporal brain lobes.
Areflexia: absent deep tendon reflexes, characteristic of lower motor neuron disorders.
Ataxia: unsteady gait characterized by a wide base of support and staggering.
Bulbar: pertaining to the cranial nerves, which exit from the medulla of the brain stem. Difficulty swallowing, slurred or nasal speech, and an impaired gag reflex are all bulbar symptoms.
Cognitive: higher skills of the cerebral cortex, such as judgment, reasoning, abstraction, and intellect.
Confusion: potentially reversible disorientation and disturbance of thought processes.
Cortical: pertaining to the cerebral cortex.
Decerebrate positioning: abnormal body position characterized by extension of both arms and legs indicating severe damage to the cerebral cortex, subcortical cerebrum, and upper brain stem.
Decorticate positioning: abnormal body position characterized by flexion and adduction of the arms and extension of the legs, indicating severe damage to the cerebral cortex.
Dementia: progressive, irreversible deterioration in mental status and cognitive functioning.
Disorientation: inability to identify self, surroundings, or time correctly.
Dysesthesia: unpleasant abnormal sensation or pain caused by stimuli that are not normally painful.
Hyperactive reflexes: abnormally increased strength of a reflex response.
Level of consciousness: degree of wakefulness and orientation. Wakefulness represents subcortical reticular system activity; orientation represents cerebral cortex activity.
Memory, immediate: ability to remember information briefly, such as looking up a phone number and remembering it long enough to dial it.
Memory, recent: ability to store and retrieve information acquired minutes, hours, or days earlier.
Memory, remote: ability to store information and retrieve it months or years later.
Neuro check: brief assessment of several key indicators of nervous system functioning, including level of consciousness, pupil size and response, verbal responsiveness, extremity strength and movement, and vital signs; used for rapid, repeated observations to detect subtle changes in the nervous system status.
Neurologic screening assessment: short examination of key nervous system functions, including level of consciousness, verbal responsiveness, brief mental status screening, motor system screening, and sensory system screening; used to gather baseline data and identify nervous system dysfunctions that need more detailed assessment.
Neuropathy: disease or disorder of a nerve.
Olfaction: sense of smell, a function of cranial nerve I (olfactory).
Paralysis: loss of ability to move. Hemiplegia is paralysis of one side of the body and characteristically results from a brain injury, such as cerebrovascular accident (stroke). Paraplegia is paralysis of the lower extremities, and quadriplegia is paralysis of all four extremities. Both result from spinal cord damage, but at different levels.
Paresis: weakness. Hemiparesis (weakness of one side of the body) usually results from a stroke.
Paresthesia: disturbance of sensation characterized by tingling, prickling, or numbness.
Proprioception: sense of position; the ability to know the position of a body part without having to look at it.
Subcortical: pertaining to regions beneath the cerebral cortex.
Vestibular: pertaining to sense of equilibrium and balance, originating in the semicircular canals of the inner ear and mediated through cranial nerve VIII (acoustic).

The chapter discusses a complete physical assessment of the nervous system as well as a briefer screening assessment. For both assessments, it describes normal and abnormal findings. It also summarizes laboratory studies that may be ordered for a client with abnormal neurologic signs. Finally, it shows how to document neurologic assessment data and how to use the information in formulating nursing diagnoses and in planning, implementing, and evaluating nursing care.

Anatomy and physiology review

The nervous system, a vast network of specialized cells, coordinates all body systems and enables the individual to respond to changes in the external and internal environment. Although the brain and spinal cord are the

(Text continues on page 470.)

Central nervous system

The central nervous system includes the brain and spinal cord. The brain is composed of the cerebrum, cerebellum, brain stem, and primitive structures that lie below the cerebrum: the diencephalon, limbic system, and reticular activating system (RAS). The spinal cord serves as the primary pathway for messages traveling between peripheral areas of the body and the brain. It also mediates the reflex arc—the natural pathway used in a reflex action.

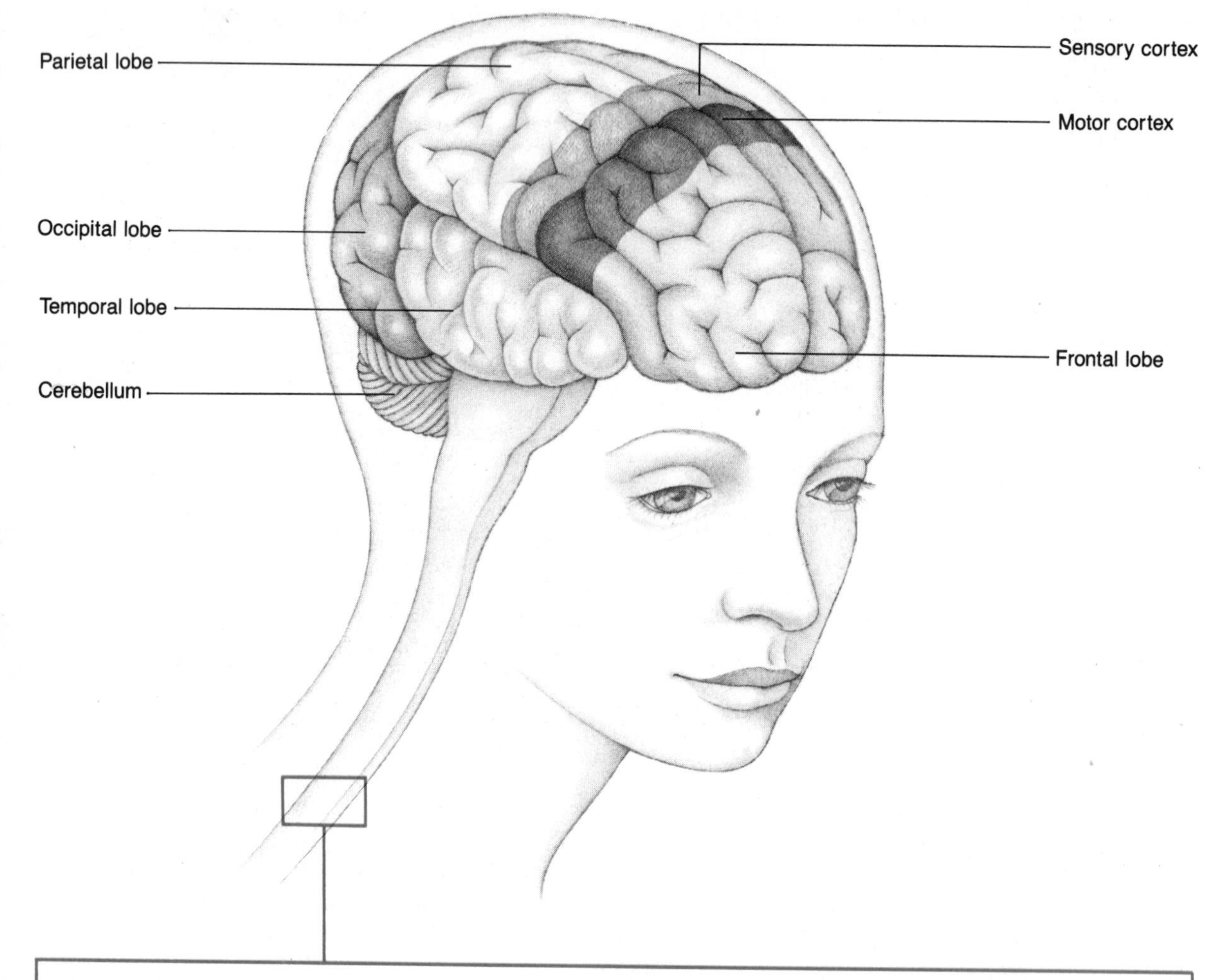

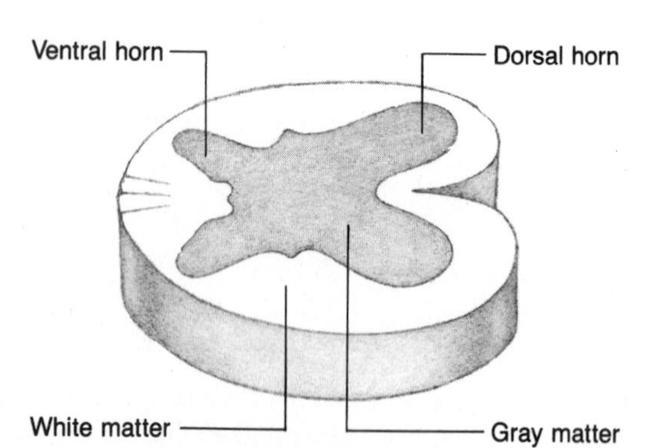

Spinal cord

The spinal cord joins the brain stem at the level of the foramen magnum and terminates near the second lumbar vertebra.

A cross section of the spinal cord reveals a central H-shaped mass of gray matter divided into dorsal (posterior) and ventral (anterior) horns. Gray matter in the dorsal horns relays sensory (afferent) impulses; in the ventral horns, motor (efferent) impulses. White matter (myelinated axons of sensory and motor nerves) surrounds these horns and forms the ascending and descending tracts.

Cerebrum

The cerebrum consists of a left and right hemisphere joined by the corpus callosum, a mass of nerve fibers that allows communication between corresponding centers in the right and left hemispheres. Each hemisphere is divided into four lobes, based on anatomical landmarks and functional differences. The lobes are named for the cranial bones that lie over them (frontal, temporal, parietal, and occipital). The cerebral cortex, the thin surface layer of the cerebrum, is composed of gray matter (unmyelinated cell bodies). The cerebrum has a rolling surface made up of convolutions (gyri) and creases or fissures (sulci).

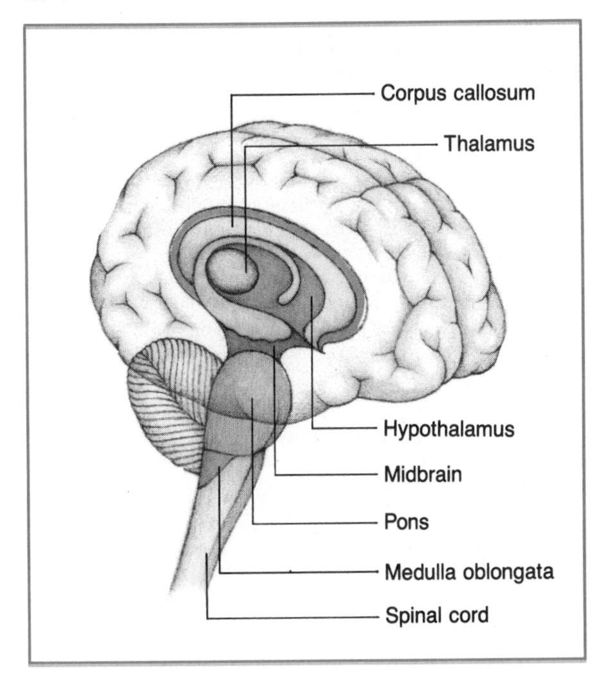

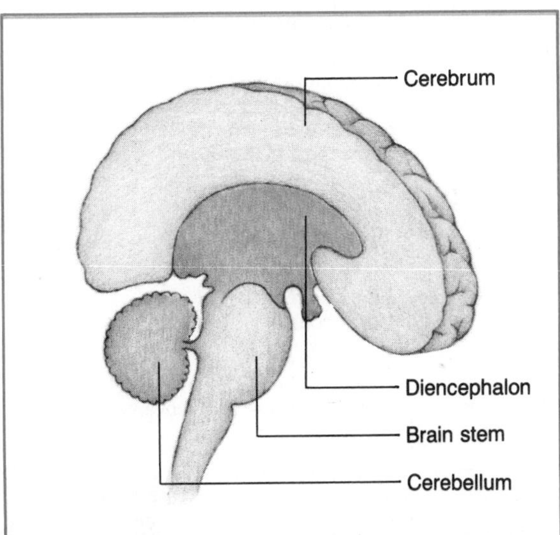

The frontal lobe influences personality, judgment, abstract reasoning, social behavior, language expression, and movement (in the motor portion). The temporal lobe controls hearing, language comprehension, and storage and recall of memories (although memories are found to be stored throughout the brain). The parietal lobe interprets and integrates sensations, including pain, temperature, and touch. It also interprets size, shape, distance, and texture. The parietal lobe of the nondominant hemisphere, usually the right, is especially important for awareness of body schema (shape). The occipital lobe functions primarily in interpreting visual stimuli.

Cerebellum

The cerebellum, which consists of two hemispheres, maintains muscle tone, coordinates muscle movement, and controls balance.

Brain stem

The brain stem is composed of the midbrain, pons, and medulla. It relays messages between upper and lower levels of the nervous system. The cranial nerves originate from the midbrain, pons, and medulla.

The pons connects the cerebellum with the cerebrum and connects the midbrain to the medulla oblongata. It contains one of the respiratory centers. The midbrain mediates the auditory and visual reflexes. The medulla oblongata regulates respiratory, vasomotor, and cardiac function.

Primitive structures

The diencephalon contains the thalamus and hypothalamus, which lie beneath the surface of the cerebral hemispheres. The thalamus relays all sensory stimuli (except olfactory) as they ascend to the cerebral cortex. Thalamic functions include primitive awareness of pain, screening of incoming stimuli, and focusing of attention. The hypothalamus controls or affects body temperature, appetite, water balance, pituitary secretions, emotions, and autonomic functions, including sleep and wake cycles.

Limbic system

The limbic system is a primitive brain area deep within the temporal lobe. Besides initiating primitive drives (hunger, aggression, and sexual and emotional arousal), the limbic system screens all sensory messages traveling to the cerebral cortex.

Reticular activating system

The RAS, a diffuse network of hyperexcitable neurons fanning out from the brain stem through the cerebral cortex, screens all incoming sensory information and channels it to appropriate areas of the brain for interpretation. RAS activity also stimulates wakefulness; when RAS activity declines, the individual falls asleep.

Peripheral nervous system

The peripheral nervous system is composed of the cranial nerves, spinal nerves, and the autonomic nervous system—which has two major divisions: the sympathetic (thoracolumbar) nervous system and the parasympathetic (craniosacral) nervous system.

Cranial nerves

The 12 pairs of cranial nerves (CNs) transmit motor or sensory messages, or both, primarily between the brain or brain stem and the head and neck. All cranial nerves, except for the olfactory and optic nerves, exit from the midbrain, pons, or medulla oblongata of the brain stem. The chart and illustration show the origin of each cranial nerve and describe its type (motor, sensory, or both) and function.

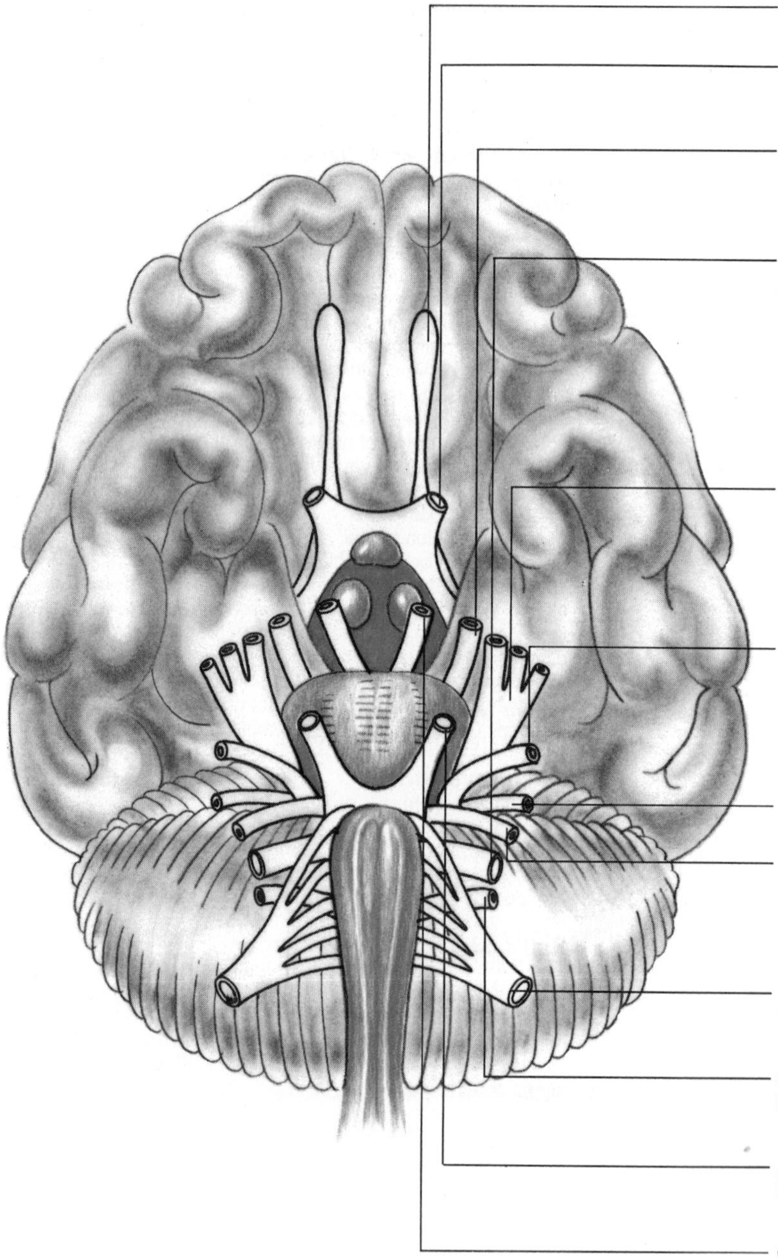

Olfactory (CN I)
Sensory: Smell

Optic (CN II)
Sensory: Vision

Trochlear (CN IV)
Motor: Extraocular eye movement (inferior medial)

Vagus (CN X)
Motor: Movement of palate, swallowing, gag reflex; activity of the thoracic and abdominal viscera, such as heart rate and peristalsis
Sensory: Sensations of throat, larynx, and thoracic and abdominal viscera (heart, lungs, bronchi, and gastrointestinal tract)

Trigeminal (CN V)
Sensory: Transmitting stimuli from face and head, corneal reflex
Motor: Chewing, biting, and lateral jaw movements

Facial (CN VII)
Sensory: Taste receptors (anterior two-thirds of tongue)
Motor: Facial muscle movement, including muscles of expression (those in the forehead and around the eyes and mouth)

Acoustic (vestibulocochlear) (CN VIII)
Sensory: Hearing, sense of balance

Glossopharyngeal (CN IX)
Motor: Swallowing movements
Sensory: Sensations of the throat; taste receptors (posterior one-third of the tongue)

Hypoglossal (CN XII)
Motor: Tongue movement

Spinal accessory (CN XI)
Motor: Shoulder movement, head rotation

Abducens (CN VI)
Motor: Extraocular eye movement (lateral)

Oculomotor (CN III)
Motor: Extraocular eye movement (superior, medial, and inferior lateral), pupillary constriction, and upper eyelid elevation

Spinal nerves

The 31 pairs of spinal nerves are each named according to the vertebra immediately below its point of exit from the spinal cord. Each spinal nerve consists of afferent (sensory) and efferent (motor) neurons, which carry messages to and from particular body regions, called dermatomes.

Autonomic nervous system

The vast autonomic nervous system (ANS) ennervates all internal organs. Sometimes known as the visceral efferent nerves, the nerves of the ANS carry messages to the viscera from the brain stem and neuroendocrine systems.

Sympathetic nervous system

Sympathetic nerves exit the spinal cord between the levels of the first thoracic and second lumbar vertebrae, hence the name thoracolumbar. Once these nerves, called preganglionic neurons, leave the spinal cord, they enter small relay stations (ganglia) near the cord. The ganglia form a chain that disseminates the impulse to postganglionic neurons. The postganglionic neurons reach many organs and glands and can produce widespread, generalized responses.

The physiologic effects of sympathetic activity include vasoconstriction; increased blood pressure; increased blood flow to skeletal muscles; increased heart rate and contractility; increased respiratory rate; smooth muscle relaxation of the bronchioles, GI tract, and urinary tract; sphincter contraction; pupillary dilation and ciliary muscle relaxation; increased sweat gland secretion; and decreased pancreatic secretion.

Parasympathetic nervous system

Also called the craniosacral system, the parasympathetic fibers leave the CNS by way of the cranial nerves from the midbrain and medulla, and also from the spinal nerves between the second and fourth sacral vertebrae (S2 to S4).

After leaving the CNS, the long preganglionic fiber of each parasympathetic nerve travels to a ganglion near a particular organ or gland; the short postganglionic fiber enters the organ or gland. This creates a more specific response involving only one organ or gland.

The physiologic effects of parasympathetic division activity include reduced heart rate, contractility, and conduction velocity; bronchial smooth muscle constriction; increased GI tract tone and peristalsis with sphincter relaxation; urinary system sphincter relaxation and increased bladder tone; vasodilation of external genitalia, causing erection; pupillary constriction; and increased pancreatic, salivary, and lacrimal secretions. The parasympathetic division has little effect on mental or metabolic activity.

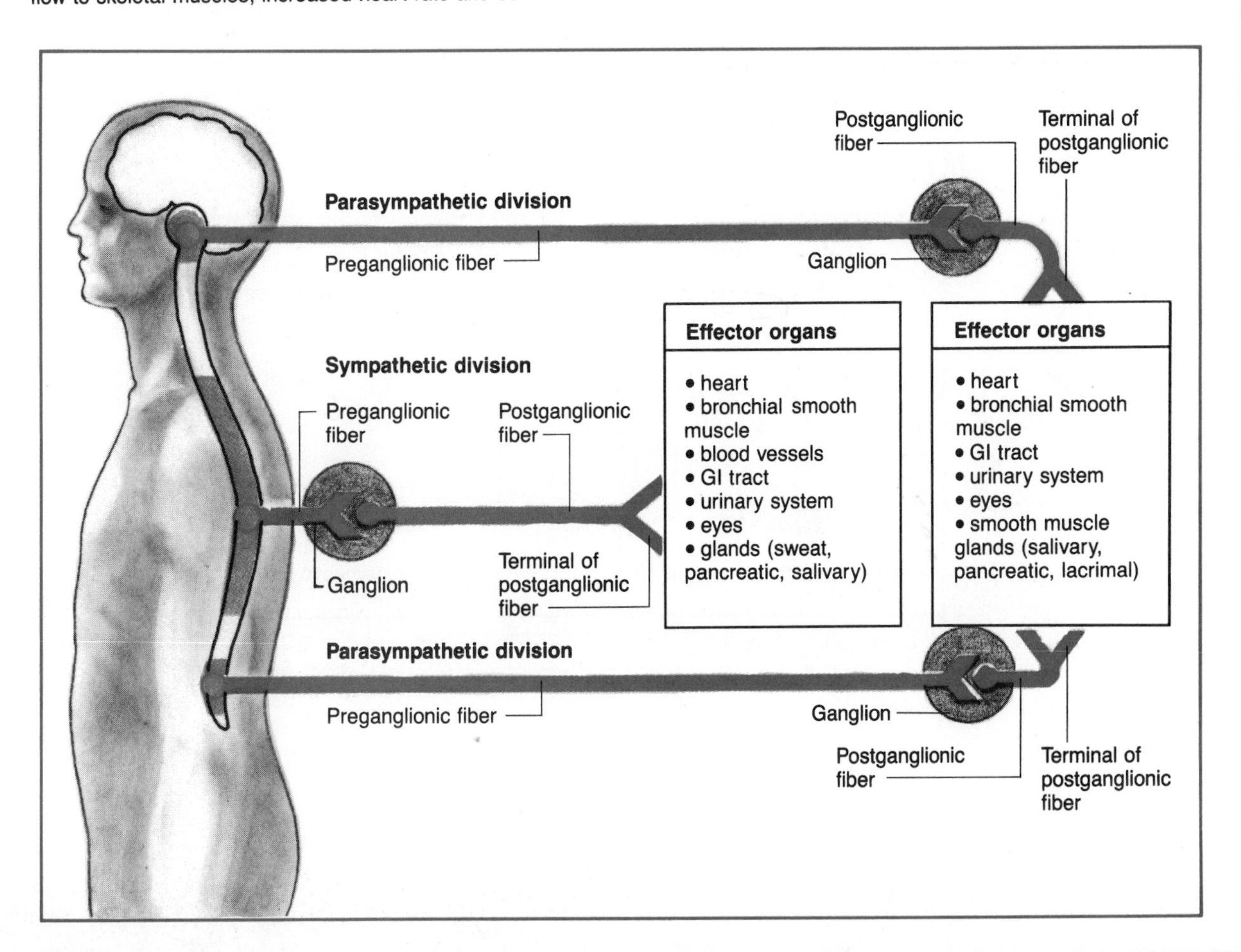

Neurotransmission and neural pathways

Neurotransmission is the conduction of impulses in the nervous system. It occurs through the actions of neurons—specialized cells that detect and transmit stimuli in the form of electrochemical messages or impulses. Stimuli can be mechanical (such as touch or pressure), thermal (heat or cold), or chemical (external chemicals or a chemical released by the body, such as histamine). On each neuron, treelike branches, called dendrites, reach out and detect stimuli and carry the impulse to the cell body of the neuron.

Then a long projection, called an axon, conducts the impulse away from the cell. Some axons are covered with a myelin sheath that allows more rapid impulse transmission.

When the impulse reaches the end of the axon, it stimulates synaptic vesicles in the presynaptic axon terminal to release a neurotransmitter substance into the synaptic cleft (the tiny space that separates one neuron from another). The neurotransmitter substance diffuses across the cleft and binds to special receptors on the cell membrane of the postsynaptic neuron. This stimulates or inhibits stimulation of the postsynaptic neuron.

Sensory impulses are carried to the brain for interpretation via the sensory (afferent or ascending) pathways. Motor impulses are transmitted from the brain to the muscles via the motor (efferent or descending) pathways.

Sensory pathways

Sensory impulses travel by two major pathways to the sensory cortex in the parietal lobe of the brain. Pain and temperature sensations enter the spinal cord through the dorsal horn, then immediately cross over to the opposite side of

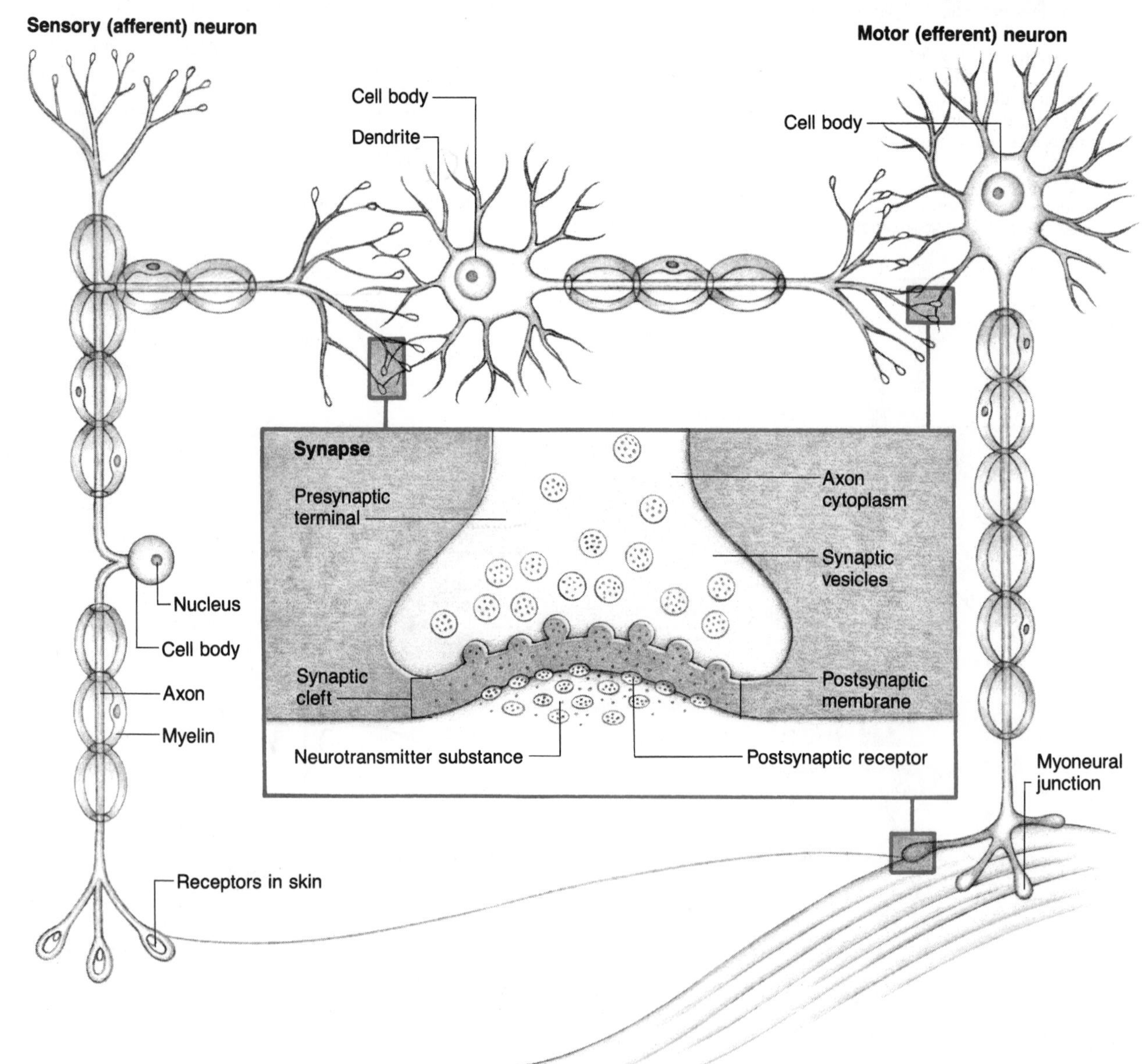

the cord. These stimuli then travel to the thalamus via the spinothalamic tract. Tactile, pressure, and vibration sensations enter the cord via the dorsal root ganglia. These stimuli then travel up the cord in the dorsal column to the medulla, where they cross to the opposite side and enter the thalamus. The thalamus relays all incoming sensory impulses, except olfactory ones, to the sensory cortex in the parietal lobe for interpretation.

Motor pathways

Motor impulses that originate in the motor cortex of the frontal lobe reach the lower motor neurons of the peripheral nervous system via upper motor neurons of the pyramidal or extrapyramidal tract. In the pyramidal tract, impulses travel from the motor cortex, through the internal capsule, to the medulla, where they cross to the opposite side and continue down the spinal cord. In the anterior horn of the spinal cord, impulses are relayed to the lower motor neurons, which carry them—via the spinal and peripheral nerves—to the muscles, producing a motor response.

Motor impulses that regulate involuntary muscle tone and control travel along the extrapyramidal tract from the premotor area of the frontal lobe to the pons of the brain stem, where they cross to the opposite side. The impulses then travel down the spinal cord to the anterior horn, where they are relayed to the lower motor neurons, which carry the impulses to the muscles.

Sensory pathway

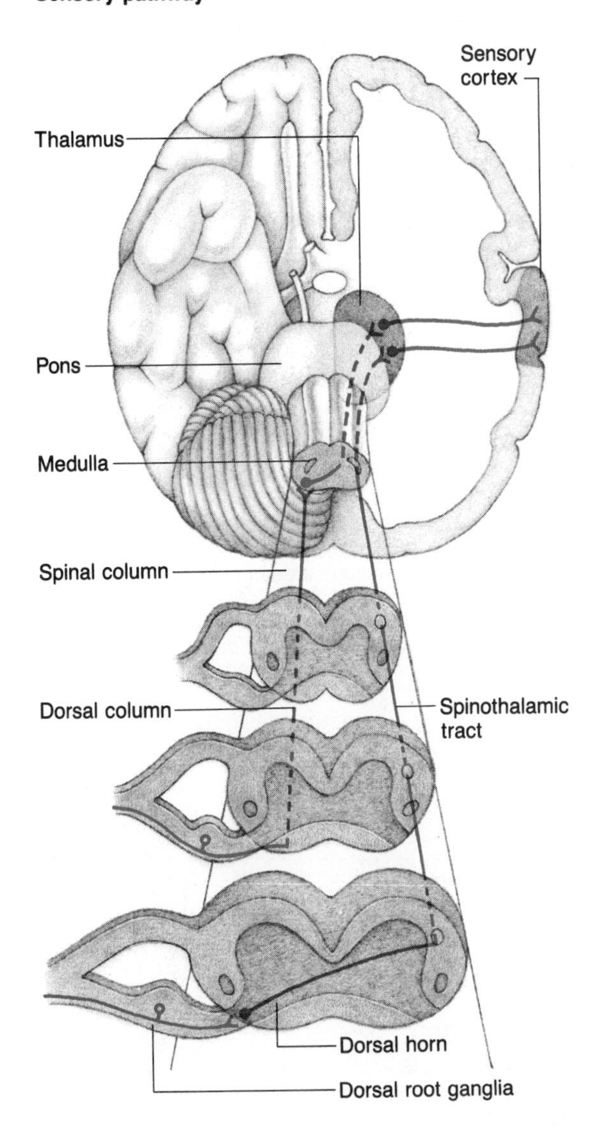

Motor pathway

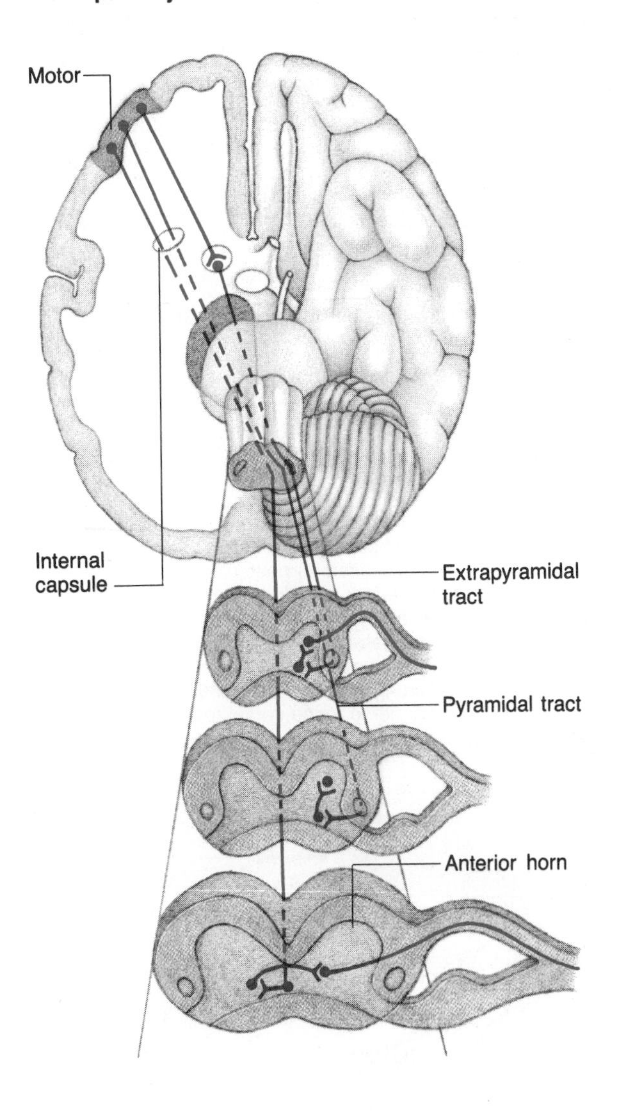

core of the nervous system, portions of the system extend to all body tissues.

Central and peripheral nervous systems

The nervous system consists of the central nervous system (CNS)—which includes the brain and spinal cord—and the peripheral nervous system (PNS)—which includes the cranial nerves, the spinal nerves, and the autonomic nervous system. (For more information, see *Central nervous system,* pages 464 and 465, and *Peripheral nervous system,* pages 466 and 467.) Bone, meninges, and cerebrospinal fluid (CSF) protect the brain and spinal cord in the CNS. The cranial bones form the skull, which completely surrounds the brain and opens at the base (the foramen magnum) to allow the spinal cord to exit. The vertebral column protects the spinal cord, and is composed of 30 vertebrae, each separated by an intervertebral disc that allows flexibility. Three layers of connective tissue—the dura mater, the arachnoid, and the pia mater—form the meninges, which cover and protect the cerebral cortex and the spinal cord.

CSF nourishes cells, transports metabolic waste, and cushions the brain. The ependymal cells that cover the surface of the choroid plexus (a tangled mass of tiny blood vessels lining the ventricles) constantly produce CSF at a rate of about 150 ml per day. CSF is a colorless fluid that circulates through the ventricular system, into the subarachnoid space of the brain and spinal cord, and back to the venous sinuses on top of the brain where it is reabsorbed.

Two major cell types, neurons and neuroglia, make up the nervous system. Neurons (nerve cells) are the conducting cells of the CNS. These specialized cells, which do not reproduce themselves, detect and transmit stimuli by electrochemical messages. (For more information, see *Neurotransmission and neural pathways,* pages 468 and 469.)

Neuroglia (glial cells, from the Greek word for *glue* because they hold the neurons together) are the supportive cells of the CNS. They nourish the neurons, remove their waste products, produce CSF and myelin (a fatlike substance that coats nerve fibers), form cerebral scars, and remove damaged tissue or other debris from the nervous system. Neuroglia form approximately 40% of the bulk of the brain.

Reflex responses

The nervous system can sense and respond to some stimuli from the environment without any brain involvement. These normal responses, called reflex responses, occur automatically to protect the body. For example, even when the brain is physiologically unable to send a

Reflex arc

Spinal nerves, which have sensory and motor portions, mediate deep tendon and superficial reflexes. A simple reflex arc requires a sensory (afferent) neuron and a motor (efferent) neuron. The knee-jerk (patellar) reflex illustrates the sequence of events in a normal reflex arc.

- A sensory receptor detects the mechanical stimulus produced by the reflex hammer striking the patellar tendon.
- The sensory (afferent) neuron carries the impulse along its axon via a spinal nerve to the dorsal root, where it enters the spinal cord.
- In the anterior horn of the spinal cord, the sensory neuron synapses with a motor neuron.
- The motor (efferent) neuron carries the impulse along its axon via a spinal nerve to the muscle.
- The motor neuron transmits the impulse to the muscle fibers via stimulation of the motor end plate. This triggers the muscle to contract and the leg to extend.

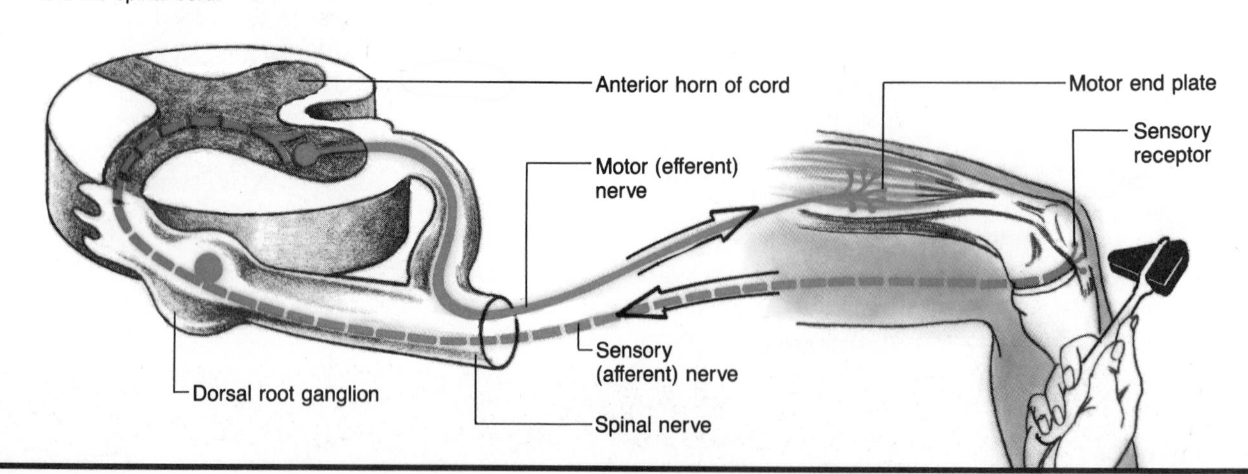

message to a muscle group (such as to a leg after a severe cervical spinal cord injury), a stimulus can still elicit reflex activity, such as the knee-jerk (patellar) reflex, provided that the spinal cord is intact at the level of the reflex. (For a description, see *Reflex arc.*)

The brain normally inhibits reflex activity. However, if damage to the CNS motor pathways prevents the brain from influencing reflex activity, reflexes become hyperactive.

Health history

To begin an accurate neurologic assessment, the nurse uses questions that focus on the health history. Ask questions in a systematic manner, proceeding from head to toe to avoid omitting information. Progress from general to specific questions, from nonthreatening to more threatening ones.

Although this health history focuses on the nervous system, use a holistic approach and inquire about the client's general well-being and overall body function. Remember, nervous system disorders can cause or result from problems in other body systems. The primary source of a neurologic disorder is not always the nervous system. For example, the impaired gas exchange associated with a chronic lung disease can affect cerebral function and produce neurologic signs and symptoms. No matter what the source, neurologic signs and symptoms can disrupt a client's vocational, social, and family life, and can interfere with the ability to perform activities of daily living (ADLs). For example, seizures may prevent a client from driving a car to work; hemiparesis may force a client to depend on others for ADLs and home maintenance.

Also remember that a client with a brain injury or disorder may have difficulty processing or recalling information. Verify any critical or questionable information with another source, such as a family member or friend, or compare the information with that in previous records. Because such a client may tire easily, consider dividing the interview into several short sessions.

The questions in this section are designed to help you evaluate the client's nervous system. They include rationales that describe the significance of the answers and, where appropriate, nursing interventions that may be incorporated into the client's care plan.

Health and illness patterns

To assess the client's health and illness patterns related to the nervous system, investigate the client's current, past, and family health status as well as any pertinent developmental considerations.

Current health status

As with any assessment, begin by obtaining information about the client's current health status. To obtain a complete description of the presenting symptom, use the PQRST method. (For information about this method, see *Symptom analysis* in Chapter 3, The Health History.) Use the following questions as a guide when conducting the interview.

Do you have headaches? If so, how would you describe them?
(RATIONALE: The pattern and characteristics of a headache can help identify its etiology. For example, vascular [migraine or cluster] headaches recur, frequently following a pattern. Early morning headaches that are present upon awakening and disappear after arising may be an early warning sign of a brain tumor in an adult.)

Have you noticed a change in your ability to remember things? If so, how would you describe this change?
(RATIONALE: Impaired recent memory is an early sign of cerebral degeneration, such as accompanies Alzheimer's disease. High stress levels and fatigue can also impair memory.)

Have you noticed any change in your mental alertness or ability to concentrate?
(RATIONALE: Decreased alertness or inability to concentrate also can be an early indicator of cerebral degeneration.)

Have you ever fainted or blacked out—even if only for a few moments? Do you have difficulty recalling blocks of time?
(RATIONALE: Transient loss of consciousness or memory may indicate a neurologic disorder such as transient cerebral ischemia [a decreased blood supply to the brain] or atypical seizures.)

How would you describe your eyesight? Do you wear eyeglasses? If so, do you need them for near-sightedness, far-sightedness, or another problem?
(RATIONALE: The location of the optic nerve makes it especially vulnerable to injury from disorders causing CNS ischemia or chronic elevation in intracranial pressure. Such disorders include CVAs, trauma, or intracranial tumors. Uncorrected vision can contribute to disorientation, especially in an elderly client.)

Do you experience blurred vision, double vision, or any other visual disturbances, such as blind spots?
(RATIONALE: Blurred or double vision can indicate disorders of cranial nerves III, IV, and VI. Blind spots suggest a localized retinal injury or damage to the optic tracts in the brain caused by a CVA or trauma. Transient blind spots or the loss of vision in one eye may signal transient cerebral ischemia and an impending stroke. Transient blind spots accompanied by flashing lights [scotomata] precede a classic migraine.)

How is your hearing? If you wear a hearing aid, does it help?
(RATIONALE: Hearing impairment may indicate a disorder of cranial nerve VIII. A gradual, progressive hearing loss in one ear may result from a neoplasm of the acoustic nerve [acoustic neuroma].)

Have you noticed any change in your sense of smell or taste? If so, how would you describe this change?
(RATIONALE: A loss of the sense of smell [olfaction], called anosmia, frequently follows a facial fracture or head injury. Occasionally, impaired olfaction can indicate a brain tumor or lesion; unusual smells can accompany temporal lobe seizures. Disorders of cranial nerves VII or IX can affect the sense of taste. A decreased sense of taste always accompanies an impaired sense of smell.)

Do you have any difficulty swallowing? If so, how would you describe it?
(RATIONALE: A dysfunction of cranial nerves IX, X, and XII can produce impaired swallowing and other bulbar symptoms that occur in such disorders as myasthenia gravis and amyotrophic lateral sclerosis [ALS]. Poor neuromuscular control from a CVA or Parkinson's disease also can impair swallowing.)

Do you have difficulty speaking or expressing the words you are thinking?
(RATIONALE: Difficulty understanding or using language indicates a language dysfunction [aphasia] from an injury to the cerebral cortex.)

How would you rate your muscle strength? Have you recently noticed any change in strength?
(RATIONALE: Degenerative neurologic disorders, such as ALS, produce progressive muscle weakness and wasting. A sudden, localized muscle weakness, such as in one arm or leg, suggests a CVA or a peripheral nerve disease or injury. Also, compression of the spinal cord or spinal nerves can cause unilateral or bilateral weakness below the lesion level.)

How would you rate your muscle coordination? Do you often drop things? Do you have difficulty walking?
(RATIONALE: Disturbed coordination implies a disease of the cerebellum, basal ganglia, or extrapyramidal tracts. An impaired gait [ataxia] is the primary sign of cerebellar dysfunction. A shuffling gait suggests disease of the basal ganglia or extrapyramidal tract.)

Do you have tremors or muscle spasms in your hands, arms, or legs?
(RATIONALE: A positive answer may indicate a disorder of the cerebellum or basal ganglia.)

Do you have problems with your balance?
(RATIONALE: Poor balance implies a cerebellar disorder or impairment of the vestibular portion of cranial nerve VIII. A client with such a problem requires assistance when walking and other safety precautions.)

Do you have dizzy spells? If so, how would you describe them?
(RATIONALE: Dizziness accompanies many neurologic disorders, and its characteristics vary. Vertigo, which is a sensation of spinning or whirling, differs from simple dizziness, which is a sensation of unsteadiness or disequilibrium accompanied by lightheadedness, giddiness, or feeling faint.)

Have you noticed any change in your ability to feel textures or any numbness, tingling, or other unusual sensations?
(RATIONALE: Altered tactile sensations can indicate a lesion in the sensory system. Numbness and tingling often signal early peripheral nerve damage and can precede total sensory loss and impaired motor function.)

What medications do you take?
(RATIONALE: Be alert for medications that can affect nervous system functioning. For information about drugs that affect neurologic function, see *Adverse drug reactions.*)

Past health status

After obtaining information about the client's current health status, ask about any previous neurologic disorders and treatments.

Have you ever had a head injury? If so, when? How would you describe what happened? Do you have any lasting effects?
(RATIONALE: Even minor head injuries can produce long-term effects. In an elderly client, a minor head injury can cause a subdural hematoma that may take weeks

Adverse drug reactions

When obtaining a health history to assess a client's neurologic status, the nurse should ask about current drug use. Many drugs affect the nervous system; some can cause permanent neurologic damage. For example, the aminoglycosides can cause eighth cranial nerve damage manifested by vestibular symptoms, auditory symptoms, or both. Other commonly used drugs and adverse reactions are listed below.

DRUG CLASS	DRUG	POSSIBLE ADVERSE REACTIONS
Adrenergics	albuterol sulfate, epinephrine, isoproterenol hydrochloride, terbutaline sulfate	Nervousness, tremors, dizziness, restlessness, insomnia
Adrenergic blockers	ergotamine tartrate, methysergide maleate	Lightheadedness, vertigo, insomnia, euphoria, confusion, hallucinations, numbness and tingling of fingers and toes
Antianginals	diltiazem hydrochloride	Headache, fatigue
	isosorbide dinitrate, nitroglycerin	Throbbing headache, dizziness, weakness, orthostatic hypotension
	nifedipine	Headache, dizziness, lightheadedness, flushing
	verapamil hydrochloride	Headache, dizziness
Antiarrhythmics	lidocaine hydrochloride	Lightheadedness, dizziness, paresthesia, tremors, restlessness, confusion, hallucinations, headache
Antimicrobials	aminoglycosides	Neuromuscular blockade; ototoxicity causing vertigo, hearing impairment, or both
	isoniazid, nitrofarantoin	Peripheral neuropathy
Anticonvulsants	carbamazepine	Dizziness, drowsiness, ataxia, confusion, speech disturbances, involuntary movements
	phenytoin sodium	Dose-related headache, confusion, ataxia, slurred speech, lethargy, drowsiness, nervousness, insomnia, blurred vision, diplopia, nystagmus
Antidepressants	amitriptyline hydrochloride	Drowsiness, weakness, lethargy, fatigue, agitation, nightmares, restlessness; confusion, disorientation (especially in elderly clients)
	monoamine oxidase inhibitors	Restlessness, insomnia, drowsiness, headache, orthostatic hypotension, hypertension
Antihypertensives	clonidine hydrochloride	Drowsiness, sedation, dizziness, headache, nightmares, depression, hallucinations
	hydralazine hydrochloride	Headache
	methyldopa	Drowsiness, sedation, decreased mental acuity, vertigo, headache, psychic disturbances, nightmares, depression
	propranolol hydrochloride	Fatigue, lethargy, vivid dreams, hallucinations, depression

continued

Adverse drug reactions continued

DRUG CLASS	DRUG	POSSIBLE ADVERSE REACTIONS
Antineoplastic agents	procarbazine hydrochloride	Paresthesis, neuropathy, confusion
	vinblastine sulfate	Paresthesis, numbness
	vincristine sulfate	Peripheral neuropathy, loss of deep tendon reflexes, jaw pain
Antiparkinsonian agents	amantadine hydrochloride	Psychic disturbances, nervousness, irritability, fatigue, depression, insomnia, confusion, hallucinations, difficulty concentrating
	levodopa	Psychic disturbances, decreased attention span, memory loss, nervousness, vivid dreams, involuntary muscle movements
Antipsychotics	haloperidol, phenothiazines	Extrapyramidal reactions, tardive dyskinesia, headache, lethargy, confusion, agitation, hallucinations
Cholinergic blockers	atropine sulfate, benztropine mesylate, glycopyrrolate	Blurred vision, headache, nervousness, drowsiness, weakness, dizziness, insomnia, disorientation
Corticosteroids	dexamethasone, hydrocortisone, methylprednisolone, prednisone	Mood swings, euphoria, insomnia, headache, vertigo, psychotic behavior
Gastrointestinal agents	cimetidine	Confusion (especially in elderly clients), depression
	metoclopramide hydrochloride	Restlessness, anxiety, drowsiness, lassitude, extrapyramidal reactions, tardive dyskinesia
Narcotic analgesics	morphine sulfate, hydromorphone hydrochloride, meperidine hydrochloride, methadone hydrochloride, oxycodone hydrochloride	Sedation, dizziness, visual disturbances, clouded sensorium
	butorphanol tartrate, nalbuphine hydrochloride, pentazocine hydrochloride	Sedation, headache, dizziness, vertigo, lightheadedness, euphoria
Nonsteroidal anti-inflammatory agents	ibuprofen, indomethacin	Headache, drowsiness, dizziness
Sedatives and hypnotics	barbiturates	Drowsiness, lethargy, vertigo, headache, depression, "hangover," paradoxical excitement in elderly clients, hyperactivity in children
	benzodiazepines	Drowsiness, dizziness, ataxia, daytime sedation, headache, confusion
Skeletal muscle relaxants	baclofen	Drowsiness
	chlorzoxazone	Drowsiness, dizziness
	cyclobenzaprine hydrochloride	Drowsiness, dizziness, headache, nervousness, confusion
Miscellaneous agents	lithium carbonate	Lethargy, tremors, headache, mental confusion, dizziness, seizures, difficulty concentrating

or months to produce symptoms. Post-concussion syndrome causes various symptoms, such as insomnia, headache, or depression, which can persist up to a year after the injury.)

Have you ever been treated by a neurologist or neurosurgeon? If so, why?
(RATIONALE: The answer to this question will help identify existing or potentially recurring neurologic problems.)

Have you ever had a seizure? If so, please describe it and indicate under what circumstances it occurred.
(RATIONALE: Besides identifying individuals at risk for seizures, the answer to this question helps differentiate between a client with a seizure disorder [recurrent seizures] and one who experiences an isolated seizure because of a metabolic disturbance.)

Have you ever had a stroke? If so, please describe it in detail.
(RATIONALE: A previous CVA predisposes a client to another one. Residual deficits [those that remain after a CVA] may be minimal and may not be obvious without specific questioning.)

Family health status

Next, ask the client about the neurologic health status of blood relatives, such as parents and siblings.

Have any family members had a neurologic disease, such as a brain tumor, degenerative disease, or senility? If so, which relative?
(RATIONALE: Some neurologic disorders—such as certain types of brain tumors, Alzheimer's disease, seizure disorders, and CVA—have a familial tendency. Many degenerative neurologic disorders, such as Huntington's chorea, are genetic and inheritable.)

Have any of your immediate family members (mother, father, or siblings) had high blood pressure or a stroke?
(RATIONALE: Hypertension has a familial tendency and can predispose the client to a CVA.)

Developmental considerations

Gathering developmental information is especially important when interviewing a child or an elderly client. A developmental health history can help identify certain neurologic abnormalities that have their roots in early life.

Pediatric client. For a young child, gather information about prenatal, perinatal, and developmental history from the child's parent or guardian. For an older child, gather information from the child as well as from the parent or guardian. Examples of possible questions include:

Were any risk factors present during the pregnancy, such as exposure to X-rays, maternal illness or injury, exposure to TORCH viruses (toxoplasmosis, other rubella virus, cytomegalovirus, and herpes simplex), poor nutrition, surgery, alcohol or drug use, or cigarette smoking?
(RATIONALE: Such factors can increase the risk of congenital neurologic defects.)

Do you have any family history of genetic or familial disorders, such as epilepsy, cerebral palsy, or Down's syndrome?
(RATIONALE: A family history predisposes the child to these disorders.)

Was the baby full term at birth or born prematurely? If premature, how early was the baby born?
(RATIONALE: The nervous system of a premature infant is not as developed as that of a full-term infant at birth; therefore, age-related developmental milestones will not be accurate for the premature infant.)

Was the labor and delivery difficult?
(RATIONALE: Difficult labor and delivery can cause neurologic birth injuries, such as cerebral palsy, paralysis, or paresis.)

Were medications used during the delivery?
(RATIONALE: Analgesics or anesthetics may decrease the neonate's responsiveness immediately after birth and therefore contribute to insufficient oxygenation [anoxia] and cerebral ischemia.)

How did the baby look right after the delivery?
(RATIONALE: A limp, gray, or mottled appearance suggests anoxia, which could produce neurologic sequelae.)

During the first month after birth, did the baby have any problems with sucking or swallowing, or any other problems, such as high bilirubin levels or a positive heel stick test for phenylketonuria?
(RATIONALE: Metabolic disorders, such as phenylketonuria, can affect nervous system functioning.)

Has the child received all recommended immunizations? Has the child recently been exposed to others with measles, chicken pox, or mumps?
(RATIONALE: Many childhood illnesses, such as measles, chicken pox, and mumps, can produce neurologic sequelae.)

Has the child had any illnesses or injuries? If so, which ones? What medications did the child receive to treat them?
(RATIONALE: Many medications can affect a child's nervous system. Previous illnesses or injuries could produce neurologic sequelae.)

Has the child reached developmental milestones, such as sitting up or walking, at the expected age? Has the child lost any functions that were previously mastered?
(RATIONALE: Delayed neuromuscular development implies an underlying neurologic disorder. Remember that premature infants are less developed neurologically at birth and therefore are behind the expected age-related developmental milestones. Loss of previously mastered skills could indicate an underlying neurologic disorder.)

When interviewing an older child and the child's parents, include the following questions:

Is the child in school? How is the child's progress in school?
(RATIONALE: Learning disabilities, such as dyslexia or attention deficit disorder [formerly called hyperactivity or minimal brain dysfunction], may have a neurologic basis. The answer to this question could also identify a visual or hearing deficit.)

Does the child have any favorite activities, such as roller skating, bicycling, or jumping rope?
(RATIONALE: Identifying the child's favorite activities provides valuable information about the child's neuromuscular skills, balance, and coordination.)

Has the child sustained any broken bones or head injuries? If so, how would you describe them?
(RATIONALE: Fractures or dislocations can produce chronic peripheral nerve compression. Even minor head injury can produce subtle changes in behavior [postconcussion syndrome] up to a year after the injury.)

Elderly client. Because visual and auditory acuity normally decrease with age, make sure the elderly client wears glasses or a hearing aid for the interview, if necessary.

During the interview, be especially alert for complaints of transient neurologic signs or symptoms (such as visual disturbance, weakness of an extremity, clumsiness, sudden falls, dizziness, or language impairment), which could reflect cerebrovascular disease and impending CVA. Also, ask the client about any family history of neurologic disorders or degenerative diseases that occur later in life, such as a CVA, senile dementia, blindness, and neuromuscular disorders. Use the following questions as a guideline.

Are you less agile than you used to be? Do you trip or fall more frequently?
(RATIONALE: These changes often occur with aging; however, an extreme change suggests a cerebellar or brain stem disorder.)

How would you describe your walking pattern? Has it changed? Have you developed tremors?
(RATIONALE: Gait changes or tremors could signify Parkinson's disease or another degenerative neurologic disorder.)

Have you noticed any change in your memory or thinking abilities, vision, hearing, or sense of smell or taste?
(RATIONALE: A change in any of these may indicate cerebral or cranial nerve changes, which may interfere with the client's life-style, health maintenance, and safety.)

Health promotion and protection patterns

As you continue the health history, ask the client about daily activities, recreational patterns, nutrition, stress and coping patterns, sleep, and personal habits. Also assess for occupational and environmental health patterns that might affect the nervous system.

What do you do with your leisure time? Do you enjoy reading or listening to music?
(RATIONALE: Vision, concentration, or language deficits can hinder reading ability; other sensory-perceptual alterations, such as hearing loss, can diminish the client's enjoyment of leisure activities, such as listening to music.)

Do you have difficulty following conversations or television programs? Do you have difficulty concentrating on activities that you once found enjoyable, such as reading or watching movies?
(RATIONALE: Difficulty following conversations or decreased attention span may be an early sign of cognitive or hearing impairment. Depression can also cause a loss of interest in previous pastimes.)

Do you eat foods every day from each of the five basic food groups—breads and cereals, vegetables, fruits, meats, and dairy products?
(RATIONALE: An inadequate diet may lead to vitamin B_{12}, folic acid, and niacin deficiencies, which can cause peripheral neuropathy.)

How would you describe an emotionally stressful siutation? How would you handle such a situation?
(RATIONALE: Some neurologic disorders produce emotional lability, causing the client to respond inappropriately or excessively. Severe stress normally impairs neuromuscular performance; brain injury or sensory-perceptual disturbances can further affect the client's response.)

Are you exposed to any toxins or chemicals, such as insecticides, petroleum distillates, or lead, in your home or on the job?
(RATIONALE: Exposure to toxins can cause neurologic signs and symptoms.)

On the job, do you perform any strenuous or repetitive activities? Do you sit, stand, or walk while performing your job?
(RATIONALE: Repetitive motions, such as on an assembly line, can cause peripheral nerve injuries from overuse. Strenuous activities or heavy lifting increases the risk of intervertebral disc injuries; prolonged sitting or standing can cause neuromuscular stiffness or discomfort.)

Do you need to rest during the day? Does your strength fluctuate during the day?
(RATIONALE: Some neurologic disorders display a distinctive variation of symptoms with time and activity. For example, symptoms of myasthenia gravis, such as muscle weakness and blurred or double vision, tend to worsen with activity and improve after rest.)

Do you use alcohol or other mood-altering drugs?
(RATIONALE: Such substances can disturb nervous system [especially cerebral] functioning.)

Role and relationship patterns

Nervous system disorders can affect the client's self-concept and impair the ability to perform self-care, to fulfill role expectations, and to continue functioning sexually. As a result, neurologic dysfunction can profoundly affect role and relationship patterns. To assess these effects, ask these questions.

How has your disability affected you? Has it made you feel differently about yourself?
(RATIONALE: Nervous system disorders that produce obvious deficits, such as paralysis, paresis, or impaired gait or coordination, or that impair the client's memory, facility with language, or other cognitive skills, can adversely affect the client's self-concept.)

Can you do the things for yourself that you would like to do?
(RATIONALE: Neurologic disorders may prevent the client from attaining personal goals or pursuing satisfying activities.)

Can you fulfill your usual family responsibilities? If not, who has assumed them?
(RATIONALE: Neurologic impairment may prevent the client from fulfilling certain roles that would then have to be assumed by another family member.)

How has your illness or disability affected members of your family emotionally and financially?
(RATIONALE: Nervous system disorders can devastate the family emotionally. Chronic or degenerative processes often require prolonged treatment, hospitalization, or special equipment, which can drain a family financially.)

Have you noticed any change in your sexuality?
(RATIONALE: Injury or damage to the nervous system, especially to the lumbosacral spinal cord, may interfere with sexual functioning. Brain injuries can also alter libido and sexual functioning.)

Physical assessment

Because the nervous system is so extensive, a complete neurologic assessment is complicated and time-consuming; it can take several hours to complete. A complete neurologic assessment provides information about five broad categories of neurologic function:
- cerebral function (including level of consciousness [LOC], mental status, and language)
- cranial nerves
- motor system and cerebellar functions
- sensory system
- reflexes.

Unless working as a nurse practitioner, the nurse probably will not perform a complete neurologic assessment.

Usually, the nurse will perform a neurologic screening assessment. This type of assessment evaluates some of the key indicators of neurologic function and helps identify areas of dysfunction. A neurologic screening assessment usually includes:

• evaluation of level of consciousness (including a brief mental status examination and evaluation of verbal responsiveness)
• selected cranial nerve assessment (usually CN II, III, IV, and VI)
• motor screening (strength, movement, and gait)
• sensory screening (tactile and pain sensations in extremities).

If the neurologic screening assessment identifies areas of neurologic dysfunction, the nurse must evaluate those areas in more detail. For this reason, the nurse must be familiar with the neurologic screening assessment as well as the components of a complete neurologic assessment.

Finally, the nurse should be able to perform a very brief neurologic assessment, called a neuro check. This assessment is used to make rapid, repeated evaluations of several key indicators of nervous system status: level of consciousness, pupil size and response, verbal responsiveness, extremity strength and movement, and vital signs. After establishing a baseline, regularly reevaluating these key indicators reveals trends in a client's neurologic functioning and helps detect transient changes that can be warning signs of problems.

This section describes the techniques used to perform a neurologic screening assessment of the client's cerebral, cranial nerve, motor and cerebellar, and sensory functions. It also includes a full description of advanced assessment skills—the additional skills needed to perform a complete neurologic assessment, including reflex evaluation.

Preparing for the assessment

Although the neurologic assessment sequence differs from other assessments, some of the techniques are the same: for example, inspection and palpation are used in parts of the neurologic assessment. The equipment needed includes a penlight, cotton, and a sharp object (or sterile needle). If a complete neurologic assessment is being performed, additional equipment will be needed, including pungent-smelling substances (peppermint, tobacco, alcohol), test tubes, salt, sugar, a sour substance (such as a lemon), a bitter substance (such as quinine), tongue depressors, a coin, paper clip, reflex hammer, and an ophthalmoscope.

Before beginning the assessment, keep in mind that some maneuvers may be difficult for the client to perform, especially an elderly client or one with a neurologic disorder affecting balance and coordination. Always be sensitive to the client's condition, and ask if the client can perform the maneuver. As with any assessment, ensure the client's privacy by performing the assessment in an appropriate setting and keeping the client draped.

Always begin with an assessment of cerebral functioning, including level of consciousness. Because the neurons of the brain are extremely sensitive to changes in the internal environment, disorders of cerebral functioning are usually the earliest signs of a developing CNS disorder.

Cerebral function

Basic assessment of cerebral function includes LOC, communication, and, briefly, mental status. Advanced assessment of cerebral function includes formal assessment of language skills and complete mental status evaluation.

Level of consciousness

Evaluation of LOC includes assessment of level of arousal and orientation.

Level of arousal. Arousal is the client's degree of wakefulness. For example, a fully awake client is alert, with open eyes, and attentive to stimuli in the environment. The less-awake client appears drowsy, has reduced motor activity, and seems less disturbed by stimuli in the environment. Decreased arousal often precedes disorientation.

Begin by quietly observing the client's behavior. Is the client awake, dozing, or asleep? Moving about or motionless? If awake, what is the client doing? Resting quietly, watching TV, conversing with a visitor, or fidgeting? If the client is dozing or sleeping, attempt arousal by providing an appropriate auditory, tactile, or painful stimulus, in that sequence. Always start with a minimal stimulus, increasing its intensity as necessary.

Speak the client's name in a normal tone of voice and note the response to an auditory stimulus. If the client does not respond, use a tactile stimulus, such as touching the client gently, squeezing the client's hand, or shaking the client's shoulder.

Use painful stimuli only to assess an unconscious client or one with a markedly decreased LOC who is unresponsive to other stimuli. Techniques to test response to painful stimuli include application of firm pressure over a nailbed with a blunt hard object, such as a pen, or a firm pinch of the Achilles tendon between your thumb and index finger. *Never* use a pin stick (which can spread infection), apply supraorbital pressure, pinch a nipple, or rub the sternum, all of which can cause bruising or other injury.

Next, note the type of stimulus and the intensity required to elicit a response. Is the response an appropriate verbal one, unintelligible mumbling, body movement, eye opening, or nothing? After you remove the stimulus, how alert is the client? Wide awake? Drowsy? Drifting to sleep?

After assessing the client's level of arousal, compare the findings with those of previous assessments. Note any trends, such as lethargy followed by several hours of drowsiness in a client who is usually awake. Also consider other factors that could affect the client's responsiveness. For example, a client who is normally awake and alert may be drowsy after being awakened at night, after a strenuous physical therapy session, or after the administration of CNS depressant medications.

Because most terms used to describe level of arousal are subjective, describe the client's action or response instead. For example, a lethargic client's response may be described as "awakened when called loudly, then immediately fell asleep."

Orientation. Orientation reflects the ability of the cerebral cortex to receive and accurately interpret sensory stimuli. Assessment of orientation includes three aspects: orientation to person, place, and time. Some authorities include purpose as a fourth aspect; however, because an individual's ability to comprehend purpose is a higher cognitive skill, this chapter includes purpose in the assessment of complete mental status.

When assessing orientation, always ask questions that require the client to provide information, rather than a yes or no answer. Remember, though, that the client cannot provide information that is not available.

Person. Is the client aware of personal identity? Ask for the client's name and note the response. Self-identity usually remains intact until late in decreasing LOC, making disorientation to person an ominous sign.

Place. Is the client able to state the location correctly? For example, when looking around the room, is the client able to interpret the environment (bed, curtains, equipment, and nurse), sounds (voices, bells or buzzers, or institutional noises), and sensations (examination procedures, or placement of a blood pressure cuff) and conclude that this is a health care facility? Or does the client think this is home and the kitchen is in the next room?

Time. Does the client know the year or month, or the day's date? Disorientation to time is one of the first indicators of decreasing LOC. People who are oriented to time can usually state the correct year, often the correct month or date, and, if in an appropriate environment, can differentiate day from night. In determining the client's orientation to time, be sure to consider the clues available in the environment. For example, if the room has a window, the client should be able to state whether it is night or day.

To minimize the subjectivity of LOC assessment and to establish a greater degree of reliability, many health care facilities use the Glasgow Coma Scale. This scale evaluates the client's LOC according to three objective behaviors: eye opening, verbal responsiveness (which includes orientation), and motor response. (For details, see *Glasgow Coma Scale*, page 480.)

Communication

Language skills reflect the ability of the brain to comprehend communication involving speech, writing, numbers, and gestures. Language skills include learning and recalling the parts of the language (such as words), organizing word relationships according to grammatical rules, and structuring message content logically. Speech involves neuromuscular actions of the mouth, tongue, and oropharynx.

Verbal responsiveness. You can obtain most of the information regarding the quantity and quality of the client's verbal responses during the interview and physical assessment. To assess verbal responsiveness, observe the client when you ask a question. If you identify or suspect a decreased LOC, call the client's name or gently shake the client's shoulder to try to elicit a verbal response.

Note the quantity of what the client says. Does the client speak in complete sentences? In phrases? In single words? Is communication spontaneous? Or does the client rarely speak?

Note the quality of the client's speech. Is it unusually loud or soft? Does the client articulate clearly, or are words difficult to understand? What is the rate and rhythm of the client's speech? What language does the client speak? (If you cannot speak the client's language, check with an interpreter or family member.)

Are the client's verbal responses appropriate? Does the client choose the correct words to express thoughts, or appear to have problems finding or articulating words? Does the client use nonsense or made-up words (neologisms)?

Can the client understand and follow commands? When given a multistep command, does the client forget what follows the first step?

If you and the client have trouble communicating, is the client aware of the difficulty? Does the client appear frustrated or angry when communication attempts fail? Or does the client continue to attempt to talk, unaware that you do not comprehend?

Glasgow Coma Scale

Originally designed as part of a tool for predicting a client's survival and recovery after a head injury, the Glasgow Coma Scale is now used to assess a client's level of consciousness (LOC). This scale minimizes the subjectivity historically accompanying LOC evaluations by testing and scoring three observations: eye response, motor response, and response to verbal stimuli. Each response receives a point value. An assessment totaling 15 points indicates that the client is alert, completely oriented to person, place, and time, and can follow simple commands. In a comatose client, the score will total 7 or less. A score of 3, the lowest possible score, indicates deep coma and a poor prognosis.

Many facilities display the Glasgow Coma Scale on neurologic flowsheets to show changes in the client's LOC over time.

OBSERVATION	RESPONSE ELICITED	SCORE
Eye response	• Opens spontaneously	4
	• Opens to verbal command	3
	• Opens to pain	2
	• No response	1
Motor response	• Reacts to verbal command	6
	• Reacts to painful stimuli	
	—Identifies localized pain	5
	—Flexes and withdraws	4
	—Assumes flexor posture	3
	—Assumes extensor posture	2
	• No response	1
Verbal response	• Is oriented and converses	5
	• Is disoriented, but converses	4
	• Uses inappropriate words	3
	• Makes incomprehensible sounds	2
	• No response	1

If observation of and interactions with the client indicate a possible language difficulty, show the client a common object, such as a cup or a book, and ask for its name, or ask the client to repeat a word that you say, such as *dog, running,* or *breakfast.*

If the client appears to have difficulty understanding spoken language, ask the client to follow a simple instruction, such as "Touch your nose." If the client can do that, then try a two-step command, such as "Touch your right knee, then touch your nose."

Also keep in mind that language performance tends to fluctuate with the time of day and the client's physical condition. Even a healthy individual may have difficulty with language when ill or fatigued. However, increasing language difficulties may indicate a deterioration of neurologic status, warranting further evaluation and notification of the physician. Impaired language function results in dysphasia (impaired ability to use or understand language) or aphasia (inability to use or understand language, or both). Speech problems include articulation difficulties and slurred speech, which may result from facial muscle paralysis or a loss of part of the tongue. Neuromuscular speech impairment is called dysarthria; voice impairment is called dysphonia.

Mental status

Many authorities recommend a brief screening examination to help identify the client with disorders of thought processes. A typical screening examination consists of 10 questions, each addressing one area of the complete mental status examination. Consider conducting a mental status screening when the client's responses seem unreliable or indicate a possible disturbance of memory or cognitive processes. (For a list of appropriate questions, see *Mental status screening questions.*) Such a screening may help identify a need for a more in-depth evaluation.

Abnormal findings

Normal cerebral function depends on the continuous activity of the reticular activating system (RAS). RAS cells are normally hyperexcitable; therefore, disorders that depress CNS function usually affect these cells first, typically making a change in LOC the earliest indication of a brain problem. Rapid deterioration of LOC (minutes to hours) usually indicates an acute neurologic problem requiring immediate intervention. A gradually decreasing LOC (weeks to months) may reflect a progressive or degenerative neurologic disorder.

A client whose disorientation arises from an organic (physiologic) problem is likely to mistake unfamiliar surroundings or people for familiar ones. For example, the client may think that the hospital room is a bedroom at home or that you are a relative. When disorientation originates from psychiatric disturbances such as schizophrenia, the client's confusion pattern is usually bizarre.

A client who is disoriented to time often incorrectly identifies the year as one that occurred earlier. For example, a client may think this is 1972. Bizarre answers, such as 1756 or 2054, indicate a possible psychiatric disturbance, but these also could be the answers of an uncooperative client.

Mental status screening questions

As part of a neurologic screening assessment, the nurse can use specific questions to help identify clients with disordered thought processes. An incorrect answer to any of these questions can indicate a need for a complete mental status examination.

QUESTION	FUNCTION SCREENED
What is your name?	Orientation to person
What is today's date?	Orientation to time
What year is it?	Orientation to time
Where are you now?	Orientation to place
How old are you?	Memory
Where were you born?	Remote memory
What did you have for breakfast?	Recent memory
Who is the U.S. president?	General knowledge
Can you count backwards from 20 to 1?	Attention and calculation skills
Why are you here?	Judgment

A client oriented to place may not be able to name the hospital, especially if admitted through the emergency department. On the other hand, a client who states the full name of the hospital and later cannot recall the name may be becoming disoriented to place and would require frequent reassessment. A hospitalized client disoriented to place most often confuses the hospital room with home or some other familiar surroundings; a nonhospitalized client disoriented to place, such as an individual suffering from Alzheimer's disease, may fail to recognize familiar home surroundings. Such an individual may wander off in search of something familiar.

The client who is disoriented to person may be unable to give any response to the question, "What is your name?" The client may look baffled, or may stammer and finally produce an unintelligible or inaccurate name.

Developmental and cultural considerations

Developmental and cultural status may affect the client's response, requiring modification of techniques for you to ensure accurate data collection.

The following considerations will help you assess LOC in a pediatric or elderly client or one with a language barrier.

Pediatric client. Because an infant or young child may be unable to respond to direct questioning, observe the child's interaction with the environment to assess orientation. Also, the child's parents can be a valuable resource because they may detect subtle changes in the child's behavior before any overt change in LOC.

To assess LOC in a young child, observe the child's behavior, noting activity, curiosity, shyness, or sleepiness. Then observe the child's response to parents or other familiar people. For example, does the child smile at the mother or appear not to recognize her? Also note the child's speech. If unable to speak yet, does the child attempt to imitate sounds or "coo" in response to the mother's voice? If able to speak, does the child use single words or short sentences? Are they appropriate to the situation?

Elderly client. When assessing an elderly client, remember that the client's ability to detect environmental stimuli accurately directly influences orientation. Decreased visual and auditory acuity related to aging can prevent the elderly client from properly recognizing or interpreting stimuli in the hospital environment. Also, keep in mind that an elderly client may process information more slowly. Before concluding that the client is disoriented, repeat the question and allow adequate response time.

Client with language barrier. A language barrier can cause an inaccurate assessment of the client's orientation. For a non-English-speaking client, consult an interpreter or ask the client's family or friends about the client's orientation, if appropriate. A client with aphasia may seem disoriented when in fact the client may not understand your questions.

To avoid inaccurate assessments, remember that orientation actually reflects the client's ability to correctly interpret and respond to surroundings. Therefore, if you cannot communicate verbally with the client, observe the client's interaction with people or things in the environment.

Advanced assessment skills

Advanced assessment of cerebral function includes assessment of communication by a formal language skills evaluation and a complete mental status assessment. A speech pathologist usually performs the language skills evaluation; a physician or specially prepared nurse conducts the complete mental status assessment. Because the nurse must know and understand the findings of a complete language and mental status examination, this section includes information about advanced assessment of cerebral function.

Formal language skills evaluation. This evaluation identifies the extent and characteristics of the client's language deficits, and it is valuable for two reasons. First, it helps pinpoint the site of a CNS lesion. For example, it can identify expressive aphasia (condition in which the client knows what he or she wants to say but cannot speak the words), which suggests a frontal lobe lesion. Second, it helps individualize the speech therapy program to meet the client's needs most effectively.

The formal language assessment includes an evaluation of the following skills:

Spontaneous speech. The client is shown a picture and asked to describe what is going on.

Comprehension. The client is asked a series of simple yes or no questions, and answers are evaluated. Questions with obvious answers are used to avoid unintentional testing of general knowledge. For example: "Does it snow in July?" or "Are your pants on fire?"

Naming. The client is shown various common objects, one at a time, and then asked to name each one. Typical objects include a comb, a ball, a cup, and a pencil.

Repetition. The client is asked to repeat words or phrases. For example: "no ifs, ands or buts."

Vocabulary. The client is asked to explain the meaning of each of a series of words.

Reading. The client is asked to read printed words on cards and perform the action described. For example: "Raise your hand."

Writing. The client is asked to write something, perhaps a story describing what is happening in a picture.

Copying figures. The client is shown several figures, one at a time, and then asked to copy them. The figures usually increase in complexity, ranging from a circle, to an X, to a square, to a triangle, and finally, to a star.

Complete mental status assessment. This assessment provides information about the client's cognitive, psychological, and intellectual skills and usually is reserved for examination of a chronically disoriented client or for a detailed evaluation after a screening assessment has revealed mental status deficits or suspicious findings.

To conduct the mental status assessment, find a quiet, private setting that will minimize distractions. Then ask a series of questions, each designed to evaluate one type of cognitive skill, and record the client's answers. Use the following guidelines to assess nine aspects of the client's mental status.

General appearance and behavior. Carefully observe the client during the interview, keeping the following questions in mind:
- How is the client's hygiene?
- Is the client's dress appropriate for age and situation?
- Is the client relaxed, or anxious and fidgety?
- How is the client's posture? Stiff? Slumped?
- How does the client interact with other people and things in the immediate environment?
- What is the quality and quantity of speech? Loud, soft, fast-paced, clear, or garbled? Is it appropriate?

Mood and affect. Observe the client's prevailing mood or attitude during the interview. Keep these questions in mind:
- Does the client appear happy or sad?
- Does the client's facial expression vary appropriately to the topics discussed?

Besides these questions, ask about the client's moods and feelings.

Cognitive functions. Assess the client's ability to think by evaluating orientation to person, place, and time, as described on page 479.

Attention. Attention is the ability to concentrate on a task over time without being distracted. Evaluate this skill by asking the client to focus on a series of numbers, using one of these two techniques: digit span or serial 7s or 3s.

To assess *digit span,* follow these steps:
- Read aloud to the client a short series of numbers, such as *5, 2* or *3, 7,* at about 1 per second.
- Have the client immediately repeat the numbers. Then read the next series, which should add a number, such as *6, 2, 4* or *9, 3, 11.* Avoid using numbers with a meaningful arrangement, such as *1, 2, 3, 4* or *2, 4, 6, 8.*
- When the client makes a mistake, offer another opportunity with a series of the same length. Stop after the second failure. Most people should be able to remember and immediately repeat 5 to 8 digits.

• Ask the client to repeat numbers in a series backwards. For example, say "2, 5, 6, 9" and ask the client to repeat this series backwards. The client should answer "9, 6, 5, 2." Again, start with a short series and gradually increase the length. Most people can recall 4 to 6 digits backwards.

To assess *serial 7s or serial 3s,* follow these steps:

• Have the client orally subtract 7 from 100, and then subtract 7 from the remainder, and so on, until the client makes a mistake. Demonstrate the task for the client if necessary.
• Observe the effort, speed, and accuracy of the client's performance. Most people can complete serial 7s in about 1½ minutes with fewer than four errors.
• If the client cannot perform serial 7s, repeat the process with serial 3s.

Memory. Because the client reveals a great deal about memory during the interview, specific questioning may not be necessary. In fact, the attention exercises indirectly test immediate memory. If the client's memory appears unreliable based on the answers to interview questions, ask specific questions to evaluate recent and remote memory. Be sure to ask questions that you know the answers to or that can be easily verified.

To assess *remote memory,* ask the following questions:

• When is your birthday?
• What was your mother's maiden name?

To assess *recent memory,* ask the following questions:

• What did you have for breakfast?
• How did you travel here today?

To evaluate recent memory further, follow these steps:

• State several words, such as "a red wagon and a doll" or "24 Willow Street."
• Have the client immediately repeat the words to make sure that the client heard them correctly; tell the client to remember them.
• Then proceed with other parts of the mental status assessment.
• After about 5 minutes, ask the client to repeat the words and evaluate the client's recall ability.

Intellectual skills. Assessing general knowledge and vocabulary can provide information about the client's intelligence level. Because intellectual skills relate to the client's educational and cultural background, be sure to ask about these factors. If needed, modify this portion of the examination in light of the client's background. Use the following guidelines to assess intellectual skills.

To assess *general knowledge,* ask the following questions:

• How many days are in a week? How many months are in a year?
• Why does water boil?
• How many states make up the United States?

To assess *vocabulary,* ask the client to define familiar words. Begin with easy words, such as *apple* or *cat,* and proceed to more difficult words, such as *shadow, plural,* or *earthquake.* Finally, ask the most difficult words, such as *chastise, egress,* or *dictatorial.*

To assess *calculation skills,* note the client's performance of the serial 7s test, which evaluates the client's ability to perform simple calculations. To assess calculation skills further ask the client to perform simple arithmetic problems such as 5 + 3 = ___. Then ask the client to solve this problem: "A loaf of bread costs 75 cents. You give the cashier one dollar. How much change should you receive?"

Abstract reasoning. An evaluation of abstract reasoning provides insight into the client's ability to think about things or situations that are not physically present. Use the following guidelines to assess abstract reasoning through the use of proverbs and similarities.

To assess the client's ability to interpret *proverbs,* repeat a proverb, such as "The squeaky wheel gets the grease." Ask the client to explain what the proverb means. Note the appropriateness of the client's interpretation and the degree of its abstractness or concreteness.

To assess the client's ability to identify *similarities,* name two objects (such as an apple and an orange, or a chair and a sofa) and ask the client to explain how they are alike. Note the client's response. A typical response begins, "They are both . . .," indicating that the client has been able to categorize or group the two objects in some way. Determine whether the comparison is accurate and realistic.

Judgment. Sound judgment enables an individual to consider various behavior options and choose an appropriate course of action. Use the following guidelines to assess judgment by observation and direct questioning.

Observe how the client responds to his or her current situation and health status. Note whether the client's actions in response to the situation imply reasonable choices.

Use direct questioning to assess the client's judgment further. Present the client with several hypothetical situations and ask for a response to each. For example, ask the client, "What would you do if you were in a crowded theater and saw a fire?" Note the client's

(Text continues on page 486.)

Integrating assessment findings

Sometimes, a cluster of assessment findings will strongly suggest a particular neurologic disorder. In the chart below, column one shows groups of presenting signs and symptoms—the ones that make the client seek medical attention. Column two shows related assessment findings that the nurse may discover during the health history and physical assessment. The client may exhibit one or more of these findings. Column three shows the possible disorder indicated by a cluster of these findings.

PRESENTING SIGNS AND SYMPTOMS	RELATED ASSESSMENT FINDINGS	POSSIBLE DISORDER
Early morning headache, subtle personality changes or dysphasia	Papilledema, possibly leading to visual loss Changes in pupil size and response Disorders of extraocular movement Focal deficits New onset of seizures	Brain tumor
Hemiparesis or hemiparalysis, loss of tactile sensation on affected side of body	Hypertension; atherosclerosis; family history of cardiovascular or cerebrovascular disease Sudden onset of symptoms with or without warning signs Intact or altered mental activity; emotional lability Hemiparesis or hemiparalysis, usually affecting the arm more than the leg Facial sagging on affected side Impaired swallowing Homonymous hemianopia (vision defect in the right halves or left halves of the visual fields in both eyes) Language disturbance and aphasia with right-sided weakness Perceptual disturbance and altered visual-spacial perceptions with left-sided weakness Loss of sensation on affected side Disturbed stereognosis, body scheme, and visual-spacial skills	Cerebrovascular accident (CVA)
Personality changes, gradual progressive decrease in level of consciousness, headache	History of trivial head injury weeks or months earlier Progressive deterioration in mental activity and level of arousal Disorientation Focal deficit	Chronic subdural hematoma
Muscle weakness that affects the lower extremities first, flaccid paralysis, little or no sensory loss	History of recent surgery, cancer, pregnancy, childbirth, infection, or vaccination Respiratory insufficiency Labile blood pressure Tachycardia Vasomotor flushes Hyperpyrexia and increased sweating Tracheobronchial secretions Paralytic ileus Blurred vision or diplopia Facial weakness; impaired swallowing Symmetrical flaccid paralysis, usually beginning in legs and progressing upward Absent deep tendon reflexes	Guillain-Barré syndrome
Sharp, severe pain in the back, which may radiate down extremity (in a pattern that reflects the nerve involved) and may be intensified by such actions as coughing, sneezing, straining, and moving	History of recurring symptoms Decreased muscle tone in affected area Mild motor weakness Paresthesia in affected area Intact, absent, or diminished brachioradialis, biceps, and triceps reflexes, depending on the level of lesion Diminished or absent patellar and Achilles reflexes	Herniated intervertebral disc

Integrating assessment findings continued

PRESENTING SIGNS AND SYMPTOMS	RELATED ASSESSMENT FINDINGS	POSSIBLE DISORDER
Headache, nuchal rigidity, elevated temperature (up to 105° F.), irritability, restlessness, photophobia, confusion	History of adjacent infection, neurosurgery, head trauma, systemic sepsis, or immunosuppression Restlessness, disorientation, lethargy, stupor, coma Decreased visual acuity or loss Brudzinski's sign, Kernig's sign Generalized seizures Opisthotonos (abnormal posture characterized by back arching and wrist flexion) as a late sign Hyperalgesia, photophobia, increased reflexes Elevated temperature Altered respiratory pattern; weak, rapid pulse Vomiting	Meningitis
Throbbing headache lasting 2 to 12 hours often preceded by a visual disturbance or scotomata lasting 15 to 20 minutes; anorexia; nausea; vomiting; diarrhea; photophobia; dizziness; syncope, scalp tenderness	History of stress, fatigue, hormonal changes, menstruation, change in amount of sleep, or other predisposing factors Ingestion of certain foods (such as aged cheese, red wine, or chocolate) or oral contraceptives that seem to trigger symptoms Perfectionist, compulsive, intelligent, rigid personality type; family emphasis on achievement Transient mood and personality changes Prodromal transient neurologic deficits such as hemiparesis, aphasia, ophthalmoplegia, and photophobia	Classic migraine
Akinesia, cogwheel rigidity, resting tremor, gait disturbance, impaired swallowing, flat affect, monotonous speech, decreased blinking, increased sweating and salivation	History of cerebral arteriosclerosis, cerebral hypoxia, trauma, toxin ingestion (carbon monoxide, manganese, or mercury), or use of illegal drugs Slow onset and gradual progression of signs and symptoms Emotional lability, depression, or paranoia Diminished facial movements, decreased blinking, impaired swallowing, and abnormal muscle tone Bradykinesia with difficulty initiating movement, intermittent "freezing," and pill-rolling tremor of hands Small, jerky, cramped handwriting (micrographia) Abnormal gait that is slow to start, includes short and shuffling steps, gradually accelerates, and is difficult to stop Low, monotonous speech; involuntary repetition of words (echolalia) or sentences (palilalia) spoken by others	Parkinson's disease
Pain and local tenderness throughout the sensory nerve root, motor weakness below level of lesion	Slow progression of sensory and motor dysfunction: initially unilateral, eventually bilateral Dysfunction of cranial nerves VIII through XII (with lesion at C4 or above) Spastic weakness or paralysis below the lesion Flaccid paralysis or weakness at level of lesion Respiratory failure or difficulty, occipital headache, nystagmus, and stiff neck with lesion at C4 or above Sensory loss below the level of the lesion Loss of pain and temperature sensation below and contralateral to lesion when only one side of cord is affected Loss of tactile, position, and vibration sensations ipsilateral to lesion Band of hyperesthesia just above level of lesion Increased deep tendon reflexes below level of lesion Absent reflexes at level of lesion; intact reflexes above lesion; positive Babinski reflex	Spinal cord tumor

response and how long it took to formulate. Determine whether the choice of action is appropriate for the situation.

Thought processes and content. Evaluation of the client's thought processes considers the overall appropriateness and coherence of the client's thinking. Note the content and organization of the client's thoughts during the interview and reflect on these questions.

- Does the client present historical data in a logical, consecutive manner without going off on a tangent?
- Does the client describe any unusual sensory-perceptual experiences or feelings that do not appear to be grounded in reality, such as hallucinations or illusions?

For some common abnormal assessment findings associated with the nervous system, see *Integrating assessment findings*, pages 484 and 485.

Developmental and cultural considerations. When assessing a client's language ability, keep in mind that developmental and cultural factors may affect the client's responses as well as your findings. Always conduct a formal language assessment in the client's primary language.

Consider the client's educational and cultural background when evaluating responses to certain questions in the complete mental status assessment. For example, performing serial 7s depends on the client's mathematical education as well as the client's ability to concentrate. Poor performance may reflect poor mathematical skills rather than poor attention. For such clients, replace that task with another exercise, such as counting from 1 to 100 or repeating the alphabet.

Another aspect of the assessment closely related to the client's social and cultural background is interpreting proverbs. A child may interpret a proverb literally. For example, a child may explain the proverb, "A rolling stone gathers no moss," by saying that "Moss won't get stuck on a stone rolling down a hill because it is going too fast." Abstract reasoning allows a person to appreciate the symbolic meaning of certain phrases, whereas concrete thinking grounds explanations in objective reality. A client from a non-Western, non-Anglo-American culture may interpret proverbs quite differently or may be unable to make any sense of certain proverbs at all because of unfamiliarity with the idiom. In a case like that, eliminate the interpretation of proverbs from the assessment.

When assessing judgment, realize that *your* cultural values can affect evaluation of the client's responses. Avoid bias and be objective when determining whether the client's response shows good or poor judgment. Do not presume that a client's choice of action must be the same as yours to show good judgment. Instead, consider whether the client's choice of action would be safe and appropriate for the situation.

Finally, general knowledge and vocabulary depend on the client's educational preparation, cultural background, and age. Like all standardized tests for evaluating intelligence, the mental status examination may contain questions or sections that are inappropriate for some clients. Eliminate such questions or parts.

Cranial nerves

Cranial nerve (CN) assessment provides valuable information about the condition of the CNS, particularly the brain stem. Because of their anatomic locations, some cranial nerves are more vulnerable than others to the effects of increasing intracranial pressure (ICP). That is why a neurologic screening assessment of the cranial nerves focuses on these key nerves: the optic (II), oculomotor (III), trochlear (IV), and abducens (VI). Evaluate the other nerves only if the client's history or symptoms indicate a potential cranial nerve disorder or when a complete nervous system assessment must be performed. However, because disorders can affect any of the cranial nerves, become familiar with methods for testing each nerve. (For a description of assessment techniques and normal findings, see *Cranial nerve assessment*, pages 488 and 489.)

Abnormal findings

The following section describes the significance of CN abnormal findings.

Olfactory nerve (CN I). The location of the olfactory nerve makes it especially vulnerable to damage from facial fractures and head injuries. Disorders of the base of the frontal lobe, such as tumors or arteriosclerotic changes, also can damage the nerve. The sense of smell remains intact as long as one of the two olfactory nerves exists; it is permanently lost (anosmia) if both nerves are affected. Anosmia also may result from non-neurologic causes, such as nasal congestion, sinus infection, smoking, or cocaine use.

Because loss of smell also impairs sense of taste, a complaint about the taste of food may signal olfactory nerve damage.

Optic nerve (CN II). CVA, head injury, or brain tumor can cause a visual field defect. The area and extent of the loss depends on the location of the lesion. In a blind client with a totally nonfunctional optic nerve, light stimulation will fail to produce either a direct or a consensual

er, a legally blind client may
ction, which causes the blind
ht. In a client who is totally
ipil of the eye with the intact
ect light stimulation, whereas
ives sensory messages from
will respond consensually.

reased ICP can put pressure
ausing a change in respon-
n the affected side. If the
the other oculomotor nerve
ng both pupils to change in
ng ICP can cause the pupils
ishly to light shortly before

n—characterized by brisk
to light followed by a pul-
n—may be normal in some
ect early oculomotor nerve

e movements (nystagmus)
e brain stem, cerebellum,
acoustic nerve (CN VIII). It can also imply drug toxicity, as from the anticonvulsant phenytoin.

An absent corneal reflex may result from peripheral nerve or brain stem damage. However, a diminished corneal reflex often occurs in clients who wear contact lenses.

Trochlear nerve (CN IV). Increased ICP can put pressure on the trochlear nerve, causing impaired extraocular eye movement inferiorly and medially.

Trigeminal nerve (CN V). Peripheral nerve damage can create a loss of sensation in any or all of the three regions supplied by the trigeminal nerve (head, face, jaw). Also, a lesion in the cervical spinal cord or brain stem can produce impaired motor or sensory function in each of the three areas. This can weaken the jaw muscles, causing the jaw to deviate toward the affected side when chewing, or allowing residual food to collect in the affected cheek.

Abducens nerve (CN VI). Increased ICP can put pressure on the abducens nerve, causing impaired extraocular eye movement laterally.

Facial nerve (CN VII). Unilateral facial weakness can reflect an upper motor neuron problem, such as a CVA or a tumor that has damaged neurons in the facial control area of the motor strip in the cerebral cortex. If the weakness originates in the cerebral cortex, the client will retain the ability to wrinkle the forehead, because the forehead receives motor messages from both hemispheres of the brain—which explains why when one side is damaged, as in a CVA, the other side takes over.

However, if the facial nerve itself is damaged, then the weakness extends to the forehead, and the eye on the affected side does not close.

An impaired sense of taste can signify damage to the facial or glossopharyngeal nerve, or may simply reflect a part of the normal aging process. Chemotherapy or head and neck radiation can also alter taste by damaging taste bud receptors.

Acoustic nerve (CN VIII). Hearing loss, nystagmus, disturbance of balance, and dizziness all can indicate acoustic nerve damage.

Glossopharyngeal (CN IX) and vagus (CN X) nerves. Glossopharyngeal neuralgia produces paroxysmal pain, which radiates from the throat to the ear. Damage to the glossopharyngeal or vagus nerves impairs swallowing. Furthermore, during swallowing, the palate fails to rise and close off the nasal passageways, allowing nasal regurgitation of fluids. A damaged vagus nerve also can cause loss of the gag reflex and a hoarse or nasal-sounding voice. Finally, because the vagus nerve innervates most viscera through the parasympathetic nervous system, vagal damage can affect involuntary vital functions, producing various disturbances, such as tachycardia, other cardiac dysrhythmias, and dyspnea.

Spinal accessory nerve (CN XI). Unilateral weakness, atrophy, or paralysis of the muscles innervated by the spinal accessory nerve suggests a peripheral nerve lesion. Symptoms include a drooping shoulder or a scapula that appears displaced toward the affected side.

Hypoglossal nerve (CN XII). A peripheral nerve lesion creates a unilateral flaccid paralysis of the tongue, atrophy of the affected side, and deviation of the tongue. A unilateral spastic paralysis of the tongue produces poorly articulated, difficult speech (dysarthria) characterized by an explosive production of words. The tongue deviates toward the unaffected side.

Developmental considerations

As in other assessment techniques, adjust the cranial nerve assessment to the client's age.

(Text continues on page 490.)

Cranial nerve assessment

The techniques for cranial nerve assessment vary according to the nerve being tested. The chart below describes these techniques and identifies normal findings.

CRANIAL NERVE	ASSESSMENT TECHNIQUE	NORMAL FINDINGS
Olfactory (CN I)	After checking the patency of the client's nostrils, have the client close both eyes. Then occlude one nostril, and hold a familiar, pungent-smelling substance, such as coffee, tobacco, soap, or peppermint, under the client's nose and ask its identity. Repeat this technique with the other nostril.	The client should be able to detect and identify the smell correctly. If the client reports detecting the smell but cannot name it, offer a choice, such as, "Do you smell lemon, coffee, or peppermint?"
Optic (CN II) and oculomotor (CN III)	To assess the optic nerve, check visual acuity, visual fields, and the retinal structures. To assess the oculomotor nerve, check pupil size, pupil shape, and pupillary response to light. (For a description of how to perform these assessments, see Chapter 9, Eyes and Ears.)	The pupils should be equal, round, and reactive to light. When assessing pupil size, be especially alert for any trends. For example, watch for a gradual increase in the size of one pupil or the appearance of unequal pupils in a client whose pupils were previously equal.
Oculomotor (CN III), trochlear (CN IV), and abducens (CN VI)	To test the coordinated function of these three nerves, assess them simultaneously by evaluating the client's extraocular eye movement. (For a description of how to perform these assessments, see Chapter 9, Eyes and Ears.)	The eyes should move smoothly and in a coordinated manner through all six directions of eye movement. Observe each eye for rapid oscillation (nystagmus), movement not in unison with that of the other eye (dysconjugate movement), or inability to move in certain directions (ophthalmoplegia). Also note any complaint of double vision (diplopia).
Trigeminal (CN V)	To assess the sensory portion of the trigeminal nerve, gently touch the right, then the left side of the client's forehead with a cotton ball while the client's eyes are closed. Instruct the client to state the moment the cotton touches the area. Compare the client's response on both sides. Repeat the technique on the right and left cheek and on the right and left jaw. Next, repeat the entire procedure using a sharp object. The cap of a disposable ballpoint pen can be used to test light touch (dull end) and sharp stimuli (sharp end). (If an abnormality appears, also test for temperature sensation by touching the client's skin with test tubes filled with hot and cold water and asking the client to differentiate between them.) To assess the motor portion of the trigeminal nerve, ask the client to clench the jaws. Palpate the temporal and masseter muscles bilaterally, checking for symmetry. Try to open the client's clenched jaws. Next, watch the client's opening and closing mouth for asymmetry. Then assess the corneal reflex. (For information about this procedure, see Chapter 9, Eyes and Ears.)	The client with a normal trigeminal nerve should report feeling both light touch and sharp stimuli in all three areas (forehead, check, and jaw) on both sides of the face. The jaws should clench symmetrically and remain closed against resistance. The lids of both eyes should close when a wisp of cotton is lightly stroked across a cornea.
Facial (CN VII)	To test the motor portion of the facial nerve, ask the client to wrinkle the forehead, raise and lower the eyebrows, smile to show teeth, and puff out the cheeks. Also, with the client's eyes tightly closed, attempt to open the eyelids. With each of these movements, observe closely for symmetry.	Normal facial movements are symmetrical.

Cranial nerve assessment continued

CRANIAL NERVE	ASSESSMENT TECHNIQUE	NORMAL FINDINGS
Facial (CN VII) (continued)	To test the sensory portion of the facial nerve, which supplies taste sensation to the anterior two-thirds of the tongue, first prepare four marked, closed containers, with one containing salt, another sugar, a third, vinegar (or lemon), and a fourth, quinine (or bitters). Then, with the client's eyes closed, place salt on the anterior two-thirds of the tongue using a cotton swab or dropper. Ask the client to identify the taste as sweet, salty, sour, or bitter. Rinse the client's mouth with water. Repeat this procedure, alternating flavors and sides of the tongue until all four flavors have been tested on both sides. Taste sensations to the posterior third of the tongue are supplied by the glossopharyngeal nerve (CN IX) and are usually tested at the same time.	Normal taste sensations are symmetrical.
Acoustic (CN VIII)	To assess the acoustic portion of this nerve, test the client's hearing acuity. (For a description of how to perform these tests, see Chapter 9, Eyes and Ears.) To assess the vestibular portion of this nerve, observe for nystagmus and disturbed balance and note reports of dizziness or the room spinning.	The client should be able to hear a whispered voice or a watch tick. The client should display normal eye movement and balance and have no dizziness or vertigo.
Glossopharyngeal (CN IX) and vagus (CN X)	To assess these nerves, which have overlapping functions, first listen to the client's voice for indications of a hoarse or nasal quality. Then watch the client's soft palate when the client says "ah." Next, test the gag reflex after warning the client. To evoke this reflex, touch the posterior wall of the pharynx with a cotton swab or tongue depressor.	The client's voice should sound strong and clear. The soft palate and the uvula should rise when the client says "ah," and the uvula should remain midline. The palatine arches should remain symmetrical during movement and at rest. The gag reflex should be intact. If the gag reflex appears decreased or the pharynx moves asymmetrically, evaluate each side of the posterior wall of the pharynx to confirm integrity of both cranial nerves.
Spinal accessory (CN XI)	To assess, press down on the client's shoulders while the client attempts to shrug against this resistance. Note shoulder strength and symmetry while inspecting and palpating the trapezius muscle. Then, apply resistance to the client's turned head while the client attempts to return to a midline position. Note neck strength while inspecting and palpating the sternocleidomastoid muscle. Repeat for the opposite side.	Normally, both shoulders should be able to overcome the resistance equally well. The neck should overcome resistance in both directions.
Hypoglossal (CN XII)	To assess, observe the client's protruded tongue for any deviation from midline, atrophy, or fasciculations (very fine muscle flickerings indicative of lower motor neuron disease). Next, ask the client to move the tongue rapidly from side to side with the mouth open, curl the tongue up toward the nose, and then curl the tongue down toward the chin. Then use a tongue depressor or folded gauze pad to apply resistance to the client's protruded tongue, and ask the client to try to push the depressor to one side. Repeat on the other side and note tongue strength. Listen to the client's speech for the sounds *d, l, n,* and *t,* which require use of the tongue. If general speech suggests a problem, have the client repeat a phrase or series of words containing these sounds.	Normally, the tongue should be midline and the client should be able to move it right to left equally. The client should be able to move the tongue up and down. Pressure exerted by the tongue on the tongue depressor should be equal on either side. Speech should be clear.

Pediatric client. To test the olfactory nerve in a child, use a substance that the child can identify, such as an orange or peanut butter. For a very young child or for a non-English-speaking or aphasic client, hold an unpleasant-smelling substance, such as acetone, under the client's nose, which should cause the client to grimace.

A child or young adult will have larger pupils than an older client. Nystagmus normally occurs in an infant immediately after birth, but should not persist for more than a few days. Persistent nystagmus can indicate blindness.

Assess an infant's sucking strength by attempting to open the infant's mouth and noting the resistance. Observe for symmetrical mouth movements when the infant cries or babbles.

To assess the facial nerve in an infant or small child, observe the child's facial movements when the child eats or cries. Ask an older child to make a "sad face," a "happy face," and a "mad face."

To assess an infant's spinal accessory nerve, raise the infant by the shoulders from a supine to a sitting position and note head control. To facilitate assessment of a young child's spinal accessory nerve, encourage the child to "show how strong you are."

To assess the hypoglossal nerve, observe tongue movements when the infant cries. The tongue normally appears midline and strongly controlled. If necessary, gently pinch the nose closed, which will stimulate the mouth to open and may cause the infant to cry.

Elderly client. With aging, the pupils normally become smaller and accommodation diminishes. However, a sudden loss of accommodation can indicate a neurologic disorder. Remember that an elderly client may have permanently irregular, and often nonreactive, pupils after cataract surgery or artificial lens implantation.

Motor system and cerebellar function

Motor system assessment evaluates the ability of the cerebral cortex to plan and initiate motor activity of the pyramidal and extrapyramidal pathways, to carry nerve impulses to the CNS, of the corticospinal tracts to carry motor messages down the spinal cord, of the lower motor neurons to carry efferent impulses to the muscles, of the muscles to carry out motor commands, and of the cerebellum and basal ganglia to coordinate and fine-tune movement.

The neurologic screening assessment of the motor system always includes assessment of the client's muscle strength (including muscle size and symmetry), arm and leg movement, and gait. Gait reflects the integrated activity of muscle strength and tone, extremity movement and coordination, balance, proprioception (sense of position), and the ability of the cerebral cortex to plan and sequence movements.

A complete neurologic assessment of the motor system includes evaluation of motor functions (muscle size, tone, strength, and movement), cerebellar functions (balance and coordination), and gait. When performing a complete assessment, proceed from head to toe (for example, moving from the neck to the shoulders, arms, trunk, hips, and finally to the legs), assessing all muscles of the major joints. Then assess the client's gait and cerebellar functions. Usually, the complete motor system assessment is reserved for clients who display a motor deficit during the screening assessment and for those who need a complete neurologic examination.

Motor function

Evaluate muscle strength (including size and symmetry) of the arms and legs, movement of the arms and legs, and gait for all clients. (For a description of how to assess these functions, see Chapter 18, Musculoskeletal System.)

When assessing arm strength, never use hand grasps. The primitive grasp reflex may return with brain dysfunction (especially with frontal lobe involvement), making hand grasps an unreliable indicator of strength and voluntary movement. Instead, assess arm strength by asking the client to push you away as you apply resistance. If this test suggests mild weakness in one arm, confirm your suspicions by evaluating for downward drift and pronation of the arm. (For a description of the evaluation procedure, see *Advanced assessment skills: Evaluating arm strength.)*

Assess the client's movement in response to a command. Instruct the client who is very weak to open and close each fist, or to move each arm without raising it off the bed or examination table. If the client fails to respond, observe for spontaneous movements of the arm. For example, note whether the client uses it for grooming, eating, personal hygiene, or positioning.

If no spontaneous movements occur, test for movement in response to tactile stimuli. Begin with a gentle touch or tickle on the arm. If the client does not move the arm, use a stronger stimulus, such as applying firm pressure over the nail bed with a blunt object like the side of a pen. Describe the client's response. Does the client attempt to withdraw the arm or try to push the stimulus away (a purposeful response)? Or does the

ADVANCED ASSESSMENT SKILLS

Evaluating arm strength

During these tests of arm strength, stand close to the client to prevent falls or have the client sit.

Ask the client to extend both arms palm up, close the eyes, and maintain this position for 20 to 30 seconds. Observe for downward drift and pronation of the arms. Pronation of one forearm, called pronator drift, may indicate a mild hemiparesis. Pronator drift may also be accompanied by downward drift of the arm, with flexion of the fingers and elbows. The client may also exhibit sideward or upward drift, which indicates loss of position sense.

Next, tap the client's arms downward. Normally, the arms return to the horizontal position, indicating proper muscle strength and coordination and sense of position; a weak arm is easily displaced and does not return to the horizontal position.

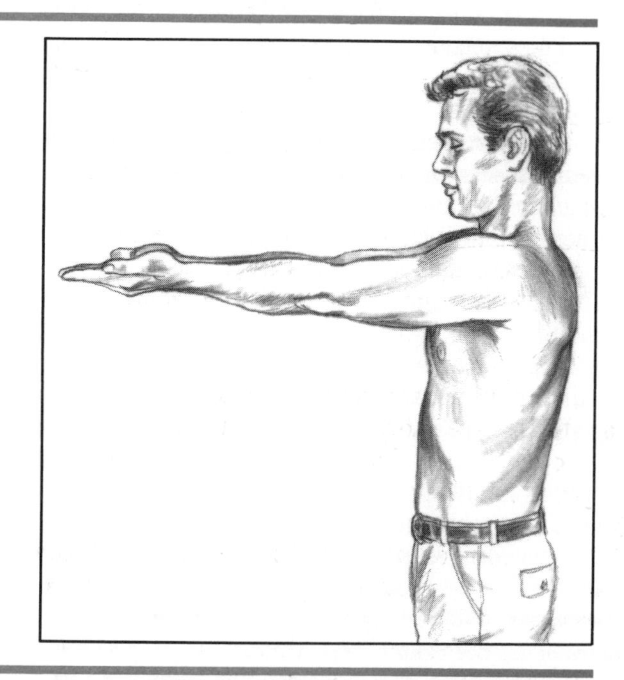

Ask the client to raise both arms overhead, palms up, and maintain this position for 20 to 30 seconds. The client normally can maintain this position well. Next, attempt to force the client's arms down to the sides while the client resists. Drifting or weakness during these tests may indicate hemiparesis.

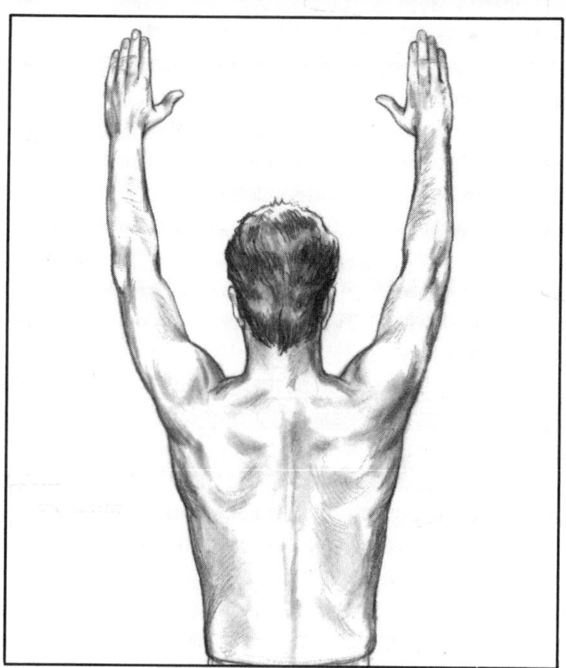

client extend or flex the arm in an abnormal or unusual position (a nonpurposeful response)?

Assess leg movement in the same manner, first asking the client to move each leg and foot. If the client fails to move the leg on command, observe for spontaneous movement. If the client cannot follow commands, if no spontaneous movements occur, and if the client requires a stimulus stronger than a light touch, press the Achilles tendon firmly between your thumb and index finger. Again, observe for purposeful or nonpurposeful movement.

Throughout the assessment, be alert for any involuntary movement of the limbs, trunk, or face. Determine whether the movement is proximal or distal and whether the movement occurs during sleep. Further assess any involuntary movements for rhythm or repetition, noting the number of repetitions per minute or second. Also note whether the involuntary movement increases, decreases, or stays the same in relation to normal movements, and whether other factors appear to exacerbate or alleviate the abnormal movement.

Abnormal findings

Abnormal findings can indicate several types of neurologic disorder. Muscle atrophy can indicate absent nerve stimulation (denervation) because of a peripheral nerve disorder (lower motor neuron disease) or can indicate disuse secondary to a lesion on the corticospinal tracts. Muscle hypertrophy may result from compensation for a weakness in other muscle groups.

Generalized muscle weakness can result from a metabolic disorder, such as electrolyte imbalance, malnutrition, prolonged illness, or bedrest. Unilateral weakness or paralysis of the arm and leg on the same side of the body (hemiparesis or hemiparalysis) suggests a lesion in the corticospinal tracts or in the motor cortex on the opposite side of the weakness or paralysis. Spasticity in the affected extremities can indicate upper motor neuron lesions, which may be caused by CVA, trauma, or brain tumor.

Bilateral paralysis or paresis suggests a lesion in the spinal cord or a disease affecting overall neuromuscular function.

Involuntary movements suggest a disorder of the basal ganglia, extrapyramidal tracts, or cerebellum. Nonpurposeful flexion or extension in response to stimuli usually indicates a severe cerebral or brain stem lesion. Disorders of the motor cortex or corticospinal tracts produce spastic hemiparesis and a characteristic gait. If the disorder involves both corticospinal tracts, as in spinal cord disease, then bilateral spastic paresis of the legs occurs, causing a scissors gait (the legs tend to cross each other). If the disorder affects the peripheral nerves or muscles, foot drop and flaccidity result (one leg appears to drag as the toes fail to lift with each step).

Developmental considerations

When assessing motor system and cerebellar function, consider the client's developmental status and adjust your techniques accordingly.

Pediatric client. To assess movement in an infant, make observations when the infant is awake and active. Note the symmetry of extremity movements. Until age 2 months, fine tremors and occasional involuntary movements normally occur. Also, increased flexor muscle tone may persist until age 3 months.

Observe an older infant's or toddler's ability to grasp and manipulate objects. Carefully watch for indications of hand preference, which normally develops after age 2. Hand preference in an infant could indicate hemiparesis.

Be discrete when assessing a child's gait and movement. If aware of observation, the child may alter normal activity. Note balance, coordination, and muscle strength as the child rolls over, sits, crawls, stands, or walks. A child normally has a wide-based gait until age 6. A wide-based gait after that age could indicate a neuromuscular or cerebellar disorder.

Elderly client. Some loss of muscle mass and strength normally occurs with age. Arthritis or other degenerative disorders can limit range of motion and reduce mobility. Fine tremors may also occur. The elderly client's gait is often slower and may be less certain and steady.

Observe for any mild unilateral weakness, such as a clumsy hand or dragging foot, which could be the result of a small CVA. A shuffling, accelerating gait accompanies Parkinson's disease, as do "pill-rolling" hand tremors and cogwheel rigidity of the limbs.

Advanced assessment skills

Muscle tone and cerebellar function evaluations are parts of the complete neurologic assessment and are advanced assessment skills. Muscle tone is the underlying tension present in the muscle at all times. (For a description of how to assess muscle tone, see Chapter 18, Musculoskeletal System.)

To evaluate cerebellar function, test the client's balance and coordination. (For illustrated procedures, see *Advanced assessment skills: Assessing cerebellar function.*)

Although formal testing of cerebellar function is impossible before age 3 months, estimate cerebellar ac-

ADVANCED ASSESSMENT SKILLS

Assessing cerebellar function

The nurse can evaluate the client's cerebellar function by assessing balance and coordination. To assess balance, have the client perform tandem-gait heel-to-toe walking, the Romberg test, and heel and toe walking. To assess coordination, evaluate the client's ability to perform rapid alternating movements, point-to-point localization, and the leg coordination test.

To assess tandem-gait (heel-to-toe) walking, ask the client to walk heel-to-toe in a straight line, as shown below. Stand close to protect a weak or elderly client from falling. Observe for normal coordination and balance. If the client leans or falls to one side, note the direction. When performing heel-to-toe walking, the client will tend to lean or fall toward the side of the lesion. If the lesion is midline, the client cannot perform heel-to-toe walking and displays a wide-based, ataxic gait.

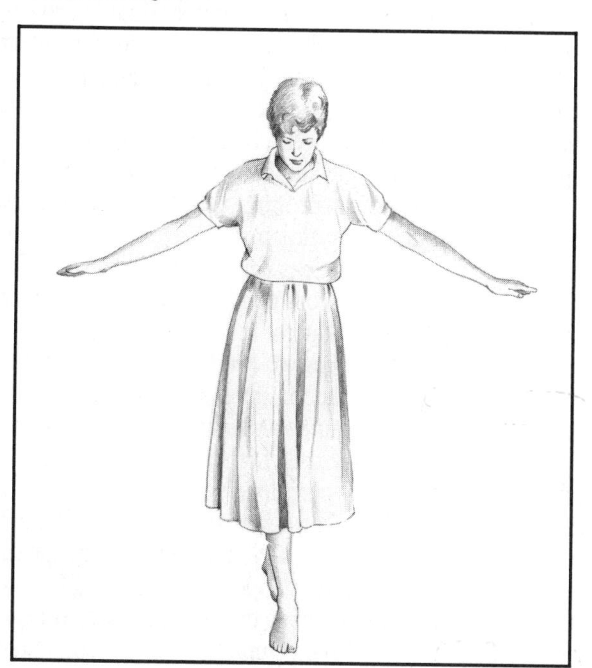

To perform the Romberg test, have the client stand with feet together, arms at sides, and without support. Observe the client's ability to maintain balance with both eyes open and then with them closed. (*Note:* Stand nearby in case the client loses balance.) Normally, a small amount of swaying occurs when the eyes are closed.

Note any abnormal problems with balance. When asked to perform the Romberg test, the client experiencing cerebellar ataxia will have trouble maintaining a steady position, with eyes opened or closed. In a positive Romberg test, the client can stand with eyes open, but loses balance with eyes closed. This indicates damage to the dorsal columns of the spinal cord, which interferes with sense of position in space. If the client has difficulty with the Romberg test, omit further balance testing.

To assess heel and toe walking, first ask the client to walk on the heels. Then have the client walk on the toes. Observe balance, coordination, and ankle strength during both procedures. Note any deviation from the normal ability to walk steadily on the heels and toes.

To assess rapid alternating movements, begin with the arms. Have the seated client pat one thigh with one hand as rapidly as possible. Test the other arm, noting speed and rhythm.

Next, have the client place an open palm on one thigh and then turn the hand over, touching the thigh with the top of the hand, as shown below. Have the client repeat this pronation and supination of the hand as rapidly as possible. Note the speed and the degree of ease or difficulty in performing the maneuver.

Have the client use the thumb of one hand to touch each finger of the same hand in rapid sequence. Repeat with the other hand. The nondominant hand will perform rapid alternating movement tasks more slowly than the dominant hand.

To assess the legs, have the client rapidly tap the floor with the ball of one foot. Test each leg separately. Note any slowness or awkwardness in performing rapid alternating movements. Such abnormalities can reflect cerebellar disease or motor weakness associated with extrapyramidal disease.

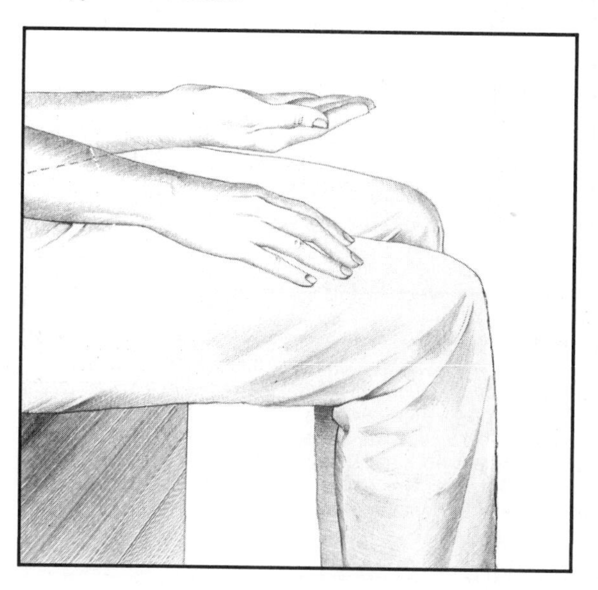

continued

ADVANCED ASSESSMENT SKILLS

Assessing cerebellar function continued

To assess point-to-point localization, have the client stand or sit with arms extended and then touch the nose. Have the client perform the test first with both eyes open, and then with them closed.

Next, hold one index finger in front of the client and ask the client to touch it with his or her index finger. Repeat the maneuver at various positions, as shown below. Evaluate the client's ability to adjust.

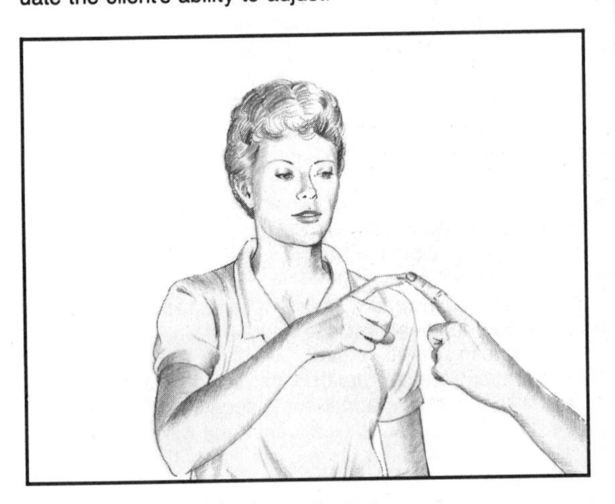

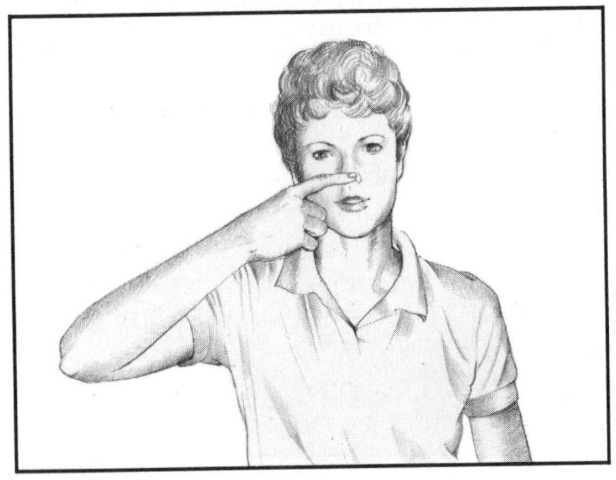

To assess leg coordination, have the client lie supine and place one heel on the shin of the opposite leg just below the knee. Then have the client slowly slide the heel along the shin toward the ankle. Repeat with the other leg. Note the client's ability to position each heel on the shin accurately as well as the ease, speed, and accuracy with which the client can move the heel down the shin.

tivity by observing the infant's sucking, swallowing, and kicking movements.

A toddler can walk but does not have the neuromuscular maturity necessary to perform most routine cerebellar tests. For example, a toddler cannot walk on tip-toes or heels and cannot stand on one leg unsupported for more than 5 or 6 seconds. Before age 7, a child usually cannot perform heel-to-toe (tandem) walking without making mistakes. Although a 7-year-old usually can walk on tip-toes or heels, the child will use more arm movements to maintain balance than an adult does. Coordination in a young child may be tested by having the child demonstrate an action, such as touching a finger to the nose.

Sensory system

Assessment of the sensory system evaluates how well the sensory receptors detect a stimulus, the afferent nerves carry sensory nerve impulse to the spinal cord, the sensory tracts in the spinal cord carry sensory messages to the brain, and the sensory, interpretive, and integrative functions of the cerebral cortex occur.

Basic neurologic screening usually consists of evaluating light-touch sensation in all extremities, and comparing both arms and legs for symmetry of sensation. Some experts also recommend assessing the client's sense of pain and vibration in the hands and feet, as well as the client's ability to recognize objects by touch (stereognosis). Those techniques are treated as part of the complete neurologic assessment in this chapter.

Because the sensory system becomes fatigued with repeated stimulation, complete sensory system testing in all dermatomes tends to give unreliable results. A few screening procedures usually can reveal any dysfunctions. If a localized deficit appears, or if the client complains of localized numbness or an unpleasant sensation (dysesthesia), perform a complete sensory assessment. Expect to perform a complete neurologic assessment for a client with motor or reflex abnormalilites or trophic skin changes, such as ulceration, atrophy, or absent sweating.

Before beginning the sensory system screening, ask the client about any areas of numbness or unusual sensations. Such areas require special attention.

To perform the assessment, have the client sit with eyes closed. Ask the client to say "yes" or "now" when you lightly touch the client's forearm with a cotton wisp. Allow time for the client's response, and then lightly touch the same area on the client's other arm.

Compare sensations on both sides of the client's body in the upper arm, back of the hand, thigh, lower leg, and top of the foot. Occasionally skip an area to test the reliabilty of the client's responses. However, be sure to check the skipped area for sensory response before concluding the assessment.

Be alert for complaints of numbness, tingling, or unusual sensations that accompany the tactile stimulus. Also note the degree of stimulation required to evoke a response. A light, brief touch should be sufficient.

Abnormal findings

The need for repeated, prolonged, or excessive contact to evoke a response indicates reduced sensory acuity.

If the client repeatedly fails to detect tactile stimuli in one body area, or if sensory acuity in one extremity appears to differ from that on the opposite side of the body, a sensory deficit may exist. Complaints of tingling or dysesthesia in one area could indicate damaged sensory nerve fibers, even if the client can correctly identify the tactile stimulus.

Advanced assessment skills

To assess sensory functioning further, perform a complete assessment of the client's sensory system and discriminative sensations. (For an illustrated procedure and a description of normal findings, see *Advanced assessment skills: Assessing the sensory system,* pages 496 and 497.) Loss of the sense of light touch, vibration, and position may suggest a disorder in the posterior tracts (dorsal columns) of the spinal cord or a peripheral nerve or root lesion. Impaired pain or temperature sensation indicates a disorder in the spinothalamic tracts of the spinal cord.

Loss of the sense of vibration often precedes the loss of other sensations in a developing peripheral neuropathy. A bilateral, symmetrical, distal sensory loss also suggests a peripheral neuropathy.

Impaired ability to recognize the distance between two points (discriminative sensation) indicates a disorder in the dorsal columns or the sensory interpretive regions of the parietal lobe of the cerebral cortex. Lesions of the sensory cortex can also impair point localization.

Developmental considerations

As with other areas of neurologic assessment, the client's developmental level affects sensory assessment.

Pediatric client. Because infants and toddlers cannot express themselves well and have poor sensory localization, sensory testing for these clients is especially difficult. To test a young child's tactile sensation, touch the nose or eyelashes with a cotton wisp. This should produce a blink response, confirming intact tactile sensation.

A child may have difficulty cooperating with complete sensory testing. Cotton wisps and vibrating tuning forks may tickle, causing the child to giggle. Some experts recommend letting the child hold the testing device, touch each extremity one at a time, and then describe the sensation. However, sensory testing results tend to vary and remain unreliable until the child has developed language skills.

Elderly client. In an elderly client, vibration sense normally diminishes or disappears in the feet and ankles. Occasionally, proprioception also diminishes or disappears in the distal lower extremities.

Reflexes

Assessment of deep tendon and superficial reflexes provides information about the intactness of the sensory receptor organ and evaluates how well the afferent nerve relays the sensory message to the spinal cord, the spinal cord or brain stem segment mediates the reflex, the lower motor neurons transmit messages to the muscles, and the muscles respond to the motor message.

Reflex assessment also indirectly provides information about the presence or absence of inhibiting brain messages. These messages travel along the corticospinal tract to modify reflex strength.

Advanced assessment skills

Evaluation of the reflexes is usually reserved for a complete neurologic assessment. (For a discussion of assessment techniques and normal findings, see *Advanced assessment skills: Assessing the reflexes,* pages 498 to 500.)

Reflexes fall into one of three groups: deep tendon reflexes, superficial reflexes, and pathologic superficial reflexes. Deep tendon reflexes, sometimes called muscle-stretch reflexes, occur when a sudden stimulus causes the muscle to stretch. When conducting deep tendon reflex assessment, be sure the client is relaxed and comfortable, because tension or anxiety may diminish the reflex. (For a description of techniques to minimize tension, see *Facilitating reflex testing,* page 502.) Also be sure to hold the reflex hammer loosely, yet securely, between your thumb and fingers so that the hammer can swing freely in a controlled direction; place the client's extremities in a neutral position, with the muscle to be tested in a slightly stretched position; and compare the reflexes on opposite sides of the body for symmetry of movement and muscle strength.

Superficial reflexes, also called cutaneous reflexes, may be elicited by light, rapid, tactile stimulation, such as stroking or scratching the tissue being tested.

ADVANCED ASSESSMENT SKILLS

Assessing the sensory system

The nurse can evaluate the client's sensory function further by assessing for superficial pain, temperature sensation, sense of position (proprioception), point localization, response to vibration, ability to recognize objects by the sense of touch (stereognosis), extinction, two-point discrimination, and number identification. All sensory testing must be performed with the client's eyes closed.

To assess superficial pain, lightly touch—but do not puncture—the client's skin using a sharp object, such as a sterile needle. Occasionally alternate sharp and blunt ends. (Remember to discard the sharp object safely after use, and never use the same object on a second client.)

Ask the client to identify the sensation as sharp or dull. Test and compare the distal and proximal portions of all extremities. If the client displays abnormal pain sensation, test for temperature sensation.

To assess temperature sensation, first fill two test tubes with water, one hot and the other cold.

Alternately touch the client's skin with the hot and cold test tubes, asking the client to differentiate between them. Test and compare distal and proximal portions of all extremities.

To assess sense of position, grasp the sides of the client's great toe between your thumb and forefinger. Move the toe upward or downward, asking the client to describe the position. Repeat on the other foot, and then perform the same technique on the client's fingers.

If the client exhibits an impaired sense of position, proceed to the next joint on the extremity and repeat the procedure. On the leg, progress from the ankle to the knee; on the arm, from the wrist to the elbow, as shown.

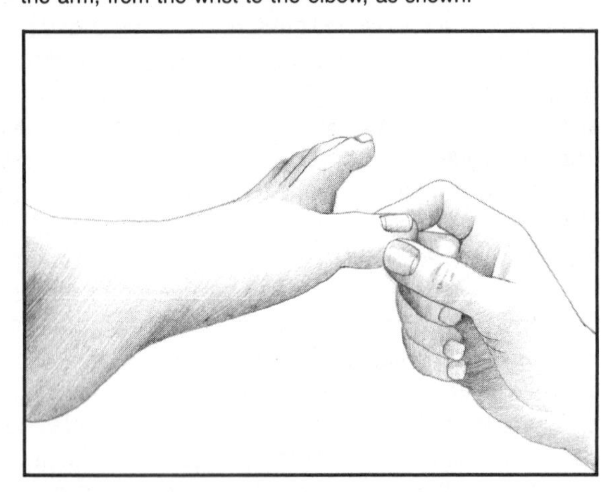

To assess point localization, have the client close both eyes while you briefly touch a point on the client's skin. Ask the client, with eyes open, to point to the place just touched. The client should be able to identify the spot.

To assess the response to vibration, tap a low-pitched tuning fork (preferably 128 cycles per second) on the heel of your hand and then place the base of the tuning fork firmly on an interphalangeal joint (any of the client's fingers or the great toe).

Ask the client to describe the sensation, differentiating between pressure and vibration, and then to state when the feeling stops. Proceed from distal to proximal areas.

If the client has intact distal vibration sensation, further testing is unnecessary. However, if the client suffers from an absence of distal vibratory sensation, test the next most proximal bony prominence. When assessing the leg, progress from the medial malleolus, to the patella, to the anterior superior iliac spine, to the spinous process of the vertebra. For the arm, progress from the wrist, to the elbow, to the shoulder.

To assess stereognosis, place a familiar object, such as a key, pencil, or paper clip, in the client's hand and ask the client to identify the object by feel—which the client should be able to do. A particularly sensitive test of stereognosis involves having the client identify the "heads" and "tails" sides of a coin. If motor impairment of the hand makes stereognosis testing impossible, evaluate number identification.

To assess extinction, touch two corresponding parts on the client (such as the forearms just above the wrist) simultaneously, as shown. Ask the client to describe the location of the touch. The client should sense the touch in both locations.

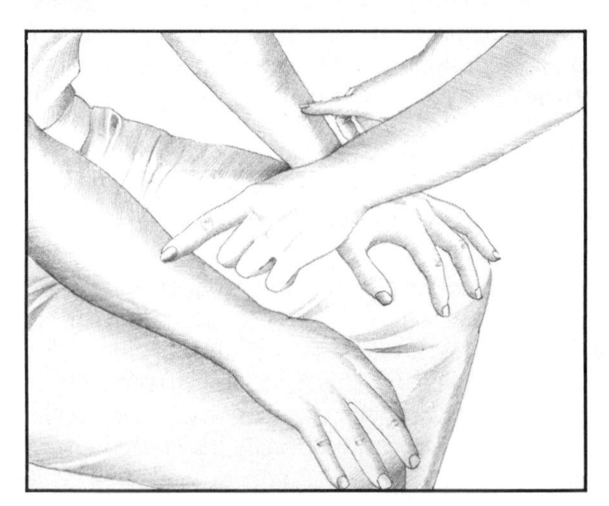

To assess two-point discrimination, alternately touch one or two sharp objects to the client's skin, as shown. First assess whether the client can feel one or two points; then assess the smallest distance between the two points at which the client can still discriminate the presence of two points. Acuity varies in different body areas. On the finger pads, an area rich in tactile sensory receptors, the average distance necessary for two-point discrimination is less than 5 mm. On the client's back, however, two-point discrimination requires a much wider distance.

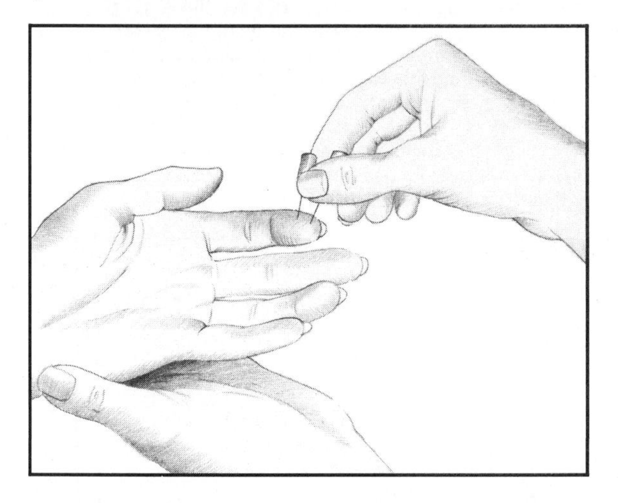

To assess number identification, trace a large number on the client's palm, using a blunt object, such as the blunt end of pen or pencil, as shown. The client should be able to identify the number.

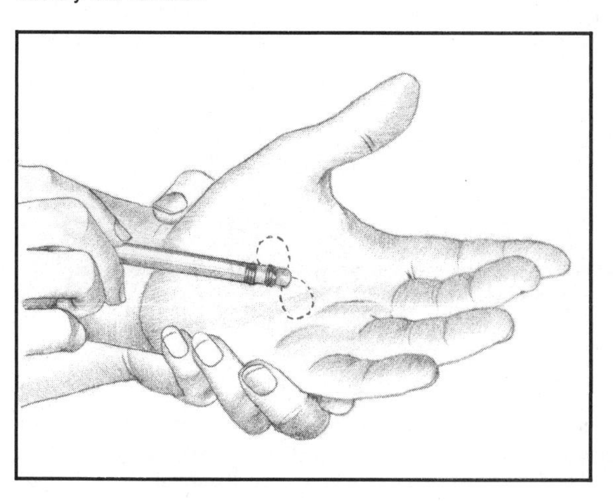

Pathologic reflexes are abnormal in adults and usually indicate an underlying nervous system disease. Sometimes called primitive reflexes, they occur normally in early infancy and then disappear with maturity.

Use a grading scale to rate each reflex. Then document the rating for each reflex at the appropriate site on a stick figure. (For more information, see *Documenting reflex findings*, page 501.)

Abnormal findings

Increased (hyperactive) reflexes occur with upper motor neuron disorders. Damaged CNS neurons in the cerebral cortex or corticospinal tracts prevent the brain from exerting its usual inhibitory control over peripheral reflex activity. This allows any small stimulus to trigger reflexes, which then tend to overrespond. Examples of hyperactive peripheral reflexes include spasticity associated with spinal cord injuries or other upper motor neuron disorders, such as multiple sclerosis.

Decreased or absent reflexes indicate a disorder of the lower motor neuron or the anterior horn of the spinal cord where the peripheral nerve originates. Examples of lower motor neuron disorders characterized by hyporeflexia (or areflexia) include Guillain-Barré syndrome and amyotrophic lateral sclerosis.

A compressed spinal nerve root can diminish the reflex associated with that cord level. For example, a herniated intervertebral disc at L3 or L4 may decrease the knee-jerk reflex.

Developmental considerations

In a very young client, certain developmental reflexes should be assessed during reflex testing; in an elderly client, aging may account for some normal changes in reflexes.

Pediatric client. An infant may display various reflexes considered abnormal in an older child or adult. All developmental reflexes normally vanish by age 2. (For additional information, see Chapter 22, Perinatal and Neonatal Assessment.) An infant also may display some deep tendon and superficial reflexes that are present in an adult. The biceps, brachioradialis, and patellar (knee-jerk) reflexes exist at birth; the Achilles (ankle-jerk) reflex appears by age 4 months; the triceps and abdominal reflexes appear by age 6 months.

Elderly client. In an elderly client, normal aging affects reflex activity. The ankle-jerk reflex frequently diminishes or disappears; occasionally, the knee-jerk reflex also decreases. The superficial abdominal reflexes also may decrease or disappear.

(Text continues on page 501.)

ADVANCED ASSESSMENT SKILLS

Assessing the reflexes

The nurse uses different procedures for testing each deep tendon, superficial, and pathologic superficial reflex, as shown below. (For information on how to assess the corneal reflex, see Chapter 9, Eyes and Ears.) Reflex assessment helps evaluate the intactness of the specific cervical (C), thoracic (T), lumbar (L), or sacral (S) spinal segments shown in parentheses below.

Assessment of deep tendon reflexes includes evaluation of the biceps, triceps, brachioradialis, quadriceps, and Achilles reflexes. Assessment of the superficial reflexes includes evaluation of the pharyngeal, abdominal, and cremasteric reflexes as well as the anal and bulbocavernous reflexes. (Assess the last two reflexes, known as the perineal reflexes, only in clients with suspected sacral spinal cord or sacral spine nerve disorders.) Pathologic reflexes include the grasp, sucking, snout, and Babinski reflexes. Although healthy adults do not display these reflexes, the nurse may assess them to detect signs of CNS damage.

To assess the biceps reflex (C5, C6), have the client partially flex one arm at the elbow with the palm facing down. Place your thumb or finger over the biceps tendon. Then tap lightly over your thumb or finger with the reflex hammer. An impulse should travel to the biceps tendon and cause brisk elbow flexion that is visible and palpable.

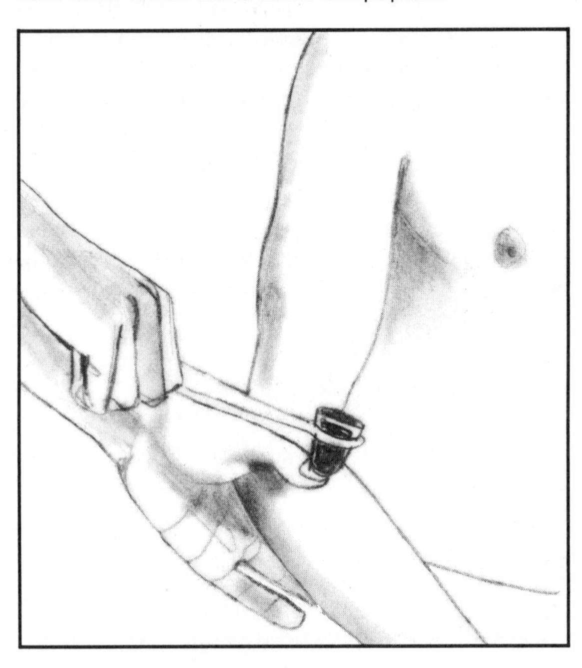

To assess the anal reflex (S3, S4, S5), gently scratch the skin at the side of the anus with a blunt instrument, such as a tongue depressor or gloved finger. Look for puckering of the anus, a normal response.

To assess the bulbocavernous reflex (S3, S4) on a male client, apply direct pressure over the bulbocavernous muscle behind the scrotum and gently pinch the foreskin or glans. This action should cause contraction of the bulbocavernous muscle.

To assess the triceps reflex (C7, C8), have the client partially flex one arm at the elbow with the palm facing the body. Support the arm and pull it slightly across the client's chest. Using a direct blow with the reflex hammer, tap the triceps tendon at its insertion (about 1″ to 2″ [2.5 to 5 cm] above the elbow on the olecranon process of the ulnar bone). Normally, this action causes brisk extension of the client's elbow with visible and palpable contraction of the triceps muscle.

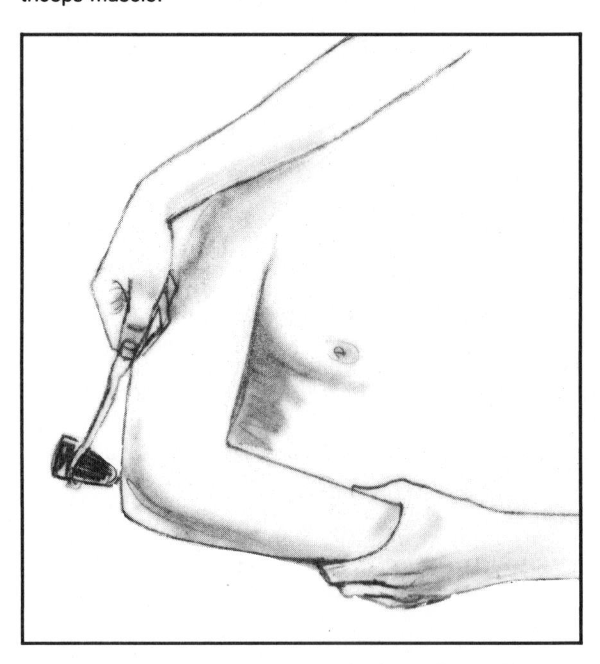

To test the pharyngeal (gag) reflex (CN IX, CN X), have the client open the mouth wide. Then touch the posterior wall of the pharynx with a tongue depressor. The normal response to this action is gagging.

To assess the cremasteric reflex (L1, L2) on a male client, use a tongue depressor to scratch the inner aspect of each thigh gently. This should cause elevation of the testicles.

To assess the brachioradialis (supinator) reflex (C5,C6), position the client with one arm flexed at the elbow, palm down, and resting in the lap, or, if the client is lying down, against the abdomen. Then tap the styloid process of the radius with the reflex hammer, about 1″ to 2″ above the wrist. Normally, this action causes flexion of the client's elbow, supination of the forearm, and flexion of the fingers and hand.

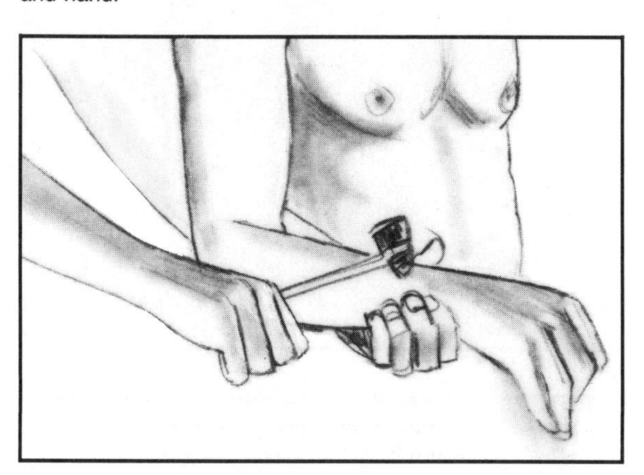

To assess the quadriceps (knee-jerk or patellar) reflex (L2, L3, L4), seat the client with one knee flexed and the lower leg dangling over the side of the examination table, or place the client in the supine position. (For the supine client, place your hand under the knee, slightly raising and flexing it.) Then tap the patellar tendon with the reflex hammer. The client's knee should extend and the quadriceps should contract.

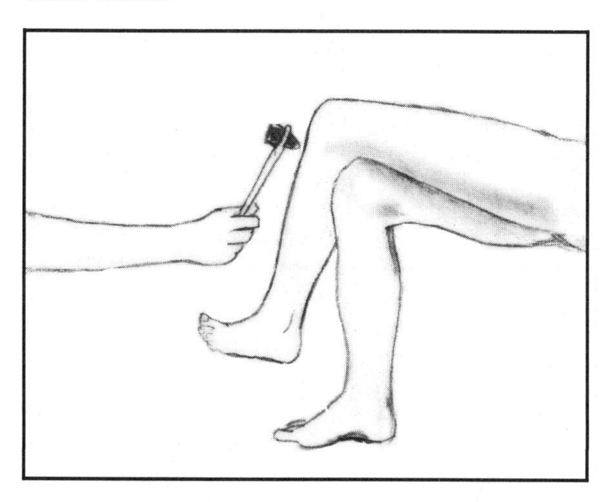

To assess the Achilles (ankle-jerk) reflex (S1, S2), first position the client with the knee bent and the ankle dorsiflexed. (The best position is with the client seated and the legs dangling over the side of the examination table.) Then tap the Achilles tendon, which should cause plantar flexion followed by muscle relaxation.

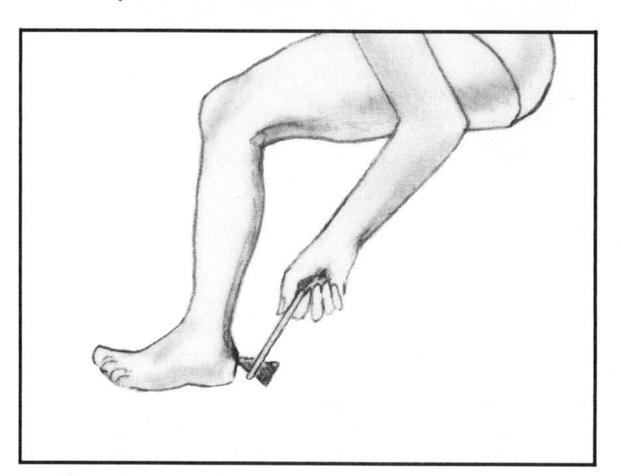

To assess the grasp reflex, stimulate the palm of the client's hand with your fingers. (*Note:* Because a lack of inhibition by the brain can cause the client to squeeze very tightly, avoid finger injury or pain by crossing your middle and index fingers before placing them in the client's palm.) In a positive grasp reflex, the client's hand will grasp yours upon stimulation, indicating frontal lobe damage, bilateral thalamic degeneration, or cerebral degeneration or atrophy.

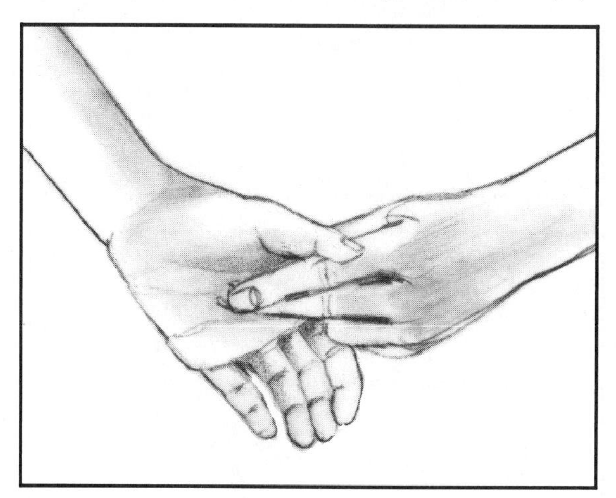

continued

ADVANCED ASSESSMENT SKILLS

Assessing the reflexes continued

To assess the sucking reflex, stimulate the client's lips with a mouth swab. A sucking movement on stimulation can indicate cerebral degeneration.

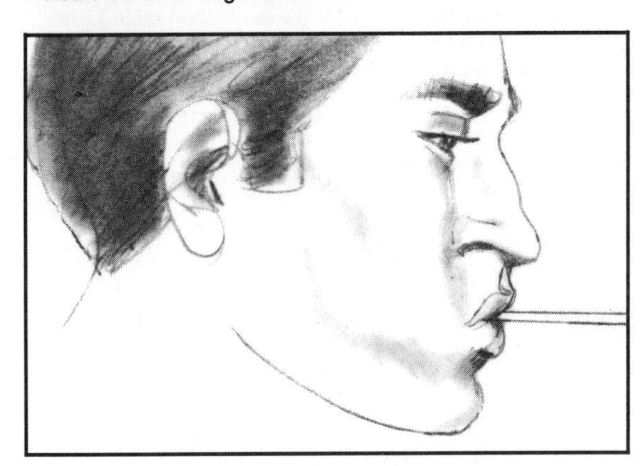

To assess the snout reflex, gently percuss the oral area with your fingers. This action may make the client's lips pucker, indicating cerebral degeneration or late-stage dementia.

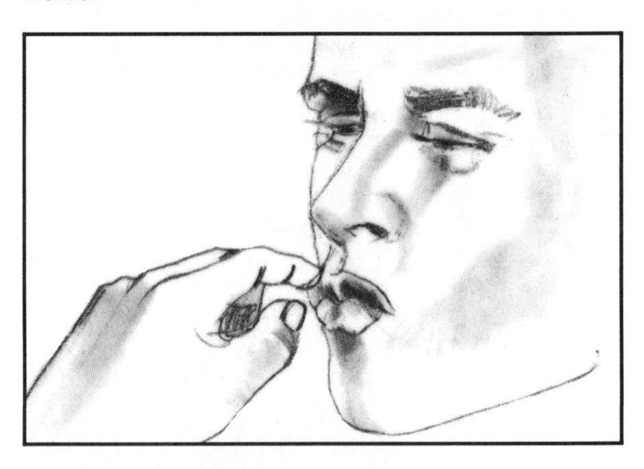

To assess the abdominal reflex (T8, T9, T10), use a fingernail or the tip of the handle of the reflex hammer to stroke one side, and then the opposite side, of the client's abdomen above the umbilicus. Repeat on the lower abdomen. Normally, the abdominal muscles contract and the umbilicus deviates toward the stimulated side.

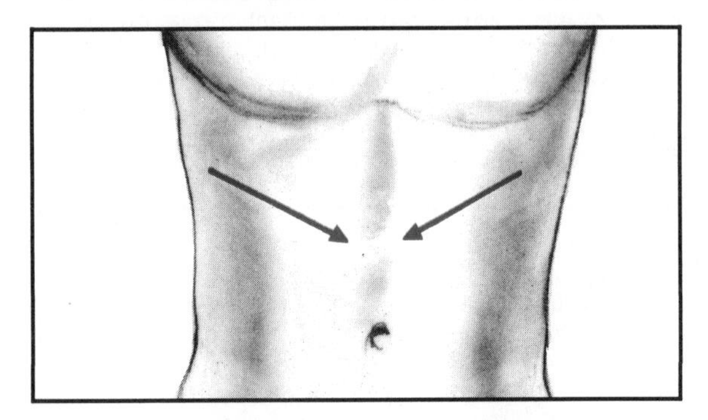

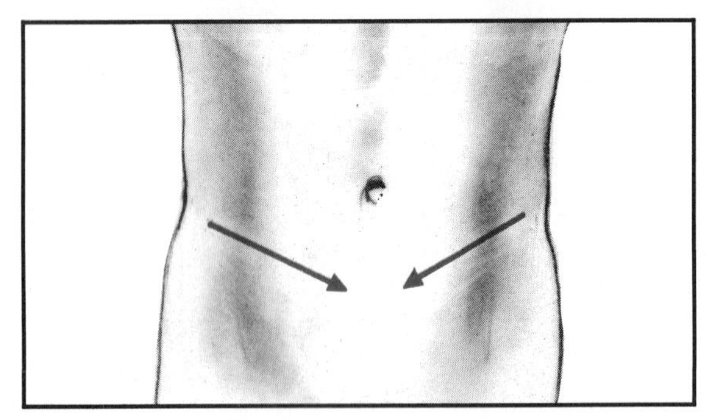

To assess the plantar reflex, stroke the lateral aspect of the sole of the client's foot. Toe flexion is the normal response. Dorsiflexion of the great toe with or without fanning—a positive Babinski's sign—indicates upper motor neuron disease.

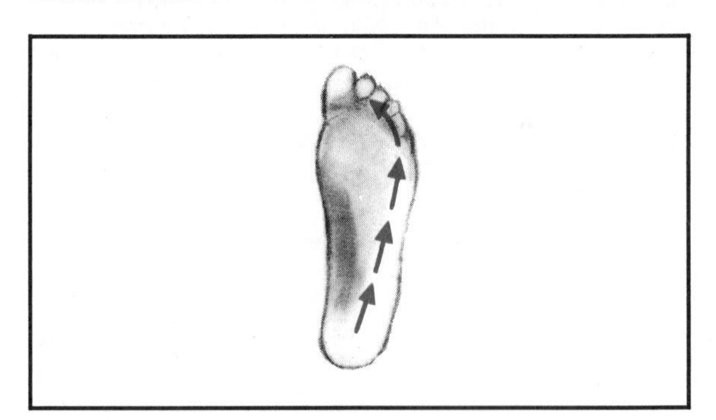

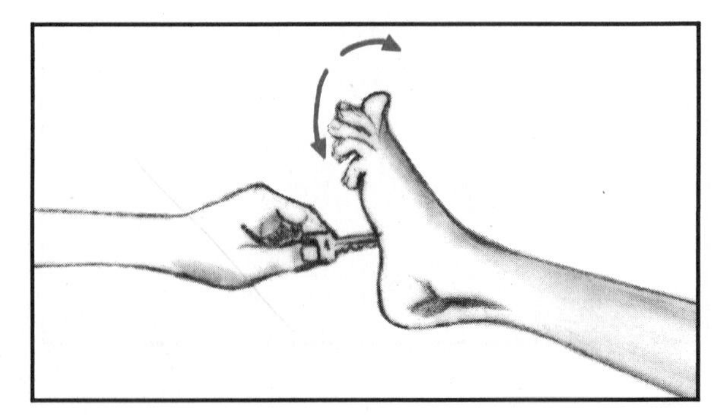

Vital signs

The CNS, primarily by way of the brain stem and autonomic nervous system, controls the body's vital functions: heart rate and rhythm; respiratory rate, depth, and pattern; blood pressure; and body temperature. However, because these vital control centers lie deep within the cerebral hemispheres and in the brain stem, changes in vital signs—temperature, pulse, respiration, and blood pressure—are not usually early indicators of CNS deterioration. Furthermore, the significance of vital sign changes must be evaluated by considering each sign individually as well as in relation to each other. (For information on assessing vital signs and on normal findings, see Chapter 4, Physical Assessment Skills.)

Temperature. Damage to the hypothalamus or upper brain stem can impair the body's ability to maintain a constant temperature, resulting in profound hypothermia (temperature below 94° F. [34.4° C.]) or hyperthermia (temperature above 106° F. [41.1° C.]). Such damage can result from petechial hemorrhages in the hypothalamus or brain stem, trauma (causing pressure, twisting, or traction), or destructive lesions.

Pulse. Because the autonomic nervous system controls heart rate and rhythm, pressure on the brain stem and cranial nerves slows the pulse by stimulating the vagus nerve.

Bradycardia (heart rate under 60 beats/minute) occurs in the later stages of increasing intracranial pressure (ICP), and usually accompanies a rising systolic blood pressure and widening pulse pressure. The pulse is often bounding. Cervical spinal cord injuries can also cause bradycardia.

In a client with acutely increased ICP or a brain injury, tachycardia (heart rate over 100 beats/minute) signals decompensation (a condition in which the body has exhausted its compensatory measures for managing ICP), which rapidly leads to death.

Respiration. Respiratory centers in the medulla and pons control the rate, depth, and pattern of respiration. Neurologic dysfunction, particularly when involving the brain stem or both cerebral hemispheres, often alters respirations. An assessment of respiration provides valuable information about the site and severity of a CNS lesion.

One of the first signs of a disorder in the cerebral hemispheres or upper brain stem is Cheyne-Stokes respirations. This is not always ominous, however; it may occur normally in an elderly client during sleep, probably the result of generalized brain atrophy from aging.

Documenting reflex findings

Use these grading scales to rate the strength of each reflex in a deep tendon and superficial reflex assessment.

Deep tendon reflex grades
0 absent
\+ present but diminished
\+ + normal
\+ + + increased but not necessarily pathologic
\+ + + + hyperactive or clonic (involuntary contraction and relaxation of skeletal muscle)

Superficial reflex grades
0 absent
\+ present

Record the client's reflex ratings on a drawing of a stick figure. The figures here show documentation of normal and abnormal reflex responses.

Normal

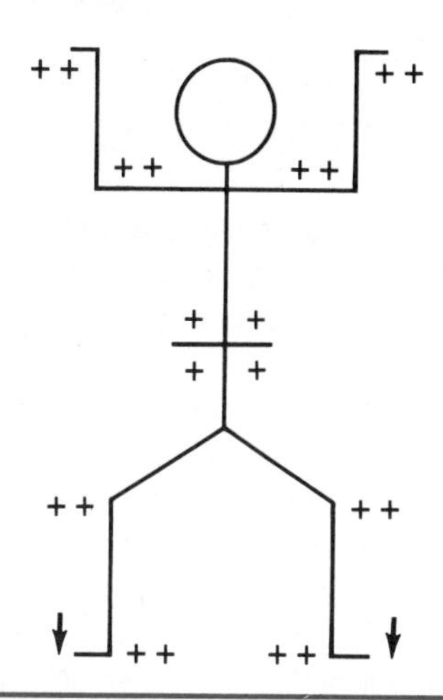

Abnormal

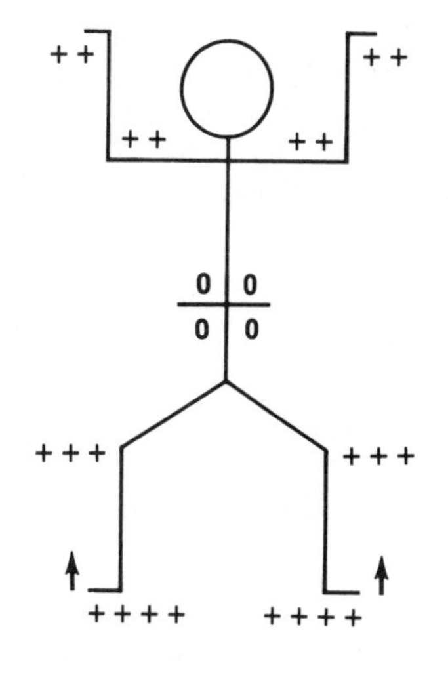

Facilitating reflex testing

Without inhibitory messages from the brain, called cognitive inhibition, peripheral reflex activity responds to any stimulus by producing involuntary muscle contractions and spasms. Although necessary for normal movement and muscle function, cognitive inhibition caused by tenseness or anxiety can suppress reflex responses. To prevent this during reflex testing, position the client comfortably and encourage the client to relax and become limp before trying to elicit a reflex response. Other guidelines follow.

Ask the client who appears to have depressed reflex activity to perform isometric muscle contractions to override the inhibitory messages from the brain and to increase reflex activity.

To improve leg reflexes, have the client clench both hands together and tense the arm muscles during the reflex assessment.

To improve arm reflex response, have the client clench his or her teeth or squeeze one thigh with the hand not being evaluated.

Both of these maneuvers force the client to concentrate on something other than the reflexes being tested, which may eliminate unintentional cognitive inhibition. If reflexes remain decreased despite these maneuvers, evaluate further.

Also, spinal cord damage above the seventh cervical vertebra weakens or paralyzes the respiratory muscles, causing varying degrees of respiratory impairment.

Blood pressure. Pressor receptors in the medulla of the brain stem constantly monitor blood pressure. In a client with no history of hypertension, rising systolic blood pressure may signal increasing ICP. If the ICP continues to rise, pulse pressure widens as the systolic blood pressure climbs and the diastolic pressure remains stable or falls. In the late stages of acutely elevated ICP, blood pressure plummets as cerebral perfusion fails, resulting in death.

Hypotension rarely accompanies a brain injury. When it does, it is an ominous sign. However, cervical spinal cord injuries may interrupt the sympathetic pathways, causing peripheral vasodilation and hypotension.

Documentation

To determine the significance of assessment findings, the nurse must carefully review and integrate the physical assessment information about the client's nervous system along with the health history findings and laboratory results. (For a summary of frequently used laboratory studies and their significance, see *Common laboratory studies.*) Based on these data, formulate appropriate nursing diagnoses, which determine how to plan, implement, and evaluate nursing care. (For a case study that shows how to apply the nursing process to a client with a neurologic disorder, see *Applying the nursing process,* pages 506 and 507.)

Proper documentation is essential to organizing assessment data and making it available to other members of the health care team. Be sure to document all data completely and specifically, including normal and abnormal findings. For example, when documenting LOC, record all aspects of that assessment category, including level of arousal and orientation to person, place, and time. If a client seems disoriented, identify exactly what the client said that led to that conclusion. Organize the documentation according to the five major divisions of the nervous system assessment.

The following sample illustrates the correct way to document normal findings of the nervous system assessment:

Vital Signs: Temperature 98.2° F., pulse 76 and regular, respirations 20 and unlabored, blood pressure 124/72.
Cerebral function: Awake, alert, and oriented to person, place, and time. Recent and remote memory intact. Thought processes coherent. Cooperative and relaxed. Language comprehension and expression intact. (Complete mental assessment not performed.)
Cranial nerves: CN II through XII intact. (CN I not tested.)
Motor system and cerebellar function: Moves all extremities on command without difficulty. Upper extremities (UE) and hand grips strong and equal bilaterally. Lower extremities (LE) strong and equal bilaterally. Muscle tone normal. No evidence of muscular atrophy or hypertrophy. No involuntary movements noted. Gait stable. Good balance and coordination. Romberg negative. Performs heel-to-toe walking without difficulty. Performs rapid alternating movements with both hands and feet smoothly and without difficulty. Right-handed.
Sensory system: Light touch, pain, vibration, and proprioception intact. Stereognosis intact. Accurately localizes touch. Distinguishes two points 3 mm apart on fingertip.
Reflexes: Deep tendon and superficial reflexes intact. Babinski reflex absent.

Common laboratory studies

For a client with neurologic signs and symptoms, various laboratory studies can provide valuable clues to the possible cause, as shown in the chart below. (*Note:* Keep in mind that abnormal findings may stem from a problem unrelated to the neurologic system.) Remember that values differ between laboratories, and check the normal value range for the specific laboratory.

TEST AND SIGNIFICANCE	NORMAL VALUES AND FINDINGS	ABNORMAL FINDINGS	POSSIBLE NEUROLOGIC AND RELATED CAUSES OF ABNORMAL FINDINGS
Blood Tests			
Electrolytes These tests provide a quantitative analysis of major extracellular electrolytes (sodium, calcium, chloride, and bicarbonates) and major intracellular electrolytes (potassium, magnesium, and phosphate).	*Sodium:* 135 to 145 mEq/liter	Above-normal level	Neuromuscular excitability, seizures, confusion, coma related to dehydration, diabetes insipidus
		Below-normal level (less than 125 mEq/liter)	Disorientation, restlessness related to syndrome of inappropriate antidiuretic hormone secretion, water intoxication
	Potassium: 3.8 to 5.5 mEq/liter	Above-normal level	Muscle weakness, flaccid paralysis, EKG changes, ventricular fibrillation or asystole related to metabolic acidosis, renal insufficiency or failure, severe burns or crushing injuries, adrenal insufficiency
		Below-normal level	Muscle weakness, muscle twitching, tetany; hypotension; hypoventilation; EKG changes
	Calcium: 4.5 to 5.5 mEq/liter	Above-normal level	Emotional lability, delirium, confusion, psychosis, stupor, coma related to excess parathyroid hormone, cancer with bone metastasis, hyperthyroidism, excess vitamin D, immobilization
		Below-normal level	Tingling (perioral), depression, dementia, psychosis, encephalopathy, laryngospasm, tetany, seizures related to vitamin D deficiency, parathyroid hormone deficiency, renal tubular disease, renal failure, acute pancreatitis
	Magnesium: 1.5 to 2.5 mEq/liter	Above-normal level (greater than 10 mEq/liter)	Absent deep tendon reflexes, muscle weakness, lethargy, flushing, diaphoresis, hypotension, respiratory depression, stupor, coma, weak bradycardia, cardiac arrest related to renal failure, adrenal insufficiency, excess magnesium
		Below-normal level	Neuromuscular irritability, tetany, tremors, leg and foot cramps, hyperactive deep tendon reflexes, cardiac dysrhythmias, seizures, malnutrition, malabsorption syndrome, impaired renal conservation, hyperparathyroidism, chronic alcoholism

continued

Common laboratory studies *continued*

TEST AND SIGNIFICANCE	NORMAL VALUES AND FINDINGS	ABNORMAL FINDINGS	POSSIBLE NEUROLOGIC AND RELATED CAUSES OF ABNORMAL FINDINGS
Cerebrospinal fluid tests			
Cerebrospinal fluid (CSF) analysis CSF analysis aids in diagnosis of acute or chronic bacterial or viral central nervous system (CNS) infections, hemorrhages, tumors, or brain abscesses.	*Color:* Clear, colorless	Cloudy (caused by increased leukocytes and proteins), xanthochromic (bloody)	Infection, such as meningitis; subarachnoid, intracerebral, or intraventricular hemorrhage; spinal cord obstruction; traumatic spinal tap (usually noted only in initial specimen)
	Glucose: 50 to 80 mg/dl (or ⅔ of blood glucose)	Above-normal level	Systemic hyperglycemia (no neurologic significance)
		Below-normal level	Bacterial, TB, or fungal meningitis; some CNS viral infections (herpes, mumps); meningeal neoplasm; meningeal sarcoidosis; post-subarachnoid hemorrhage; brain abscess; degenerative disease
	Protein: 15 to 45 mg/dl	Above-normal level (greater than 60 mcg/dl)	Peripheral neuropathy involving nerve roots, brain tumor, encapsulated brain abcess, bacterial meningitis, viral CNS infections, degenerative CNS diseases (multiple sclerosis, neurosyphilis), Guillain-Barré syndrome, subarachnoid hemorrhage, blood in CSF from traumatic tap
		Below-normal level	Rapid CSF production
	Gamma globulin: 3% to 12% of total protein	Above-normal level	Herpes encephalitis, Guillain-Barré syndrome, neurosyphilis
	Cell count: No red blood cells	Presence	Hemorrhage (subarachnoid, intracerebral), bleeding into ventricular system, CNS trauma, traumatic tap
	0 to 5 white blood cells	Increase (greater than 10)	Meningitis, CNS infections, infectious mononucleosis, subarachnoid hemorrhage, thrombosis

The following sample illustrates the correct way to document abnormal findings of the nervous system assessment:

Vital signs: Temperature 98.4° F.; pulse 82 and irregular; respirations 22 and unlabored, Cheyne-Stokes pattern with 15-second periods of apnea occurring approximately once a minute; blood pressure 162/50.
Cerebral function: Lethargic, falls asleep when left alone. Opens eyes when name called loudly. Oriented to person, but can only give first name. Disoriented to place ("my house") and time ("1967"). Complete mental status examination reveals severe impairment of recent memory. Remote memory relatively intact. Attention span severely impaired: difficulty repeating more than a single digit. Unable to perform serial 7s. Intellectual skills (vocabulary, general knowledge) greatly reduced. Poor judgment. Concrete thinking. Thought content wanders. Speaks to persons not present: questionable auditory and visual hallucinations. Language: does not initiate conversation. Responses to many questions inappropriate or unintelligible. Speech slurred

and garbled. Reading, writing, and copying skills not evaluated.
Cranial nerves:
CN I: Unable to identify peppermint, coffee, or orange odors. Pungent odor (acetone) does not produce facial grimacing, withdrawal, or other signs of detection.
CN II: Visual acuity corrected with glasses OS, legally blind OD.
CN III, IV, and VI: Right pupil 3 mm, round, reacts sluggishly. Left pupil 7 mm, round, nonreactive. Extraocular movements: upward, lateral, and nasal gazes intact (III, VI). Unable to direct eye downward and nasally (IV). Reports diplopia in lower, medial portion of both visual fields.
CN V: Unable to detect light touch on right side of forehead or right cheek. Touch sensation intact over right jaw and on left side of face. Jaw clench weak on right, strong on left. Mouth deviates to left with jaw opening and closing. Corneal reflex absent.
CN VII: Facial movement decreased on right side: unable to puff right cheek, wrinkle forehead on right, or close eyelid tightly. Smile droops on the right. Left-sided facial movement intact. Unable to differentiate sweet from salt on left anterior two-thirds of tongue; sense of taste intact on right side.
CN VIII: Auditory acuity decreased in right ear; intact in left ear. Complains of vertigo and nausea. Balance poor: falls to left side when sitting without support.
CN IX and X: Taste sensation absent posterior one-third of tongue bilaterally. Left side of soft palate does not rise, uvula deviates to the right. Voice sounds nasal. Gag reflex absent.
CN XI: Decreased strength in left sternocleidomastoid; right intact.
CN XII: Tongue deviates to left. Fasciculations noted.
Motor system and cerebellar function: Muscle atrophy noted in bilateral UE, most pronounced in hand. Moves all extremities on command. Decreased UE strength, more pronounced on right: overcomes gravity with difficulty. LE strong bilaterally. Gait shuffling and unsteady, leans forward while walking. Romberg positive: stable with eyes open, falls to left when eyes closed. Performs heel-to-toe walk with difficulty, falls to left, requires support. Unable to perform heel or toe walking, shallow knee bends and hopping in place.
Sensory system: Light touch absent in left arm, left leg, and left side of face. Reports dysesthesias characterized by intense burning sensation in response to light touch on right forearm. Paresthesia in feet and lower legs. Pain and temperature sensation diminished in left arm and leg. Proprioception and vibration absent in distal extremities; intact at knee and elbow bilaterally.
Reflexes: UE (triceps, biceps, brachioradialis) reflexes intact. Achilles and patellar reflexes hyperactive. Superficial reflexes absent. Babinski present.

Chapter summary

This chapter introduces the nurse to nervous system assessment. Careful observation and information from the health history, physical assessment, and laboratory studies form the basis of a thorough evaluation. They also establish a baseline of neurologic functioning, which ensures accurate interpretation of future observations. Here are the important points discussed in Chapter 17.

- The two major anatomical divisions of the nervous system are the central nervous system—composed of the brain and spinal cord—and the peripheral nervous system—composed of the cranial nerves, the spinal nerves, the peripheral nerves, and the autonomic nervous system.
- The neuron is the functional unit of the conduction network of the nervous system. It has an electrical potential that makes it capable of transmitting impulses.
- When collecting the health history, the nurse should ask questions that assess health and illness patterns, health promotion and protection patterns, and role and relationship patterns. During the history, the nurse should be sure to ask about medications the client takes. Many medications may produce adverse neurologic effects.
- Because many neurologic disorders have a familial tendency, the health history should also include information about the health status of the client's family.
- A neurocheck evaluates LOC, pupil size and response, verbal responsiveness, extremity strength and movement, and vital signs. A neurologic screening assessment consists of evaluation of LOC and verbal responsiveness as well as a brief mental status screening, motor system screening, and sensory system screening. The complete

(Text continues on page 508.)

Applying the nursing process

Assessment findings form the basis of the nursing process. Using them, the nurse formulates the nursing diagnoses and develops appropriate planning, implementation, and evaluation of the client's care.

The table below shows how the nurse can use nervous system assessment data in the nursing process for the client described in the case history (shown at right). In the first column, history and physical assessment data appear, followed by a paragraph of mental notes. These notes help the nurse make important mental connections among assessment findings, aiding in the development of the nursing diagnoses and planning.

The second column presents several appropriate nursing diagnoses; however, the information in the remaining columns is based on the *first* nursing diagnosis. Although it is not part of the nursing process, documentation appears in the last column because of its importance. Documentation consists of an initial note using all components of the SOAPIE format and a follow-up note using the appropriate SOAPIE components.

ASSESSMENT	NURSING DIAGNOSES	PLANNING	IMPLEMENTATION
Subjective (history) data • Client states, "I have spells when I can hardly move my right hand or arm. It feels numb and tingling, like it is asleep. When I try to tell my wife what is happening, I can't seem to find the right words, or else they get jumbled and won't come out right." • Client reports that these spells started about 8 months ago. The spells begin suddenly, last 10 to 20 minutes, and resolve spontaneously. • Client states that, initially, the spells occurred about once a month, but during the last 2 weeks they have increased to at least one every other day. • Client reports that he has had high blood pressure "for 40 years." He had been taking an antihypertensive medication but reports that he stopped taking it "last year" since he was "feeling good." • Client's father died of a stroke at age 82. **Objective (physical) data** • Vital signs: Temperature 98.8° F., pulse 78 and regular, respirations 22 and even and unlabored, blood pressure 182/96. • Awake, alert, oriented to person, place, and time. Remote and recent memory intact. Speech slightly slurred but intelligible. Occasionally seems to have trouble finding words. • Pupils round, equal, and reactive to light. • Right-handed. Moves all extremities on command without difficulty. Arms and legs strong. Right grasp slightly weaker than left. Mild paresis indicated by downward drift of right arm when extended by client with eyes closed. Gait slow and steady, unassisted. • Light touch, pain, and temperature sensation absent in right hand and forearm, but intact in left arm and both legs. **Mental notes** *Mr. Collins' presenting signs and symptoms strongly suggest cerebral ischemia. Transient neurologic deficits, caused by transient ischemic attacks (TIAs), are the classic warning signs of impending stroke. His failure to report his "spells" sooner probably reflects a knowledge deficit but may also reflect denial as a coping mechanism. His rationales for discontinuing antihypertensive medications ("feeling good," "no headache") also suggest a lack of knowledge about high blood pressure and its treatment.*	• Knowledge deficit related to warning signs of stroke and importance of adhering to antihypertensive regimen. • Sensory-perceptual alteration: tactile, related to right arm paresthesias. • Impaired physical mobility related to right arm weakness and clumsiness. • Potential self-care deficit related to right arm paresis and sensory loss, especially because client is right-handed. • Impaired verbal communication related to difficulty in word-finding and slurred speech.	**Goals** Before leaving the hospital, the client will: • state why for his health maintenance he must continue taking antihypertensive medications even without physical symptoms • define a TIA in his own words, state why it is a warning sign of stroke, and explain the meaning this has for his health • name five warning signs of cerebral ischemia associated with TIAs that he should report to help limit further injury.	• Explain that antihypertensive medications control, but do not cure, high blood pressure. • Emphasize the importance of scheduling regular checkups to monitor blood pressure. • Define TIAs in simple terms. For example, "TIAs are temporary changes in nervous system functioning that occur when certain brain cells do not receive enough oxygen for a brief period. They often warn of a stroke." • Teach the client some of the warning signs of TIAs: sensory changes (tingling or numbness), muscle weakness, visual disturbances, difficulty talking or understanding speech, and dizziness.

CASE HISTORY

Joseph Collins, age 73, comes to the clinic because his right arm feels "heavy and clumsy" and, unlike previous episodes, this sensation has not gone away.

EVALUATION	DOCUMENTATION BASED ON NURSING PROCESS DATA			
		Initial		**Follow-up**
Before leaving the hospital, the client: • accurately stated why he must have regular blood pressure checks and why he must continue antihypertensive medications unless they are discontinued by the physician • defined a TIA in simple words and named five warning signs that he should report to the physician or health clinic nurse • explained the importance of scheduling regular follow-up appointments.	**S**	Client states that right arm is "heavy and clumsy." Reports having "spells" of being unable to move right hand or arm, feels numb and tingling. Having difficulty finding appropriate words. Episodes started 8 months ago, now occur every other day and last 10 minutes. Client has had hypetension "for 40 years." Stopped taking prescribed antihypertensive medication last year because he was feeling good. Father died of a stroke at age 82.	**S**	"My right arm feels as good as my left one. My speaking is fine, too. The words come just like they used to. I've been taking those pills like you told me."
	O	T 98.8° F.; P 78, regular; R 22, even and unlabored; BP 182/96. Alert and oriented. Remote and recent memory intact. Speech slightly slurred. Pupils round, equal, and reactive to light. Motor: right-handed. Moves all extremities on command without difficulty. Upper and lower extremities strong bilaterally; right grasp slightly weaker than left. Right arm drifts. Sensory: light touch, pain, temperature sensation absent in right hand and forearm; intact in left arm and both legs.	**O**	T 98.6° F.; P 74 and regular; R 20 and regular; BP 152/84. Motor: arm and grasp strength equal bilaterally; sensory response equal bilaterally. Client speaks clearly and expresses himself without difficulty or hesitation.
	A	Knowledge deficit related to warning signs of stroke and importance of adhering to antihypertensive regimen. Correlates hypertension medications with feeling bad and having headaches.	**A**	Right arm sensory and motor deficits completely resolved.
	P	Teach client importance of following antihypertensive regimen and warning signals of TIAs. Encourage client to keep appointments.	**P**	Review therapeutic regimen and instructions.
	I	Taught client about antihypertensive regimen and importance of adherence. Explained TIAs and associated warning signs that should be reported. Gave client printed material for reinforcement. Discussed importance of regular checkups to monitor blood pressure and TIAs.	**E**	Client correctly explained why he must adhere to antihypertensive regimen and stated date and time for scheduled follow-up visit. Correctly named warning signs of stroke and stated, "Next time, I'll report signs right away."
	E	Client repeats some information and states that he will make a follow-up appointment.		

neurologic assessment has five components: (1) assessment of cerebral function, including LOC, communication, and mental status; (2) cranial nerve evaluation; (3) assessment of motor system and cerebellar function; (4) assessment of the sensory system; and (5) evaluation of reflexes.
• LOC assessment includes two aspects: orientation, which reflects cerebral cortical functioning, and level of arousal, which reflects the activity of the subcortical reticular activating system.
• A complete mental status examination includes evaluation of the client's cognitive skills: orientation, attention (concentration), memory, intellectual skills, abstract reasoning, judgment, thought processes, and content.
• The cognitive tests in the mental status examination must be interpreted in light of the client's educational, socioeconomic, and cultural background.
• Formal assessment of language includes evaluation of spontaneous speech, comprehension, naming, repetition, vocabulary, reading, writing, and copying figures.
• Cranial nerve evaluation can provide important clues about brain stem condition because most of these nerves originate at the brain stem. The 12 cranial nerves have distinct functions and require different assessment techniques.
• A complete motor system examination should include assessment of muscle strength, size, and symmetry; gait; coordination; and balance. Disturbances in gait (ataxia), coordination, or balance signal cerebellar disorders.
• Complete sensory system testing should assess the client's ability to detect touch, pain, temperature, vibration, and position.
• A return of developmental reflexes, such as the Babinski or sucking reflex, often reflects central nervous system damage.
• Vital signs, temperature, pulse, respirations, and blood pressure provide important information about neurologic function. The hypothalamus, the midbrain, and the pons and medulla of the brain stem contain centers for controlling body temperature, cardiac rate and rhythm, blood pressure, and respiratory rate, rhythm, and depth.
• The nurse should check available laboratory study results, including electrolytes and cerebrospinal fluid analysis. Disorders in other body systems can produce changes in neurologic functioning that alter these test results.
• The nurse should document the health history and physical assessment concisely, avoiding subjective terms when describing observations, and describing activity level, behaviors, or complaints in the client's own words.

Study questions

1. Thomas Wilson, age 28, has just been brought to the emergency department after a motorcycle accident. Despite wearing a helmet, Mr. Wilson sustained a head injury and was unconscious for approximately 20 minutes at the scene of the accident. He is now awake, but restless and disoriented.

Mr. Wilson needs a rapid assessment of the nervous system; however, his condition does not allow a complete examination of all cranial nerves. Considering the nature of his injuries, which cranial nerves are essential to assess? (For each cranial nerve, identify its name, describe which function(s) require evaluation, and explain why the assessment is essential.)

2. Joseph Jones, age 83, is a farmer from rural North Carolina. Over the past two months, Mr. Jones's family has become concerned over subtle changes in his behavior. They brought him to the clinic, where he is now being evaluated.

According to the health history, Mr. Jones has had no formal education beyond the second grade. Although he needs a complete mental status examination (MSE), you realize that the usual MSE will need to be adapted to the client's socioeconomic and educational background to elicit meaningful information.

How would you modify each of the following aspects of the complete MSE for Mr. Jones's assessment? What questions or procedures would you use to test each of the cognitive functions listed below?
• vocabulary
• general knowledge
• abstract reasoning
• calculations
• attention span.

3. You are performing a complete assessment of Mary Kelly, age 93. You know that nervous system anatomy and physiology change with age, which, in turn, affects neurologic function.

When assessing the following neurologic functions, what normal changes would you expect to see in this client?
• proprioception (position) sense
• vibration sense
• auditory acuity
• superficial abdominal reflexes

- pupil size
- muscle size
- muscle strength
- recent memory
- coordination
- sense of taste.

4. Mrs. Wilkins brings her daughter, Beth, age 14, to the hospital for evaluation of difficulty walking. Beth's gait is unsteady, she cannot walk without assistance, and her mother reports that she has already fallen twice at home. At this time, the etiology of Beth's problem is unknown.

Which five specific aspects of a complete nervous system assessment are especially important to emphasize when evaluating Beth?

5. Elizabeth Jamison, age 37, is the mother of two small children and the vice president of a branch office of a well-known bank. She has been experiencing recurrent severe headaches lasting 18 to 36 hours, usually accompanied by nausea and dizziness. Most distressing to her is that the headaches make work and care of her children impossible. How would you document the following information related to your assessment of Mrs. Jamison?
- history (subjective) assessment
- physical (objective) assessment
- assessment techniques and any special equipment
- two appropriate nursing diagnoses
- documentation of your findings.

Selected references

Adams, R., and Victor, M. (1989). *Principles of neurology* (4th ed.). New York: McGraw-Hill.

Andrews, L. (1990). Neurovascular assessment. *Advancing Clinical Care,* 5(6), 5-7.

Carpenito, L. (1991). *Handbook of nursing diagnoses* (4th ed.). Philadelphia: Lippincott.

Guyton, A. (1991). *Textbook of medical physiology* (8th ed.). Philadelphia: Saunders.

Hickey, J. (1985). *The clinical practice of neurological and neurosurgical nursing* (2nd ed.). Philadelphia: Lippincott.

Kaufman, J. (1990). Nurse's guide to assessing the 12 cranial nerves. *Nursing90,* 20(6), 56-58.

McHugh, J., and McHugh, W. (1990). How to assess deep tendon reflexes. *Nursing90,* 20(8), 62-64.

Neurologic care. (1986). Clinical Pocket Manual Series. Springhouse, PA: Springhouse Corp.

Nursing92 drug handbook. (1992). Springhouse, PA: Springhouse Corp.

Price, M., and DeVroom, H. (1985). A quick and easy guide to neurological assessment. *Journal of Neurosurgical Nursing,* 17(5), 313-320.

Silver, B. (1989). How to assess neurologically impaired patients. *Advancing Clinical Care,* 4(6), 6-9.

Sullivan, J. (1990). Neurologic assessment. *Nursing Clinics of North America,* 25(4), 795-809.

Weiner, H. and Levitt, L. (1989). *Neurology for the house officer* (4th ed.). Baltimore: Williams & Wilkins.

Nursing research

Grant, J. (1990). Altered level of consciousness: Validity of a nursing diagnosis. *Journal of Neuroscience Nursing,* 22(6), 250.

Martin, K. (1987). Predicting short-term outcome in comatose head-injured children. *Journal of Neuroscience Nursing,* 19(1), 9-13.

Miller, E., and Williams, S. (1987). Alteration in cerebral perfusion: Clinical concept or nursing diagnosis? *Journal of Neuroscience Nursing,* 19(4), 183-190.

Segatore, M., and Villenueve, M. (1988). Spinal cord testing: Development of a screening tool. *Journal of Neuroscience Nursing,* 20(1), 30-33.

Parsons, L., and Kidd, P. (1989). Neurologic nursing research. *Annual Review of Nursing Research,* 7, 3-25.

Pasquarello, M. (1990). Measuring the impact of an acute stroke program on patient outcomes. *Journal of Neuroscience Nursing,* 22(2), 76-82.

18

Musculoskeletal System

Objectives

After reading and studying this chapter, you should be able to:

1. Describe the normal anatomy and physiology of musculoskeletal structures.
2. Identify developmental musculoskeletal system variations.
3. Discuss the health history questions required to elicit information about a client's musculoskeletal system.
4. Discuss appropriate modifications of a musculoskeletal physical assessment for a child and for an elderly client.
5. Explain overall body symmetry, posture, gait, muscle and joint function, and range of motion.
6. Describe systematic palpation of muscles, bones, and joints.
7. Describe normal findings for posture, gait, and muscle and joint functions.
8. Identify representative adverse drug reactions in the musculoskeletal system.
9. Document musculoskeletal system assessment findings using the nursing process.

Introduction

Assessing the musculoskeletal system entails examination of muscles, bones, and joints. Because the central nervous system coordinates muscle and bone function, the examiner must understand how the two systems interrelate. (For information about the central nervous system, see Chapter 17, Nervous System.)

Usually, the musculoskeletal system assessment is a small fraction of the overall physical assessment, especially for the client who has other complaints. However, where the general assessment reveals an abnormality or the symptom history suggests musculoskeletal involvement, a complete assessment of the system is necessary. This chapter presents the components of a comprehensive musculoskeletal assessment, beginning with a brief review of anatomy and physiology followed by a list of pertinent health history questions.

Clients with musculoskeletal complaints can be found in hospitals, emergency departments, and outpatient clinics. Accidents and sports activities cause musculoskeletal injuries in all age groups, especially in school-age children and adolescents. Normal aging changes, such as osteoarthritis, commonly cause musculoskeletal problems in elderly clients.

The physical assessment portion of this chapter describes systematic procedures for evaluating general body symmetry, posture, gait, and muscle and joint function. It emphasizes how the nurse performs various tests and describes normal, variations from normal, and abnormal findings. Then the chapter discusses information about relevant laboratory studies. Documentation samples represent normal and abnormal findings. The chapter also presents a case study that shows how to integrate musculoskeletal assessment findings into the nursing process.

Glossary

Abduction: limb movement away from the body's midline.
Adduction: limb movement toward the body's midline.
Ankylosis: fixation and immobilization of a joint.
Ataxia: impaired ability to coordinate movement.
Atony: lack of normal tension in a muscle; flaccidity.
Atrophy: decrease in size; often used to describe change in muscle size.
Crepitus: abnormal crackling or grating sound or sensation produced, in the musculoskeletal system, when irregular bone edges rub together.
Dorsiflexion: backward bending of a joint.
Effusion: collection of fluid not normally present.
Extension: movement that increases the angle between two articulating bones.
Fasciculation: involuntary twitching of muscle fiber bundles.
Fasciculi: bundles of skeletal muscle fibers.
Flaccid: weak, soft, and flabby; often used to describe muscles that lack tone.
Flexion: movement that decreases the angle between two articulating bones.
Goniometer: instrument used to measure joint range of motion.
Hypertrophy: increase in size of a cell or group of cells, such as muscles.
Kyphosis: exaggerated dorsal convexity of the thoracic spine.
Lordosis: exaggerated dorsal concavity of the lumbar spine.
Osteocyte: bone cell.
Osteoporosis: bone condition resulting in quantitative loss of bone mass although, qualitatively, the mineral-to-matrix ratio remains normal.
Range of motion: amount of movement measured in degrees of a circle through which a joint can be extended or flexed.
Scoliosis: abnormal lateral curvature of the spine.
Subluxation: partial or incomplete dislocation.
Tonus: normal muscle tone maintained by partial contraction and relaxation of muscle fibers.
Valgus: abnormal position in which a part of a limb is bent or twisted outward or away from midline.
Varus: abnormal position in which a part of a limb is turned inward toward midline.

Anatomy and physiology review

The musculoskeletal system consists of muscles, tendons, ligaments, bones, cartilage, joints, and bursae. These structures work together to produce skeletal movement.

Muscles

The body contains three major muscle types: visceral (involuntary, smooth), skeletal (voluntary, striated), and cardiac. This chapter discusses only skeletal muscle, which is attached to bone. (For information on visceral muscles, see Chapter 13, Gastrointestinal System; on cardiac muscle, see Chapter 11, Cardiovascular System.)

Viewed through the microscope, skeletal muscle looks like long bands or strips (striations). Skeletal muscle is voluntary because its contraction can be controlled at will. (For illustrations of skeletal muscles and muscle fibers, see *Muscular system,* pages 512 and 513.)

Muscle develops when existing muscle fibers hypertrophy. Exercise, nutrition, sex, and genetic constitution account for variations in muscle strength and size among individuals.

Tendons

These bands of fibrous connective tissue attach muscles to the periosteum (fibrous membrane covering the bone). Tendons enable bones to move when skeletal muscles contract.

Ligaments

These dense, strong, flexible bands of fibrous connective tissue tie bones to bones. The ligaments of concern in a musculoskeletal system assessment connect the joint (articular) ends of bones, serving either to limit or to facilitate movement as well as to provide stability.

Bones

Classified by shape and by location, bones may be long (such as the humerus, radius, femur, and tibia), short (such as the carpals and tarsals), flat (such as the scapula, ribs, and skull), irregular (such as the vertebrae

Muscular system

The human body has about 600 skeletal muscles classified by the kind of movement for which they are responsible (for example, flexors permit flexion; adductors, adduction; circumductors, circumduction; and external rotators, external rotation).

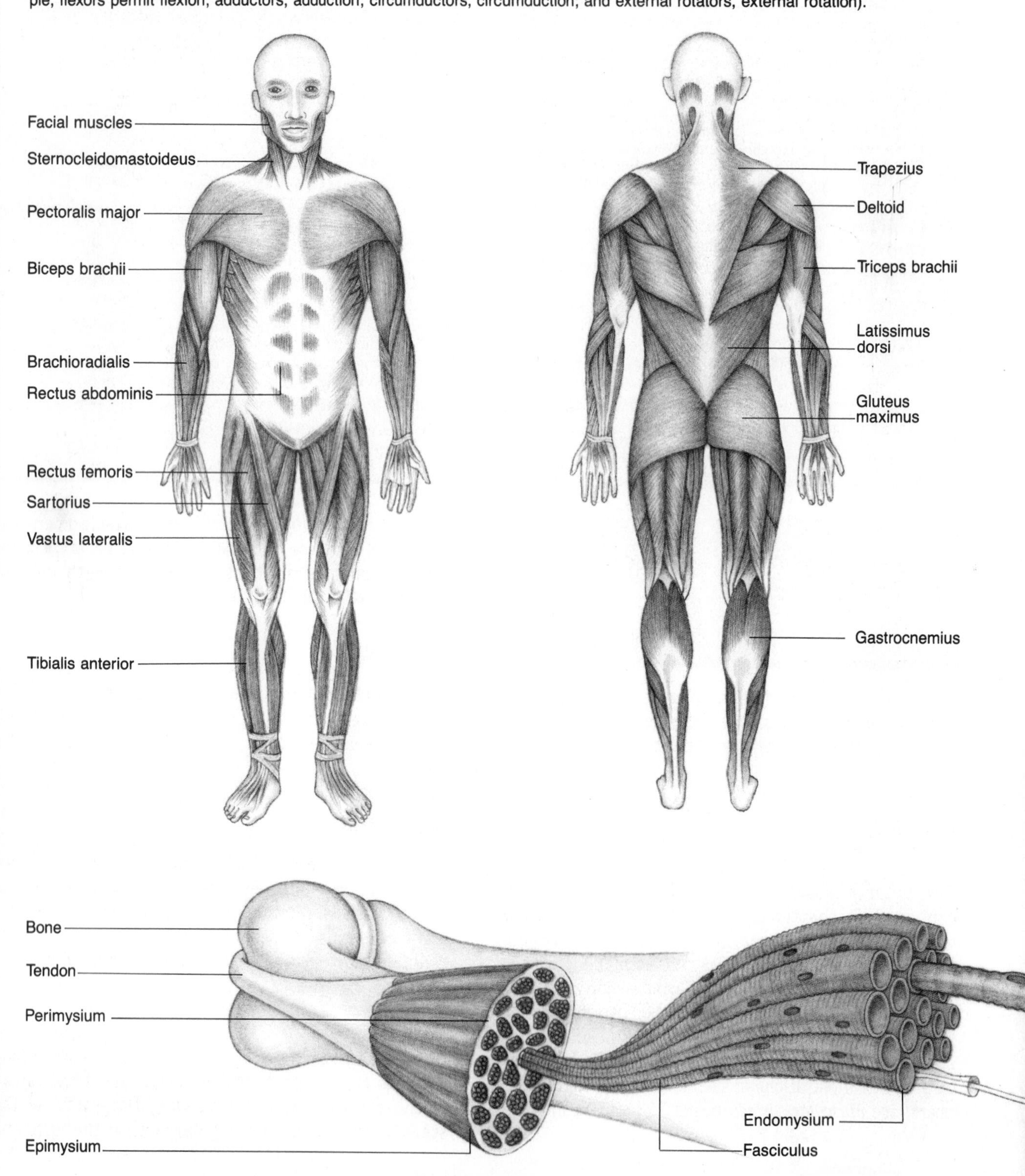

Muscle structure

Each muscle contains cell groups called muscle fibers that extend the length of the muscle. The perimysium—a sheath of connective tissue—binds the fibers into a bundle, or fasciculus. A stronger sheath, the epimysium, binds fasciculi together to form the fleshy part of the muscle. Extending beyond the muscle, the epimysium becomes a tendon.

Each muscle fiber is surrounded by a plasma membrane, the sarcolemma. Within the sarcoplasm (cytoplasm) of the muscle fiber lie tiny myofibrils. Arranged lengthwise, myofibrils contain still finer fibers—about 1,500 myosin (thick) fibers and about 3,000 actin (thin) fibers.

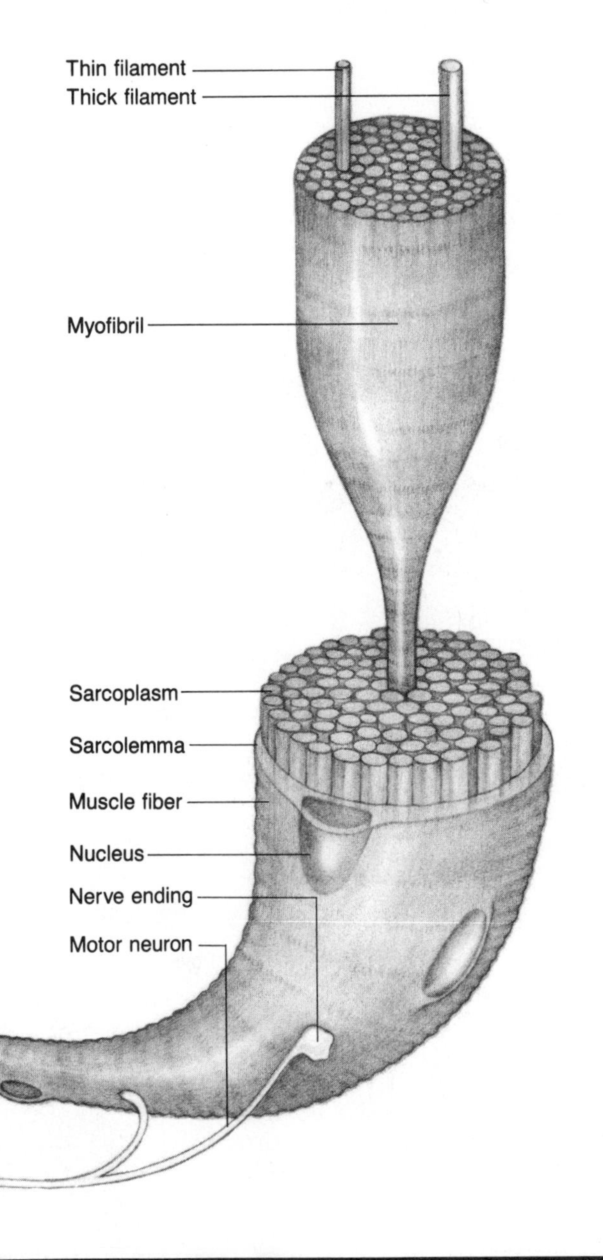

and mandible), sesamoid (such as the patella), of the axial skeleton (such as the facial and cranial bones, hyoid bone, vertebrae, ribs, and sternum), or of the appendicular skeleton (such as the clavicle, scapula, humerus, radius, ulna, metacarpals, pelvic bone, femur, patella, fibula, tibia, and metatarsals). (For illustrations of the bones of the skeletal system and a cross section of bone, see *Skeletal system*, pages 514 and 515.)

Bone function

The 206 bones of the human skeleton have anatomic (mechanical) and physiologic functions. They:

- protect internal tissues and organs (for example, the 33 vertebrae that surround and protect the spinal cord)
- stabilize and support the body
- provide a surface for muscle, ligament, and tendon attachment
- move through "lever" action when contracted
- produce red blood cells in the bone marrow (hematopoiesis)
- store mineral salts (for example, approximately 99% of the body's calcium).

Bone formation

Cartilage composes the fetal skeleton at 3 months in utero. By about 6 months, the fetal cartilage has been transformed into bony skeleton. However, some bones harden (ossify) after birth, most notably the carpals and tarsals. The change results from endochondral ossification, a process by which bone-forming cells (osteoblasts) produce a collagenous material (osteoid) that ossifies.

Two types of osteocytes—osteoblasts and osteoclasts—are responsible for remodeling, which is the continuous process by which bone is created and destroyed. These cells are located in small spaces (lacunae) between the concentric layers of lamellae (thin bone layers). Osteoblasts deposit new bone, and osteoclasts increase long-bone diameter through reabsorption of previously deposited bone. These activities promote longitudinal bone growth, which continues until the epiphyseal growth plates, located at the bone ends, close in adolescence.

The role of the endocrine system in bone formation, especially through estrogen secretion, currently interests scientists who know that estrogen plays a significant role not only in calcium uptake and release, but also in osteoblastic activity regulation. Although the process is not totally understood, scientists think that decreased estrogen levels lead to diminished osteoblastic activity.

A client's age, race, and sex affect bone mass and its structural integrity (ability to withstand stress) and bone loss. For example, Blacks may have denser bones

Skeletal system

The human skeletal system contains 206 bones: 80 form the axial skeleton (the head and trunk) and 126 form the appendicular skeleton (the extremities).

Bones

Bone consists of layers of calcified matrix containing spaces occupied by osteocytes (bone cells). Bone layers (lamellae) are arranged concentrically about central canals (haversian canals). Small cavities (lacunae) lying between the lamellae contain osteocytes. Tiny canals (canaliculi) connect the lacunae. They form the structural units of bone and provide nutrients to bone tissue. A typical long bone has a diaphysis (main shaft) and an epiphysis (end). The epiphyses are separated from the diaphysis with cartilage at the epiphyseal line. Beneath the epiphyseal articular surface lies the articular cartilage, which cushions the joint. Each bone consists of an outer layer of dense compact bone containing haversian systems and an inner layer of spongy (cancellous) bone composed of thin plates, called trabeculae, that interlace to form a latticework. Red marrow fills the spaces between the trabeculae of some bones.

Cancellous bone does not contain haversian systems. Compact bone is located in the diaphyses of long bones and the outer layers of short, flat, and irregular bones. Cancellous bone fills central regions of the epiphyses and the inner portions of short, flat, and irregular bones. Periosteum—specialized fibrous connective tissue—consists of an outer fibrous layer and an inner bone-forming layer. Endosteum (tissue) lines the medullary cavity (inner surface of bone, which contains the marrow).

Blood reaches bone by way of arterioles in haversian canals; vessels in Volkmann's canals, which enter bone matrix from the periosteum; and vessels in the bone ends and within the marrow. In children, the periosteum is thicker than in adults and has an increased blood supply to assist new bone formation around the shaft.

Anterior view

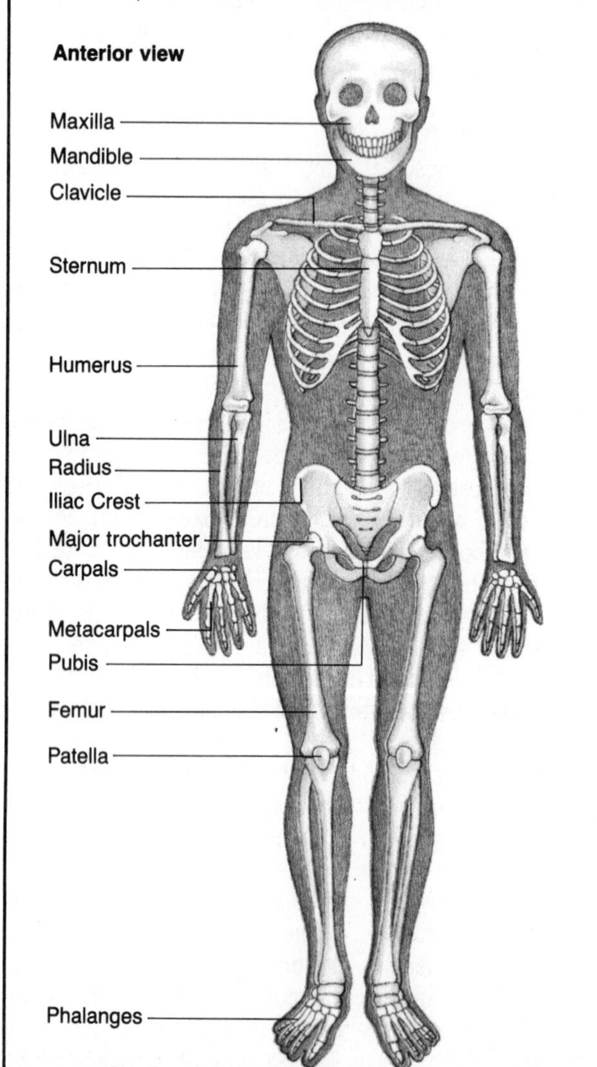

Posterior view

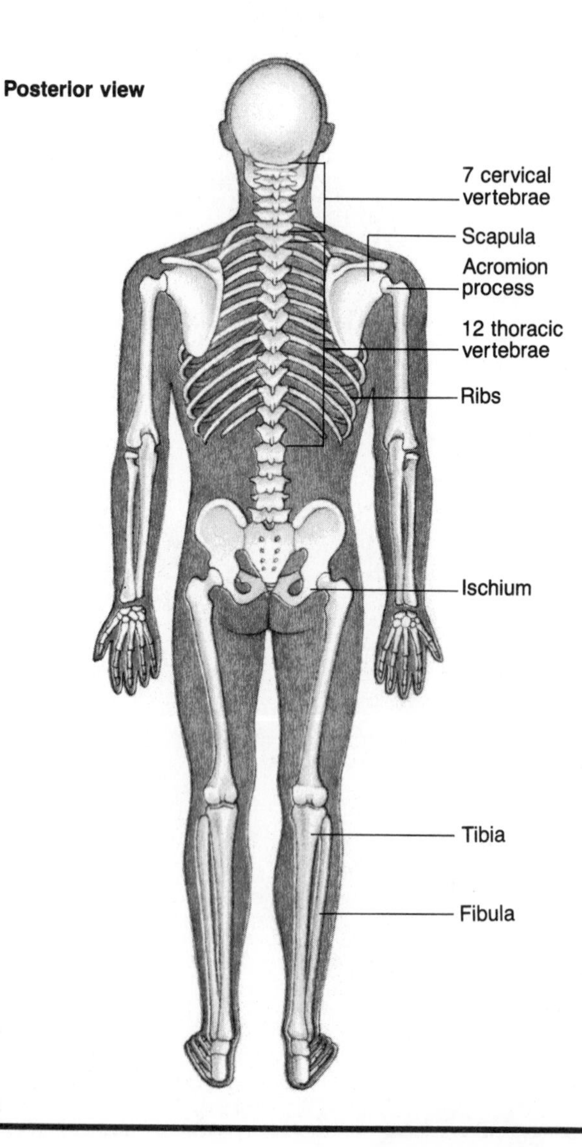

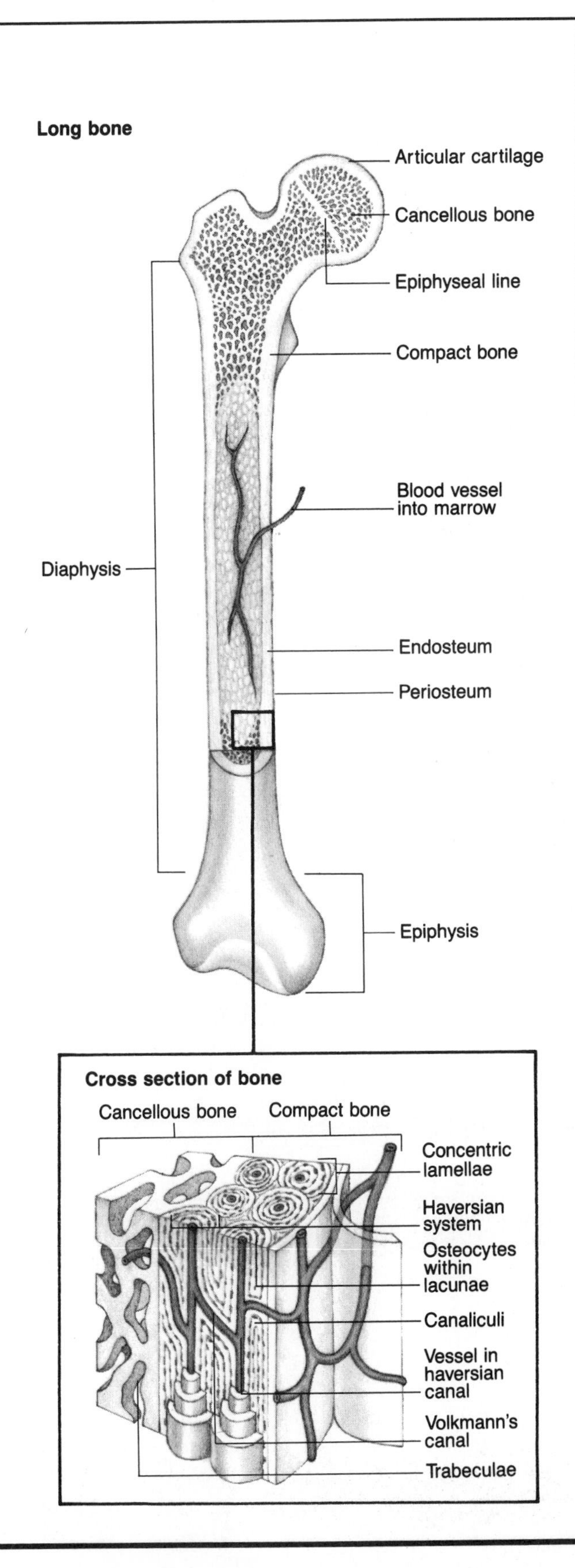

than Caucasians, and women may have less bone density than men. Bone density and structural integrity decrease after age 30 in women and age 45 in men. Thereafter, a relatively steady quantitative loss of bone matrix occurs.

Cartilage

This dense connective tissue consists of fibers embedded in a strong, gel-like substance. Avascular, cartilage also lacks nerve innervation.

Cartilage may be fibrous, hyaline, or elastic. Fibrous cartilage forms the symphysis pubis and the intervertebral disks. Hyaline cartilage covers the articular bone surfaces (where one or more bones meet at a joint); connects the ribs to the sternum; and appears in the trachea, bronchi, and nasal septum. Elastic cartilage is located in the auditory canal, the external ear, and the epiglottis.

Cartilage supports and shapes various structures (for example, the auditory canal), and some cartilage (for example, the intervertebral disks) cushions and absorbs shock that otherwise would be transmitted directly to bone.

Joints

Two or more bones meet at a joint. The body contains three major types of joints, classified by extent of movement. Synarthrodial joints, such as cranial sutures, permit no movement. This joint type separates bones with a thin layer of fibrous connective tissue. Amphiarthrodial joints, such as the symphysis pubis, allow slight movement. This joint type separates bones with hyaline cartilage. Diarthrodial joints, such as the ankle, wrist, knee, hip, or shoulder, permit free movement. In this joint type, a cavity exists between the bones forming the joint. The cavity is lined with a synovial membrane that secretes a viscous lubricating substance called synovial fluid. The membrane is encased in a fibrous joint capsule. The joint is stabilized by this capsule as well as by the ligaments, tendons, and muscles connecting the bones of the joint. Joints are further classified by shape and by motion; for example, ball and socket, hinge and pivot.

Bursae

These small synovial fluid sacs are located at friction points around joints between tendons, ligaments, and bones. They act as cushions, thereby decreasing stress to adjacent structures. The subacromial bursa (in the shoulder) and the prepatellar bursa (in the knee) are two examples.

Body movement

Skeletal muscles help facilitate joint movements by exerting force on tendons, which, in turn, pull on the bones to which they are attached. During movement, bones act as levers; joints, as fulcrums.

The diarthrodial joints allow 13 different angular and circular movements that are the basis of musculoskeletal system assessment. The shoulder demonstrates circumduction; the elbow, flexion and extension; the hip, internal and external rotation; the arm, abduction and adduction; the hand, supination and pronation; the foot, eversion and inversion; and the jaw, retraction and protraction.

Retraction: moving backward
Protraction: moving forward

Circumduction: moving in a circular fashion

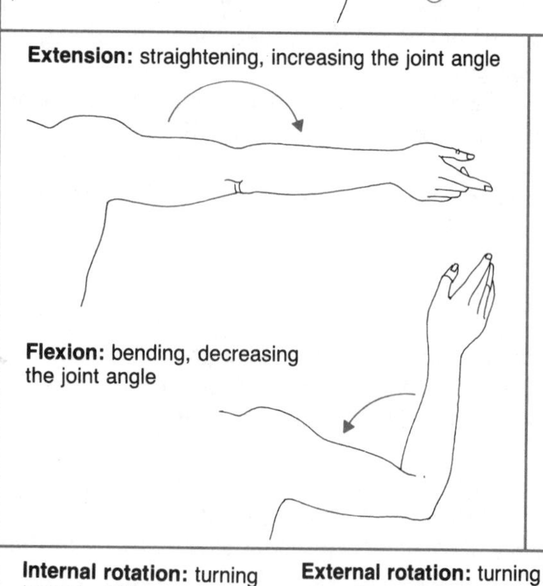

Extension: straightening, increasing the joint angle

Flexion: bending, decreasing the joint angle

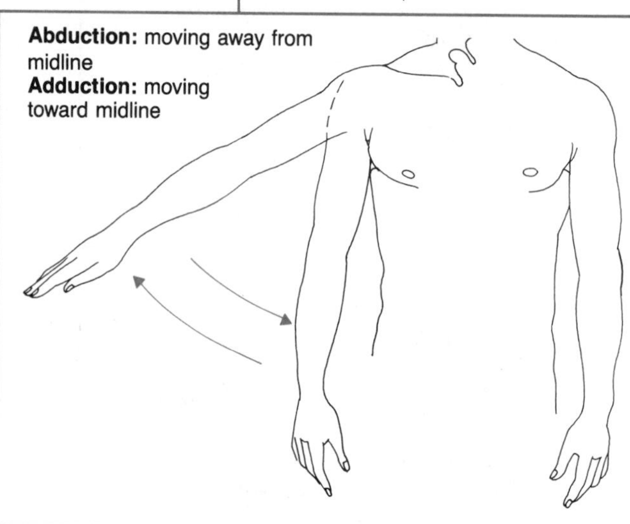

Abduction: moving away from midline
Adduction: moving toward midline

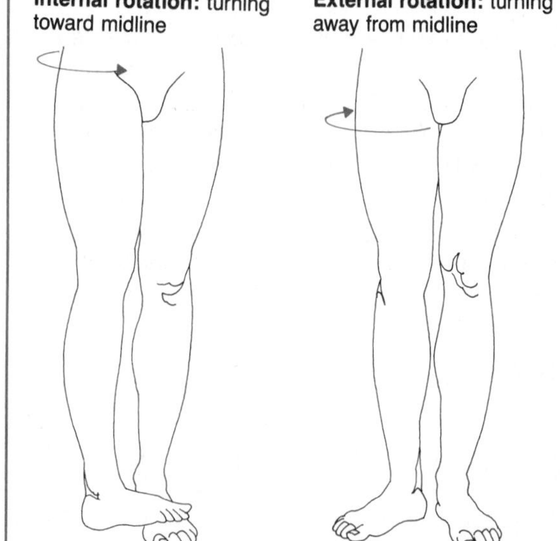

Internal rotation: turning toward midline

External rotation: turning away from midline

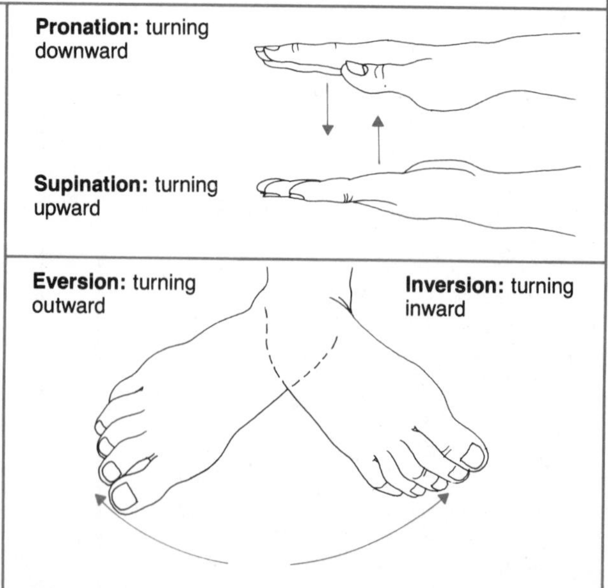

Pronation: turning downward

Supination: turning upward

Eversion: turning outward

Inversion: turning inward

Skeletal movement

Skeletal movement results primarily from muscle contractions. Other musculoskeletal structures also play a role. To contract, skeletal muscle, which is richly supplied with blood vessels and nerves, needs an impulse from the nervous system and oxygen and nutrients from the circulatory system.

When a skeletal muscle contracts, force is applied to the tendon (the cordlike structure that connects the muscle to the bone). Then one bone is pulled toward, moved away from, or rotated around a second bone, depending on the type of muscle contracted. Usually, one bone moves less than the other (or remains more stationary). The muscle tendon attachment to the more stationary bone is called the origin. The muscle tendon attachment to the more movable bone is called the insertion site. The origin usually lies on the proximal end of the bone and the insertion site on the distal end.

In skeletal movement, the bones act as levers and the joints act as fulcrums, or fixed points. Each bone's function is partially determined by the location of the fulcrum, which establishes the relationship between resistance (a force to be overcome) and effort (a force to be resisted). Most movement uses groups of muscles rather than one muscle. (For more information, see *Body movement.*)

Health history

Obtaining a thorough and accurate client health history is crucial to the nurse's assessment of the musculoskeletal system. Information about the client's musculoskeletal system is obtained from questions such as: Does the client's occupation require heavy lifting or other strenuous physical activity that increases the risk of injuring muscles, bones, tendons, or ligaments? Is the risk of developing osteoporosis increased because the client sits at a desk most of the day?

As the musculoskeletal health history interview progresses, the nurse clarifies exactly what the client means by certain subjective complaints. For example, do the client's "stiffness" complaints refer to initial stiffness in extending and flexing the joints upon waking, or to more serious chronic stiffness that hinders mobility and the activities of daily living?

The questions in this section are designed to help you evaluate the client's musculoskeletal system. They include rationales that describe the significance of the answers and, where appropriate, nursing interventions that may be incorporated into the client's care plan.

Health and illness patterns

To assess important health and illness patterns, explore the client's current, past, and family health status as well as developmental considerations.

Current health status

Because the client is most concerned with current health status, the health history interview begins with questions that explore this topic. Using the PQRST method, ask the client to describe completely the current musculoskeletal complaint, and any others. (For a detailed explanation of the PQRST method, see *Symptom analysis* in Chapter 3, The Health History.) The following questions about musculoskeletal function may be used to investigate the client's complaint thoroughly.

Are you having any pain? Can you point to the area where you feel pain?
(RATIONALE: The client's response will validate your understanding of the client's verbal description.)

How would you describe the pain—for instance, aching, burning, stabbing, or throbbing?
(RATIONALE: Frequently, the client's description provides clues to identify the tissue affected; for example, "sore or aching" points to muscle pain; "throbbing," to bone pain.)

When you have this pain, do you also have pain in any other location?
(RATIONALE: An affirmative response requires further assessment to check for referred pain. For example, pain felt in the leg may result from lumbosacral nerve root irritation.)

When did this pain begin? What were you doing at the time it began?
(RATIONALE: These questions establish whether onset was gradual or sudden. Certain activities increase the potential for injury and pain; for example, lifting heavy or awkward loads can strain ligaments and vertebral disks, causing acute, immediate pain.)

What activities seem to decrease or eliminate the pain?
(RATIONALE: Resting and elevating the affected body part usually decrease pain.)

What activities seem to increase the pain?
(RATIONALE: Weight bearing usually increases pain if the client has a degenerative disease of the hip, knee, or vertebrae.)

Do you have any other unusual sensations, such as tingling, with the pain?
(RATIONALE: Paresthesias—sensations of tingling, burning, or prickling—can accompany compression of nerves or blood vessels serving a body area.)

Will you describe your weakness? When did you first notice muscle weakness? Did the weakness begin in the same muscles where you now notice it?
(RATIONALE: Muscle weakness associated with certain diseases migrates, traveling from muscle to muscle or to groups of muscles. Knowing the symptom patterns and when they occur helps identify the disease process, if any, responsible for pain.)

When did you first notice swelling? Did you injure this area? Is the area tender? Does the overlying skin ever look red or feel hot?
(RATIONALE: These findings may indicate infection or recent trauma to the area.)

What have you tried to reduce the swelling; for example, have you tried heat or ice applications?
(RATIONALE: The client's response may help identify remedies that can be continued or may uncover inappropriate client actions.)

When did the stiffness begin? Has the stiffness increased since it began? Do you feel stiff only upon awakening or all the time?
(RATIONALE: Remission and exacerbation periods occur with some diseases. Some diseases, such as osteoarthritis and rheumatoid arthritis, cause stiffness upon awakening that decreases with activity.)

Is pain associated with the stiffness, or do you sometimes hear a grating sound or feel a grating sensation as if your bones are scraping together?
(RATIONALE: Pain, stiffness, and a crackling noise [crepitus] indicate rough, irregular articular cartilage, as found in osteoarthritis.)

What methods have you tried to reduce the stiffness?
(RATIONALE: The stiffness of rheumatoid arthritis usually decreases if the client exercises the affected joints.)

When did you first notice your movement was impaired; for instance, raising your arm, turning your head, kneeling, bending over (or whatever motion may relate to the client's complaint)*? Do you think your motion is limited by pain or something else? What else do you think might be causing this problem?*
(RATIONALE: The client's response establishes whether the problem with mobility is acute or chronic. Impaired movement can result from pain, tumors, scar tissue, bony overgrowths, and other causes.)

Are you taking any prescription or nonprescription drugs or using any home remedies to treat the problem? If so, which ones, at which strengths, for how long, and with what results?
(RATIONALE: Many prescription and nonprescription drugs can adversely affect musculoskeletal function. For information on the most common of these drugs, see *Adverse drug reactions*. The client's response will also reveal which nonprescription medications have been effective against musculoskeletal aches and pains.)

Have you noticed any other symptoms; for instance, fever, rash, numbness, tingling, or swelling?
(RATIONALE: Many musculoskeletal diseases present with multiple symptoms. In polymyositis, for example, muscle weakness, fever, and a dusky red lesion in the periorbital area are common.)

Are you having any problems with elimination?
(RATIONALE: Constipation related to lack of exercise can present problems for the client with musculoskeletal disease.)

Do you have problems with personal hygiene because of limited mobility?
(RATIONALE: The question gives the client an opportunity to detail physical concerns and limitations.)

Are you having any problems with written communication?
(RATIONALE: The client with severe rheumatoid arthritis may have great difficulty using writing implements.)

Past health status

In this portion of the health history interview, ask the following questions to gather additional information related to the musculoskeletal system.

Have you ever had any injury to a bone, muscle, ligament, cartilage, joint, or tendon? If so, what was the injury and how and when did it occur? How was it treated? Have you experienced any aftereffects?
(RATIONALE: The client's answers provide useful guides to physical assessment activities, particularly evaluating muscle strength and joint range of motion.)

Adverse drug reactions

When obtaining a health history to assess a client's musculoskeletal system, the nurse should ask about current drug use. Many drugs can seriously affect the musculoskeletal system. For example, adrenocorticosteroids can increase the risk of vertebral compression fractures.

DRUG CLASS	DRUG	POSSIBLE ADVERSE REACTIONS
Adrenocorticosteroids	prednisone	Muscle weakness, muscle wasting, osteoporosis, vertebral compression fractures, aseptic necrosis of humeral or femoral heads
Adrenocorticotropic hormone (ACTH)	corticotropin	Muscle weakness, muscle wasting, osteoporosis, vertebral compression fractures, aseptic necrosis of humeral or femoral heads
Anticoagulants	heparin sodium	Bleeding into joints with high dosages
Anticonvulsants	phenytoin sodium	Ataxia, osteomalacia (softening of the bones), rickets
Antidepressants	trazadone hydrochloride	Musculoskeletal aches and pains
Antigout agents	colchicine	Myopathy with prolonged administration
Antilipemic agents	clofibrate	Acute flulike muscular syndrome characterized by myalgia (muscle pain) or myositis with symptoms of muscle cramps, weakness, and arthralgia
Benzodiazepines	diazepam	Ataxia
Central nervous system stimulants	amphetamine sulfate	Increased motor activity
Diuretics	bumetanide, furosemide	Muscle cramps
Phenothiazines	chlorpromazine hydrochloride	Extrapyramidal symptoms (dystonic reactions, motor restlessness, and Parkinsonian signs and symptoms)
Miscellaneous skin agents	isotretinoin	Bone or joint pain, general muscle aches

Have you had surgery or other treatment involving bone, muscle, joint, ligament, tendon, or cartilage? What was the outcome?
(RATIONALE: The answers to these questions also provide useful guides to physical assessment.)

Have you had X-rays of your bones? What was X-rayed and when? What were the results?
(RATIONALE: X-ray studies show bone and joint integrity as well as previous injuries.)

Have you had blood or urine tests because of a muscle or bone problem? If so, when? What were the results of these tests?
(RATIONALE: Certain test results can point to specific musculoskeletal problems; for example, hypercalciuria and urine positive for Bence-Jones protein may indicate multiple myeloma [malignant neoplasm of the bone marrow] that has infiltrated bone.)

Have you had joint fluid removed or a biopsy performed?
(RATIONALE: Synovial fluid analysis and tissue biopsy usually provide important diagnostic information.)

What immunizations have you had and when did you have them?
(RATIONALE: Tetanus and polio vaccines are especially important to the musculoskeletal system. Tetanus and polio can cause musculoskeletal signs and symptoms that mimic

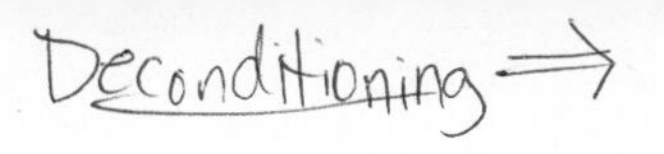

those of other disorders and may lead to an incorrect diagnosis. Tetanus, especially in an elderly client, may be diagnosed as arthritis because of joint stiffening. The muscle weakness of polio may also prompt an incorrect diagnosis. Immunization information can aid in differential diagnosis.)

Family health status

After assessing current and past musculoskeletal health status, investigate possible familial tendencies toward musculoskeletal problems by asking the following question.

Has anyone in your family had osteoporosis, gout, arthritis, or tuberculosis?
(RATIONALE: A family history of certain diseases or a history of infectious tuberculosis increases the possibility that the client may have or be at risk for these conditions.)

Developmental considerations

If the client is young, female, pregnant, or elderly, investigate developmental considerations by exploring the areas described below.

Pediatric client. When assessing a child, try to involve the child as well as the parent or guardian in the interview. Of course, the parent or guardian will answer for an infant or very young child, but any child old enough to speak can participate. A complete musculoskeletal assessment of a child should include the following questions (directed to a parent or guardian):

Was labor and delivery difficult?
(RATIONALE: Birth injuries may include fractures or nerve damage. A neonate's difficult breathing at birth may cause hypoxia leading to decreased muscle tone.)

At what age did your child first hold up his (or her) head, sit, crawl, and walk?
(RATIONALE: The answers to these questions help determine whether the child is achieving appropriate developmental milestones or if a musculoskeletal problem is preventing normal development.)

Have you noted any lack of coordination? Can your child move about normally? Would you describe your child's strength as normal for his (or her) age?
(RATIONALE: Poor coordination may point to a serious musculoskeletal problem, such as cerebral palsy, or may indicate something less serious, such as a vision problem. Muscle weakness may signify muscular dystrophy.)

Has your child ever broken a bone? If so, which one and when? Did any complications occur during the healing?
(RATIONALE: The answers to these questions help guide subsequent physical assessment.)

Female client. The following questions complete the female client's musculoskeletal health history:

At what age did you begin menstruating? If you have undergone menopause, at what age did it occur? Are you taking estrogen?
(RATIONALE: Late menarche and early menopause allow fewer years for exposure to estrogen levels that provide for bone mass, placing a woman at risk for osteoporosis.)

Pregnant client. Ask the following questions of a pregnant client:

Are you having back pains or spasms?
(RATIONALE: Often, the forward abdominal tilt during pregnancy strains the lower back.)

Are you experiencing weakness, pain, or tingling in one or both hands?
(RATIONALE: A pregnant client is at increased risk for carpal tunnel syndrome—compression neuropathy of the median nerve in the wrist—from the hand and wrist edema that occurs during the last trimester of pregnancy.)

Elderly client. Ask the following questions of an elderly client:

Have you broken any bones recently? If so, how?
(RATIONALE: Bones lose density with age. The vertebrae, hips, and wrists are particularly susceptible to fractures in an elderly client. Some fractures result from trauma; others result from a pathological (nontraumatic) cause.

Have you noticed any change in agility, in the speed at which you can move, or in endurance?
(RATIONALE: Decreased agility, reaction time, and endurance occur normally with aging.)

Do you exercise regularly? If not, why not?
(RATIONALE: Regular exercise slows the musculoskeletal deterioration attributed to aging. Encourage the client to engage in regular exercise appropriate to ability.)

Health promotion and protection patterns

As the next step in the health history interview, explore the client's personal habits, sleep and wake patterns, and typical daily activities. The following questions can help identify potential musculoskeletal problems:

How much alcohol do you drink daily? How much coffee, tea, or other caffeine-containing beverages?
(RATIONALE: High alcohol or caffeine consumption may increase the risk of osteoporosis.)

Does your current problem prevent you from falling asleep?
(RATIONALE: Many musculoskeletal problems can interfere with sleep. For example, a client with osteoarthritis may have difficulty getting comfortable.)

Does the problem cause you to wake up during the night?
(RATIONALE: This is common if the problem is tendinitis or bursitis. Pain may frequently awaken the client with a rotator cuff injury of the shoulder.)

Do you follow an exercise schedule? If so, describe it. How has your current problem affected your usual exercise routine?
(RATIONALE: Routine exercise helps maintain strength, muscle tone, bone density, and flexibility.)

Have any of your usual activities, such as dressing, grooming, climbing stairs, or rising from a chair, become difficult or impossible for you to do?
(RATIONALE: The client's response helps establish the degree of weakness and assesses its impact on daily living.)

Are you now using or do you think you would be helped by an assistive device, such as a cane, walker, or brace?
(RATIONALE: The answer shows how the client feels about an assistive device and its effects on daily life.)

What is your typical diet over 24 hours?
(RATIONALE: A client's nutritional status—especially normal caloric, calcium, protein, and vitamins A, C, and D intake—profoundly affects the musculoskeletal condition.)

Do you supplement your diet with vitamins, calcium, protein, or other products? If so, which ones and in what amounts?
(RATIONALE: Although controversy surrounds the use of dietary supplements, an affirmative answer indicates an interest in nutritional status. The amount and type of supplements the client takes are important to know because they could be helpful or detrimental.)

What is your current weight? Is this your normal weight?
(RATIONALE: Obesity adds stress to weight-bearing joints, such as the knees, putting the client at greater risk for such musculoskeletal disorders as osteoarthritis.)

Does your current problem affect your ability to prepare food and to eat? For instance, do you have difficulty opening cans or cutting meat?
(RATIONALE: Finger stiffness that accompanies osteoarthritis or rheumatoid arthritis can interfere with such tasks, possibly compromising the client's nutritional status.)

Do weather changes seem to affect the problem in any way; for example, does pain increase in cold or damp weather?
(RATIONALE: A low temperature with increased humidity tends to exacerbate muscle pain in inflammatory conditions and joint pain in osteoarthritis.)

Role and relationship patterns

Because musculoskeletal problems can profoundly affect role and relationship patterns, explore this area by asking the following questions.

Has this problem adversely affected your hobbies, leisure pursuits, and social life?
(RATIONALE: An affirmative answer indicates the need to help identify new activities within the client's capabilities.)

Do you feel any stress because of your current problem?
(RATIONALE: Certain musculoskeletal problems can interfere with life-style and self-image. For example, finger flexion associated with Dupuytren's contracture [progressive thickening and tightening of subcutaneous tissue of the palm] severely limits a client's dexterity. Pronounced scoliosis [lateral curvature of the spine] can cause self-consciousness and low self-esteem in a child or adolescent.)

What effect, if any, does this problem have on your sexual relationship?
(RATIONALE: Chronic back pain or other musculoskeletal problems can interfere with sexual desire and performance.)

Physical assessment

Physical assessment of the musculoskeletal system may be divided into observing posture, gait, and coordination; and inspecting and palpating muscles, joints, and bones.

lumbar lordosis

The nurse may perform a head-to-toe assessment, simultaneously evaluating muscle and joint function of each body area.

Preparing for the assessment

General physical assessment rules apply to musculoskeletal assessment: provide the client with warmth, privacy, and respect. The client may wear underwear or swimwear, removing it only when necessary. The examination table should be positioned to allow barrier-free access for the nurse and full range of motion for the client.

Observation, inspection, and palpation are the primary techniques used during a musculoskeletal assessment. Equipment consists of a tape measure and a goniometer, or a protractor, for measuring angles. Most of the assessment data collected will be objective. However, record client complaints about pain and other sensations related to a maneuver or test as subjective data.

As the assessment proceeds, physical findings may uncover a need to ask further history questions. For instance, when inspection reveals a scar over a joint, ask the client about surgeries or injuries to that joint. Record the new information in the health history.

Because a complete musculoskeletal assessment may exhaust a client with compromised health and strength, pace the assessment with adequate rest periods or schedule additional appointments. Some musculoskeletal tests can be performed with the client sitting, which is less tiring than standing. To enhance client comprehension, accuracy, and compliance, demonstrate the activity or movement to the client while giving instructions in language appropriate to the client's cognitive and developmental level.

Always compare both sides of the body for characteristics such as size, strength, movement, and complaints of tenderness.

Observing posture, gait, and coordination

Musculoskeletal system physical assessment begins the instant you see the client. Even before the formal assessment begins, use observation to obtain a wealth of information, such as approximate muscle strength, facial muscle movement symmetry, and obvious physical or functional deformities or abnormalities. Observation skills are particularly important in assessing children who are often unable or unwilling to follow directions.

Assess the client's overall body symmetry as the client assumes different postures and makes diverse movements. Planning more detailed assessments later, initially note marked dissimilarities in side-to-side size, shape, and motion.

Posture

Evaluating posture—the attitude, or position, that body parts assume in relation to other body parts and to the external environment—involves inspecting spinal curvature and knee positioning.

Spinal curvature. To assess spinal curvature, instruct the client to stand as straight as possible. Standing to the client's side, back, and front, respectively, inspect the spine for alignment and the shoulders, iliac crests, and scapulae for symmetry of position and height. Then have the client bend forward from the waist with arms relaxed and dangling. Stand behind the client, and inspect the straightness of the spine, noting flank and thorax position and symmetry.

Normally, convex curvature prevails in the thoracic spine, whereas concave curvature is normal in the lumbar spine when the client is standing.

Normal findings include a midline spine without lateral curvatures; a concave lumbar curvature that changes to a convex curvature in the flexed position; and iliac crests, shoulders, and scapulae at the same horizontal level. Race may cause differences in spinal curvatures; for example, some Blacks have a pronounced lumbar lordosis.

Knee positioning. Another important aspect of posture is knee position. To assess this, have the client stand with the feet together. Note the relationship of one knee to the other. The knees should be bilaterally symmetrical and located at the same height in a forward-facing position. Normally, the knees are less than 1″ (2.5 cm) apart and the medial malleoli (ankle bones) are less than 1⅛″ (3 cm) apart.

Gait

Gait consists of two main phases: stance and swing. (For illustrations, see *Components of gait,* pages 524 and 525.)

To assess gait, direct the client to walk away, turn around, and walk back. Observe and evaluate the client's posture, movement (such as pace and length of stride), foot position, coordination, and balance. During the stance phase, the foot on the floor should flatten completely and be able to bear the weight of the body. As the client pushes off, the toes should be flexed. In the swing phase, the foot in midswing should clear the floor and pass the opposite leg in its stance phase. When the swing phase ends, the client should be able to control the swing as it stops, as the foot again contacts the floor.

Other normal findings include smooth, coordinated movements, the head leading the body when turning, and erect posture with approximately 2″ to 4″ (5 to 10 cm) of space between the feet. (*Note:* Remain close to an elderly or infirm client and be prepared to help if the client stumbles or starts to fall.)

Coordination

Assessing coordination involves evaluating how well a client's muscles produce movement. Coordination results from neuromuscular integrity. A lack of muscular or nervous system integrity, or both, can impair the client's ability to make voluntary and productive movements.

Assess gross motor skills with such tests as lifting the arm to the side or other range-of-motion exercises (any body action involving the muscles and joints in natural directional movements). (For additional information, see *Assessing muscle strength and joint range of motion,* pages 526 through 536.) Fine motor coordination can be assessed by asking the client to remove a small object from a desk or table.

Abnormal findings

Abnormal gait results from joint stiffness and pain, muscle weakness, deformities, and orthopedic devices, such as leg braces. Other abnormal findings may include an abnormally wide support base (which, in adults, may indicate central nervous system dysfunction), toeing in or out, arms held out to the side or in front, jerky or shuffling motions, and the ball of the foot striking the floor instead of the heel.

Examples of coordination problems associated with voluntary movement include ataxia (impaired movement coordination, characterized by unusual or erratic muscular activity); spasticity (awkward, jerky, and stiff movements); and tremor (muscular quivering). (For more information, see Chapter 17, Nervous System.)

Developmental considerations

To assess accurately the posture, gait, and coordination of a pediatric, pregnant, or elderly client, modify assessment techniques according to the client's developmental stage and evaluate structure and abnormalities in terms of normal ranges for the client's age group.

Pediatric client. For an infant's or small child's assessment, the parent's lap can serve as an examination surface. With a child who cannot follow directions well, observe active and passive motions as a way to assess strength. Palpate any affected part last to facilitate the child's cooperation with the rest of the assessment.

The neonate has a generalized convexity (C-shape) of the spine. When the infant begins to hold up its head, a concave cervical curve develops. Then a lumbar concavity (lordosis), which may appear exaggerated, develops when the infant begins to walk. The school-age child usually stands with the normal adult spinal curvature, which should continue until old age.

A toddler's gait normally involves a wide support base—that is, with feet wide apart.

Common knee deviations in children include knock-knees (genu valgum) and bowlegs (genu varum). In a child with genu valgum, the knees touch and the medial malleoli are ¾″ to 1⅛″ (2 to 3 cm) or more apart when the child is standing. (This is common during the first year the child walks.)

In a child with genu varum, the knees are more than 1″ (2.5 cm) apart and the medial malleoli touch when the child stands. This is normal in children from ages 2 to 3½ and may persist until age 6.

Lateral curvature (scoliosis) may become apparent during adolescence, with a higher incidence among girls. The spine will not grow straight and the shoulders and iliac crests will not be the same height. To assess the difference between a functional scoliosis (one related to posture) and a true scoliosis, ask the client to flex the spine by bending over. A functional scoliosis will disappear, but a true scoliosis will remain, its appearance emphasized by a thoracic hump.

Pregnant client. Posture and gait change gradually during pregnancy. The enlarging fetus and the forward shift in the woman's center of gravity cause increased lordosis and a compensatory forward cervical flexion. In preparation for delivery, the sacroiliac joints and the symphysis pubis become more mobile and unstable, contributing to the characteristic waddling gait.

Elderly client. A dorsal kyphosis (exaggerated convexity of the thoracic curvature) typically accompanies aging.

An elderly client may have an abnormal gait with uneven rhythm, wide support base, and short steps. Some contributing factors include loss of muscle strength and coordination, fear of falling, painful arthritic joints, peripheral neuropathy, and poor vision.

Inspecting and palpating muscles

Although inspection and palpation are performed separately in many assessments, they are performed simultaneously during the musculoskeletal assessment.

Muscle assessment includes evaluating muscle tone, mass, and strength. Palpate the muscles with gentleness, never forcing movement when the client reports pain or when you feel resistance. Watch the client's face and body language for signs of discomfort; a client may suffer silently.

Components of gait

Each phase of gait has several components.

Stance phase
This phase begins when the heel strikes the floor (the heel strike). Next, the foot is completely flattened and bearing the weight of the body. In midstance, the opposite foot is lifted, while the flattened foot begins to push off with the toes flexed and the heel lifting from the floor.

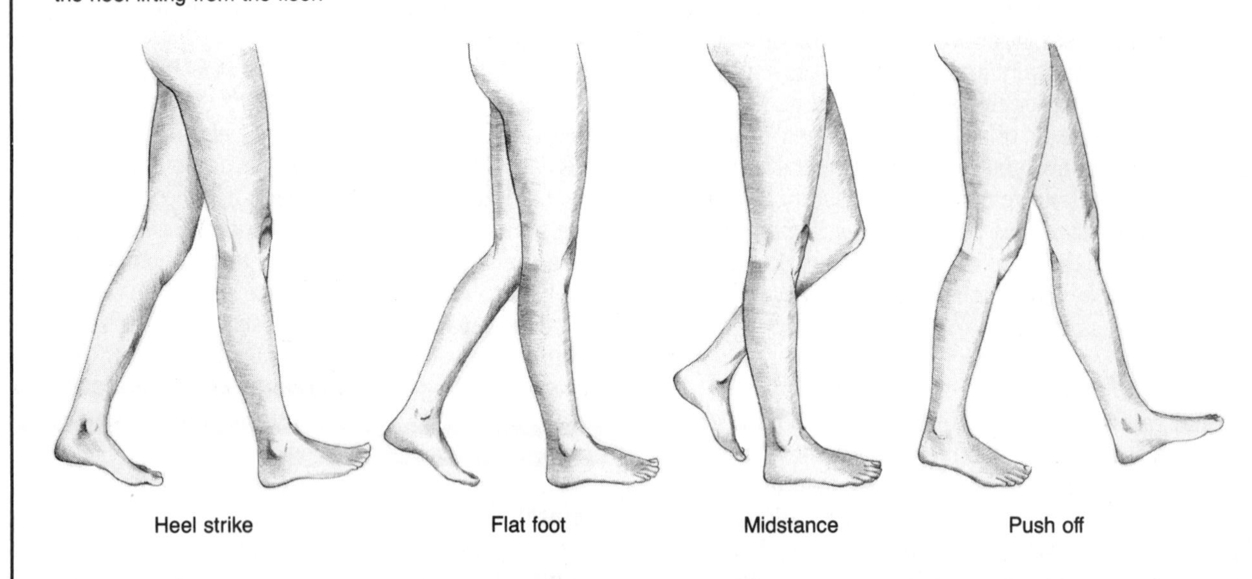

Tone and mass. Assess muscle tone—the consistency or tension in the resting muscle—by palpating a muscle at rest and during passive range of motion. Palpate a muscle at rest from the muscle attachment at the bone to the edge of the muscle. Normally, a relaxed muscle should feel soft, pliable, and nontender; a contracted muscle, firm.

Muscle mass is the actual size of a muscle. Assessment of muscle mass usually involves measuring the circumference of the thigh, the calf, and the upper arm. When measuring, establish landmarks to ensure measurement at the same location on each area.

When measuring the upper midarm circumferences to assess muscle size, be sure to ask the client which side is dominant (that is, whether the client is right- or left-handed). Expect symmetry of size (greater than a ½" [1-cm] circumferential difference between opposite thighs, calves, and upper arms is considered abnormal unless the increased muscle size results from specific physical activities).

Abnormal findings include decreased muscle size or wasting (atrophy), excessive muscle size (hypertrophy) without a history of muscle-building exercises, flaccidity (atony), weakness (hypotonicity), spasticity (hypertonicity), and fasciculations (involuntary twitching of muscle fibers).

Strength. To evaluate muscle strength, have the client perform active range-of-motion movements as you apply resistance. Note the strength that the client exerts against resistance. If the muscle group is weak, lessen the resistance to permit a more accurate assessment. Record findings according to a five-point scale. (For information on how to test and grade muscle strength, see *Assessing muscle strength and joint range of motion,* pages 526 through 536.)

Inspecting and palpating joints and bones

Assessment of the joints and bones includes measuring the client's height and the length of the extremities (arms and legs), and evaluating joint and bone characteristics and joint range of motion.

During joint assessment, never force joint movement if you feel resistance or if the client complains of pain. General deviations from normal include pain, swelling, stiffness, deformities, altered range of motion, crepitation (a grating sound or sensation accompanying joint movement), ankylosis (joint fusion or fixation), and contracture (muscle shortening).

Swing phase
In the acceleration portion of this phase, the foot begins moving forward. In midswing, the foot clears the floor, continuing past the opposite leg. In the deceleration phase, the swing stops, and the foot moves toward the floor with control until the heel strikes the floor.

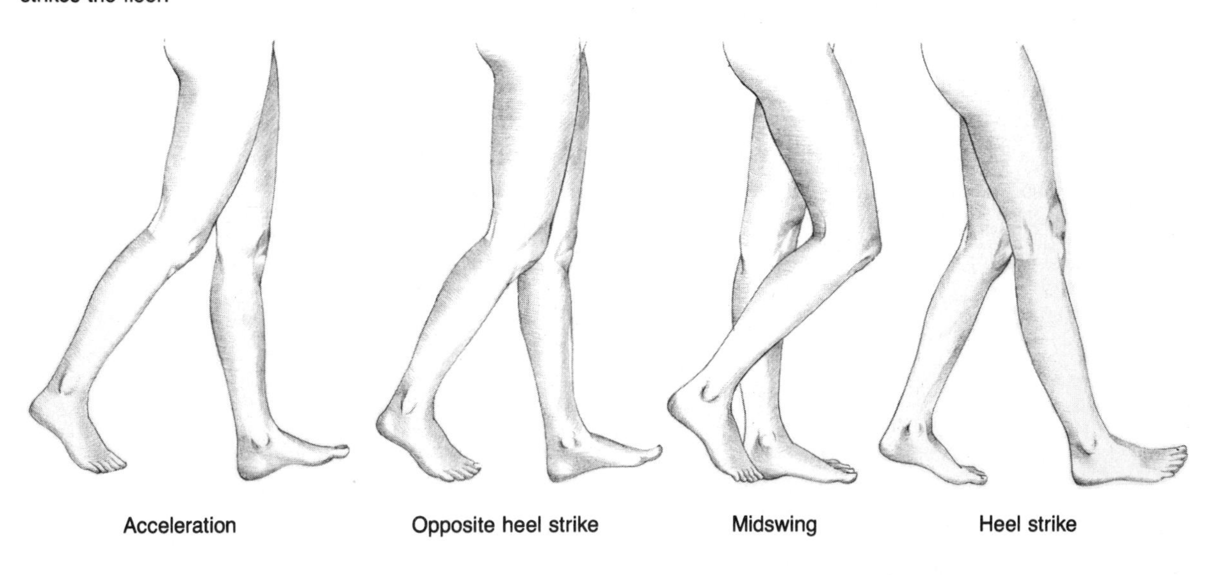

Begin the assessment with measurements; then assess bone and joint characteristics. (For more information, see *Assessing muscle strength and joint range of motion*, pages 526 through 536.)

Measurements. Measure the height of the client as well as the length of the extremities for comparison. (For a description of how to measure height, see Chapter 4, Physical Assessment Skills.)

To measure the extremities, place the client in the supine position on a flat surface with the arms and legs fully extended and the shoulders and hips adducted. Measure each arm from the acromion process to the tip of the middle finger. Measure each leg from the anterior superior iliac spine to the medial malleolus with the tape crossing at the medial side of the knee. More than 3/8" (1 cm) disparity in the length between each limb is abnormal.

Cervical spine. Inspect the cervical spine from three viewpoints: from behind, from the side, and facing the client. The client may sit or stand.

Observe the alignment of the head with the body. The nose should be in line with the midsternum and extend beyond the shoulders when viewed from the side.

Flexion → head forward

The head should align with the shoulders. Normally, the seventh cervical and first thoracic vertebrae are more prominent than the others.

AB Abnormal findings include arthritis, which often affects the cervical joints, with audible crepitus on movement, pain, stiffness, or sensory changes in the arm and hand; loss of a normal cervical curve; abnormally protruded vertebrae; and bony enlargements.

Clavicles. Inspect and palpate the length of the clavicles, including the sternoclavicular and acromioclavicular joints. Normal findings include firm, smooth, and continuous bone.

Abnormal findings include pain, crepitus, noncontinuous bone (a fracture, for example), asymmetrical size or contour, and masses. ABN.

Scapulae. To inspect and palpate the scapulae, sit directly behind the client, who sits with shoulders thrust backward. Normally, the scapulae are located over thoracic ribs 2 through 7. Check for an equal distance from the medial scapular edges to the midspinal line.

(Text continues on page 536.)

Assessing muscle strength and joint range of motion

Assessment of joint range of motion (ROM) tests the joint function; assessment of muscle strength against resistance tests the function of the muscles surrounding the joint. To assess joint ROM, ask the client to move specific joints through the normal ROM. If the client cannot do so, move the joints through passive ROM. To assess muscle strength, apply pressure to a point at or near the muscles surrounding a joint. Normally, the client can move joints a certain distance in degrees and can easily resist pressure applied against movement. If two sides are assessed, strength should be symmetrical.

The following pages show each joint and surrounding muscle group and describe and illustrate the tests for muscle strength and ROM, including the expected degree of motion for each joint.

Grading muscle strength

When evaluating muscle strength, use the scale below. Column 1 describes the possible muscle response and its significance. Column 2 grades the response.

MUSCLE RESPONSE AND SIGNIFICANCE	GRADE RATING
No visible or palpable contraction • Paralysis	0
Slightly palpable contraction • Paresis, severe weakness	1
Passive range of motion (ROM) maneuvers when gravity is removed • Paresis, moderate weakness	2
Active ROM against gravity alone or against light resistance • Mild weakness	3 to 4
Active ROM against full resistance • Normal	5

CERVICAL SPINE AND NECK

Posterior view of upper spine

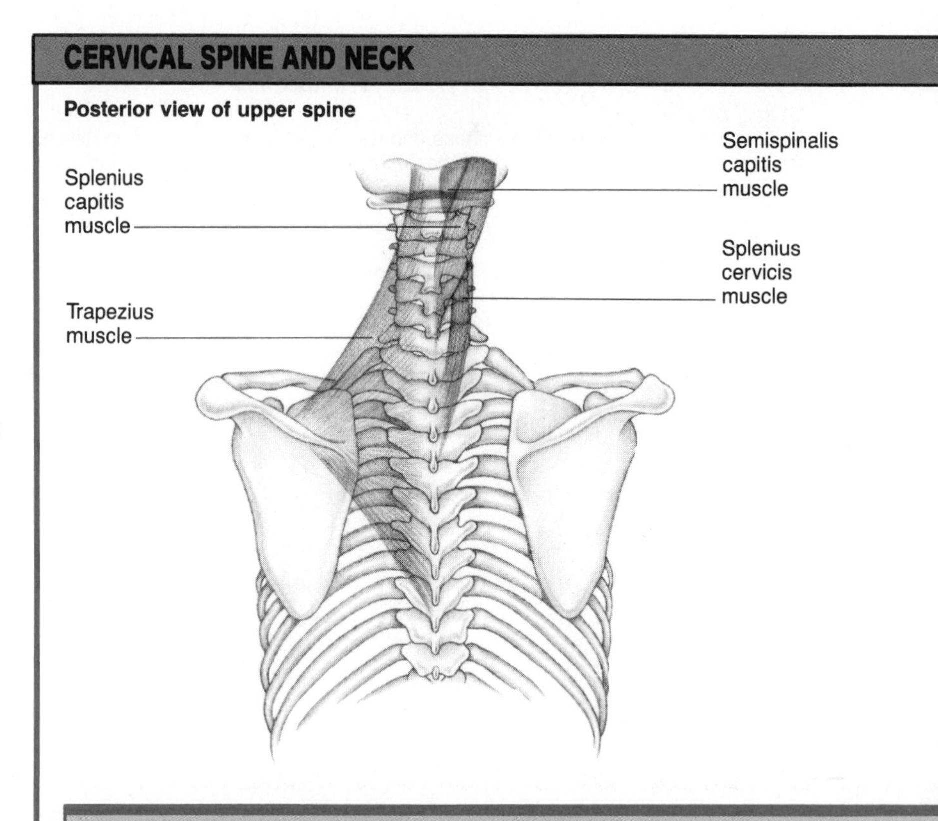

Muscle strength

To assess flexion of the cervical spine, place your hand on the client's forehead, applying pressure. Ask the client to bend the head forward and touch the chin to the chest.

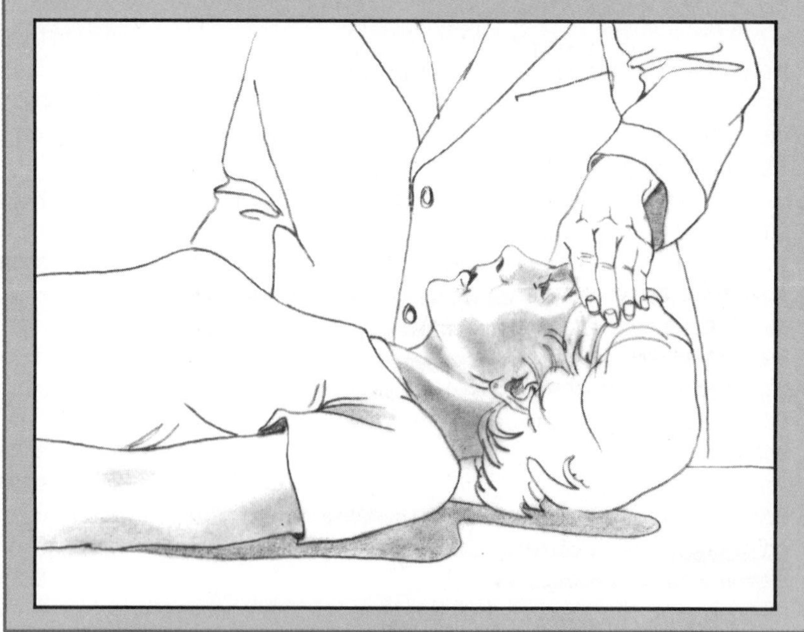

Range of motion

Ask the client to flex the neck (attempt to touch the chin to the chest), then extend the neck (bend the head backward).

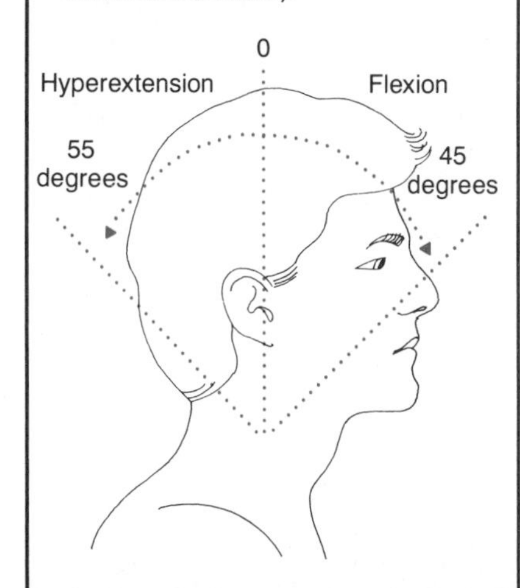

Next, ask the client to bend laterally, touching the ears to the shoulders.

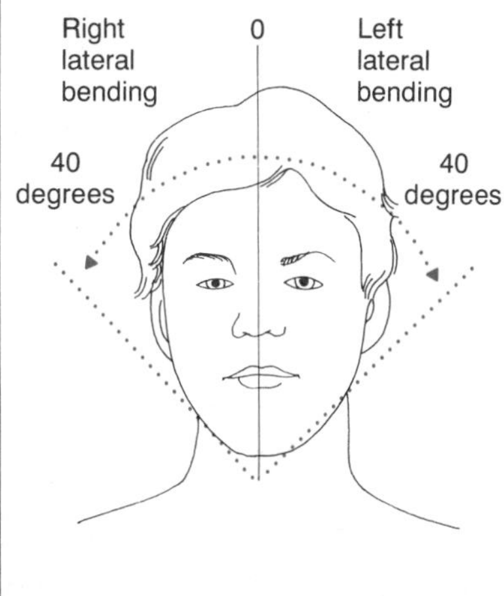

Then, ask the client to rotate the head from side to side.

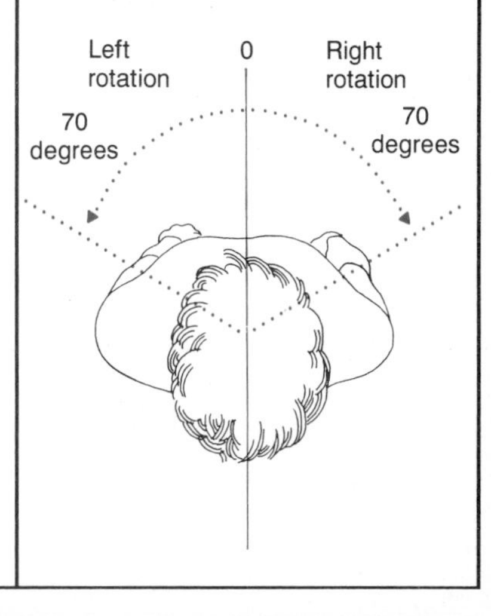

To assess rotation of the cervical spine, ask the client to push laterally against your hand positioned firmly against the left side of the face to prevent movement. At the same time, palpate the sternocleidomastoid muscle on the opposite side. Repeat the procedure on the right side.

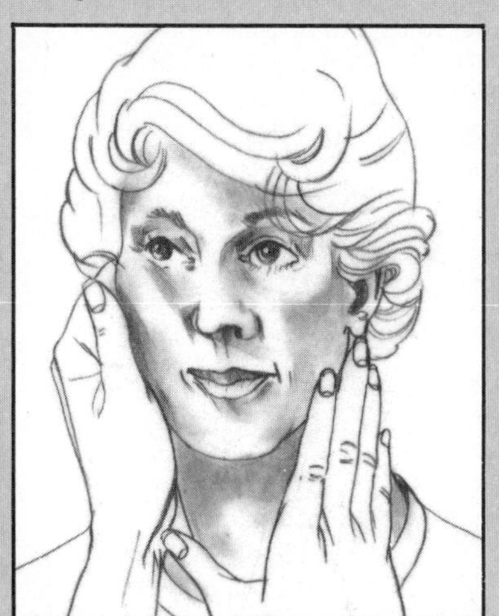

To assess extension of the cervical spine, apply pressure with your hand on the client's occipital bone. Ask the client to bend the head backward as far as possible.

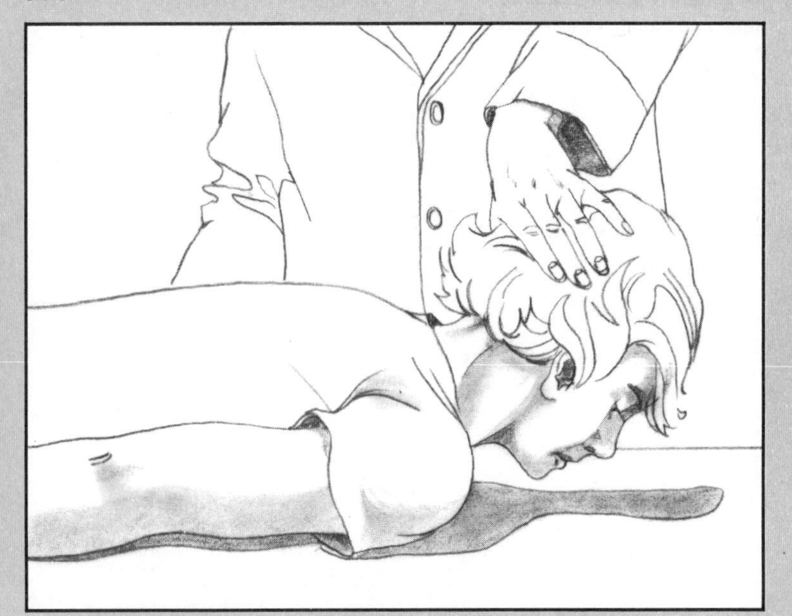

continued

Assessing muscle strength and joint range of motion continued

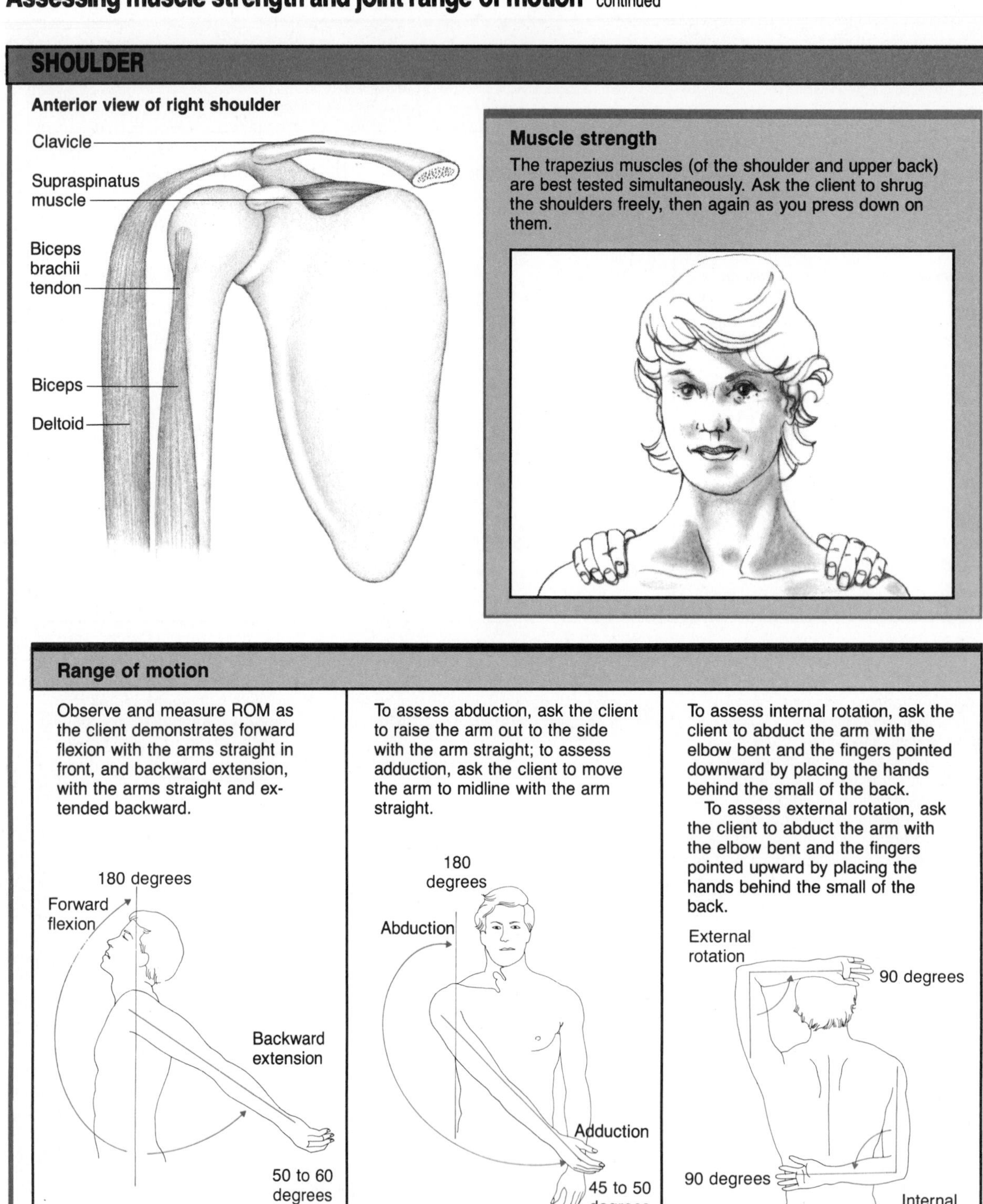

UPPER ARM AND ELBOW

Anterior view of left arm

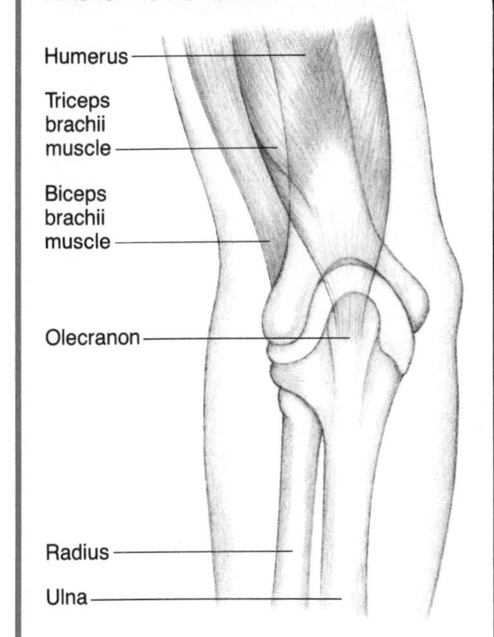

Range of motion

Ask the client to sit or stand. Then, assess flexion by having the client bend the arm and attempt to touch the shoulder. To assess extension, ask the client to straighten the arm.

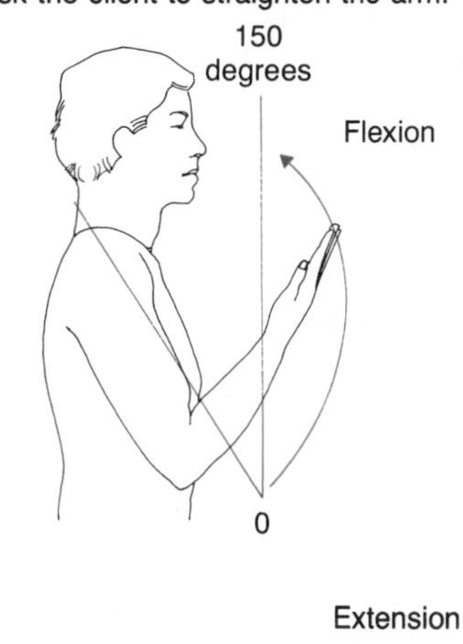

Assess pronation by holding the client's elbow in a flexed position while the client rotates the arm until the palm faces the floor.

Assess supination by holding the client's elbow in a flexed position while the client rotates the arm until the palm faces upward.

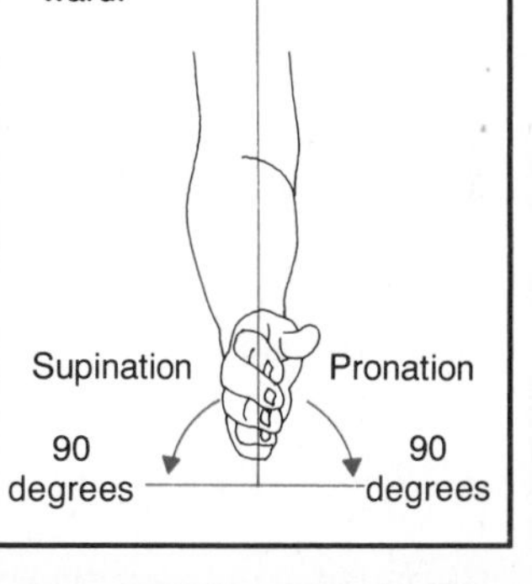

Muscle strength

To test triceps strength, try to flex the client's arm while the client tries to extend it.

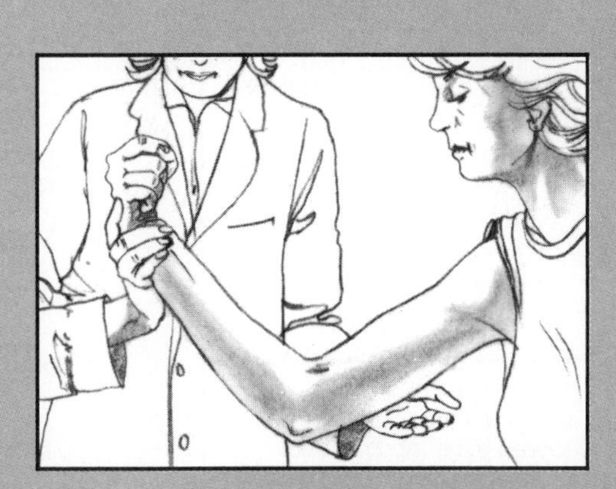

To test deltoid strength, push down on the client's arms (abducted to 90 degrees) while the client resists.

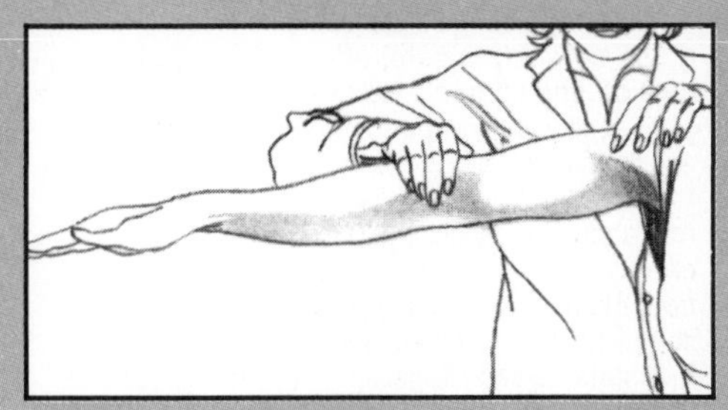

To assess biceps strength, try to pull the client's flexed arm into extension while the client resists.

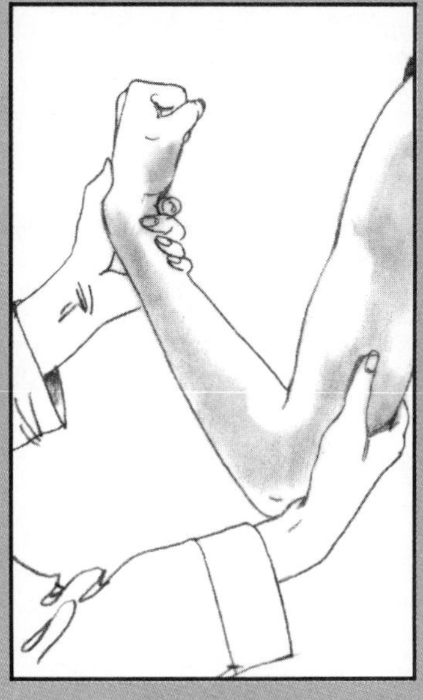

continued

Assessing muscle strength and joint range of motion continued

WRIST AND HAND

Lateral view of left hand and wrist

Extensor digiti minimi muscle
Metacarpophalangeal joint
Proximal interphalangeal joint
Ulna
Radius
Extensor indicis proprius muscle
Distal interphalagneal joint

Range of motion

To assess flexion, ask the client to bend the wrist downward; assess extension by having the client straighten the wrist. To assess hyperextension or dorsiflexion, ask the client to bend the wrist upward.

70 degrees
Hyperextension (dorsiflexion)
Extension
0
Flexion
80 degrees

To assess the metacarpophalangeal joints, ask the client to hyperextend (dorsiflex), extend (straighten), and flex (make a fist) the fingers.

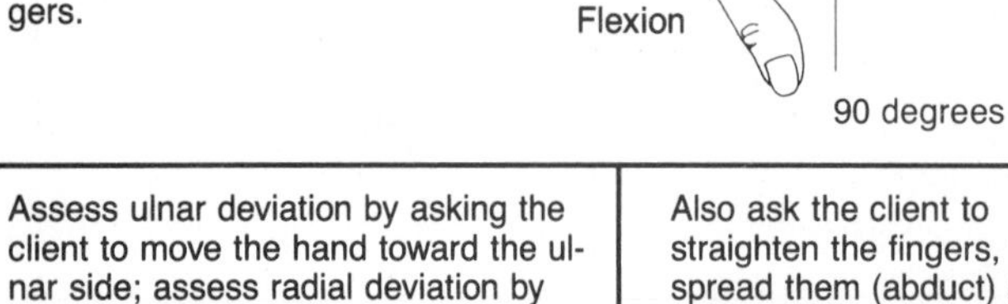

Assess ulnar deviation by asking the client to move the hand toward the ulnar side; assess radial deviation by asking the client to move the hand toward the radial side.

Radial deviation
20 degrees
0
Ulnar deviation
30 to 50 degrees

Also ask the client to straighten the fingers, then spread them (abduct) and bring them together (adduct). Abduction should be 20 degrees between fingers; adduction, the fingers touch.

To assess palmar adduction, ask the client to bring the thumb to the index finger; assess palmar abduction by asking the client to move the thumb away from the palm. Assess opposition by having the client touch the thumb to each fingertip.

Muscle strength

Test muscle strength and movement of both hands simultaneously by having the client squeeze the first two fingers of your hand, make a fist, resist your efforts to straighten a flexed wrist, and resist your efforts to flex a straightened wrist. (Normally, the dominant hand may be slightly stronger.)

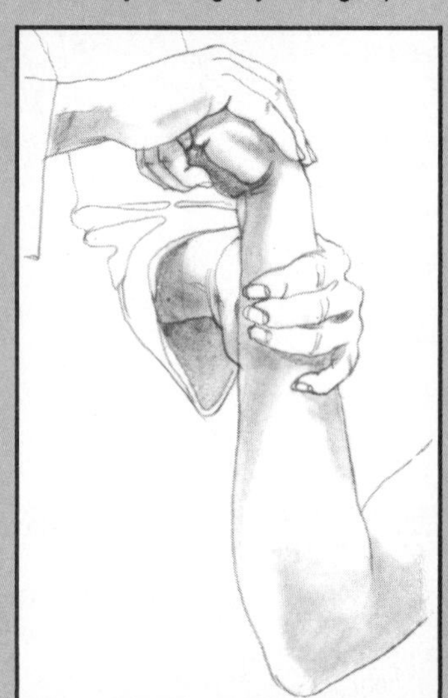

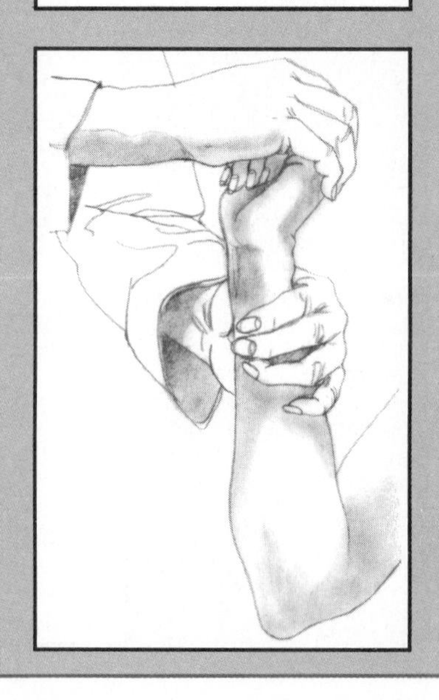

THORACIC AND LUMBAR SPINE

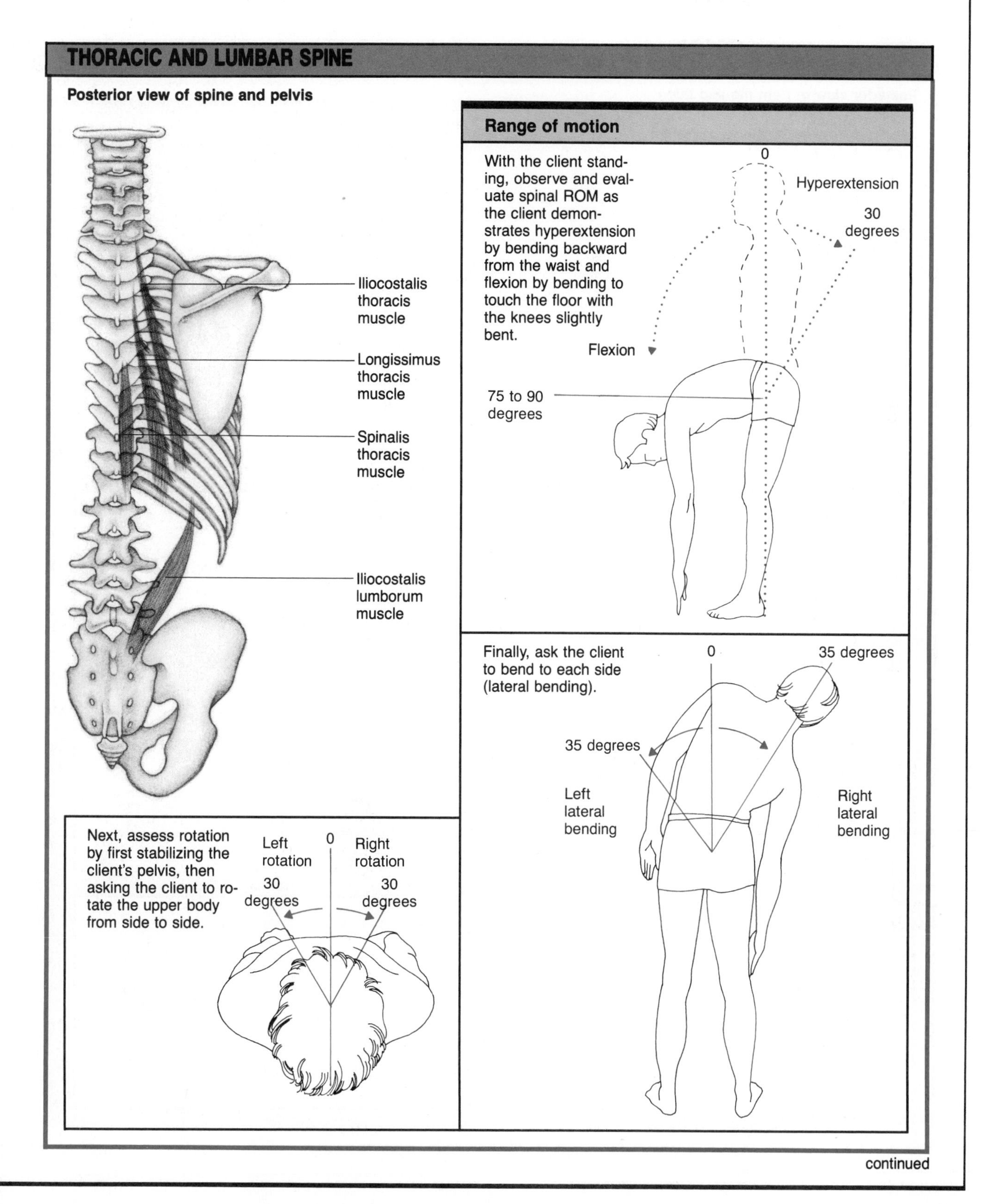

With the client standing, observe and evaluate spinal ROM as the client demonstrates hyperextension by bending backward from the waist and flexion by bending to touch the floor with the knees slightly bent.

Next, assess rotation by first stabilizing the client's pelvis, then asking the client to rotate the upper body from side to side.

Finally, ask the client to bend to each side (lateral bending).

continued

Assessing muscle strength and joint range of motion continued

HIP AND PELVIS

Posterior view of right hip and thigh

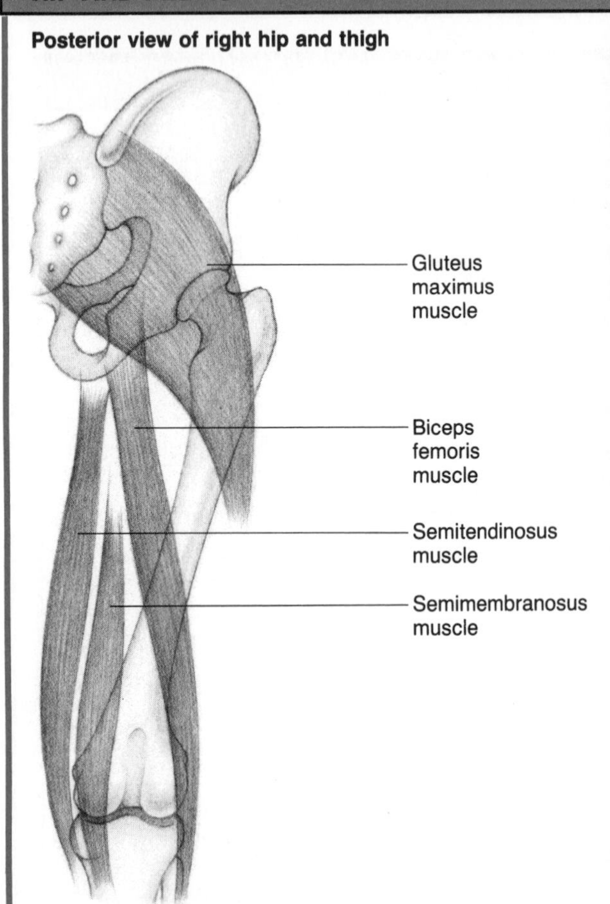

Muscle strength

With the client lying (prone and, later, supine), then sitting, evaluate muscle strength and palpate muscles as you carry out the following tests.

To assess hip extensors, ask the prone client to hyperextend the leg backward (toward the ceiling) as you try to push the leg downward.

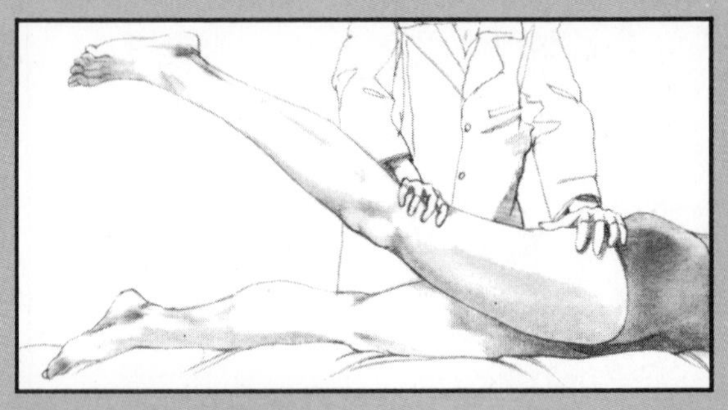

To assess hip flexors, ask the client to sit and raise the knee to the chest as you apply downward pressure proximal to the knee.

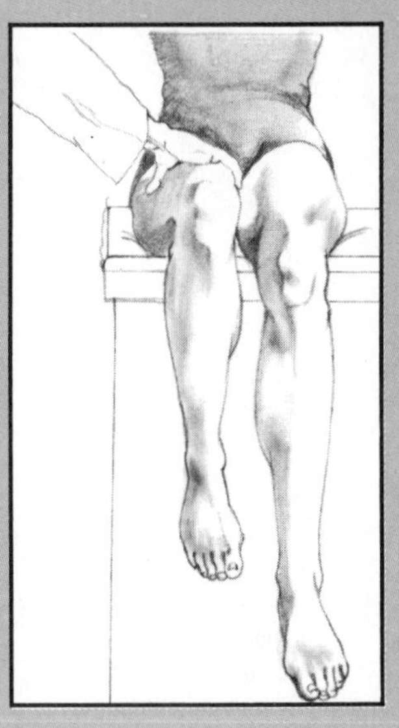

To assess hip abductors, ask the supine client to move the straightened leg away from midline as you attempt to push the client's leg toward midline.

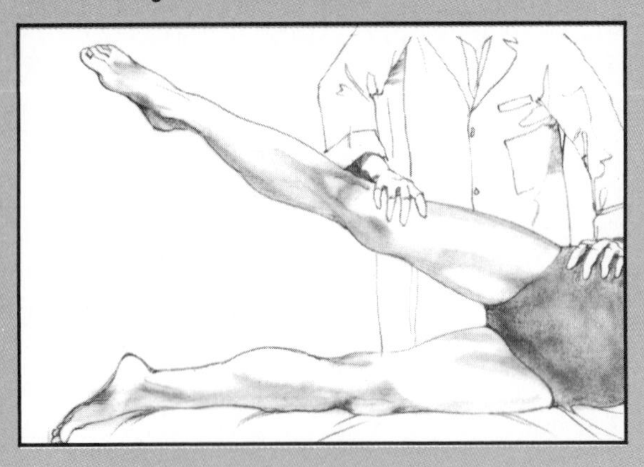

To assess hip adductors, ask the supine client to move the leg toward midline as you try to pull the leg away from midline.

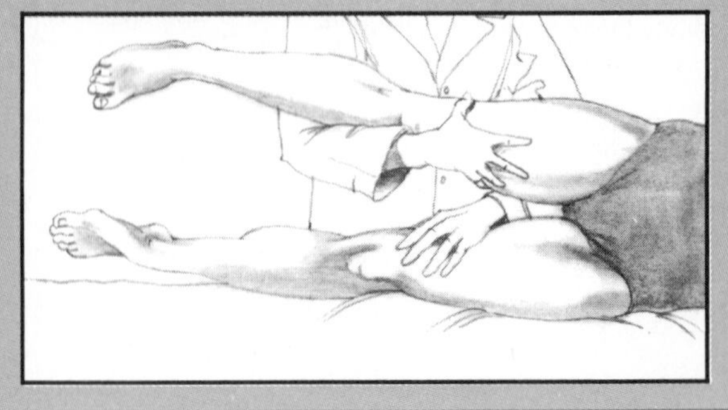

Greater Trochanter

Range of motion

With the client supine or standing, observe and evaluate ROM as the client demonstrates flexion by bending the knee to the chest with the back straight. *Caution:* Do not perform this movement on a client who has undergone total hip replacement without the surgeon's permission because the motion can cause the prosthesis to dislocate.

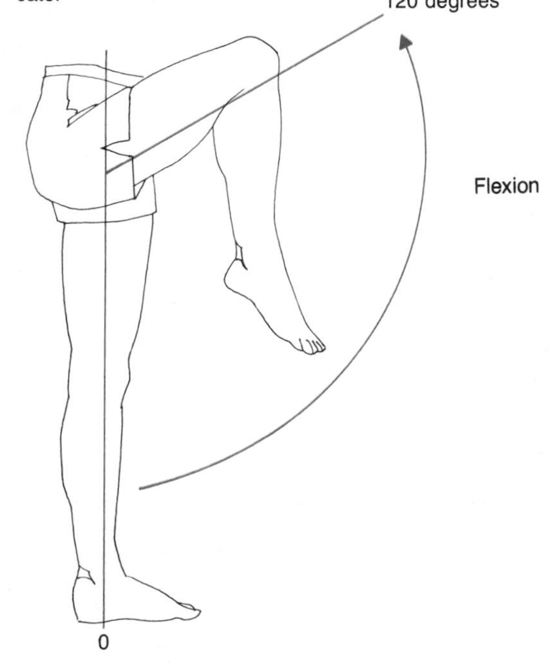

Next, evaluate extension by asking the client to straighten the knee and hyperextension by asking the client to extend the leg backward with the knee straight. *Note:* This motion can be performed with the client prone or standing.

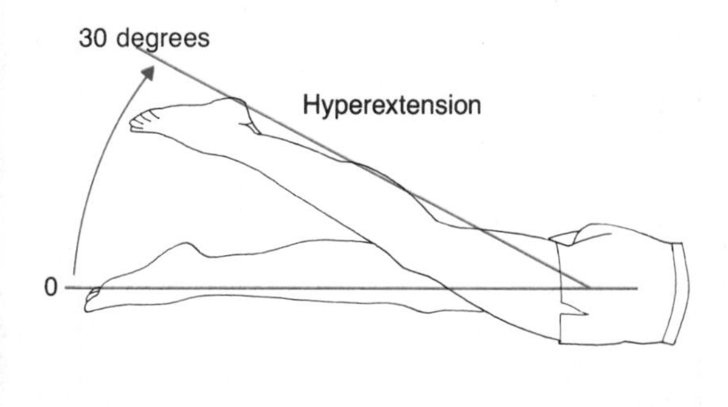

To assess abduction, have the client move the straightened leg away from midline; assess adduction by having the client move the straightened leg toward midline. *Caution:* This motion can displace a hip prosthesis.

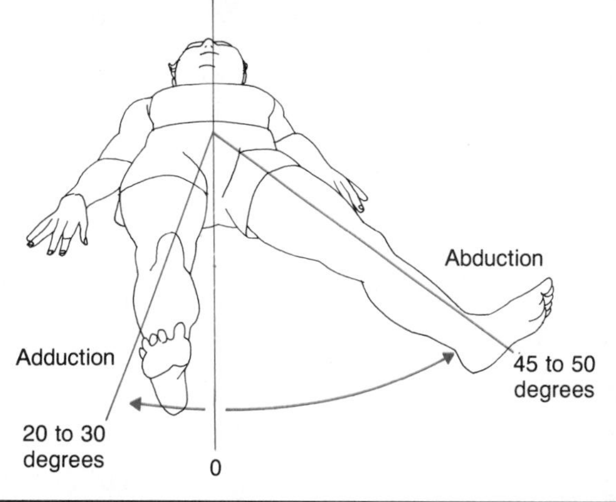

Finally, assess internal and external rotation by asking the client to bend the knee and turn the leg inward and outward, respectively.

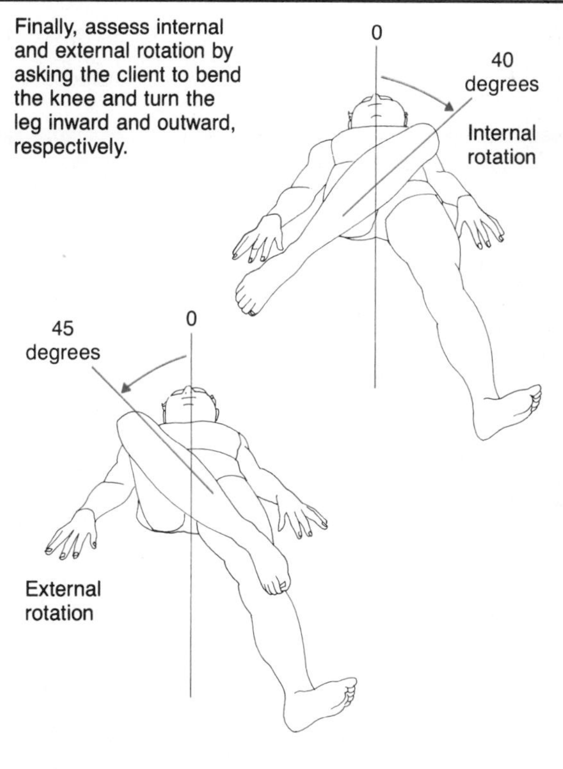

continued

Assessing muscle strength and joint range of motion continued

KNEE

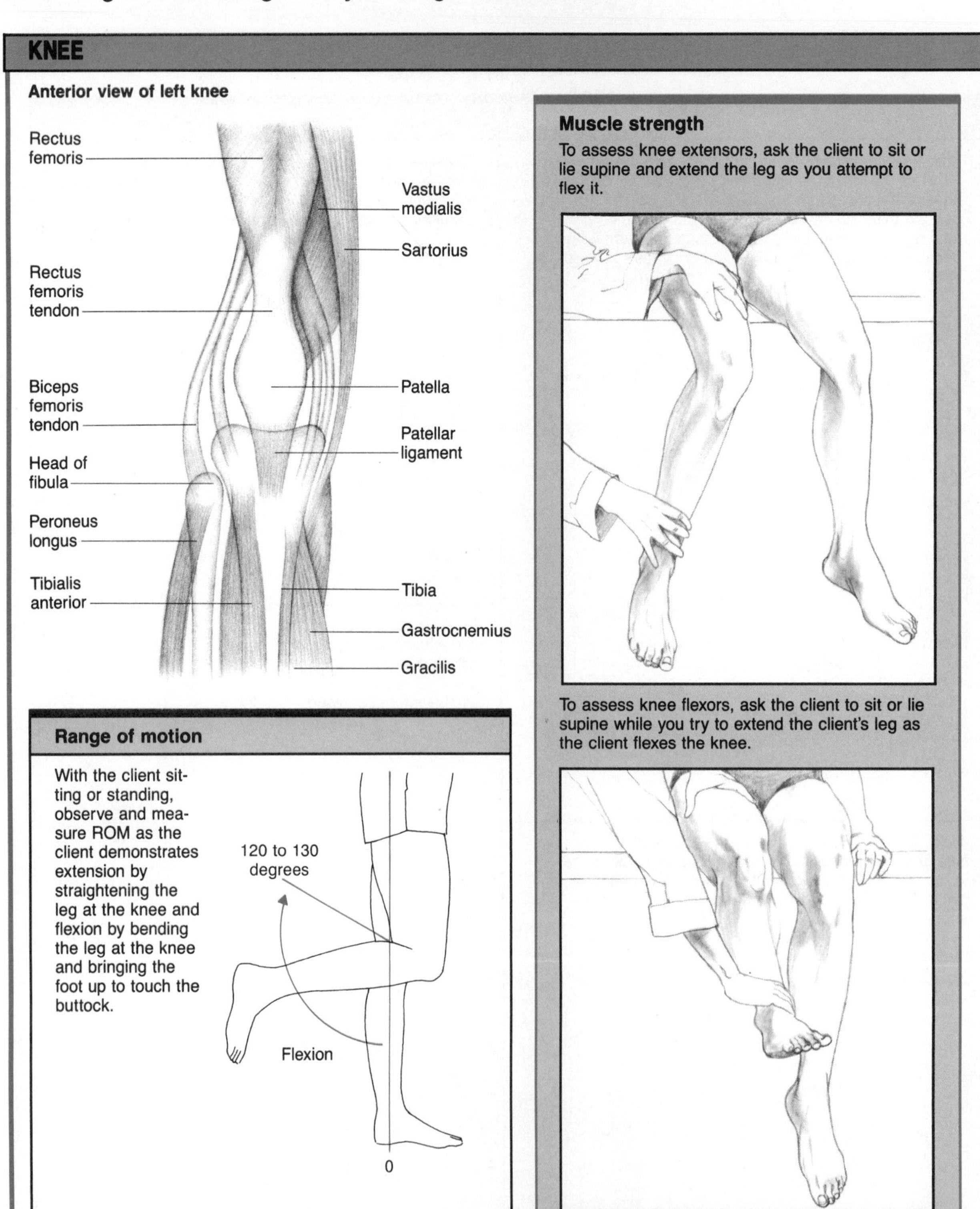

Range of motion

With the client sitting or standing, observe and measure ROM as the client demonstrates extension by straightening the leg at the knee and flexion by bending the leg at the knee and bringing the foot up to touch the buttock.

Muscle strength

To assess knee extensors, ask the client to sit or lie supine and extend the leg as you attempt to flex it.

To assess knee flexors, ask the client to sit or lie supine while you try to extend the client's leg as the client flexes the knee.

ANKLE AND FOOT

Anterior view of right ankle and foot

Tibialis posterior muscle
Tibia
Metatarsophalangeal joint
Tarsometatarsal joint
Proximal phalanx
Distal phalanx
Fibula
Peroneus brevis muscle

Muscle strength

To assess dorsiflexion of the ankle joint, apply pressure with your hand to the dorsal surface of the client's foot as the client attempts to bend the foot up.

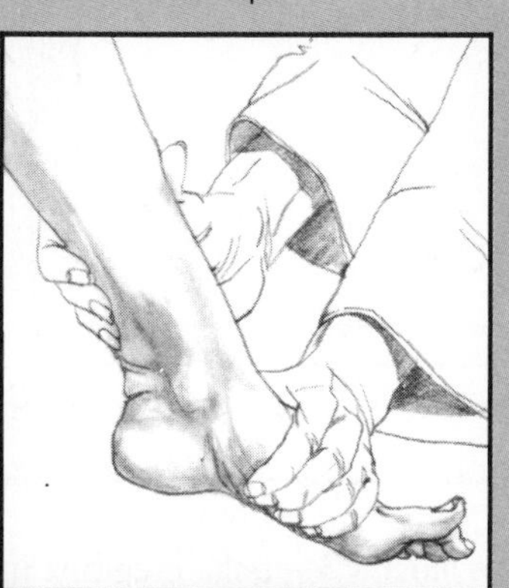

To assess plantar flexion, apply pressure with your hand to the plantar surface of the client's foot as the client attempts to bend the foot down.

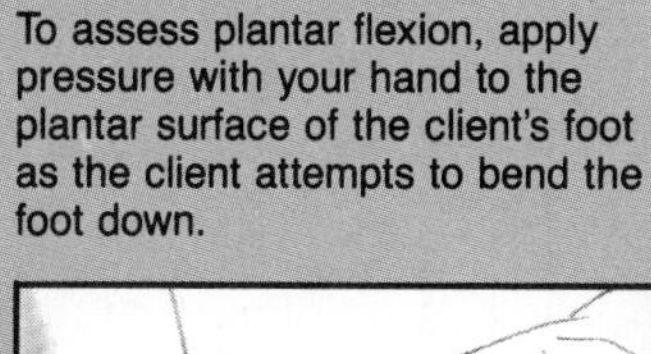

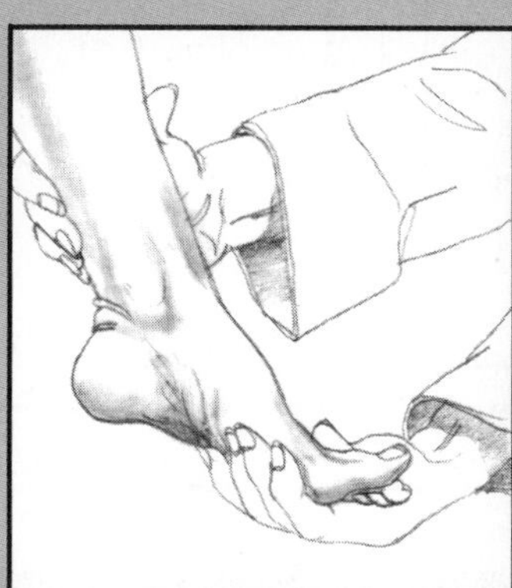

To assess inversion, apply pressure with your hand to the medial surface of the client's first metatarsal bone as the client attempts to move the toes inward. Assess eversion by placing your hand on the lateral surface of the fifth metatarsal bone and apply pressure as the client attempts to move the toes outward.

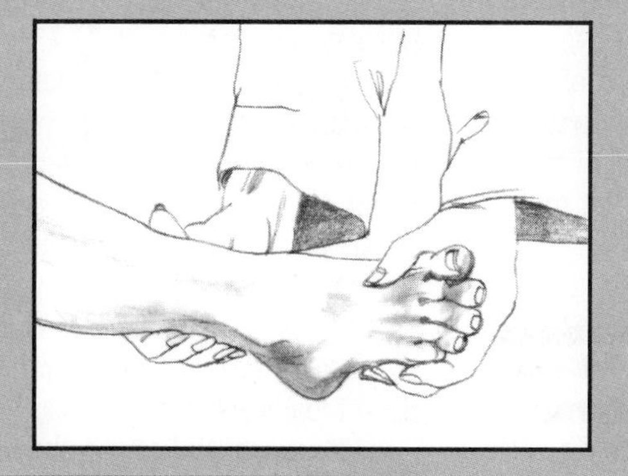

Range of motion

Ask the client who is sitting, lying, or standing to demonstrate plantar flexion by bending the foot downward and plantar dorsiflexion by bending the foot upward.

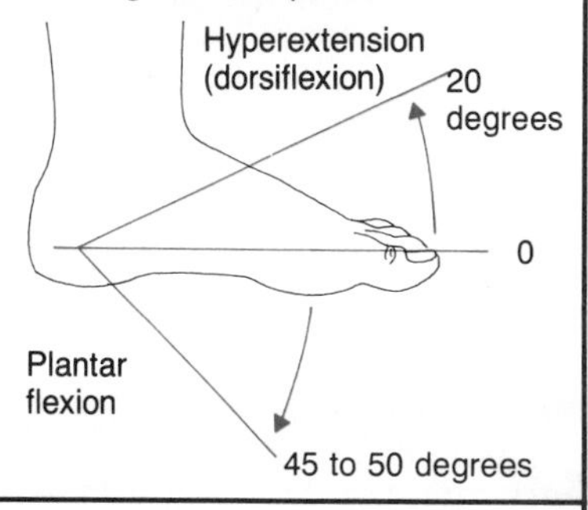

Then ask the client to invert the foot by pointing the toes and turning the foot inward and to evert the foot by pointing the toes and turning the foot outward.

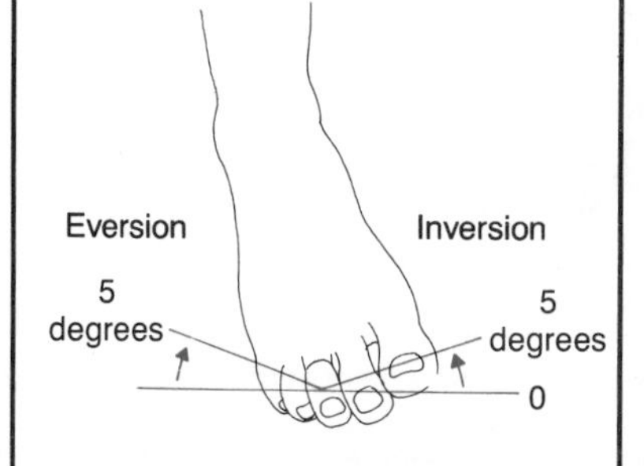

To assess forefoot adduction and abduction, stabilize the client's heel while the client turns the forefoot inward and outward, respectively.

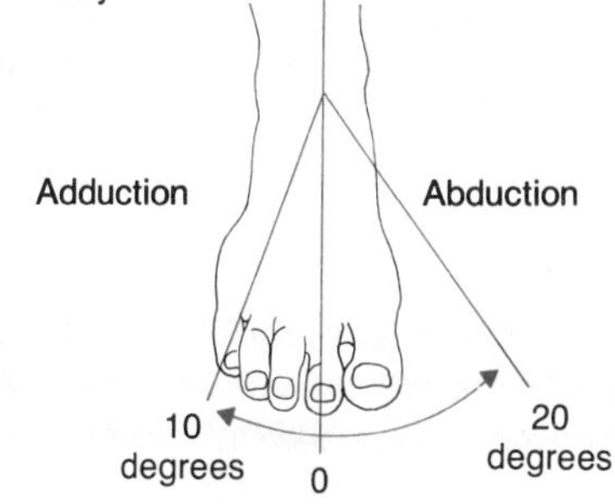

continued

Assessing muscle strength and joint range of motion continued

TOES

Anterior view of left foot

Lower extensor retinaculum

Extensor digitorum brevis

Range of motion

To assess the metatarsophalangeal joints, ask the client to extend (straighten) and flex (curl) the toes. Then, ask the client to hyperextend the toes by straightening and pointing them upward.

40 degrees
Hyperextension (dorsiflexion)
0
Flexion
40 degrees

Muscle strength

To assess flexion, apply pressure with your finger to the plantar surface of the client's toes as the client attempts to bend the toes downward.

To assess extension, apply pressure with your finger to the dorsal surface of the client's toes as the client attempts to point the toes upward.

Abnormal findings of the scapulae include asymmetrical placement, muscular development, or contour, as well as pain during palpation.

Scapular winging (an outward prominence of the scapulae) is an abnormality best seen with the client in an upright position with shoulders thrust back. Outward scapular displacement signifies dysfunction of the muscles and nerves serving this structure.

Ribs. After assessing the scapulae, inspect and palpate the anterior, posterior, and lateral surfaces of the ribs. Normal findings include firm, smooth, continuous bones.

Abnormal findings include pain or crepitus during palpation; noncontinuous, unstable ribs (a fracture, for example); abnormally prominent ribs (scoliosis secondary to vertebral rotation, for example); and masses.

Shoulders. Palpate the moving joints for crepitus. Inspect the skin overlying the shoulder joints for erythema, masses, or swelling.

Palpate the acromioclavicular joint and the area over the greater humeral tuberosity. Shoulder joint palpation begins with the client's arm at the side. Ask the client to move the arm across the chest (adduction). Then, place your thumb on the anterior portion of the client's shoulder joint and your fingers on the posterior portion of the joint. Ask the client to move the arm backward. Palpate the shoulder joint as the client's arm moves backward.

Next, stand behind the client. With your fingertips placed over the greater humeral tuberosity, instruct the client to rotate the shoulder internally by moving the arm behind the back. Besides palpating the bony structures of the shoulder joint, you can also palpate a portion of the musculotendonous rotator cuff in this way.

Abnormal findings include pain or crepitus from movement or palpation; less than normal range of motion; asymmetrical movements, sizes, or contours; swelling; nodularities; erythema; or increased temperature of skin overlying the joints.

If shoulder joint palpation produces client complaints of pain in the greater humeral tuberosity area, suspect that calcium deposits or trauma-related inflammation may be the cause. If the client has difficulty abducting the arm and, during palpation, complains of pain in the deltoid muscle or over the supraspinatus tendon insertion site, suspect a rotator-cuff tear.

Elbows. Inspect joint contour and the skin over each elbow. Palpate the joint at rest and during movement.

Abnormal findings are pain from movement or palpation, less than normal range of motion, erythema, nodules, swelling, or crepitus.

Wrists. Inspect the wrists for masses, erythema, skeletal deformities, and swelling. Palpate the wrist at rest and during movement by gently grasping it between your thumb and fingers.

Abnormal findings include pain from movement or palpation, less than normal range of motion, erythema, swelling, crepitus, nodules, and asymmetry of movement.

A positive Tinel's sign (tingling sensations in the thumb, index, and middle fingers), which is elicited by briskly tapping the client's wrist over the median nerve, may indicate carpal tunnel sydrome (painful disorder of the wrist and hand caused by compression of the median nerve between the carpal ligament and other structures within the carpal tunnel); similar tingling sensations in response to Phalen's test, in which the client holds the wrists in acute flexion for 60 seconds, also indicate this disorder. As the syndrome progresses, the thenar eminence (mound at the base of the thumb or the palm of the hand) atrophies.

Fingers and thumbs. On each hand, inspect the fingers and thumb for nodules, erythema, spacing, length, and skeletal deformities. Palpate fingers and thumb at rest and during movement for crepitus, heat (inflammation), and pain.

Abnormal findings include pain during movement or rest, decreased range of motion, asymmetry of movement, crepitus, swelling, erythema, nodules (for example, Heberden's nodes of osteoarthritis), and deformities (for example, webbing, extra digits, abnormal digital length or spacing, ulnar deviation of chronic rheumatoid arthritis, or contractures).

Thoracic and lumbar spine. Besides evaluating the curvatures of the thoracic and lumbar spine during the postural assessment, palpate the length of the spine for tenderness and vertebral alignment. To check for tenderness, percuss each spinous process (directly over the vertebral column) with the ulnar side of your fist.

Normal spinal assessment findings include the client's ability to perform movements with a full range of motion, while maintaining balance, smoothness, and coordination.

Abnormal findings include scoliosis, kyphosis, or lordosis (except in toddlers and some Blacks). With the client in the upright position, scoliosis appears as a lateral curvature of the spine; in the flexed position, as one shoulder more prominent than the other. Kyphosis is an exaggerated dorsal convexity of the spine. Other abnormal findings include shoulders and iliac crests misaligned horizontally; decreased range of motion; pain during movement, palpation, or percussion; fasciculations (localized, uncoordinated, uncontrollable, and visible twitching of a single muscle group innervated by a single motor nerve fiber); crepitus; and loss of balance during range-of-motion maneuvers.

Hips and pelvis. Inspect and palpate over the bony prominences: iliac crests, symphysis pubis, anterior spine, ischial tuberosities, and greater trochanters. Palpate the hip at rest and during movement.

Abnormal findings include decreased range of motion, pain or crepitus during movement (common in elderly people who have osteoarthritis of the hip), pain during palpation of bony prominences, and flexion of the opposite hip when flexion is tested.

Knees. Inspect the knees with the client seated. Palpate the knees at rest and during movement. Inspect and palpate the popliteal spaces (behind the knee joint). Knee movements should be smooth.

Abnormal findings include decreased range of motion, pain during palpation or movement, erythema, nodules, swelling, asymmetrical movement, and swellings, crepitus, or lumps in the popliteal space.

Ankles and feet. Inspect and palpate the ankles and feet at rest and during movement. Abnormal findings include decreased range of motion, pain, crepitus, swelling, nodules, erythema, ulcerations, calluses, asymmetrical movement, and deformities such as pes varus (inverted foot), pes valgus (everted foot), pes planus (flatfoot, with low, longitudinal arch), and pes cavus (exaggerated arch, or high instep).

(Text continues on page 541.)

ADVANCED ASSESSMENT SKILLS

Assessing musculoskeletal abnormalities

The nurse who suspects an abnormality of a client's spine, hip, or knee can perform special techniques to assess the injury or dysfunction further. Some guidelines follow.

Spine

1 The client who complains of low back pain or pain radiating down a leg, or both, may have a herniated lumbar disk. To assess, place the client in a supine position.

2 Raise the client's leg in a straightened position and dorsiflex the foot. Low back pain resulting from this maneuver and intensifying with dorsiflexion is a positive sign for a herniated disk.

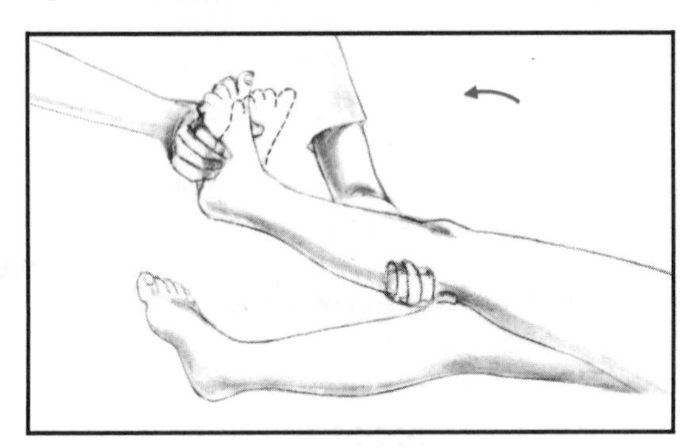

Hip

1 When assessing hip range of motion, perform the Thomas test, which can uncover flexion contractures of the hip that are hidden by excessive lumbar lordosis. Place the client in a supine position with both legs extended. Have the client flex one leg, bringing the knee to the chest. If the other extended leg lifts off the table, the client has a hip flexion contracture of the extended leg. Repeat with the opposite leg.

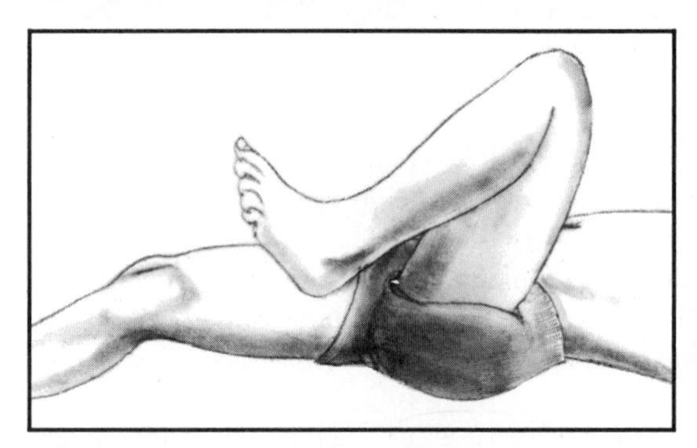

2 Use the Trendelenburg test to check for hip dislocation. While the client balances first on one foot and then on the other, assess the iliac crest levels. If the iliac crest on the side opposite of the weight-bearing leg stays at the same level or drops when the client's weight is shifted (as opposed to rising slightly), suspect a hip dislocation.

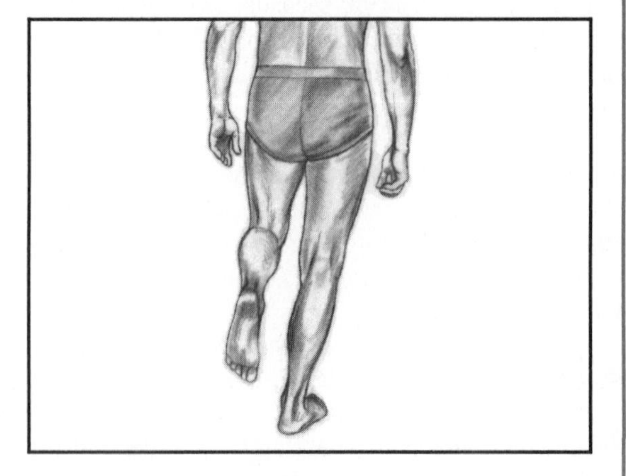

Knee

1 Assess for effusion (fluid collection) in the knee joint with the client seated on the examination table and the legs dangling over the edge. Using your hand, compress the area just above the client's patella. If an effusion exists, a bulge will appear to the sides or immediately below the patella, or in both places.

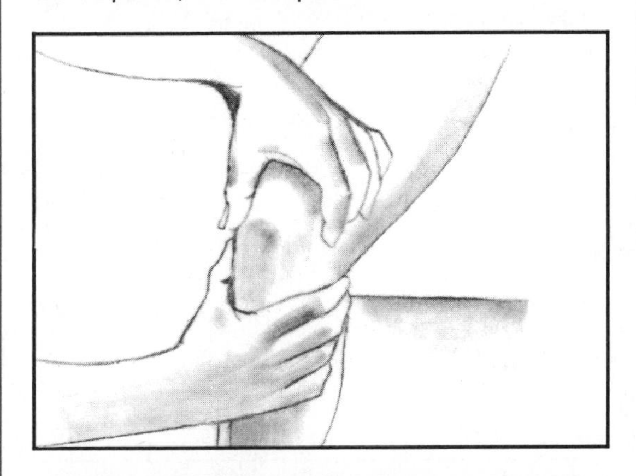

2 When the client complains that the knee "gives way" or "buckles," assess anterior, posterior, medial, and lateral knee stability with the drawer test. To test medial and lateral stability, have the client extend the knee and place your hands as shown. Attempt to abduct and adduct the knee; it normally shows no medial or lateral movement. To test stability in the anteroposterior plane, position the client supine with the involved knee in approximately 90-degree flexion. Stabilize the foot (an attendant can help). Then grasp the leg just below the knee and gently attempt to produce anterior and posterior movement; such movement is abnormal.

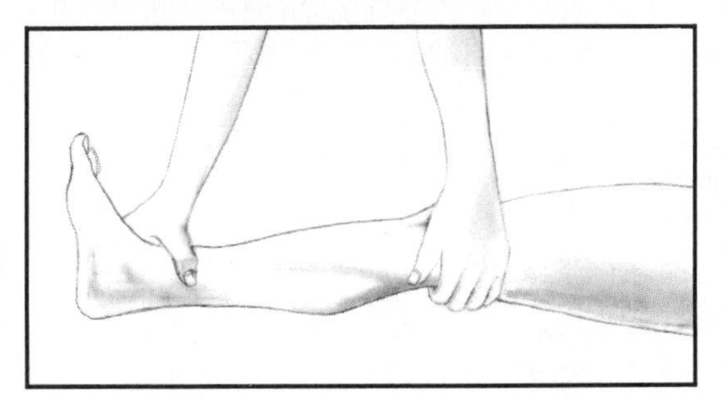

3 To test collateral ligament integrity, position the client supine and the knee in slight flexion. Place your hand on the client's lower leg. Place your other hand over the head of the fibula and apply pressure in a medial direction. Then, by reversing your hands, apply lateral pressure beside the medial condyle of the tibia. If impaired collateral ligaments are causing loss of stability, this motion will create a palpable medial or lateral gap in the joint.

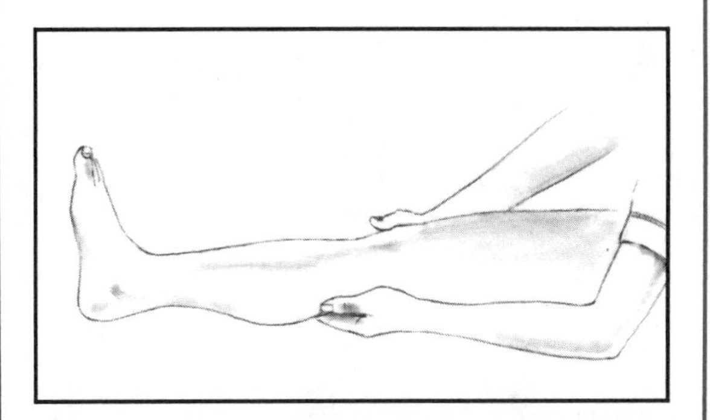

4 The client with a torn meniscus (curved fibrous cartilage in the knee) usually complains that the knee "locks." Use McMurray's test if you suspect this injury. Position the client supine with the knee maximally flexed so that the foot rests flat on the examination table near the buttocks. Hold the client's heel and stabilize the knee with your other hand. Internally rotate the tibia on the femur at this angle first, then move through 90 degrees and into full extension. Repeat the maneuver using external rotation. McMurray's test is positive if the knee responds with an audible or palpable click or if the client cannot extend the leg.

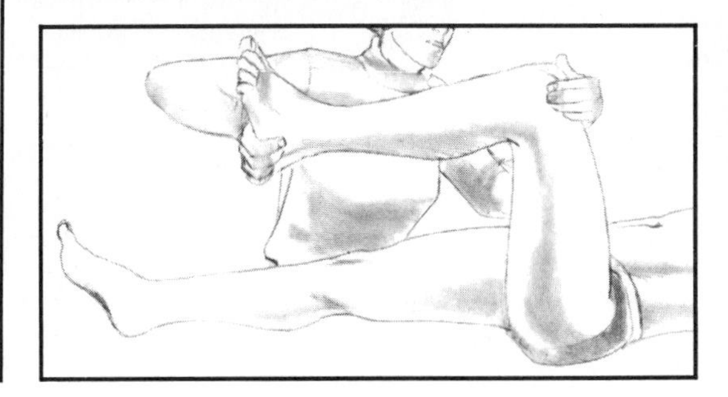

Integrating assessment findings

Sometimes, a cluster of assessment findings will strongly suggest a particular musculoskeletal disorder. In the chart below, column one shows groups of presenting signs and symptoms—the ones that make the client seek medical attention. Column two shows related assessment findings that the nurse may discover during the health history and physical assessment. The client may exhibit one or more of these findings. Column three shows the possible disorder indicated by a cluster of these findings.

PRESENTING SIGNS AND SYMPTOMS	RELATED ASSESSMENT FINDINGS	POSSIBLE DISORDER
Low back ache, decreased joint range of motion (ROM) and muscle stiffness, joint swelling, and redness	Deformity and immobility; progressively limited back movement and chest expansion; in severe cases, fusion of entire spine Male ages 10 to 30 Familial disorder; genetic predisposition Decreased spinal ROM; abnormal vertebral alignment; flattened lumbar curve; dorsal kyphosis Decreased chest expansion Cardiac conduction disturbances (with severe and long-standing disease) Atrophy of trunk muscles Fever Fatigue Weight loss	Ankylosing spondylitis (Marie-Strümpell disease)
Pain that worsens after manual activity (especially involving wrist rotation) or at night; radiates up the arm, may be intermittent or constant; numbness, burning, or tingling of the thumb, index, and middle fingers	History of predisposing factors such as wrist trauma or injury, rheumatoid arthritis, gout, myxedema, diabetes mellitus, leukemia, acromegaly, edema of the hand associated with pregnancy Atrophy of thenar eminences (mass of tissue on the lateral side of the palm) Positive Tinel's sign (tingling during wrist percussion) Muscle weakness Dry skin over thumb and first two fingers Inability to oppose thumb and little finger	Carpal tunnel syndrome
Pain with coughing, sneezing, straining, bending, or lifting; increases with sitting; accompanied by mild to severe low back, buttock, or leg pain; may be associated with spasms	Decreased sensation; paresthesias; absent or diminished deep-tendon reflexes of affected dermatomes Voiding (particularly urinary retention) or defecating difficulties History of predisposing factors such as recent spinal trauma; heavy or awkward lifting or occupational stress on back; lack of exercise; obesity; degenerative changes Decreased spinal ROM Unequal limb circumferences Abnormal posture, scoliosis Diminished deep-tendon reflexes of knee and ankle Positive straight-leg–raising test	Lumbosacral disk herniation
Pain aggravated with movement	Fractures of involved bones; collapse of vertebrae; increasing kyphosis History of predisposing factors such as endocrine disorders, inadequate dietary intake of calcium and vitamin D, malabsorption, inadequate exercise, prolonged immobility, decreased estrogen levels (in women), excessive smoking or alcohol and caffeine intake, family history of osteoporosis, small stature Postmenopausal woman Evidence of fracture: loss of height, wedging of dorsal vertebrae or anterior vertebrae, uneven shoulder and iliac crest levels, lateral curvature of spine with rotational deformity, thoracic and flank deformities (humps)	Osteoporosis

Toes. The client may be sitting or lying supine for toe assessment. Inspect all toe surfaces. Palpate toes at rest and during movement.

Abnormal findings include decreased range of motion, pain with movement or palpation, crepitus, erythema, swelling, calluses, and bunions (indicates chronic irritation or pressure).

Other abnormal findings include deformities such as claw toe (hyperextension of metatarsophalangeal joint with flexion of proximal and distal toe joints); hallux malleus, or hammer toe (hyperextension of metatarsophalangeal joint with flexion of proximal toe joint); and hallux valgus (lateral deviation of the great toe, possibly causing it to underlap the second toe). For a summary of the implications of some abnormal findings, see *Integrating assessment findings.*

Developmental considerations

To assess accurately the bones and joints of a pediatric or elderly client, the nurse must know the normal variations for these age groups.

Pediatric client. Expect to find these musculoskeletal variables in a pediatric client:

- A concave cervical spine does not develop until an infant gains head control (about age 3 or 4 months).
- A fractured clavicle is a relatively common birth and playground injury.
- Wrist palpation may be difficult because of soft tissue and uncalcified carpal bones.
- External hip rotation (160 to 175 degrees) is greater than in adults (normally about 45 degrees).
- Hip dislocation or subluxation in an infant causes uneven gluteal folds and external hip rotation of less than 160 degrees.
- In a child with rheumatic fever, the wrist is a common site for migratory arthritis, characterized by tenderness, pain, and inflammation.
- An infant will not develop a longitudinal arch of the foot until walking begins. A slight degree of forefoot adduction, related to in utero positioning, is common among neonates.
- A toddler will normally have lumbar lordosis when learning how to walk.

If a young child fails to use the arm and if assessment reveals forearm pronation (rotation of the forearm with the palm of the hand facing downward and backward), a partially flexed elbow, and an abnormal carrying angle (the normal angle is 5 degrees in children), suspect a subluxation (partial dislocation) of the radial head (nursemaid's elbow). A common injury of children under age 5, the dislocation occurs when a child is lifted or forcefully tugged by the hand.

Elderly client. In an elderly client, the head and neck may be thrust forward and the head tilted backward.

As the body ages, the normal convexity of the thoracic spine increases, thrusting the head and cervical spine (neck vertebrae) forward. The pronounced convex curvature may prevent an elderly client from looking upward because the back of the head cannot tilt beyond the thoracic vertebrae.

A partially adducted and flexed hip joint is often noted in an elderly client, as is reduced range of motion during rotation and hyperextension.

Arthritic changes of the knees and wrist, including crepitus, pain, stiffness, and joint enlargement, are common in an elderly client.

Advanced assessment skills

To quantify joint range of motion (for example, when assessing a client's progress after joint injury or surgery), use a goniometer. (For an explanation of how to use the goniometer, see Chapter 4, Physical Assessment Skills.)

As you gain expertise with basic musculoskeletal assessment skills, learn and use more specific tests. (For examples of these tests and the significance of findings, see *Advanced assessment skills: Assessing musculoskeletal abnormalities,* pages 538 and 539.)

Documentation

Because the musculoskeletal system assessment is so extensive, the nurse may have difficulty remembering all assessment findings until the assessment concludes. To cope with this problem, record your findings in a brief form as the assessment progresses. Then review information from the health history and physical assessment, and remember to examine the client's record for laboratory test results. (For more information on these tests and what abnormal results may indicate, see *Common laboratory studies,* page 544.)

Once you have reviewed the assessment data, formulate appropriate nursing diagnoses, which will help you plan, implement, and evaluate the client's nursing care. (For a case study that shows how to apply the nursing process to a client with a musculoskeletal disorder, see *Applying the nursing process,* pages 542 and 543.)

(Text continues on page 544.)

Applying the nursing process

Assessment findings form the basis of the nursing process. Using them, the nurse formulates nursing diagnoses and develops appropriate planning, implementation, and evaluation of the client's care.

The table below shows how the nurse can use musculoskeletal system assessment data in the nursing process for the client described in the case history (shown at right). In the first column, history and physical assessment data appear, followed by a paragraph of mental notes. These notes help the nurse make mental connections among assessment findings, aiding in development of the nursing diagnoses and planning.

The second column presents several appropriate nursing diagnoses; however, the information in the remaining columns is based on the *first* nursing diagnosis. Allthough it is not part of the nursing process, documentation appears in the last column because of its importance. Documentation consists of an initial note using all components of the SOAPIE format and a follow-up note using the appropriate SOAPIE components.

ASSESSMENT	NURSING DIAGNOSES	PLANNING	IMPLEMENTATION
Subjective (history) data • Client states, "My pain and stiffness are much worse in the morning." • Client complains that pain, stiffness, and loss of strength limit the use of her hands. • Client also reports "pain in both feet," which increases on weight bearing. • Client reports that arthritis, diagnosed at age 32, is becoming progressively more "crippling." For about 4 years, the achiness was controlled with aspirin. At age 36, she began to experience increased pain and stiffness. • Wrists, elbows, knees, and ankles stiff and sore in the morning. Client rates them a 2 on the 1-to-10 pain scale; hands and feet, 7 or 8. **Objective (physical) data** • Hands: hyperextension of distal phalanges, flexion of proximal phalanges, and ulnar deviation of fingers. Interphalangeal joints swollen, slightly red, and warm to the touch. Pain when joints are palpated or moved. Hand muscle atrophy apparent. Poor ability to grip examiner's hand; unable to form a tight fist (rating of 2 for strength). Markedly reduced range of motion (ROM): flexion of distal interphalangeal joints, 20 degrees; flexion of proximal interphalangeal joints, 40 degrees. Findings are symmetrical. • Toes: metatarsophalangeal joints edematous. Pain with joint movement. ROM markedly reduced bilaterally: flexion of first metatarsophalangeal joints, 10 degrees; flexion of distal interphalangeal joints, 20 degrees; flexion of proximal interphalangeal joints, 10 degrees; flexion of metatarsophalangeal joints, 5 degrees; hyperextension of metatarsophalangeal joints, 5 degrees. • X-rays show joint space narrowing and marked bilateral erosion of finger and toe articular joint cartilages. • White blood cell (WBC) count slightly elevated, 12,500/mm^3. • Erythrocyte sedimentation rate (ESR) elevated, 30 mm/hour. **Mental notes** *Client demonstrates significant strength and motion loss in hands and feet. She needs help modifying her environment; possibly suggest a home visit by an occupational therapist. Otherwise, pain management should be top priority. With pain controlled, the client's mobility and coping ability should improve.*	• Alteration in comfort: pain in hand and foot joints related to inflammatory changes. • Impaired physical mobility related to pain and decreased muscle strength. • Ineffective coping related to management of pain and musculoskeletal limitations. • Knowledge deficit related to lack of information about management and control of rheumatoid arthritis. • Disturbance in self-concept: body image, related to decreased function and deformities of hands.	**Goals** Within 2 weeks, the client will: • experience pain relief or control • verbalize symptom relief • demonstrate increased ROM.	• Assess such pain characteristics as severity and timing. • Develop an appropriate schedule for administering pain medication. • Provide the client with such medication information as action, dosage, whether to take with or without food, and possible adverse effects. • Describe use and benefits of heat and cold to affected joints. • Encourage the client to relieve symptoms with hot bath, shower, or soaks. • Suggest using pain relief interventions before exercising and at bedtime. • Encourage client to adopt such alternative pain management strategies as distraction. • Discuss importance of adequate hydration and nutrition to decrease inflammation and to prevent further muscle wasting. • Encourage regular exercise to maintain muscle integrity. • Promote regular attendance at prescribed physical and occupational therapy sessions.

CASE HISTORY

Mrs. Linda Jackson, age 40, was referred to the clinic for pain management related to moderately advanced rheumatoid arthritis. She recently resigned her job as a 3rd grade teacher when arthritis limited her ability to function. Her reason for coming to the clinic at this time is pain management.

EVALUATION		DOCUMENTATION BASED ON NURSING PROCESS DATA: Initial		Follow-up
At the next follow-up visit, the client: • reported minimal improvement in pain relief and in ROM of hand and foot joints.	**S**	Client states, "My pain and stiffness are much worse in the morning." Client also reports limited use of hands and "pain in both feet," which increases on weight bearing. Client reports that arthritis was diagnosed at age 32 and is progressively more "crippling."	**S**	Client reports only minimal pain relief. States, "I revised my schedule, substituting a warm shower in the morning for the soaks," and "The heating pad wasn't very effective, so I stopped using it."
	O	Distal phalangeal hyperextension, proximal phalangeal flexion, and ulnar deviation of fingers noted. Joints are swollen, slightly red, warm to the touch, and painful when palpated. Atrophy of hand muscles noted. Grip poor; client cannot form a tight fist. Muscle strength rating is 2. ROM markedly reduced: flexion of distal interphalangeal joints, 20 degrees; flexion of proximal interphalangeal joints, 40 degrees. Findings are symmetrical. Metatarsophalangeal joints are swollen and painful with joint movement. Marked reduction of ROM bilaterally: flexion of first metatarsophalangeal joints, 10 degrees; flexion of distal interphalangeal joints, 20 degrees; flexion of proximal interphalangeal joints, 10 degrees; flexion of metatarsophalangeal joints, 5 degrees; hyperextension of metatarsophalangeal joints, 5 degrees. X-rays show joint space narrowing and marked bilateral erosion of finger and toe articular joint cartilages. WBC count slightly elevated (12,500/mm³). ESR elevated (30 mm/hour).	**O**	Hand and foot joint ROM marginally improved (less than 10 degrees in any joint). Pain level has not decreased measurably.
	A	Alteration in comfort: pain in hand and foot joints related to inflammatory changes.	**A**	Pain level and joint ROM have not changed measurably in 2 weeks.
	P	Help client control and relieve pain. Assess pain. Develop an appropriate pain medication schedule. Teach client to apply heat and cold to joints. Encourage regular ROM exercise.	**P**	Schedule ibuprofen every 4 hours for the next week. Change meal and exercise times accordingly. Have occupational or physical therapist fit client for resting hand splints.
	I	Emphasize importance of medication and exercise schedule.	**I**	A new schedule was arranged for activities and medication. An appointment with the therapist was made for hand splint fitting.
			E	Initial interventions to decrease pain and increase joint ROM were ineffective. Will evaluate success of new plan in 1 week.

After completing the assessment, document all normal and abnormal findings. The following example shows how to document some normal physical assessment findings:

Weight: 185 lb
Height: 5′10″.
Posture erect, gait with normal stance and swing phases.
Left triceps, biceps, and deltoid: normal contour, tone, and strength; no pain or fasciculations.
Left elbow range of motion (ROM): extension, 0 degrees; flexion, 150 degrees; pronation, 90 degrees; supination, 90 degrees. Client reports no pain with movement.
Right triceps, biceps, and deltoid: normal contour, tone, and strength; no pain or fasciculations.
Right elbow ROM: extension, 0 degrees; flexion, 150 degrees; pronation, 90 degrees; supination, 90 degrees. Client reports no pain with movement.
No evidence of erythema of overlying skin and no swelling, nodules, or masses of joints or muscles in either arm.

The following example shows how to document some abnormal physical assessment findings:

Weight: 134 lb
Height: 6′3″.
Posture slumped, gait rolling with toes striking floor before heel in swing phase.
Left triceps, biceps, and deltoid: normal contour, tone, and strength; no pain or fasciculations.
Left elbow ROM: extension, 0 degrees; flexion, 150 degrees; pronation, 90 degrees; supination, 90 degrees. Client reports no pain with movement.
Right biceps: normal contour, tone, and strength; no pain or fasciculations. Right triceps: normal contour and tone, slight weakness (4 rating; scale 1 to 10), no pain or fasciculations.
Right deltoid: flattened contour, reduced strength (3 rating), hypotonicity. Client complains of pain during movement, although not during palpation.
Right elbow ROM: extension, 10 degrees; flexion, 120 degrees; pronation, 90 degrees; supination, 45 degrees. Client complains of discomfort in right elbow during all ROM movements (pain rating, 4). Crepitus felt with extension and flexion but not with pronation or supination.

Besides recording assessment findings, remember to document the other nursing process steps—nursing diagnosis, planning, implementation, and evaluation—as they apply to the client with a musculoskeletal disorder.

Chapter summary

To assess a client's musculoskeletal system effectively, the nurse relies on health history data, physical assessment findings, and laboratory test results. Chapter 18 describes how to gather and integrate this information. Chapter highlights follow:

- The musculoskeletal system consists of skeletal muscles, ligaments, tendons, bones, cartilage, joints, and bursae.
- Because the client's health history is a crucial data base component for formulating a care plan, the collected information must be inclusive. To promote client cooperation, the nurse first focuses on the chief complaint.
- As the assessment progresses, the nurse remains alert for findings not initially identified during history taking and asks additional questions as necessary.
- The musculoskeletal system physical assessment should be conducted in a way that conserves client strength and ensures client comfort.
- Physical assessment begins with general observations regarding symmetry of shape, size, position, and movement of body parts. Finer evaluations of posture, gait, and coordination follow.
- Physical assessment continues with testing and evaluation of muscle strength, mass, and tone.
- The nurse also assesses joint and bone characteristics, then tests and evaluates joint range of motion.
- Specific musculoskeletal problems, such as scapular winging or meniscal tears in the knee, require advanced assessment skills.
- To complete the musculoskeletal system assessment, the nurse evaluates any laboratory test results.
- The nurse documents all assessment findings, using them in the nursing process to plan, implement, and evaluate the client's care.

Study questions

1. After you have assessed 82-year-old Joseph Dolan, a Black retired accountant, your documented findings include:
- dorsal kyphosis of the thoracic spine
- short, shuffling walk

(Questions continue on page 546.)

Common laboratory studies

For a client with musculoskeletal signs and symptoms, various laboratory studies can provide valuable clues to the possible cause, as shown in the chart below. (*Note:* Keep in mind that abnormal findings may stem from a problem unrelated to the musculoskeletal system.) Remember that values differ among laboratories, and check the normal value range for the specific laboratory.

TEST AND SIGNIFICANCE	NORMAL VALUES OR FINDINGS	ABNORMAL FINDINGS	POSSIBLE MUSCULOSKELETAL OR RELATED CAUSES OF ABNORMAL FINDINGS
Blood tests			
Serum glutamic-pyruvic transaminase (SGPT) Also called alanine aminotransferase, this test reflects muscle tissue damage when the enzyme, found in skeletal muscle, exceeds normal levels.	*Males:* 10 to 32 units/liter *Females:* 9 to 24 units/liter *Infants:* twice the adult values	Above-normal level	Skeletal muscle damage
Serum glutamic oxaloacetic transaminase (SGOT) Also called aspartate aminotransferase (AST), this test reflects muscle damage when the enzyme, found in skeletal muscle, exceeds normal levels.	*Adults:* 8 to 20 units/liter *Infants:* four times adult values	Above-normal level	Primary muscle disease, such as muscular dystrophy or muscle trauma
Creatine phosphokinase (CPK) enzyme with isoenzyme (CPK-MM) This test indicates skeletal muscle damage.	*CPK males:* 23 to 99 units/liter *CPK females:* 15 to 57 units/liter *CPK-MM:* 5 to 70 IU/liter	Above-normal level	Muscle trauma from injury or intramuscular injections, dermatomyositis, muscular dystrophy
Rheumatoid factor (RF) This test is an immunologic study specific for rheumatoid arthritis.	Nonreactive test with titer value less than 1:20	Above-normal level	Positive titer values above 1:80 are diagnostic for rheumatoid arthritis
Alkaline phosphatase This test reflects the enzyme that influences bone calcification.	*Males:* 90 to 239 units/liter *Females under age 45:* 76 to 196 units/liter *Females over age 45:* 87 to 250 units/liter	Above-normal level	Osteomalacia, metastatic bone tumors, Paget's disease, bone fracture healing
Calcium This test reflects the electrolyte that promotes and regulates bone growth.	4.5 to 5.5 mEq/liter	Above-normal level	Paget's disease, multiple myeloma, multiple fractures, metastatic carcinoma with bony involvement
		Below-normal level	Rickets
Urine tests			
Uric acid This test reflects excretion of uric acid.	250 to 750 mg/24 hours	Above-normal level	Multiple myeloma
		Below-normal level	Gout
Bence Jones protein This test reflects glomerular filtration of this low-weight protein.	Absence of Bence Jones protein in urine	Presence of Bence Jones protein	Multiple myeloma

• right shoulder crepitus and pain with movement
• a weak (rating 3) effort resisting nurse's effort to push down on arms abducted to 90 degrees
• a hard, bony ridge on the left clavicle, 2″ (5 cm) lateral to the sternoclavicular joint.

For each physical finding, state whether the deviation from normal is related to developmental, sexual, or racial factors.

What are the anatomic and physiologic bases for each finding?

2. Jenny Nice, a 16-year-old Caucasian high school student, has an appointment at the outpatient clinic. Her reason for the visit is left arm pain.

List 10 questions you should ask Jenny to obtain a thorough history. How would you word these questions so that Jenny can understand them?

3. Michael Birdsong, a 35-year-old Native American psychiatrist, has just had a long leg cast removed after 4 months. The cast was applied after torn right knee ligaments were repaired. His stated concerns are: "I can't bend my knee as far as I used to, and I can't straighten it completely. My leg is stiff, sore, and weak. It feels like it won't support my weight." You need to obtain a baseline assessment before Dr. Birdsong begins physical therapy.

How would you document the following information related to your nursing assessment of Dr. Birdsong?
• history (subjective) assessment data
• physical (objective) assessment data
• assessment techniques and equipment
• two appropriate nursing diagnoses
• documentation of your findings.

4. You have three clients who are to have selected body areas and characteristics assessed. The clients are Sandy Jones, age 2; George Hurd, age 30; and Agnes Friend, age 92. What findings would you expect for each in gait, posture, and arm and hand strength?

5. For these clients, what differences would you plan in your overall examination and assessment techniques?

Selected references

Carroll-Johnson, R. (Ed.). (1991). *Classification of nursing diagnoses: Proceedings of the ninth NANDA conference.* Philadelphia: Lippincott.

Doenges, M., Jeffries, M., and Moorhouse, M. (1989). *Nursing care plans: Guidelines in planning patient care* (2nd ed.). Philadelphia: Davis.

Henry, J. (1991). *Clinical diagnosis and management by laboratory methods* (18th ed.). Philadelphia: Saunders.

Jones-Walton, P. (1990). Orthopaedic nursing assessment. *Advancing Clinical Care,* 5(3), 22.

Kee, J. (1991). *Laboratory and diagnostic tests with nursing interventions.* East Norwalk, CT: Appleton & Lange.

Killam, P. (1989). Orthopedic assessment of young children: Developmental variations. *Nurse Practitioner,* 14(7), 27-28, 30, 32+.

Mason, K. (1989). Pediatric orthopaedics: Developmental norms. *Orthopedic Nursing,* 8(4), 45-50.

McEvoy, G. (Ed.). (1992). *American Hospital Formulary Service drug information.* Bethesda, MD: American Society of Hospital Pharmacists.

Olson, E., Johnson, B., and Thompson, L. (1990). The hazards of immobility. *AJN,* 90(3), 43-44, 46-48.

Pagana, K., and Pagana, T. (1990). *Diagnostic testing and nursing implications* (3rd ed.). St. Louis: Mosby.

Phipps, W., Long, B., and Woods, N. (1991). *Medical-surgical nursing: Concepts and clinical practice* (4th ed.). St. Louis: Mosby.

Schoen, D. (1986). *The nursing process in orthopedics.* East Norwalk, CT: Appleton & Lange.

Spence, A., and Mason, E. (1987). *Human anatomy and physiology* (3rd ed.). Menlo Park, CA: Benjamin-Cummings.

Thompson, J., McFarland, G., Hirsch, J., Tucker, S., and Bowers, A. (1989). *Clinical nursing* (2nd ed.). St. Louis: Mosby.

Nursing research

Estok, P., and Rudy, E. (1987). Marathon running: Comparison of physical and psychosocial risks for men and women. *Research in Nursing and Health,* 10(2), 79-85.

Stewart, N. (1986). Perceptual and behavioural effects of immobility and social isolation in hospitalized orthopedic patients. *Nursing Papers,* 18(3), 59-74.

Strickler, T., Malone, T., and Garrett, W. (1990). The effects of passive warming on muscle injury. *American Journal of Sports Medicine,* 18(2), 141-145.

19

Immune System and Blood

Objectives

After reading and studying this chapter, you should be able to:

1. Identify the elements that constitute blood and describe their functions.
2. Name the immune system structures and describe their functions.
3. Explain the body's general defense system.
4. Describe the specific defenses of the immune system.
5. Write interview questions that elicit information about the client's immune system and blood.
6. Perform a physical assessment of the lymph nodes and spleen.
7. Differentiate between normal and abnormal assessment findings of the immune system and blood.
8. Describe representative laboratory studies used to assess the immune system and blood.
9. Identify representative adverse reactions to drugs that might affect the immune system or blood.
10. Using the nursing process, document assessment findings for the immune system and blood.

Introduction

This chapter reviews the structures and functions of the immune system and blood, describing the cellular components and explaining their interrelated development and actions. The main purpose of the immune system is to defend the body from assault by microorganisms. Blood, the body's major transportation fluid, performs a vital function by maintaining homeostasis (natural, physiologic equilibrium of the body's internal environment). Through its lymphatic channels, the immune system also performs a transport function.

Unlike other body systems, the immune system and blood are not composed of simple organ groups. The immune system consists of billions of circulating cells and specialized structures, such as lymph nodes, that are located thoughout the body. The blood includes fluid (plasma) and formed elements (blood cells and platelets) that circulate throughout the body. The spleen assists the blood and immune system by serving as a reservoir for blood and producing blood cells. The spleen also aids in defense against microorganisms. Because of their diffuse nature, the immune system and the blood can affect, and be affected by, every other body system; for this reason, assessing the immune system and blood is complex. Sometimes, immune or blood disorders produce characteristic signs or symptoms, such as the butterfly rash of systemic lupus erythematosus (SLE). Usually, though, they cause vague symptoms, such as fatigue or dyspnea (shortness of breath), that initially seem related to other body systems.

The nurse should consider assessing the immune system and blood whenever a client reports symptoms such as frequent or recurring infections, slow wound healing, or blood clotting problems.

Chapter 19 explains how to gather pertinent health history data and conduct a physical assessment of the immune system and blood. It describes normal and abnormal physical findings and explains relevant laboratory studies.

Glossary

Agglutination: aggregation or clumping of insoluble particles as a result of their interaction with specific antibodies called agglutins.

Agranulocyte: a nongranular leukocyte having a nucleus without lobes. Agranulocytes include monocytes and lymphocytes.

Anemia: abnormal decrease in red blood cells (RBCs) per cubic millimeter (mm^3) of blood, hemoglobin quantity, or volume of packed RBCs per deciliter of blood. Anemia occurs when balance between blood loss (through bleeding or RBC destruction) and blood production is disrupted.

Antibody: immunoglobulin synthesized by lymphoid tissue in response to an invasive antigen. An antibody can bind with a specific antigen.

Antigen: any substance capable of eliciting an immune response; a foreign substance that stimulates the body to secrete specific antibodies or to proliferate activated T cells specific to the introduced antigen.

Autoimmunity: abnormal response of the body to its own tissue, possibly from an inability to differentiate resident self antigens from foreign antigens.

Basophil: least common granulocyte, having cytoplasmic granules containing serotonin and histamine and irregularly shaped, two-lobed, segmented nucleus.

B cell or **B lymphocyte:** white blood cell (WBC), originating in the bone marrow, that produces antibodies; responsible for humoral immunity.

Cell-mediated immunity or **cellular immunity:** acquired specific immunity in which T cells play a major role, responding to infections caused by certain bacteria, fungi, and viruses; possibly, cancer; hypersensitivity reactions; certain autoimmune diseases and allograft rejection; and allergens.

Chemotaxis: process by which leukocytes are directed toward an attractor (chemotactant).

Diapedesis: process by which blood cells migrate from the intravascular compartment to tissue sites.

Differentiation: process that allows blood cells to acquire different characteristics from the original cell; progressive diversification.

Ecchymosis: flat, purple-blue, hemorrhagic bruise on the skin or mucous membranes caused by blood escaping into tissue from a blood vessel.

Eosinophil: granulocyte with two lobes that responds phagocytically to allergens and parasites.

Erythrocyte or **red blood cell:** rounded, biconcave disk-shaped nonnuclear cell that contains hemoglobin and transports oxygen and carbon dioxide throughout the body.

Granulocyte: WBC characterized by prominent cytoplasmic granules and a single multilobed nucleus. According to the staining characteristics of their specific granules, granulocytes are known individually as neutrophils, eosinophils, or basophils, collectively as polymorphonuclear leukocytes.

Hematocrit (HCT): concentration of RBCs in total blood volume, expressed as a percentage.

Hematopoiesis: formation and development of blood cells from precursors.

Hemoglobin (Hb): oxygen-carrying RBC pigment; formed by the developing erythrocyte in bone marrow. A conjugated protein carrying four heme groups and globin, hemoglobin can carry and release oxygen. It is expressed as grams of hemoglobin per deciliter of blood.

Hemostasis: process that terminates bleeding by a complex mechanism including vasoconstriction and coagulation.

Humoral immunity: acquired specific immunity in which B cells and immunoglobulins play a major role, responding to antigens such as bacteria and foreign tissue.

Hypersensitivity: exaggerated response of the body to a foreign substance.

Immunity: ability to resist or overcome disease-carrying microorganisms or the toxic effects of other antigens.

Immunodeficient disease: disorder reflecting impairment of one or more immunity mechanisms.

Immunoglobulin: antibody, one of a class of proteins that interacts specifically with antigens, usually at the cell surface.

Immunoproliferative disease: disorder characterized by abnormal proliferation of cells that normally provide immunity, such as leukocytes and lymphocytes.

Immunosuppression: induced suppression of the immune response by such agents as radiation or drugs.

Leukocyte or **white blood cell:** cell that constitutes an important part of the body's defense and immune system. Leukocytes may be subdivided into two groups, granulocytes and agranulocytes, or into five cell types: neutrophils, eosinophils, basophils, monocytes, and lymphocytes.

Lymphadenopathy: lymph node condition characterized by hypertrophy or proliferation of lymphoid tissue.

Lymphocyte: mononuclear leukocyte produced chiefly by lymphoid tissue. The smallest of the WBCs, lymphocytes give rise to T cells and B cells, which are instrumental in cell-mediated and humoral immunity, respectively.

Lymphokines: mediator substances released by sensitized T cells (T lymphocytes) on contact with antigens. Lymphokines play a role in macrophage activation, lymphocyte transformation, and cell-mediated immunity.

Macrophage: large, mononuclear, highly phagocytic WBC that stimulates antibody production. Found in blood vessel walls (adventitious cells) and in loose connective tissue (histiocytes, phagocytic reticular

Glossary continued

cells), macrophages derive from monocytes and form part of the reticuloendothelial system.

Megakaryocyte: large, multilobed bone marrow cell that releases thrombocytes (platelets).

Monocyte: mononuclear phagocytic leukocyte, the largest of the WBCs. When monocytes enter peripheral tissues, they swell and transform into fixed populations of cells called tissue macrophages.

Multipotential stem cell: bone marrow cell that gives rise to five distinct cell types, each committed to develop and function differently.

Neutrophil: granulocyte with single, multilobed nucleus. Neutrophils account for 50% to 70% of circulating WBCs and migrate to infection sites by diapedesis. They are phagocytic.

Opsonization: process of preparing alien bacteria and other microorganisms and cells for phagocytosis by coating (marking) them with an antibody (opsonin) that attracts phagocytes.

Petechia: tiny, flat, round, red or purple spot on skin caused by minute submucosal or intradermal hemorrhage.

Phagocytosis: process by which a cell engulfs and destroys foreign material; involves recognizing the material as foreign, engulfing it, and digesting it.

Polycythemia: abnormal increase of RBCs in the blood.

Primary immune response: response (usually undramatic) after first exposure to an antigen.

Purpura: any of several hemorrhagic states characterized by purplish or brownish red patches on skin caused by blood escaping into tissues, skin, or mucous membranes. Small purpurae are petechiae; large purpurae are ecchymoses.

Reticulocyte: immature RBC characterized by a meshlike network. Released into circulation by the bone marrow, reticulocytes mature into RBCs in about 1 day. The reticulocyte release rate about equals the rate of RBC removal by the spleen, so the reticulocyte count reflects the blood cell activity rate in the bone marrow.

Secondary immune response: response to second or subsequent exposure to an antigen; qualitatively and quantitatively different from the primary immune response.

T cell or **T lymphocyte:** thymic lymphocyte responsible for cell-mediated immunity.

Thrombocyte or **platelet:** disk-shaped blood cell essential for coagulation. Formed in a megakaryocyte, thrombocytes are released in clumps into the blood, where they contribute to hemostasis.

Anatomy and physiology review

The body's immune system consists of specialized cells—lymphocytes and macrophages—and structures, including lymph nodes, spleen, thymus, bone marrow, tonsils, adenoids, and appendix. The blood includes plasma and numerous kinds of blood cells. Although they are distinct entities, the immune system and blood are closely related. For example, their cells share a common origin in the bone marrow; and the immune system uses the bloodstream to transport its components.

Origin

The cells of the immune system and blood develop from multipotential stem cells formed in the bone marrow by a process called hematopoiesis. (For a diagram of this process, see *Hematopoiesis: Development of blood and immune cells,* pages 550 and 551.)

In the embryo, multipotential stem cells develop in the yolk sac, liver, spleen, lymph nodes, and bone marrow. In the neonate, all bone marrow has hematopoietic potential, but hematopoiesis occurs only in a few bone marrow sites. In the adult, hematopoiesis can occur only in the marrow of particular bones—for example, in the flat bones of the cranium, vertebral column, pelvis, ribs, and sternum, and the proximal ends of some long bones, such as the femur.

Differentiation of the precursor cells occurs almost exclusively in the bone marrow. Under normal conditions, cells are not released into circulation until they are nearly or completely mature. However, bone marrow activity varies among individuals.

Immune system

Immunity is the body's capacity to resist invading organisms and toxins and thereby prevent tissue and organ damage. The body accomplishes this through the immune system, a complex network of specialized cells and organs. (For more information, see *Organs of the immune system,* pages 552 and 553.) Designed to recognize, respond to, and eliminate such foreign substances (anti-

(Text continues on page 553.)

Hematopoiesis: Development of blood and immune cells

Hematopoiesis produces all of the body's blood cells, including those for immunologic defense. The process occurs in the bone marrow, where multipotential stem cells give rise to five distinct cell types known as unipotential stem cells. Each unipotential cell can differentiate (diversify) into one of the following: an erythrocyte, a granulocyte (neutrophil, eosinophil, or basophil), an agranulocyte (lymphocyte or monocyte), or a thrombocyte, as shown in the chart below.

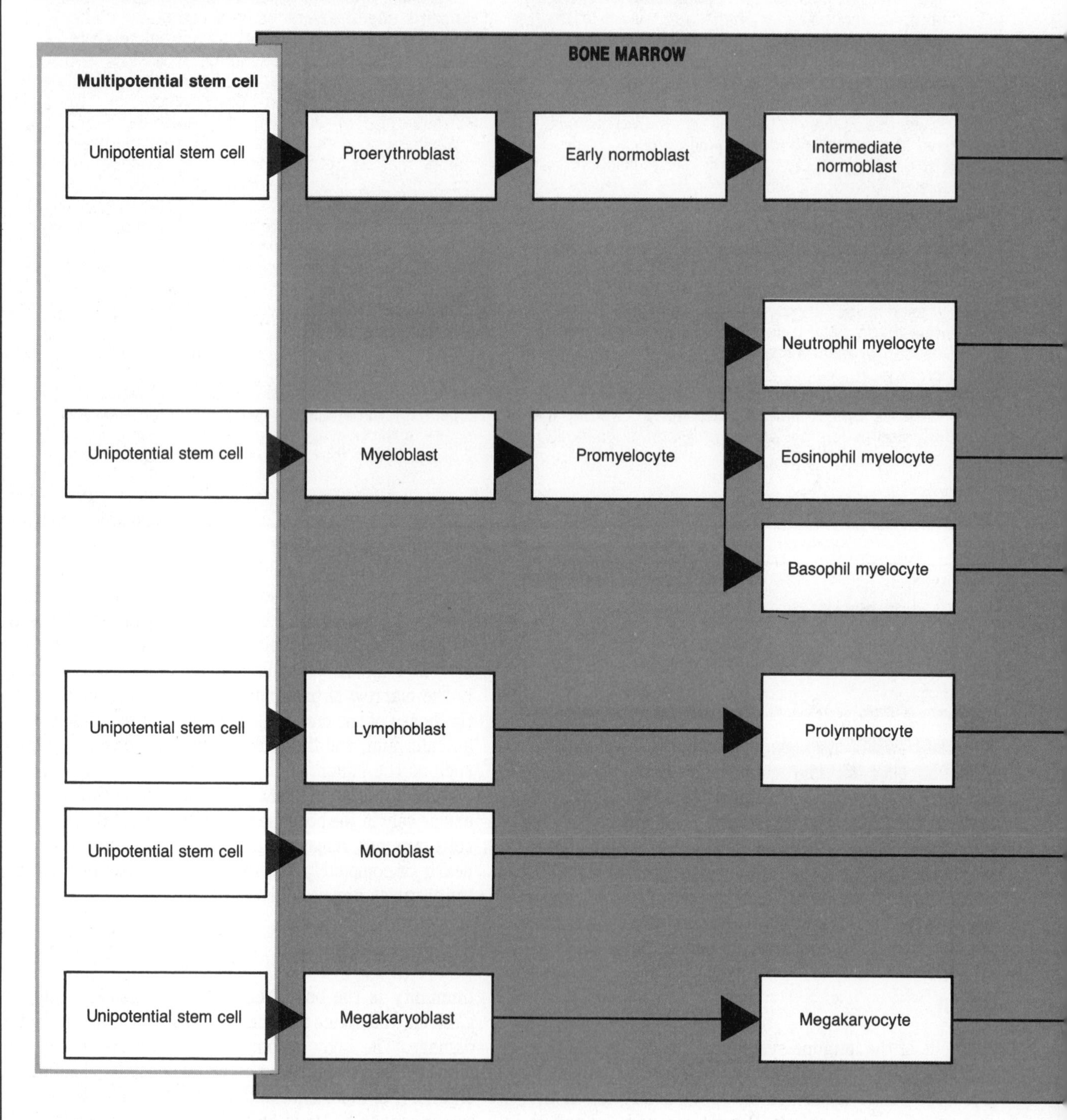

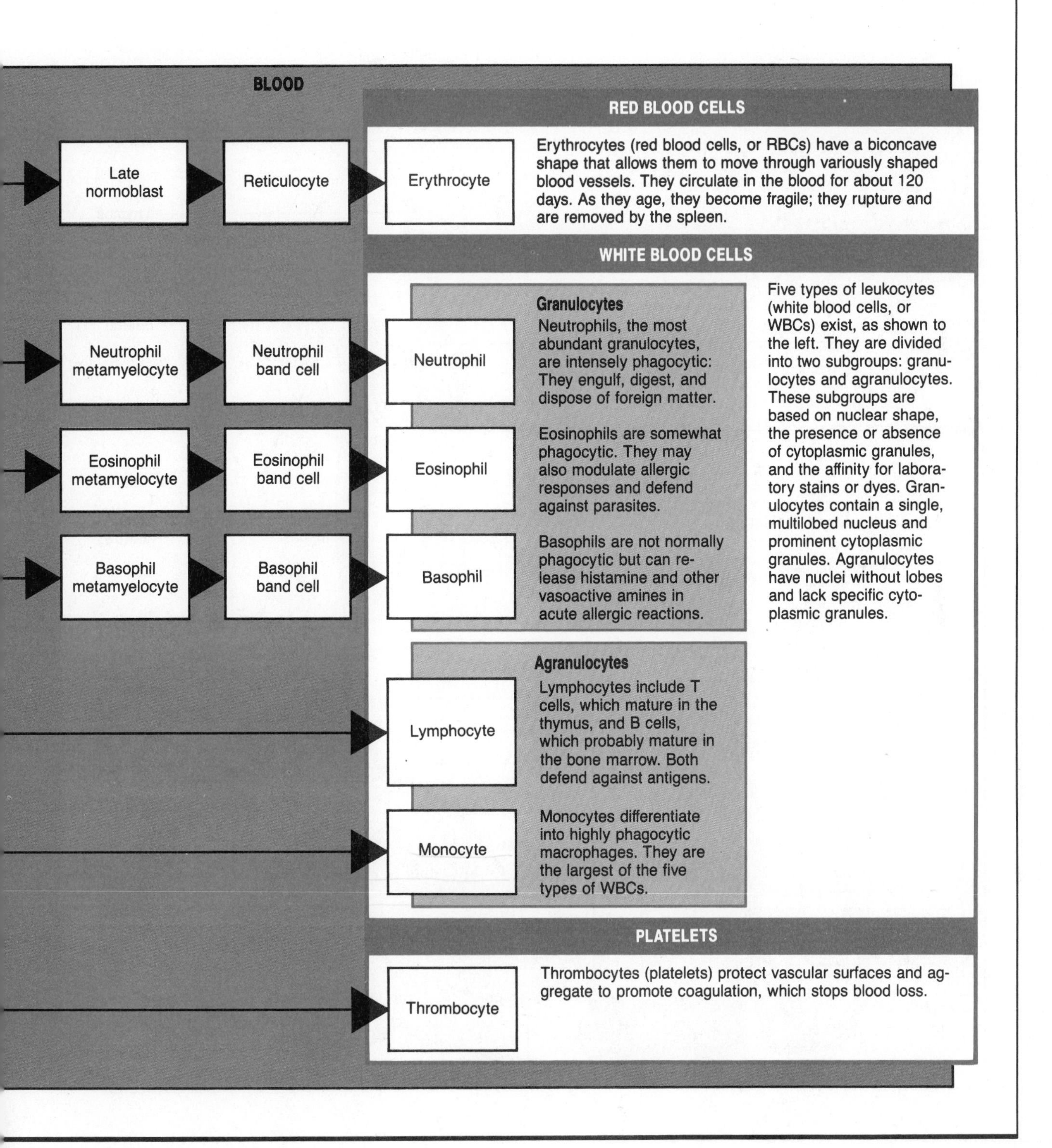
BLOOD
RED BLOOD CELLS
Late normoblast
Reticulocyte
Erythrocyte
Erythrocytes (red blood cells, or RBCs) have a biconcave shape that allows them to move through variously shaped blood vessels. They circulate in the blood for about 120 days. As they age, they become fragile; they rupture and are removed by the spleen.
WHITE BLOOD CELLS
Neutrophil metamyelocyte
Neutrophil band cell
Neutrophil
Eosinophil metamyelocyte
Eosinophil band cell
Eosinophil
Basophil metamyelocyte
Basophil band cell
Basophil
Granulocytes
Neutrophils, the most abundant granulocytes, are intensely phagocytic: They engulf, digest, and dispose of foreign matter.
Eosinophils are somewhat phagocytic. They may also modulate allergic responses and defend against parasites.
Basophils are not normally phagocytic but can release histamine and other vasoactive amines in acute allergic reactions.
Five types of leukocytes (white blood cells, or WBCs) exist, as shown to the left. They are divided into two subgroups: granulocytes and agranulocytes. These subgroups are based on nuclear shape, the presence or absence of cytoplasmic granules, and the affinity for laboratory stains or dyes. Granulocytes contain a single, multilobed nucleus and prominent cytoplasmic granules. Agranulocytes have nuclei without lobes and lack specific cytoplasmic granules.
Lymphocyte
Monocyte
Agranulocytes
Lymphocytes include T cells, which mature in the thymus, and B cells, which probably mature in the bone marrow. Both defend against antigens.
Monocytes differentiate into highly phagocytic macrophages. They are the largest of the five types of WBCs.
PLATELETS
Thrombocyte
Thrombocytes (platelets) protect vascular surfaces and aggregate to promote coagulation, which stops blood loss.

Organs of the immune system

The immune system includes organs and tissues in which lymphocytes predominate, as well as cells that circulate in peripheral blood. Central lymphoid organs include the bone marrow and thymus. Peripheral lymphoid organs include the lymph nodes and vessels, spleen, tonsils, adenoids, appendix, and intestinal lymphoid tissue (Peyer's patches).

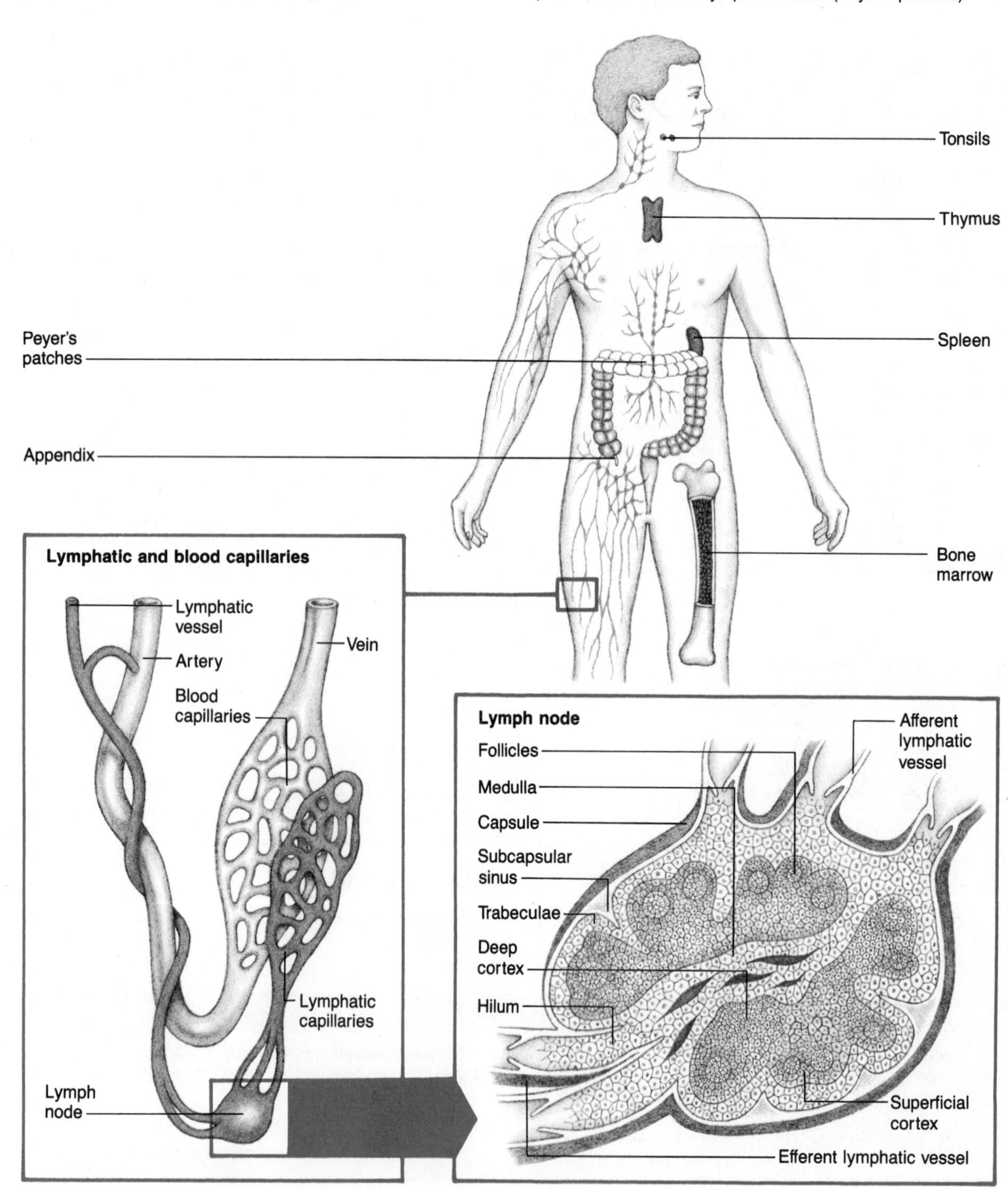

The bone marrow and thymus play a role in developing the primary cells of the immune system: B cells and T cells. Both cell types probably originate in the bone marrow. B cells may also mature and differentiate from multipotential stem cells in the bone marrow. T cells mature and differentiate in the thymus, a bilobular endocrine gland located in the upper mediastinum. B and T cells are distributed throughout the tissue of the peripheral lymphoid organs, especially the lymph nodes and spleen.

Lymph nodes

Most abundant in the head, neck, axillae, abdomen, pelvis, and groin, lymph nodes are small, oval-shaped structures located along a network of lymph channels. They help remove and destroy antigens circulating in the blood and lymph.

Each lymph node is surrounded by a fibrous capsule that extends bands of connective tissue (trabeculae) into the node, dividing it into three compartments: superficial cortex, deep cortex, and medulla.

The superficial cortex of the node contains follicles made up predominantly of B cells. During an immune response, the follicles enlarge and develop a germinal area with large proliferating cells. The deep cortex consists mostly of T cells as do the interfollicular areas. The medulla contains numerous plasma cells that actively secrete immunoglobulins during an immune response.

Afferent lymphatic vessels carry lymph into the subcapsular sinus of the node. From here, it flows through cortical sinuses and smaller radial medullary sinuses. Phagocytic cells in the deep cortex and medullary sinuses attack the antigen. The antigen may also be trapped in the follicles of the superficial cortex.

Cleansed lymph leaves the node through efferent lymphatic vessels at the hilum. These vessels drain into specific lymph node chains, which, in turn, drain into large lymph vessels known as trunks that empty into the subclavian vein of the vascular system. In most parts of the body, lymphatic vessels and lymphatic capillaries assist veins and blood capillaries to function by draining many body tissues and increasing the return of blood to the heart.

Lymph usually travels through more than one lymph node since numerous nodes line the lymphatic channels that drain a particular region. For example, axillary nodes filter drainage from the arms; femoral nodes (located in the inguinal region) filter drainage from the legs. This arrangement prevents organisms that enter peripheral body areas from migrating unchallenged to central areas. Lymph nodes are also a principal source of circulating lymphocytes that provide specific immune responses.

Spleen

This lymphoid organ is located in the left upper quadrant of the abdomen beneath the diaphragm. Major splenic functions include gathering and isolating worn-out erythrocytes and storing blood and 20% to 30% of platelets. The spleen filters and removes foreign materials, worn-out cells, and cellular debris.

Accessory organs

Other lymphoid tissues—the tonsils, adenoids, appendix, thymus, and Peyer's patches (intestinal lymphoid tissue)—also remove foreign debris in much the same way as lymph nodes do. They are positioned in food and air passages—likely areas of microbial access.

gens) as bacteria, fungi, viruses, and parasites, the immune system also preserves the internal environment by scavenging dead or damaged cells and by performing surveillance.

Immunocompetent cells are stationed strategically and travel throughout the body scouting for aberrant cells that could develop malignant characteristics. To perform these functions efficiently, the immune system uses three basic defense strategies: protective surface phenomena, general host defenses, and specific immune responses.

Protective surface phenomena

Strategically placed physical, chemical, and mechanical barriers work to prevent organism entry. Intact and healing skin and mucous membranes provide the first line of defense against microbial invasion, preventing attachment of microorganisms. Skin desquamation (normal cell turnover) and low pH further impede bacterial colonization. Seromucous surfaces, such as the conjunctiva of the eye and the oral mucous membranes, are protected by antibacterial substances such as the enzyme lysozyme, found in tears, saliva, and nasal secretions.

The respiratory system requires special protection because microorganisms enter it easily from outside. Nasal hairs and turbulent airflow through the nostrils filter foreign materials. Nasal secretions contain an immunoglobulin (naturally produced antibody) that discourages microbe adherence. Lining the respiratory tract is a mucous layer that is continuously disposed of and replaced. This mucous layer, coupled with ciliary action, traps and expels inhaled particles and microbes before they can damage delicate alveolar tissues.

In the gastrointestinal (GI) system, saliva, swallowing, peristalsis, and defecation mechanically remove bacteria. Furthermore, the low pH of gastric secretions is bactericidal, rendering the stomach virtually free of viable bacteria. The remainder of the GI system is protected by a process known as colonization resistance: Bacteria that normally reside there prevent colonization by other microorganisms.

The urinary system is sterile except for the distal end of the urethra and the urinary meatus. Working together, urine flow, low urine pH, an immunoglobulin, and the bactericidal effects of prostatic fluid (in men) impede bacterial colonization; and a series of sphincters inhibits bacterial migration.

General host defenses

Once an antigen penetrates the skin or mucous membrane, the immune system launches nonspecific cellular responses in an attempt to identify and remove the invader.

The first cellular line of defense, these nonspecific responses are activated by exposure to an antigen. Although the responses differentiate self from nonself, that is the limit of their recognition capability. They cannot identify specific antigens or respond to them differently. Therefore, the initial response is the same for bacteria, fungi, viruses, or any other foreign substance.

Inflammation, the first of these defensive responses against an antigen, causes four characteristic signs and symptoms: heat, redness, swelling, and pain. (For more information, see *The inflammatory response.*)

Phagocytosis usually occurs after inflammation or in chronic infections. At that point, macrophages and lymphocytes assume command. These cells move to the site of insult and infection by diapedesis (process by which blood cells migrate from the intravascular compartment to tissue sites) and chemotaxis (movement toward a chemical attractor).

The inflammatory response

The inflammatory response to an antigen involves vascular and cellular changes that eliminate dead tissue, microorganisms, toxins, and inert foreign matter. This nonspecific immune response facilitates tissue repair by the following steps:

1. Soon after microorganisms invade damaged tissue, basophils release heparin, histamine, and kinins.
2. These substances promote vasodilation and increase capillary permeability.
3. Blood flow increases to the affected tissues and fluid collects in them.
4. Granulocytes—predominantly neutrophils—promptly migrate to the invasion site.
5. At the invasion site, these cells engulf and destroy the microorganisms, foreign materials, and debris from dying cells.
6. Tissue repair occurs.

Specific immune responses

In contrast to the general host defenses, in which all foreign substances elicit the same response, specific immune responses are activated by particular microorganisms or molecules and initially involve a limited number of specific immune cells. The primary function of a specific immune response, therefore, is to produce *specific* responses directed against *specific* antigens. The specific responses of the immune system are humoral or cell-mediated immunity. Lymphocytes (B cells and T cells) are responsible for these specific immune responses.

Humoral immunity. In this specific response, B cells, primarily, produce antibodies (native proteins of the immunoglobulin class). An invasive antigen causes the B cells to divide and differentiate into plasma cells that produce and secrete antigen-specific antibodies. The five types of antibodies, or immunoglobulins, are IgA, IgD, IgE, IgG, and IgM. Each type serves a particular function: IgA, IgG, and IgM protect against viral and bacterial invasion; IgD acts as an antigen receptor of B cells; IgE causes allergic response.

After the body's initial exposure to an antigen, a time lag occurs during which little or no antibody can be detected. During this time, the B cell recognizes the antigen, and the sequence of division, differentiation, and antibody formation begins. This *primary antibody response* occurs 4 to 10 days after first-time antigen exposure, during which immunoglobulin increases, then quickly dissipates, and IgM antibodies form.

Subsequent exposure to the same antigen initiates a *secondary antibody response.* In this situation, memory B cells manufacture antibodies (now mainly IgG), achieving peak levels in 1 to 2 days. These elevated levels persist for months and then fall slowly. The secondary immune response is, therefore, faster, more intense, and more persistent; and it amplifies with each subsequent exposure to the same antigen.

An antigen-antibody complex, which forms after the antibody reacts to the antigen, serves several functions. First, a macrophage processes the antigen and presents it to antigen-specific B cells. Then the antibody activates the nine-factor complement system, causing an enzymatic cascade that destroys the antigen. The activated complement system bridges humoral and cell-mediated immunity and results in the arrival of phagocytic neutrophils and macrophages at the antigen site. This combination of humoral and cell-mediated immune response is common.

Cell-mediated immunity. T-cell activity characterizes cell-mediated immunity, which protects the body against bacterial, viral, and fungal infections and resists transplanted cells and tumor cells. In cell-mediated response, a macrophage processes the antigen, which is then presented to T cells. Some T cells become sensitized and destroy the antigen; others release lymphokines, which activate macrophages that destroy the antigen. Sensitized T cells then travel through the blood and lymphatic systems, providing ongoing surveillance in their quest for specific antigens.

Blood

Blood, a tissue, consists of various formed elements (blood cells) suspended in a fluid called plasma. It transports gases, nutrients, metabolic wastes, blood cells, immune cells, and hormones throughout the body. To accomplish this task, the blood, which is confined to the vascular system, constantly interacts with the body's extracellular fluid for exchange and transfer.

Formed elements in the blood include erythrocytes (red blood cells), thrombocytes (platelets), and leukocytes (white blood cells). Red blood cells and platelets function entirely within blood vessels; leukocytes act mainly in the tissues outside the blood vessels. Thus, leukocytes found in circulation are in transit between various activity sites.

Erythrocytes

Red blood cells (RBCs) transport oxygen and carbon dioxide to and from body tissues. These minute cells lose their nuclei during the maturation process, thus developing a biconcave shape and needed flexibility to travel through different-sized blood vessels. RBCs contain hemoglobin, the oxygen-carrying substance that gives blood its red color.

Typically, RBCs constitute about 40% of blood volume: 4.5 to 6.2 million/mm^3 of blood for an adult male, 4.2 to 5.4 million/mm^3 of blood for an adult female. Usually, RBCs are quantified as concentrations (rather than as absolute numbers) in relation to plasma: hemoglobin (Hb) and hematocrit (HCT). Hemoglobin is expressed as grams per deciliter of blood, and hematocrit as the volume percentage of RBCs in whole blood. Thus, an HCT of 30% means that RBCs account for 30% of the blood volume. Because this value represents a concentration, it may change without an alteration in the actual number of RBCs—for example, in response to dehydration.

Constant circulation wears out RBCs, which have an average 120-day life span. The spleen sequesters, or isolates, the old, worn-out RBCs, thus removing them from circulation. This process requires that the body manufacture billions of new cells daily to maintain RBCs at normal levels.

Bone marrow releases RBCs into circulation in immature form as reticulocytes. The reticulocytes mature into RBCs in about 1 day. The rate of reticulocyte release usually equals the rate of old RBC removal. Polycythemia occurs when the hemoglobin amount or the number of RBCs markedly increases. Anemia occurs when the hemoglobin amount, the number of RBCs, or the hematocrit concentration falls below normal levels. When RBC depletion occurs—for example, with hemorrhage—the bone marrow increases reticulocyte production to maintain the normal balance of RBCs in circulation.

The RBC surface carries antigens, and these antigens determine a person's blood group, or blood type.

Blood group compatibilities. All blood falls into one of four blood types. In type A blood, the A antigen is present on the RBCs. In type B blood, the B antigen appears. Type AB blood contains both antigens. Type O blood has neither antigen.

Blood from any of these types may also include the Rh antigen. With the Rh antigen, the blood is called Rh positive (Rh^+); without the Rh antigen, the blood is Rh negative (Rh^-).

Plasma may contain antibodies that can interact with these antigens, causing the cells to agglutinate (clump); but plasma would not contain antibodies to its own cell antigen, or it would destroy itself. Thus, type A blood has A antigen but no anti-A antibodies; however, it does have anti-B antibodies. This principle is important for blood transfusions, where a donor's blood must be compatible with a recipient's blood. Incompatibility can be fatal to the recipient. That explains why precise blood typing and cross matching (mixing and observing for agglutination of donor cells) are essential.

The following blood groups are compatible: Type A with Type A or O; Type B with Type B or O; Type AB with Type A, B, AB, or O; and Type O with Type O only.

Thrombocytes

Thrombocytes (platelets) play a major role in hemostasis (termination of bleeding). Produced in the bone marrow, platelets bud from a large cell called a megakaryocyte (giant cell with a multilobed nucleus). Like RBCs, platelets are round or oval biconcave disks, having no nucleus.

In the peripheral blood, platelets are sticky and contribute to hemostasis in three ways: They clump together to plug small defects in small blood vessel walls; they congregate at an injury site in a larger vessel to help close the wound so that a blood clot can form; and they release substances that fortify clot stabilization—for example, serotonin, which reduces blood flow by vasoconstriction, and thromboplastin, an enzyme essential to blood clot formation.

Platelets circulate in massive numbers, ranging from 130,000 to 370,000/mm^3 of blood, and have an average life span of 8 to 12 days. Thrombocytopenia is

Blood clotting

Through a three-part process, the circulatory system protects itself from excessive blood loss. In this process, vascular injury activates a complex chain of events—vasoconstriction, platelet aggregation, and coagulation—leading to clotting, that stops the bleeding without hindering blood flow through the injured vessel.

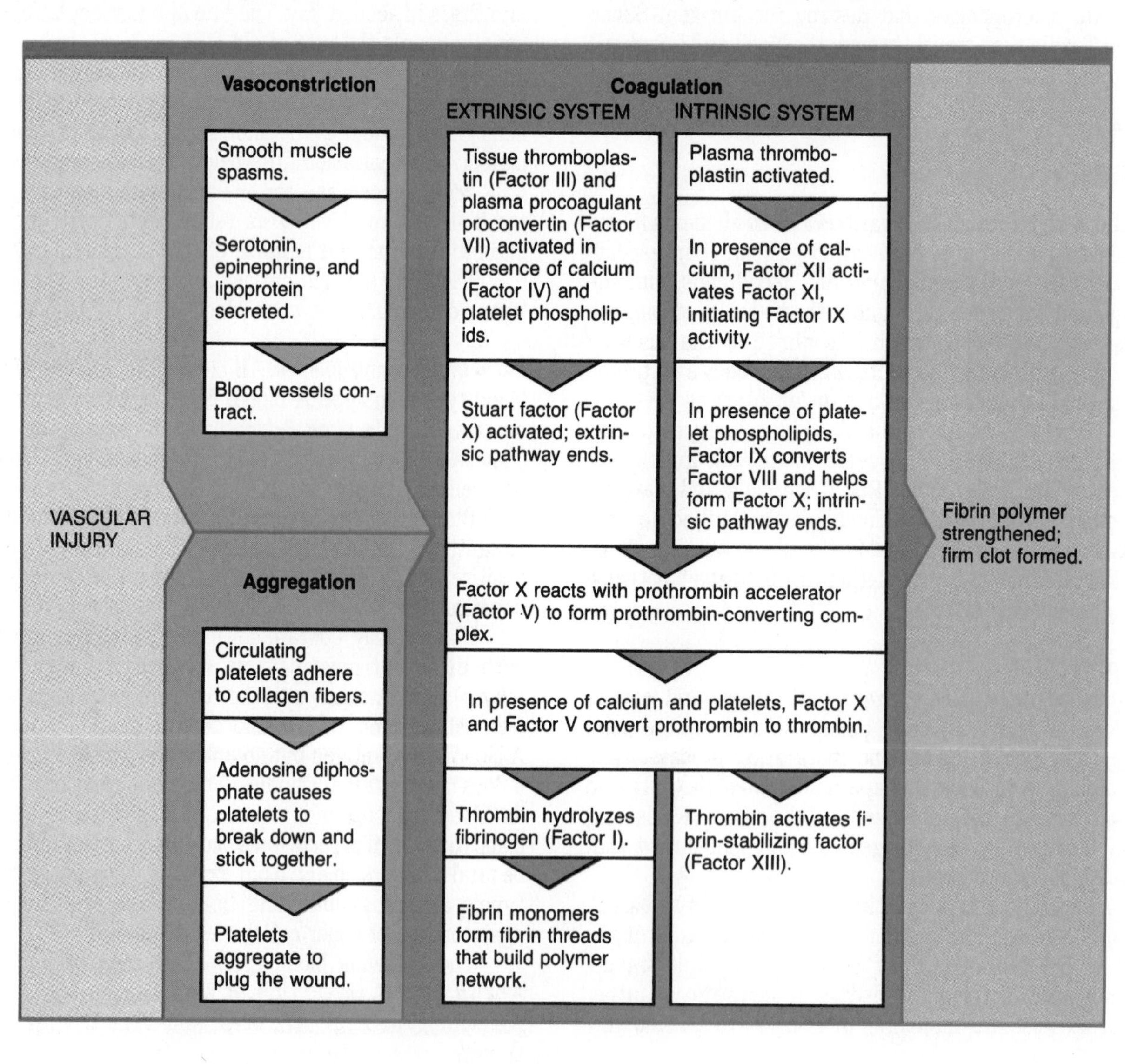

a platelet count below 50,000/mm³ of blood. Spontaneous bleeding may occur if the platelet count falls below 20,000/mm³ of blood.

Platelets are not the only blood components involved in coagulation (blood clotting). Coagulation requires the interaction of plasma components and plasma and tissue clotting factors with calcium ions. (For more information about the process, see *Blood clotting.*) The absence of any clotting factors (as in hemophilia) may interfere with this vital response and trigger bleeding.

Leukocytes

Five types of leukocytes (white blood cells, or WBCs) participate in the body's defense and immune systems: neutrophils, eosinophils, basophils, monocytes, and lymphocytes. These are grouped as granulocytes and agranulocytes, depending on their nucleus shape, the presence or absence of cytoplasmic granules, and affinity for laboratory stains or dyes. The total WBC count typically ranges from 4,100 to 10,900/mm³ of blood.

Granulocytes. All granulocytes contain a single multilobed nucleus and prominent cytoplasmic granules. Cell types in this category include neutrophils, eosinophils, and basophils. Collectively, these cells are known as polymorphonuclear leukocytes. However, each cell type exhibits different properties and each is activated by different stimuli.

The most abundant granulocytes, neutrophils account for 47.6% to 76.8% of circulating WBCs. Neutrophils are phagocytic; that is, they can engulf, ingest, and digest foreign materials. (For an illustration of this process, see *Phases of phagocytosis.)* Neutrophils can leave the bloodstream by diapedesis and migrate to and accumulate at infection sites. Worn-out neutrophils form the main component of pus. Immature neutrophils, called bands, are produced by bone marrow to replace worn-out neutrophils. In response to infection, bone marrow must produce many immature cells and release them into circulation, elevating the band count.

Less common than neutrophils, eosinophils account for 0.3% to 7% of circulating WBCs. These granulocytes also migrate from the bloodstream by diapedesis, but in response to different stimuli. During allergic responses, eosinophils accumulate in loose connective tissue where they are highly phagocytic to antigen-antibody complexes. Eosinophil percentages also rise in response to certain parasitic infestations, such as hookworm.

The least common granulocytes, basophils usually constitute fewer than 2% of circulating WBCs. They possess little or no phagocytic ability. However, their

Phases of phagocytosis

When microorganisms or other foreign materials (antigens) invade the skin or mucous membranes, the immune system and blood remove them by the defense mechanism phagocytosis. Primarily, macrophages and neutrophils carry out this process of chemotaxis, opsonization, ingestion, digestion, and release.

Chemotaxis
In response to invasion, macrophages are attracted to the microorganism site.

Microorganism
Macrophage
Opsonizing antibodies

Opsonization
Antibodies coat the microorganisms, enhancing macrophage binding to them.

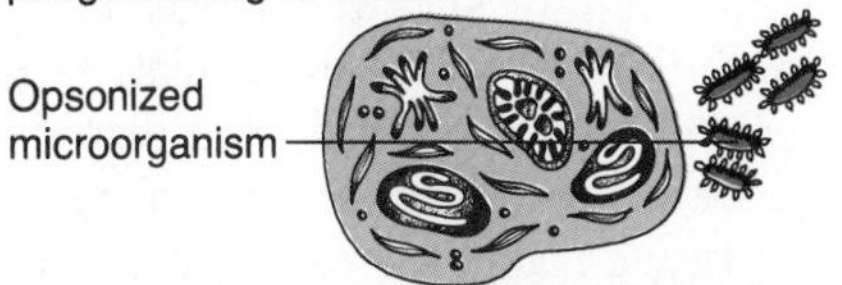

Ingestion
Then the macrophage forms pseudopods (footlike extensions), extending its membrane around the opsonized microorganisms, engulfing and ingesting them within a vacuole (phagosome).

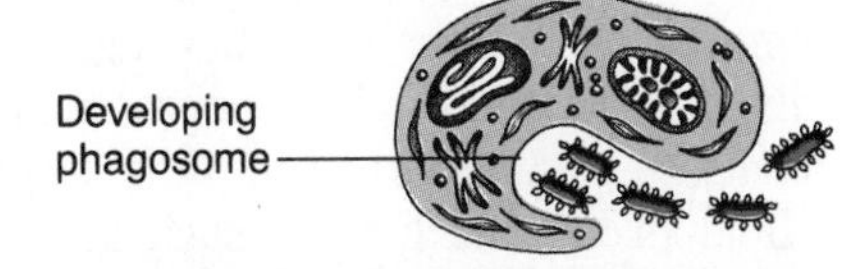

Digestion
The phagosome digests the microorganisms and merges with lysosomes, forming a phagolysosome, which releases enzymes that help iodine, bromide, and chloride bind to the cell wall to destroy the microorganisms.

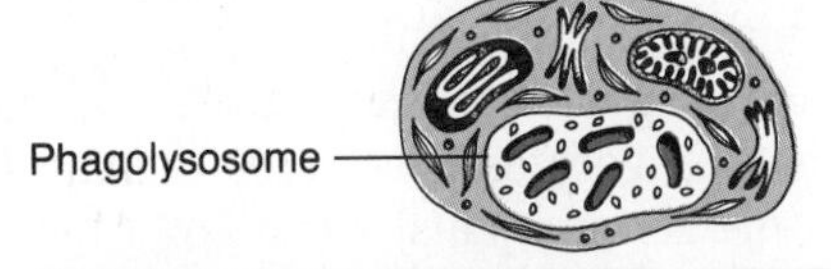

Release
The macrophage releases digestive debris, including lysosomes, and continues to mediate the immune response.

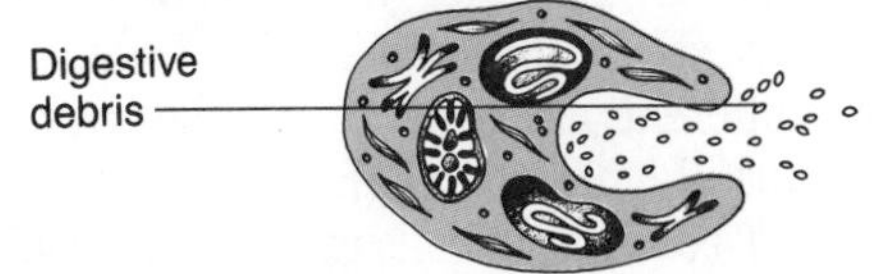

cytoplasmic granules secrete heparin and histamine in response to certain inflammatory and immune stimuli, increasing vascular permeability and easing fluid passage from capillaries into body tissues.

Because of their phagocytic capabilities, granulocytes—especially neutrophils—serve as the body's first line of cellular defense against foreign organisms. Noting the numbers of these cells in circulation (rather than just the percentage) helps the nurse assess the client's susceptibility or resistance to infection. For example, a client with a total granulocyte count of 1,000/mm³ of blood, or less, would be considered granulocytopenic (poor in granulocytes) and at risk for infection. The lower the granulocyte count, the more profound the risk for infection.

Agranulocytes. WBCs in this category—monocytes and lymphocytes—lack specific cytoplasmic granules and have nuclei without lobes.

Monocytes are the largest of the WBCs, but constitute only 0.6% to 9.6% of WBCs in circulation. Like neutrophils, monocytes are phagocytic and diapedetic. Once outside the bloodstream, monocytes enlarge and mature, becoming tissue macrophages, or histiocytes.

As macrophages, monocytes may roam freely through the body when stimulated by inflammation. Usually they remain immobile, populating most organs and tissues. Collectively, they are components of the reticuloendothelial system (a functional, rather than anatomic, body system responsible for defending against infection and for disposing of cell breakdown products). Macrophages concentrate in structures that filter large amounts of body fluid (blood and lymph), such as the liver, spleen, and lymph nodes, where they defend against invading organisms. Macrophages exhibit different physical characteristics and are referred to by different names, depending on their organ location. Examples of these tissue macrophages include Kupffer's cells in the hepatic sinuses, microglia in the central nervous system, and alveolar macrophages in the lung alveoli. Macrophages are efficient phagocytes of bacteria, cellular debris (including worn-out neutrophils), and necrotic tissue. When mobilized at an infection site, they phagocytize cellular remnants and promote wound healing.

Lymphocytes, the smallest of the WBCs and the second most numerous (16.2% to 43%), derive from a multipotential stem cell. Unlike other blood cells, they mature in two different locations: T lymphocytes (T cells) in the thymus, B lymphocytes (B cells) in the bone marrow, probably. T cells and B cells produce antibodies for specific immune responses. T cells are involved in cell-mediated immunity and B cells are involved in humoral immunity.

Developmental considerations

The immune system and the blood undergo important transformations in a pediatric or elderly client.

Pediatric client

A neonate has the most RBCs of any age-group—from 4.4 to 5.8 million/mm³ of blood. A neonate also has immunity established before birth when, as a fetus, it receives significant amounts of IgG from the mother during pregnancy. For the first 3 to 6 months after birth, the neonate is immune to antigens to which the mother was exposed when pregnant. During this period, the neonate begins to produce IgG, reaching 40% of adult levels by age 1.

However, by age 6 months, the neonate's acquired immunity disappears. Therefore, immunizations must be administered. Although the infant begins to produce IgA, IgD, and IgE, these antibodies do not reach adult levels until early childhood—which explains why a child may experience numerous colds and minor infections when exposed to new antigens.

The toddler's antibody production is well established. At age 2, the toddler's IgG production reaches adult levels, and the toddler can neutralize microorganisms as effectively as the adult.

Elderly client

Evidence suggests that bone marrow activity decreases as age increases. This results in a decrease of formed elements in the marrow and a slowed response to the body's need for these elements.

An elderly adult is at increased risk for intravascular thrombus formation, resulting in blood vessel occlusion in the extremities and brain. This is attributed to development of a rough layer of atherosclerotic plaque that causes blood vessel defects and injuries, stimulating platelets to overproduce components of coagulation.

Advancing age also affects the immune system. The protective surface phenomena of the respiratory tract wane because of decreasing ciliary action and cough ability, which may increase respiratory infection incidence in an elderly client.

T cells are dependent on the thymus, which undergoes fatty deterioration with age. In an elderly adult, thymic mass is only about 10% that of a younger person. Because of this thymic regression, cell-mediated immunity may wane with advancing age, increasing the incidence of infections like herpes zoster (shingles).

Health history

The nurse who is preparing to collect health history data about the client's immune system and blood should review these interview guidelines:

Establish a comfortable interview environment that ensures client comfort and privacy. Allow time to conduct the interview at a comfortable, uninterrupted pace so that the client and other participants do not feel rushed and omit important information.

Use familiar terms. For example, ask about bruises, not ecchymoses. If you use medical terms, explain them and make sure the client understands them.

Obtain full biographic data, including age, sex, race, and ethnic background, because some immune and blood disorders occur more frequently in certain groups. For example, some autoimmune diseases appear more often in young women than in men. Sickle cell anemia occurs primarily in Blacks; pernicious anemia typically affects those of Northern European descent.

Focus the health history on detecting the most common signs and symptoms of immune and blood disorders: abnormal bleeding, lymphadenopathy (hypertrophy of lymphoid tissue, often called swollen glands), fatigue, weakness, fever, and joint pain. Focus on blood and immune system concerns, but maintain an holistic approach by inquiring about the status of other systems and about health-related concerns. Blood and immune system problems may result from problems in other systems, may cause problems in other systems, or may impair other aspects of the client's life. For example, the client at severe risk for infection may need protective isolation, which can disrupt family and social life and lead to sensory deprivation.

The questions in this section include rationales that describe the significance of the answers and, where appropriate, nursing interventions that may be incorporated into the client's nursing care plan.

Health and illness patterns

To assess important health and illness patterns, explore the client's current and past health status, developmental status, and family health status.

Current health status

Because current health status usually is foremost in the client's mind, begin the interview with this topic. Carefully document the chief complaint in the client's own words. Then, using the *PQRST* method, encourage a complete description of this complaint and any others. (For a detailed explanation of this method, see *Symptom analysis* in Chapter 3.)

The client with an immune or blood disorder may report vague signs and symptoms, such as lack of energy, light-headedness, or frequent bruising. Sometimes, such signs and symptoms as pallor and declining energy are attributed to aging. Signs and symptoms with a rapid onset usually indicate a disorder; those that begin insidiously or increase gradually may be related to hidden or chronic illness. To avoid overlooking important clues, remember that any change from the client's usual status could be significant and requires investigation.

To assess the client's current health status, ask the following questions:

How have you been feeling lately? Have you noticed any changes in your usual health? If so, please tell me more about them.
(RATIONALE: Because immune and blood disorder symptoms may be vague, open-ended questions usually elicit more information than a checklist might. The client may discuss seemingly insignificant health deviations when comparing current and past health status. Draw the client out about difficult-to-pinpoint, vague complaints. The more specific the information, the better the probability of identifying interrelationships among the client's discomforts.)

Have you noticed any unusual bleeding—for example, frequent nosebleeds or bruises that you don't remember getting?
(RATIONALE: With low platelet counts or clotting factor deficiencies, a client's unusual bleeding or unexplained ecchymoses can occur secondary to minimal trauma. The extremities are most prone to such injuries, but no body part is exempt.)

Have you ever bled for a long time after accidentally cutting yourself?
(RATIONALE: Prolonged bleeding may indicate a platelet or clotting mechanism deficiency, which can occur with certain immune disorders. If it occurs regularly, it can lead to anemia.)

Have you noticed any bleeding from your gums?
(RATIONALE: Because oral mucosal tissues are highly vascular [and visible], the client may note bleeding from these tissues before noting abnormal bleeding in other areas. Gingivae may bleed after the client chews coarse

foods or roughage, or after daily oral hygiene; they may bleed vigorously after dental hygiene or repair.)

Have you noticed any rash or skin discolorations? If so, on which part of your body?
(RATIONALE: Petechiae, pinpoint accumulations of blood in the skin or mucous membranes, may appear to the client as a rashlike discoloration. Petechiae occur when small vessels leak under pressure and platelet numbers are insufficient to stop the bleeding. They are likely to appear where clothing constricts circulation, such as at the waist and wrists.)

Have you noticed any swelling in your neck, armpits, or groin? If so, are the swollen areas sore, hard, or red? Do they appear on one or both sides?
(RATIONALE: Lymphadenopathy may signal inflammation, infection, or elevated lymphocyte production associated with certain leukemias. Primary lymphatic tumors usually are not painful; nontender, swollen lymph nodes may occur in Hodgkin's disease.)

Do you ever feel tired? If so, are you tired all the time or only after exertion? Do you need frequent naps, or do you sleep an unusually long time at night?
(RATIONALE: Fatigue is a prominent symptom of many hematologic disorders. The change may be subtle [the client requires more sleep at night] or dramatic [the client can no longer climb a flight of stairs comfortably or requires a longer time to do so]. The client may complain of *always* feeling tired.)

Do you ever feel weak? If so, are you weak all the time or only at certain times? Does weakness ever interfere with your ability to perform your usual daily tasks, such as cooking or driving a car?
(RATIONALE: Although weakness is different from fatigue, these symptoms often occur together in a client with an immune or blood disorder. Exertional fatigue and weakness suggest moderate anemia; constant or extreme fatigue and weakness, severe anemia or neuropathy from an autoimmune disorder. *Note:* Instead of reporting weakness, the client may complain of heavy extremities, "as if my ankles and wrists had weights around them.")

Have you had a fever recently? If so, how high was it? Was it constant or intermittent? Did it follow any particular pattern?
(RATIONALE: A fever that recurs every few days, for example, Pel-Ebstein fever, may indicate Hodgkin's disease; a temperature that rises and falls within 24 hours suggests an infection. Frequently recurring fevers may signal immune system impairment or rapid blood cell proliferation.)

Do you ever have joint pain? If so, which joints are affected? Do swelling, redness, or warmth accompany the pain? Do your bones ache?
(RATIONALE: Pain in the knees, wrists, or hands may indicate an autoimmune process or hemarthrosis [blood in a joint] from a blood disorder. Pain accompanied by swelling, redness, or warmth typically suggests inflammation, which may be relieved by heat application or salicylates. Aching bones may result from the pressure of expanding bone marrow [from blood cell proliferation and subsequent crowding].)

Have you noticed any change in your skin's texture, color, or other characteristics?
(RATIONALE: Hard, thickened skin may indicate scleroderma; dry skin, Hashimoto's disease; sallow skin, SLE.)

Have you noticed any sores that heal slowly?
(RATIONALE: With too few WBCs to control infection and promote healing, a client may have delayed wound healing from compromised hematopoietic or immune functions.)

Have you developed any vision problems recently? If so, can you describe them?
(RATIONALE: Double vision or increased sensitivity to light can indicate SLE.)

Has your hearing changed recently?
(RATIONALE: Ear infections or Hashimoto's disease can impair hearing.)

Have you recently developed wheezing, runny nose, or difficulty breathing?
(RATIONALE: Wheezing, rhinitis, and dyspnea may signify an allergy. Dyspnea may also be caused by anemia, connective tissue disease, or infection.)

Do you ever experience heart palpitations?
(RATIONALE: Palpitations may indicate tachycardia, which can result from an infection in a client with an immunodeficiency.)

Are you bothered by a persistent or recurrent cough or cold? Do you cough up sputum? Do you feel chest pain when you cough, breathe deeply, or laugh?

(RATIONALE: Immunodeficiency increases the risk of persistent or recurrent respiratory infections, especially pneumonia. Sputum color and consistency may suggest the underlying disorder. For example, greenish sputum suggests bacterial infection; rust-colored sputum suggests pneumococcal pneumonia. Pleuritic pain [a sharp, knifelike pain that increases with coughing, deep breathing, or laughing] commonly occurs with pneumonia.)

Has your appetite changed recently? Do you experience nausea, flatulence, or diarrhea?
(RATIONALE: Such effects may result when anemia causes gastric hypoxia. The severity of these manifestations may reflect the severity of the hypoxia.)

Have you vomited recently? If so, how would you describe the vomitus?
(RATIONALE: Hematemesis [vomiting blood] may produce bright-red, brown, or black vomitus that is the color and consistency of coffee grounds. This sign may be caused by thrombocytopenia or a clotting factor disorder.)

Have you noticed any blood in your bowel movements or have you had any black, tarry bowel movements? Do you experience any discomfort when defecating?
(RATIONALE: Hematochezia [passing bloody stools] can cause bright-red, blood-streaked, or dark-colored stools. It may be caused by thrombocytopenia or a clotting factor deficiency. It may also result from tears in the rectal mucosa caused by straining or hemorrhoidal irritation. In either case, the rectal mucosa is predisposed to infection in the client with an immune or blood disorder because macrophages that normally inhabit the area are absent.)

Have you noticed any change in how your urine looks or in your urination pattern?
(RATIONALE:The urine may appear pink or grossly bloody from bladder capillary hemorrhages in a client who has a coagulation disorder. It may appear cloudy and malodorous in a client who has an external genitalia inflammation caused by a WBC deficiency, immunodeficiency, or a urinary tract infection. Such a client may also experience changes in usual urinary patterns, such as nocturia [urination at night], dysuria [painful urination], urinary frequency, urinary urgency, or urinary incontinence.)

Do you have any difficulty walking, or do you experience a pins-and-needles sensation?
(RATIONALE: These neurologic effects may result from pernicious anemia.)

Sex-specific questions

When interviewing a female client, ask these questions:

Have your menstrual periods changed recently? For example, do they last longer or occur more frequently? Have your periods become irregular? Has the volume or nature of your menstrual flow increased or changed?
(RATIONALE: A menstrual pattern change may be the initial sign of a bleeding disorder stemming from inadequate platelet numbers or function or from deficient clotting factors.)

Do you experience any pain or discomfort during sexual intercourse?
(RATIONALE: In a client with a white blood cell deficiency or an immunodeficiency, a genital inflammation may develop, causing dyspareunia [painful or difficult intercourse].)

Have you recently suffered from emotional instability, headaches, irritability, or depression?
(RATIONALE: These effects commonly occur with SLE and other chronic immune disorders.)

For a female client, some additional questions will help complete the health history assessment. (For these questions and rationales, see *Sex-specific questions.*)

Past health status

In compiling data on the client's past health status, ask the following questions:

In the past, have you had any of the problems we've just discussed?
(RATIONALE: The client may have experienced problems related to hematopoiesis, coagulation, or immune function in the past.)

Did you have sore throats frequently in the past?
(RATIONALE: Frequent sore throats suggest poor immune response to infecting organisms.)

Do you recall being seriously ill as a child or having a long illness requiring frequent visits to a physician?
(RATIONALE: Information about childhood illnesses can provide clues to immune or blood disorders. For example, Hodgkin's disease, sarcoma, and acute lymphocytic leukemia, which occur mostly in childhood and adolescence, require aggressive bone marrow suppression therapy with drugs or radiation. Some chemotherapeutic agents, known as alkylating agents, may induce bone marrow dysfunction or leukemia.)

Adverse drug reactions

When obtaining a health history to assess a client's immune system and blood, the nurse must ask about medication use. Many drugs can increase or decrease the numbers of certain types of blood cells and can suppress immune system functioning; some drugs can cause other immune or blood disorders. The commonly used drugs listed below may cause adverse reactions affecting the immune system and blood.

DRUG CLASS	DRUG	POSSIBLE ADVERSE REACTIONS
Anticonvulsants	carbamazepine	Aplastic anemia (characterized by decreased levels of all formed elements of blood), leukopenia (decreased leukocyte levels), agranulocytosis (increased agranulocyte levels), eosinophilia (increased eosinophil levels), leukocytosis (increased leukocyte levels), thrombocytopenia (decreased thrombocyte levels)
	phenytoin	Thrombocytopenia, leukopenia, granulocytopenia (decreased granulocyte levels), pancytopenia (decreased levels of all blood cells), macrocytosis (enlarged erythrocytes), megaloblastic anemia (characterized by increased, immature, enlarged erythrocytes)
Antidiabetics	acetohexamide, chlorpropamide, glipizide, glyburide, tolbutamide	Leukopenia, thrombocytopenia, pancytopenia, agranulocytosis, aplastic anemia, hemolytic anemia (characterized by premature erythrocyte destruction)
Antihypertensives	captopril	Neutropenia (decreased neutrophil levels), agranulocytosis
	hydralazine	Positive ANA (antinuclear antibodies) titer that occurs when the immune system creates antibodies against some of the body's own cells; systemic lupus erythematosus-like syndrome
	methyldopa	Positive Coombs' test, indicating that some type of immunoglobulin coats the red blood cells
Anti-infectives	cephalosporins	Positive Coombs' test; hypothrombinemia (decreased thrombin levels), with or without bleeding
	chloramphenicol	Bone marrow depression, pancytopenia, aplastic anemia
	penicillins	Eosinophilia, hemolytic anemia, leukopenia, neutropenia, thrombocytopenia, positive Coombs' test
	pentamide isethionate	Leukopenia, thrombocytopenia
	sulfonamides	Granulocytopenia, leukopenia, eosinophilia, hemolytic anemia, aplastic anemia, thrombocytopenia, methemoglobinemia (increased levels of an oxidative compound of hemoglobin), hypoprothrombinemia (prothrombin, or Factor II, deficiency)
Antineoplastics	busulfan	Severe leukopenia, anemia, severe thrombocytopenia
	chlorambucil	Leukopenia, thrombocytopenia, anemia

Adverse drug reactions continued

DRUG CLASS	DRUG	POSSIBLE ADVERSE REACTIONS
Antineoplastics (continued)	cisplatin, cyclophosphamide, doxorubicin hydrochloride, fluorouracil	Leukopenia, granulocytopenia, thrombocytopenia, anemia
	methotrexate	Leukopenia, thrombocytopenia, anemia, hemorrhage
	mitomycin	Thrombocytopenia, leukopenia
Antipsychotic agents	chlorpromazine hydrochloride, thioridazine hydrochloride	Agranulocytosis, mild leukopenia
Cardiac agents	procainamide hydrochloride	Positive ANA titer; systemic lupus erythematosus-like syndrome
	quinidine	Thrombocytopenia, hypoprothrombinemia, acute hemolytic anemia, agranulocytosis, aplastic anemia, and leukopenia can occur as hypersensitivity reactions
Gold compounds	auranofin, gold sodium thiomalate	Leukopenia, thrombocytopenia, anemia, eosinophilia
Nonsteroidal anti-inflammatory agents	ibuprofen	Neutropenia, agranulocytosis, aplastic anemia, hemolytic anemia, thrombocytopenia, decreased hemoglobin and hematocrit
Miscellaneous agents	furosemide	Anemia, leukopenia, neutropenia, thrombocytopenia
	lithium	Leukocytosis

Do you have any allergies? If so, what causes them and which symptoms are most bothersome?
(RATIONALE: Multiple allergies to foods, drugs, insects, or environmental pollutants are common. A description of the allergic reaction symptoms helps differentiate between a food intolerance or an adverse drug reaction and a true allergic reaction that indicates an immune system dysfunction.)

Have you ever had asthma?
(RATIONALE: A history of asthma may indicate immunopathology.)

Do you have an autoimmune disease, such as AIDS? Have you tested positive for human immunodeficiency virus (HIV)?
(RATIONALE: An autoimmune disease history may mean the client is predisposed to other diseases because the immune system does not function properly.)

Have you had any other disorders or health problems?
(RATIONALE: Hepatitis or tuberculosis promote bone marrow failure. Liver failure or cirrhosis can disrupt normal production of prothrombin and fibrinogen needed for blood coagulation. A history of peptic ulcer with excessive bleeding may suggest anemia.)

Are you currently taking any prescription or over-the-counter medications? Have you taken any of these medications in the past few weeks? If so, which ones? How often do you take them?
(RATIONALE: Many drugs produce adverse reactions in the immune system and blood. For more information, see *Adverse drug reactions.*)

Have you ever had surgery? If so, what kind and when? What follow-up care did you receive?
(RATIONALE: Surgery can exert a negative effect on the immune system and blood. For example, gastric surgery can contribute to malabsorption of nutrients and vita-

mins needed for blood formation. A splenectomy places the client at increased risk for disseminated infection.)

Have you had an organ transplant?
(RATIONALE: Organ transplants usually require prolonged treatment with immunosuppressant agents to prevent organ rejection. Such therapy compromises the immune system, predisposing the client to numerous disorders, such as infections and lymphoreticular cancers.)

Have you ever had a blood transfusion? If so, when? How many units did you receive?
(RATIONALE: Blood products can transmit infectious agents, such as hepatitis virus [non-A, non-B, and B], cytomegalovirus, plasmodia that cause malaria, and the Epstein-Barr virus. Donor blood has been screened for hepatitis B for many years. Donor blood is now screened for HIV, which causes AIDS, but before March 1985, it was not routinely tested and could have transmitted this virus.)

Have you ever been rejected as a blood donor?
(RATIONALE: A blood donation refusal may stem from chronic anemia or a history of hepatitis or jaundice from an unknown cause.)

Family health status

Investigate the immune system and blood status of the client's family by asking the following:

How would you describe the health of your blood relatives? How old are your living relatives? How old were those who died? What caused their deaths? Do or did any of them have immune, blood, or other problems of the kinds we have discussed?
(RATIONALE: Several blood and immune disorders, such as hemophilia, sickle cell anemia, and hemolytic anemia, are transmitted genetically. To determine the client's risk of developing such disorders, trace the occurrence of these disorders on a family genogram. [For more information on genograms, see *Developing a genogram* in Chapter 3.])

Developmental considerations

During the health history, the following questions may provide valuable information about a child or an elderly client:

Pediatric client. Involve the child who is old enough in the interview. If not, direct your questions to the child's parent or guardian.

Is the infant breast-fed or bottle-fed? If the infant is bottle-fed, what type of formula do you use?
(RATIONALE: Breast-feeding introduces immunoglobulins into the infant's GI tract, conferring some immunity. If the infant is bottle-fed, the formula should be iron-fortified to prevent anemia.)

Does your child ever seem pale or lethargic? Does the child sleep too much? Has the child been gaining weight at a normal rate?
(RATIONALE: Pallor, lethargy, fatigue, and failure to gain weight are common signs of anemia.)

Did the mother have any obstetric bleeding complications? Was parental blood Rh compatible?
(RATIONALE: Obstetric bleeding complications or Rh incompatibility of the parents may lead to clotting disorders in the child.)

Does the child have frequent or continuous severe infections?
(RATIONALE: Constant severe infections may suggest thymic deficiency or bone marrow dysfunction.)

Does the child have any allergies? If so, to what? Does anyone else in the family have allergies?
(RATIONALE: Children are more susceptible to allergies than adults, but a family history of infections and allergic or autoimmune disorders may suggest a pattern of immunodeficiencies.)

Which immunizations has the child received?
(RATIONALE: Immunizations can prevent many common communicable diseases. However, immunization timing is important. Every effort should be made to follow the recommended immunization schedule.)

Elderly client. In an elderly client, virtually the same immune and blood disorder signs and symptoms appear as in a younger adult. However, some effects, such as cerebral and cardiac effects, may be more pronounced. The following questions will help elicit additional useful information from an elderly client:

Do you take walks? If so, for how long?
(RATIONALE: A disorder that impairs the oxygen-carrying capacity of the blood [such as anemia] can cause weakness, dyspnea, and light-headedness. All of these effects can be pronounced in an elderly client, preventing the client from taking even short walks.)

Do you have any difficulty using your hands?
(RATIONALE: Weakness and numbness in the hands and impaired fine finger movement may suggest a blood disorder, such as anemia. Joint pain in the hands and other

areas may indicate an autoimmune disorder, such as rheumatoid arthritis.)

Do you ever have headaches, faintness, vertigo, ringing in the ears, or confusion?
(RATIONALE: These symptoms are especially probable in an elderly client with anemia.)

Have you ever had arthritis, osteomyelitis, or tuberculosis?
(RATIONALE: These disorders can predispose the client to anemia related to chronic illness.)

What do you eat on a typical day? Do you cook for yourself?
(RATIONALE: Because of limited income, resources, and mobility, an elderly client may consume a diet deficient in protein, calcium, and iron—nutrients essential for hematopoiesis. Even with an adequate diet, nutrients may not be metabolized because an elderly client has fewer digestive enzymes, which explains why about 40% of people over age 60 have iron-deficiency anemia.)

Health promotion and protection patterns

To continue the health history, determine the client's personal habits and activities that may affect the immune system and blood.

What is your typical daily diet? What types and amounts of food do you eat at each meal? What do you eat between meals?
(RATIONALE: Certain foods, such as beef, liver, milk, and kidney beans, contain iron, vitamin B_{12}, and folic acid—the nutrients required for RBC development. A diet lacking these foods may lead to anemia. Inadequate caloric and protein intake alter the immune response by compromising antibody formation, antigen recognition and processing, and phagocytosis. When this happens, the client runs a higher risk of developing infections.)

Do you drink alcoholic beverages? If so, what kind, how much, and how often do you drink?
(RATIONALE: Alcohol, especially when combined with decreased food intake, may cause folic acid-deficiency anemia.)

How would you rate your stress level? In the past 2 years, have you experienced death of a loved one, a job change, divorce, marriage, or other major change?
(RATIONALE: Persistently high levels of stress can reduce the client's resistance to infection. Researchers are exploring the possible connection between high stress and immune system suppression.)

Occupational hazards

During the interview, the nurse should investigate the client's occupational health history. Some occupations expose workers to agents that increase the risk of specific immune and blood disorders, as shown in the chart below.

OCCUPATION	HAZARDOUS AGENT	POSSIBLE DISORDER
Painting, glue and varnish work, shoemaking, plastic work, rubber cement work, rubber tire manufacturing, shoe manufacturing	Benzene	Leukemia, aplastic anemia
Chemical work	Epichlorohydrin	Leukemia, aplastic anemia
Hospital work, research laboratory work, beekeeping, fumigating	Ethylene oxide	Leukemia, aplastic anemia
Uranium mining, radiology, radiography, luminous dial painting	Ionizing radiation	Lymphoma, leukemia, aplastic anemia
Chemical work, steelwork, ceramic work, incandescent lamp making, nuclear reactor work, gas mantle making, metal refining, vacuum tube making	Thorium dioxide	Lymphoma, leukemia, aplastic anemia
Plastic factory work, vinyl chloride polymerization plant work	Vinyl chloride	Leukemia, lymphoma
Farming	Insecticides	Leukemia

Have you ever used intravenous (I.V.) drugs? If so, which ones and under what conditions?
(RATIONALE: All I.V. drugs compromise intact skin, one of the body's first defenses against invasion by microorganisms. However, illegal I.V. drugs are most likely to be unsanitary, which promotes transmission of infectious agents, such as HIV or hepatitis virus.)

Have you ever been in military service? If so, when and where did you serve?
(RATIONALE: A client who served in Vietnam in the 1960s may have been exposed to such dioxin-containing defol-

iants as Agent Orange. These agents may be oncogenic and are linked to the development of leukemia and lymphoma.)

What type of work do you do? In what kind of environment do you work?
(RATIONALE: On the job, many workers are exposed to substances that increase the risk of blood and immune disorders. For information about specific substances, see *Occupational hazards,* page 565. Emphasize safety regulations for a client in a hazardous occupational setting and investigate specific health-related problems.)

Role and relationship patterns

Ask the following questions to assess the client's role and relationship patterns related to immune and blood disorders:

How supportive are your family members and friends? How do they perceive and cope with your illness?
(RATIONALE: Chronic autoimmune disorders, such as multiple sclerosis, and immunodeficiency diseases, such as AIDS, are devastating. If the client receives little support from friends and family members, or if these people have difficulty coping with the client's illness, plan to refer the client to a supportive agency.)

Are you sexually active? If so, are you involved in a monogamous relationship?
(RATIONALE: A client who has multiple sexual partners may acquire or transmit infectious organisms, such as HIV. Barrier contraceptives such as condoms are effective in reducing this risk.)

Have you noticed any change in your usual pattern of sexual functioning? If so, can you describe this change?
(RATIONALE: Any chronic illness or pain can profoundly affect sexual performance and satisfaction. For example, anemia may cause such severe cellular hypoxia and fatigue that the client has loss of sexual desire or difficulty with erection or ejaculation.)

What is your sexual preference? Do you or have you engaged in anal intercourse?
(RATIONALE: The AIDS virus can be transmitted by intimate sexual contact, especially that associated with the rectal mucosal trauma that occurs during anal intercourse.)

Physical assessment

To assess the client's immune system and blood, the nurse evaluates factors that reflect changes (for example, vital signs); related body structure status (for example, the skin and respiratory system); and, of course, the spleen and lymph nodes (the only accessible immune system structures). Often nonspecific, the initial complaints and findings may involve several body systems. Use the following guidelines for assessment.

Preparing for immune system and blood assessment

Before assessing the immune system and blood, obtain the following equipment: a flashlight (for transillumination), a ruler, a nonstretchable tape measure, and a gown and drapes for the client's comfort and privacy.

Make sure the examination room is well lighted. Adjust the examination table to an appropriate height for supine and sitting positions. Have the client void for comfort, then undress and dress in a gown and drapes that provide adequate access and prevent unnecessary exposure.

Required physical assessment techniques include inspection and palpation. Only superficial lymph nodes can be assessed by inspection and palpation. Usually, you will incorporate the immune system and blood assessment in the assessment of body systems where lymph nodes are located. For example, during head and neck assessment the cervical lymph nodes may be palpated.

The following section discusses all regional lymph nodes. Whatever the assessment routine, be sure to integrate all physical findings for an overall picture of the client's health status.

General appearance and vital signs

Because signs and symptoms of immune and blood disorders typically are nonspecific, begin the assessment by observing the client's general physical appearance. Look for signs of acute illness, such as grimacing or profuse perspiration, and of chronic illness, such as emaciation and listlessness. Determine whether the client's stated age and appearance agree. Chronic disease and nutritional deficiencies related to immune and blood disorders may make a client look older than the stated age.

Also observe the client's facial features. Note any edema, grimacing, or lack of expression. Edema may indicate Hashimoto's disease (thyroid disease in which lymphoid tissue replaces epithelial tissue).

Next, measure the client's height and body weight. Compare the findings with normal values for the client's structure. (For height and weight tables, see Chapter 6, Nutritional Status.) Weight loss may result from anorexia and other GI problems related to immune and blood disorders.

Observe the client's posture, movements, and gait. Abnormalities can indicate joint, spinal, or neurologic changes caused by an immune or blood disorder.

Finally, assess the client's vital signs, noting especially whether they vary from the client's normal baseline measurements. (For procedural information about assessing vital signs, see Chapter 4, Physical Assessment Skills.)

An elevated temperature, with or without a chill, suggests infection; a subnormal temperature usually occurs with gram-negative infections. Other inflammation signs, such as redness, swelling, or tenderness, may accompany a fever. Caused by phagocytosis, these effects may be absent if the client has a WBC deficiency, such as leukopenia (a decrease in total WBCs), granulocytopenia (a decrease in circulating granulocytes), or neutropenia (an absolute neutrophil count below 500/mm^3 of blood).

Assess the client's heart rate by checking the pulse. The heart pumps blood harder and faster to compensate for decreased oxygen-carrying capacity in anemia or for decreased volume from active or slow bleeding. This compensation results in tachycardia (a rapid, but regular, heart rate of 100 to 150 beats per minute) or other dysrhythmias.

Check the client's respiratory rate and character. Particularly note tachypnea (an abnormally rapid breathing rate), air hunger (as evidenced by gasping for air), or labored breathing—especially on exertion. These abnormal respiratory signs may occur as the respiratory system tries to meet the body's oxygen needs when a disorder compromises the blood's oxygen-carrying capacity.

With the client in the supine, seated, and standing positions, measure blood pressure. After the client changes position, blood pressure usually rises or falls only slightly. A decrease of 20 mm Hg or more after changing position suggests orthostatic hypotension, which can result from hypovolemia (decreased volume of circulating plasma).

Assessing related body structures

Because immune and blood disorders affect so many body systems, your assessment must include physical effects in such areas as the skin, hair, and nails; head and neck; eyes and ears; respiratory system; cardiovascular system; GI system; urinary system; nervous system; and musculoskeletal system. The following guidelines describe how to perform this assessment.

Skin, hair, and nails. Observe the color of the client's skin. Normally, the skin has a slightly rosy undertone, even in dark-skinned clients. Notice any pallor, cyanosis (blueness), or jaundice. Pallor may indicate anemia or another blood disorder that disrupts oxygen delivery. Cyanosis suggests hypoxia in cutaneous blood vessels, which appears in some anemias. Pallor and jaundice may accompany hemolytic anemia. Also check for erythema (redness), indicating a local inflammation, and plethora (red, florid complexion), appearing with polycythemia.

Because skin appearance may be the first indicator of a bleeding disorder, such as thrombocytopenia, also observe for petechiae or ecchymoses. Carefully check body areas prone to pressure, such as the elbow, waistline, or upper arm where a blood pressure cuff is applied. For a dark-skinned client, check for petechiae or ecchymoses on the oral mucosa or conjunctiva.

Evaluate skin integrity. Look for signs of inflammation or infection: redness, swelling, heat, or tenderness. Also note other infection signs, such as poor wound healing, wound drainage, induration (tissue hardening), or lesions. Pay close attention to sites of recent invasive procedures, such as venipunctures, bone marrow biopsies, or surgery, for evidence of wound healing.

Also check for rashes and note their distribution. For example, a butterfly-shaped rash over the nose and cheeks may indicate SLE; palpable, nonpainful, purplish lesions on the lower extremities may be Kaposi's sarcoma, which occurs with AIDS.

Observe hair texture and distribution, noting any alopecia (hair loss) on the arms, legs, or head. Alopecia in these areas and broken hairs above the forehead (lupus hairs) occur with SLE.

Inspect the client's nail color and texture, which should appear pink, smooth, and slightly convex. Pale nail beds may reflect compromised oxygen-carrying capacity (in anemia). Longitudinal striations also indicate anemia. Koilonychia (spoon-shaped nails) may occur in a client with iron-deficiency anemia. Onycholysis (nail separation from the nail bed) may result from Hashimoto's disease. In fact, the nail angle may change from 160 degrees to 180 degrees or more. This abnormality, known as finger clubbing, indicates chronic hypoxia, which sometimes occurs with an immune or blood disorder. (For more information about these assessments, see Chapter 7, Skin, Hair, and Nails.)

Head and neck. An immune or blood disorder may affect the nose and mouth. Using a pencil-thin flashlight, assess the nasal cavity. Tilt up the client's nose slightly and look for mucous membrane ulceration, which may indicate SLE, and pale, boggy turbinates, which suggest chronic allergy.

Next, inspect the oral mucous membranes. They should be pink, moist, smooth, and lesionless. Red mucous membranes suggest polycythemia; petechiae and ecchymoses suggest bleeding disorders. Fluffy white patches scattered throughout the mouth may be candidiasis, a fungal infection. Lacy white plaques on the buccal mucosa may be caused by hairy leukoplakia, associated with AIDS. Such lesions occur in a client who has immunosuppressive disorders or who receives chemotherapy.

Observe the gingivae (gums). They should be pink, moist, and slightly irregular with no spongy or edematous areas. Gingival swelling, redness, oozing, bleeding, or ulcerations can signal bleeding disorders. Also inspect the tongue. Pink and slightly rough, it should fit comfortably into the floor of the mouth. The tongue may appear smooth and beefy red in folic-acid deficiency states or enlarged in Hashimoto's disease and multiple myeloma. It may lack papillae in pernicious anemia. (For more information, see Chapter 8, Head and Neck.)

Eyes and ears. First, test the client's eye muscle strength using the six cardinal positions of gaze and the convergence tests. The client with myasthenia gravis may exhibit transient eye muscle weakness, especially when fatigued.

Next, inspect the color of the client's conjunctivae (normally pink) and sclerae (normally white). Conjunctival pallor may accompany anemia or a bleeding disorder. Scleral icterus may occur with blood disorders that cause jaundice—for example, hemolytic anemia—or with liver dysfunction, and may be noted before skin color changes. Also observe the eyelids for drooping, which occurs in myasthenia gravis, and for signs of infection or inflammation, such as swelling, redness, or lesions.

Assess the fundus with an ophthalmoscope. The retina should be light yellow to orange, and the background should be free of hemorrhages, aneurysms, and exudates. Inspection may reveal vessel tortuosity, which may accompany sickle cell anemia, or hemorrhage or infiltration, which may occur in hemorrhagic leukemia, vasculitis, or thrombocytopenia.

Test the client's hearing acuity with the whispered or spoken voice test and the watch tick test. A client with reduced auditory function may have Hashimoto's disease.

Using an otoscope, observe the tympanic membrane for erythema, bulging, indistinct landmarks, and a displaced light reflex. These are signs of otitis media, an infection that may affect a client with an immune disorder. (For more information about these procedures, see Chapter 9, Eyes and Ears.)

Respiratory system. Besides observing the client's respiratory rate, rhythm, and energy expenditure related to respiratory effort, note the position the client assumes to ease breathing. During an asthma attack, the client may sit up to use every accessory muscle of respiration. Chest expansion may be limited in a client with scleroderma. Exertional dyspnea, tachypnea, and orthopnea (difficulty breathing except in an upright position) commonly accompany the cardiac effort needed to supply oxygen to hypoxic tissues.

Percuss the client's anterior, lateral, and posterior thorax, comparing one side with the other. A dull sound indicates consolidation, which may occur with pneumonia; hyperresonance may result from trapped air, which occurs with bronchial asthma.

Auscultate over the lungs to assess for adventitious (abnormal) sounds. Wheezing suggests asthma or an allergic response. Crackles may denote a respiratory infection, such as pneumonia, which may affect a client with an immunodeficiency. (For more information about these procedures, see Chapter 10, Respiratory System.)

Cardiovascular system. Besides assessing the pulse rate and rhythm for anemia-related tachycardia or other dysrhythmias, palpate and auscultate the heart and vessels for other signs of immune or blood disorders.

First, palpate the point of maximal impulse (PMI), normally located in the fifth intercostal space at the midclavicular line. The PMI may be broadened, displaced, or less distinct because of ventricular enlargement, the body's compensatory mechanism for severe anemia.

Auscultate for heart sounds over the precordium. Normally, auscultation reveals only the first and second heart sounds (*lub-dub*). Any auscultated apical systolic murmurs may signify severe anemia; mitral, aortic, and pulmonic murmurs, sickle cell anemia; pericardial friction rub, endocarditis or pericardial effusion—which occurs in about 50% of clients with SLE.

Finally, assess the client's peripheral circulation. Begin by inspecting for Raynaud's phenomenon (intermittent arteriolar vasospasm of the fingers or toes and sometimes of the ears and nose). This phenomenon, which may be caused by SLE or scleroderma, produces blanching in the affected area followed by cyanosis, pallor, and, then, reddening. Next, palpate the peripheral pulses, which should be symmetrical and regular. Weak, irregular pulses may indicate anemia. (For more information about these procedures, see Chapter 11, Cardiovascular System.)

Gastrointestinal system. Use auscultation, percussion, palpation, and inspection of the GI system to assess for signs and symptoms of blood and immune disorders.

First, auscultate the abdomen for bowel sounds. In autoimmune disorders that cause diarrhea, such as ulcerative colitis, bowel sounds increase. In scleroderma and in autoimmune disorders that cause constipation, bowel sounds decrease.

Next, percuss the client's liver. Normally, the liver produces a dull sound over a span of 2½" to 4¾" (6 to 12 cm). Hepatomegaly (liver enlargement) may accompany many immune disorders, such as hemolytic anemia.

Then, palpate the abdomen to detect enlarged organs and tenderness. An enlarged liver that feels smooth and tender suggests hepatitis; one that feels hard and nodular suggests a neoplasm. Hepatomegaly may occur in immune disorders that cause congestion by blood cell overproduction or by excessive demand for cell destruction. Abdominal tenderness may result from infections, commonly seen in clients with immunodeficiency disorders.

Finally, inspect the anus, which should be pink and puckered without inflammation or breaks in the mucosal surface. Defer internal examination of the anus and rectal vault if you suspect or know that the client has insufficient platelets (less than 50,000/mm^3 of blood) or granulocytes (less than 1,000/mm^3 of blood). (For more information about these procedures, see Chapter 13, Gastrointestinal System.)

Urinary system. Because the urinary system also may be affected by blood and immune dysfunctions, obtain a urine specimen and evaluate its color, clarity, and odor. Normal urine appears clear and amber or straw colored. Slightly aromatic, it may look pink or grossly bloody from bladder capillary hemorrhages in a client with a coagulation disorder. Cloudy, malodorous urine may result from a urinary tract infection.

Inspect the client's urinary meatus. In a client with a WBC deficiency or immunodeficiency, the external genitalia may be focal points for inflammation. Discharge or bleeding related to infection may be noted, too. (For more information about this assessment, see Chapter 14, Urinary System.)

Nervous system. Evaluate the client's level of consciousness and mental status. The client should be alert, responding appropriately to questions and directions. Impaired neurologic function may occur secondary to hypoxia, fever, or, more drastically, from intracranial hemorrhage related to a coagulation defect. Thus, an anemic client may not be able to concentrate or may become confused; this likelihood increases for an elderly client. Hemorrhage also compromises oxygen supply to nerve tissues, resulting in similar symptoms. If bleeding occurs within the cranial vault, disorientation, progressive loss of consciousness, changes in motor and sensory capabilities, changes in pupillary responses, and seizures may result. (These responses depend on the hemorrhage site.)

Other neurologic effects may occur in a client with an immune disorder. For example, a client with SLE may experience altered mentation, depression, or psychosis; a client with rheumatoid arthritis may have peripheral neuropathies, such as numbness or tingling of fingers. (For more information about performing neurologic assessment procedures, see Chapter 17, Nervous System.)

Musculoskeletal system. Ask the client to perform simple maneuvers, such as standing up, walking, and bending over. The client should be able to perform these maneuvers effortlessly. Then test joint range of motion, particularly in the hand, wrist, and knee. Palpate the joints to assess for swelling, tenderness, and pain. Autoimmune disorders, such as SLE, rheumatoid arthritis, and hemarthrosis, can limit range of motion and cause joint enlargement. If palpation reveals bone tenderness in the sternum, the cause may be bone marrow hyperactivity, a compensatory mechanism for oxygen-carrying deficits prevalent in anemias. Bone tenderness may also result from a leukemic or immunoproliferative disorder, such as plasma cell myeloma, that causes cell packing in the marrow. Skeletal pain also may be from direct disease invasion of the marrow in some leukemias or immunoproliferative disorders—for example, plasma cell myeloma. (For more information about musculoskeletal assessment, see Chapter 18, Musculoskeletal System.)

Inspection

The first step in regional lymph node assessment is to inspect areas where the client reports "swollen glands" or "lumps" for color abnormalities and visible lymph node enlargement. Then inspect all other nodal regions. Proceed from head to toe to avoid missing any region. Normally, lymph nodes cannot be seen.

Visibly enlarged nodes suggest a current or previous inflammation. Nodes covered with red-streaked skin suggest acute lymphadenitis (lymph node inflammation).

(Text continues on page 572.)

Palpating the lymph nodes

When assessing a client for signs of an immune or blood disorder, the nurse should palpate the superficial lymph nodes of the head and neck, axillary, epitrochlear, inguinal, and popliteal areas, using the pads of the index and middle fingers. Always palpate gently; begin with light pressure and gradually increase the pressure.

Head and neck nodes

Head and neck nodes are best palpated with the client in a sitting position.

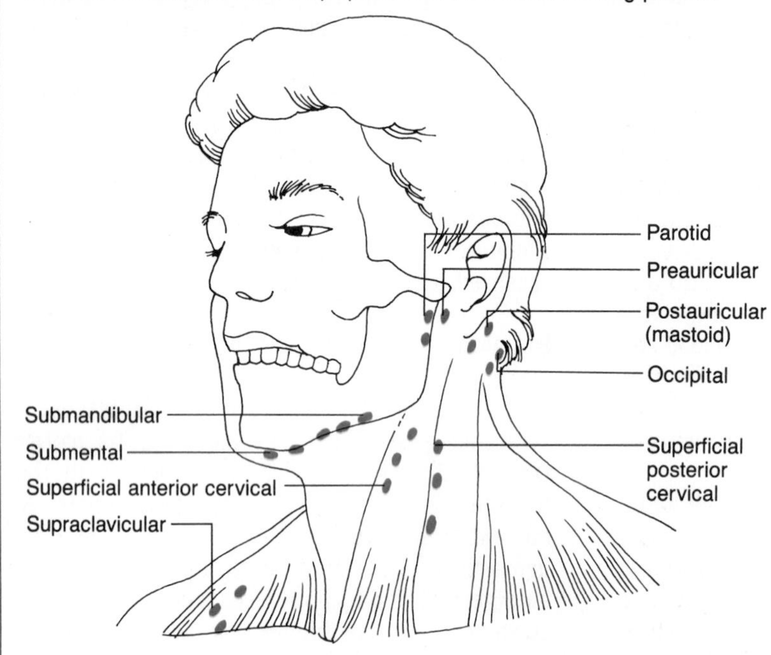

To palpate the submandibular, submental, anterior cervical, and occipital nodes, position your fingers as shown. Palpate over the mandibular surface and continue moving up and down the entire neck. Flex the head forward or to the side being examined. This relaxes the tissues and makes enlarged nodes more palpable. Reverse your hand position to palpate the opposite side.

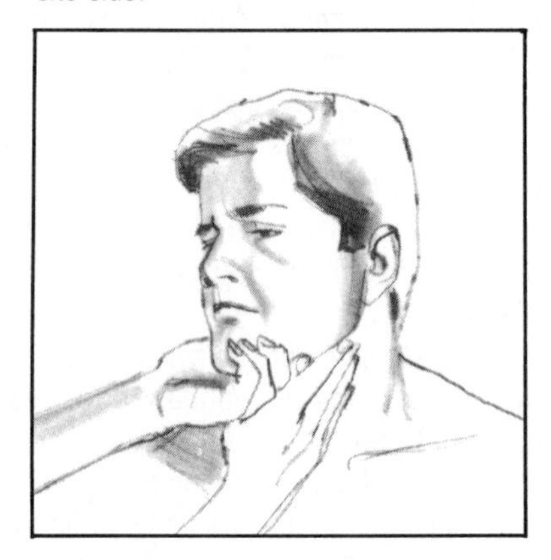

To palpate the preauricular, parotid, and mastoid nodes, position your fingers as shown.

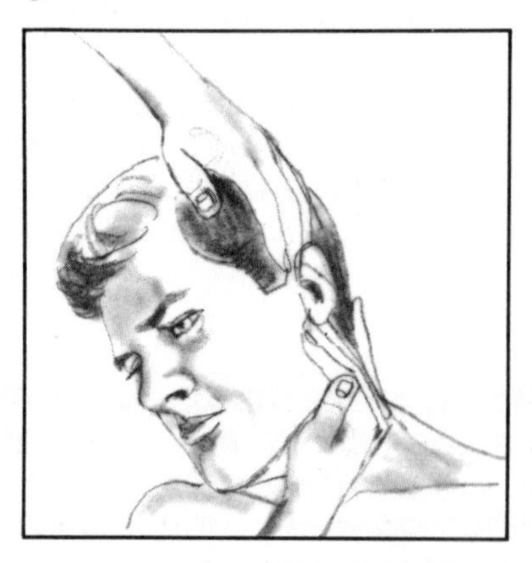

To palpate the posterior cervical nodes and spinal nerve chain, place your fingertip pads along the anterior surface of the trapezius muscle. Then move your fingertips toward the posterior surface of the sternocleidomastoid muscle.

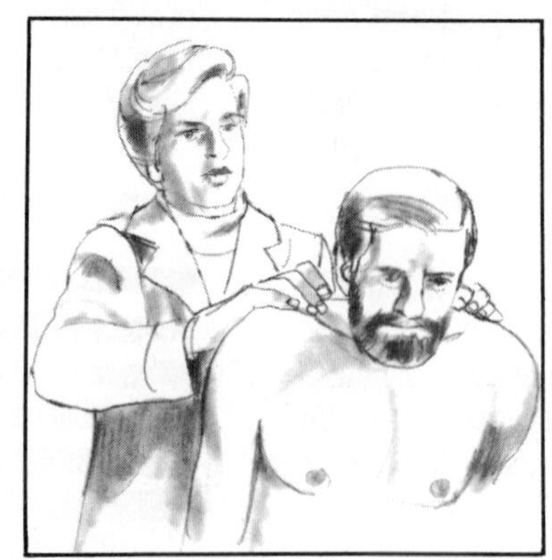

To palpate the supraclavicular nodes, encourage the client to relax so the clavicles drop. To relax the soft tissues of the anterior neck, flex the client's head slightly forward with your free hand. Then hook your left index finger over the clavicle lateral to the sternocleidomastoid muscle. Rotate your fingers deeply into this area to feel these nodes.

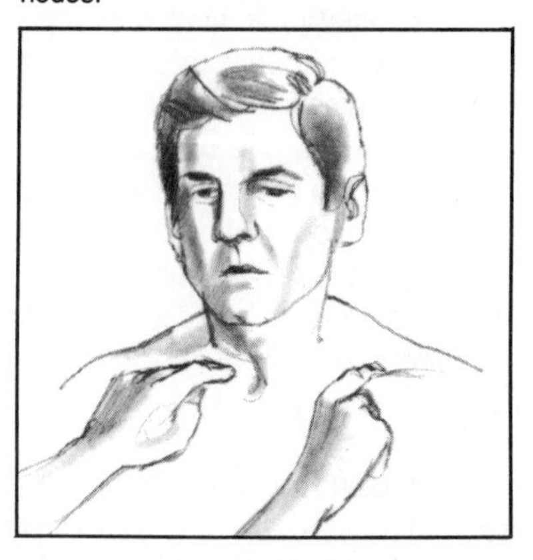

Axillary and epitrochlear nodes

Axillary and epitrochlear nodes are best palpated with the client in a sitting position. Axillary nodes may also be palpated with the client lying supine.

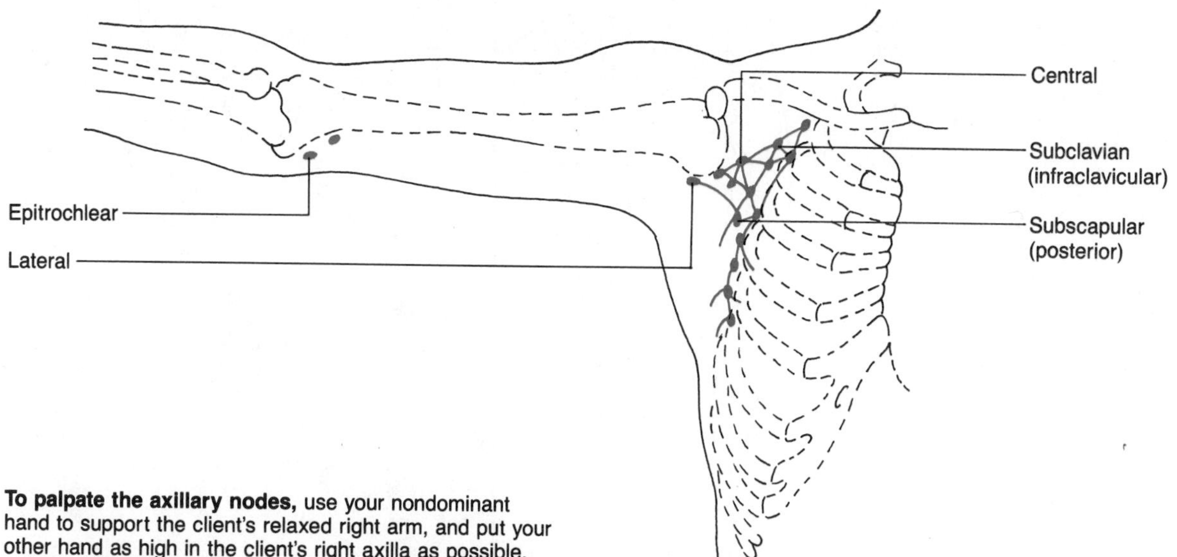

To palpate the axillary nodes, use your nondominant hand to support the client's relaxed right arm, and put your other hand as high in the client's right axilla as possible.

Then palpate the axillary nodes, gently pressing the soft tissues against the chest wall and the muscles surrounding the axilla (the pectorals, latissimus dorsi, subscapular, and anterior serratus). Repeat this procedure for the left axilla.

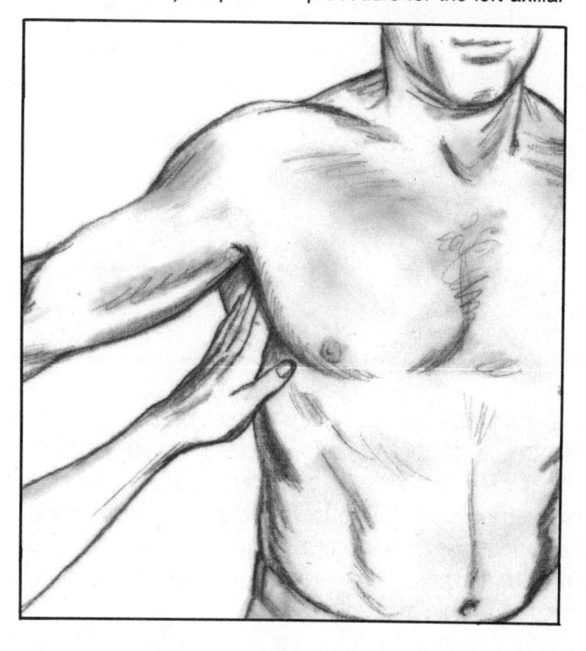

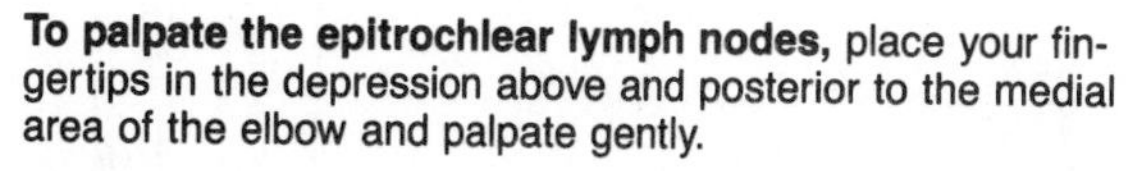

To palpate the epitrochlear lymph nodes, place your fingertips in the depression above and posterior to the medial area of the elbow and palpate gently.

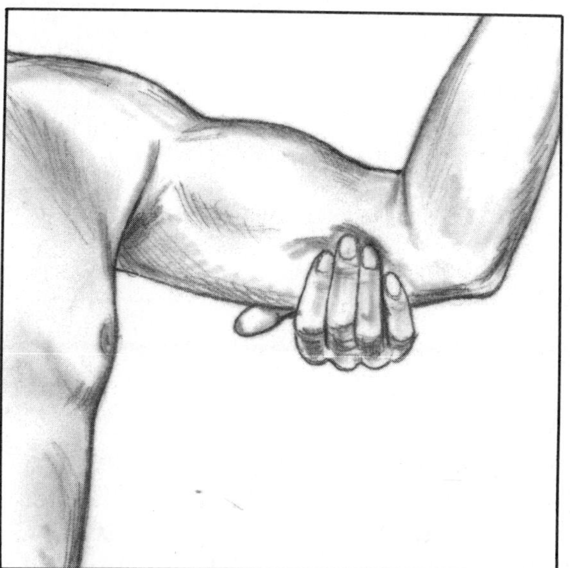

continued

Palpating the lymph nodes continued

Inguinal and popliteal nodes
Inguinal and popliteal nodes are best palpated with the client lying supine. Popliteal nodes may also be assessed with the client sitting or standing.

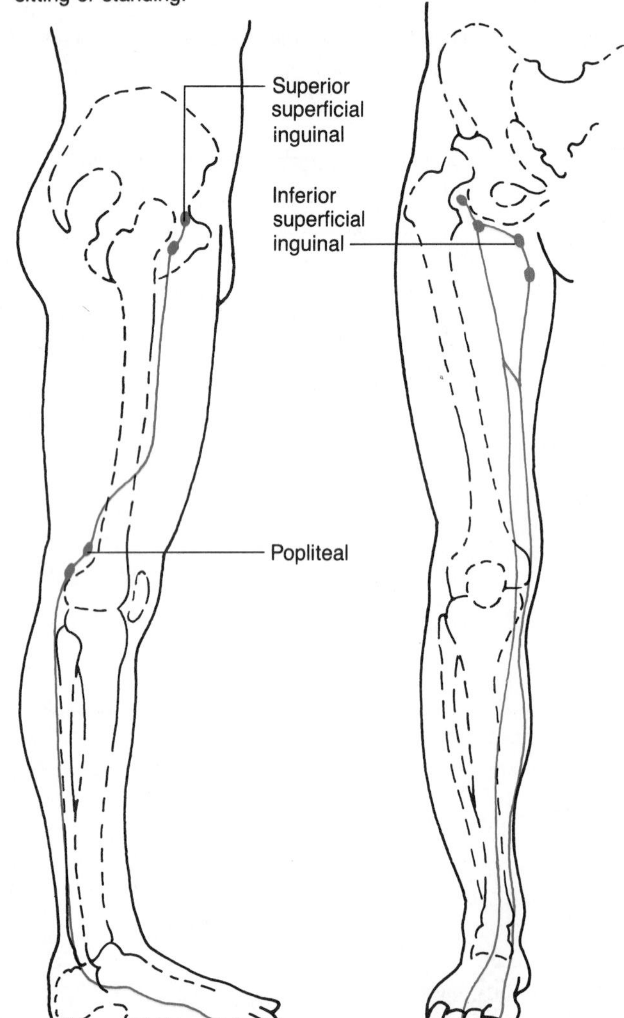

To palpate the inferior superficial inguinal (femoral) lymph nodes, gently press below the junction of the saphenous and femoral veins.

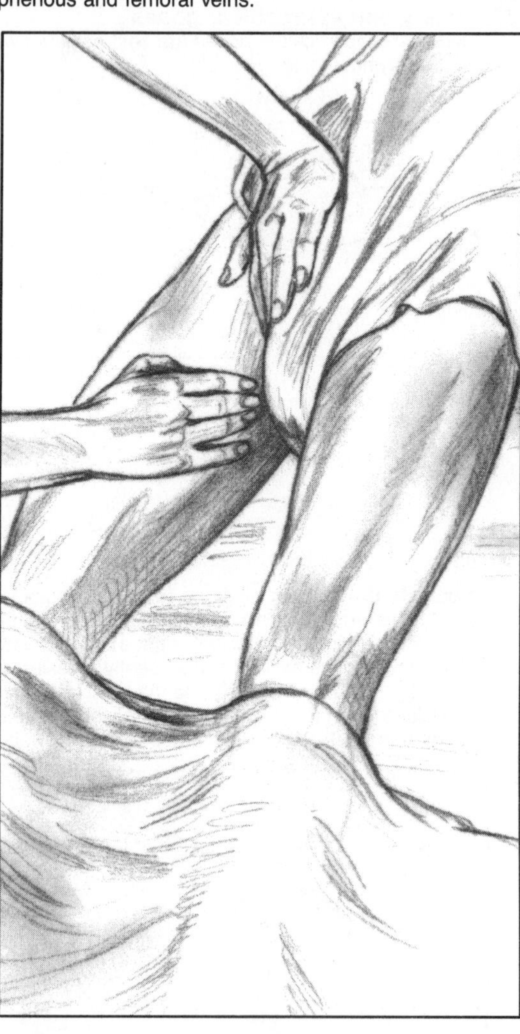

Palpation

Use the pads of your index and middle fingers to palpate the client's superficial lymph nodes in the head and neck, axillary, epitrochlear, inguinal, and popliteal areas. Apply gentle pressure and rotary motion to feel the underlying nodes without obscuring them by pressing them into deeper soft tissues. (For an illustrated procedure, see *Palpating the lymph nodes,* pages 570 to 573.)

Normally, lymph nodes cannot be felt in a healthy client. The number of nodes varies from client to client.

If palpation reveals nodal enlargement or other abnormalities, note the following characteristics: location, size, shape, surface, consistency, symmetry, mobility, color, tenderness, temperature, pulsations, and vascularity of the node.

To describe the location of the node, use reference points such as body axis and lines to pinpoint the site, or sketch the location, if appropriate. Then indicate the

To palpate the superior superficial inguinal lymph nodes, press along the course of the saphenous veins from the inguinal area to the abdomen.

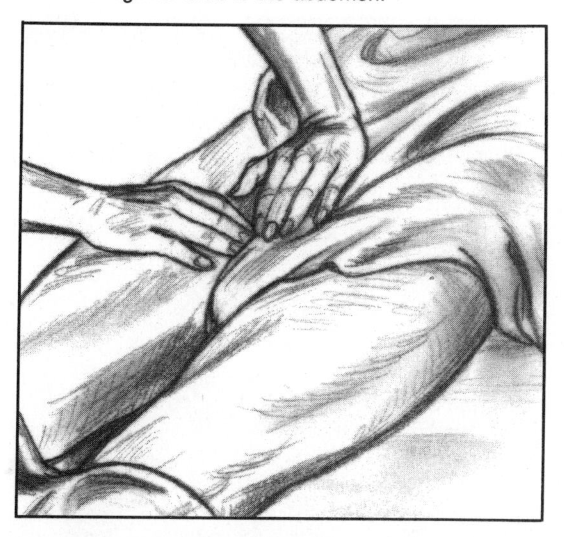

To palpate the popliteal nodes, press gently along the posterior muscles at the back of the knee.

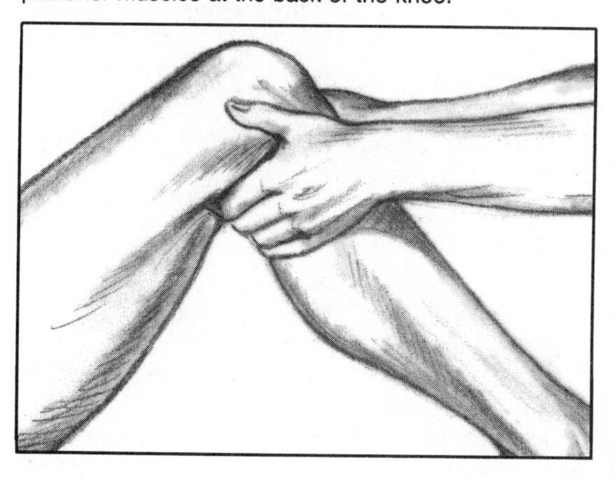

nodal length, width, and depth in centimeters, and describe or sketch its shape. Accurately describe its surface as smooth, nodular, or irregular. Identify the consistency of the node, as hard, soft, firm, resilient, spongy, or cystic. Evaluate its symmetry, comparing the node with similar structures on the other side of the body. Describe the node's degree of mobility. If it is immobile, indicate whether it is fixed to overlying tissues, underlying tissues, or both. During palpation, use the *PQRST* method to help the client describe any tenderness. Note whether the tenderness was elicited by palpation, movement, or rebound phenomenon (tenderness that occurs after the pressure of the palpating fingerpads is released). Describe any color change, such as pallor, erythema, or cyanosis, in overlying skin. Note whether the site feels warm. Be alert for pulsations in the mass; plan to auscultate a pulsating mass for a bruit. If the node exhibits increased vascularity, describe any changes in the overlying blood vessels.

Use a flashlight to assess further an abnormal lump in an area that can be transilluminated, such as the scrotum. Describe the results of transillumination along with the other characteristics. A lump that allows light to pass through it indicates fluid, which usually defines a cyst rather than a node.

Abnormal findings

Enlarged lymph nodes may result from an increase in the number and size of lymphocytes and reticuloendothelial cells that normally line the node or from infiltration by cells not normally part of the structure (as in metastasized cancers). The clinical significance of a palpated node depends on its location, the client's age (a child with a mild infection may have swollen nodes, whereas nodal enlargement in an adult is usually more significant), and even the client's working and living environment (exposure to chemicals, pollutants, animals, or insects).

Red streaks in the skin, palpable nodes, and lymphedema may indicate a lymphatic disorder. Enlarged nodes suggest current or recent inflammation. Tender nodes usually denote infection. In acute infection, nodes are large, tender, and discrete; in chronic infection, they become confluent (run together). Metastasized cancer usually affects nodes unilaterally, causing them to become discrete, nontender, firm or hard, and fixed. Generalized lymphadenopathy (involving three or more node groups) can indicate an autoimmune (for example, SLE), an infectious, or a neoplastic disorder. In SLE, nodal enlargement may be localized or generalized. (For assessment findings associated with some common immune system and blood disorders, see *Integrating assessment findings,* page 574.)

Developmental considerations

Although blood and immune system physical assessment techniques are essentially the same for all ages, normal findings are different for a child or an elderly client.

Pediatric client

Often, in a client under age 12, lymph nodes can be palpated. For instance, cervical and inguinal nodes, measuring from 1 to 3 cm (about an inch or less), may be

Integrating assessment findings

Sometimes, a cluster of abnormal assessment findings will strongly suggest a particular immune or blood disorder. In the chart below, column one shows groups of presenting signs and symptoms—the ones that make the client seek medical attention. Column two shows related assessment findings that the nurse may discover during the health history and physical assessment. The client may exhibit one or more of these findings. Column three shows the possible disorder indicated by a cluster of of these findings.

PRESENTING SIGNS AND SYMPTOMS	RELATED ASSESSMENT FINDINGS	POSSIBLE DISORDER
Fatigue, weakness, fever, severe joint pain in multiple sites, dyspnea, bone pain, chest or abdominal pain, painless hematuria, recurrent infection	Black race (most common in Black Americans of African descent) Presence of two hemoglobin S genes Failure to thrive Tachycardia Cardiac hypertrophy Cardiac murmur Pulmonary infarctions Tachypnea Hepatomegaly Joint swelling Jaundice or pallor	Sickle cell anemia
Swollen neck glands, night sweats, pruritus, weight loss of 10% of body weight, increased susceptibility to infection	Age (incidence rises sharply after age 10, peaks around age 25, then declines until after age 50 when it rises again with age) Enlarged, rubbery, painless lymph nodes Splenomegaly Pallor Sternberg-Reed cells found on lymph node biopsy	Hodgkin's disease
Abnormal bleeding, such as epistaxis, spontaneous bruising, or bleeding ulcers; fatigue; weakness; possible joint pain; headaches; dizziness; tinnitus; vertigo; blurred vision; pruritus; chest pain; dyspnea; gastrointestinal distress; intermittent claudication	Jewish culture Male sex Middle to old age Plethora (ruddy cyanosis of the face, hands, and mucous membranes) Ecchymoses Engorged conjunctival and retinal veins Enlarged, firm, nontender spleen Hypertension Thrombosis Emboli	Primary polycythemia (polycythemia vera)
Fatigue, weakness, fever, painless lymphadenopathy, occasional abnormal bleeding, joint pain at multiple sites, anorexia, weight loss, malaise, muscle pain, cough, photosensitivity	Female sex (most common in females aged 10 to 35) Butterfly rash on cheeks and bridge of nose Pigmentation changes Alopecia Raynaud's phenomenon Pericarditis, pleural effusion, myocarditis, nephritis Hepatomegaly Splenomegaly Mental status alterations Convulsive disorders	Systemic lupus erythematosus (SLE)
Fatigue, weakness, lymphadenopathy, cough, weight loss	Infection with unusual pathogen Recurrent infections Homosexual or bisexual preference Use of intravenous drugs History of hemophilia (with blood transfusions before 1985) Engagement in unsafe sexual practices Weight loss greater than 10% of body weight	Acquired immunodeficiency syndrome (AIDS)

ADVANCED ASSESSMENT SKILLS

Percussing and palpating the spleen

To assess the spleen, the nurse can use percussion to estimate its size and palpation to detect tenderness and enlargement.

Percussion
To percuss the spleen, follow these steps:

1 Percuss the lowest intercostal space in the left anterior axillary line; percussion notes should be tympanic.

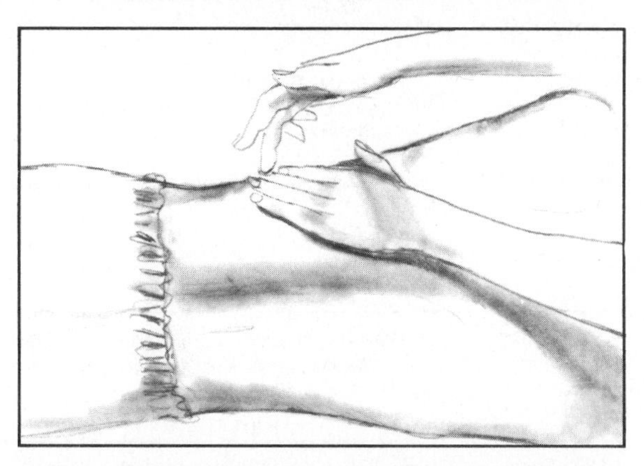

2 Ask the client to take a deep breath, then percuss this area again. If the spleen is normal in size, the area will remain tympanic. If the tympanic percussion note changes on inspiration to dullness, the spleen is probably enlarged.

3 To estimate spleen size, outline the spleen's edges by percussing in several directions from areas of tympany to areas of dullness.

Palpation
To palpate the spleen, follow these steps:

1 Stand on the right side of the supine client. Then reach across the client to support the posterior lower left rib cage with your left hand. Place your right hand below the left costal margin and press inward.

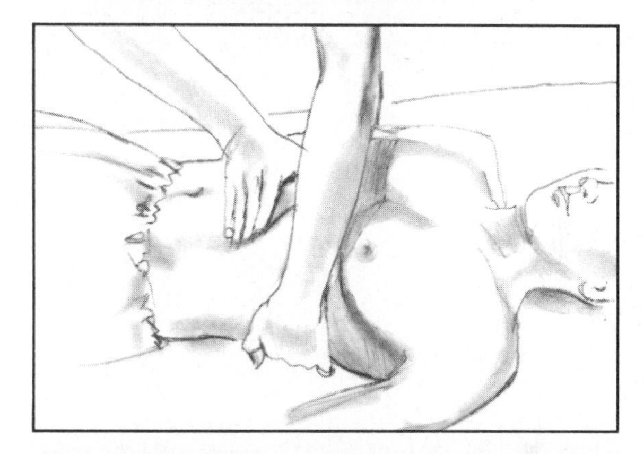

2 Instruct the client to take a deep breath. The spleen normally should not descend on deep inspiration below the ninth or tenth intercostal space in the posterior midaxillary line. If the spleen is enlarged, you will feel its rigid border. Do not overpalpate the spleen; an enlarged spleen can rupture easily.

felt. Moderate numbers of cool, firm, movable, and painless nodes indicate past infection. The liver (1 to 2 cm below the right costal margin) or a spleen tip (at the left costal margin), too, may be palpable in a child. Of course, neither should be tender.

Elderly client

When assessing an elderly client, remember that immune system and blood-forming activities decline with age. The number and size of nodes also decrease with age, as lymphoid capabilities decline and fatty degeneration and fibrosis take place. This reduces the febrile response to infection.

Advanced assessment skills

To assess the immune system and blood further, percuss and palpate the spleen. (For an illustrated procedure, see *Advanced assessment skills: Percussing and palpating the spleen.)*

First, percuss the spleen to estimate its size. On percussion, the spleen normally produces tympany in the left anterior axillary line between the sixth and tenth ribs. Spleen enlargement (splenomegaly) may indicate an immune disorder, such as hemolytic anemia.

Next, palpate the spleen to detect tenderness and confirm splenomegaly. The spleen must be enlarged approximately three times normal size to be palpable. Splenic tenderness may result from infections, commonly seen in a client with an immunodeficiency disorder. Splenomegaly may occur in immune disorders that cause congestion by cell overproduction or by excessive demand for cell destruction.

(Text continues on page 581.)

Common laboratory studies

For a client with signs and symptoms of an immune or blood disorder, various laboratory studies can provide valuable clues to the possible cause, as shown in the chart below. (*Note:* Keep in mind that abnormal findings may stem from a problem unrelated to the immune system or blood.) Remember that values differ among laboratories. Check the normal value range for the specific laboratory.

TEST AND SIGNIFICANCE	NORMAL VALUES OR FINDINGS	ABNORMAL FINDINGS	POSSIBLE IMMUNE, BLOOD, OR RELATED CAUSES OF ABNORMAL FINDINGS
Bone marrow test			
Bone marrow aspiration This test evaluates hematopoiesis by showing blood elements and precursors as well as abnormal or malignant cells.	*Normoblasts, total* Adult: 25.6% Child: 23.1% Infant: 8%	Above-normal level	Polycythemia vera
		Below-normal level	Vitamin B_{12} or folic acid deficiency; iron-deficiency anemia; hemolytic, hypoplastic, or aplastic anemia
	Neutrophils, total Adult: 56.5% Child: 57.1% Infant: 32.4%	Above-normal level	Acute myeloblastic or chronic myeloid leukemia
		Below-normal level	Lymphoblastic, lymphatic, or monocytic leukemia; aplastic anemia
	Eosinophils Adult: 3.1% Child: 3.6% Infant: 2.6%	Above-normal level	Bone marrow carcinoma, lymphadenoma, myeloid leukemia, eosinophilic leukemia, pernicious anemia in relapse
	Basophils Adult: 0.01% Child: 0.06% Infant: 0.07%	Above-normal level	Chronic myelocytic leukemia, polycythemia vera
	Lymphocytes Adult: 16.2% Child: 16% Infant: 49%	Above-normal level	Lymphatic leukemia, lymphosarcoma, lymphoblastic or follicular lymphoma, mononucleosis, aplastic anemia, macroglobulinemia
	Plasma cells Adult: 1.3% Child: 0.4% Infant: 0.02%	Above-normal level	Myeloma, collagen disease, infection, antigen sensitivity, malignancy
	Megakaryocytes Adult: 0.1% Child: 0.1% Infant: 0.05%	Above-normal level	Advanced age, chronic myeloid leukemia, polycythemia vera, megakaryocytic myelosis, infection, idiopathic thrombocytopenic purpura, thrombocytopenia
		Below-normal level	Pernicious anemia
	Myeloiderythroid ratio Adult: 2:3 Child: 2:9 Infant: 4:4	Above-normal level	Myeloid leukemia, infection, leukemoid reactions, depressed hematopoiesis
		Below-normal level	Agranulocytosis, hematopoiesis after hemorrhage or hemolysis, iron-deficiency anemia, polycythemia vera
Blood tests			
Peripheral blood smear This test shows maturity and morphology of red blood cells (RBCs) and determines qualitative abnormalities.	Anucleated biconcave RBC disks 6 to 8 microns in diameter and uniform in size, shape, and	Macrocytic (abnormally large) cells	Pernicious anemia
		Microcytic (abnormally small) cells	Iron-deficiency anemia, thalassemia

Common laboratory studies continued

TEST AND SIGNIFICANCE	NORMAL VALUES OR FINDINGS	ABNORMAL FINDINGS	POSSIBLE IMMUNE, BLOOD, OR RELATED CAUSES OF ABNORMAL FINDINGS
Peripheral blood smear (continued)	staining characteristics	Sickling cells	Sickle cell anemia
		Target cells	Thalassemias, hemoglobinopathies, liver disease
		Spherocytes	Hereditary spherocytosis, hemolytic conditions (mechanical injury)
		Schistocytes	Microangiopathic hemolytic anemia, anemias associated with uremia and hypertension, hemolysis from physical agents or toxins
Complete blood count (CBC) This test determines the actual number of blood elements in relation to volume and quantifies abnormalities.	*Erythrocyte (RBC) count* Man: 4.5 to 6.2 million/mm³ Woman: 4.2 to 5.4 million/mm³ Child: 4.6 to 4.8 million/mm³ Full-term neonate: 4.4 to 5.8 million/mm³	Above-normal level	Primary or secondary polycythemia, dehydration
		Below-normal level	Anemia, fluid overload, recent hemorrhage
	Hematocrit (HCT or packed RBC volume) Man: 42% to 54% Woman: 38% to 46% Child: 36% to 40% Neonate: 55% to 68%	Above-normal level	Polycythemia, hemoconcentration related to blood loss, dehydration
		Below-normal level	Anemia, hemodilution
	Hemoglobin (Hb) Man: 14 to 18 g/dl; 12.4 to 14.9 g/dl (after middle age) Woman: 12 to 16 g/dl; 11.7 to 13.8 g/dl (after middle age) Child: 11 to 13 g/dl Neonate: 17 to 22 g/dl	Above-normal level	Hemoconcentration from polycythemia or dehydration
		Below-normal level	Anemia, recent hemorrhage or fluid retention causing hemodilution
Red blood cell indices These tests provide information about the size (MCV), hemoglobin weight (MCH), and hemoglobin concentration (MCHC) of an average RBC.	*Mean corpuscular volume (MCV)* 84 to 99 μm³/RBC	Above-normal level of MCV	Macrocytic anemias related to megaloblastic anemias, folic acid or vitamin B_{12} deficiency, inherited DNA synthesis disorders, reticulocytosis
	Mean corpuscular hemoglobin (MCH) 26 to 32 pg/RBC	Below-normal level of MCV and MCHC	Microcytic, hypochromic anemias related to iron-deficiency anemia, pyridoxine-responsive anemia, thalassemia

continued

Common laboratory studies continued

TEST AND SIGNIFICANCE	NORMAL VALUES OR FINDINGS	ABNORMAL FINDINGS	POSSIBLE IMMUNE, BLOOD, OR RELATED CAUSES OF ABNORMAL FINDINGS
Red blood cell indices (continued)	*Mean corpuscular hemoglobin concentration (MCHC)* 30% to 36%		
Leukocyte (WBC) count This test, along with the differential white cell count, establishes the quantity and maturity of white blood cell (WBC) elements in the blood.	4,100 to 10,900/ mm^3	Above-normal level (leukocytosis)	Infection (usually); leukemia; tissue necrosis from burns, myocardial infarction (MI), or gangrene
		Below-normal level (leukopenia)	Bone marrow depression related to viral infections, toxic reactions (from antineoplastic or other drugs), typhoid fever, radiation, alcoholism, diabetes, multiple myeloma
Differential white cell count This test evaluates WBC distribution and morphology, providing more information about the body's ability to resist and overcome infection than the WBC count alone. It classifies cells by type and subtype into granulocytes (neutrophils, eosinophils, and basophils) and agranulocytes (monocytes and lymphocytes). The test also determines the percentage of each blood cell type. To determine the absolute number for each type, multiply the percentage by the total WBC number.	*Neutrophils* 47.6% to 76.8%	Above-normal level (neutrophilia)	Bacterial and parasitic infections, metabolic disturbances (gout, diabetic or uremic coma, eclampsia)
		Above-normal level of mature cells	Hemolysis, use of certain drugs (diuretic mercurials, sulfonamides), tissue breakdown (burns, MI, tumors, gangrene, hemolytic transfusion reaction, or after surgery for liver, GI tract, bone marrow cancers)
		Below-normal level (neutropenia)	Acute viral infections, blood diseases, toxic agents, hormonal diseases, massive overwhelming infection in debilitated client
	Eosinophils 0.3% to 7%	Above-normal level (eosinophilia)	Hyperimmune, allergic, and degenerative reactions; antigen-antibody reactions in allergies, parasitic disease, Addison's disease, lung and bone cancer, chronic skin infections, myelogenous leukemia, Hodgkin's disease, polycythemia, subacute infections, polyarteritis nodosa, various tumors
		Below-normal level (eosinopenia)	Increased adrenal steroid production from stress, infectious mononucleosis, hypersplenism; congestive heart failure; Cushing's syndrome; aplastic and pernicious anemias; use of ACTH, epinephrine, or thyroxine; infections (with neutrophilia)
	Basophils 0.3% to 2%	Above-normal level (basophilia)	Granulocytic and basophilic leukemia and myeloid metaplasia (usually), chronic inflammation, polycythemia vera, postsplenectomy, healing phase of inflammation, postradiation
		Below-normal level	Acute allergic reactions, hyperthyroidism, stress reactions as in MI and bleeding peptic ulcer, hypersensitivity reactions, prolonged steroid therapy

Common laboratory studies continued

TEST AND SIGNIFICANCE	NORMAL VALUES OR FINDINGS	ABNORMAL FINDINGS	POSSIBLE IMMUNE, BLOOD, OR RELATED CAUSES OF ABNORMAL FINDINGS
Differential white cell count (continued)	*Monocytes* 0.6% to 9.6%	Above-normal level	Viral infections, bacterial and parasitic infestations, collagen diseases, hematologic disorders
	Lymphocytes 16.2% to 43%	Above-normal level	Infections such as pertussis, brucellosis, syphilis, tuberculosis, hepatitis, infectious mononucleosis, mumps, rubella, and cytomegalovirus; thyrotoxicosis; hypoadrenalism; ulcerative colitis; immune diseases; lymphocytic leukemia
		Below-normal level	Severe debilitating illness such as congestive heart failure, renal failure, and advanced tuberculosis; defective lymphatic circulation; high levels of adrenal corticosteroid related to immunodeficiency or immunosuppressive drugs
Erythrocyte (osmotic) fragility This test measures RBC resistance to hemolysis on exposure to a series of increasingly dilute saline solutions to confirm morphologic abnormalities and diagnose hereditary spherocytosis.	Normal curve as plotted against known normals	High osmotic fragility (cells burst easily)	Hereditary spherocytosis; spherocytosis associated with autoimmune hemolytic anemia, severe burns, chemical poisoning, and hemolytic disease of the newborn (erythroblastosis fetalis)
		Low osmotic fragility (cells resist bursting)	Thalassemia, iron-deficiency anemia, sickle cell anemia, other RBC disorders in which target cells and wafer cells are found; postsplenectomy
Erythrocyte sedimentation rate (ESR) This test measures the time required for RBCs in a whole blood sample to settle to the bottom of a verticle tube, displacing the plasma upward, which retards settling of other blood elements. The ESR is a sensitive, but nonspecific, early indicator of occult inflammatory or malignant diseases.	0 to 20 mm/hour Rates gradually increase with age.	Above-normal level	Pregnancy, acute or chronic inflammation, tuberculosis, paraproteinemias, rheumatic fever, rheumatoid arthritis, some cancers, anemias
		Below-normal level	Polycythemia, sickle cell anemia, hyperviscosity, low plasma protein levels
Platelet (thrombocyte) count This test assesses the number of platelets in a blood sample. It evaluates production of platelets, which are vital to coagulation; assesses the effects of chemotherapy and radiation on platelet production; and aids diagnosis of platelet disorders.	130,000 to 370,000/ mm^3	Above-normal level (thrombocytosis)	Primary thrombocytosis, myelofibrosis with myeloid metaplasia, polycythemia vera, chronic myelogenous leukemia, hemorrhage, infectious disorders, carcinomas, iron-deficiency anemia, recent surgery, splenectomy, pregnancy, inflammatory disorders
		Below-normal level (thrombocytopenia)	Aplastic or hypoplastic bone marrow; infiltrative bone marrow disease (such as carcinoma or leukemia); megakaryocytic hypoplasia; folic acid or vitamin B_{12} deficiency; disseminated intravascular coagulation (DIC); increased platelet destruction from drugs, immunotherapy, or mechanical injury

continued

Common laboratory studies *continued*

TEST AND SIGNIFICANCE	NORMAL VALUES OR FINDINGS	ABNORMAL FINDINGS	POSSIBLE IMMUNE, BLOOD, OR RELATED CAUSES OF ABNORMAL FINDINGS
Activated partial thromboplastin time (APTT) This test evaluates the clotting factors of the intrinsic pathway, except for Factors VII and XIII, by measuring the time required for fibrin clot formation after adding calcium and phospholipid emulsion to a plasma sample.	25 to 36 seconds	Prolonged time	Deficiency of plasma clotting factors other than VII and XIII; presence of heparin; presence of fibrin split products, fibrinolysins, or circulating antibodies that are specific to the clotting factors
Prothrombin time (PT) Although less sensitive than the APTT, this test aids in evaluating thrombin generation (extrinsic clotting mechanism). It indirectly measures prothrombin by measuring the time required for a fibrin clot to form in a citrated plasma sample after the addition of calcium and tissue thromboplastin.	Male: 9.6 to 11.8 seconds Female: 9.5 to 11.3 seconds	Prolonged time	Deficiencies in fibrinogen, prothrombin, Factors V, VII, or X, or vitamin K; hepatic disease; oral anticoagulant therapy
		Time exceeding 2½ times normal	Abnormal bleeding related to causes above
Plasma thrombin time (thrombin clotting time) This test estimates plasma fibrinogen levels by measuring how quickly a clot forms when thrombin is added to plasma samples from client and a normal control.	10 to 15 seconds	Prolonged time (>1.3 times the control time)	Effective heparin therapy, hepatic disease, DIC, hypofibrinogenemia, macroglobulinemia, multiple myeloma
Plasma fibrinogen (Factor I) This test measures the level of plasma protein fibrinogen available for coagulation. In this test, thrombin is added to a citrated plasma sample, a clot forms and is then dissolved, and its proteins assayed.	195 to 365 mg/dl	Above-normal level	Hemostatic stress; nonspecific stresses such as inflammation, pregnancy, or autoimmune disorders; stomach, breast, or kidney carcinomas
		Below-normal level	Congenital afibrinogenemia; hypofibrinogenemia; dysfibrinogenemia; DIC; fibrinolysis; severe hepatic disease; carcinoma of the prostate, pancreas, or lung; lesions that occupy or replace bone marrow; acute illness that consumes excessive amounts of fibrinogen, such as trauma or obstetric complications
Fibrin split products (fibrinogen degradation products, FDP) This test detects the breakdown products of fibrin and fibrinogen that occur in response to the activity of plasmin, the fibrin-dissolving enzyme that prevents excessive clotting. Fibrin split products have anticoagulant activity, so excessive levels inhibit clot formation.	*Screening assay* <10 mcg/ml *Quantitative assay* <3 mcg/ml	Above-normal level	Primary and secondary fibrinolytic states, alcoholic cirrhosis, postcesarean birth, preeclampsia, abruptio placentae, congenital heart disease, sunstroke, burns, intrauterine death, pulmonary embolus, deep-vein thrombosis, MI, portacaval shunt, acute leukemia, incompatible blood transfusions, hypoxia, after thoracic or cardiac surgery and renal transplant

Common laboratory studies continued

TEST AND SIGNIFICANCE	NORMAL VALUES OR FINDINGS	ABNORMAL FINDINGS	POSSIBLE IMMUNE, BLOOD, OR RELATED CAUSES OF ABNORMAL FINDINGS
Direct antiglobulin test (DAGT, direct Coombs' test) This test demonstrates the presence of IgB antibodies (such as antibodies to the Rh factor) or complement on circulating RBCs.	Negative (neither antibodies nor complement appear on RBCs)	Positive (antibodies or complement appear on RBCs)	Autoimmune hemolytic anemic (idiopathic, drug-induced, or related to underlying disease); certain diseases (sepsis) or medications (cephalothin, penicillin) in clients who do not demonstrate hemolysis; hemolytic disease of the newborn
Immunoelectrophoresis This test identifies immunoglobulins IgG, IgA, and IgM in a serum sample by nephelometry. It assesses the effectiveness of chemotherapy or radiation therapy, detects hypogammaglobulinemias and hypergammaglobulinemias, and diagnoses paraproteinemias.	*IgG* 6.4 to 14.3 mg/ml *IgA* 0.3 to 3 mg/ml *IgM* 0.2 to 1.4 mg/ml	Above-normal levels of all three	Hepatic disorders such as hepatitis; other disorders such as rheumatoid arthritis and systemic lupus erythematosus
		Below-normal levels of all three	Immunoglobulin disorders such as lymphoid aplasia and agammaglobulinemia; myelomas and leukemias such as heavy chain disease and chronic lymphocytic leukemia
		Combinations of normal, above-normal, and below-normal levels of all three	Immunoglobulin disorders, myelomas, leukemias, hepatic disorders, other disorders
Enzyme-linked immunosorbent assay (ELISA) This test identifies antibodies to bacteria, viruses, DNA, and allergens as well as substances such as carcinoembryonic antigens and immunoglobulins.	Negative for antibodies	Positive for antibodies	Exposure to human immunodeficiency virus (HIV)

Documentation

Before documenting, the nurse evaluates what the assessment findings indicate by reviewing and integrating the physical assessment data about the client's vital signs, immune system and blood, and related systems with the client's health history.

The final step in immune system and blood assessment includes evaluating the client's laboratory study results. (For a summary of frequently used studies and their significance, see *Common laboratory studies*, pages 576 to 581.) Together with the physical assessment and health history data, these results should clarify the client's clinical status.

Assessment data collection is the first step in the nursing process. Based on these data, appropriate nursing diagnoses allow you to plan, implement, and evaluate holistic, individualized client care. (For a case study that integrates immune system and blood assessment findings into the nursing process, see *Applying the nursing process*, pages 582 and 583.)

After completing the assessment, document the data completely, including normal and abnormal findings. The following example shows how to document some normal physical assessment findings:

Height: 5′10″
Weight: 157 lb
Vital signs: Blood pressure 126/60, temperature 98.0° F. (36.7° C.), pulse 54 and regular, respirations 16 and regular.

Oriented to person, place, and time. Eye examination normal. Skin color and integrity normal, without petechiae or ecchymoses. Other body systems normal, with recent pneumonia completely resolved. Spleen and liver not palpable. Percussion

(Text continues on page 584.)

Applying the nursing process

Assessment findings form the basis of the nursing process. Using them, the nurse formulates the nursing diagnoses and develops appropriate planning, implementation, and evaluation of the client's care.

The table below shows how the nurse can use immune system and blood assessment data in the nursing process for the client described in the case history (shown at right). In the first column, history and physical assessment data are followed by a paragraph of mental notes. These notes help the nurse make important mental connections among assessment findings, aiding in development of the nursing diagnoses and planning.

The second column presents several appropriate nursing diagnoses; however, the information in the remaining three columns is based on the *first* nursing diagnosis. Although it is not part of the nursing process, documentation appears in the last column because of its importance. Documentation consists of an initial note using all components of the SOAPIE format and a follow-up note using the appropriate SOAPIE components.

ASSESSMENT	NURSING DIAGNOSES	PLANNING	IMPLEMENTATION
Subjective (history) data • Client states: "I'm tired all the time. I have to make an effort to go to work each morning." • Client reports prolonged menses lasting 9 days. • Client reports intermittent, localized, dull sternal pain. • Clients says her appetite is poor; she has lost 15 pounds (6.75 kg) over the past 3 weeks. Client denies alcohol use. • Client denies recent acute illness, headache, or dyspnea. Recalls mild gingival bleeding after tooth brushing, but no other unusual bleeding. **Objective (physical) data** • Vital signs: blood pressure 126/84 mm Hg, temperature 100° F. (37.8 ° C.), pulse 100 and regular, respirations 22 and regular. • Skin pale. Scattered ecchymoses noted on legs bilaterally. Petechiae seen at site of recent blood pressure cuff placement. Petechiae also appear around the waist and lower border of breasts bilaterally. • Oral examination reveals markedly reddened and inflamed gingivae as well as petechiae on the buccal mucosa. • Complete blood count (CBC): hematocrit (HCT) 29%, hemoglobin (Hb) 10 g/dl, platelet count 32,000/mm^3, and white blood cell (WBC) count 3,000/mm^3. • WBC differential: neutrophils 30%, basophils 2%, eosinophils 0%, lymphocytes 60%, monocytes 2%. **Mental notes** *The client's weight loss may result from her inability to prepare meals because of fatigue. Signs of bleeding show the need for bleeding precautions to ensure client safety. Oral assessment suggests the client's need to consult a dentist and use a soft bristle toothbrush. Laboratory values are low; the client may benefit from infection precautions.*	• Potential for infection related to alteration in protective mechanisms. • Potential for injury related to decreased platelet count. • Activity intolerance related to fatigue. • Altered nutrition: less than body requirements, related to loss of appetite.	**Goals** By the time of discharge, the client will: • be free of infection • tolerate mild activity • demonstrate infection-prevention routine • be free of gingival bleeding and petechiae.	• Instruct all staff and visitors to use strict handwashing procedures to decrease infection risk. • Take the client's vital signs every 4 hours to detect early signs of infection. • Teach the client to perform mouth care with a soft bristle toothbrush to prevent mucosal injury. • Teach the client to lubricate her lips as needed. • Advise the client's friends and family that no fresh flowers are permitted in the client's room to prevent introducing organisms. • Teach the client to eat a cooked food diet (no raw food) to minimize acquisition of organisms. • Minimize invasive procedures, such as venipunctures, blood drawing for laboratory studies, and rectal examinations. • Provide a stool softener or a gentle daily cathartic to maintain regular bowel movements and prevent rectal injury from straining at stool. • Give the client literature about infection prevention to supplement teaching sessions.

CASE HISTORY

Ms. Delaney, age 38, who was admitted to the hospital this morning, is an unmarried, Caucasian woman who enjoyed good health until 3 weeks ago when she began to suffer chronic fatigue. She lives alone and works as a real estate broker.

EVALUATION	DOCUMENTATION BASED ON NURSING PROCESS DATA			
		Initial		**Follow-up**
At discharge, the client: • explained and demonstrated infection precautions and rationales for each • had no gingival bleeding or petechiae • had returned to normal activities of daily living without fatigue.	**S**	Client states, "I'm tired all the time. I have to make an effort to go to work each morning." Client reports recent prolonged menses lasting 9 days; intermittent, localized, dull sternal pain; and poor appetite; 15-lb (6.75 kg) weight loss over past 3 weeks. Client denies recent acute illness, headache, and dyspnea.	**S**	Client reports: "I'm not as tired, but I still don't feel like myself." Client denies cough, dysuria, or other infection signs.
	O	Temperature 100° F. (37.8° C.), pulse 100 and regular, respirations 22 and regular, blood pressure 126/84. CBC: HCT 29%, Hb 10 g/dl. Pale skin with scattered, bilateral ecchymoses on legs and petechiae on upper arm, around waist, and under breasts bilaterally. Markedly red and inflamed gingivae. Petechiae on buccal mucosa.	**O**	Blood pressure 126/80; temperature 98.6° F. (37° C.), pulse 88, respirations 20. Oral appearance improved with decreased inflammation, some gingival pallor. Bleeding persists after oral hygiene. CBC: HCT 32%, Hb 12 g/dl; platelet count 46,000/mm^3 after transfusion, WBC count 2,800/mm^3.
	A	Potential for infection related to alteration in protective mechanisms. Client appears pale and lethargic. CBC results show low hemoglobin and hematocrit.	**A**	Client adhering to infection precautions.
	P	Teach client how to prevent infection. Also teach family and friends to avoid infecting the client. Teach client to use soft toothbrush. Monitor laboratory results.	**P**	Teach client how to prevent infection. Teach family and friends to avoid infecting the client.
	I	Instructed client about personal hygiene techniques that reduce infection risk. Monitor blood transfusion ordered by physician.	**I**	Instructed client about personal hygiene techniques that reduce infection risk.
	E	Client demonstrates regular use of soft toothbrush.	**E**	Client demonstrates regular use of soft toothbrush. Client reports making a dental appointment.

reveals approximate size of right lobe of liver as 3" (7.5 cm); left lobe, 2" (5 cm). Lymph nodes not palpable.

The following example shows how to document some abnormal physical assessment findings:

Height: 5'1"
Weight: 96 lb
Vital signs: Blood pressure 140/90, temperature 99.2° F. (37.3° C.), pulse 120 and regular, respirations 28 and regular.

Client is alert but listless and lethargic. Buccal mucosa and palpebral conjunctivae are pale. Skin tone: pallor. Functional systolic murmur, grade 2, noted at aortic and pulmonic sites. Liver palpated 1" (3 cm) below right costal margin. Spleen tip palpated at left costal margin. Cervical nodes enlarged ¾" (2 cm), nontender, and freely movable. Inguinal nodes present, ½" (1 cm) across.

Be sure to document the other nursing process steps: nursing diagnosis, planning, implementation, and evaluation, as you care for the client with an immune system or blood disorder.

Chapter summary

To care for a client with an immune or blood disorder, the nurse relies on health history data, physical assessment findings, and laboratory study results. Chapter 19 explains how to gather and integrate this data. Here are the chapter highlights:

- The immune system, a complex network of specialized cells and organ tissues, recognizes and defends against attacks by foreign invaders. It preserves the body's internal environment by scavenging dead or damaged cells and by recognizing its own elements (self) as distinct from a foreign substance (nonself). Its three main defense strategies include protective surface phenomena, general host defenses, and specific immune responses.
- Immune system organs include the bone marrow and thymus (where the B and T cells mature) as well as the lymph nodes, spleen, and accessory organs (tonsils, appendix, and Peyer's patches). Lymph nodes are small oval-shaped structures located along lymph channels that collect fluids and proteins and filter waste materials and microbes before returning the useful materials to vascular circulation. All lymph travels through one or more nodes (in chained arrangements) that drain a specific region.
- Protective surface phenomena include such activities as pH changes and defensive secretions at accessible entry sites.
- General host defenses are nonspecific, responding alike to all invaders. They stimulate phagocytosis and inflammatory responses.
- Specific immune responses exhibit memory for and response to specific microorganisms via humoral and cell-mediated immunity. Humoral immunity requires B cells; cell-mediated immunity, T cells.
- Blood cells arise from multipotential stem cells in the bone marrow. During hematopoiesis, the following cells develop from the multipotential stem cells: erythrocytes (red blood cells, or RBCs), thrombocytes (platelets), and five kinds of leukocytes (white blood cells, or WBCs).
- Blood, a tissue composed of formed elements (blood cells) suspended in a fluid medium (plasma), transports gases, nutrients, wastes, and other substances to and from the body's cells and tissues.
- RBCs contain hemoglobin, which allows them to transport oxygen and carbon dioxide. Antigens on RBC surfaces determine blood group or type. The major blood groups are A, B, AB, and O.
- Platelets contribute to hemostasis by controlling bleeding and maintaining intravascular integrity. Four major plasma components and several plasma and tissue clotting factors participate in the coagulation process.
- WBCs play an important part in the body's defense against invasive miroorganisms. Identified by their nuclear and cytoplasmic characteristics, WBCs are categorized as granulocytes (neutrophils, eosinophils, and basophils) and agranulocytes (lymphocytes and monocytes).
- Granulocytes, migratory and mainly phagocytic, engulf, ingest, and digest foreign materials, or assist with this function. They constitute the body's first line of cellular defense.
- Agranulocytes are also part of the immune system. Monocytes are phagocytic and may be migratory or fixed. Outside the bloodstream, in tissues that filter large amounts of body fluids, monocytes are called macrophages. They defend against invading organisms. Lymphocytes differentiate into two cell types, B cells and T cells, which function in humoral and cell-mediated immunity, respectively.
- Immune and blood disorders typically cause abnormal bleeding, lymphadenopathy, fatigue, weakness, fever, and joint pain. The nurse should assess for these effects during the health history interview. The nurse also

should evaluate effects on other body structures and systems because immune and blood disorders cause multisystem effects.

- The health history should explore the client's medication history because over-the-counter and prescription drugs can induce hematopoietic problems, blood dyscrasias, and impaired immune responses.
- Physical assessment of the immune system and blood should incorporate assessment of related body structures and systems, such as the skin and oral mucosa and the respiratory and neurologic systems.
- The physical assessment should also include inspection and palpation of the superficial lymph nodes. Red streaks, palpable nodes, and lymphedema may indicate a lymphatic disorder, whereas enlarged nodes suggest current or recent inflammation. Tender nodes usually indicate infection; hard or fixed nodes, malignant tissue. General lymphadenopathy can result from an inflammatory or neoplastic process.
- To complete the assessment, the nurse reviews the laboratory test results—for example, blood and bone marrow studies and immunocompetence studies.
- The nurse documents all assessment findings and uses them in the nursing process to formulate nursing diagnoses that enable individualized planning, implementation, and evaluation of client care.

Study questions

1. What are the organs and tissues that make up the immune system? What are their functions?

2. The body's first line of defense against microorganisms is a series of physical, chemical, and mechanical barriers known as protective surface phenomena. How would placement of an indwelling urinary catheter compromise this defense?

3. How do normal lymph node palpation findings differ for a child under age 12, an adult, and an adult age 75?

4. Why is an individual with decreased circulating WBCs, particularly granulocytes, unable to manifest the characteristic signs and symptoms of infection?

5. Ms. Polly Wagner, age 30, comes to the clinic this morning complaining of fatigue, weakness, and intermittent epistaxis (nosebleed), which is not active at present. You take her vital signs and find that her temperature is 100.2° F. (38.9° C.); pulse rate is 100 beats/minute; respiratory rate is 22 breaths/minute; and blood pressure is 96/64 mm Hg. The physician orders a complete blood count, which reveals a hemoglobin of 10 g/dl, a hematocrit of 29%, and a platelet count of 25,000/mm^3. How would you report the following information related to Ms. Wagner?

- history (subjective) assessment data
- physical (objective) assessment data
- assessment techniques and any special equipment used
- two appropriate nursing diagnoses
- documentation of your findings.

Selected references

Galluci, B. (1987). The immune system and cancer. *Oncology Nursing Forum,* 14(6), 3-12.

Griffin, J. (1986). *Hematology and immunology concepts for nursing.* East Norwalk, CT: Appleton & Lange.

Gurevich, I. (1985). The competent internal immune system. *Nursing Clinics of North America,* 20(1), 151-161.

Henry, J. (1991). *Clinical diagnosis and management by laboratory methods* (18th ed.). Philadelphia: Saunders.

Immune disorders. (1985). Nurse's Clinical Library Series. Springhouse, PA: Springhouse Corp.

McEvoy, G. (Ed.). (1992). *American Hospital Formulary Service drug information.* Bethesda, MD: American Society of Hospital Pharmacists.

Selekman, J. (1990). The multiple faces of immune deficiency in children. *Pediatric Nursing,* 16(4), 351-355, 361.

Nursing research

Holmes, S. (1991). Preliminary investigations of symptom distress in two cancer patient populations: Evaluation of a measurement instrument. *Journal of Advanced Nursing,* 16(4), 439-446.

Pepler, C., and Lynch, A. (1991). Relational messages of control in nurse-patient interactions with terminally ill patients with AIDS and cancer. *Journal of Palliative Care,* 7(1), 18-29.

Pickard-Holley, S. (1991). Fatigue in cancer patients: A descriptive study. *Cancer Nursing,* 14(1), 13-19.

20

Endocrine System

Objectives

After reading and studying this chapter, you should be able to:
1. Identify the endocrine glands and their anatomic locations.
2. Identify the hormone secreted by each endocrine gland, and describe its target site and specific actions.
3. Discuss how the hypothalamus regulates endocrine function.
4. Gather appropriate health history information for a client with an endocrine disorder.
5. List representative adverse reactions to drugs that affect endocrine function.
6. Differentiate between normal and abnormal endocrine system findings revealed during physical assessment.
7. Demonstrate how to palpate the thyroid gland and how to elicit Chvostek's sign and Trousseau's sign, and describe the significance of the findings.
8. Describe the common laboratory tests used to evaluate endocrine function.
9. Use the nursing process to document endocrine assessment findings.

Introduction

The endocrine system, together with the nervous system, regulates important body functions, including growth and development of body tissue, reproduction, energy production, metabolism, and the ability to adapt to stress. For this reason, endocrine dysfunction can affect virtually every body system and profoundly influence a person's health and sense of well-being.

Such systemic signs and symptoms as fatigue and weakness, weight changes, abnormalities of sexual maturity or function, mental status changes, frequent urination (polyuria), or extreme thirst (polydipsia) should alert the nurse to the need for an endocrine system assessment. Although their relationship to the endocrine system may be less apparent, symptoms involving multiple body systems, such as headache, extreme hunger (polyphagia), nervousness, and depression, also may warrant a complete endocrine assessment.

Chapter 20 begins by reviewing endocrine system anatomy and physiology, including a description of hormonal regulation. It then discusses appropriate health history questions to ask the client during an endocrine system assessment. The chapter continues with a section on physical assessment of the endocrine system, describing normal and abnormal findings. Included is information about laboratory studies used to assess the endocrine system; a case study shows the nurse how to use the nursing process to document endocrine system assessment findings.

Anatomy and physiology review

The endocrine system consists of three major components: glands, which are specialized cell clusters; hormones, which are chemical substances secreted by glands

Glossary

Acromegaly: endocrine condition characterized by gradual, marked enlargement and elongation of the bones of the face, jaw, hands, and feet, caused by excess production of growth hormone in adults.

Addison's disease: endocrine disorder of the adrenal cortex, caused by decreased cortisol and aldosterone secretion, characterized by a bronze coloration of the skin and potentially life-threatening crises.

Amines: hormones derived from tyrosine (an amino acid synthesized in the body and found in food).

Catecholamines: epinephrine and norepinephrine—the functioning units of the autonomic nervous system.

Cretinism: endocrine disorder of the thyroid gland, caused by deficient thyroid hormone secretion in a pediatric client, characterized by a lack of physical growth.

Cushing's syndrome: endocrine disorder, caused by excess corticosteroid production, characterized by hirsutism, obese trunk and abdomen, and thin extremities.

Diabetes insipidus: endocrine disorder of the posterior lobe of the pituitary gland, caused by ineffective or decreased vasopression secretion.

Diabetes mellitus: endocrine disorder of the pancreas involving chronically elevated blood glucose levels resulting from insufficient or ineffective insulin production, decreased insulin receptors, or post-receptor defects.

Endocrine glands: glands that release hormones directly into the bloodstream.

Feedback mechanism: return of information on hormone levels that signals specific endocrine gland response.

Glands: specialized cell clusters that synthesize and release chemical substances that regulate body processes.

Goiter: thyroid enlargement.

Hirsutism: increased hair in masculine pattern in females.

Hormone: chemical substance produced by an endocrine gland that exerts a specific regulatory effect on the activity of a certain organ or organs.

Hyperglycemia: excessive blood glucose levels.

Hyperparathyroidism: endocrine disorder of the parathyroid glands, caused by excess parathyroid hormone secretion and characterized by back pain and fractures.

Hyperthyroidism: endocrine disorder of the thyroid gland, caused by excess thyroid hormone secretion and characterized by heat intolerance, anxiety, and weight loss.

Hypoglycemia: insufficient blood glucose levels.

Hypoparathyroidism: endocrine disorder of the parathyroid glands, caused by decreased or ineffective use of parathyroid hormone and characterized by neuromuscular irritability and increased deep tendon reflexes.

Hypothyroidism: endocrine disorder of the thyroid gland, caused by deficient or ineffective thyroid hormone levels and characterized by fatigue, dry skin, and puffy face.

Inhibiting factor: tropic hypothalamic hormone that inhibits release of the anterior pituitary hormones.

Panhypopituitarism: endocrine disorder of the pituitary gland, caused by decreased pituitary hormone secretion; characterized in children by retarded growth and in adults by decreased libido, extreme fatigue, and apathy.

Pheochromocytoma: rare tumor of the adrenal medulla that secretes excessive catecholamines at inappropriate times.

Polypeptide: type of hormone formed as a protein with a defined genetically coded structure.

Receptor mechanism: mechanism in which hormones bind to macromolecules on the cell membranes or in the cells so that hormonal action can take place at the cellular level.

Releasing factor: tropic hypothalamic hormone that stimulates release of the anterior pituitary hormones.

Steroid: type of hormone formed as a protein derived from cholesterol.

Syndrome of inappropriate antidiuretic hormone secretion (SIADH): endocrine disorder of the posterior lobe of the pituitary gland, caused by continued secretion of antidiuretic hormone (vasopressin) despite contrary regulatory signals.

Target sites: locations of hormonal action in the body.

in response to nervous system stimulation; and receptors, which are protein macromolecules that determine the activity of a hormone at its target cell.

Glands

The glands of the endocrine system, which collectively weigh less than 7 ounces, include the pituitary, thyroid, parathyroid, pineal, and adrenal glands, the gonads (ovaries and testes), the thymus, and selected areas of the pancreas known as the islets of Langerhans. (For a description of these glands, see *Endocrine system,* pages 588 and 589. For information about the ovaries and testes, see Chapter 15, Female Reproductive System, and Chapter 16, Male Reproductive System, respec-

(Text continues on page 590.)

Endocrine system

The endocrine system consists of eight glands: the pituitary gland, thyroid gland, parathyroid glands, adrenal glands, pancreas, gonads (testes in males and ovaries in females), thymus, and pineal gland.

Pituitary gland

Also known as the hypophysis, the pituitary rests in the sella turcica—a depression in the sphenoid bone at the base of the brain. The pea-sized gland weighs less than 0.75 g and has three regions. The largest, the anterior pituitary lobe (adenohypophysis), produces six hormones: somatotropin, or growth hormone (GH); thyrotropin, or thyroid-stimulating hormone (TSH); corticotropin, or adrenocorticotropic hormone (ACTH); follicle-stimulating hormone (FSH); luteinizing hormone (LH); and mammotropin, or prolactin (PRL).

The posterior pituitary lobe (neurohypophysis), which makes up about 25% of the gland, stores and releases oxytocin and vasopressin (also called antidiuretic hormone [ADH]). Produced by the hypothalamus, these hormones travel down nerve endings to the posterior pituitary, where they are stored for future use.

The pars intermedia, a narrow tissue band between the anterior and posterior pituitary regions, produces only one known hormone: melanocyte-stimulating hormone (MSH). However, because the pars intermedia produces ACTH in other mammals, some experts believe it plays the same role in humans.

Thyroid gland

The thyroid gland lies directly below the larynx, partially in front of the trachea. Two lobes, one on either side of the trachea, join with a narrow tissue bridge called the isthmus to give the thyroid its butterfly-like shape. The lobes function as one unit to produce the hormones thyroxine (T_4), triiodothyronine (T_3), and thyrocalcitonin. T_4 and T_3 are referred to collectively as thyroid hormone.

Parathyroid glands

Four parathyroid glands lie embedded on the posterior surface of the thyroid, one in each corner. Like the thyroid lobes, the parathyroid glands work together as a single gland, producing parathyroid hormone (PTH).

Adrenal glands

Sometimes called the suprarenal glands, the two adrenal glands sit atop the two kidneys. Each gland contains two distinct endocrine glands with separate functions. The inner portion—the medulla—produces the catecholamines epinephrine and norepinephrine. Because these hormones play important roles in the autonomic nervous system, the

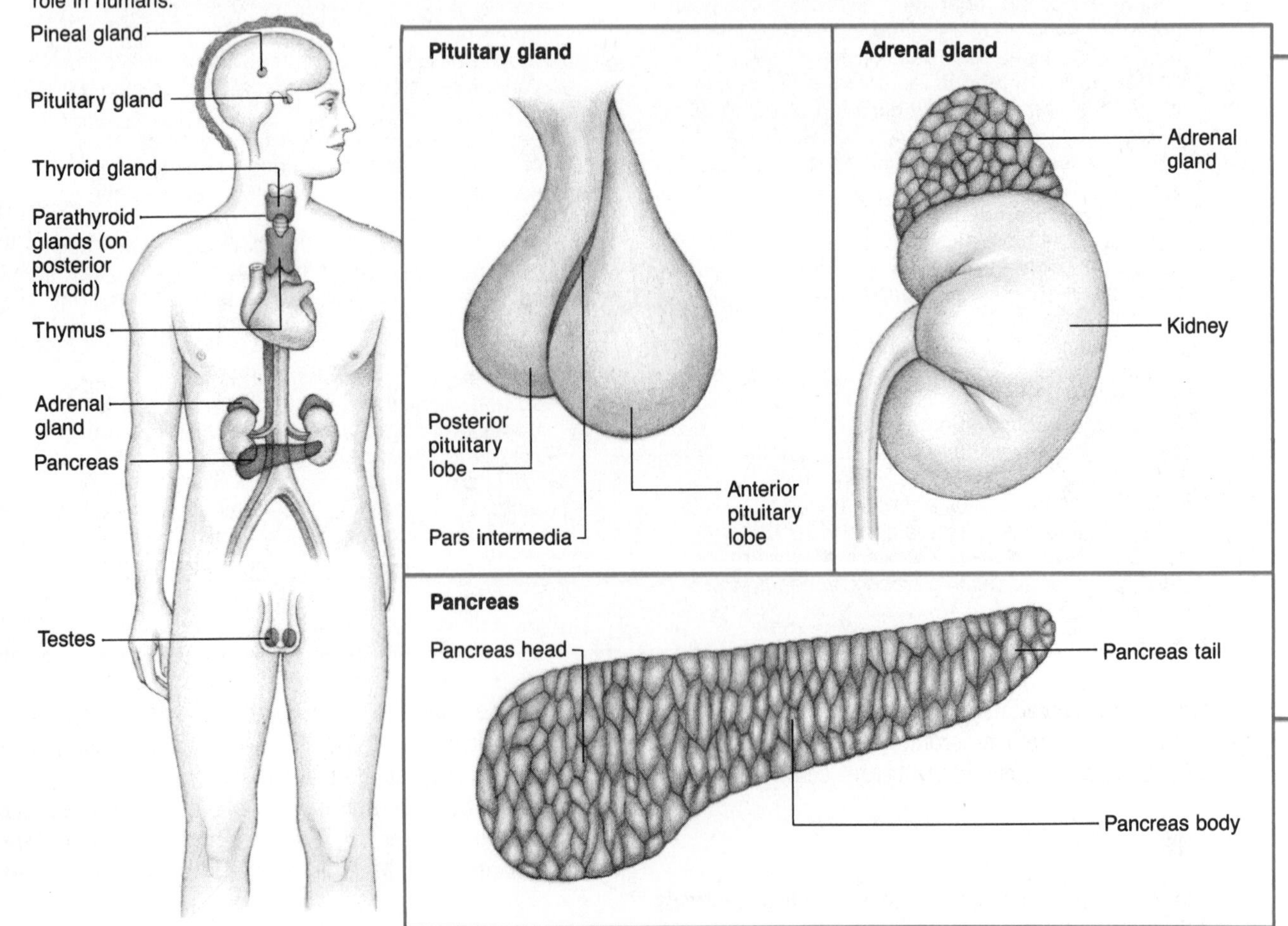

adrenal medulla is also considered a neuroendocrine structure.

The much larger, outer adrenal portion—the cortex—has three zones. The outermost zone, the zona glomerulosa, produces mineralocorticoids, primarily aldosterone. The zona fasciculata, the middle and largest zone, produces the glucocorticoids cortisol (hydrocortisone), cortisone, and corticosterone as well as small amounts of the sex hormones androgen and estrogen. The inner zone, the zona reticularis, produces glucocorticoids and sex hormones.

Pancreas

The pancreas lies across the posterior abdominal wall, in the upper left quadrant behind the stomach. The islets of Langerhans, which perform the endocrine function of this gland, contain alpha, beta, and delta cells. Alpha cells produce glucagon, beta cells produce insulin, and delta cells produce somatostatin.

Gonads

Males have two testes enclosed within the scrotum that contain interstitial cell clusters called Leydig's cells, which produce the male sex hormone testosterone.

Females have two ovaries in the abdominal cavity, one on either side of the uterus. Ovaries produce the estrogens estrone and estradiol as well as progesterone. (For more information about the testes and ovaries, respectively, see Chapter 16, Male Reproductive System, and Chapter 15, Female Reproductive System.)

Thymus

The thymus gland, located below the sternum, contains lymphatic tissue. Although the thymus produces the hormones thymosin and thymopoietin, its major role seems related to the immune system because it produces T cells, important in cell-mediated immunity.

Pineal gland

The tiny pineal gland—only about ¼″ (8 mm) in diameter—lies at the back of the third ventricle of the brain. Although the pineal gland produces the hormone melatonin, its precise role in endocrine function has not been clearly identified.

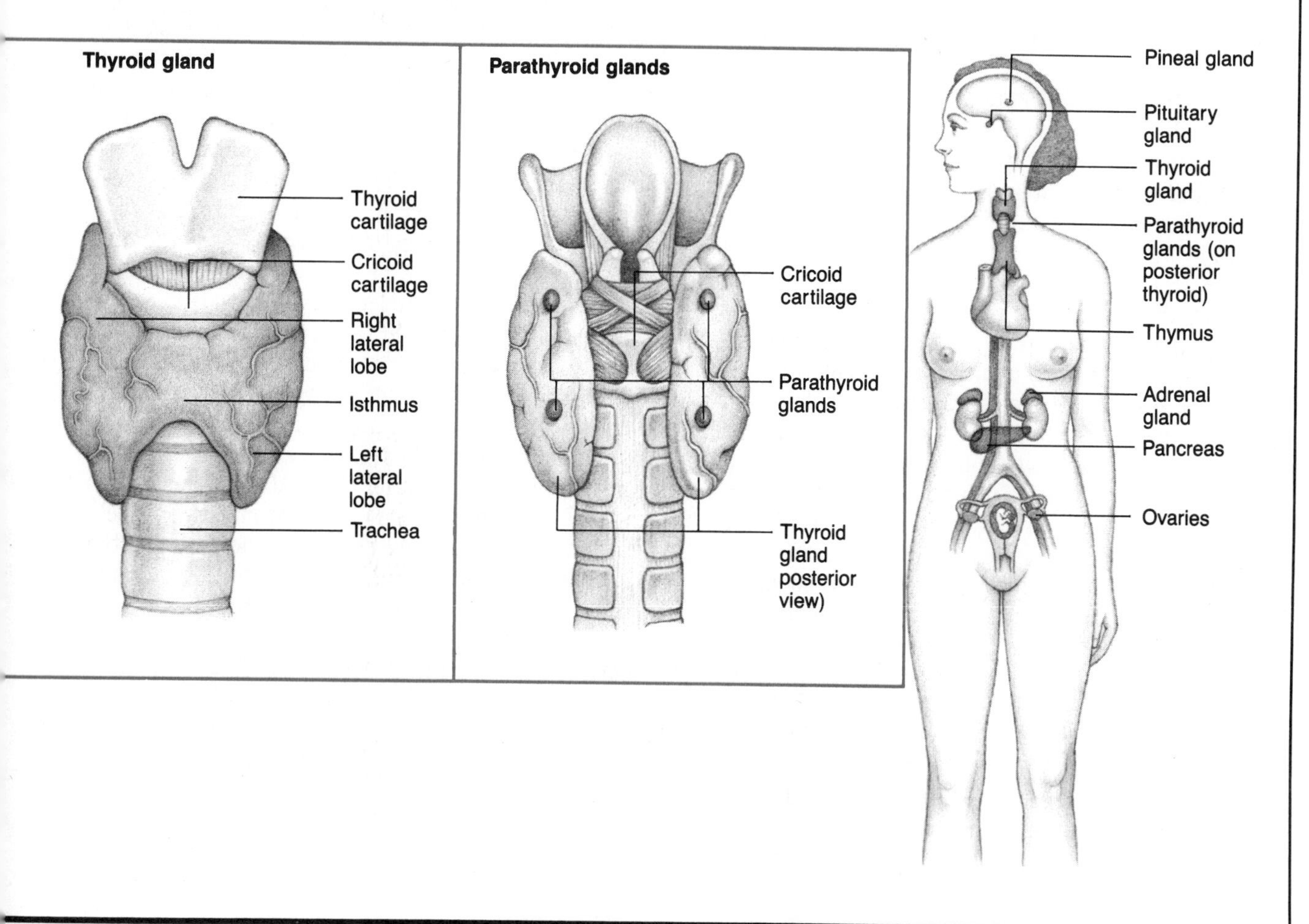

tively.) Endocrine glands release hormones into the bloodstream for transport to specific target sites. At each target site, hormones combine with specific receptors to trigger specific physiologic changes.

Hormones

Structurally, hormones can be classified into three types: polypeptides, steroids, and amines. Polypeptides, proteins with a defined, genetically coded structure, include anterior pituitary hormones (growth hormone, thyroid-stimulating hormone, adrenocorticotropic hormone, follicle-stimulating hormone, luteinizing hormone, interstitial-cell–stimulating hormone, and prolactin), posterior pituitary hormones (antidiuretic hormone and oxytocin), parathyroid hormone, and pancreatic hormones (insulin and glucagon). Steroids, derived from cholesterol, include the adrenocortical hormones secreted by the adrenal cortex (aldosterone and cortisol) and the sex hormones (estrogen and progesterone in females and testosterone in males) secreted by the gonads. Amines are derived from tyrosine (an essential amino acid found in most proteins). They include thyroid hormones (thyroxine and triiodothyronine) and catecholamines (epinephrine, norepinephrine, and dopamine).

Hormonal release and transport

Although all hormone release results from endocrine gland stimulation, release patterns of hormones vary greatly. For example, adrenocorticotropic hormone (ACTH), secreted by the anterior pituitary, and cortisol, secreted by the adrenal cortex, are released in irregular spurts in response to body rhythm cycles, with levels peaking in the morning. In contrast, secretion of parathyroid hormone (by the parathyroid gland) and prolactin (by the anterior pituitary) occurs fairly evenly throughout the day. Insulin, secreted by the pancreas, has both steady and sporadic release patterns. Pancreatic beta cells secrete small amounts of insulin continuously but secrete additional insulin in response to food intake.

After their release into the bloodstream, hormones travel either unbound or bound to plasma proteins. Catecholamines and most polypeptides circulate unbound; thyroid hormones and most steroids travel bound. The amount of bound steroid or thyroid hormone is significant; binding inactivates the hormone, inhibiting its action at the target site.

Hormonal action

Once a hormone reaches its target site, it binds to a specific receptor on the cell membrane or within the cell. Polypeptides and some amines bind to cell wall receptor sites; the smaller, more lipid-soluble steroids and thyroid hormone diffuse through the cell membrane and bind to intracellular receptors.

After binding occurs, each hormone produces unique physiologic changes, depending on its target site and its specific action at that site. A particular hormone may have different effects at different target sites.

Hormonal regulation

To maintain the body's delicate homeostatic balance, a feedback mechanism involving hormones, blood chemicals, and the nervous system regulates hormone secretion. *Feedback* refers to information sent to endocrine glands that signals changes in hormone levels, either increasing or decreasing hormone production and release. Four basic mechanisms control hormone release: pituitary-target gland axis, hypothalamic-pituitary-target gland axis, chemical regulation, and nervous system regulation.

Pituitary-target gland axis. The pituitary gland regulates other endocrine glands—and their hormones—through the secretion of tropic hormones, including ACTH, thyroid-stimulating hormone (TSH), and luteinizing hormone (LH). ACTH regulates the adrenal cortex hormones, TSH regulates the thyroid hormones thyroxine (T_4) and triiodothyronine (T_3), and LH regulates gonadal hormones. Tropic hormones get feedback about their target glands by continuously monitoring levels of hormones produced by these glands. If a change occurs, the tropic hormone corrects it in one of two ways: by stimulating its target gland, causing an increase in tropic and target gland hormones, or by stopping its target gland stimulation, inhibiting tropic and target gland hormones.

A tropic hormone increases or decreases its stimulation from moment to moment by continuously monitoring its feedback and changing its own level in the opposite direction from its target gland hormone. For example, if the cortisol level rises, ACTH decreases its own level to reduce adrenal cortex stimulation, which, in turn, decreases cortisol secretion. Conversely, if the cortisol level drops, the ACTH level rises, stimulating the adrenal cortex to produce more cortisol.

Hypothalamic-pituitary-target gland axis. The hypothalamus, in the diencephalon of the brain, also produces tropic hormones. Known as releasing and inhibiting factors, these hormones regulate anterior pituitary hormones. (For more information, see *Hypothalamic-pituitary-target gland axis*.) By controlling pituitary hormones, which control the target gland hormones, the hypothalamus indirectly affects target glands as well.

Chemical regulation. Endocrine glands not controlled by the pituitary gland are controlled by specific substances that trigger gland secretions. For example, serum glucose level is a major regulator of glucagon and insulin release. An elevated serum glucose level stimulates the pancreas to increase insulin secretion and suppress glucagon secretion. Conversely, a depressed serum glucose level triggers increased glucagon secretion and suppresses insulin secretion.

Similarly, calcium level regulates parathyroid hormone (PTH) and calcitonin. A calcium decrease stimulates the parathyroid glands to increase parathyroid hormone secretion, making the calcium level rise. However, decreased calcium also suppresses calcitonin secretion, which prevents further calcium reduction. A serum calcium increase suppresses parathyroid hormone and stimulates calcitonin secretion.

Sodium and potassium regulate aldosterone similarly. Decreased extracellular sodium and increased serum potassium stimulate the adrenal cortex to release more aldosterone, which promotes sodium retention and potassium excretion. Increased extracellular sodium and decreased serum potassium have the opposite effect.

Antidiuretic hormone (ADH) regulation occurs mainly through changes in plasma osmolality (the osmotic pressure of a solution expressed in milliosmols [mOsm] representing the concentration of particles in a solution), although other factors also affect ADH levels. Increased plasma osmolality (indicating dehydration) stimulates ADH to promote water retention; decreased osmolality (indicating fluid overload) suppresses ADH secretion to promote diuresis.

Nervous system regulation. The central nervous system helps regulate hormone secretion in several ways. The hypothalamus controls pituitary hormones, as described earlier, as well as the catecholamine secretion of the adrenal medulla. Because hypothalamic nerve cells stimulate the production of the posterior pituitary hormones ADH and oxytocin, these hormones are controlled directly by the central nervous system. Nervous system stimuli such as hypoxia, nausea, pain, stress, and certain pharmacologic agents also affect ADH levels.

The relationship between the hypothalamus and the pituitary underscores the importance of the nervous

Hypothalamic-pituitary-target gland axis

Several endocrine glands fall under the regulatory influence of the hypothalamic-pituitary-target gland axis. Through a feedback mechanism (illustrated by the arrows on the diagram below), the hormone or hormone-induced action of the target gland provides information on hormone levels to other endocrine glands, such as the adrenals and thyroid, which then act on this information.

Action begins when an impulse from the central nervous system stimulates the hypothalamus to secrete hormones that stimulate the pituitary gland. Hypothalamic hormones that stimulate the anterior pituitary include corticotropin-releasing factor (CRF), thyrotropin-releasing hormone (TRH), gonadotropin-releasing hormone (GnRH), and growth-hormone-releasing hormone (GHRH). Each releasing factor or hormone is named for the anterior pituitary hormone it regulates.

The hypothalamus regulates anterior pituitary hormones through the same feedback mechanism that the pituitary gland uses. Thus, the hypothalamus continuously monitors anterior pituitary target hormones and, when necessary, increases or decreases pituitary stimulation. For example, if adrenocorticotropic hormone (ACTH) or cortisol levels drop, CRF release increases, stimulating the anterior pituitary to produce more ACTH. This, in turn, stimulates the adrenal cortex to increase cortisol secretion. Consequently, if hypothalamic stimulation stops, levels of the involved hormones decrease.

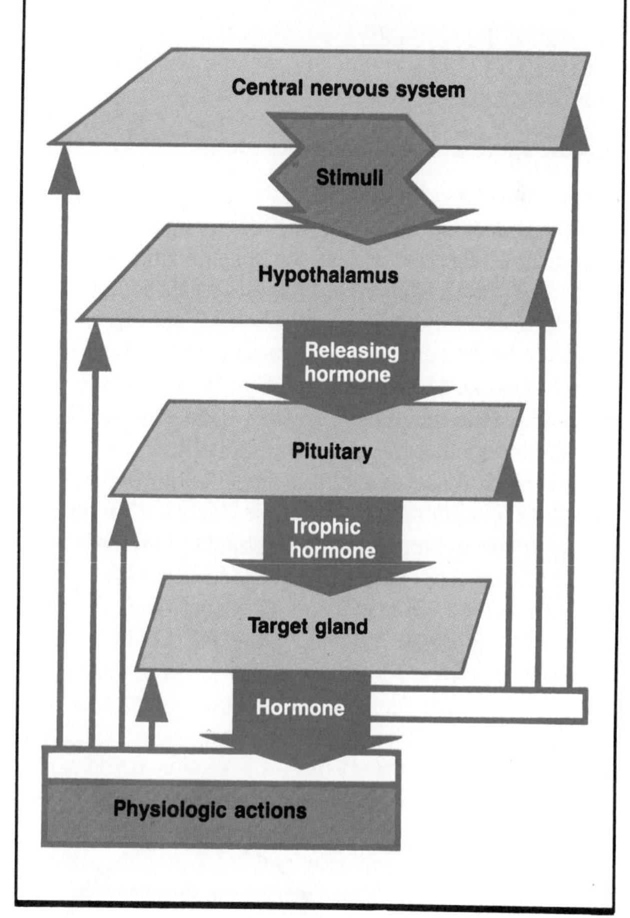

system to endocrine function. Because the hypothalamus also controls the autonomic nervous system, it directly regulates the hormones of the sympathetic branch—epinephrine and norepinephrine.

The nervous system also modifies other endocrine hormones. For example, stress, which leads to sympathetic stimulation, causes the pancreas to release insulin as part of the fight or flight reaction. Although the nervous and endocrine systems are thought to share other regulatory mechanisms, these are not well understood.

Hormonal imbalance

Endocrine dysfunction takes one of two forms: hyperfunction, resulting in excessive hormone secretion, or hypofunction, causing hormone deficiency. Hormonal imbalance also may be classified according to disease site. Primary hyperfunction or hypofunction results from disease within an endocrine gland—for example, Addison's disease (adrenal hypofunction); secondary hyperfunction or hypofunction, from disease in a tissue that affects the target tissue; and functional hyperfunction or hypofunction, from disease in a nonendocrine tissue or organ.

Health history

When collecting health history information about a client's endocrine function, the nurse should keep in mind that endocrine system components function interdependently with each other and with other body organs. Therefore, assessment requires a holistic approach. Complaints related to endocrine dysfunction may result from, or be the cause of, problems in other body systems. The nurse also should remember that endocrine problems can alter a client's life-style dramatically. For example, a client with diabetes mellitus must make lifelong adjustments to maintain blood glucose levels within normal limits; a young woman with Cushing's syndrome may have difficulty coping with her altered appearance.

Often, the systemic effects of endocrine dysfunction are readily apparent, related to the effects of hormone deficiency or excess regardless of the cause or location of the original defect. Sometimes, however, endocrine dysfunction manifests itself in nonspecific ways—particularly in early phases. The questions in this section are designed to help you evaluate the client's endocrine system by assessing health and illness patterns, health promotion and protection patterns, and role and relationship patterns. They include rationales that describe the significance of the client's answers and, where appropriate, nursing interventions that you may incorporate into the client's care plan.

Health and illness patterns

To assess important health and illness patterns, explore the client's current, past, and family health status; the status of each physiologic system; and developmental considerations.

Current health status

Begin the interview by asking about the client's current health status, carefully documenting the chief complaint in the client's own words and using the PQRST method to elicit a complete description of the problem and any others. (For a detailed explanation of this method, see *Symptom analysis* in Chapter 3, The Health History.) Common chief complaints associated with endocrine disorders include fatigue, weakness, weight changes, mental status changes, polyuria, polydipsia, and abnormalities of sexual maturity.

Do you feel tired, lethargic, or weak?
(RATIONALE: Decreased energy level may result from hypopituitarism, hypothyroidism, or altered blood glucose levels from excessive or insufficient insulin.)

If you feel weak, is the weakness generalized or confined to a specific area or areas?
(RATIONALE: Generalized weakness occurs in various endocrine disorders, including diabetes mellitus, hyperparathyroidism, and Addison's disease. Weakness in a specific area seldom results from an endocrine disorder.)

Have you noticed any muscle twitching?
(RATIONALE: Muscle twitching may result from increased secretion of antidiuretic hormone or decreased secretion of parathormone or aldosterone.)

Do you feel any numbness or tingling in your arms or legs?
(RATIONALE: These sensations may indicate sensory peripheral neuropathy, an abnormal condition characterized by biochemical abnormalities and degeneration of the peripheral nerves that often occurs in diabetes mellitus.)

Have you recently gained or lost weight unintentionally? If so, how much and over what time period?
(RATIONALE: Weight gain may result from hypothyroidism, syndrome of inappropriate antidiuretic hormone secretion [SIADH], or Cushing's syndrome. Weight loss may be seen in panhypopituitarism, hyperthyroidism, Addison's disease, and hyperglycemia.)

Have you recently experienced any changes in your normal behavior, such as nervousness or mood swings?
(RATIONALE: Endocrine disorders that alter thyroid hormone, insulin, or corticosteroid levels can alter behavior and cause emotional lability.)

How would you rate your memory and attention span?
(RATIONALE: Memory loss can result from hypothyroidism or hypoparathyroidism; shortened attention span, from hyperthyroidism or hyperparathyroidism.)

Have you noticed an increase in the amount of urine you pass, or have you been feeling unusually thirsty lately?
(RATIONALE: Increased urination [polyuria] and increased thirst [polydipsia] are classic signs of diabetes mellitus and diabetes insipidus.)

Do you often feel hot or cold when other people in the same room are comfortable?
(RATIONALE: Heat intolerance often is associated with hyperthyroidism; cold intolerance, with hypothyroidism.)

Are you currently taking any prescription or over-the-counter drugs? If so, which ones and at what dosages?
(RATIONALE: Some drugs can mask or simulate symptoms of endocrine disorders. For more information, see *Adverse drug reactions,* pages 594 and 595.)

Past health status

Careful assessment of the client's past health status may help identify insidious and vague symptoms of endocrine dysfunction that may go unreported. The following questions can help uncover some of the most common unnoticed or unreported symptoms.

Have you ever had a skull fracture or experienced repeated fractures in other areas of the body?
(RATIONALE: A fracture at the base of the skull may cause midbrain injury, resulting in pituitary and hypothalamic dysfunction. Repeated fractures in any area may lead to thyroid or parathyroid underproduction of calcitonin and parathormone, which control the balance of bone calcium.)

Have you ever had surgery? If so, when and what for? Did you experience any complications after the surgery?
(RATIONALE: Surgery involving any of the endocrine glands may cause abnormalities in gland function. Stress from any surgical procedure can precipitate a crisis from an underlying endocrine disorder.)

Have you ever had radiation treatments? If so, what for?
(RATIONALE: Radiation exposure can cause endocrine glands to atrophy, resulting in dysfunction.)

Have you ever had a brain infection, such as meningitis or encephalitis?
(RATIONALE: These infections can cause hypothalamic disturbances, which can disrupt the hypothalamic-pituitary-target gland axis.)

What was your growth pattern? Were you considered tall or short for your age? Did you have any growth spurts? If so, when and to what degree?
(RATIONALE: A slow growth rate could indicate hypopituitarism or hypothyroidism; a rapid growth rate, hyperpituitarism, hyperthyroidism, or gonadal hormone excess.)

Have you ever been diagnosed as having an endocrine, or glandular, problem? If so, what was the problem, when was it diagnosed, and how has it been treated?
(RATIONALE: Most endocrine disorders are chronic, requiring lifelong treatment.)

Family health status

Because certain endocrine disorders are inherited and others have strong familial tendencies, a thorough family history is essential. Ask the following question when assessing the client's family health status.

Does anyone in your family have diabetes mellitus, thyroid disease, hypertension (high blood pressure), or elevated blood fats?
(RATIONALE: Diabetes mellitus [particularly Type II] and thyroid disease show familial tendencies. Pheochromocytoma, a rare tumor of the adrenal medulla that secretes excessive amounts of catecholamines and elevates blood pressure, may result from an autosomal dominant trait. Lipid abnormalities are often inherited.)

Status of physiologic systems

Endocrine dysfunction can produce signs and symptoms related to almost any body system. For this reason, conduct a complete body systems review, asking the client the following questions about systems not already addressed in the questions on current health status.

Have you noticed any changes in your skin, such as acne, increased or decreased oiliness or dryness, or changes in color?
(RATIONALE: Many endocrine problems produce cutaneous manifestations. For example, in adults, acne may

Adverse drug reactions

When obtaining a health history to assess a client's endocrine system, the nurse should ask about drug use. Many drugs can increase or decrease hormone levels and cause endocrine system dysfunctions; some drugs can mask signs and symptoms of endocrine dysfunctions. The commonly used drugs listed below may cause adverse reactions affecting the endocrine system.

DRUG CLASS	DRUG	POSSIBLE ADVERSE REACTIONS
Anticonvulsants	carbamazepine	Syndrome of inappropriate antidiuretic hormone secretion (SIADH)
	phenytoin	Osteomalacia (bone disorder caused by inadequate phosphorus and calcium in the blood); at high doses, hyperglycemia (increased blood glucose) and glycosuria (abnormal presence of glucose in urine)
Antifungals	ketoconazole	Transient depression of serum testosterone levels, inhibited adrenal steroid production, decreased adrenocortical response to corticotropin (ACTH)
Antihypertensives	clonidine hydrochloride, methyldopa	Sodium and water retention (transient with clonidine)
	minoxidil	Sodium and water retention and increased plasma renin activity resulting in limited usefulness of the drug
Antineoplastics	busulfan	Addisonian-like syndrome (with long-term use), hyperuricemia (increased uric acid levels in blood)
	cyclophosphamide	Hyperuricemia, SIADH
	tamoxifen citrate	Hypercalcemia (increased serum calcium levels)
	vinblastine sulfate	Hyperuricemia, SIADH
Antipsychotics	chlorpromazine hydrochloride, haloperidol	Increased serum prolactin levels, decreased vasopressin and corticotropin secretion, impaired glucose tolerance
Beta blockers	nadolol, propranolol hydrochloride, timolol maleate, atenolol, labetalol hydrochloride, metoprolol tartrate, pindolol	Masking of signs and symptoms of hypoglycemia (decreased serum glucose levels) and hyperthyroidism, impaired glucose tolerance, inhibited insulin release, hyperglycemic reactions
Corticosteroids	methylprednisolone, prednisone	Adrenocortical and ACTH suppression, cushingoid fat distribution, decreased glucose tolerance, sodium retention, hypocalcemia, hypercholesterolemia (increased cholesterol levels in blood)
Diuretics	bumetanide, furosemide, thiazides	Hypokalemia, impaired glucose tolerance
Oral contraceptives	estrogen-progestin combinations, conjugated estrogens	Decreased glucose tolerance, hypercholesterolemia

Adverse drug reactions continued

DRUG CLASS	DRUG	POSSIBLE ADVERSE REACTIONS
Miscellaneous agents	chlorpropamide	SIADH, water intoxication
	clofibrate	SIADH
	lithium carbonate	Mild asymptomatic hyperparathyroidism (parathyroid gland hyperactivity), hypothyroidism (thyroid gland hypoactivity), goiter
	metoclopramide hydrochloride	Increased serum prolactin levels, transient increase in plasma aldosterone levels

result from Cushing's syndrome. Increased oiliness may be related to acromegaly or androgen excess. Dry, thick skin may result from hypothyroidism; scaly skin, from hypoparathyroidism. Patchy loss of pigmentation [vitiligo] is associated with hypothyroidism and Addison's disease. Purplish striae, especially on the abdomen and breasts, typically occur in Cushing's syndrome. Pallor may be associated with panhypopituitarism, Addison's disease, or hyperthyroidism.)

Do you bruise more easily than you used to?
(RATIONALE: Abnormal susceptibility to bruising may be associated with hypothyroidism or Cushing's syndrome.)

Have you noticed any increase in the size of your hands or feet? For instance, have you had to stop wearing your rings or buy wider shoes?
(RATIONALE: In adults, widening of the hand and foot bones may result from acromegaly.)

Do your fingernails and toenails seem brittle? Have they thickened or separated from your fingers and toes?
(RATIONALE: Nail brittleness may result from hypoparathyroidism or hypothyroidism. Separation of the distal end of the nail from the nail bed [onycholysis] may occur in hyperthyroidism.)

Have you noticed any change in the amount and distribution of your body hair?
(RATIONALE: An overall decrease in hair growth can be related to hyperthyroidism. In males, decreased axillary and pubic hair growth often points to androgen deficiency. In females, excessive androgen levels can cause increased hair growth in a masculine pattern [hirsutism].)

Has your voice deepened or otherwise changed recently?
(RATIONALE: Vocal hoarseness can result from hypothyroidism. Deepening of the voice in females may indicate excess testosterone or, in both sexes, excess growth hormone.)

Do you ever experience neck pain? Does your neck seem larger than normal? For instance, have you noticed that your shirts or blouses are tighter at the neck?
(RATIONALE: Neck pain could be related to thyroid inflammation [thyroiditis]; an enlarged neck, to thyroid hyperplasia [goiter] or adenoma.)

Are you experiencing any visual problems, especially double vision (diplopia) or blurred vision?
(RATIONALE: Diplopia may point to a pituitary adenoma putting pressure on the optic nerve or to Graves' ophthalmopathy, a disorder commonly associated with hyperthyroidism. Blurred vision can be an early sign of hyperglycemia.)

Do your eyes burn or feel "gritty" when you close them?
(RATIONALE: Such sensations often occur with exophthalmos [protruding eyeballs], a common manifestation of Graves' disease.)

Have you ever felt as though your heart was racing, even when you hadn't been exerting yourself?
(RATIONALE: Tachycardia [a heart rate in excess of 100 beats/minute] may be associated with hyperthyroidism, diabetes insipidus, or Addison's disease.)

Have you ever been told that you have high blood pressure?
(RATIONALE: Excessive catecholamine levels resulting from pheochromocytoma often cause episodic hypertension.)

Has your appetite increased or decreased recently?
(RATIONALE: Increased appetite [polyphagia] may indicate hyperthyroidism or diabetes mellitus. Decreased appetite [anorexia] often occurs in hypothyroidism and Addison's disease.)

Do you often experience constipation or frequent stools?
(RATIONALE: Constipation can result from hypopituitarism, hypothyroidism, decreased ADH, hyperparathyroidism, or pheochromocytoma. Frequent defecation often occurs in hyperthyroidism.)

Do you have less interest in people, things, and activities that once interested you? Do you ever feel depressed for no particular reason?
(RATIONALE: Apathy and depression may be related to hypopituitarism, hypothyroidism, hyperthyroidism, or increased or decreased levels of ADH, glucocorticoids, insulin, or PTH.)

Do you have any numbness or tingling around your mouth or in your hands or feet?
(RATIONALE: Paresthesias may result from hypothyroidism, hypoparathyroidism, or diabetic sensory neuropathy. Periaural numbness often occurs in hypoglycemia.)

How good is your sense of smell?
(RATIONALE: Inability to smell [anosmia] may result from a pituitary tumor.)

Have you ever had seizures? If so, what type, and under what circumstances?
(RATIONALE: Seizures may be associated with hypopituitarism, hypothyroidism, hypoparathyroidism, Addison's disease, antidiuretic hormone excess, or hypoglycemia.)

Do you often have headaches? Do you ever have sudden, severe headaches that gradually go away?
(RATIONALE: Headaches can indicate pituitary problems or excessive catecholamine levels. Acute, severe headaches that gradually resolve may indicate pituitary hemorrhage or infarction.)

Developmental considerations

If the client is young or pregnant, investigate developmental status by exploring the areas described below.

Pediatric client. When assessing a child, try to involve the child and a parent or guardian in the interview. Of course, with an infant, pose questions to the parent or guardian. With any client who can understand and speak, invite that person's participation in the interview, using age-approppriate terms. To help perform a thorough endocrine system assessment, ask the following questions.

Has the child's activity level changed? If so, describe a typical day before this change and a typical day now.
(RATIONALE: The answer to this question will help distinguish a quiet or hyperactive child from one with altered endocrine function.)

Have you ever been told that the child's growth and development are above or below normal rates?
(RATIONALE: Altered growth and development may indicate a disturbance in growth, thyroid, or gonadal hormone levels.)

Has the child had a recent history of weight loss and excessive thirst, hunger, and urination?
(RATIONALE: These classic signs of Type I diabetes mellitus commonly occur in children.)

Pregnant client. When assessing a pregnant client, keep in mind that some symptoms during pregnancy (for example, mood changes and fatigue) are also symptoms of endocrine disorders. The following questions can help your assessment of a pregnant client's endocrine status.

Have you ever been told you had diabetes during this or any previous pregnancy?
(RATIONALE: Women who have had gestational diabetes mellitus [diabetes associated only with pregnancy] have an increased risk of developing Type II diabetes mellitus later in life.)

Have you ever given birth to an infant weighing more than 10 lb (4.5 kg)?
(RATIONALE: A high-birth-weight infant may indicate a maternal predisposition to diabetes mellitus.)

Health promotion and protection patterns

Continue the health history by asking questions to determine how the client feels about and practices health care.

Have you been sleeping more or less than usual?
(RATIONALE: Sleep disturbances often occur in endocrine disorders. Disorders such as hyperthyroidism, Cushing's syndrome, pheochromocytoma, diabetes mellitus, and diabetes insipidus may lead to restlessness and insomnia or an inability to sleep related to nocturia.)

What type of exercise do you engage in? How regularly do you exercise? Have you had any difficulty exercising lately?
(RATIONALE: Weakness and fatigue related to endocrine dysfunction can decrease stamina. Also, in a client with diabetes mellitus, exercise patterns will have an effect on where and when insulin is injected if required. For example, if the client injects insulin into the thigh before jogging, the insulin will be absorbed more rapidly because of muscle motion that increases blood flow.)

Have you been feeling under more stress lately? Can you talk about what may be causing this stress? Does your current problem seem to be related to this stress?
(RATIONALE: Many endocrine disorders, such as diabetes mellitus, can be exacerbated by stress. Also, treatment of certain endocrine disorders—for instance, diabetes mellitus, Addison's disease, and hypothyroidism—may require lifelong hormone replacement therapy and changes in life-style [such as activity restrictions and dietary changes], which may increase stress. Adapting to such life-style changes may be particularly difficult for an adolescent or an elderly client.)

What is your approximate yearly or monthly household income? Do you have health insurance?
(RATIONALE: Lifelong hormone replacement therapy for some endocrine disorders can be costly. A client without adequate financial resources or health insurance coverage may have trouble affording certain treatments and may need referral to a social worker.)

What type of work do you do? What are your normal work or school hours? Do you have enough time for breaks and meals?
(RATIONALE: Scheduling of hormone replacement therapy attempts to mimic the body's natural rhythms. A client with irregular sleep-wake cycles, such as one who performs shift work, may have problems adjusting to hormone therapy.)

Role and relationship patterns

Conclude the health history with questions that help evaluate the client's self-perception and view of the social support system.

What is your image of yourself? Do you think that the problem you are experiencing will get better or worse? What bothers you most about your problem?
(RATIONALE: A client with an endocrine disorder often has a poor self-image related to such effects as altered metabolism, increased susceptibility to and inability to cope with stress, and disfigurement or disability. Identifying the client's concerns about self-image will help you plan interventions that help the client understand and cope with transient or permanent problems.)

Do you have family members or close friends that you can ask for help when you need it?
(RATIONALE: A client receiving treatment for an endocrine disorder may need another person's help in administering prescribed medications, complying with life-style changes, or performing normal activities of daily living. For example, a client with Addison's disease may need someone to administer intramuscular injections of cortisone during crises; a client with diabetes mellitus may need someone to inject glucagon to treat hypoglycemia or to help in drawing up and injecting insulin correctly.)

Physical assessment

Because of the interrelationship of the endocrine system with all other body systems, physical assessment of a client with a known or suspected endocrine problem must include a total body evaluation, focusing on the areas described in the following sections. It also must include a complete neurologic assessment because of the role of the hypothalamus in regulating endocrine function through the pituitary gland. (For detailed information on neurologic assessment steps, see Chapter 17, Nervous System.)

During the physical assessment, the nurse should obtain most of the objective findings through inspection, augmented at some points by palpation and auscultation.

Before beginning, gather a tape measure, scale with height-measuring device, stethoscope, watch with a second hand, glass of water with a straw, a gown, and drapes. Make sure the examination room is warm and well-lit.

Vital signs, height, and weight

Begin the assessment by measuring the client's vital signs, height, and weight. Compare the findings with the client's baseline measurements, if available. (For more information on assessing vital signs, height, and weight, see Chapter 4, Physical Assessment Skills, and Chapter 6, Nutritional Status.)

Abnormal findings

Vital sign changes may provide important clues to the presence and nature of an endocrine disorder. For example, hypertension develops in many endocrine disorders, particularly pheochromocytoma, Cushing's syndrome, and hyperthyroidism. Hypotension commonly occurs in hypothyroidism. Fever may be related to excessive glucocorticoid levels or insufficient insulin levels; hypothermia may develop in hypoglycemia. Bradycardia (a heart rate of less than 60 beats/minute) occurs in myxedema and hypopituitarism. Tachycardia occurs in thyroid tumors and hyperthyroidism.

Weight gain unexplained by overeating or lack of exercise may point to Cushing's syndrome or hypothyroidism. In Cushing's syndrome, excessive cortisol secretion stimulates the appetite and frees glucose for fat synthesis, causing excessive fat deposition on the face, neck, trunk, and abdomen. In hypothyroidism, a decreased thyroxin level slows metabolic rate and decreases nutrient use, leading to weight gain.

In children, height that is consistently above or below normal for a sustained time could point to an increase or decrease in growth hormone production by the anterior pituitary.

In hyperthyroidism, an increased metabolic rate can accelerate the body's use of nutrients and lead to weight loss. Weight loss can also accompany uncontrolled diabetes mellitus as a result of osmotic diuresis. A weight gain or loss of 2 to 3 pounds within 48 hours may result from altered ADH levels. Weight gain occurs from oversecretion of ADH; weight loss, from insufficient secretion with resultant alterations in fluid balance.

Inspection

After measuring the client's vital signs, height, and weight, proceed to a systematic inspection that begins with general appearance and continues to an assessment of all body areas. Focus on the steps and areas discussed below.

General appearance. Assess the client's overall physical appearance and mental and emotional status. Note such factors as overall affect, speech, level of consciousness and orientation, appropriateness and neatness of dress and grooming, and activity level. Evaluate general body development, including posture, body build, proportionality of body parts, and distribution of body fat. (For more information on how to perform a general survey, see Chapter 4, Physical Assessment Skills.)

Skin, hair, and nails. Assess the client's overall skin color, and inspect the skin and mucous membranes for any lesions or areas of increased, decreased, or absent pigmentation. As you do so, be sure to consider racial and ethnic variations. In a dark-skinned client, color variations are best assessed in the sclera, conjunctiva, mouth, nail beds, and palms. Next, assess skin texture and hydration.

Inspect the client's hair for amount, distribution, condition, and texture. Assess scalp and body hair, looking for abnormal patterns of growth or loss. Again, remember to consider normal racial and ethnic—as well as sexual—differences in hair growth and texture. Then, check the client's fingernails for cracking, peeling, separation from the nail bed (onycholysis), and clubbing, and the toenails for fungal infection, ingrown nails, discoloration, length, and thickness. (For more information on assessing these features and on normal findings, see Chapter 7, Skin, Hair, and Nails.)

Head and neck. Assess the client's face for overall color and presence of erythematous areas, especially in the cheeks. Note facial expression—is it pained and anxious, dull and flat, or alert and interested? Note the shape and symmetry of the eyes and look for eyeball protrusion, incomplete eyelid closure, or periorbital edema. Have the client extend his or her tongue, and inspect it for color, size, lesions, positioning, and any tremors or unusual movements.

Standing in front of the client, examine the neck first with it held straight, then slightly extended, and finally while the client swallows water. Check for neck symmetry and midline positioning and for symmetry of the trachea. (For more information on assessing these structures and on normal findings, see Chapter 8, Head and Neck.)

Chest. Evaluate the overall size, shape, and symmetry of the client's chest, noting any deformities. In females, assess the breasts for size, shape, symmetry, pigmentation (especially on the nipples and in skin creases), and nipple discharge (galactorrhea). In males, observe for bilateral or unilateral breast enlargement (gynecomastia) and nipple discharge. (For more information, see Chapter 12, Female and Male Breasts.)

Genitalia. Inspect the client's external genitalia—particularly the testes and clitoris—for normal development. (For more information on assessing the genitalia and on normal findings, see Chapter 15, Female Reproductive System, and Chapter 16, Male Reproductive System.)

Extremities. Inspect the client's arms and hands for tremors. To do so, have the client hold both arms outstretched in front with the palms down and fingers separated. Then place a sheet of paper on the outstretched fingers and watch for any trembling. Note any muscle wasting, especially in the upper arms, and have the client grasp your hands to assess the strength and symmetry of the client's grip.

Next, inspect the legs for muscle development, symmetry, color, and hair distribution. Then, assess muscle strength by having the client sit on the edge of the examination table and extend the legs horizontally. A client who can maintain this position for 2 minutes usually exhibits normal strength. Examine the feet for size, and note any lesions, corns, calluses, or marks made from socks or shoes. Inspect the toes and the spaces between them for maceration and fissures. (For more information on assessing the extremities and on normal findings, see Chapter 18, Musculoskeletal System.)

Abnormal findings

Inspection may reveal abnormalities indicative of endocrine disease.

General appearance. Initial observation may identify the effects of a major endocrine disorder, such as hyperthyroidism or hypothyroidism, dwarfism, or acromegaly. Evaluation of the client's overall affect, clarity and quality of speech, and activity level may provide more insight. For example, a client with hyperthyroidism may speak rapidly, perhaps incoherently at times; a client with hypothyroidism may speak slowly and deliberately; and a client with myxedema may slur words and sound hoarse. In an adult male client, a high-pitched voice may point to hypogonadism; in an adult female, an abnormally deep voice may point to excessive androgen secretion related to Cushing's syndrome, acromegaly, congenital adrenal hyperplasia or tumors, polycystic ovaries, or ovarian tumors.

A client's body development also may provide important clues to the presence and nature of an endocrine problem. For example, an outward-curved spine (kyphosis) may indicate compression fractures related to osteoporosis, which often occurs with hyperparathyroidism. Osteoporosis also may manifest itself as a sharp angular deformity caused by collapsed vertebrae. In a client with Cushing's syndrome, fat deposits typically concentrate on the face (moon facies), neck, interscapular area (buffalo hump), trunk, and pelvic girdle.

Even the client's dress may provide clues to an endocrine problem. For instance, inappropriately heavy clothing in warm weather may indicate cold sensitivity from hypothyroidism, and a lack of outer garments in cold weather may indicate heat intolerance from hyperthyroidism.

Skin, hair, and nails. Hyperpigmentation of joints, genitalia, buccal mucosa, palmar creases, recent scars, and sun-exposed body areas occurs in most clients with Addison's disease. In a client who has undergone adrenalectomy, this hyperpigmentation usually indicates an ACTH-producing pituitary tumor or may indicate growth hormone excess. Gray-brown pigmentation of the neck and axillae (acanthosis nigricans) may occur in a client with polycystic ovaries, growth hormone excess, or Cushing's syndrome. Yellow pigmentation in the palmar creases can indicate hyperlipidemia; a yellowish cast to the skin may point to hypothyroidism. An overall decrease in skin pigmentation typically occurs in panhypopituitarism.

Dry, coarse, rough, and scaly skin can indicate hypothyroidism or hypoparathyroidism. Coarse, leathery, moist skin and enlarged sweat glands usually occur in acromegaly. Warm, moist, tissue-thin skin may point to hyperthyroidism. In an adult client, acne frequently develops in Cushing's syndrome or from androgen excess. Yellowish nodules on extensor surfaces of the elbows and knees and on the buttocks typically occur in severe hypertriglyceridemia. Purple striae, typically on the abdomen, and bruises (ecchymoses) are common signs of Cushing's syndrome. Edema often occurs in hypothyroidism and Cushing's syndrome. Dry mucous membranes and poor skin turgor may occur in diabetes mellitus.

Coarse, dry, brittle hair usually is associated with hypothyroidism; fine, silky, thinly distributed hair, with hyperthyroidism. In an adult female client, excessive facial, chest, abdominal, or pubic hair (hirsutism) may point to growth hormone or androgen excess. Hair loss or thinning in the axillae, pubic area, and the outer third of the eyebrows may indicate hypopituitarism, hypothyroidism, or hypogonadism.

Thick, brittle nails may suggest hypothyroidism; thin, brittle nails may result from hyperthyroidism. Increased nail pigmentation occurs in Addison's disease.

Head and neck. Eyelid tremors may indicate hyperthyroidism. Eyeball protrusion (exophthalmos) and incomplete eyelid closure, usually bilateral, are associated with Graves' disease, a common cause of severe hyperthyroidism, or thyrotoxicosis. A visible increase in tongue size may indicate hypothyroidism or acromegaly; in acromegaly, the enlarged tongue may have a furrowed appearance. A fine, rhythmic tremor of the tongue may occur in hyperthyroidism; fine, fascicular (twitching) tremors, in hyperparathyroidism. A mass at the base of the neck or a visible thyroid gland may indicate thyroid hyperplasia.

Chest. In an adult male client, gynecomastia may be related to hypogonadism, hypothyroidism, thyrotoxicosis, estrogen excess from an adrenal tumor, or Cushing's syndrome. (Keep in mind, however, that transient gynecomastia may develop during puberty.) In a nonlactating female, nipple discharge could indicate prolactin or estrogen excess, hypothyroidism, diabetes mellitus, or Cushing's syndrome. Breast (areolar) hyperpigmentation may accompany excess ACTH production, as in Cushing's disease or an ACTH-secreting pituitary tumor.

Genitalia. In an adult male, abnormally small testes suggest hypogonadism. In an adult female, an enlarged clitoris may indicate masculinization. Vaginitis occurs in uncontrolled diabetes mellitus.

Extremities. Muscle atrophy in the arms and legs usually occurs in Cushing's syndrome, hypothyroidism, and hyperthyroidism. A fine rhythmic tremor of the extremities also may occur in hyperthyroidism. Muscle atrophy between the thumb and index finger (thenar wasting) and contracture of the palmar fascia (Dupuytren's contracture) may develop in long-term diabetes mellitus. Abnormally large fingers and hands may indicate acromegaly; finger clubbing may be associated with thyroid abnormalities. In the lower legs, dependent redness or bluish coloration and absence of hair may indicate vascular insufficiency related to diabetes mellitus.

Palpation

The following guidelines are for assessing the thyroid gland and testes, the only endocrine glands accessible to palpation. (For information on how to perform these two techniques, see *Palpating the thyroid*, and *Testicular self-examination* in Chapter 16, Male Reproductive System.)

Usually, you will not be able to palpate the client's thyroid, but you may feel the isthmus (center portion connecting the two lobes of the thyroid). You may, however, see or feel a normal thyroid in a client with an extremely thin neck. An enlarged thyroid may feel well-defined and finely lobulated. Thyroid nodules feel like a knot, protuberance, or swelling; a firm, fixed nodule may be a tumor. Be careful not to confuse thick neck musculature with an enlarged thyroid or goiter.

In a client with suspected hypocalcemia (low calcium levels in the blood) related to deficient or ineffective parathormone secretion from hypoparathyroidism or surgical removal of the parathyroid glands, attempt to elicit

Palpating the thyroid

Using these techniques, the nurse can palpate the thyroid from in front of or behind the client.

Anterior approach

1. To palpate from the front, face the client and locate the cricoid cartilage with the pads of your index and middle fingers. Ask the client to swallow as you palpate the thyroid isthmus just below the cricoid cartilage, using the same two fingers. (Swallowing raises the larynx, the trachea, and the thyroid gland, but not the lymph nodes or other structures.)

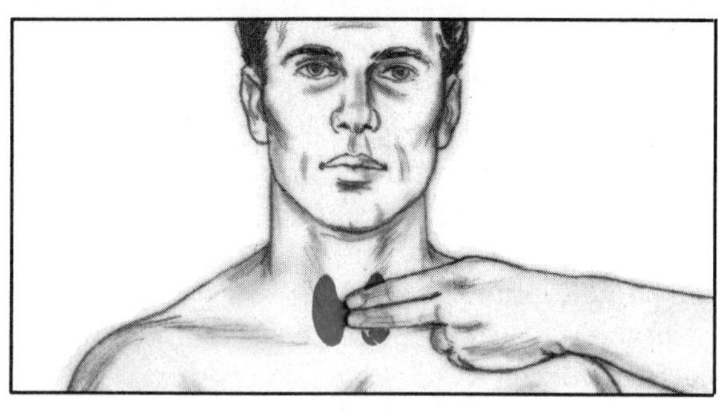

2. To palpate the anterior of the right lobe, displace the client's trachea to the right with your right hand and palpate with the fingers of your left hand.

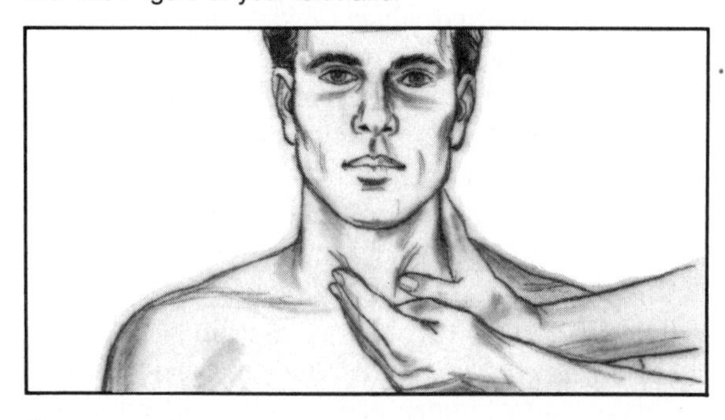

3. Grasp the sternocleidomastoid muscle with your left hand (place the tips of your index and middle fingers behind the muscle, your thumb in front), and palpate for the posterior of the right lobe of the thyroid between your left fingers.

To palpate the left lobe, use your left hand to move the thyroid cartilage and your right hand to palpate.

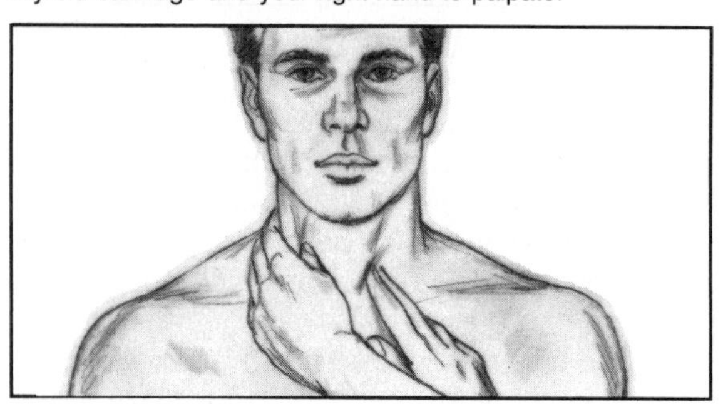

Posterior approach

1. To palpate the thyroid from behind the client, gently place the fingers of both hands on either side of the trachea, just below the cricoid cartilage. Ask the client to swallow as you palpate the thyroid isthmus.

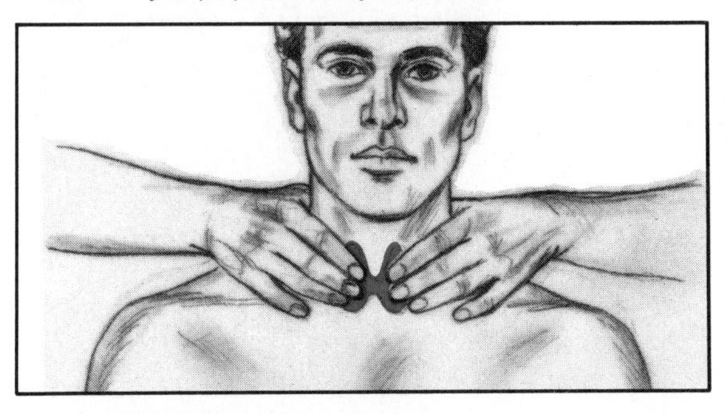

2. Palpating one lobe at a time, ask the client to lower the chin and flex the neck slightly to the side you are assessing. To palpate the anterior right lobe, place your left hand on the client's neck and move the thyroid cartilage to the right; palpate with the fingers of your right hand.

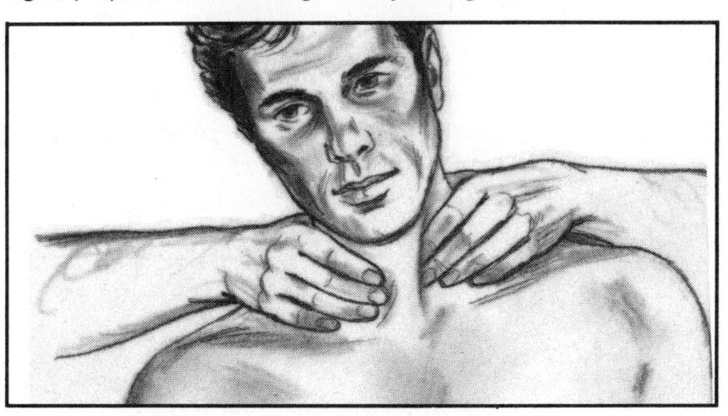

3. Grasp the sternocleidomastoid muscle with your right hand while placing your middle fingers deep into and in front of the muscle; palpate for the right lateral border of the right lobe.

For the left lobe, use your right hand to move the cartilage to the left and your left hand to palpate.

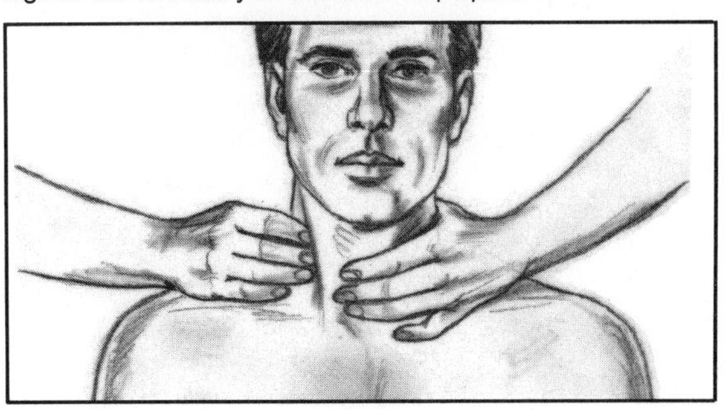

Chvostek's sign and Trousseau's sign. To elicit Chvostek's sign, tap the facial nerve in front of the ear with a finger; if the facial muscles contract toward the ear, the test is positive for hypocalcemia. To elicit Trousseau's sign, place a blood pressure cuff on the client's arm and inflate it above the client's systolic pressure. In a positive test, the client will exhibit carpal spasm (ventral contraction of the thumb and digits) within 3 minutes.

Auscultation

If you palpate an enlarged thyroid gland, auscultate it. In a client with an enlarged thyroid, auscultation may detect systolic bruits. Such bruits, caused by vibrations produced by accelerated blood flow through the thyroid arteries, may indicate hyperthyroidism. To auscultate for bruits, place the bell of the stethoscope over one of the lateral lobes of the thyroid, then listen carefully for a low, soft, rushing sound. To ensure that tracheal sounds do not obscure any bruits, have the client hold his or her breath while you auscultate. To distinguish a bruit from a venous hum, listen for the rushing sound, then gently occlude the jugular vein with your fingers on the side you are auscultating and listen again. A venous hum (produced by jugular blood flow) disappears during venous compression; a bruit does not. (For some common abnormal assessment findings associated with endocrine disorders, see *Integrating assessment findings,* pages 602 and 603.)

Developmental considerations

When assessing a child's body development, keep in mind that the normal growth rate averages roughly 3" per year between ages 1 through 7, and 2" per year between ages 8 through 15. Hypopituitary dwarfism related to growth hormone deficiency usually becomes apparent at about age 2. Thyroid hormone deficiency in infants (cretinism) is characterized by a stocky build.

To evaluate a child's body proportions, have the child stand with arms outstretched to the left and right. Then measure the span between the tips of the middle fingers on both hands. Normally, this distance should approximate the child's height. Short arms and legs may indicate gonadal dysfunction. Keep in mind that normal body proportions in children differ from those in adults, in whom the distance from the top of the head to the pubis and from the pubis to the bottom of the feet is approximately equal. In contrast, the distance from the top of the head to the pubis at birth is normally 70% of overall height; at age 2, 60% of overall height; and at age 10, 52% of overall height.

Integrating assessment findings

Sometimes, a cluster of assessment findings will strongly suggest a particular endocrine system disorder. In the chart below, column one shows groups of presenting signs and symptoms—the ones that make the client seek medical attention. Column two shows related assessment findings that the nurse may discover during the health history and physical assessment. The client may exhibit one or more of these findings. Column three shows the possible disorder indicated by a cluster of these findings.

PRESENTING SIGNS AND SYMPTOMS	RELATED ASSESSMENT FINDINGS	POSSIBLE DISORDER
Lethargy, easy fatigue; weight changes (usually loss); general loss of secondary sex characteristics; amenorrhea; impotence; somnolence; coma	History of predisposing factors, such as congenital abnormalities, acute infections, vascular problems, pituitary tumor Skin changes, such as yellowing, wrinkling, thinning, drying Slow pulse rate Hypotension Decreased growth, genital atrophy Loss of teeth Brittle nails Anorexia, constipation	Hypopituitarism
Fatigue, weakness, and lethargy; need for increased sleep; weight gain; diminished sexual functioning; menorrhagia; impotence; abnormal tranquility; depression	History of predisposing factors, such as surgery or radioiodine treatment for hyperthyroidism Insidious onset Sparse (especially at eyebrows), brittle, coarse hair Muscle stiffness Diminished hearing Sensitivity to cold Constipation Hoarseness Inappropriate answers to questions Slowed cognitive activities	Hypothyroidism
Progressive fatigue and weakness; weight loss caused by poor appetite, food idiosyncrasies, nausea, vomiting, diarrhea; loss of secondary sex characteristics and libido in females; depression, irritability, restlessness	Insidious onset History of predisposing factors, such as tuberculosis, treatment with exogenous steroids, and family history of adrenal insufficiency Fasting hypoglycemia Hypotension and syncope Poor coordination Bronze skin pigmentation Abdominal pain Salt craving	Addison's disease (primary adrenal insufficiency)
Fatigue; loss of strength; weight loss; in chronic illness, bloating, fullness; impotence; polyuria and polydipsia (classic symptoms)	History of predisposing factors, such as long-standing obesity, pancreatic disease, family history of diabetes, and, in females, delivery of large infants Mild long-standing symptoms (in Type II) Dry skin and mucous membranes Blurred vision Light-headedness Pruritus	Diabetes mellitus
Lethargy; irritability, emotional lability, impaired memory, confusion, depression; changes in level of consciousness	History of predisposing factors, such as injury to parathyroids during removal of thyroid; tetany; twitching of muscles; numbness; tingling in fingers, toes, and around lips Chvostek's and Trousseau's signs Laryngeal stridor, dyspnea Malformed, pitted nails; thinning hair, alopecia Coarse, dry skin Dysplasia of tooth enamel Diplopia, cataracts, photophobia (light sensitivity) Convulsions Abdominal pain, nausea, vomiting	Hypoparathyroidism

Integrating assessment findings continued

PRESENTING SIGNS AND SYMPTOMS	RELATED ASSESSMENT FINDINGS	POSSIBLE DISORDER
Extreme weakness; increased fatigue; weight loss despite increased appetite; short, scanty menstrual periods; decreased fertility; temporal recession of hairline in females; anxiety; nervousness; difficulty concentrating; agitation; paranoid tendencies; polyuria with increased thirst	History of predisposing factors, such as recent emotional crisis, infection, physical stress; family history of Graves' disease Thin, brittle hair and nails Palpable thyroid Systolic bruit over thyroid Tender supraclavicular lymph nodes Palpitations, tachycardia Increased heat production with excessive perspiration and decreased heat tolerance Exophthalmos and lid lag Muscle atrophy Decreased subcutaneous fat	Hyperthyroidism, thyrotoxicosis
Fatigue and weakness; weight gain; increased fat distribution on neck, face, abdomen, girdle; hirsutism; gynecomastia in males; irritability, emotional lability, depression, psychosis; polyuria or polydipsia with other symptoms of hyperglycemia	History of predisposing factors, such as steroid treatment and adrenal tumors Female (most common in women) Hypertension Osteoporosis with spontaneous fractures, height reduction, and backache Purple striae on arms, breasts, abdomen, and thighs Petechiae, excessive bruising Decreased healing ability Loss of muscle mass Clitoral hypertrophy	Cushing's syndrome

With age, a person normally loses about 3″ in height by age 70. For this reason, an elderly client's arm span typically will exceed the person's height. When assessing an elderly client, also keep in mind that dry, thin skin, slower responses and reflexes, and decreased body temperature may be normal physiologic effects of aging and not necessarily indicative of endocrine disorders.

Documentation

Before documenting assessment findings, the nurse carefully reviews and integrates health history and physical assessment data, along with the results of any diagnostic or laboratory tests. (For a summary of frequently used laboratory studies and their significance, see *Common laboratory studies*, pages 604 and 605.) Based on these data, the nurse formulates appropriate nursing diagnoses and then plans, implements, and evaluates the client's nursing care. (For a case study that shows how to apply the nursing process to a client with an endocrine disorder, see *Applying the nursing process,* pages 606 and 607.)

Proper documentation is essential in organizing assessment data and making information available to other members of the health care team. Document all data completely, including normal and abnormal findings.

The following sample illustrates the proper way to document some normal physical assessment findings related to the endocrine system:

> *Weight:* 150 lb
> *Height:* 5′7″
> *Vital signs:* Temperature 98.6° F., pulse 72 and regular, respirations 18 and regular, blood pressure 130/70.
> Client is a well-developed, healthy male who appears to be his stated age of 35. Oriented to person, place, and time; speech clear. No visible abnormalities in skin, hair, nails, or facial characteristics. Neck supple, trachea midline. Thyroid palpable: firm, smooth, freely movable, and nontender. Breasts

Common laboratory studies

For a client with signs and symptoms of an endocrine disorder, various laboratory studies can provide the nurse with valuable clues to the possible cause, as shown in the chart below. (*Note:* Keep in mind that abnormal findings may stem from a problem unrelated to the endocrine system.) Remember that values differ between laboratories; check the normal range for the specific laboratory.

TEST AND SIGNIFICANCE	NORMAL VALUES OR FINDINGS	ABNORMAL FINDINGS	POSSIBLE ENDOCRINE OR RELATED CAUSES OF ABNORMAL FINDINGS
Blood tests			
Cortisol This test evaluates the status of adrenocortical function.	8 a.m. 7 to 28 mcg/dl 4 p.m. 2 to 18 mcg/dl (The 4 p.m. level is usually half the 8 a.m. level.)	Above-normal level Below-normal level.	Cushing's disease, Cushing's syndrome Addison's disease, hypopituitarism
Catecholamines Epinephrine, basal supine Epinephrine, standing Norepinephrine, basal supine Norepinephrine, standing This test assesses adrenal medulla function.	 0 to 110 pg/ml 0 to 140 pg/ml 70 to 750 pg/ml 200 to 1,700 pg/ml	Above-normal level	Pheochromocytoma
Parathyroid hormone (PTH) This test evaluates parathyroid function.	210 to 310 pg/ml	Above-normal level Below-normal level	Hyperparathyroidism Hypoparathyroidism
Total calcium This test helps detect bone and parathyroid disorders.	8.9 to 10.1 mg/dl	Above-normal level Below-normal level	Hyperparathyroidism Hypoparathyroidism
Phosphorus This test helps detect parathyroid disorders and renal failure.	2.5 to 4.5 mg/dl	Above-normal level Below-normal level	Hypoparathyroidism, renal failure Hyperparathyroidism
Oral glucose tolerance test This test detects diabetes mellitus and hypoglycemia.	160 to 180 mg/dl 30 to 60 min after oral glucose dose; fasting levels or lower in 2 to 3 hr	Above-normal level Below-normal level	Diabetes mellitus Hypoglycemia
Glycosylated hemoglobin (GHB, glycohemoglobin) This test monitors the degree of glucose control in diabetes mellitus over 3 months.	5.5% to 9% of total hemoglobin	Above-normal level	Uncontrolled diabetes mellitus
HGH (RTA) This test evaluates growth hormone oversecretion.	Male: <5 ng/ml Female: <10 ng/ml	Above-normal level	Acromegaly
Insulin-induced hypoglycemia This test detects hypopituitarism.	Rise in growth hormone 2- to 3-fold over baseline	Below-normal level of growth hormone	Hypopituitarism
Thyroid stimulating hormone (TSH) This test detects primary hypothyroidism.	<15 μIU/ml	Above-normal level	Primary hypothyroidism

Common laboratory studies continued

TEST AND SIGNIFICANCE	NORMAL VALUES OR FINDINGS	ABNORMAL FINDINGS	POSSIBLE ENDOCRINE OR RELATED CAUSES OF ABNORMAL FINDINGS
Gonadotropins (FSH, LH) This test distinguishes a primary gonadal problem from pituitary insufficiency.	*Females* FSH: follicular phase 5 to 20 mIU/ml; mid-cycle peak 15 to 30 mIU/ml; luteal phase 5 to 15 mIU/ml; postmenopausal 50 to 100 mIU/ml LH: follicular phase 5 to 25 mIU/ml; mid-cycle peak 30 to 60 mIU/ml; luteal phase 5 to 15 mIU/ml; postmenopausal >50 mIU/ml *Males* FSH: 5 to 20 mIU/ml LH: 5 to 20 mIU/ml	Above-normal level Below-normal level	Primary gonadal failure Pituitary insufficiency
T_4 radioimmunoassay (RIA) This test evaluates thyroid function and monitors iodine or antithyroid therapy.	5 to 13.5 mcg/dl	Above-normal level	Hyperthyroidism
T_3 RIA This test detects hyperthyroidism if T_4 levels are normal.	90 to 230 ng/dl	Above-normal level	Hyperthyroidism
Urine studies			
17-Ketosteroids (17-KS) This test evaluates adrenocortical and gonadal function.	Males: 6 to 21 mg/24 hr Females: 4 to 17 mg/24 hr	Above-normal level Below-normal level	Congenital adrenal hyperplasia Adrenal insufficiency
17-Hydroxycorticosteroids (17-OHCS) This test evaluates adrenal function.	Males: 4.54 to 12 mg/24 hr Females: 2.5 to 10 mg/24 hr	Above-normal level Below-normal level	Hyperadrenalism Hypopituitarism, adrenal disease

symmetrical, nipples everted. Abdomen slightly rounded, with no scars or striae. Upper extremities strong; no tremors noted. Lower extremities strong, with normal color and hair distribution.

The following example shows how to document some abnormal assessment findings:

Weight: 164 lb
Height: 5′2″
Vital signs: Temperature 96.8° F., pulse 52 and regular, respirations 14 and deep, blood pressure, 130/70.
Client is a well-developed male who appears older than his stated age of 52. Oriented to person, place, and time, but lethargic. Speech slow and hoarse; skin and hair, dry and coarse; nails, thick and brittle. Nonpitting edema present on lower extrem-

(Text continues on page 608.)

Applying the nursing process

Assessment findings form the basis of the nursing process. Using them, the nurse formulates the nursing diagnoses and develops appropriate planning, implementation, and evaluation of the client's care.

The table below shows how the nurse can use endocrine system assessment data in the nursing process for the client described in the case history (shown at right). In the first column, history and physical assessment data appear, followed by a paragraph of mental notes. These notes help the nurse make important mental connections among assessment findings, aiding in development of the nursing diagnoses and planning.

The second column presents several appropriate nursing diagnoses; however, the information in the remaining columns is based on the *first* nursing diagnosis. Although it is not part of the nursing process, documentation appears in the last column because of its importance. Documentation consists of an initial note using all components of the SOAPIE format and a follow-up note using the appropriate SOAPIE components.

ASSESSMENT	NURSING DIAGNOSES	PLANNING	IMPLEMENTATION
Subjective (history) data: • Client states, "I hope my blood sugar is down. I don't know if I can give myself insulin." • Client reports that he continues to urinate frequently and drinks a lot of fluid. He states that he is frequently sleepy and asks if this has anything to do with his blood sugar. • Client also states that his mother died shortly after she started taking insulin, and that he fears "the same thing will happen to me." **Objective (physical) data:** • Blood sugar 310 mg/dl, urine and glucose ketones negative. • Height 5′9″, weight 210 lb. • Skin is flushed and dry; turgor, poor—as evidenced by tenting. • Urine appears dilute. **Mental notes** *When considered along with assessment and laboratory findings, the client's complaints point to ineffective dietary and medication control of blood glucose. Oral hypoglycemic agents may control blood glucose levels for a period of time and then become ineffective, causing secondary failure. Obesity and stress increase insulin requirements. Client seems to have excessive anxiety about self-injection of insulin.*	• Anxiety related to self-injection of insulin. • Knowledge deficit related to insulin injection and necessary dietary and activity measures. • Altered nutrition: more than body requirements, related to decreased exercise and frequent dining out. • Altered family processes related to recent death of spouse. • Altered health maintenance related to inability of pancreas to increase insulin secretion or peripheral tissues to use insulin. • Fear of dying related to mother's death from diabetic complications.	**Goals** Before leaving the clinic today, the client will: • exhibit less fear about self-injection of insulin • verbalize reason for taking insulin and identify the type, amount, onset, peak, and duration of insulin • demonstrate correct self-injection of insulin • describe care and storage of insulin • list the signs and symptoms of an insulin reaction • describe steps to treat an insulin reaction. At the next follow-up visit, the client will: • reveal rotation pattern used for insulin injection • demonstrate how to mix insulins in one syringe, if required • self-administer insulin with no anxiety or fear.	• Encourage the client to verbalize fears and concerns regarding self-injection of insulin. • Show the client an insulin syringe and needle, and explain the parts of the syringe. • Teach the client how to draw up insulin. • Obtain a syringe magnifier or magnifying glass, if the client has difficulty seeing the syringe markings. • Instruct the client on proper rotation of injection sites and importance of rotating sites within one anatomical area. • Demonstrate proper injection technique, using normal saline if an insulin injection is not scheduled. • Have the client give himself an injection, using normal saline if an insulin injection is not scheduled. • Explain insulin reactions, including their causes, signs and symptoms, and treatments. • Give the client written, pictorial, or video instructions on insulin injection techniques.

CASE HISTORY

Jacob Smith, age 52, has Type II diabetes mellitus. Until recently, when Mr. Smith experienced stress related to his wife's death, his diabetes was well controlled by diet and chlorpropamide (Diabinese), 500 mg every a.m. Mr. Smith has come for a follow-up evaluation of his blood glucose level, which was 260 mg/dl at his last visit.

EVALUATION

- By the end of the initial clinic visit, the client:
  - drew up insulin correctly
  - injected himself with insulin correctly
  - verbalized the reason for taking insulin and correctly identified the type, amount, onset, peak, and duration of his insulin
  - described care and storage of insulin
  - identified the signs and symptoms of an insulin reaction and appropriate treatment measures
  - stated that injecting insulin was not as difficult as expected and that he no longer feels nervous when thinking about it.

At the next follow-up visit, the client:
- handled the syringe and insulin vial without difficulty or hesitancy
- mixed two types of insulin in one syringe.

DOCUMENTATION BASED ON NURSING PROCESS DATA

Initial

S Client states, "I'm urinating a lot, drinking a lot, and I'm always hungry." Client also states, "I hope my blood sugar is down. I can't give myself insulin...my hands shake every time I pick up the needle. The thought of sticking the needle in my leg makes me want to vomit."

O Weight loss of 6 lb in past 2 weeks. Fasting blood glucose level 310 mg/dl. Urine glucose and ketones negative. Skin flushed and dry. Poor skin turgor noted, as evidenced by tenting. Urine is dilute in appearance.

A Anxiety related to self-injection of insulin. Client has lost weight and is dehydrated.

P Allow time for client to verbalize fear about self-injection of insulin. Teach client about drawing up insulin into a syringe, injecting insulin, rotating injection sites, storing and caring for insulin and syringes, identifying signs and symptoms of low blood glucose levels, and identifying treatment measures.

I Spent time with client, allowing him to express his fears and anxiety about self-injection of insulin. Gave client printed information about insulin injection and hypoglycemia to take home. Client viewed film on insulin injection before leaving. Taught client self-injection of insulin.

E Client self-injected 10 units of saline S.Q. in right lower abdominal quadrant after drawing it up correctly. Although nervous, client stated, "That didn't really hurt. I can't believe I did it!" Client stated that film was good reinforcement.

Follow-up

S Client states, "I can't believe I was so upset about giving myself insulin. It isn't so bad after all. Now, it's just another habit like brushing my teeth in the morning."

O Blood glucose level 160 mg/dl fasting. Skin turgor good—skin returns to normal position after pinching between fingers. Weight gain of 3 lb in 1 week.

A Client successfully self-administering insulin. Blood glucose level normal. Hydration improved. Anxiety alleviated.

P Follow-up visit scheduled in 2 weeks; if blood glucose level normal, follow-up in 6 weeks and 3 months thereafter.

ities. Thyroid palpable: firm, smooth, freely movable, enlarged left lobe contains a firm, fixed, pea-sized nodule.

• The nurse should document all assessment findings and use them in the nursing process to plan, implement, and evaluate the client's care.

Chapter summary

To assess the endocrine system effectively, the nurse must rely on health history data, physical assessment findings, and laboratory studies. Chapter 20 describes how to gather and integrate this information. Here are the major points:

• The endocrine system includes the pituitary gland, thyroid gland, parathyroid glands, adrenal glands, islets of Langerhans in the pancreas, gonads (ovaries and testes), thymus, and pineal gland.

• Hormones, the functional units of the endocrine system, regulate most major body functions and maintain homeostasis with nervous system actions mainly through the hypothalamus.

• Once secreted by the endocrine glands, hormones travel to specific body areas to perform their individualized actions.

• When obtaining a health history, the nurse should use a holistic approach because endocrine system problems may affect any body system.

• During the health history, the nurse should ask about the client's medication use, which may indicate that the client is being treated for an endocrine disorder. Many drugs affect hormone levels and may cause endocrine dysfunction.

• Physical assessment of the endocrine system involves measuring the client's height, weight, and vital signs and using inspection, sometimes augmented by palpation and auscultation.

• When inspecting a client with an endocrine system problem, the nurse should focus on the client's general appearance, speech, and body development; skin, hair, and nails; head and neck; chest; genitalia; and extremities.

• If a thyroid disorder is suspected, the nurse should palpate and auscultate the thyroid gland.

• To complete the endocrine system assessment, the nurse should check the results of any laboratory studies ordered to assess endocrine function. Frequently ordered studies include electrolytes, blood chemistries, hematology and urine tests, and measurements of individual hormones.

Study questions

1. Which glands make up the endocrine system? What are the major functions of each gland?

2. What are five skin abnormalities that should alert you to possible endocrine disorders, and what specific endocrine disorders are usually associated with each abnormality?

3. What are the essential steps in palpating the thyroid gland? What palpation findings should you expect in a normal thyroid? What findings would be considered abnormal?

4. When assessing a client for a potential endocrine problem, why should you assess body systems, such as the nervous and reproductive systems?

5. Mrs. Maria DelaCruz, age 74, was admitted with complaints of polyuria, polydipsia, and polyphagia. Her skin turgor is poor as evidenced by tenting, she is obese, and she states that her mother has diabetes. On admission, her blood glucose level measured 436 mg/dl. After receiving insulin to lower her blood glucose level, she was started on low-dose oral hypoglycemic therapy. How should you document the following information related to a nursing assessment of Mrs. DelaCruz?

• history (subjective) assessment data
• physical (objective) assessment data
• assessment techniques and equipment used
• two appropriate nursing diagnoses
• documentation of your findings.

Selected references

Baxter, J., Frohman, L., Broadus, A., and Felig, P. (1987). Introduction to the endocrine system. In P. Felig, J. Baxter, A. Broadus, and L. Frohman (Eds.), *Endocri-*

nology and metabolism (2nd ed.). New York: McGraw-Hill.

Becker, K. (1990). *Principles and practice of endocrinology and metabolism.* Philadelphia: Lippincott.

Endocrine problems. (1986). NurseReview Series. Springhouse, PA: Springhouse Corp.

Gambert, S. (1985). A typical presentation of thyroid disease in the elderly. *Geriatrics,* 40(2), 63-69.

Garofano, C. (1991). Assessment of the endocrine system. In D. Ignatavicius and M. Bayne (Eds.), *Medical-surgical nursing: A nursing process approach.* Philadelphia: Saunders.

Greenspan, F., and Forsham, P. (1990). *Basic and clinical endocrinology* (3rd ed.). East Norwalk, CT: Appleton & Lange.

Guyton, A. (1991). *Textbook of medical physiology* (8th ed.). Philadelphia: Saunders.

Haas, L. (1987). Nursing assessment: Endocrine system. In S. Lewis and K. Collier (Eds.), *Medical-surgical nursing: Assessment and management of clinical problems* (2nd ed.). New York: McGraw-Hill.

Halloran, T. (1990). Nursing responsibilities in endocrine emergencies. *Critical Care Nursing Quarterly,* 13(3), 74-81.

Henry, J. (1991). *Clinical diagnosis and management by laboratory methods* (18th ed.). Philadelphia: Saunders.

Hershman, J. (1988). *Endocrine pathophysiology: A patient-oriented approach* (3rd ed.). Philadelphia: Lea & Febiger.

McConnell, E. (1985). Assessing the thyroid. *Nursing85,* 15(5), 60-62.

McEvoy, G. (Ed.). (1992). *American Hospital Formulary Service drug information.* Bethesda, MD: American Society of Hospital Pharmacists.

Nursing research

Grey, M., Cameron, M., and Thurber, F. (1991). Coping and adaptation in children with diabetes. *Nursing Research,* 40(3), 144-149.

Krug, L., Haire, J., and Heady, S. (1991). Exercise habits and exercise relapse in persons with non-insulin-dependent diabetes mellitus. *Diabetes Educator,* 17(3), 185-188.

McCargar, L., Tauton, J., and Pare, S. (1991). Benefits of exercise training for men with insulin-dependent diabetes mellitus. *Diabetes Educator,* 17(3), 179-184.

UNIT FIVE

Special Assessments

The previous unit explored assessment of specific body structures and systems. This unit builds on that information, explaining how to integrate it into a complete, partial, prenatal, postpartum, or neonatal assessment.

To perform any of these assessments, the nurse must know how to obtain a thorough health history and must possess excellent physical assessment skills. Chapters 21 and 22 describe how to develop these basic skills to an advanced degree and use them skillfully in special assessments.

Although all nurses may perform special assessments, nurse practitioners and nurse midwives are especially likely to perform them. These assessments may be needed in settings that range from public health centers to physicians' offices to hospital nurseries.

Chapter 21
Complete and Partial Assessments

Chapter 21 begins by comparing complete and partial assessments, pointing out the differences in their uses and in the areas examined. Then it discusses the complete assessment in depth. It reviews how to obtain a complete health history, including biographic data, health and illness patterns, health promotion and protection patterns, role and relationship patterns, and a summary of health history data. It also discusses how to perform a complete physical assessment, from the general survey to vital sign measurements to an integrated head-to-toe assessment of all body structures and systems. As an aid to the nurse, the chapter provides a head-to-toe physical assessment guide. It also illustrates how to document normal findings by body system.

The second part of Chapter 21 highlights the most frequently done evaluation—the partial assessment. It explains how to get the most health history information in the shortest time by focusing on key aspects of the client's health, such as the reason for seeking health care. It also explains how to use health history information to guide the partial physical assessment. Although specific assessment areas will differ between clients with different signs and symptoms, some areas, such as vital signs and heart sounds, must be assessed for all clients. Chapter 21 includes a partial assessment checklist for all of these common assessment areas.

Chapter 22
Perinatal and Neonatal Assessments

This chapter actually presents three different assessments: prenatal, postpartum, and neonatal assessments. The prenatal section begins with the health history, focusing particularly on behaviors that may influence the health of the fetus and on signs and symptoms of pregnancy-related problems. It continues with physical assessment, highlighting the physiologic changes that occur during pregnancy. It concludes by describing how to document the physical assessment.

In the postpartum assessment section, the health history provides questions that evaluate maternal-child bonding and other factors, such as feeding. Then it moves to the postpartum physical assessment, identifying normal changes after giving birth. It also includes a brief example of postpartum documentation.

The neonatal assessment explains how to perform a neonatal physical assessment, including tests for neonatal reflexes. It concludes with an illustration of proper documentation for a neonatal assessment.

21

Complete and Partial Assessments

Objectives

After reading and studying this chapter, you should be able to:

1. Explain the uses of complete and partial assessments.
2. Differentiate between a complete and a partial health history.
3. Prepare for the complete physical assessment.
4. Perform a complete physical assessment.
5. Describe how to modify the complete physical assessment for a pediatric client.
6. Describe how to modify the complete physical assessment for an elderly client.
7. Document findings obtained during a complete physical assessment.
8. Perform a partial physical assessment.
9. Document findings obtained during a partial physical assessment.

Introduction

The main elements of the nurse's assessment include the health history, physical assessment, and review of laboratory and other diagnostic studies. They provide the information needed to formulate nursing diagnoses, which in turn serve as the basis for planning, implementing, and evaluating client care. This chapter describes how the nurse can carry out these tasks efficiently by performing a complete assessment effectively and by performing a properly focused partial assessment.

After reviewing how to obtain a complete health history, the chapter shows how to perform the complete physical assessment by integrating assessment components in a format of brevity, accuracy, and consistency. Then it explains how to document assessment data completely. By using this complete assessment, you can manage time efficiently while obtaining a comprehensive view of a client.

Chapter 21 also describes the partial assessment. It explains how to modify health history questions and physical assessment techniques in cases where time is limited, where the client tires easily, or where the assessment is a follow-up to a complete assessment.

Complete assessment

The nurse's complete assessment includes three essential components: the health history, physical assessment, and review of laboratory or diagnostic studies.

Health history

The client's health history is the most important part of the complete assessment. It provides information about the client's physical and environmental background and investigates the client's cultural, social, emotional, intellectual, philosophical, and religious views. Also, it tells you whether a complete or partial physical assessment is necessary.

A complete health history should take about ½ hour to 1 hour to obtain, depending on the type and completeness of the history, your interviewing skills, and the client's physical, mental, and developmental status. To obtain health history information consistently and efficiently, many health care facilities use standardized forms. These forms may be checklists or questionnaires with space for short answers. If you use such forms, review them after they are completed, especially if they are completed by the client, and ask questions for clarification, as needed.

The complete history consists of five basic components: biographic data, health and illness patterns, health promotion and protection patterns, role and relationship patterns, and a summary of health data. Each component seeks information about a different aspect of the client's life and health. To obtain a complete health history, explore each component with the client during the interview. (For a detailed discussion of health history components and interviewing skills, see Chapter 3, The Health History.)

Physical assessment

The preceding chapters described how to assess each body system separately. This section of Chapter 21 will show how to integrate different body system assessments into a complete physical assessment.

A complete physical assessment may be needed during a client's first visit to an outpatient setting (if the client does not need emergency or urgent care) or as a periodic checkup. To perform a complete physical assessment for routine screening, follow the guidelines below. Keep in mind that this physical assessment format is just one of many possible formats. Modify it, as needed, to meet the client's needs and abilities.

Preparing for the complete physical assessment

For the complete physical assessment, plan to use all four assessment techniques: inspection, palpation, percussion, and auscultation. Also employ the gentle art of listening to the client. Throughout the examination, be sensitive to the client's needs. Provide proper instruction and information to help the client feel comfortable with the examination, and drape the client appropriately, exposing only the body area to be examined.

Before beginning the complete assessment, check the room to make sure it has an examination table with stirrups, stool, gooseneck lamp, desk with two chairs, counter or stand to hold supplies, scale, and sink. (If the assessment takes place in the client's home, adapt available furnishings, as needed.) Then gather the following supplies and equipment:

- thermometer
- watch with a second hand
- stethoscope with diaphragm and bell heads
- sphygmomanometer
- visual acuity chart, page of newsprint, and color perception pages or plates
- ophthalmoscope
- otoscope or an ophthalmoscope with an otoscopic tip
- nasoscope, an ophthalmoscope with a nasal tip, or a nasal speculum and a penlight
- penlight
- transilluminator
- ruler and measuring tape
- marking pencil
- gloves
- tongue depressors
- cotton balls
- cotton-tipped swabs
- 4" x 4" gauze pads
- tuning fork
- reflex hammer
- vaginal speculum and Papanicolaou (Pap) smear materials
- lubricant
- fecal testing materials
- goniometer
- test tubes of hot and cold water (optional)
- test tubes of odorous materials, such as coffee, chocolate, or other familiar substances (optional)
- substances for taste assessment, such as sugar, salt, vinegar, and quinine (optional)
- coin
- paper clip
- pin and cotton to test sharp and dull sensations
- gown and drapes.

After gathering the necessary equipment, warm the room and the instruments. Instruct the client to empty the bladder (and provide a urine specimen, if needed), remove all clothing, and put on the gown. Ensure privacy by closing the examination room door or pulling the bed curtains closed, and draping the client appropriately. To prevent contamination of the client, yourself, or another client, wear gloves during examination of the mucous membranes, genitals, rectum, and any area with lesions or signs of infection or infestation.

General survey

Make a general survey to obtain fundamental information about the client's overall health and mental status. Observe the client and listen closely to develop an overall picture that will guide subsequent assessment.

To obtain general survey information, begin by noting the client's sex, race, and approximate age. Then check for obvious signs of physical or emotional distress and adjust your assessment accordingly.

If the client is not in severe distress, continue the general survey by observing the client's face for expression, contour, and symmetry; noting the client's body type, posture, and movement; assessing the client's speech for tone, clarity, strength, vocabulary, sentence structure, and pace; and noting the client's dress, grooming, and personal hygiene. Finally, assess the client's mental state, especially noting level of consciousness and behavior. (For more information about the general survey, see Chapter 4, Physical Assessment Skills.)

Height, weight, and vital signs

First, measure the client's height and weight, which should fall within the norms for adults and children. (For details, see Chapter 6, Nutritional Status.) Keep in mind that body weight not only provides information about nutrition, but also is a valuable indicator of fluid balance and hydration. For an infant, also measure the head and chest circumference and compare the findings to a chart of standard measurements.

Next, assess the client's vital signs, which include temperature, pulse, respirations, and blood pressure. (For details about assessing and evaluating vital signs, see Chapter 4, Physical Assessment Skills.)

Body structures and systems

To begin the "hands on" part of the assessment, make sure the client is seated comfortably. Then assess each body structure and system in an integrated fashion, using a body region approach rather than a body system approach. For example, assess the posterior thorax—which includes portions of the respiratory, urinary, and musculoskeletal systems—and then assess the anterior thorax—which includes portions of the respiratory, cardiovascular, musculoskeletal, and gastrointestinal systems as well as the breasts. After the physical assessment, however, plan to organize and document your findings by body system.

Many health care professionals use a head-to-toe approach when performing a complete assessment. However, most health care professionals develop their own variations. Whether you perform a head-to-toe assessment or some other type, take a systematic approach that will provide consistency and aid documentation. It should minimize the number of changes in nurse-client positioning, avoid tiring the client unnecessarily, allow you to work most efficiently, and ensure that no assessment area is overlooked. (For an illustrated procedure of a modified head-to-toe assessment, see *Performing physical assessments,* pages 614 to 631.)

Documentation

To understand the significance of assessment findings and form a clear picture of the client's health status, carefully review the physical assessment information as well as the health history findings and the results of any laboratory studies and diagnostic tests that may have been ordered. Laboratory studies will depend on the client's condition, but usually include blood and urine tests. Based on these data, formulate appropriate nursing diagnoses, which determine how to plan, implement, and evaluate nursing care.

The ability to organize data is essential for proper documentation. To document a complete physical examination, organize and record assessment findings by body system. This provides easier access to more concise assessment data for the entire health care team. Remember to document all data completely, including normal and abnormal findings, and to be specific. Be sure to document negative findings, rather than not mentioning them.

The following documentation sample illustrates the proper way to document normal and abnormal physical assessment findings for an adult.

> *Height:* 5′3″
> *Weight:* 120 lb
> *Vital signs:* Temperature 98.6° F. (oral), pulse 82 (radial) and regular, respirations 16 and regular, blood pressure 120/80 L sitting.
> *General survey:* Caucasian female, age 34, well-dressed, well-nourished, in no apparent distress. Relaxed facial expression, clear, strong, non-pressured speech. Moves well. Dress and grooming appropriate. Alert and oriented to person, place, time, situation. Emotional status slightly anxious, but appears in good mood; no suicidal ideation.
> *Skin, hair, and nails:* Skin warm and dry with good turgor. Few freckles over bridge of nose; small (5 mm) round, brown maculopapular mole above right breast; 2-cm scar beneath right knee (from a fall as a child). Hair auburn, clean, fine-textured. Scalp free of lesions.
> Nails pink, firm, well-trimmed, without lesions or clubbing. Right fourth toe has 1-cm corn.
> *Head and neck:* Skull and face symmetrical; facial sensation intact to pin and cotton. Smiles, grimaces, wrinkles forehead, and closes eyelids tightly. No

(Text continues on page 632.)

Performing physical assessments

The chart on the following pages provides guidelines for the complete assessment. It presents an approach that moves systematically from head to toe, and concludes with the reproductive system—the most potentially embarrassing or sensitive part of the assessment. It groups assessment techniques by body region and nurse-client positioning to make the assessment as efficient as possible and to avoid tiring the client. In the first column, the chart describes the assessment technique to be used. The second column lists the normal findings for adults. The third column reviews special considerations, including the purpose of the technique as well as nursing and developmental considerations. Where a change in nurse-client positioning is essential, it appears as the first item under special considerations. Before beginning, take and record the client's vital signs, height and weight.

TECHNIQUE	NORMAL FINDINGS	SPECIAL CONSIDERATIONS
Head and neck		
Inspect the hair and scalp color and condition.	Normal hair color (black, brown, red, blond, gray) and texture with full distribution over scalp; pink, smooth, mobile scalp without lesions	• This assessment can provide information about the client's personal care activities and may provide information about other body sytems, such as the endocrine system. • An elderly client may have thin hair. • An infant commonly has fine, thin hair or no hair.
Inspect the client's head. Then palpate from the client's forehead to the posterior triangle of the neck for the posterior cervical lymph nodes. (For an illustration, see page 570.)	Symmetrical, rounded normocephalic head positioned at midline and erect with no lumps or ridges	• This technique can detect asymmetry, size changes, enlarged lymph nodes, and tenderness. • Wear gloves for palpation if the client has lesions or a suspected infection. • Inspect and gently palpate the fontanelles and sutures in an infant. Fontanelles should feel soft, yet firm, and be flush with the scalp; sutures should be smooth and not override one another or feel separated. • A neonate's head may be asymmetrical from molding during vaginal delivery. • Measure head circumference of an infant.
Palpate in front of and behind the ears, under the chin, and in the anterior triangle for the anterior cervical lymph nodes. (For an illustration, see page 570.)	Nonpalpable lymph nodes or small, round, soft, mobile, nontender lymph nodes	• This technique can detect enlarged lymph nodes. • If nodes are enlarged, note their size, location, consistency, tenderness, temperature, and mobility. • A client under age 12 may normally have palpable lymph nodes that may range from ⅛" to ⅜" (3 mm to 1 cm) across. • Palpate only one side of the anterior neck at a time to avoid pressing both carotid arteries and reducing blood supply to the brain.
Palpate the left and then the right carotid artery. (For an illustration, see page 312.)	Bilateral equality in pulse amplitude and rhythm	• This technique evaluates circulation through the carotid pulse. • Palpate gently using the index and middle fingers. Check only one side of the neck at a time.
Auscultate the carotid arteries. (For an illustration, see page 319.)	No bruit on auscultation	• Auscultation in this area can detect a bruit, a sign of turbulent blood flow.
Palpate the trachea. (For an illustration, see page 264.)	Straight, midline trachea	• This technique evaluates the position of an important respiratory system structure. • Palpate by placing a thumb or forefinger on either side of the trachea at the sternocleidomastoid inner border above the suprasternal notch.
Palpate the suprasternal notch.	Palpable pulsations with an even rhythm	• Palpation in this area allows evaluation of aortic arch pulsations. • Palpate gently using only one index finger.

Performing physical assessments continued

TECHNIQUE	NORMAL FINDINGS	SPECIAL CONSIDERATIONS
Palpate the supraclavicular area.	Nonpalpable lymph nodes	• This technique can detect enlarged lymph nodes.
Palpate the thyroid gland. (For an illustration, see pages 600 and 601.)	Thin, mobile thyroid isthmus; nonpalpable thyroid lobes	• Palpation can detect thyroid gland enlargement, tenderness, or nodules. • Palpate gently with the pads of your index and middle fingers, assessing the left lobe with your right hand and the right lobe with your left hand. Palpate inside of the sternocleidomastoid muscle and below the cricoid and thyroid cartilages. • If the client's thyroid is difficult to palpate, try palpating from behind the client or asking the client to drink some water while you feel for thyroid movement. The thyroid normally rises with swallowing. • If the thyroid is enlarged, auscultate for bruits.
Have the client touch the chin to the chest and to each shoulder, each ear to one shoulder, then tip the head back as far as possible.	Symmetrical strength and movement of neck muscles	• These maneuvers evaluate range of motion (ROM) in the neck. • Increased cervical flexion may make head tilting difficult for an elderly client. Have such a client move only to the point of discomfort. Record the degree of motion or limitation.
Place your hands on the client's shoulders while the client shrugs the shoulders against this resistance.	Symmetrical strength and movement of neck muscles	• This procedure checks cranial nerve XI (accessory nerve) functioning and trapezius muscle strength.
Place your hand on the client's left cheek while the client pushes against this resistance. Repeat this procedure on the client's right side.	Symmetrical strength of neck muscles	• This procedure checks cranial nerve XI (accessory nerve) functioning and sternocleidomastoid muscle strength.
Inspect the client's facial structures.	Symmetrical structures without edema, deformities, or lesions	• Face the client. • This technique evaluates the overall condition of the face.
Have the client smile, frown, wrinkle the forehead, and puff out the cheeks.	Symmetrical smile, frown, and forehead wrinkles; equal puffing out of the cheeks	• This maneuver evaluates the motor portion of the cranial nerve VII (facial nerve).
Inspect the external appearance of the nose.	Symmetrical nose without edema, deformity, drainage, discoloration, or nostril flaring	• This technique evaluates the overall condition of the nose. • The external appearance of the nose can vary between individuals. • An infant's nose usually is slightly flattened.
Occlude one nostril externally with your finger, while the client breathes through the other. Repeat this procedure on the client's other nostril.	Patent nostrils	• This technique checks patency of the nasal passages.
Inspect the internal nostrils, using an ophthalmoscope handle with a nasal attachment.	Moist, pink-to-red nasal mucosa without lesions or polyps	• This technique can detect excessive drainage, edema, inflammation, and other abnormalities. • Use nasal speculum instead, if desired. • Steady the client's head with your opposite hand. • The nasal mucosa normally appears slightly enlarged in a pregnant client. • Use only a flashlight to inspect an infant's or toddler's nostrils; a nasal speculum is too sharp.

continued

Performing physical assessments continued

TECHNIQUE	NORMAL FINDINGS	SPECIAL CONSIDERATIONS
Palpate the nose.	Nose without bumps, lesions, edema, or tenderness	• This technique assesses for structural abnormalities in the nose. • Palpate gently with the pads of your index and middle fingers. • Nose deviation to one side may be caused by asymmetrical bones or cartilages, which can be palpated. Such deviation may be normal if the nostrils are patent.
Palpate and percuss the frontal and maxillary sinuses. (For illustration, see page 194.)	No tenderness on palpation or percussion	• These techniques are used to elicit tenderness, which may indicate sinus congestion or infection. • When percussing the sinuses, use immediate percussion. • In a client under age 8, the frontal sinuses commonly are too small to assess. • If palpation and percussion elicit tenderness, assess further by transilluminating the sinuses.
Palpate the temporomandibular joints as the client opens and closes the jaws. (For an illustration, see page 192.)	Smooth joint movement without pain; good approximation (bones line up where they meet)	• This action assesses the temporomandibular joints and the motor portion of the cranial nerve V (trigeminal nerve). • Use the middle three fingers of each hand to palpate properly.
Inspect the oral mucosa, gingivae, teeth, and salivary gland openings, using a tongue depressor and a penlight.	Pink, moist, smooth oral mucosa without lesions; pink, moist slightly irregular gingivae without sponginess or edema; 32 bright white to ivory-colored teeth with smooth edges and correct occlusion; small, white-rimmed salivary gland openings without tenderness or inflammation	• Have the client open the mouth and remove any dentures. • Wear examination gloves. • This technique evaluates the condition of several oral structures. • Move the tongue depressor from the molar area to the front of the mouth, being careful not to bump the frenula. • The oral mucosa normally appears bluish or patchily pigmented in a dark-skinned client. • A child may have up to 20 temporary (baby) teeth. • Slight gingival swelling may be normal during pregnancy.
Observe the tongue and hard and soft palates.	Pink, slightly rough tongue with a midline depression and comfortable fit in floor of mouth; pink to light red palates with symmetrical lines	• Observation provides information about the client's hydration and the condition of these oral structures. • If necessary, flatten the top of the tongue with the tongue depressor. • Mucous membrane inspection is especially important to assessing hydration in a child.
Ask the client to stick out the tongue.	Midline tongue without tremors	• This procedure tests cranial nerve XII (hypoglossal nerve), which controls the motor function of the tongue.
Ask the client to say "Ahh" while sticking out the tongue. Inspect the visible oral structures.	Symmetrical rise in soft palate and uvula during phonation; pink, midline, cone-shaped uvula; +1 tonsils (both tonsils behind the pillars)	• Phonation ("Ahh") checks portions of the cranial nerves IX and X (glossopharyngeal and vagus nerves). It also lowers the tongue, providing a good view of the anterior and posterior uvula, pillars, and tonsils.
Test the client's gag reflex using a tongue depressor.	Gagging	• Gagging during this procedure indicates that cranial nerves IX and X are intact. • Use this procedure cautiously in a client with nausea; it may cause vomiting. • Use a light touch on the back of the tongue to elicit this reflex.

Performing physical assessments continued

TECHNIQUE	NORMAL FINDINGS	SPECIAL CONSIDERATIONS
Place the tongue depressor at the side of the tongue while the client pushes it to the left and right with the tongue.	Symmetrical ability to push tongue depressor to left and right	• This action tests cranial nerve XII (hypoglossal nerve). • If the client reports impaired taste, test cranial nerves VII and IX using moist cotton swabs flavored with sugar, salt, vinegar, and quinine.
Test the client's sense of smell using a test tube of coffee, chocolate, or another familiar substance.	Correct identification of all smells in both nostrils	• This action tests cranial nerve I (olfactory nerve). • Make sure the client keeps both eyes closed as you test one nostril at a time.
Eyes and ears		
Perform visual acuity test using the standard Snellen eye chart.	20/20 vision	• Stand 20′ away from the seated client. • This test assesses the client's distance vision (central vision) and evaluates the cranial nerve II (optic nerve). • Note whether the client's visual acuity was tested with or without corrective lenses. • For an infant, check the blink reflex because visual acuity assessment is not possible. For a child age 30 to 42 months, assess visual acuity with a Denver Eye Screening Examination (DESE); age 7 and under, with the Snellen E chart or the DESE. • Visual acuity varies with age. For example, 20/30 is normal for a toddler. • In an elderly client, decreased lens elasticity commonly causes presbyopia, which reduces near vision. • Refer client with decreased or increased acuity to an ophthalmologist or optometrist for evaluation.
Hold a page of newsprint 12″ to 14″ (30.5 to 35.5 cm) from the client while the client reads it aloud.	Correct reading of newsprint without difficulty	• Sit directly in front of the seated client. • This test assesses the client's near vision. • Make sure that a client who normally wears corrective lenses for reading does so for this test. • For an illiterate client, use the Snellen E chart.
Ask the client to identify the pattern in a specially prepared page of color dots or plates.	Correct identification of pattern	• This test assesses the client's color perception. • Early detection of color blindness is important for a child. It allows the child to compensate for the difficulty and alerts teachers to the child's needs.
Perform the six cardinal positions of gaze test. (For illustrations, see page 218.)	Bilaterally equal eye movement without nystagmus	• This test evaluates the function of each of the six extraocular muscles and tests cranial nerves III, IV, and VI (oculomotor, trochlear, and abducens nerves). • A child who fails this test requires immediate referral to an ophthalmologist to evaluate and possibly correct strabismus (crossed eyes). • An adult client who fails this test and one of the other extraocular muscle tests requires immediate referral to an ophthalmologist.
Perform the cover-uncover test. (For an illustration, see page 219.)	Steady eyes without movement, wandering, or jerking	• This extraocular muscle function test assesses the fusion reflex, which makes binocular vision possible. • A child who fails this test requires immediate referral to an ophthalmologist to correct strabismus (crossed eyes). • An adult client who fails this test and one of the other extraocular muscle tests requires immediate referral to an ophthalmologist.

continued

Performing physical assessments continued

TECHNIQUE	NORMAL FINDINGS	SPECIAL CONSIDERATIONS
Perform the corneal light reflex test. (For an illustration, see page 219.)	Light reflection by cornea in exactly the same place in both eyes	• This test checks the ability of extraocular muscles to hold the eyes steady, or parallel, when fixed on an object. • A child who fails this test requires immediate referral to an ophthalmologist to correct strabismus (crossed eyes). • An adult client who fails this test and one of the other extraocular muscle tests requires immediate referral to an ophthalmologist.
Test client's peripheral vision by comparing it to your own. (For an illustration, see page 220.)	A field of vision that is 50 degrees from the top, 60 medially, 70 downward, and 110 laterally	• This test assesses the peripheral vision portion of cranial nerve II (optic nerve) and measures the ability of the retina to receive stimuli from the periphery of the client's vision. • The nurse must have normal vision; otherwise, the test will be inaccurate. • This test discovers only large peripheral vision defects, such as blindness in one quarter of the visual field. • Peripheral vision normally decreases in an elderly client.
Inspect the external structures of the eyeball (eyelids, eyelashes, and lacrimal apparatus).	Bright, clear, symmetrical eyes without nystagmus; ability to close eyelids completely over the sclera; eyelids that match the client's complexion and are free from edema, scaling, and lesions; equally distributed eyelashes that curve outward; smooth lacrimal apparatus without signs of inflammation	• This portion of the assessment allows the nurse to detect common problems, such as ptosis (lid lag), ectropion (outward-turning eyelids), entropion (inward-turning eyelids), and styes (purulent infection of sebaceous gland of the eyelid). • An Asian client may have epicanthal folds (skin folds over the inner canthus) in the eyelids. • An elderly client may have thin eyelashes and lackluster eyes.
Palpate the lacrimal apparatus.	No tenderness or masses on palpation	• This technique evaluates the condition of the tear ducts. • Palpate gently by pressing your index finger against the lower orbital rim near the nose. • If palpation causes excessive tearing or expresses purulent material, suspect a blockage or infection.
Inspect the conjunctiva and sclera. (For an illustration, see page 221.)	Pink palpebral conjunctiva and clear bulbar conjunctiva without swelling, drainage, or hyperemic blood vessels; white, clear sclera	• This technique detects conjunctivitis and the scleral color changes that may occur with systemic disorders. • A dark-skinned client may have small, dark spots on the sclera. • An elderly client may have a thickened bulbar conjuctiva on the nasal side (pinguecula).
Inspect the cornea, iris, and anterior chamber by shining a penlight tangentially across the eye.	Clear, transparent cornea and anterior chamber; illumination of total iris	• This technique assesses anterior chamber depth and the condition of the cornea and iris. • An elderly client may exhibit a thin, grayish ring in the cornea (arcus senilis). • A black client may have a gray-blue cornea.
Examine the pupils for equality of size, shape, reaction to light, and accommodation.	Pupils equal, round, reactive to light, and accommodation (PERRLA), directly and consensually	• Testing the pupillary response to light and accommodation assesses cranial nerves III, IV, and VI. • A client over age 85 may show almost no pupil reaction to accommodation.

Performing physical assessments continued

TECHNIQUE	NORMAL FINDINGS	SPECIAL CONSIDERATIONS
Observe the red reflex using an ophthalmoscope. (For an illustration, see pages 226 and 227.)	Sharp, distinct orange-red glow	• Presence of the red reflex indicates that the cornea, anterior chamber, and lens are free from opacity and clouding. • For information about the complete ophthalmoscopic examination, see Chapter 9.
Inspect the ear.	Nearly vertical–positioned ears that line up with the eye, match the facial color, are similarly shaped, and are in proportion to the face; no drainage, nodules, or lesions	• Sit or stand at the client's side facing the ear. • This technique determines the general condition and positioning of the ears. • Ear size and shape vary greatly. Obtain information about other family members' ears for comparison. • In an elderly client, the external ear structure may have lost adipose tissue and the cartilage may be harder. • A dark-skinned client may have darker orange or brown cerumen (earwax); a fair-skinned client will have yellow cerumen.
Palpate the ear and mastoid process.	No pain, swelling, nodules, or lesions	• These techniques can detect any areas of tenderness or edema, which may indicate an inflammation or infection. They may also uncover other abnormalities, such as nodules or lesions. • If the client has pain or swelling on palpation, use extreme care when performing an otoscopic examination. If otitis externa is present, this examination may not be possible.
Perform the whispered voice test or the watch-tick test on one ear at a time.	Whispered voice heard at a distance of 1′ to 2′ (30.5 to 61 cm); watch-tick heard at a distance of 5″ (12.7 cm)	• Stand 1′ to 2′ (30.5 to 61 cm) behind the client. • Record the number of feet or inches you stand away from the client during the test. • Perform a complete otoscopic examination. (See Chapter 9.)
Perform Weber's test using a 512 or 1024 cycles/second (CPS) tuning fork.	Tuning fork vibrations heard equally in both ears or in the middle of the head	• This test helps differentiate any conductive or sensorineural hearing loss. • The sound is heard best in the ear with a conductive loss.
Perform the Rinne test using a 512 or 1024 CPS tuning fork.	Tuning fork vibrations heard in front of the ear for at least as long as they are heard on the mastoid process	• This test helps differentiate any conductive or sensorineural hearing loss.
Posterior thorax		
Observe the skin, bones, and muscles of the spine, shoulder blades, and back as well as symmetry of expansion and accessory muscle use.	Even skin tone; symmetrical placement of all structures; bilaterally equal shoulder height; symmetrical expansion with inhalation; no accessory muscle use	• Stand behind the seated client, slightly to the client's right if you are right-handed or to the client's left if you are left-handed. • Expose the posterior thorax. • Ensure that your hands and the stethoscope are warm. • Observation provides information about lung expansion and accessory muscle use during respiration. It may also detect a deformity that can alter ventilation, such as scoliosis.
Assess the anteroposterior and lateral diameters of the thorax.	Lateral diameter up to twice the anteroposterior diameter (2:1)	• This assessment may detect abnormalities, such as an increased anteroposterior diameter (barrel chest as low as 1:1) associated with chronic obstructive pulmonary disease (COPD).

continued

Performing physical assessments continued

TECHNIQUE	NORMAL FINDINGS	SPECIAL CONSIDERATIONS
Anteroposterior and lateral diameters (continued)		• An infant's anteroposterior diameter may equal or exceed the lateral diameter; a toddler's should be smaller than the lateral diameter. • An elderly client's anteroposterior diameter may increase in relation to the lateral diameter, creating a rounded chest. • Measure an infant's chest circumference at the nipple line. Compare this measurement against a standard growth chart to assess development.
Palpate down the spine.	Properly aligned spinous processes without lesions or tenderness; firm, symmetrical, evenly spaced muscles	• This technique detects pain in the spine and paraspinous muscles. It also evaluates their consistency. • Use the pads of your middle three fingers to palpate the spine.
Palpate over the posterior thorax. (For an illustration, see page 265.)	Smooth surface; no lesions, lumps, or pain	• This technique helps detect musculoskeletal inflammation and other abnormalities. • Use the palmar surfaces of your fingertips and hands to palpate the posterior thorax.
Percuss the costovertebral area. (For an illustration, see page 402.)	Thudding sensation without pain or tenderness	• This action evaluates the condition of the kidneys. • Perform blunt percussion in this area using the ulnar surface of your fist.
Assess the client's respiratory excursion. (For an illustration, see pages 266 and 267.)	Symmetrical expansion and contraction of the thorax	• This technique checks for equal expansion of the lungs. • Assess for respiratory excursion in two locations posteriorly: at T10 and at the level of the axilla just below the scapula.
Palpate for tactile fremitus as the client repeats *ninety-nine.*	Equally intense vibrations of both sides of the chest	• Palpation provides information about the content of the lungs; vibrations increase over consolidated or fluid-filled areas and decrease over gas-filled areas. • Use the ulnar or palmar surface of your hands to detect fremitus. • Palpate at the apices, inside the scapulae, down the back, and under the axillae, using a systematic palpation sequence and comparing each side to the other. • Vibration intensity varies with chest thickness and underlying thoracic structures.
Percuss over the posterior and lateral lung fields. (For an illustration, see page 268.)	Resonant percussion note over the lungs that changes to a dull note at the diaphragm	• This technique helps identify the density and location of the lungs, diaphragm, and other anatomic structures. • Use mediate percussion in all areas of the posterior and lateral thorax. • Follow a systematic percussion sequence and compare each side to the other. • Percussion is unreliable in an infant because of the relative size of the infant's chest and the adult's fingers. • Percussion may produce hyperresonant sounds in a client with COPD or an elderly client because of hyperinflation of lung tissue.
Percuss for diaphragmatic excursion on each side of the posterior thorax. (For an illustration, see page 278.)	Excursion from 1¼" to 2¼" (3 to 6 cm)	• This technique evaluates diaphragm movement during respiration. • Keep in mind that the diaphragm normally is slightly higher on the right side than on the left.

Performing physical assessments continued

TECHNIQUE	NORMAL FINDINGS	SPECIAL CONSIDERATIONS
Auscultate the lungs through the posterior thorax as the client breathes slowly and deeply through the mouth. Also auscultate lateral areas.	Bronchovesicular sounds (soft, breezy sounds) between the scapulae; vesicular sounds (soft, swishy sounds about two notes lower than bronchovesicular sounds) in the lung periphery	• Lung auscultation helps detect abnormal fluid or mucus accumulation as well as obstructed passages. It also helps determine the condition of the alveoli and surrounding pleura. • Use the diaphragm of the stethoscope for an adult. For a pediatric client, use the bell of an adult stethoscope (if you do not have a pediatric one), pressing it firmly to create a small diaphragm. • Follow the same systematic sequence as for percussion. • For a client with significant hair growth over the area to be auscultated, wet the hair to decrease sound blurring. • Auscultate a child's lungs before performing other assessment techniques that may cause crying, which increases the respiratory rate and interferes with clear auscultation. • Auscultate at fewer sites for a pediatric client. • Because a child's chest is thinner and more resonant than an adult's, breath sounds are normally harsher or more bronchial.
Anterior thorax		
Observe the skin, bones, and muscles of the anterior thoracic structures as well as symmetry of expansion and accessory muscle use.	Even skin tone; symmetrical placement of all structures; symmetrical costal angle of less than 90 degrees; symmetrical expansion with inhalation; no accessory muscle use	• Stand in front of the seated client and expose the anterior thorax. • Observation provides information about lung expansion and accessory muscle use during respiration. It may also detect a deformity that can prevent full lung expansion, such as pigeon chest. • Women tend to use their upper chest muscles to breathe; men and children tend to breathe diaphragmatically.
Inspect the anterior thorax for lift, heaves, or thrusts and for the point of maximum impulse (PMI).	PMI not usually visible; no lifts, heaves, or thrusts	• PMI may be visible in a thin or young client.
Palpate over the anterior thorax. (For an illustration, see page 265.)	Smooth surface; no lesions, lumps, or pain	• This technique helps detect musculoskeletal inflammation and other abnormalities. • Use the palmar surfaces of your fingertips and hands to palpate the anterior thorax. • Compare the left side to the right side during palpation.
Assess the client's respiratory excursion. (For an illustration, see pages 266 and 267.)	Symmetrical expansion and contraction of the thorax	• This technique checks for equal expansion of the lungs. • Assess for respiratory excursion in three locations anteriorly: at the second, fifth, and 10th intercostal spaces. • For a client with pendulous breasts, do not assess respiratory excursion at the 10th intercostal space anteriorly. Instead check posterior excursion at this level.
Palpate for tactile fremitus as the client repeats *ninety-nine.*	Equally intense vibrations of both sides of the chest, with more vibrations in the upper chest than in the lower chest	• Palpation provides information about the content of the lungs; vibrations increase over consolidated or fluid-filled areas and decrease over gas-filled areas. • Use the ulnar or palmar surface of your hands to detect fremitus.

continued

Performing physical assessments continued

TECHNIQUE	NORMAL FINDINGS	SPECIAL CONSIDERATIONS
Tactile fremitus palpation (continued)		• Use a systematic palpation sequence and compare each side to the other. • Vibration intensity varies with chest thickness and underlying thoracic structures.
Percuss over the anterior thorax. (For an illustration, see page 268.)	Resonant percussion note over lung fields that changes to a dull note over ribs and other bones	• This technique helps identify the density and location of the lungs, diaphragm, and other anatomic structures. • Use mediate percussion in all areas of the anterior thorax. • Follow a systematic percussion sequence and compare each side to the other. • Percussion is unreliable in an infant because of the relative size of the infant's chest and the adult's fingers. • Percussion may produce hyperresonant sounds in an elderly client because of hyperinflation of lung tissue.
Auscultate the anterior thorax as the client breathes slowly and deeply through the mouth.	Bronchovesicular sounds (soft, breezy sounds) on either side of sternum at the second to fourth intercostal space; vesicular sounds (soft, swishy sounds about two notes lower than bronchovesicular sounds) in the lung periphery	• Lung auscultation helps detect abnormal fluid or mucus accumulation as well as obstructed passages. It also helps determine the condition of the alveoli and surrounding pleura. • Use the diaphragm of the stethoscope for an adult. For a pediatric client, use the bell of an adult stethoscope (if you do not have a pediatric one), pressing it firmly to create a small diaphragm. • Follow the same systematic sequence as for percussion. • For a client with significant hair growth over the area to be auscultated, wet the hair to decrease sound blurring. • Auscultate a child's lungs before performing other assessment techniques that may cause crying, which increases the respiratory rate and interferes with clear auscultation. • Auscultate at fewer sites for a pediatric client. • Because a child's chest is thinner and more resonant than an adult's, breath sounds are normally harsher or more bronchial.
Inspect the breasts and axillae with the client's hands resting at his or her side, placed on the hips, and raised above the head.	Symmetrical, convex, similar-looking breasts with soft, smooth skin and bilaterally similar venous patterns; symmetrical axillae with varying amounts of hair, but no lesions; nipples at same level on chest, and same color	• This technique evaluates the general condition of the breasts and axillae, and detects such abnormalities as retraction, dimpling, and flattening. • If the client's breasts are large or pendulous, observe them with the client leaning forward. • Some women have a congenital anomaly in which extra breast tissue, nipples, or breasts appear along the milk lines. • Assess the breasts of a female adolescent according to the stage of breast development. • Reassure a young male adolescent that gynecomastia (male breast enlargement) normally disappears within a year. • Expect to see enlarged breasts with darkened nipples and areola and purplish linear streaks in a pregnant client. • On the breasts of a lactating client, check for abnormalities, such as cracks, fissures, redness, tenderness, blisters, and petechiae.

Performing physical assessments continued

TECHNIQUE	NORMAL FINDINGS	SPECIAL CONSIDERATIONS
Palpate the axillae with the client's arms resting against the side of the body. (For an illustration, see page 345.)	Nonpalpable nodes	• This technique detects nodular enlargements and other abnormalities. • Assess the central axilla as well as the anterior and posterior axillary folds and the lateral nodes. • Palpate deep in the axilla, using the fingerpads.
Palpate the breasts and nipples. (For an illustration, see page 346.)	Smooth, relatively elastic tissue without masses, cracks, fissures, areas of induration (hardness), or discharge	• Help the client lie down and place her hands above her head. Stand at the right side if you are right-handed; at the left, if you are left-handed. • Place a small pad or pillow under the client's shoulder on the side to be assessed to spread the breast tissue evenly. • This technique evaluates the consistency and elasticity of the breasts and nipples, and may detect nipple discharge. • Employ circular or wedge palpation, using your fingerpads and overlapping the finger movements. • Make a cytologic smear of any nipple discharge not caused by pregnancy or lactation. • Some neonates exhibit palpable breast enlargement and nipple discharge ("witch's milk"). • A mature breast may feel more granular or stringy than a youthful breast. • Premenstrually, the client may exhibit breast tenderness, nodularity, and fullness. • A pregnant client may discharge colostrum from the nipple and may exhibit nodular breasts with prominent venous patterns. • A lactating client may have breast engorgement, with hard, warm, reddened breasts.
Inspect the neck for jugular vein distention. (For an illustration, see page 310.)	No visible pulsations	• Help the client into a supine position at a 45-degree angle. • This technique roughly assesses right-sided heart pressure. • Note the angle at which the client is reclining when you inspect. (A 45-degree angle is most common.)
Palpate the precordium for the PMI. (For an illustration, see page 311.)	PMI in the apical area (fifth intercostal space at the midclavicular line)	• This technique helps evaluate the size and location of the left ventricle.
Auscultate the aortic, pulmonic, tricuspid, and mitral areas for heart sounds. (For an illustration, see page 318.)	S_1 and S_2 heart sounds with a regular rhythm and an age-appropriate rate	• Auscultation over the precordium with the bell and diaphragm evaluates the heart rate and rhythm and can detect extra sounds, murmurs, and other abnormal heart sounds. • Note any extra heart sounds (S_3 or S_4), murmurs, clicks, snaps, or rubs. • If you detect a murmur, recheck it with the client sitting leaning forward or lying on one side. If a murmur is still present, document its timing (in systole, diastole, or both), location, intensity, pitch, radiation, and quality. • A child may have functional (innocent) heart murmurs.

continued

Performing physical assessments continued

TECHNIQUE	NORMAL FINDINGS	SPECIAL CONSIDERATIONS
Abdomen		
Observe the abdominal contour.	Symmetrical flat or rounded contour	• Stand on the client's right if you are right-handed; on the left, if you are left-handed. • Expose the abdomen from the breast to the groin. Keep a female client's breast covered, and place a drape at the pubic hair line. • Normal abdominal contour may vary with body type. • An infant or toddler will have a rounded abdomen. • An emaciated client will have a scaphoid abdomen.
Inspect the abdomen for skin characteristics, symmetry, contour, peristalsis, and pulsations.	Symmetrical contour with no lesions, striae, rash, or visible peristaltic waves	• A slender client may have a flat or concave abdomen. • To detect an incisional or umbilical hernia, observe for a protrusion while the supine client lifts his or her head. • Expect to see a pot belly in a child under age 4.
Auscultate all four quadrants of the abdomen. (For an illustration, see page 367.)	Normal bowel sounds in all four quadrants	• Abdominal auscultation can detect abnormal bowel sounds and other abnormal sounds. • Always auscultate the abdomen before palpating and percussing it to avoid creating unusual sounds or rupturing an aneurysm. • Apply the diaphragm of the stethoscope lightly to the abdomen. You may need to listen for up to 5 minutes to detect bowel sounds. • Note any bruits, especially over the aorta, iliac arteries, and femoral arteries. • Promote cooperation in an infant or young child by auscultating with the child on the parent's lap.
Percuss from below the right breast to the inguinal area down the right midclavicular line. (For an illustration, see page 375.)	Dull percussion note over the liver; tympanic note over the rest of the abdomen	• Percussion in this area helps evaluate the size of the liver. • Gas in the colon or consolidation in the right lower lung lobe can mask liver border dullness.
Percuss from below the left breast to the inguinal area down the left midclavicular line. (For an illustration, see page 575.)	Tympanic percussion note	• Percussion in this area that elicits a dull note can detect an enlarged spleen. • If percussion elicits a dull note, turn the client on the right side and percuss along the left midaxillary line between the sixth and 11th ribs to assess the degree of splenic dullness. • Percussion sounds may be difficult to assess in an obese client.
Palpate all four quadrants of the abdomen, moving from the upper quadrants to the inguinal areas down the midclavicular lines.	Nontender organs without masses	• Ask the client to bend his or her knees while remaining supine. This helps relax the abdominal muscles for palpation and percussion. • Palpation provides information about the location, size, and condition of the underlying structures. • Palpate in a systematic sequence, using light palpation first and repeating the process with deep palpation, which may be done with one or two hands. • Plan to palpate and percuss any painful area last to prevent guarding. • Have a ticklish client place his or her hand over yours during palpation as a distraction. • If palpation reveals bladder distention above the symphysis pubis, percuss and palpate the bladder.

Performing physical assessments continued

TECHNIQUE	NORMAL FINDINGS	SPECIAL CONSIDERATIONS
Palpate for the kidneys on each side of the abdomen. (For an illustration, see page 403.)	Nonpalpable kidneys or solid, firm, smooth kidneys (if palpable)	• This technique evaluates the general condition of the kidneys. • Keep in mind that the right kidney lies lower than the left, and that it may be palpable in a thin client or a client with reduced abdominal muscle mass. • If you cannot feel the kidneys, try capturing the kidney, an advanced palpation technique.
Palpate the liver at the right costal border. (For an illustration, see page 375.)	Nonpalpable liver or smooth, firm, nontender liver with a rounded, regular edge (if palpable)	• This technique evaluates the general condition of the liver. • Perform deep palpation with one or both hands while the client takes a deep breath. • The liver may be palpable in a thin client. • An alternative technique requires "hooking" your fingerpads under the costal margin to palpate the liver. This technique may give the client pain. • In a child, the liver is proportionally larger and easier to palpate.
Palpate for the spleen at the left costal border. (For an illustration, see page 575.)	Nonpalpable spleen	• This procedure detects any splenomegaly (spleen enlargement). • Perform deep palpation with one or both hands while the client takes a deep breath. • An alternative technique requires "hooking" your fingerpads under the edge of the costal margin to palpate the spleen. This technique may give the client pain.
Palpate the femoral pulses in the groin area. (For an illustration, see page 312.)	Strong, regular pulse	• This technique assesses vascular patency. • This is an important pulse point in a child.
Upper extremities		
Observe the skin and muscle mass of the client's upper extremities.	Uniform color and texture with no lesions; elastic turgor; muscle mass equal bilaterally	• Stand in front of the seated client. • Beginning the assessment with the hands puts the client at ease. • The skin provides information about hydration, circulation, and the status of body systems, such as the urinary system. • Continue to observe the client's skin throughout the assessment. • If lesions are present, note their size, shape, color, location, and elevation. • An elderly client may have dry, thin skin with reduced turgor. • An infant can become dehydrated quickly, so assessing turgor is important.
Ask the client to extend the arms forward and then rapidly turn the palms up and down.	Steady hands with no tremors or pronator drift	• This maneuver tests proprioception and cerebellar function.
With the client's palms up, place your hands on the client's forearms while the client pushes up against resistance. Then place your hands under the forearms while the client pushes down against resistance.	Symmetrical strength and ability to push up and down against resistance	• This procedure checks the muscle strength of the arms.

continued

Performing physical assessments continued

TECHNIQUE	NORMAL FINDINGS	SPECIAL CONSIDERATIONS
Inspect and palpate the fingers, wrists, and elbow joints.	Smooth, freely movable joints with no swelling	• This procedure provides information about the status of the joints. • An elderly client may exhibit osteoarthritic changes that cause the joints to be enlarged, stiff, and painful.
Palpate the client's hands to assess skin temperature.	Warm, moist skin with bilaterally even temperature	• Skin temperature assessment provides data about circulation to the area. • Particularly note cool, clammy skin or warm, dry skin.
Palpate the radial and brachial pulses. (For an illustration, see page 313.)	Bilaterally equal rate and rhythm	• Palpation of pulses helps evaluate peripheral vascular status.
Inspect the color, shape, and condition of the client's fingernails, and test for capillary refill.	Pink nail beds with smooth, rounded nails; 160-degree angle where nail meets the cuticle; brisk capillary refill	• Nail assessment provides data about the integumentary, cardiovascular, and respiratory systems.
Place two fingers in each of the client's palms while the client squeezes your fingers.	Bilaterally equal hand strength	• This maneuver tests muscle strength in the hands.
Lower extremities		
Inspect the legs and feet for color, lesions, varicosities, hair growth, nail growth, edema, and muscle mass.	Skin color that matches rest of complexion; symmetrical hair and nail growth; no lesions, varicosities, or edema; muscle mass equal bilaterally	• Stand near the supine client. • Inspection assesses adequate circulatory function.
Test for pitting edema in the pretibial area midway between the knee and ankle and in the pedal area. (For an illustration, see page 399.)	No pitting edema	• This test checks for and evaluates pitting edema, which results from excess sodium and water in interstitial spaces. • If edema is present, grade it according to the scale approved by your health care facility.
Palpate for pulses and skin temperature in the posterior tibial area behind the ankle and the dorsalis pedis area on the foot. (For an illustration, see page 313.)	Bilaterally even pulse rate, rhythm, and skin temperature	• Palpation of pulses and temperature in these areas helps evaluate the client's peripheral vascular status. • Keep in mind that both pulses are located on the great-toe side of the foot. • If the posterior tibial and the dorsalis pedis pulses are normal, you do not need to check the popliteal pulse. If they are abnormal, ask the client to bend the knees slightly. Then palpate the popliteal pulse.
Perform the straight leg test on one leg at a time.	Painless leg lifting	• Stand to one side of the client. • This test checks for vertebral disk problems. • Remind the client to keep the knee straight and the foot comfortably dorsiflexed. • If the client has difficulty with this test, you may help by steadying the leg being raised.
Palpate for crepitus as the client abducts and adducts the hip. Repeat this procedure on the opposite leg.	No crepitus	• Place one hand on the client's hip and the other on the knee. • This test assesses ROM of the hip. • To assess hip movement, have the client bring the knee over the abdomen as far as possible. • Help the client cross the knee over the abdomen and away from you. • Perform Ortolani's maneuver on an infant to assess hip abduction and adduction.

Performing physical assessments continued

TECHNIQUE	NORMAL FINDINGS	SPECIAL CONSIDERATIONS
Ask the client to raise his or her thigh against the resistance of your hands. Repeat this procedure on the opposite thigh. (For an illustration, see page 532.)	Each thigh lifts easily against resistance	• Help the client sit up. Place both hands on the client's thigh. • This maneuver tests the motor strength of the upper legs. • Have a preschooler or school-age child hop on each foot to test motor strength in the legs.
Ask the client to push outward against the resistance of your hands. (For an illustration, see page 532.)	Each leg pushes easily against resistance	• Place one hand on each leg in the tibial area below the knee. • This maneuver tests the motor strength of the lower legs. • Have a preschooler or school-age child hop on each foot to test motor strength in the legs.
Ask the client to pull backward against the resistance of your hands. (For an illustration, see page 532.)	Each leg pulls easily against resistance	• Place one hand on each calf. • This maneuver tests the motor strength of the lower legs. • Have a preschooler or school-age child hop on each foot to test motor strength in the legs.
Nervous system		
Lightly touch the ophthalmic, maxillary, and mandibular areas on each side of the client's face with a cotton swab and a pin. Ask what the client feels with each touch.	Correct identification of sensation and location	• Have the client remain seated with eyes closed. • This test evaluates the function of cranial nerve V (trigeminal nerve). • Test the three different areas randomly so that the client does not notice a pattern, but be sure to check all three areas with both the pin and the swab. • Temperature sensitivity does not need to be tested if the client exhibits pain sensitivity. (Pain and temperature travel on the same tracts in the nervous system.) If pain sensitivity is not elicited, test temperature sensitivity using test tubes of warm and cold water.
Touch several areas on the dorsal and palmar surfaces of the arms, hands, and fingers with the cotton swab and pin. Ask what the client feels with each touch.	Correct identification of sensation and location	• This test evaluates the function of the ulnar, radial, and medial nerves (the dermatomes). • Do not break the skin with the pin. • The wooden end of a broken cotton swab will serve instead of a pin, if desired. • Do not perfom this test on a young child, who may be frightened by the pinpricks.
Touch several nerve distribution areas on the legs, feet, and toes with the cotton swab and pin. Ask what the client feels with each touch.	Correct identification of sensation and location	• This test evaluates the function of the dermatome areas randomly. • If the client does not perceive a sensation in a particular area, evaluate that area in greater detail. • Do not perform this test on a young child, who may be frightened by the pinpricks. • This test may take more time for an elderly client.
Tap on your fingers above the client's wrist, using a reflex hammer. Repeat this procedure on the opposite arm.	Normal reflex reaction	• Have the client place both hands thumbs up in his or her lap. Place two fingers of one of your hands over the client's radius about 1⅛" to 2" (3 to 5 cm) above the wrist. As an alternate position, hold the client's thumb up and away from the body, and have the client "let go" of the weight in the arm during the procedure. • This procedure elicits the brachioradialis deep tendon reflex (DTR).

continued

Performing physical assessments continued

TECHNIQUE	NORMAL FINDINGS	SPECIAL CONSIDERATIONS
Finger tap with reflex hammer (continued)		• Manipulate the client's hand and tap in several areas over the wrist, if necessary, to elicit the reflex. • If you have difficulty eliciting this DTR, ask the client to squeeze both thighs together during this procedure. This should distract the client's attention from the area being assessed.
Tap on your fingers over the client's antecubital fossa, using a reflex hammer. Repeat this procedure on the opposite arm.	Normal reflex reaction	• Have the client place both hands in his or her lap and relax both arms. Place two fingers of one of your hands in the client's antecubital fossa. • This procedure elicits the biceps DTR. • Manipulate the joint and tap in several areas, if necessary, to elicit the reflex. • If you have difficulty eliciting this DTR, ask the client to squeeze both thighs together during the procedure. This should distract the client's attention from the area being assessed.
Tap on your fingers over the client's triceps tendon area, using a reflex hammer. Repeat this procedure on the opposite arm.	Normal reflex reaction	• Have the client place both hands on his or her hips. Place two fingers of one of your hands over the client's triceps tendon area. As an alternate position, hold the client's upper arm in a flexed position and have the client "let go" of the weight in the arm during the procedure. • This procedure elicits the triceps DTR. • Manipulate the joint and tap in several areas, if necessary, to elicit the reflex. • If you have difficulty eliciting this DTR, ask the client to squeeze both thighs together during the procedure. This should distract the client's attention from the area being assessed.
Tap just below the patella, using a reflex hammer. Repeat this procedure on the opposite patella.	Normal reflex reaction	• Have the client sit at the edge of the table, knees flexed. • This procedure elicits the patellar DTR. • Manipulate the joint and tap in several areas, if necessary, to elicit the reflex. • If you have difficulty eliciting this DTR, ask the client to link both hands together tightly and try to pull them apart against resistance. This should distract the client's attention from the area being assessed.
Tap over the Achilles tendon area, using a reflex hammer. Repeat this procedure on the opposite ankle.	Normal reflex reaction	• Crouch in front of the seated client. Hold the client's dorsiflexed foot in your hand. As an alternate position, have the client kneel on a stable chair, with both feet dangling over the edge. • This procedure elicits the Achilles DTR. • Manipulate the joint and tap in several areas, if necessary, to elicit the reflex. • If you have difficulty eliciting this DTR, ask the client to link both hands together tightly and try to pull them apart against resistance. This should distract the client's attention from the area being assessed.
Stroke the sole of the client's foot using the end of the reflex hammer handle. Stroke on the little toe side from the heel to the toe; then stroke across the ball of the foot.	Plantar reflex	• This procedure elicits a superficial reflex, known as the plantar reflex, which is plantar flexion of all toes. Babinski's sign occurs as dorsiflexion of the great toe with or without fanning of the other toes. Expect Babinski's sign in children under age 2 and under; later, it is abnormal.

Performing physical assessments continued

TECHNIQUE	NORMAL FINDINGS	SPECIAL CONSIDERATIONS
Ask the client to dorsiflex both feet against the resistance of your hands.	Both feet lift easily against resistance	• Place your hands on the dorsal surfaces of the client's feet. • This procedure tests foot strength and ROM.
Ask the client to plantarflex both feet against the resistance of your hands.	Both feet push down easily against resistance	• Place your hands, palms up, on the plantar surfaces of the client's feet. • This procedure tests foot strength and ROM. • Wash your hands or remove your gloves when you complete assessing the client's feet.
Inspect the feet and toes for lesions. Palpate for dorsalis pedis pulses.	No lesions or lumps; equal bilateral pulses	• Pulses and hair distribution help evaluate peripheral vascular status.
Trace a one-digit number in the palm of the client's hand using your finger. Ask the client to identify the number. (For an illustration, see page 496.)	Correct identification of number	• Stand in front of the seated client. Have the client close both eyes. • This procedure evaluates the client's tactile discrimination through graphesthesia.
Place a familiar object, such as a key or a coin, in the client's hand. Ask the client to identify it.	Correct identification of object	• This procedure evaluates the client's tactile discrimination through stereognosis.
Observe the client walk across the room in four ways: with a regular gait, on the toes, on the heels, and heel-to-toe. (For an illustration, see page 494.)	Steady gait, good balance, and no signs of muscle weakness or pain in any style of walking	• Ask the client to stand up. Stand several feet away from the client. • This technique evaluates the cerebellum and motor system, and checks for vertebral disk problems.
Inspect the scapulae, spine, back, and hips as the client bends forward as far as possible; bends backwards, and bends from side to side.	Full ROM, easy flexibility, and no signs of scoliosis or varicosities	• Stand in back of the client. • Open the client's gown in the back. • Inspection evaluates the client's ROM and detects musculoskeletal abnormalities, such as scoliosis.
Perform the Romberg test. Ask the client to stand straight with both eyes closed and both feet together.	Steady stance with minimal weaving	• Stand facing the client. • This test checks cerebellar functioning and evaluates balance and coordination. • Do not touch the client unless the client is about to lose balance. • If the client begins to lose balance, stop the test.
Male reproductive system		
Inspect the client's penis.	Loose, wrinkled skin over the shaft and taut, smooth skin over the glans penis with no lesions, ulcers, or breaks; appropriate size of penis for developmental age	• Stand facing the standing male client. • Put on surgical gloves. • Minimize client embarrassment by explaining each assessment step before doing it and projecting a professional demeanor. • This technique assesses the general condition of the penis and detects abnormalities such as lesions and ulcers. • Lift the penis to inspect its dorsal and ventral surfaces, or alternatively, ask the client to lift his penis. • If lesions are present, document their location, size, color, and presence of any exudate. Obtain an exudate sample to culture, if necessary. • If the client is uncircumcised, have him retract the foreskin to allow inspection of the glans penis.

continued

Performing physical assessments continued

TECHNIQUE	NORMAL FINDINGS	SPECIAL CONSIDERATIONS
Penis inspection (continued)		• An infant's penis usually appears pink and smooth. An uncircumcised infant's foreskin usually is tight for 2 to 3 months after birth and does not retract easily. • During childhood, the penis remains completely hairless. During puberty, the genitals enlarge and secondary sex characteristics appear.
Palpate the penis.	Palpable dorsal vein and ridges of internal structures; no lumps, induration, or tender areas	• This technique allows detection of structural abnormalities or lumpy, indurated, or tender areas. • To palpate the penis properly, gently grasp the shaft between the thumb and first two fingers and palpate its length.
Inspect the urethral meatus. (For an illustration, see page 401.)	Opening at tip of the glans penis free of redness or discharge	• Inspection evaluates the overall condition of the urethral meatus and detects signs of infection. • If a discharge is present, obtain a sample to culture. If necessary, have the client "milk" his penis to obtain a sample. To maintain asepsis, avoid touching the culture plate with your gloved (contaminated) hand.
Inspect the scrotum.	Symmetrical distribution of pubic hair over the symphysis pubis and scrotum; scrotal skin free of lesions, ulcers, or redness; appropriate size of scrotum for the client's developmental age, with the left testicle slightly lower than the right	• Inspection of these structures checks for male sex characteristics and hair distribution patterns. • A child's scrotum should be hairless. • An elderly client may have gray or white pubic hair. His scrotal skin may be less taut, giving the scrotum a pendulous appearance.
Palpate the scrotum.	Rough, rugated skin; symmetrical, smooth, freely movable, oval-shaped testes; palpable ridge of tissue lying vertically on the testicular surface (epididymis); smooth, freely movable vas deferens	• This technique allows detection of lumps or tender areas. • To palpate a testicle properly, place your thumb in front and your first two fingers behind the scrotal sac. • Absence of one or both testes (undescended testes) in an infant over a few months old should be referred to a physician. When the cremasteric muscle relaxes, the testes resume their normal position. • Transilluminate any lumps, nodular areas, or areas of swelling.
Inspect and palpate the inguinal area. (For an illustration, see page 573.)	Smooth skin without visible bulges or palpable lymph nodes	• These techniques can detect femoral hernias and enlarged inguinal lymph nodes. • To make a suspected hernia more visible, ask the client to bear down as if passing a stool. • Keep in mind that the hand used for palpation is contaminated.
Palpate the groin as the client coughs or bears down. (For an illustration, see page 456.)	No palpable lumps	• This procedure can detect a hernia, which will feel like a bump, mass, or bulge when the client coughs or bears down. • To palpate for an inguinal hernia in an adult, gently insert the middle or index finger into the inguinal canal and up to Hesselbach's triangle. • To palpate for an inguinal hernia in a child, use your little finger. • To palpate for a femoral hernia, palpate near the femoral artery. • If you have had special preparation, perform a prostate examination. (See Chapter 16.)

Performing physical assessments continued

TECHNIQUE	NORMAL FINDINGS	SPECIAL CONSIDERATIONS
Female reproductive system		
Inspect the vulva and other visible structures.	Female hair distribution pattern; skin without lesions	• Help the client into the lithotomy position. Sit on a stool at the base of the examination table. • Drape the client appropriately. • Focus the light before you put on gloves. • If necessary, call in an assistant before proceeding with this part of the assessment. • Inspection evaluates the development of female sex characteristics. • Compare a pediatric client's development to her developmental stage. • An elderly client may have little pubic hair.
Palpate the vulva and labia. (For an illustration, see page 430.)	Smooth surfaces free of lumps and lesions	• This technique checks the vulva and labia for abnormalities, such as lumps and lesions. • To palpate properly, use your dominant thumb and index finger. • Do not palpate a child's vulva and labia unless abuse is suspected. • An elderly client may have decreased fat in the labia and mons pubis.
Palpate the Bartholin's glands. (For an illustration, see page 430.)	No swelling	• Palpation can detect signs of infection, such as swelling or discharge. • To palpate properly, use your thumb (at the posterior-lateral area of the vaginal opening) and index finger (in the vagina). • If a discharge is present, obtain a sample for culture. • Do not palpate a child's Bartholin's glands unless abuse is suspected.
Inspect the structures inside the labia minora.	Pink urethral meatus without redness or swelling; intact clitoris; vaginal orifice free of swelling, redness, or discharge	• To perform this inspection, turn your palm up with your index finger still in the vagina. Part the labia with your middle finger and thumb. • For a pediatric client, inspect the orifice for lesions.
Withdraw the index finger from the vagina while gently "stripping down" the urethra about ¾" (2 cm). (For an illustration, see page 430.)	No discharge	• This procedure checks for discharge from the Skene's glands and urethra. • If a discharge is present, obtain a sample for culture. • Do not perform this procedure on a pediatric client unless abuse is suspected.
Press your fingers down just inside the vaginal introitus as the client bears down.	Pressure on finger, but no protrusion of bladder	• This maneuver checks for cystocele. • To palpate properly, use your index and middle fingers.
Withdraw the fingers as the client bears down. Have the client to a comfortable position. Then leave the examination room to allow the client to dress in private.	Gentle tightening of the vaginal walls; no bulges or masses	• This manuever checks for uterine prolapse and rectocele. • Ask the client to bear down more than once, if necessary. • Glove both hands if the client is heavy. • Do not perform this procedure on a child unless abuse is suspected or unless she is sexually active. • If you have had special preparation, perform a complete pelvic examination. (See Chapter 15.)

maxillary or frontal sinus tenderness on palpation or percussion. Clenches jaw without pain. Bilateral tonsillar nodes, 1 cm, nontender, mobile, discrete. Nonpalpable occipital, postauricular, preauricular, submaxillary, submental, posterior cervical, anterior cervical, and supraclavicular lymph nodes. Trachea midline. Carotid pulses bilaterally full and equal; no bruits. No jugular vein distention. Thyroid without masses, enlargement, tenderness; rises with swallowing. Full range of motion (ROM) of neck with equal, bilateral strength to resistance.

Nose: Straight septum without lesions; patent nostrils. Nasal mucosa free of lesions with scant clear discharge; bright pink, nonswollen turbinates.

Mouth and throat: 32 teeth, clean and in good repair; gums intact. Tongue and uvula midline. Palate rises with phonation. Gag reflex present. Tonsils absent. Tongue, palate, mucosa, and throat without lesions or exudate. Tongue pushes easily against resistance of tongue depressor.

Eyes: Symmetrical and free of lesions, discharge, pain, exophthalmos. Visual acuity with Snellen—left eye 20/25, right eye 20/20, both eyes 20/20 with corrective lenses. Lids and lashes intact. Sclera white; bulbar conjunctiva and corneas clear; palpebral conjunctiva deep pink; irises equally round and brown; pupils equal, round, reactive to light and accommodation. Extraocular movement intact without nystagmus. Visual fields grossly intact by confrontation. Ophthalmoscopic examination: red reflex present; background pink without lesions; optic disks creamy white with sharp margins; cup less than half of disk; vessels show no narrowing or A-V nicking; A-V ratio 2:3; bright foveal reflection in macula.

Ears: Pinna symmetrical without lesions or tenderness. Gross hearing intact. Weber heard equally in both ears; Rinne air conduction > bone conduction. Small amount of reddish cerumen in ear canals. Tympanic membranes pearly gray; light reflexes and landmarks appropriately placed bilaterally.

Respiratory system: Respirations unlabored. No bony abnormalities or tenderness. Anteroposterior diameter 1:2. Respiratory expansion equal; diaphragmatic excursion 5 cm bilaterally. No increased fremitus. Lung fields resonant. Breath sounds vesicular through most of lung fields.

Breasts: Left breast slightly larger than right (has been this way since puberty). No skin changes, tenderness, masses, nipple discharge, or axillary or supraclavicular adenopathy. Does breast self-examination about once a month.

Cardiovascular system: No lifts or heaves. Point of maximum impulse visible and palpable at left midclavicular line at the 5th intercostal space. S_1 and S_2, regular rate and rhythm. No murmurs, extra sounds, or rubs on auscultation. No pretibial edema or varicosities. Radial, posterior tibial, and dorsalis pedis pulses normal amplitude and equal. Normal hair distribution on feet and toes.

Abdomen: Contour flat without lesions or pulsations. Bowel sounds auscultated in all four quadrants. No bruits. No masses, tenderness, hepatomegaly, or splenomegaly. Tympany throughout abdomen on percussion. Liver span of 8 cm percussed at right midclavicular line from costal angle to 6th ICS. No costovertebral angle tenderness. Femoral pulses equal bilaterally. One 1-cm, mobile, nontender node in right inguinal area.

Musculoskeletal system: Spine without abnormalities; full ROM. Fingers, wrists, elbows, shoulders, hips, knees, and ankles full ROM. No joint abnormalities or pain palpated. Muscle size and strength equal bilaterally.

Nervous system: Reasoning intact and judgment appropriate. (Answers questions appropriately and can list alternatives for a stressful situation, choosing appropriate action.) Immediate, recent, and remote memory intact. Intellect appears superior to educational level; can do serial sevens. Cranial nerves II through XII intact. Deep tendon reflexes—brachioradialis, biceps, triceps, patellar, Achilles, 2+ and equal. Plantar reflex intact. Sensory function intact to pin and cotton over face, hands, forearms, lower legs, and feet. Motor function adequate with equal hand, arm, leg, and foot strength. Gait intact. Cerebellar function intact—Romberg negative, heel-to-toe intact, no pronator drift.

Female reproductive system: Vulva and Bartholin's glands, urethral meatus, and Skene's glands without lesions, discharge, or atrophy. Normal female hair distribution. Vaginal wall with rugae and small amount of whitish, thin, nonodorous discharge. No cystocele or rectocele. Cervix nontender and without lesions. Squamocolumnar junction on exocervix. Slightly friable with Pap. Uterus firm, midline, anteflexed, mobile, nontender, and nonpregnant in size. Adnexae have no masses or tenderness. Ovaries nonpalpable.

No rectal lesions or masses; confirms bimanual examination; brown stool; guaiac negative.

Partial assessment

Like the complete assessment, the nurse's partial assessment includes a health history, a physical examination, and a review of the results of laboratory and diagnostic studies. However, the partial assessment focuses on a specific client concern or problem. More commonly performed than a complete assessment, it may be done in many different health care settings.

Health history

For an outpatient, an inpatient (as in the emergency department), or a distressed client, expect to take a partial history, or episodic write-up. For this type of health history, obtain full biographic data and detailed information only about the reason for seeking health care. (Use the PQRST method.)

Combine other health history components, such as past health status, family health status, status of physiologic systems, and health promotion and protection patterns, as needed. For example, combine past history and family history by asking the client, "Have you or anyone in your family had any of the following disorders?" Then list specific disorders. Be sure to determine the presence or absence of five prevalent diseases (alcoholism, cancer, diabetes, heart disease, and hypertension) and others appropriate to the client or culture.

Physical assessment

Although you might perform a complete physical assessment on the client's first visit or during a periodic checkup, most of the time you will perform episodic (partial) physical assessments to evaluate the specific symptoms reported in the health history.

Use the health history information as a guide when assessing a client with a specific problem or when tracking the progress of a regular client. For example, partial assessment techniques for a child with an allergic reaction to a medication might include temperature assessment; skin inspection; evaluation of breathing and respirations; auscultation of the lungs and heart; and evaluation of the ears, nose, and throat. Partial assessment techniques for a client recovering from abdominal surgery might include vital sign measurements, weight measurement, inspection of the incision, auscultation of bowel sounds, and abdominal palpation. (For examples of assessment of clients with specific symptoms, see Appendices 1 through 4.)

No matter what the client's condition, however, a partial assessment should include a general survey, vital sign measurements, and evaluation of certain body structures and systems.

Partial assessment checklist

When a client needs a partial assessment, use the following checklist to evaluate basic structures and systems. Then list any additional areas that need to be assessed based on the client's reason for seeking health care.

- ☐ Make a general survey.
- ☐ Assess level of consciousness.
- ☐ Take temperature.
- ☐ Assess pulse rate and rhythm.
- ☐ Assess the respiratory rate and rhythm.
- ☐ Measure blood pressure.
- ☐ Observe skin color, texture, and turgor.
- ☐ Test gross motor coordination.
- ☐ Assess cardinal positions of gaze.
- ☐ Examine the pupils (PERRLA).
- ☐ Assess gross vision and hearing.
- ☐ Examine oral structures as client says "Ahh."
- ☐ Auscultate breath sounds in the posterior thorax.
- ☐ Auscultate breath sounds in the anterior thorax.
- ☐ Auscultate the heart for apical rate.
- ☐ Auscultate the abdomen.
- ☐ Percuss the abdomen.
- ☐ Palpate for pretibial edema.
- ☐ Palpate the dorsalis pedis pulse.
- ☐ Additional areas for assessment based on reason for seeking health care: ____________________

____

General survey and vital signs

Make a general survey by assessing the client's mental status during the health history interview and by observing the client walk into the room and sit down (or move around in bed). Assess any additional mental status elements by talking with the client during the physical examination.

Next, evaluate the client's vital signs, combining assessments when possible. For example, take the client's blood pressure while an oral thermometer registers the client's temperature. (For detailed information about the general survey and vital signs, see Chapter 4, Physical Assessment Skills.)

Body structures and systems

During this part of the physical assessment, evaluate certain basic structures and systems. (For information about these assessments, see *Performing physical assessments,* pages 614 to 631, and *Partial assessment checklist,* page 633.) Then, based on the client's needs and health history data, assess additional pertinent areas.

Documentation

If laboratory or diagnostic studies have been ordered for a client, consider the results along with the health history and partial physical assessment findings. As with the complete assessment, use this information as the basis for nursing diagnoses, which in turn are the foundation for planning, implementing, and evaluating the client's care.

Finally, document all partial assessment findings, using the same concise, accurate documentation style as for a complete assessment. (For documentation samples based on partial assessments of clients with specific symptoms, see Appendices 1 through 4.)

Chapter summary

The main elements of the complete and partial assessments are the health history, physical assessment, and review of laboratory and other diagnostic studies. Chapter 21 describes how to perform these assessments, which provide the information needed for client care. Here are the highlights of the chapter:

- The health history is the most important part of the assessment. It provides information about the client and helps the nurse decide which areas to assess.
- The complete health history includes these basic components: biographic data, health and illness patterns, health promotion and protection patterns, role and relationship patterns, and a summary of health data. In many health care facilities, history information may be recorded on a standardized checklist or questionnaire.
- The nurse may perform a complete physical assessment during a client's first visit to an outpatient setting or as a periodic checkup.
- After making a general survey and obtaining the client's height, weight, and vital signs, the nurse begins the "hands on" part of the complete physical assessment. The nurse assesses each body structure and system in an integrated fashion, using a body region approach and keeping in mind the structures and functions of the body systems involved.
- A systematic head-to-toe approach when the nurse performs a complete assessment provides consistency and aids documentation. It also minimizes the number of changes in nurse-client position, avoids tiring the client unnecessarily, allows the nurse to work most efficiently, and ensures that no assessment area is overlooked.
- More commonly performed than a complete assessment, the partial assessment focuses on a specific client concern or problem. It may be done in many different health care settings.
- A partial history is appropriate for an outpatient, an inpatient, or a distressed client. It requires full biographic data and detailed information about the reason the client seeks health care. If needed, information about other health history topics may be combined.
- Usually, the nurse performs episodic (partial) physical assessments to evaluate the specific symptoms reported in the health history. Such assessments include a general survey, vital sign measurements, and assessment of certain body structures and systems. Additional systems are assessed as indicated by the client's condition. This type of assessment is especially useful when the nurse tracks the progress of a client with a particular problem.
- Proper documentation is essential for organizing complete or partial assessment data. To document the physical examination, the nurse organizes and records assessment findings by body system.

Study questions

1. When should you perform a complete and a partial health history? What information should you obtain during each type of history?

2. What body systems and structures should you evaluate when performing a complete physical assessment of the anterior thorax, posterior thorax, and abdomen?

3. What organizational approach would you take to a complete physical assessment? How does this compare with the organizational approach you would use to document physical assessment findings?

4. During the complete physical assessment, which physical assessment techniques are used on which parts of the body?

5. Assessment of pediatric and elderly clients requires certain modifications from the usual adult assessment. For instance, one area involving major differences is the eyes. What are the important special considerations to keep in mind when performing an eye assessment in pediatric and elderly clients?

Selected references

Andresen, G. (1989). A fresh look at assessing the elderly. *RN,* 52(6), 28-40.

Gastrointestinal Problems. (1988). NurseReview Series. Springhouse, PA: Springhouse Corp.

Dychtwald, K. (1986). *Wellness and illness promotion for the elderly.* Rockville, MD: Aspen Systems.

Grabbe, L. (1989). Fine-tuning your percussion techniques. *Nursing89,* 19(11), 32J, 32L.

Kennedy, C., Gyr, P., and Garst, K. (1991). A nursing tool to assess children upon hospital admission. *MCN,* 16(2), 78-82.

Kennedy, W. (1990). Vital signs: Reading the essentials. *JEMS,* 15(5), 26-30, 34, 36-39.

McEwan, R. (1989). Issues in evaluation: Evaluating assessments of elderly people using a combination of methods. *Journal of Advanced Nursing,* 14(2), 103-110.

Moschella, S., and Hurley, H. (1986). *Dermatology* (2nd ed.). Philadelphia: Saunders.

Perry, A., and Potter, P. (1990). *Clinical nursing skills and techniques: Basic, intermediate, and advanced.* St. Louis: Mosby.

Phillips, S. (1989). Monitoring vital sign changes in children. *Nursing89,* 19(10), 48-49.

Rice, E. (1989). Geriatric assessment. *Advancing Clinical Care,* 4(3), 8-15.

Richard, C. (1986). *Comprehensive nephrology nursing.* Boston: Little, Brown.

Wandel, J. (1990). The use of postural vital signs in the assessment of fluid volume status. *Journal of Professional Nursing,* 6(1), 46-54.

Witkowski, A. (1985). *Pulmonary assessment: A clinical guide.* Philadelphia: Lippincott.

Wong, D., and Whaley, L. (1990). *Clinical handbook of pediatric nursing* (3rd ed.). St. Louis: Mosby.

Nursing research

Asiain, M., Montes, Y., Costa-Ramos, M., and Imizcoz, P. (1990). Blood pressure measurement: An evaluation of direct and indirect methods. *Intensive Care Nursing,* 6(3), 111-117.

McElmurry, B. (1986). Health appraisal of low-income women. In D. Kjervik and I. Martinson (Eds.), *Women in health and illness: Life experiences and crises.* Philadelphia: Saunders.

Utley, R. (1990). Mid-arm circumference: Estimating patients' weight. *DCCN,* 9(2), 75-81.

22

Perinatal and Neonatal Assessment

Objectives

After reading and studying this chapter, you should be able to:

1. Gather appropriate health history information for a pregnant client.
2. Identify normal prenatal assessment findings.
3. Document prenatal assessment findings.
4. Gather appropriate health history information for a postpartum client.
5. Identify normal postpartum assessment findings.
6. Document postpartum assessment findings.
7. Identify normal neonatal assessment findings, including neonatal reflexes.
8. Document neonatal assessment findings.

Introduction

Complete and accurate assessment forms the basis for developing the nurse's individualized care plans for a client during pregnancy and after delivery, and for the neonate. This chapter discusses the essentials of perinatal assessment—including prenatal and postpartum evaluations—and neonatal assessment. (It does not include intrapartal assessment.) It covers health history questions, physical assessment steps, and documentation of findings.

Because pregnancy affects a woman's entire body, the prenatal assessment must be comprehensive. It should evaluate common complaints and include a complete assessment of each body system. It should also assess the client's emotional status, including her acceptance of the pregnancy, her preparation for motherhood, and the pregnancy's impact on the family.

For postpartum assessment, collect data on the client's response to delivery and to the neonate as well as her adjustment to the puerperium (the 6 weeks after childbirth). Also, teach the client about the changes occurring in her body.

Neonatal assessment begins immediately after birth and continues for the duration of the neonate's nursery stay. The nurse is usually the first health care professional to examine the neonate in the delivery room. To conduct such an examination, you will need to know how to calculate an Apgar score and how to make general—but crucial—observations about the neonate's appearance and behavior. This information, coupled with pertinent maternal and fetal history data, provides an initial data base for nursery personnel and pediatricians to use during subsequent examinations.

Prenatal assessment

Prenatal assessment begins when the client first seeks medical care because she suspects she may be pregnant, and continues until labor and delivery. The nurse's assessment of the client involves a thorough health history and physical examination. (For detailed assessment information, see *Prenatal physical assessment,* page 639, and *Assessing the fundus,* page 640.)

Glossary

Chloasma: brownish pigmentation of facial skin in some pregnant women. Also known as the mask of pregnancy.

Colostrum: secretion from the breast before the onset of lactation, containing mainly serum and white blood cells.

Fontanel: an unossified space, or soft spot, between the cranial bones of the neonate.

Involution: gradual reduction in size of the uterus after delivery.

Lanugo: fine, downy body hair on the neonate, predominantly covering the face, shoulders, and back.

Linea nigra: black line or discoloration of the abdomen running from the umbilicus to the pubis, often developing in the third trimester of pregnancy.

Lochia alba: yellow-white uterine discharge consisting mainly of plasma and white blood cells that appears after delivery, following the lochia serosa and continuing for about a week.

Lochia rubra: uterine discharge of blood, mucus, and tissue that occurs the first 6 days after delivery.

Lochia serosa: brownish uterine discharge that appears after delivery, following the lochia rubra and continuing for 3 to 4 days.

Meconium: first feces of a neonate, greenish black to dark brown and of tarry consistency, normally passed within 24 to 48 hours after birth.

Milia: tiny white papules commonly occurring on a neonate's nose, cheeks, and chin, caused by unopened sebaceous glands.

Ophthalmia neonatorum: severe purulent conjunctivitis in the neonate.

Puerperium: 6-week period after childbirth, during which the uterus and vagina return to their prepregnant state.

Striae gravidarum: stretch marks; these pinkish-white or red lines commonly appear on the breasts, abdomen, thighs, and buttocks during pregnancy.

Vernix caseosa: white, cheeselike, sebaceous deposit often covering the just-born neonate.

Health history

Help put the client at ease by conducting the health history interview in a quiet, comfortable, and private environment. Proceed at an unhurried pace to allow the client time to answer all questions thoroughly and accurately. Begin by obtaining all relevant biographic data. Then ask questions about the pregnancy and the client's health status.

Health and illness patterns

To assess important health and illness patterns that may affect the pregnancy, explore the client's current, past, and family health status.

Current health status. To assess the client's current health status, ask the following questions:

When was the first day of your last menstrual period?
(RATIONALE: Knowing the date of the last menstrual period helps diagnose pregnancy and determine the approximate delivery date.)

Was this menstrual period like the previous ones?
(RATIONALE: A pregnant client may seem to have a period, but with different characteristics. The client could interpret as a period changes that include spotting [scant bloody discharge from the vagina], which could indicate an ectopic pregnancy, a cervical infection, or a problem with hormonal support of the endometrium.)

How would you describe your energy level?
(RATIONALE: Fatigue during the first stages of pregnancy is normal; however, complaints of extreme fatigue or lethargy may call for further investigation.)

How is your overall health? Have you experienced any problems during this pregnancy?
(RATIONALE: These questions allow the client to discuss her general health status and any specific complaints related to pregnancy or other conditions.)

Past health status. When compiling information on the client's past health status, ask the following questions to explore her medical and obstetric history:

Have you had uterine or pelvic surgery or injury?
(RATIONALE: Previous uterine or pelvic surgery or injury may necessitate cesarean delivery.)

Have you ever had a sexually transmitted disease? If so, which one and when? What treatment did you receive?
(RATIONALE: An untreated sexually transmitted disease places the fetus at risk for infection during passage through the birth canal.)

Have you been pregnant before? If so, how would you describe the pregnancy and its outcome? How long did the pregnancy and labor last? What type of delivery was it? Did you suffer any complications during pregnancy, labor, or delivery or have any problems after delivery? What was the birth weight and overall health of the infant?
(RATIONALE: Knowing the history of the client's previous pregnancies can help identify any potential problems with the current pregnancy.)

Have you ever had an abortion?
(RATIONALE: Abortion may result in cervical incompetency or adhesions that could cause problems during pregnancy and delivery.)

If you have given birth before, have you breast-fed or bottle-fed your infant(s)?
(RATIONALE: This question allows the client to discuss her plans for feeding her infant and any problems she might have experienced with feeding previous infants.)

Is your blood Rh negative? If so, did you receive Rh_o immunoglobulin (RhoGAM) after your first delivery?
(RATIONALE: An Rh-negative woman who has delivered an Rh-positive infant becomes sensitized to the Rh factor and needs RhoGAM to prevent complications with subsequent deliveries.)

Family health status. Investigate the client's family health status related to pregnancy and childbirth by asking the following questions:

Has anyone in your family experienced any complications during pregnancy, labor, or delivery? If so, what were the complications and how were they resolved?
(RATIONALE: A family history of pregnancy or childbirth complications—such as spontaneous abortion, multiple births, or difficult labor—suggests a predisposition to such problems.)

Has anyone in your family had hypertension, diabetes mellitus, gestational diabetes (diabetes during pregnancy only), obesity, or heart disease?
(RATIONALE: Such familial conditions can adversely affect the health of a pregnant client or her fetus.)

Health promotion and protection patterns

Continue the history by assessing personal habits and activities that may affect the client's pregnancy.

Are you currently taking any prescription or over-the-counter medications? If so, which ones? How often do you take them and how much do you take?
(RATIONALE: A client's use of certain drugs can adversely affect the developing fetus or lead to complications during pregnancy. If the client uses any drugs, check to make sure they are considered safe during pregnancy.)

Are you currently using any street drugs or alcohol? If so, which ones, in what amounts, and for how long?
(RATIONALE: During pregnancy, a client's use of illicit drugs—such as cocaine and heroin—can cause severe drug withdrawal symptoms and possible long-term neurologic effects in the neonate. Alcohol abuse during pregnancy can cause fetal birth defects.)

Did you use a contraceptive before this pregnancy? If so, which type? When did you stop using it?
(RATIONALE: The answer to this question provides information about the effectiveness of contraception and pregnancy planning.)

Do you smoke cigarettes? If so, how many do you smoke per day and how long have you been smoking?
(RATIONALE: Smoking during pregnancy is associated with fetal growth retardation and increased fetal and neonatal morbidity and mortality.)

When did you last have a Papanicolaou (Pap) test? What were the results?
(RATIONALE: The answer provides information about the client's health promotion and protection patterns. It also indicates whether the Pap test was normal.)

What is your typical daily diet? Which types and what amounts of food do you eat at each meal and between meals?
(RATIONALE: This question helps assess the client's nutritional status. It also gives the client an opportunity to discuss any concerns about food and gives you an opportunity to clear up any misconceptions she may have, such as "eating for two.")

Do you exercise regularly? If so, which type of exercise and how often?
(RATIONALE: Unless contraindicated, regular moderate exercise can improve or maintain muscle tone, which can help ease delivery and speed the body's return to its prepregnant state.)

How much sleep do you usually get per day? Do you feel well rested?
(RATIONALE: A pregnant client may require more sleep, particularly during the first and third trimesters. Inadequate sleep can cause increased stress and stress-related problems.)

Prenatal physical assessment

Pregnancy affects almost all body systems and major organs. The nurse who assesses a pregnant client needs to know these effects, along with normal findings.

Throughout the prenatal assessment, keep in mind that pregnancy can be a stress-filled time as the client and her family adjust to many physical and emotional changes. Always observe and listen for clues about the client's positive or negative adjustment. For example, does the client indicate by words and actions, such as preparing the infant's room, that she is happily pregnant? Alternatively, does she cry and express only negative feelings about having a child?

Skin

First, inspect the client's skin, particularly noting any color changes. During pregnancy, melanotropin (a hormone secreted by the anterior pituitary) normally increases, causing hyperpigmentation of several skin structures. Examples include a brownish hyperpigmentation of the facial skin (chloasma, also called melasma, or the mask of pregnancy) and a brownish black pigmented line on the abdominal midline (the linea nigra). The areolae, nipples, and vulva also may darken from hyperpigmentation. Most of these color changes fade gradually after delivery.

Thyroid gland

When assessing the head and neck, be sure to palpate the thyroid. (For a description of this technique, see Chapter 20, Endocrine System.) In about 50% of all pregnant women, the thyroid gland enlarges because of increased vascularity and hyperplasia of this glandular tissue.

Respiratory system

As you observe the client's chest, note the breathing pattern and respiratory rate. During pregnancy, the thoracic (rib) cage shortens, widening at the base. The growing fetus elevates the diaphragm, causing an increased maternal respiratory rate. The pregnant client may change from abdominal breathing to thoracic breathing as pregnancy progresses. Some shortness of breath commonly occurs in the later weeks of pregnancy, particularly during exertion.

Cardiovascular system

Auscultate the client's cardiovascular system, keeping in mind that a 30% to 50% increase in blood volume occurs during pregnancy, commonly accentuating heart sounds. In fact, systolic murmurs occur in about 90% of pregnant women. The heart is displaced upward and laterally, secondary to the pressure exerted by the gravid (pregnant) uterus on the diaphragm, sometimes causing the point of maximum impulse (PMI) to be displaced laterally. (For a description of how to assess PMI and heart sounds, see Chapter 11, Cardiovascular System.)

Obtain the client's blood pressure, which should remain within the normal range for the client's nonpregnant state. However, the blood pressure may drop during midpregnancy. Any elevations of 30 mm Hg (systolic) or 15 mm Hg (diastolic), or both, over the client's baseline blood pressure are abnormal, requiring further assessment.

Observe the condition of the client's veins. Pelvic congestion predisposes the client to venous varicosities in the legs and vulva. Edema in the arms and legs is also common.

Breasts

Inspect and palpate the breasts. In about the 8th week, they enlarge. The nipples become larger and more erect. Montgomery's tubercles (sebaceous glands on the areolae) become more prominent. Colostrum, the precursor of milk, can be expressed as early as the 24th gestational week. Initially clear to yellowish, colostrum becomes cloudy later in the pregnancy. Striae (streaks or stretch marks caused by rapidly increasing skin tension) on the breast may become more visible as vascularity and venous engorgement increase.

Abdomen

Inspect and auscultate the abdomen. Striae gravidarum, varying from one pregnant woman to another, appear as the skin stretches to accommodate the growing uterus. Caused by separation of the underlying connective tissue, they usually fade gradually after delivery. The umbilicus may flatten or protrude. Peristalsis (rhythmic motion of smooth-muscle bowel) slows during pregnancy, so bowel sounds may decrease. (For a description of how to assess bowel sounds, see Chapter 13, Gastrointestinal System.) The gravid uterus displaces the colon laterally upward and posteriorly, thereby repositioning the appendix and making the diagnosis of appendicitis more difficult.

Auscultate the fetal heart, which can be heard with a Doppler system as early as the 10th gestational week. In early pregnancy, the fetal heart beats loudest (area of maximum intensity) just above the mother's symphysis pubis at midline. Later in pregnancy, the fetal heart is best heard through the fetal back.

Musculoskeletal system

Observe the client's posture and gait during the assessment. Posture and gait changes result from the gravid uterus thrusting forward and changing the woman's center of gravity. To compensate for these changes, the woman throws her shoulders backward and hyperextends the vertebral column. The abnormal lordosis (curve of the spine) will return to normal after delivery. During the third trimester, the pelvic joints and ligaments relax in preparation for delivery. The pelvis becomes slightly broader.

Assessing the fundus

To estimate the size of the uterus—and fetal growth—palpate and measure the fundus. Before the 12th gestational week, when the gravid uterus moves into the abdominal cavity, estimate uterine size by bimanual assessment. After the 12th week, use fundal palpation to determine fundal height.

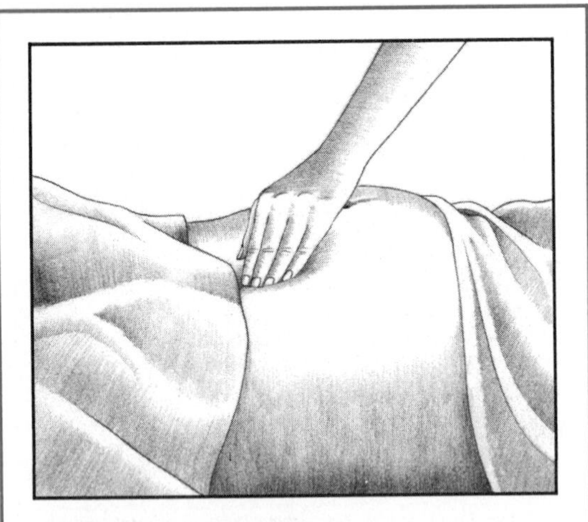

Palpating fundal height
Stand at the supine client's right side and place the palm of your left hand about 1⅛" to 1⅝" (3 to 4 cm) above where the fundus should be. Palpating toward the symphysis pubis, find the point where the soft abdomen ends and the firm, round fundal edge begins.

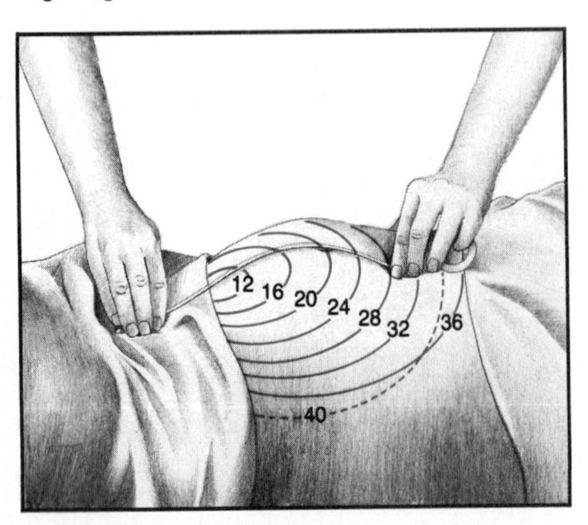

Measuring fundal height
Next, using a measuring tape, determine the distance along the anterior abdominal wall from the top of the fundus to the notch at the inferior edge of the symphysis pubis. At 12 to 13 weeks, the fundus can be felt just above the symphysis pubis; at 16 weeks, the fundus is about midway between the symphysis pubis and the umbilicus; at 20 weeks, it can be felt at the umbilical level.

How would you describe your stress level? Is anything in your life increasing stress?
(RATIONALE: Increased stress can cause various physiologic and psychological problems that can complicate pregnancy and delivery. This question provides an opportunity to assess the client's stress level and to discuss appropriate stress-reduction techniques.)

What type of work do you do? What sort of environment do you work in?
(RATIONALE: Certain jobs and work environments may expose a pregnant woman to unsafe conditions, such as pollutants or excessive physical or psychological stress.)

Have you thought about what type of delivery you would like? Have you attended any prenatal classes?
(RATIONALE: These questions help assess the client's preparation for labor and delivery as well as her attitudes toward the pregnancy. They also provide an opportunity to explain available learning resources.)

Do you have any questions about any aspect of pregnancy or childbirth?
(RATIONALE: This open-ended question gives the client an opportunity to discuss any concerns and explore any areas not yet covered in the interview.)

Role and relationship patterns

Conclude the health history by asking the following questions to assess the client's role and relationship patterns related to pregnancy and childbirth.

How do you feel about being pregnant? How do you feel about having and caring for your baby? Is the pregnancy (or the anticipated baby) causing any problems in such areas as family relationships, finances, career, or living accommodations? Do you feel that you are receiving sufficient support from your family and friends during your pregnancy?
(RATIONALE: These questions provide an opening for the client to express her concerns.)

Have you been engaging in sexual intercourse during this pregnancy? How do you feel about sexual activity during pregnancy?
(RATIONALE: Normally, sexual activity need not be restricted during pregnancy. The client may experience increased sexual desire after the first trimester as a result of pelvic vasocongestion.)

Are you familiar with the community agencies and services that can provide financial, educational, and health care support during your pregnancy and after delivery?

(RATIONALE: This question provides an opportunity to teach the client about available prenatal and postnatal support services.)

Physical assessment

Physical assessment of the pregnant client involves assessment of all body systems as well as an assessment of fetal growth and well-being.

Documentation

To complete the prenatal assessment, document your history and physical assessment findings as well as the results of any laboratory studies that may have been ordered. The following example shows how to document some normal assessment findings:

> *Height:* 5′6″
> *Weight:* 136 lb
> The client, a 23-year-old primigravida, states that she has not had a period in 2 months. She reports nausea and vomiting upon awakening and complains of tenderness and fullness in her breasts. Physical assessment reveals brownish discoloration around the areolae of both breasts. The client reports tenderness when the breasts are palpated. The breasts feel firm and full. Abdominal palpation finds the uterus at the level of the symphysis pubis. Gynecologic assessment shows dark-blue discoloration of the vaginal mucosa.

Postpartum assessment

The postpartum period represents a time of great change in the mother, the neonate, and the family. The nurse's postpartum assessment of the client evaluates the physiologic and psychological changes that occur as her body returns to its prepregnant state. It also assesses the client's and family's adjustment to these changes.

Health history

The postpartum health history collects data on the client's responses to delivery and to the neonate as well as on her adjustment to the puerperium. Take this opportunity to teach the client about the changes in her body.

Health and illness patterns

Begin the postpartum interview by asking the following questions about the client's physical condition, comfort, and mental and emotional status.

How do you feel? Are you experiencing any specific problems you would like to discuss?
(RATIONALE: The client's physical health and comfort can directly affect her mental and emotional adjustment. These questions also give the client a chance to discuss any issues that she may be reluctant to bring up.)

How is your energy level?
(RATIONALE: Postpartum fatigue normally results from disrupted sleep patterns and the emotional stress of adjusting to the neonate and to motherhood.)

Do you have any pain or discomfort in your abdominal or genital areas?
(RATIONALE: For 2 or 3 days after delivery, periodic uterine contractions commonly produce afterpains. Vaginal bruising and edema caused by vaginal delivery also may produce discomfort for several days. Pain or discomfort also is likely if the client had an episiotomy.)

Do you have any discomfort in your breasts or nipples?
(RATIONALE: Breast milk production, which begins around the third day after delivery, commonly causes painful breast engorgement. In a breast-feeding woman, the nipples may be tender for the first few days of nursing.)

Do you have difficulty urinating or feel any pain or discomfort in your bladder or urinary tract?
(RATIONALE: Bladder trauma during birth can cause overdistension and incomplete bladder emptying during voiding. These effects may persist for several days.)

Have you had a bowel movement yet?
(RATIONALE: After delivery, decreased bowel motility, fluid loss, and perineal discomfort commonly delay resumption of normal bowel function for up to a week.)

Do you have any weakness or decreased sensations in your legs and feet?
(RATIONALE: A transient decrease in leg muscle strength may result from the muscle strain and exertion associated with labor and delivery. Use of regional anesthesia during labor and delivery may lead to diminished sensations in the legs and feet for up to 24 hours.)

Health promotion and protection patterns

To continue the postpartum health history, ask the following questions about personal habits and activities

Postpartum physical assessment

Postpartum physical assessment begins with the client supine. Throughout the assessment, the nurse collects data on the client's responses to delivery and to the neonate, as well as on her adjustment to the puerperium (the 6 weeks after childbirth). The nurse also teaches the client about her physical changes. Usually, postpartum physical assessment proceeds from head to toe.

Breasts

Inspect the nipples for signs of infection, bleeding, or crusting. On palpation, the breasts should be soft and nontender. However, many women experience engorgement secondary to the increased breast vascularity that occurs in preparation for lactation. Engorged breasts become enlarged, firm, and usually tender. Look for any reddened or warm areas, which could indicate mastitis.

Abdomen

After delivery, the abdomen is soft, lacking appreciable muscle tone, but muscle tone usually returns to the prepregnant level by 6 weeks postpartum.

Because urine in the bladder causes the fundus to rise above the previously assessed level or to be displaced from the midline, instruct the client to urinate before you begin the fundal height assessment. Without causing the client discomfort, assess fundal height. Immediately after delivery, the fundus should be firm and positioned at the umbilicus. As normal involution (decrease in uterine size) progresses, the fundus gradually moves from below the umbilicus to just above the symphysis pubis. The fundus can be palpated after childbirth for 10 to 14 days, when the uterus again becomes a nonpalpable pelvic organ.

Throughout the postpartum period, the uterus should remain rounded and firm. If the fundus is nonpalpable or feels boggy (soft and mushy), gently massage it and simultaneously observe for the lochia drainage (postpartum vaginal discharge). Blood clots or products of conception can interfere with the normal, postpartum involutional contractions. To massage the fundus, place one hand on the client's symphysis pubis, then grasp the fundus with the other hand and massage gently. Massaging will not only help the uterus return to its normal size, but will also help remove any clots and other matter that remain.

Assessing fundal height

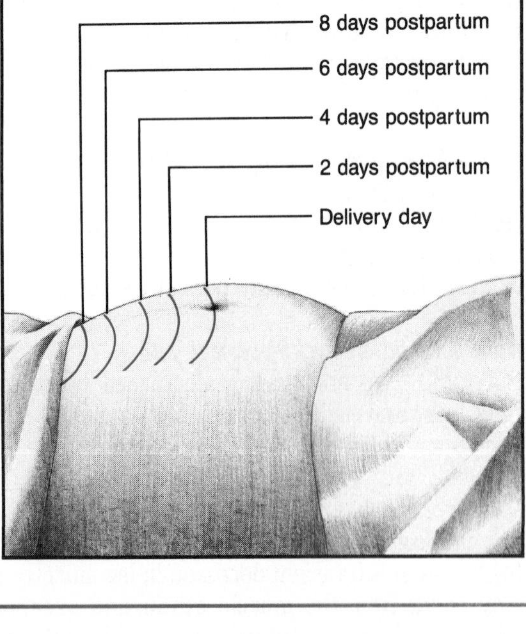

8 days postpartum
6 days postpartum
4 days postpartum
2 days postpartum
Delivery day

Perineum and rectum

Inspect the perineum and episiotomy (incision made in the perineum to enlarge the vaginal opening for delivery) site for signs of erythema, edema, ecchymoses (bruising), or hematoma (blood clot).

Assess the lochia for consistency, amount, color, and odor. Lochia rubra, the dark-red vaginal drainage occurring the first 3 days after delivery, contains red blood cells, placental and decidual debris, and plasma. As the placental site heals, fewer red blood cells are shed and the lochia becomes serosanguineous. Called lochia serosa (pale pink or brown), the serosanguineous matter continues sloughing for 4 to 10 days after delivery. After about 10 days, the lochia is called lochia alba (yellow or white) and consists mostly of plasma and leukocytes.

After assessing the perineum, assess the rectum for hemorrhoids, which may result from engorged pelvic tissue during pregnancy and pressure on the rectum during vaginal delivery.

Extremities

Assess the arms and legs for signs of edema, varicosities, or thrombophlebitis. Homans' sign (pain in the calf with dorsiflexion of the foot, indicating thrombophlebitis) should be absent. Edema in the legs requires a complete assessment of leg pulses and skin temperature.

that may affect the client's recovery from childbirth and adjustment to the neonate.

What is your typical daily diet? Which types and what amounts of food do you eat at each meal and between meals?
(RATIONALE: When caring for the neonate, the client may ignore her own health. Encourage the client to eat properly, especially if she is breast-feeding.)

How much sleep are you getting? Do you feel well rested or tired?
(RATIONALE: A woman often has difficulty sleeping after delivery; excitement, discomfort, and problems of adjusting to the neonate's demands may seriously disrupt sleep patterns.)

Have you been walking? If not, why not?
(RATIONALE: Early ambulation in the postpartum period can help promote healing and decrease the risk of thrombophlebitis.)

Do you feel that the baby is increasing your stress?
(RATIONALE: A neonate may seriously disrupt the tranquility of a household. Assess the client's ability to cope with this disruption and teach stress-management techniques, if appropriate.)

Do you know the signs and symptoms of postpartum problems that require immediate medical attention?
(RATIONALE: Make sure that the client and her family can recognize the warning signs and symptoms of serious postpartum complications, such as hemorrhage, infection, thromboembolism, and hypertension.)

Are you aware of community agencies and other resources that could help you care for the baby at home?
(RATIONALE: Social service and other agencies may provide assistance in caring for the neonate at home.)

Have you scheduled a follow-up examination?
(RATIONALE: A maternal follow-up examination should be performed 4 to 6 weeks after delivery.)

Do you have a car seat to take the baby home from the hospital?
(RATIONALE: Most hospitals require that the parents have an approved car seat for transporting the neonate home.)

Role and relationship patterns

To assess role and relationship patterns, ask about the client's and her family's adjustment to the neonate.

How do you feel about the new baby and your role as mother?
(RATIONALE: The client may experience "postpartum blues" during the first 10 days or so after delivery. Symptoms include crying, irritability, loss of appetite, and difficulty sleeping. Usually, this condition is transient; persistence for more than 2 weeks may indicate postpartum depression.)

Is your partner supportive and is he taking an active role in caring for the baby?
(RATIONALE: A new father may feel ignored and may withdraw as the client focuses her attention on the neonate.)

Do you feel that you are receiving enough help and support from family and friends?
(RATIONALE: The client's psychological well-being depends heavily on how her family and friends respond to the neonate.)

Physical assessment

Postpartum physical assessment focuses on the client's vital signs, breasts, abdomen, reproductive system, perineum, rectum, and extremities. (For more information, see *Postpartum physical assessment.*)

Documentation

To complete the postpartum assessment, document your health history and physical assessment findings as well as any laboratory studies that may have been ordered. The following example shows how to document some normal postpartum assessment findings.

> *Height:* 5′4″
> *Weight:* 140 lb
> Client is a 35-year-old multigravida, 2 days after her third delivery. Temperature 99° F., pulse 86 and regular, respirations 20 and regular. Breasts swollen and tender, breast milk flow scanty. Uterus at level of umbilicus. Lochia rubra present.

Neonatal assessment

Neonatal assessment begins immediately after delivery and continues throughout the nursery stay. The nurse's complete neonatal assessment includes a perinatal his-

(Text continues on page 646.)

Neonatal physical assessment

Knowing the perinatal history and observing astutely are essential skills for the nurse's complete neonatal assessment. Systematic inspection of the neonate usually proceeds from head to toe, beginning with observing the pulse and respiratory rates while the neonate sleeps. Use a radiant warmer or take other precautions, such as exposing only those areas of the neonate that are being assessed, to ensure thermoregulation.

Respirations and pulse rate

Immediately after the neonate's birth, assess respirations. The normal irregular and shallow respiratory rate ranges from 30 to 60 breaths/minute. Brief (15-second) apnea (absence of respiration), also called periodic breathing, occurs characteristically. The chest and abdomen should rise simultaneously with respiration. Auscultated breath sounds are bronchial and loud. (For a description of how to assess breath sounds, see Chapter 10, Respiratory System.)

Then evaluate the pulse rate and heart sounds. The pulse rate changes and usually follows a pattern similar to the respiratory rate. Auscultated apically with a stethoscope for a full minute, normal pulse rate is 120 to 160 beats/minute, increasing to 180 beats/minute during crying and motor activity. During deep sleep, the pulse rate may drop to 100 beats/minute. A slower heartbeat should be reported to the physician. Neonatal heart sounds have a higher pitch, shorter duration, and greater intensity than adult heart sounds.

General appearance

Assess overall skin color. Is the neonate jaundiced (yellow), pale, cyanotic (blue), or ruddy? To determine muscle tone and level of consciousness, observe position and motor activity. Is the neonate crying? What type of cry? Is it high-pitched, weak, or lusty? Is the neonate moving all extremities? Are movements symmetrical? Continue these observations throughout the assessment.

Weight ranges from 5 lb, 8 oz to 8 lb, 13 oz (2,500 to 4,000 g). To weigh the neonate, calibrate the scale at zero, drape a protective covering on the weighing platform, and place the unclothed neonate on it. Weigh at the same time each day. A neonate may lose up to 10% of birth weight within the first 3 or 4 days of life. Height assessment usually accompanies weight assessment. Measure the neonate from crown to heel. The normal range is 18″ to 22″ (45 to 55 cm).

Skin and hair

Observe the skin for color and condition. Large amounts of vernix caseosa (a gray-white, cheeselike, protective skin covering) is normally seen immediately after birth, diminishing after several days. Vernix residues cling to the neck and groin creases and to the genital region. Skin tones range from pink in Caucasian neonates to creamy tan in darker-skinned, Black, Hispanic, or Asian neonates. Acrocyanosis (blue and red discoloration), resulting from sluggish peripheral circulation or from chilling, commonly appears during the first 24 hours. Also, when the neonate is cold, mottling (a patchy, purplish skin discoloration) may appear. Milia, white papules caused by accumulated sebum in the sebaceous glands, frequently occur across the nose, cheeks, and chin. These disappear within 2 to 3 weeks.

Note the type and amount of hair. The full-term neonate should have some head hair, but the amount varies. Lanugo (downy fetal hair) normally covers the face, shoulders, and back.

Head

Within a couple of hours of the neonate's birth, measure the head circumference at its greatest diameter, usually the occipitofrontal circumference. The normal size range is about 12¾″ to 14½″ (32 to 36 cm).

Next, palpate, inspect, and measure the fontanels. The diamond-shaped anterior fontanel normally measures 1⅛″ to 1⅝″ (3 to 4 cm) long and ¾″ to 1⅛″ (2 to 3 cm) wide and may enlarge as molding resolves. The triangle-shaped posterior fontanel may be closed at birth (from molding) but can remain palpable for about 3 months. The anterior fontanel is flat and should remain open for about 18 months.

Inspect the face for overall appearance and symmetry. Features should be appropriately placed and proportionate. Structures, muscle tone, and expression should be symmetrical.

Eyes, symmetrically sized and shaped, should be framed by eyebrows and eyelashes. Eyeballs should be round and firm. Watch for the neonate to focus momentarily, follow an object to the midline, and face toward a speaking voice. Nystagmus (involuntary oscillating eye movements) and strabismus (crossed eyes) are common in the first 2 to 3 months. Because of immature lacrimal glands, tears or discharge may appear. Occasionally, an exudate or swelling results from prophylactic drugs used to prevent ophthalmia neonatorum (neonatal conjunctivitis).

Check the ears for proper placement. The pinnas should intercept an imaginary line from the outer canthus of the eyes (see Chapter 9, Eyes and Ears). Palpate for cartilage in the pinnas, and confirm hearing by eliciting the neonatal startle response to a sudden loud noise.

The nose should be midline, usually flat and broad. Some mucus may appear but no drainage. Because a neonate is an obligatory nose breather, check nostril patency by occluding one nostril at a time and observe for respiratory distress signs, such as sternal retraction.

Chest

Measure the chest at the nipple line. The average chest circumference is 12″ to 13″ (30 to 33 cm) or ¾″ to 1½″ less than the head circumference. (For a description of how to measure the head and chest, see Chapter 6, Nutritional Status.)

Palpate the normally rounded chest for signs of fracture, such as asymmetrical movement and crepitus. Symmetrical, the nipples normally measure less than ½″ (5 to 10 mm) in diameter in a full-term neonate. Related to maternal estrogen in utero, breast engorgement may occur in either sex.

Abdomen

Inspect, auscultate, and palpate the abdomen, which should be rounded and dome-shaped, and soft with no masses. Bowel sounds should exist 1 to 2 hours after birth. Meconium (the thick, sticky, green or black first stool) should pass within the first 24 to 48 hours, indicating an intact and functioning gastrointestinal tract.

The umbilical stump falls midline at the lower abdomen. The umbilical cord—at birth moist, soft, and creamy white—should be securely clamped, nonbleeding, and free of signs of infection. It should remain dry and odorless. Then it progressively shrinks, turns black, and detaches in approximately 2 weeks.

Back

To inspect the back, turn the neonate to a prone position with the head to the side to prevent occluding the nostrils. Look first for a straight spine and planar alignment of shoulders, scapulae, and iliac crests; then palpate the spine. It should be intact, without indentations or dimpling.

Extremities

Note positions and movements of the arms and legs. The neonate usually assumes a position reflecting its normal position in utero. Motor activity should include a full range of motion with all four extremities moving spontaneously and equally. Often the fist is clenched with the thumb under the fingers. Fingernails and toenails should extend slightly beyond the tips of the fingers and toes. The legs should be equally long with comparable gluteal folds. Because the lateral muscles are more developed than the medial muscles, the legs should appear bowed.

Test hip joint stability by using Ortolani's maneuver. With the neonate supine, flex the hips and knees at right angles; abduct them until the lateral aspects of the knees touch the examination table; next, bring the knees together, keeping the hips and knees flexed, and attempt to rotate the hips clockwise and counterclockwise to evaluate symmetry of movement. You may hear and feel a click or popping sound if the joint is unstable.

Anus and genitalia

Take the temperature rectally to assess anal patency in either sex.

In the male neonate, palpate the two pendulous and wrinkled scrotal sacs for evidence of a testis in each. Then observe that the prepuce (the foreskin, which does not retract easily) covers the glans penis and that the urinary meatus appears as a slit at the penile tip.

In the female neonate, the external genitalia usually look edematous and hyperpigmented. The labia majora dominate and cover the labia minora. The clitoris, also edematous, is noticeable. A grayish white mucus discharge (smegma), which is normal, or a blood-tinged discharge (pseudomenstruation), caused by maternal hormones in utero, may be present. The urinary meatus, positioned beneath the clitoris, is difficult to see.

Assess urination in both sexes. Because the fetal kidneys function, the neonate commonly voids within 24 hours of birth. Urine voided in the first few days may be scant and infrequent (two to six times daily); however, as dietary intake increases, the frequency of daily voidings also increases (15 to 20 times daily).

Ortolani's maneuver

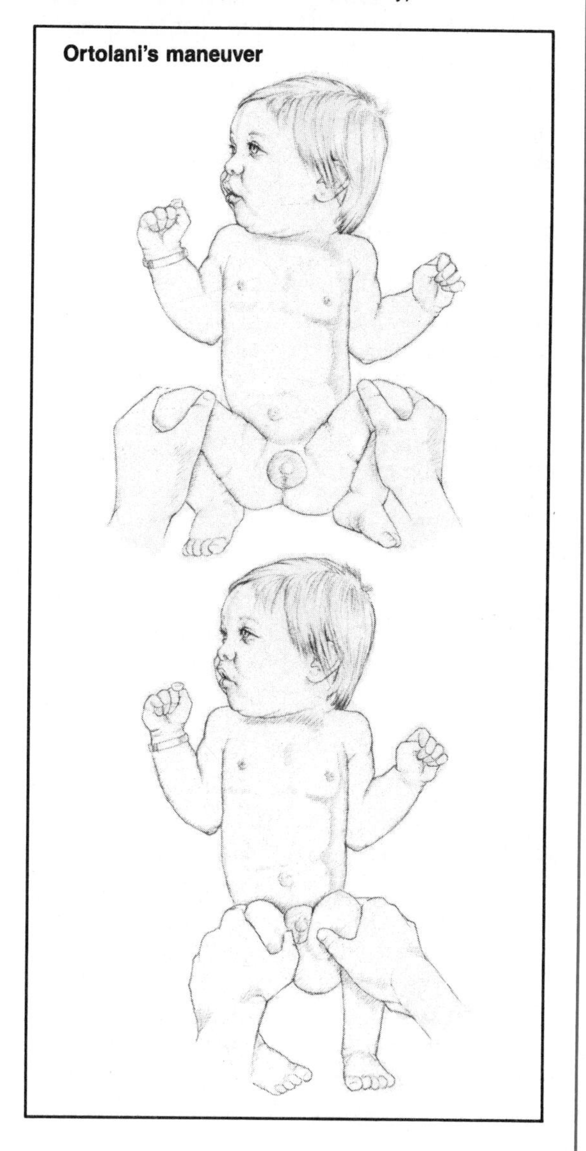

tory (covering such factors as maternal health history, duration of labor, use of analgesia or anesthesia during labor, and any complications of labor and delivery), determination of gestational age, behavioral assessment, and physical assessment. This section briefly covers the behavioral and physical assessment of the neonate. (For a discussion of the specific steps involved in physical assessment, see *Neonatal physical assessment,* pages 644 and 645.)

Behavioral assessment

Begin the assessment by observing the neonate's interactions with the environment. To do this, observe the state of alertness: Is the neonate sleeping deeply or lightly? Is the neonate drowsy or alert? Are the eyes open? Is the neonate crying? The time that the neonate spends in each state and the ease of transition from one state of alertness to another varies between individuals. Recording the state of alertness is an important part of the collected neonatal assessment data.

Physical assessment

Physical assessment of the neonate requires a systematic, head-to-toe approach. Before beginning, make sure the examination room is warm, quiet, and well lit. If possible, let the parents observe the assessment so that they can become better acquainted with their child. (For descriptions of the major neonate reflex tests, see *Neonatal reflex assessment.)*

Documentation

To complete the neonatal assessment, document your findings, including the results of any laboratory studies that may have been ordered. The following example shows how to document some normal neonatal assessment findings.

> *Length:* 19″
> *Weight:* 6 lb 8 oz
> A 2-day-old Caucasian male infant of ruddy complexion has lanugo on back and some skin peeling over bridge of the nose. Anterior and posterior fontanels soft and flat. Eyelids edematous and closed. Short, thick neck with round thorax. Abdomen slightly protuberant, no masses noted on palpation. Cord stump intact, bluish white, and moist. Urethral opening at tip of penis; testes palpable in scrotal sac. Anus patent. Appropriate number and size of digits on hands and feet.

Neonatal reflex assessment

The nurse assesses several reflexes to help determine whether the neonate's neuromuscular system is intact. Keep in mind that gestational age and neonatal muscle tone can alter the reflex responses, and that some reflexes are not as age-specific as others.

REFLEX	ELICITING THE REFLEX	NORMAL RESPONSE
Sucking or rooting	Touch neonate's lip, cheek, or corner of mouth.	Neonate will turn head toward stimulation and open mouth; sucking activity noted.
Extrusion	Touch or depress tongue.	Neonate will force tongue outward.
Tonic neck or "fencing"	Turn head of supine neonate from midline to one side.	Extremities will extend on side toward which neonate is turned; opposite extremities will reflex.
Palmar grasp	Apply pressure to palm of hand.	Neonate's fingers will curl around examiner's finger.
Plantar	Apply pressure to base of toes.	Neonate will hyperextend the toes, dorsiflex the great toe, and fan the toes outward.
Moro or "startle"	Apply a sudden stimulus, such as a hand clap, when neonate is lying quietly.	Neonate will draw up legs and bring arms up in an embracing motion; extremity movements should be symmetrical.
Stepping or "walking"	Hold neonate vertically; allow soles of feet to touch table surface.	Neonate will step, simulating walking.

Chapter summary

Chapter 22 covers the essentials of prenatal, postpartum, and neonatal assessment, including health history questions, physical assessment steps, and documentation of assessment findings. Here are the chapter highlights:

- Prenatal assessment begins when the client first suspects she may be pregnant and continues until labor and delivery. The nurse's assessment includes a thorough health history, focusing on questions related to the pregnancy and the client's overall health status, and physical assessment, covering all maternal body systems as well as an evaluation of fetal growth and well-being.

• Postpartum assessment involves assessing the physiologic and psychological changes that occur as the client's body returns to its prepregnant state as well as evaluating the client's and family's adjustments to these changes.

• Neonatal assessment begins immediately after delivery and continues throughout the neonate's time in the nursery. The nurse's complete neonatal assessment includes a perinatal history, determination of gestational age, physical assessment—including evaluation of neonatal reflexes—and behavioral assessment.

Study questions

1. Mrs. Graves, age 28, is 7 months pregnant. She expresses distress about the stretch marks on her abdomen. What information should you give her?

2. Which prenatal health history questions help assess both maternal and fetal health?

3. How would you compare normal prenatal changes in the abdomen and breasts with postpartum changes?

4. Which aspects of general appearance are vital to the neonatal physical assessment?

5. Which reflexes help assess the neonate's neuromuscular system and how are they elicited?

Selected references

Cohen, S., Kenner, C., and Hollingsworth, A. (1991). *Maternal, neonatal, and women's health nursing.* Springhouse, PA: Springhouse Corp.

Gates, D., and O'Neill, N. (1990). Promoting maternal-child wellness in the workplace. *AAOHN Journal,* 38(6), 258-263, 291-293.

Gorrie, T. (1986). Postpartal nursing diagnosis. *JOGNN,* 15(1), 52-56.

Hans, A. (1986). Postpartum assessment: The psychological component. *JOGNN,* 15(1), 49-51.

Jones, M. (1989). Identifying signs that nurses interpret as indicating pain in newborns. *Pediatric Nursing,* 15(1), 76-79.

Kenner, C. (1990). Measuring neonatal assessment. *Neonatal Network,* 9(4), 17-22.

Key, T., and Resnick, R. (1990). Maternal changes in pregnancy. In D. Danforth and J. Scott (Eds.), *Danforth's obstetrics and gynecology* (6th ed.). Philadelphia: Lippincott.

Reeder, S., Martin, L., and Koniak, D. (1987). *Maternity nursing* (17th ed.). Philadelphia: Lippincott.

Shapiro, C. (1989). Pain in the neonate: Assessment and intervention. *Neonatal Network,* 8(1), 7-21.

Nursing research

Albrecht, S., and Rankin, M. (1989). Anxiety levels, health behaviors, and support systems of pregnant women. *MCN,* 18(1), 49-60.

Ferketich, S., and Mercer, A. (1990). Effects of antepartal stress on health status during early motherhood. *Scholarly Inquiry for Nursing Practice,* 4(2), 127-149.

Freda, M., Andersen, H., Damus, K., Poust, D., Brustman, L., Merkatz, I. (1990). Lifestyle modification as an intervention for inner city women at risk for preterm birth. *Journal of Advanced Nursing,* 15(3), 364-372.

Green, J., Coupland, V., and Kitzinger, J. (1990). Expectations, experiences, and psychological outcomes of childbirth: A prospective study of 825 women. *Birth,* 17(1), 15-24.

Jacoby, A. (1988). Mothers' views about information and advice in pregnancy and childbirth: Findings from a national study. *Midwifery,* 4(3), 103-110.

LaFoy, J., and Geden, E. (1989). Postepisiotomy pain: Warm versus cold sitz baths. *JOGNN,* 18(5), 399-403.

Leatherman, J., Blackburn, D., and Davidhizar, R. (1990). How postpartum women explain their lack of obtaining adequate prenatal care. *Journal of Advanced Nursing,* 15(3), 256-267.

Loos, C., and Julius, L. (1989). The client's view of hospitalization during pregnancy. *JOGNN,* 18(1), 52-56.

Morales-Mann, E. (1989). Comparative analysis of the perceptions of patients and nurses about the importance of nursing activities in a postpartum unit. *Journal of Advanced Nursing,* 14(6), 478-484.

Waldenstrom, U. (1989). Early discharge as voluntary and involuntary alternatives to a longer postpartum stay in the hospital—Effects on mothers' experiences and breast-feeding. *Midwifery,* 5(4), 189-196.

APPENDICES

1: Adult client with altered cardiac output
2: Adult client with impaired gas exchange
3: Pediatric client with altered comfort
4: NANDA nursing diagnoses grouped into Gordon's functional health patterns

For an acutely ill client, the nurse may decide that a complete head-to-toe assessment is impractical or dangerous. In such a situation, the nurse would perform only essential assessment techniques focusing on the client's presenting signs and symptoms.

The first three appendices review assessment skills for adult clients with altered cardiac output and impaired gas exchange, and for a pediatric client with altered comfort. Each offers a short case history that serves as the basis for the assessment and then provides a chart that lists important history questions to ask the client and appropriate assessment activities; a rationale for each history question or physical assessment activity; and appropriate documentation for each activity. The health history documentation paraphrases the client's response to each question; the physical assessment documentation shows the proper recording of findings.

Appendix 1: Adult client with altered cardiac output

CASE HISTORY
Mrs. Jane Parnell, age 75, is a Black widowed female who lives alone in a two-story row home. She has been admitted to an acute care facility after a checkup in which she complained of fatigue and shortness of breath after light activity.

ASSESSMENT ACTIVITY	RATIONALE	DOCUMENTATION
Health history		
What activities tire you? Do you become more tired as the day progresses?	An early symptom of congestive heart failure (CHF), fatigue is caused by reduced cardiac output and decreased perfusion of skeletal muscle tissue.	Light housework (dusting and washing dishes) causes fatigue that worsens by evening. (Fatigue assessed at 2 to 4 metabolic equivalents of a task [METs].)
Do you ever feel lightheaded or pass out?	Reduced cardiac output leads to decreased cerebral oxygenation, which can cause lightheadedness, syncope, or dysrhythmia.	Lightheadedness on exertion.

continued

Appendix 1: Adult client with altered cardiac output continued

ASSESSMENT ACTIVITY	RATIONALE	DOCUMENTATION
Health history continued		
Palpation continued		
Do you become short of breath easily? If so, does it worsen with exertion? Does it improve with position changes?	Pressure from left heart failure forces fluid backward from the pulmonary capillaries into the alveoli, causing pulmonary congestion. In turn, this congestion causes impaired gas exchange, which results in dyspnea.	Mild dyspnea with light activity; dyspnea worsens with exertion and is relieved by sitting upright.
Do you have a cough? If so, do you cough up any mucus?	A nonproductive cough results from accumulated fluid irritating the alveoli. A productive cough (usually with frothy, pink-tinged mucus caused by capillary rupture) typically occurs with pulmonary congestion.	No daytime cough; moist, nonproductive cough at night.
Do you ever have chest pain?	Decreased cardiac output leads to decreased coronary artery perfusion, which can cause chest pain.	No chest pain.
Does your heart ever seem to race, flutter, or jump or skip a beat?	Ventricular ischemia caused by decreased myocardial perfusion can produce the compensatory tachycardia and premature ventricular contractions that cause palpitations.	Rapid heart rate with exertion. "Once my heart felt as if it was turning over in my chest."
Do your feet, legs, or other parts of your body ever feel cold?	Low cardiac output causes vasoconstriction and shunting of blood away from peripheral circulation to the vital organs, resulting in cool, diaphoretic extremities.	Cold feet at night, even when wearing wool socks; occasional cold hands and nose.
Do you ever have leg pain when walking?	Muscles need more oxygen during exertion. Low cardiac output causes muscle ischemia and resultant claudication.	No leg pain on ambulation.
Do your feet or ankles seem swollen, or do your shoes feel tight? Have you gained any weight over the past week?	Edema, a classic sign of chronic right-sided CHF, results from increased pulmonary venous pressure. As blood backs up into the systemic circulation, fluid shifts from the capillaries into the interstitial spaces, producing edema.	Shoes and clothes feel tight; 5-lb weight gain in the past week despite decreased appetite.
What prescription and over-the-counter medications do you take?	The answer to this question helps evaluate the therapeutic and adverse effects of drugs, the client's compliance with her prescribed drug regimen, and the need for client teaching.	Takes "blood pressure and water pills" every day but does not know the names or dosages of the drugs. She used to feel that these drugs helped, but not so much during the past week. No adverse drug reactions.
What heart or circulatory problems have you had?	The answer to this question can help identify problems related to the CHF and provide information that could affect the nursing diagnosis.	Hypertension for 20 years; CHF was diagnosed 5 years ago. Hospitalized four times over past 5 years for related problems but has been stable since last 5-day hospitalization 6 months ago until this episode.
Does anyone in your family have heart or blood pressure problems?	A positive family history may correlate with the client's current problem or may indicate a predisposition to future problems.	One brother has hypertension; thinks father died of stroke and mother of heart failure.

Appendix 1: Adult client with altered cardiac output continued

ASSESSMENT ACTIVITY	RATIONALE	DOCUMENTATION
Do you have any other health problems?	Problems in other body systems can contribute to CHF, and vice versa.	On last hospital admission, was diagnosed as having borderline diabetes, which was treated with dietary modifications. Reports no GI symptoms, except for recent anorexia; no GU symptoms, except for recent nocturia; and no respiratory symptoms, except for cardiac-related dyspnea.
Have you ever smoked tobacco or used alcohol?	Tobacco and alcohol may contribute to or exacerbate health problems.	Does not use tobacco or alcohol because of religious convictions.
Is your sleep ever interrupted because you have to get up to urinate or because you feel short of breath?	A client with CHF may experience sleep pattern disruption because of paroxysmal nocturnal dyspnea (PND) and nocturia. PND results from increased venous return and resultant increased pulmonary vascular pressure. Nocturia develops from the improved kidney perfusion that occurs when the client is at rest.	Normally sleeps 7 hours a night, but is often awakened by nocturia or PND. Has slept with head elevated on two pillows for the past few years; however, in the past week this hasn't eased breathing, so has been sleeping in a recliner chair.
Physical assessment		
Inspection		
Mental status: signs of restlessness or anxiety, attention span, orientation	Reduced cardiac output related to CHF may impair cerebral circulation and alter level of consciousness. Anxiety and restlessness can result from dyspnea.	Client appears restless and anxious, fully oriented, with attention span intact.
Jugular veins	With client in a semi-Fowler's position, jugular vein distention may indicate right-sided CHF.	With client at 45-degree elevation, jugular veins filled; in upright position, jugular veins distended.
Chest: respiratory rate, rhythm, client positioning for respiratory comfort, use of accessory muscles of respiration	Pulmonary congestion causes impaired gas exchange, which increases respiratory rate and can cause abdominal breathing and use of accessory muscles. A client with left-sided CHF related to pulmonary congestion is comfortable only in orthopnea position.	Respirations 30/minute, labored, shallow. Client comfortable only in orthopnea position. Primarily chest breathing with some abdominal breathing and use of accessory muscles of neck and shoulders noted.
Palpation		
Heart: point of maximum impulse (PMI) and right ventricular impulse (RVI)	In a client with left ventricular hypertrophy, PMI is enlarged and displaced from the fifth intercostal space (ICS) at the midclavicular line (MCL). In a client with right ventricular hypertrophy, RVI may be present and displaced to the epigastric area.	PMI enlarged to 3 cm, displaced laterally 2 cm past the MCL and down to the sixth left ICS. RVI present at sternal border. Heave noted.
Pulses: rate, rhythm, amplitude, symmetry, contour, and strength	Tachycardia is a compensatory mechanism to increase cardiac output. Dysrhythmias are often related to ventricular irritability. Alternating weak and strong pulses may be caused by ineffective pump action. Decreased peripheral pulses are related to low cardiac output, which results in vasoconstriction and edema of extremities.	Pulse 120 and regular. Peripheral pulses +2 and equal bilaterally, except for dorsalis pedis and posterior tibialis, which are +1.

continued

Appendix 1: Adult client with altered cardiac output *continued*

ASSESSMENT ACTIVITY	RATIONALE	DOCUMENTATION
Physical assessment continued		
Palpation continued		
Blood pressure: systolic, diastolic, and pulse pressure	Decreased stroke volume reduces the systolic blood pressure. Compensatory vasoconstriction maintains a constant diastolic pressure and, along with the decreased systolic pressure, decreased pulse pressure.	BP 120/92. Pulse pressure below 30 mm Hg.
Skin: edema, temperature changes, turgor, and color	Edema in dependent areas (ankles and feet; and in bedridden clients, the sacral area) indicates excess fluid volume and fluid displacement related to increased backward pressure in CHF. Peripheral vasoconstriction related to chronic CHF causes cool extremities. Dusky peripheral extremities indicates increased carboxyhemoglobin.	2+ pitting edema of dorsal surfaces and ankle at malleolus bilaterally. Extremities cool and slightly diaphoretic. Hands dusky from nail beds to wrist area.
Abdomen	Ascites related to fluid displacement may occur in client with right-sided CHF.	Abdomen distended. Ascites noted; fluid wave present on palpation.
Liver and spleen	Hepatomegaly, splenomegaly, and hepatojugular reflux related to excess fluid may develop in a client with right-sided CHF.	Spleen palpable just below left costal border. Liver palpable, smooth, and slightly tender, located 2 cm below right costal border.
Percussion		
Lungs	Increased pulmonary congestion can cause pleural effusion, detected by dullness on percussion.	Chest dullness on percussion in posterior lung bases bilaterally.
Abdomen	Ascites related to right-sided CHF may produce dullness on percussion.	Abdominal dullness on percussion.
Liver and spleen	Hepatomegaly and splenomegaly are related to backward CHF.	Splenic dullness on percussion just below left costal border, during inspiration. Liver dullness on percussion 2 cm below right costal border.
Auscultation		
Lungs	Crackles, caused by fluid-filled alveoli, are related to pulmonary congestion from left-sided CHF. Extensive crackles, gurgles, and wheezes are caused by upper airway obstruction related to pulmonary edema.	Faint crackles at posterior lung bases bilaterally.
Heart: S_1, S_2, S_3, S_4; summation gallop	S_1 and S_2 correspond with rapid pulse rate. S_3 (ventricular gallop) at the apex of the heart is a classic early sign of CHF. A deficit between the apical rate and radial pulse rate commonly occurs in CHF. S_4 (atrial gallop) typically indicates a stressed heart (caused by such disorders as hypertension, myocardial infarction, or coronary artery disease), which may cause the CHF. Summation gallop (S_3 and S_4 with a rapid rhythm) also occurs in CHF.	Apical heart rate and radial pulse both 120/minute and regular. S_1 and S_2 heard. Summation gallop present.

Appendix 2: Adult client with impaired gas exchange

CASE HISTORY
Ronald Jones, age 63, has been admitted to the medical-surgical unit complaining of severe shortness of breath and persistent cough. His medical history shows chronic obstructive pulmonary disease (COPD), which was diagnosed about a year ago.

ASSESSMENT ACTIVITY	RATIONALE	DOCUMENTATION
Health history		
Are you coughing up any mucus? (If client answers yes, perform a symptom analysis. [See Chapter 3.]) How much? What is the consistency? Does the mucus have an odor? What color is it?	Persistent cough commonly accompanies respiratory and cardiovascular disorders. Sputum production is a valuable clue to assessing COPD; a client with Type A COPD (emphysema) typically produces little sputum, but a client with Type B COPD (chronic bronchitis) usually produces large amounts of sputum, especially in the early morning. With both types of COPD, increased sputum and any change in its color or odor commonly indicate infection.	The client has had a productive morning cough with white sputum for several years. It worsened when the weather changed about a week ago. Now coughing up large amounts of thick, greenish, foul-smelling sputum, mostly in the morning and occasionally throughout the rest of the day.
When do you have the most difficulty breathing? Does anything seem to make breathing easier? (Perform a complete symptom analysis.)	Dyspnea, especially on exertion, is a common symptom of respiratory and cardiovascular disorders; its severity often depends on the degree of tissue hypoxia. Paroxysmal nocturnal dyspnea (PND) may indicate cardiac involvement related to a chronic respiratory problem. A client with PND may assume an upright position when sleeping (by sleeping in a chair or on several pillows) to ease the respiratory effort.	The client has had dyspnea on exertion for several years. It has worsened in the past week. Now experiencing dyspnea at rest, and difficulty performing activities of daily living (ADLs) because of easy fatigability. Dyspnea increases with coughing and decreases with position changes (sitting upright and leaning forward). Sleeps on two pillows because of PND; has used three pillows the past few nights and has tried sleeping in a chair. Often awakened by coughing.
Do you have any allergies? Have you ever smoked? If so, how much? Are you exposed to dust, fumes, or tobacco smoke at home or at work?	Allergies or exposure to air pollutants (including tobacco smoke) may indicate the source of bronchial and alveolar irritation, which can exacerbate COPD.	A retired steelworker, client has lived in an urban environment near heavy industry and a major highway for 30 years. Had smoked cigarettes for 45 years (one pack a day for 10 years, plus two packs a day for 25 years, plus three packs a day for 10 years, for a total of 90 pack-years) until a year ago, when COPD was diagnosed.
Which prescription and nonprescription drugs do you take? How often do you take these drugs, and how much do you take?	Noncompliance with a prescribed drug regimen or misuse of nonprescription drugs may exacerbate symptoms or promote resistance to conventional treatment.	Complies with prescribed drug regimen: theophylline (Theo-Dur), 1 tablet a.m. and p.m.; and isoproterenol sulfate (Medihaler-Iso), 1 or 2 inhalations q.i.d. and 1 inhalation during acute episodes of dyspnea, repeated every 2 to 5 minutes times three. Tried over-the-counter antihistamines, which did not relieve symptoms.

continued

Appendix 2: Adult client with impaired gas exchange continued

ASSESSMENT ACTIVITY	RATIONALE	DOCUMENTATION
Health history continued		
Have you gained weight or noticed ankle swelling recently?	Cor pulmonale (right ventricular hypertrophy related to pulmonary hypertension) may develop in chronic respiratory disease. This leads to right-sided congestive heart failure (CHF), causing fluid retention, venous congestion, dependent edema, and weight gain.	5-lb weight gain in past week. Pants and shoes often feel tight; ankles sometimes swell over tops of shoes.
Do any family members have respiratory problems?	A family history of COPD may reflect a familial or genetic tendency.	No family history of respiratory problems.
Physical assessment		
Inspection		
Mental status: orientation to person, place, and time; anxiety	A change in mental status such as restlessness is a common early sign of hypoxia. Dyspnea often increases anxiety, which in turn increases dyspnea.	Client is alert and oriented to person, place, and time. Anxiety level moderate, as evidenced by restlessness, fidgeting, and rapidly shifting gaze.
Respirations: rate, rhythm, and other characteristics such as use of accessory muscles and client positioning for breathing	A client with COPD may have labored, shallow respirations and may breathe through pursed lips (which helps improve gas exchange by increasing the length of expiration). Nasal flaring, retraction of neck muscles during respiration, and tripod position for breathing may indicate acute respiratory distress, respiratory failure, or airway obstruction.	Respirations 32/minute, labored and shallow with pursed-lip breathing. Respiratory effort tires client and limits his ability to speak. Client exhibits nasal flaring and use of accessory muscles of neck and shoulder, with slight retraction of neck muscles.
Skin and oral mucosa: color	A client with Type A COPD usually has pink skin and oral mucosa because of relatively normal blood gas levels; a client with Type B COPD usually has a bluish-gray tint to the skin and oral mucosa, caused by severe cyanosis, hypercapnia, and polycythemia.	Blue-gray skin and oral mucosa.
Jugular veins	Distended jugular veins often indicate right-sided CHF, possibly related to cor pulmonale.	With client positioned at a 60- to 90-degree angle, jugular vein distention noted, with visible pulsations 4 to 5 cm above the sternal angle.
Chest: anterior-posterior diameter and retraction or bulging	A client with COPD may develop "barrel chest" (equal anterior-posterior and lateral chest diameters). This abnormality results from chronic lung hyperinflation caused by trapped air and secretions blocking the airways. Retraction on inspiration or bulging on expiration results from the increased respiratory effort needed to overcome blocked airways.	Anterior-posterior chest diameter equals lateral chest diameter. Retraction occurs on inspiration.
Palpation		
Skin and mucus membranes	Palpation helps evaluate the client's hydration status and venous congestion as evidenced by dependent edema (edema in ankles and feet, and if the client is bedridden, in the sacral area). Poor hydration can cause thickening sputum and exacerbation of dyspnea.	Dry oral mucosa; poor skin turgor (skin tents when pinched) on trunk and arms; pitting edema (2+) on ankles and pretibial areas.
Respiratory excursion	Airway obstruction traps air in the lungs, causing limited movement in the lung bases and · decreased respiratory excursion.	Respiratory excursion symmetrical but decreased bilaterally at anterior and posterior lung bases.

Appendix 2: Adult client with impaired gas exchange continued

ASSESSMENT ACTIVITY	RATIONALE	DOCUMENTATION
Tactile fremitus	Airway obstruction traps air in the lungs, causing limited movement in lung bases and decreased tactile fremitus.	Decreased fremitus at anterior and posterior lung bases.
Heart: point of maximal impulse (PMI) and second heart sound (S_2) at cardiac bases	Pulmonary hypertension and right ventricular hypertrophy related to COPD may displace the PMI from the fifth intercostal space (ICS) in the midclavicular line toward the epigastric area. Pulmonary hypertension related to COPD may increase the intensity of S_2, making it easily palpable.	PMI displaced toward lower left sternal border into epigastric area. S_2 palpable, with increased intensity at left sternal border.
Liver	Hepatomegaly – marked by an easily palpated liver edge – may result from downward liver displacement caused by right-sided CHF or hyperinflated lungs.	Smooth liver edge palpated 2 cm below costal margin.
Percussion		
Lung bases	Hyperinflation can trap air in the lungs, causing hyperresonance on percussion.	Bilateral hyperresonance noted to T11 over posterior chest. Hyperresonance noted over anterior chest to sixth ICS on right side and to second ICS on left side.
Level of diaphragm and respiratory excursion	In COPD, lung hyperinflation may produce a flattened diaphragm extending to T12, with little or no movement on inspiration or expiration.	Diaphragm percussed at T12 bilaterally. No movement noted on deep inspiration or expiration.
Liver	Hepatomegaly may result from right-sided CHF related to COPD. Percussion will detect edge of enlarged liver.	Percussion reveals liver edge extending 2 cm beyond costal margin.
Auscultation		
Lungs	Decreased breath sounds – particularly in the lung bases – may result from decreased air flow caused by mucus accumulation or bronchospasm. Prolonged expiration may occur throughout the lung fields in an attempt to deflate the lungs. Abnormal breath sounds associated with COPD may include crackles, caused by air moving through fluid in small airways; rhonchi (gurgles), caused by excessive mucus production; and wheezes, related to narrowed airways.	Prolonged expiration. Vesicular lung sounds normal throughout most of the lung fields, but diminished at the bases. Abnormal breath sounds noted: bibasilar crackles unaffected by coughing and gurgles in the anterior and posterior upper airways that do not clear fully after coughing.
Heart	In COPD, lung hyperinflation may muffle heart sounds, and poor tissue oxygenation may lead to tachycardia.	Heart sounds distant; apical rate 110 with regular rhythm.

Appendix 3: Pediatric client with altered comfort

CASE HISTORY
Joey Anderson, age 8, has just been admitted to the pediatric unit. He is accompanied by his parents and complaining of acute abdominal pain. His medical diagnosis is acute abdomen.

ASSESSMENT ACTIVITY	RATIONALE	DOCUMENTATION
Health history (Questions for Joey)		
What hurts?	The child's answer can help locate the pain, providing important clues to its cause.	Child's "stomach hurts real bad."
Please show me where the pain started and where it hurts now. Does it hurt in other places, too?	Appendicitis typically begins with generalized or periumbilical pain that descends and localizes in the right lower quadrant (RLQ). Low back pain may indicate a retrocecal (behind the cecum) appendix.	Pain is "all over my stomach." Guarding RLQ with his hands.
When did the pain start? Does anything seem to make it worse?	No specific factors precipitate appendicitis; however, movement may exacerbate the abdominal pain.	Pain woke child last night. Riding over bumpy roads to the hospital made the pain worse. It worsens when child moves or inhales.
Does anything make your stomach hurt less?	Positioning with the right leg flexed or extended may help relieve irritation of the iliopsoas muscle, which often occurs in appendicitis.	Lying still with legs bent; position "makes it feel a little better."
How does the pain feel? For instance, is it sharp and burning or dull and achy?	The characteristics of abdominal pain vary with the cause. For example, aching or burning pain may result from an ulcer; sharp pain, from an inflammation, such as appendicitis.	Pain feels "hot and sticking, like squeezing and letting go."
How strong is the pain? Does it feel like when you scrape your knee, or is it worse? If this picture of a thermometer had a red line inside showing how bad it hurts, how far up would the line go?	This question helps assess the severity of the pain, which is typically severe in appendicitis and intensifies as the disorder progresses. A child may require a more graphic pain-assessment tool than the scale of 1 to 10 normally used for adults; the thermometer image, or something similar, may prove useful.	Pain described as "the worst pain ever. It would fill the thermometer all the way up and run over the top."
Did the pain start suddenly, or did it hurt a little when you woke up and get worse later?	This question assesses the timing of the pain. In appendicitis, the onset of abdominal pain may be gradual or sudden. In a small child, the pain may occur suddenly, abate somewhat, and then recur more intensely.	Pain described as sudden. Medication mother gave child did not relieve pain.
Health history (Questions for Joey's parents)		
Before this episode, did Joey have a fever, eat any specific foods, or experience any change in bowel habits or pain with bowel movements or urination?	Epigastric pain followed by vomiting and localizing pain are the classic symptoms of appendicitis. However, in a child, the symptoms (vomiting, constipation or diarrhea, anorexia, and fever) are less diagnostic. Specific food intolerances suggest other GI problems, not appendicitis. Pain on defecation may indicate retrocecal appendix; pain on urination may result from peritonitis or an inflamed appendix that irritates the right ureter.	Pain with fever (100.8° F.) on awakening. Despite medication (acetaminophen [Tylenol] 300 mg), the pain continued and seemed to worsen. At about 3 a.m., child vomited "a large amount" of brownish-green emesis. No bowel movement that day; no pain on defecation previously. General anorexia from onset of pain but no specific food intolerance.

Appendix 3: Pediatric client with altered comfort continued

ASSESSMENT ACTIVITY	RATIONALE	DOCUMENTATION
When did Joey last eat?	Information on recent food intake helps determine the safety of general anesthesia in case the child requires emergency surgery.	Last full meal at 6 p.m. and snack of milk and cookies at 9 p.m. the previous day.
Does Joey have any allergies to medications?	This question identifies potential problems if the child requires emergency surgery.	Child does not have any known medication allergies.
Has Joey had any previous stomach or intestinal problems or abdominal surgery?	This question helps identify potential causes of the condition. For example, the child may have had diverticulitis or mesenteric lymphadenitis, which produces similar symptoms.	Generally in excellent health. Rarely sick except for occasional colds, minor stomachaches, and, one time, influenza with diarrhea and vomiting.
Do any family members have stomach or intestinal problems?	This information helps rule out any familial gastrointestinal disorders.	Child's paternal uncle has stomach ulcers.
Does Joey engage in rough play? For example, does he participate in contact sports? Did he suffer abdominal trauma recently—even a minor injury?	This information helps rule out or confirm abdominal injury as the cause of pain. It also aids discharge planning, by indicating what postoperative activity restrictions may be needed to prevent incisional stress.	Child actively engages in sports, particularly football and baseball, and generally "plays hard" with a lot of running, jumping, and climbing. Parents cannot recall any recent incident that might have caused abdominal injury.
Physical assessment		
Note: In a client with appendicitis, excessive abdominal manipulation may increase the risk of perforation. For this reason, a physican usually performs—and does not repeat—abdominal palpation and percussion in a child with suspected appendicitis.		
Height, weight, and vital signs	Height and weight measurements help determine proper drug dosages. Blood pressure, pulse rate, and respiratory rate may increase with severe pain. Pulse rate may increase with fever and increased metabolic rate associated with inflammation.	Height 53"; weight 68 lb, temperature 101°F.; pulse 122 and regular; respirations 32 and shallow; blood pressure 130/79.
Inspection		
General survey: facial expression, skin color, and hydration	Facial expression may help assess severity of pain, particularly in a young child, who may have difficulty describing pain. Facial flushing often occurs with fever; pallor, with pain; diaphoresis, with pain; dehydration, with nausea and vomiting.	Crying and grimacing during assessment. Pallor, dry lips and oral mucosa, and beads of sweat on brow and upper lip.
Body position (particularly right leg position)	Peritonitis or an inflamed or perforated appendix may cause the child to flex or rigidly extend the right leg to decrease the pain.	Child lying motionless and rigid on his right side with knees flexed to abdomen and hands guarding the RLQ; winces on any movement.
Chest: respiratory rate, rhythm, depth, and muscle use	An increased respiratory rate may result from increased metabolism caused by fever. The child may breathe irregularly or pant as pain increases. Shallow respirations often result from the child's attempt to splint (tighten) the abdominal muscles to reduce pain on breathing.	Respirations 32/minute, regular and shallow. Child demonstrates thoracic breathing.

continued

Appendix 3: Pediatric client with altered comfort *continued*

ASSESSMENT ACTIVITY	RATIONALE	DOCUMENTATION
Physical assessment *continued*		
Inspection *continued*		
Abdomen: respiratory and peristaltic movements, shape and symmetry, scars	In child with severe abdominal pain, abdominal respiratory movements may not be visible; abdominal muscles are tightened to reduce pain. Paralytic ileus may cause abdominal distention; ileus and peritonitis, decreased peristalsis.	No abdominal respiratory movements noted; child covering abdomen with hands. No visible peristaltic movements. Abdomen flat to concave; no scars. Guarding on palpation.
Auscultation		
Abdomen: bowel sounds	Decreased bowel sounds commonly accompany appendicitis. Absence of bowel sounds may indicate peritonitis or paralytic ileus.	Bowel sounds decreased in all four quadrants.
Chest: lung and heart sounds	This information helps assess the child's cardiopulmonary status to determine the safety of anesthesia and surgery, if necessary.	Normal lung sounds; no adventitious sounds noted. Heart rate 122/minute with normally split S_2 at base and S_3 at apex in left lateral decubitus position; no murmurs or rubs noted.
Palpation		
Abdomen: light palpation	This technique helps assess the location and severity of abdominal pain and determine the presence of abdominal guarding and rigidity. In a child with appendicitis, pain often begins in the periumbilical or epigastric areas; as inflammation progresses, the pain localizes in the RLQ at McBurney's point (midway between the umbilicus and the anterior iliac crest). Peritonitis may produce diffuse abdominal pain. In a very young child, however, the pain of appendicitis may be poorly localized because of the undeveloped omentum (serous membrane that covers the abdominal organs). In all clients, abdominal muscle guarding increases as the severity of pain increases, and rigidity may indicate peritonitis.	Diffuse abdominal pain on light palpation with increased tenderness in RLQ at McBurney's point. Widespread abdominal muscle guarding and rigidity.
Abdomen: deep palpation	Rebound tenderness (intense pain elicited by deep palpation and quick release of pressure) often occurs in appendicitis. Pressure applied in left lower quadrant (LLQ) that produces tenderness in RLQ (Rovsing's sign) also suggests appendicitis.	Direct and referred rebound tenderness; positive Rovsing's sign.
Percussion		
Abdomen	Tenderness in all four quadrants may accompany appendicitis and peritonitis.	Diffuse and RLQ tenderness on percussion.
Advanced assessment skills		
Iliopsoas sign	Increased abdominal pain elicited by passive hyperextension of the thigh (iliopsoas sign) results from irritation of the iliopsoas muscle by an inflamed extrapelvic appendix.	Positive iliopsoas sign.
Obturator sign	RLQ pain elicited by flexing the child's right thigh at the hip and then rotating the leg at the hip (with the child's right knee bent) laterally and medially points to irritation of the obturator muscle by an inflamed intrapelvic appendix.	Positive obturator sign.

Appendix 4: NANDA nursing diagnoses grouped into Gordon's functional health patterns

Below is a list of NANDA-approved nursing diagnoses arranged under Gordon's functional health patterns.

Health-perception – health-management pattern
- Altered health maintenance
- Health-seeking behaviors (specify)
- Ineffective management of therapeutic regimen (individual)
- Noncompliance (specify)
- High risk for infection
- High risk for injury
- High risk for trauma
- High risk for poisoning
- High risk for suffocation
- Altered protection

Nutritional-metabolic pattern
- Altered nutrition: high risk for more than body requirements
- Altered nutrition: more than body requirements
- Altered nutrition: less than body requirements
- Interrupted breast-feeding
- Ineffective breast-feeding
- Effective breast-feeding
- Ineffective infant feeding pattern
- Impaired swallowing
- High risk for aspiration
- Altered oral mucous membrane
- Potential fluid volume deficit
- Fluid volume deficit
- Fluid volume excess
- Potential impaired skin integrity
- Impaired skin integrity
- Impaired tissue integrity
- High risk for altered body temperature
- Ineffective thermoregulation
- Hyperthermia
- Hypothermia

Elimination pattern
- Constipation
- Colonic constipation
- Perceived constipation
- Diarrhea
- Bowel incontinence
- Altered urinary elimination
- Functional incontinence
- Reflex incontinence
- Stress incontinence
- Urge incontinence
- Total incontinence
- Urinary retention

Activity-exercise pattern
- High risk for activity intolerance
- Activity intolerance
- Fatigue
- Impaired physical mobility
- High risk for peripheral neurovascular disorder
- High risk for disuse syndrome
- Feeding self-care deficit
- Bathing or hygiene self-care deficit
- Dressing or grooming self-care deficit
- Toileting self-care deficit
- Diversional activity deficit
- Impaired home maintenance management
- Ineffective airway clearance
- Ineffective breathing pattern
- Inability to sustain spontaneous ventilation
- Dysfunctional ventilatory weaning response
- Impaired gas exchange
- Decreased cardiac output
- Altered tissue perfusion (specify)
- Dysreflexia
- Altered growth and development

Sleep-rest pattern
- Sleep-pattern disturbance

Cognitive-perceptual pattern
- Pain
- Chronic pain
- Sensory-perceptual alterations (specify – visual, auditory, kinesthetic, gustatory, tactile, olfactory)
- Unilateral neglect
- Knowledge deficit (specify)
- Altered thought processes
- Decisional conflict (specify)

Self-perception – self-concept pattern
- Fear
- Anxiety
- Hopelessness
- Powerlessness
- Self-esteem disturbance
- Chronic low self-esteem
- Situational low self-esteem
- Body image disturbance
- Personal identity disturbance
- High risk for self-mutilation

Role-relationship pattern
- Anticipatory grieving
- Dysfunctional grieving
- Altered role performance
- Social isolation
- Impaired social interaction
- Altered family processes
- Potential for altered parenting
- Altered parenting
- Parental role conflict
- Impaired verbal communication
- High risk for violence: self-directed or directed at others

Sexuality-reproductive pattern
- Sexual dysfunction
- Altered sexual patterns
- Rape-trauma syndrome
- Rape-trauma syndrome: compound reaction
- Rape-trauma syndrome: silent reaction

Coping – stress-tolerance pattern
- Ineffective individual coping
- Defensive coping
- Ineffective denial
- Impaired adjustment
- Post-trauma response
- Caregiver role strain
- High risk of caregiver role strain
- Family coping: potential for growth
- Ineffective family coping: compromised
- Ineffective family coping: disabling
- Relocation stress syndrome

Value-belief pattern
- Spiritual distress (distress of the human spirit)

Adapted with permission from Gordon, M. *Manual of Nursing Diagnosis, 1991-1992.* New York: McGraw-Hill Book Co., 1991.

Acknowledgments for photographs and equipment continued from page iv

p. 53PG Varicose veins, Keith
p. 54PG Peripheral cyanosis and clubbing, 1990 National Medical Slide Bank
p. 59PG Nipple retraction, 1990 National Medical Slide Bank
Eczema-like nipple changes, National Medical Slide Bank
p. 66PG Striae, National Medical Slide Bank
p. 72PG Cervical polyps, 1991 Michael English, MD
Uterine prolapse, 1991 Michael English, MD
Venereal warts, George Moore, MD, PhD
Inguinal mass, 1989 Michael English, MD
p. 75PG Venereal warts, 1991 Steven J. Nussenblatt
Ulcerative lesion, 1991 Steven J. Nussenblatt
p. 91PG Pediatric client – lumbar concavity, 1991 National Medical Slide Bank
Scoliosis, 1991 National Medical Slide Bank
Heberden's nodes, 1991 Lee Samsami
p. 92PG Hallux malleus, 1991 National Medical Slide Bank
Hallux valgus, National Medical Slide Bank
p. 104PG Goiter, 1991 National Medical Slide Bank
Buffalo hump, National Medical Slide Bank
p. 105PG Skin, 1991 National Medical Slide Bank
Abdomen – striae, National Medical Slide Bank
p. 106PG Palpation – fundus, Linda Steimark
Auscultation – ultrasound stethoscope, Linda Steimark

Medichrome

p. 5PG Hemangioma simplex, Dr. Wolfin
p. 6PG Nevus flammeus, Dr. Wolfin
Acne, Dr. Wolfin
p. 8PG Skin lesion configuration – annular, Len Barbiero
p. 9PG Skin lesion distribution – generalized, Harry J. Przekop, Jr.
p. 53PG Venous insufficiency, Michael English, MD
Arterial obstruction, Michael English, MD
p. 66PG Symmetrical abdominal distention, Steve Lissau
p. 92PG Gouty deformities, Michael English, MD
p. 100PG Kaposi's sarcoma
Discoid lesions, Michael English, MD
p. 106PG Auscultation – fetoscope, Jeffrey Reed

Arthur S. Miller, DMD

p. 11PG Structures of the upper mouth
Structures of the lower mouth
p. 14PG Elderly client – gingival recession

Photo Researchers, Inc.

p. 7PG Vertiligo, J. Wilson, MD
Jaundice, SPL
Albinism in light-skinned client, John Watney
Albinism in dark-skinned client, Nancy Hamilton
p. 8PG Primary lesion, Gregory K. Scott
Secondary lesion, Martin M. Rotker
Skin lesion distibution – localized, Biophoto Assoc.
p. 9PG Skin lesion distribution – regional, SPL
Skin lesion configuration – linear, N.M. Hauprich
Nail discoloration, SPL
p. 14PG Pediatric client – head circumference, SPL
p. 15PG Nasal polyps, Biophoto Assoc.
Leukoplakia, SPL
Inflamed tonsils, SPL
Glossitis, SPL
p. 26PG Entropion, SPL
p. 27PG Inflamed conjunctiva, SPL
Red, swollen eyelid gland, SPL
Eyelid nodule, John Watney
p. 54PG Pitting edema – finger pressure, SPL
Pitting edema – small depression, John Watney
p. 66PG Incisional hernia, Biophoto Assoc.
p. 75PG Chancre, Biophoto Assoc.
p. 92PG Rheumatoid nodules, SPL
p. 100PG Raynaud's phenomenon, Biophoto Assoc.
p. 104PG Exophthalmos, Biophoto Assoc.
p. 107PG Capillary hemangioma, Biophoto Assoc.
p. 111PG Extrusion, Petit Format
p. 112PG Plantar reflex, Petit Format

PHOTOTAKE

p. 59PG Asymmetrical breasts
Gynecomastia
p. 75PG Inguinal mass
p. 100PG Wasting syndrome
p. 104PG Acromegaly

Wills Eye Hospital

p. 24PG Optic disk and retina – fair-skinned client
Optic disk and retina – dark-skinned client
p. 25PG Elderly client's pupils
p. 26PG Asymmetrical corneal reflex
Ptosis
Ectropion
p. 29PG Hard exudates

Equipment

Nasal speculum and otoscope in the Photo Gallery, courtesy of Welch Allyn, Inc., Skaneateles Falls, New York

Examination table in the Photo Gallery, courtesy of Enochs Examining Room Furniture, Indianapolis

Medical equipment depicted in Chapter 4, Physical Assessment Skills, courtesy of Jack Kahan, Numedco, Inc., Philadelphia

INDEX

A

Abdomen
  abnormalities of, 66PG, 368t
  acute, 659-661
  assessment of, 625-626t
    neonatal, 108PG, 645
    pregnant client and, 105PG, 639
  auscultation of, 367i
  distention of, 66PG, 355, 369
  landmarks of, 61PG, 366i
  palpation of, 65PG
  percussion of, 63PG
    for fluid wave, 64PG
    for shifting dullness, 64PG
Abdominal pain, 376i, 377
  pediatric client with, 659-661
Abdominal reflex, 85PG, 500i
Abducens nerve, 466i, 487
  assessment of, 488t
Abduction, 109PG, 511, 516i
Abortion, 414
Absorption, of nutrients, 125
Abstract reasoning, assessment of, 483, 486
Acceptance, demonstration of, 38
Accommodation reflex, 22 PG, 207, 222
Accountability, as collaborative strategy, 28-29
Acculturation, 35
Achilles reflex, 84PG, 499i
Acid-base balance, 253, 386
Acid phosphatase levels,
  male reproductive disorder and, 459t
Acini cells, 55PG, 337i, 338
Acne, 6PG
Acoustic nerve, 232i, 233i, 466i, 487
  assessment of, 489t
Acquired immunodeficiency syndrome (AIDS)
  assessment findings in, 574t
  high-risk client and, 452
Acromegaly, 104PG, 587
Acromion process, 87PG, 514i
Activities of daily living (ADLs), 104-110
  developmental considerations for, 110
  documentation of, 110
  factors affecting, 105-107
  importance of, 104-105
Activity pattern, assessment of, 53
Adaptation syndrome, stress assessment and, 54
Addison's disease, 587
  assessment findings in, 602t
Adduction, 109PG, 511, 516i
Adenohypophysis, 588i
Adenoids, 553i
Adipose layer, 55PG, 156i, 157i
ADLs. *See* Activities of daily living.
Adolescent client
  female reproductive assessment for, 423-424, 428
  male reproductive assessment for, 450
Adrenal cortex, 589i
Adrenal glands, 101PG, 388i, 588-589i
Adrenal insufficiency, 587
  assessment findings in, 602t
Adrenal medulla, 588-589i
Adrenocorticotropic hormone, 588i
Adverse drug reactions
  breast disorders and, 340t
  cardiovascular disorders and, 299t
  ear disorders and, 234t
  endocrine disorders and, 594-595t
  eye disorders and, 214-215t
  female reproductive disorders and, 421-422t
  gastrointestinal disorders and, 361-362t
  head trauma and, 189-190t
  immune disorders and, 562-563t
  male reproductive disorders and, 449t
  musculoskeletal disorders and, 519t
  nervous system disorders and, 473-474t
  nutritional disorders and, 130t
  respiratory disorders and, 257-258t
  urinary disorder and, 394-395t
Affect, 35
Affective function, family assessment of, 62
Affective skills
  care plan for, 16
  nursing process and, 3
Afterload, cardiac, 283
Age
  activities of daily living and, 105
  cardiac risk and, 294
  sleep patterns and, 112, 113
  vital signs and, 95t, 100
Agglutination, 548
Agranulocyte, 548, 558
  hematopoiesis and, 551
AIDS. *See* Acquired immunodeficiency syndrome.
Air pressure, differences in, respiration and, 251i
Airways, respiratory, 245, 246i
Albinism
  in dark-skinned client, 7PG
  in light-skinned client, 7PG
Albumin, urinary disorders and, 406t
Albuminuria, 386
Alcohol, sleep patterns and, 113
Aldosterone, 386
  kidneys and, 391
  source of, 589i
Alimentary canal, 354, 356-357i
Alkaline phosphatase
  gastrointestinal disorders and, 380t
  musculoskeletal disorders and, 544t
Alopecia, 154, 171
Alpha cells, pancreatic, 589i
Alpha-fetoprotein
  gastrointestinal disorders and, 380t
  male reproductive disorders and, 459t
Alveoli
  breast, 337i, 338
  lung, 246i, 249i
Alveolus, 34PG
Amblyopia, 207, 219
American Medical Association
  founding of, 25
  Sheppard-Towner Act and, 26
American Nurses' Association
  collaborative concerns of, 29-30
  nursing code of, 29
  nursing definition of, 23
Amines, 587, 590
Amino acids, 124
  protein metabolism and, 126
Amphiarthrodial joints, 515
Amylase, gastrointestinal disorders and, 380t
Anabolism, 124, 125
Anal canal, 357i
Anal reflex, 498i
Anatomic lines, 36PG-37PG
Androgens, 443
Anemia, 548, 555
Aneurysm, aortic, 296t
Angina, 283
  assessment findings in, 321t
  chest pain in, 296t
Angle of Louis, 45PG, 244, 246i
Anhidrosis, 154, 170
Ankle-jerk reflex, assessment of, 499i
Ankles, assessment of, 535i, 537
Ankylosing spondylitis, assessment findings in, 200t, 540t
Ankylosis, 511
Anorexia nervosa, 124
  assessment findings in, 141t
Anosmia, 463, 486
Anovulation, 414
Anthropometric measurements, 101
  for nutritional disorders, 137, 142-144, 142i, 143i
Antibody, 548
Antidiuretic hormone, 386
  kidneys and, 387, 391
  storage site for, 588i
Antigen, 548
  carcinoembryonic, 380t
Antigen-antibody complex, 555
Antiglobulin test, 581t
Anthelix, 30PG, 232i
Antitragus, 30PG
Anus, imperforate
  assessment findings in, 371t
  neonatal, inspection of, 110PG
Anxiety, 35
  stress vs., 54
Aorta, 44PG, 285

i refers to an illustration; t, to a table; PG, to Photo Gallery (a photograph)

Aortic valve, 284, 287i
Aphasia, 463
Apical impulse, 309, 311
Apnea
  respiratory pattern for, 98i
  sleep, 105, 115
Apneusis, respiratory pattern for, 98i
Apocrine glands, 158i
Appendicitis, 659-660
Appendix, 60PG, 93PG, 356i, 553i
Aqueous humor, 207, 210i
Arachnoid, 470
Arciform, 154
Arcus senilis, 25PG, 225
Areflexia, 463
Areola mammae, 55PG, 335, 336i
Arm measurements, 143i
Arm strength, assessment of, 490, 491i, 529i
Arrector pili muscle, 1PGi, 156i, 158i
Arteries, 44PG, 67PG, 289i
  auscultation of, 14PG, 319
  blood analysis of, 279t
  blood flow in, 307
  obstruction of, 53PG
  pulse in, 96, 69i
Arterioles, 249i, 289i
Arthritis, assessment findings in, 200t
Articular cartilage, 514i
Ascending colon, 60PG, 356i, 357i
Ascites, 355, 369, 370
  urinary disorders and, 400
Assessment. *See also specific body systems.*
  complete, 611-633
  data collection for, 6-7
  neonatal, 105PG-106PG
  nursing process and, 5-7
  partial, 633-634
  perinatal, 107PG-112PG
  types of, 5-6
Assimilation, 35
Asthma, assessment findings in, 272t
Astigmatism, 207
Ataxia, 463
Atherosclerosis, 283
Atony, 511
Atria, 284, 287i
Atrial gallop, 283, 324i
  auscultation of, 324
  implications of, 320t
Atrioventricular node, 290, 290i
Atrioventricular valves, 284, 287i
Atrophy, 172i, 511
Auditory screening, 235
Auricle, 30PG, 230, 232i
Auscultation, 72, 86
  abdominal, 62PG, 367i
  arterial, 14PG, 319i
  bowel sounds, 62PG
  breath sounds, 42PG-43PG
Auscultation *(continued)*
  cardiac, 50PG-52PG, 316-319, 318i
    client positioning for, 50PG, 317i
  endocrine assessment and, 103PG, 601
  gastrointestinal, 62PG, 367-368
  head assessment and, 14PG, 193
  heart sounds and, 316-319, 320t, 323-326, 328
  in prenatal assessment, 106PG
  respiratory, 43PG, 269-270, 274i
  thorax, 41PG-42PG
  urinary, 401
  vascular sounds, 2PG
Auscultatory gap, 100
Autoimmunity, 548
Autonomic nervous system, 467i
Axillae
  lymph nodes of, 94PG, 552i
  temperature of, 94
Axon, 468i

B

Babinski
  reflex, assessment of, 112PG
  sign, 500i
Balance, assessment of, 81PG
Ballottement, 72, 84i
Barrel chest, 262, 253i
  cardiovascular disorders and, 309
Bartholin's glands, 71PG, 416i
Basal cell, epidermal, 1PGi, 156i
Basal metabolic rate, 125
Basement membrane, 157i
Basophils, 548, 551, 557-558
B cells, 548
B_1 deficiency, assessment findings in, 141t
Beau's lines, 171
Behavioral considerations, health history and, 38
Bence Jones proteins, musculoskeletal disorders and 545t
Benzene, 565t
Beta cells, pancreatic, 589i
Beverages, caffeine content of, 131t
Biceps brachii muscle, 86PG, 512i
Biceps femoris muscle, 512i
Biceps reflex, 84PG, 498i
Bicep strength, assessment of, 529i
Bile, 358
Bile ducts, 357i
Bilirubin, gastrointestinal disorders and, 380t, 381t
Bimanual palpation, 84i
  female genitalia and, 433-436i
Biographic data, 36, 44-45
Biological rhythms, 105, 107
Biot's respirations, 98i
Birthmark, 2PG
Blackhead (comedo), 170, 172i
Bladder, 67PG, 388i, 389i
  palpation of, 70PG, 403i
  percussion of, 69PG, 402i
Blanching, 167
Bleeding, breakthrough, 414
Blood. *See also* Immune system.
  clotting of, 556-557
  formed elements in, 555-558
  hematopoiesis and, 551
Blood cells
  development of, 550-551
  immune disorders and, 577-579t
Blood groups, compatibility of, 555
Blood pressure, 72, 98, 99i, 100-101
  cardiovascular disorders and, 306
  immune disorders and, 567
  diastolic, 98, 100
  factors affecting, 100
  measurement of, 98
  neurologic dysfunction and, 502
  normal ranges for, 100-101
  systolic, 98, 100
Blood pressure cuff, 73, 76
Blood smear, immune disorders and, 577t
Blood tests
  for endocrine disorders, 604-605t
  for gastrointestinal disorders, 380-381t
  for immune disorders, 577-581t
  for male reproductive disorders, 459t
  for musculoskeletal disorders, 544t
  for nervous system disorders, 503t
  for nutritional status, 145-146t
  for respiratory disorders, 279t
  for urinary disorders, 406-407t
Blood urea nitrogen (BUN), urinary disorders and, 406t
B lymphocytes, 548
Body hair distribution, 2PG
Body image, 35
Body language, 37
Body movements, 516i
Body position, urinary disorders and, 398
Body temperature, 94-95
Body weight. *See* Weight.
Bone, types of, 514i
Bone conduction, hearing pathway and, 232i, 233i
Bone marrow, 93PG, 514i, 552i, 553i
  aspiration of, 576t
  hematopoiesis and, 550
  immune disorders and, 576t
Bones
  anatomy of, 514i
  classification of, 511, 513
  formation of, 513, 515
    endocrine system and, 513
  function of, 513

i refers to an illustration; t, to a table; PG, to Photo Gallery (a photograph)

Borborygmi, 355
Bowel sounds, 368t
  auscultation of, 62PG
Bowlegs, 523
Bowman's capsule, 388i, 390i
Brachioradialis muscle, 86PG, 412i
Brachioradialis reflex, 85PG, 499i
Bradycardia, 72
Bradypnea, 72, 98i
Brain, 464-465i
Brain tumor, assessment findings in, 484t
Brain stem, 76PG, 464i, 465i
Breast disorders
  adolescents and, 348
  adverse drug reactions and, 340t
  assessment findings in, 349t
  child with, 341, 348
  documentation of 349, 351t
  eczema-like nipple changes, 59PG
  elderly client and, 341, 348
  health history of, 338-343
  lactation and, 348
  locations of, 352i
  nursing process for, 350-351t
  nursing research on, 353
  physical assessment of, 343-348
  pregnancy and, 341, 348
Breast-feeding, nutritional status for, 132
Breasts
  abnormalities of, 59PG
  anatomy of, 55PG, 336-337i
  assessment of, 57PG-58PG, 338-348
    after childbirth, 643
    pregnant client and, 105PG, 639
  asymmetrical, 59PG
  cancer of, assessment findings in, 349t
  ducts, 55PG
  inspection of, 57PG
  lactation and, 335, 338
  lesions of, 348
  lymphatic drainage of, 337i
  palpation of, 58PG
  pregnancy and, 335
  puberty and, 335, 338i
  quadrants of, 56PG
  self-examination of, 342i
Breathing, mechanics of, 248, 250-251i
Breath odor, implications of, 199
Breath sounds
  abnormal, 269, 271t
  adventitious, 270, 271t
  locations of, 42PG
  normal, 269, 270i
Bronchi, 34PG, 245, 246i, 248
Bronchial sounds, 43PG, 269, 270i
Bronchioles, 34PG, 246i, 248
Bronchitis, 656
  assessment findings in, 272t
Bronchophony, 244
Bronchovesicular sounds, 43PG, 269, 270i
Brown, Esther, 23
Bruit, 283, 319
Bruxism, 105, 115
Buddhism, beliefs of, 60
Buffalo hump, 104PG
Bulbocavernous reflex, 498i
Bulimia, 124
  assessment findings in, 141t
Bulla, 172t
Bundle branches, 290, 290i
Bundle of His, 290, 290i
Bursae, 515
Butler, Robert, developmental theory of,52t

C

Caffeine
  beverages containing, 131t
  sleep patterns and, 113
  intake of, 129
Calcium levels, musculoskeletal disorders and, 545t
Calculus, 386
Calorics test, cold, 491i
Calorie, 124
Calorimetry, 125
Canaliculi, 514i
Canal of Schlemm, 210i
Candidiasis, assessment findings in, 429t
Canthus, 16PG, 208i
Capillaries, 289i
Capillary hemangioma, 107PG
Capillary refill, 175
  assessment of, 4PG
  cardiovascular disorders and, 308
Carbohydrate metabolism, 126
Cardiac auscultation, positions for, 50PG
Cardiac cachexia, assessment of, 306
Cardiac circulation, 285, 288-289i
Cardiac conduction system, 285, 290i
Cardiac cycle, 290, 292, 292i
Cardiac landmarks, 45PG
Cardiac output, 283, 649-652
Cardiac structures, 284-285, 286-287i
Cardiac veins, 291i
Cardinal positions of gaze test, 18PG-19PG
Cardiomyopathies, assessment findings in, 322t
Cardiovascular system
  abnormalities of, 53PG-54PG,
  anatomy of, 44PG, 284, 286-287i
  assessment of, 45PG-52PG, 293, 295, 298, 300-320, 323-325, 328
    immune disorders and, 568
    pregnant client and, 639
Cardiovascular system *(continued)*
  disorders of
    adverse drug reactions and, 299t
    assessment findings in, 321-322t
    child with, 292, 319-320
    documentation of, 327t, 328, 330
    elderly client and, 293, 320, 323
    health history of, 293, 295, 298, 300-305
    laboratory studies for, 329t
    nursing process for, 326-327t
    nursing research on, 333
    physical assessment of, 305-320, 323-325, 328
    pregnancy and, 292-293, 320
    prevalence of, 282
    risk factors and, 294-295
    sex-specific questions for, 300
    pregnant client and, 639
  physiology of, 284-285, 288-289i, 290, 291-292, 292i
Care plans, nursing, 15-17
Carina, 246i
Caring, 21
Carotid arteries, 10PG, 44PG
  auscultation of, 52PG
Carotid pulse
  assessment of, 96, 312i
  location of, 96i
Carpals, 86PG
Carpal tunnel syndrome, assessment findings in, 540t
Cartilage, 515
Caruncle, 16PG, 208i, 209i
Catabolism, 124, 125
Cataract, 207, 222
  assessment findings in, 223t
Catecholamines, 587
  endocrine disorders and, 604t
Cecum, 60PG, 356i, 357i
Cell-mediated immunity, 548, 555
Cell metabolism, 125-128
Cellulitis, periorbital, 223
Centigrade, conversion of, 94
Central nervous system (CNS), 464-465i
  assessment of, 77PG-85PG
  structures of, 76PG
Cerebellar function, 80PG-81PG
Cerebellum, 76PG
  assessment of, 80PG-81PG, 492, 493-494i
Cerebrum, 76PG
  assessment of, 478-483, 486
Cerebrospinal fluid, 470
  neurologic disorders and, 504t
Cerebrovascular accident (CVA), assessment findings in, 484t
Cervical spine, assessment of, 88PG, 90PG, 525, 526-527i

i refers to an illustration; t, to a table; PG, to Photo Gallery (a photograph)

Cervix, 71PG, 417i
 cancer of, 432
 developmental changes in, 418i
 ectropion of, 414, 428-429
 lymph nodes of, 184i, 552i
Chadwick's sign, 431i
Chancre, 75PG
Cheilitis, 183
Cheilosis, 183
Chemical dot thermometer, 73, 74i, 94
Chemotaxis, 548, 557i
Cherry angioma, 170
Chest. *See also* Thorax.
 assessment of, 38PG, 262, 264-265, 265i, 267, 268i, 269-270
  endocrine disorder and, 598, 600
  neonatal, 108PG, 644
 circumference of, 108PG, 142i
 contours of, age-group and, 253i
 deformities of, 262, 263i
  cardiovascular disorders and, 309
 pain in, 296-297t
Cheyne-Stokes respirations, 98i
 cardiovascular disorders and, 307
Chloasma, 105PG, 637
Choanae, 183, 184i
Cholecystitis, assessment findings in, 372t
Cholesterol, 127-128
 gastrointestinal disorders and, 380t
Choroid, 210i
Christianity, beliefs of, 60
Chronic obstructive pulmonary disease (COPD), 656-658
Chvostek's sign, 601
Chylomicrons, 124, 127
Chyme, 124, 355, 358
Cigarette smoking, cardiac disease and, 294
Ciliary body, 210i
Circadian rhythm, 107
Circulatory system, 285, 288-289i
Circumcision, 443
Circumduction, 516i
Cirrhosis, assessment findings in, 372t
Clarification, as interviewing technique, 35, 40
Clavicles, 86PG, 184i
 assessment of, 525
Claw toe, 541
Client goals, 13-15
Client records, 28t
Client health beliefs, assessment of, 57
Client expectations, health history and, 38
Climacteric, 414, 415
 reproductive assessment of, 424-425
Clitoris, 71PG, 416i
Clubbing, 244, 261i
Clustering, client assessment and, 10
Coagulation, 556-557
Coccyx, 87PG
Cochlea, 232i, 233i
Cognition, 35
 developmental theories on, 48, 51, 52t
Cognitive abilities, assessment of, 48, 51
Cognitive function, 105
 effect of, activities of daily living and, 106
Cognitive skills
 care plan for, 16
 nursing process and, 3
Collaboration, 21, 27-31
 American Nurses' Association on, 29-30
 health care, 20-31
 National Joint Practice Commission on, 27, 28t
 nursing process for, 30-31
 problems with, 30-31
 strategies for, 27-29
Collagen, 157i
Collecting tubule, 388i, 390i
Colon, 60PG, 356i, 357i
Color blindness, 217
Color perception, testing of, 217
Colostrum, 335
Comedo, 170, 172i
Comfort, altered, pediatric client with, 659-661
Commands, response to, 490
Communication
 collaborative strategy for, 27-28
 nurse-client, 37-39
Complete assessment, 611-633
 documentation of, 613, 632-633
 health history in, 611-612
 physical assessment in, 612-613, 614-632t
Concha, 30PG, 232i
Condylomata acuminata, 432
Confucianism, beliefs of, 60
Conjunctivae, 208i, 209i
 assessment of, 21PG, 221i
 inflamed, 27PG
Conjunctivitis, 222
 assessment findings in, 223t
 bulbar, 208i, 209i
  assessment of, 221i
Consensual reaction, 207
Consensual validation, 40
Constipation, 355
Contraceptives, cardiac disease and, 295
Contractility, 283
Coombs' test, 581t
Coordination
 assessment of, 80PG, 494, 493-494i
 neuromuscular integrity and, 523
COPD. *See* Chronic obstructive pulmonary disease.
Coping strategies, 54
Corium, 156i, 157i
Cornea, 210i
 assessment of, 21PG, 221
Corneal abrasions, 28PG, 222
 assessment findings in, 223t
Corneal light reflex, test for, 17PG, 217, 219i
Corneal reflex
 asymmetrical, 26PG
 test for, 21PG
Corona, 73PG, 444i, 445i
Coronary circulation, 285, 291i
Cor pulmonale, 657
Corpus callosum, 76PG
Corpus cavernosum, 73PG, 444i
Corpus luteum, cysts of, 429t
Corpus spongiosum, 73PG, 444i
Corrigan's pulse, 283, 314i
Cortical, 463
Corticosterone, 589i
Corticotropin, source of, 588i
Cortisol
 endocrine disorders and, 604t
 source of, 589i
Cortisone, 589i
Costal angle, 244, 262
 assessment of, 264
Cover-uncover test, 17PG, 217, 219i
Crackles, 244, 271t
Cranial bones, 186i
Cranial nerves, 466i
 assessment of, 77PG-80PG, 486, 488-489t, 490
Craniosacral system, 467i
Cranium, sutures in, 183, 186i
Creatine phosphokinase
 musculoskeletal disorders and, 545t
 cardiovascular disorders and, 329t
Creatinine, urinary disorders and, 406t
Cremasteric reflex, 498i
Crepitus, 266, 511
Cretinism, 587
Cricoid cartilage, 10PG, 34PG, 102PG, 184i, 185i
Crohn's disease, assessment findings in, 372t
Crust, 172i
Cryptorchidism, 443, 445
Cultural considerations
 health history and, 38-39
 neurologic assessment and, 481, 486
Cultural identity, assessment of, 57-58
Cultural influences, assessment of, 57-58
 activities of daily living and, 105-106
Cultural relativism, 35
Culture specimens, female reproductive assessment and, 437t
Cumming, Elaine, developmental theory of, 52t
Cushing's syndrome, 587
 assessment findings in, 104PG, 603t
 facial characteristics in, 193
Cutaneous reflexes, 495, 498i, 500i
Cuticles, 1PGi, 158i
Cyanosis, 260, 657
 cardiovascular disorders and, 307
 peripheral, 54PG

i refers to an illustration; t, to a table; PG, to Photo Gallery (a photograph)

Cyst, 172i
Cystic adenosis, assessment findings in, 349t
Cystic mastitis, assessment findings in, 349t
Cystitis, assessment findings in, 404t
Cystocele, 414
Cytoplasm, 513i

D

Data collection, 6-7
  health history and, 44-65
Deafness. *See* Hearing loss.
Decerebrate positioning, 463
Decorticate positioning, 463
Deep tendon reflexes, assessment of, 84PG
Defense mechanisms, 54
Defensive responses, 41
Deglutition, 355
Delta cells, pancreatic, 589i
Delta sleep, 112
Deltoid muscle, 87PG, 512i
  assessing strength of, 529i
Demarcation, 154
Dementia, 463
Dendrites, 468i
Dependent intervention, 16
Dermal papilla, 156i, 157i
Dermatome, 154, 155, 467i
Dermis, 1PGi, 156i, 157i
Descending colon, 356i, 357i
Development, definition of, 35
Developmental considerations
  activities of daily living and, 105
  for breast assessment, 341, 348
  for cardiovascular assessment, 292-293, 319-320, 323
  for ear assessment, 33PG, 233-234, 236
  for eliciting abdominal pain, 377
  for endocrine assessment, 596, 601, 603
  for eye assessment, 25PG, 213, 215, 224-225
  for female reproductive assessment, 423-425, 428
  for gastrointestinal assessment, 363-364, 370, 373-374, 377
  for head and neck assessment, 14PG, 188, 190, 200-201
  for immune assessment, 558, 564-565, 573
  for male reproductive assessment, 450, 457-458
  for musculoskeletal assessment, 91PG, 520, 523, 541
  for neurologic assessment, 475-476, 481, 486, 487, 490, 492, 495, 497, 501
  for nutritional assessment, 129, 131-133, 142, 144
  for respiratory assessment, 253-254, 256, 258, 270-271, 273, 274i, 275
  for skin assessment, 5PG-6PG, 155, 157, 160-164, 175, 177
  for sleep pattern assessment, 120
  health history and, 47-48, 51
Diabetes insipidus, 587
Diabetes mellitus, 587
  assessment findings in, 602t
  risk of, cardiac disease and, 294
Diagnoses
  medical vs. nursing, 7, 12, 24
  nursing. *See* Nursing diagnoses.
Diapedesis, 548
Diaphonography. *See* Transillumination.
Diaphragmatic excursion, 244
  measurement of, 275, 278
  percussion to assess, 41PG
Diaphysis, 514i
Diarrhea, 355
Diarthroidal joints, 515
Diastasis recti, 355, 373
Diastole, 292i
Diencephalon, 464i, 465i
Diet, sleep patterns and, 113
Dietary history, 133, 136
Diet, cardiac disease and, 294
Differentiation, definition of, 548
Diffuse, definition of, 154
Diffusion, 252-253
Digestion, 125, 355, 358
Diopter, 72, 77
Diplopia, 207
Disabled client
  considerations for, 92
  health history and, 65
  physical assessment of, 90
Disorientation, 463
Distress, signs of, 90
Diverticulitis, assessment findings in, 372t
Documentation, 6-7
  activities of daily living, 110
  breast assessment, 349, 351t, 352
  cardiovascular assessment, 327t, 328, 330
  complete assessment, 613, 632-633
  ear assessment, 240
  endocrine assessment, 603, 605, 607t, 608
  eye assessment, 229t, 230
  female reproductive assessment, 436-437, 439t, 440
  gastrointestinal assessment, 377, 379t, 382
  general survey, 93
  hair assessment, 177, 179t, 180
  head and neck assessment, 201-204
  health history, 66-68
  immune assessment, 575, 581, 583t, 584
  male reproductive assessment, 455t, 460
  musculoskeletal assessment, 541, 543t, 545
  neonatal assessment, 646
  neurologic assessment, 501, 502, 504-505, 507t
  nutritional assessment, 139t, 144, 146
  partial assessment, 634
Documentation *(continued)*
  postpartum assessment, 643
  prenatal assessment, 641
  pulse amplitude, 97
  respiratory assessment, 277t, 278, 280
  skin assessment, 177, 179t, 180
  sleep assessment, 119t, 120
  SOAPIE method of, 66
  urinary assessment, 405, 409, 411t
  vital signs, 101
Doll's eyes reflex, 491i
Dorsal horn of spinal cord, 464i, 465i
Dorsalis pedis pulse, 96i
  palpation of, 313i
Dorsiflexion, 511
Draping, physical assessment and, 88i
Drawer test, 539i
Dreaming, 105, 111, 112
Dress, observation of, general survey and, 91
Drugs. *See specific drug names.*
  adverse reactions to. *See* Adverse drug reactions.
Dullness, as percussion sound, 83, 86t, 269
Duodenum, 60PG
Dupuytren's contractures, 600
Dura mater, 470
Duvall, Evelyn, developmental theory of, 52t
Dysesthesia, 463
Dysmenorrhea, 414
Dyspareunia, 414
Dyspepsia, 355
Dysphagia, 355
Dyspnea, 244, 295, 656
  paroxysmal noctural, 651, 656

E

Ear
  abnormalites of, 33PG
  anatomy of, 30PG, 230, 232-233i
  assessment of, 231, 233-236, 239-240, 619-620t
    immune disorders and, 568
  disorders of
    adverse drug reactions and, 234t
    assessment findings in, 237t
    bulging tympanic membrane, 33PG
    canal drainage, 33PG
    child with, 233-234, 236
    ethnic considerations for, 236, 239
    documentation of, 240
    elderly client and, 234, 236
    health history of, 231, 233-235
  external, 232i
  inner, 233i
  middle, 232-233i
  physical assessment of, 235-236, 239-240
  physiology of, 230-231
Eardrum, 230, 232i, 233i

Ecchymosis, 154, 170, 548
Eccrine glands, 156i, 158i
Economic means, family assessment of, 62
Ectropion, 26PG, 222
Eczema, 154
Edema
  cardiovascular disorders and, 307-308, 650, 652
  COPD and, 657
  nonpitting, signs of, 400
  pitting, evaluation of, 54PG, 399i
  types of, 400
Effusion, 511
Egophony, 244, 278
Ejaculation, 443
Ejaculatory duct, 73PG, 444i
Elastance, 244
Elastic cartilage, 515
Elastin, 157i
Elbows, assessment of, 529i, 537
Elderly client
  cardiovascular assessment of, 293, 320, 323
  ear assessment of, 234, 236
  endocrine assessment of, 603
  eye assessment of, 215, 224-225
  female reproductive assessment of, 428
  gastrointestinal assessment of, 364, 373-374, 377
  general survey considerations for, 92
  head and neck assessment of, 188, 190, 201
  health history for, 65
  immune assessment of, 558, 564-565, 573
  male reproductive assessment of, 450, 458
  musculoskeletal assessment of, 520, 523, 541
  nail changes in, 157
  neurologic assessment of, 476, 481, 490, 492, 495, 497, 501
  nutritional assessment of, 132-133, 144
  physical assessment for, 89
  respiratory assessment of, 254, 258, 273-274
  skin assessment of, 163-164
  skin changes in, 157
  urinary assessment of, 396, 405
Electrolyte levels
  gastrointestinal disorders and, 380-381t
  neurologic disorders and, 503t
  urinary disorders and, 406-407t
Elimination, 358
Emotional factors, sleep patterns and, 114
Emotional status, assessment of, 63
Empathy, nurse-client communication, 37
Empedocles, 25
Emphysema, 656
  assessment findings in, 272t
Encopresis, 355
Endocarditis, assessment findings in, 322t
Endocardium, 286i
Endochondral ossification, 513
Endocrine glands, 588-589i
Endocrine system
  abnormalities of, 104PG
  anatomy of, 101PG-102PG, 586-587, 588-589i
  assessment of, 102PG-103PG, 592-593, 595-601, 603
  disorders of
    adverse drug reactions and, 594-595t
    assessment findings in, 602-603t
    child with, 596
    documentation of, 603, 605, 607t, 608
    elderly client with, 603
    health history of, 592-593, 595-597
    laboratory studies for, 604-605t
    nursing process for, 606-607t
    nursing research on, 609
    physical assessment of, 597-601, 603
    pregnant client with, 596
  dysfunction of, 592
  physiology of, 588-589i, 590-592, 591i
Endogenous, 154
Endometriosis, assessment findings in, 429t
Endometrium, 71PG, 416i, 417i
  cancer of, assessment findings in, 429t
Endosteum, 514i
Energy, 124, 125
Enterocele, 414
Entropion, 26PG, 222
Enuresis, 105, 115, 386
Environmental factors
  health assessment of, 55
  sleep patterns and, 113-114
Enzyme-linked immunosorbent assay (ELISA), 581t
Eosinophils, 548, 551, 557
Epicanthal folds, 24PG, 192, 225
Epicardium, 286i, 287i
Epichlorohydrin, 565t
Epidermis, 1PGi, 155, 156-157i
Epididymis, 73PG, 444-445i
Epiglottis, 34PG, 246i
Epiglottitis, assessment findings in, 273t
Epimysium, 513i
Epinephrine, 588i
Epiphyses, 514i
Epispadias, 443
Erb's point, 45PG
Erection, 443
Erikson, Erik, developmental theories of, 52t
Erosion, 173i
Erythema, 170
Erythema toxicum neonatorum, 176i
Erythrocytes, 548, 551, 555
  immune disorders and, 579t
Erythrocyte sedimentation rate, 579t
Esophagus, 34PG, 60PG, 356i, 357i
  disorders of, chest pain and, 297t
Esophoria, 219
Esotropia, 207, 219
Estradiol, 589i
Estrogens, 589i
Estrone, 589i
Ethics, professional, 1
Ethmoidal sinuses, 194i
Ethnic considerations, health history and, 38-39
Ethnicity, 35
Ethnocentrism, 35
Ethylene oxide, 565t
Eupnea, 244
  respiratory pattern in, 98i
Eustachian tube, 232i, 233i
  assessment findings in, 237t
Eversion, 516i
Exanthem, 154
Excretion, 125
Exercise
  assessment of, 53
  sleep patterns and, 113
Exophoria, 219
Exophthalmos, 104PG 207
Exotropia, 207, 219
Extension, 511, 516i
Extraocular muscles, 208i, 209i
  assessment of, 17PG-19PG, 217, 218, 219i
Extraocular nerves, 209
Extrapyramidal tract, 469i
Extremities
  assessment of, 626-627t
    endocrine disorders and, 599, 600
    neonatal, 109PG, 643, 645, 645i
  measurement of, 89PG, 525
Extrusion reflex, assessment of, 111PG
Exudates
  hard, 29PG
  soft, 29PG
Eye
  abnormalities of, 26PG-29PG
  anatomy of, 16PG, 207, 208-209i, 209
  assessment of, 211-213, 215-227, 230
    anterior chamber, 22PG
  cardiovascular disorders and, 308
  developmental considerations, 25PG
  disorders of, adverse drug reactions and, 214-215t
    assessment findings in, 223t
    child with, 213, 215, 224
    documentation of assessment data for, 229t, 230
    elderly client with, 215, 224-225
    ethnic considerations for, 225
    health history of, 211-213, 215-216

i refers to an illustration; t, to a table; PG, to Photo Gallery (a photograph)

Eye *(continued)*
nursing process for, 228-229t
physical assessment of, 216-227, 230, 618-619t
ethnic considerations, 24PG
immune disorders and, 568
lens of, 210i
opacities in, 29PG
nutritional disorders and, 137
urinary disorders and, 398-399
Eye charts, 76
Eyelid, 16PG, 208i, 209i
assessment of, 220
glands, 27PG
nodule, 27PG

F

Face
anatomy of, 183
assessment of, 12PG, 191-193, 616-617t
characteristics of, health factors and, 90
hyperpigmentation of, 155, 157
muscles of, 86PG, 512i
assessment of, 192
nerves of, 466i, 487
assessment of, 78PG, 488-489t, 490
Fahrenheit degrees, conversion of, 94
Fallopian tubes, 71PG, 416i, 417i
Family
functions of, 58
assessment of, 47, 62
role patterns in, 59
Family responsibilities, assessment of, 108
Fasciculation, 511
Fat
emulsification of, 355
metabolism of, 126, 128
Feces, occult blood test for, 382t
Feedback mechanism, 587
Female reproductive system
abnormalities of, 72PG
anatomy of, 71PG, 414, 416-417i
assessment of, 418-420, 422-436, 631-632t
disorders of
adolescents and, 423-424, 428
adverse drug reactions and, 421-422t
assessment findings in, 429t
assessment of, 436-437, 439t, 440
child with, 423, 428
climacteric and, 424-425
elderly client and, 428
health history of, 418-420, 422-425
nursing process for, 438-439t
nursing research on, 441
physical assessment of, 425, 436
Femoral hernia, 455
palpation for, 456i
Femoral pulse
assessment of, 96, 312i
location of, 96i
Femur, 86PG, 514i
Fenestra ovalis, 232i
Fenestra rotunda, 232i, 233i
Fibrinogen degradation products, immune disorders and, 581t
Fibrin split products, immune disorders and, 581t
Fibroadenoma, breast, assessment of, 349t
Fibrocystic disease, assessment of, 349
Fibrous septa, 55PG
Fibula, 87PG, 514i
Fimbria, 71PG
Fingernails
color and attachment of, 3PG
consistency of, 3PG
inspection of, 37PG
Fingers
assessment of, 537
clubbing of, 171, 261i
immune disorders and, 567
Fissure, 173i
Fist percussion, 374
Flail chest, 264
Flatus, 355
Flexion, 511, 516i
Fluid loss, insensible, 386
Fluid status
skin turgor and, 166
urinary disorders and, 398
Fluid wave test, 64PG
Follicle cysts, assessment findings in, 429t
Follicle-stimulating hormone, 588i
Fontanels, 183, 186i
assessment of, 200-201
palpation of, 110PG
Food groups, 133
Foot
abnormalities of, 92PG
assessment of, 535i
Foreskin, 444-445i
Fovea centralis, 211i
Freckles, 2PG
Frenulum, 183, 184-185i
Freud, Sigmund, developmental theories of, 52t
Friction rub, 368t
Frontal lobes, 76PG, 464i
Frontal sinus, 10PG, 184i, 194i
Functional health patterns
health history and, 34
nursing diagnoses and, 25
Fundus, assessment of
after childbirth, 643i
palpation of, 106PG
in pregnant client, 640i
Funnel chest, 262, 263i
cardiovascular disorders and, 309
Futcher's line, 173

G

Gag reflex, 498i
Gait, 89PG, 522-523, 524-525i
Gallbladder, 60PG, 356i, 357i, 359
Gamma glutamyl transpeptidase, 381t
Ganglia, 467i, 469i
Gas exchange
impaired, 656-658
mechanism of, 249i
Gastric dysfunction, chest pain and, 297t
Gastritis, assessment findings in, 371t
Gastrocnemius muscle, 87PG, 512i
Gastrointestinal system
abnormalities of, 66PG
accessory organs of, 356i, 357i, 358-359
anatomy of, 354-355, 356-357i, 60PG
assessment of, 62PG-65PG, 359-360, 362-370, 373-377
disorders of
adverse drug reactions and, 361-362t
assessment findings in, 371-372t
assessment of, 377, 379t, 382
elderly client and, 364, 373-374
health history of, 359-360, 362-365
immune, 568-569
laboratory studies for, 380-382t
nursing process for, 378-379t
nursing research on, 384
physical assessment of, 365-370, 373-377
pregnant client and, 364, 373
physiology of, 355, 358-359
General survey, 90-93
body types and, 90-91
child and, 92
cultural considerations for, 92-93
disabilities and, 92
distress in, signs of, 90
documentation of, 93
elderly client and, 92
facial characteristics in, 90
grooming and, 91
posture and, 91
psychological state and, 91-92
Genitalia
endocrine disorders and, 598, 600
female, 416-417i
neonatal, 110PG, 645
Genogram, 35, 47, 48i
Genu valgum, 523
Genu varum, 523
Gilligan, Carol, developmental theories of, 52t
Gingivae, 11PG, 183, 185i
recession of, 14PG
Gingivitis, 183
assessment findings in, 200t
signs of, 199
Glans penis, 73PG, 444i
Glasgow Coma Scale, 480t
Glaucoma, 207, 219, 226
assessment findings in, 223t

i refers to an illustration; t, to a table; PG, to Photo Gallery (a photograph)

Glial cells, 470
Glomerular filtrates, 386
Glomerulonephritis, assessment findings in, 404t
Glomerulus, 388i, 390i
Glossitis, 15PG
  assessment findings in, 200t
Glossopharyngeal nerve, 466i, 487
  assessment of, 79PG, 489t
Glottis, 246i
Glucagon, 589i
Glucocorticoids, 589i
Glucose tolerance test, 604t
Gluteal folds, 109PG
Gluteus maximus, 87PG, 512i
  neonatal, 109PG
Glycerides, 127
Glycogenesis, 124
Glycogenolysis, 124
Goiter, 104PG, 587
Gonadotropin, 445, 447i
  endocrine disorders and, 605t
  test for, 437, 440
Gonads, 588i, 589i
Goniometer, 81i, 511
Gonorrhea, assessment findings in, 457t
Gout
  cardiac disease and, 295
  deformities from, 92PG
Granulocyte, 548, 557-558
  hematopoiesis and, 551
Grasp reflex, 85PG, 499i
Graves speculum, 426
Gravida, 414
Gray matter, 464i, 465i
Grooming, observation of, 91
Growth hormone, 588i
Guarding, 91
Guillain-Barré syndrome, assessment findings in, 484t
Gurgles (rhonchi), 245, 271t, 658
Gynecologic assessment
  bimanual palpation in, 433-436i
  equipment for, 426
  guidelines for, 426-427
Gynecomastia, 59PG, 335, 348

H

Hair. *See also* Skin.
  anatomy of, 1PGi, 156i, 158i
  assessment of, 2PG, 167, 173, 615t
    cardiovascular disorders and, 308
    endocrine disorders and, 598, 599
    immune disorders and, 567
    neonatal, 107PG, 644
  growth of, 158i
  loss of, 154, 171
Hallux malleous, 92PG
Hallux valgus, 92PG, 541
Hammer toe, 541
Hands
  assessment of, 530i, 614t
Hard palate, 185i
  assessment of, 196
Harvey, William, 25
Haversian canals, 514i
Havighurst, Robert, developmental theories of, 52t
Head. *See also* Neck.
  abnormalities of, 15PG
  anatomy of, 10PG, 183, 184-185i
  assessment of, 12PG, 615-620t
    endocrine disorders and, 598, 599
    immune disorders and, 567-568
    neonatal, 107PG, 644
  circumference of, 142i, 14PG
  common abnormalities, 15PG
  developmental considerations, 14PG
  physical assessment of, 191-201
Head disorders, 187-190
  adverse drug reactions and, 189-190t
  child with, 188
  documentation of, 201-204
  nursing process for, 202-203t
  pregnant client with, 201
Head molding, 107PG
Head trauma
  adverse drug reactions and, 189-190t
  assessment findings in, 200t
  assessment of, 201-204
  child with, 188, 200-201
  elderly client with, 188, 190, 201
  health history for, 187-188, 190-191
  physical assessment of, 191-199
  pregnant client with, 201
Health beliefs, 51-52
Health history, 34-70, 611-612, 633
  child and, 63-64
  disabled client and, 65
  documentation of, 66-68
  elderly client and, 65
  format of, 34-37
  in breast assessment, 338-343
  in cardiovascular assessment, 293, 295, 298, 300-305
  in ear assessment, 231, 233-235
  in endocrine assessment, 592-593, 595-597
  in eye assessment, 211-213, 215-216
  in female reproductive assessment, 418-420, 422-425
  in gastrointestinal assessment, 359-365
  in head assessment, 187-188
  in immune assessment, 559-561, 563-566
  in male reproductive assessment, 446-448, 450-452
  in mouth assessment, 446-448, 450-452
  in musculoskeletal assessment, 517-521
  in neck assessment, 187-188
Health history *(continued)*
  in neurologic assessment, 471-472, 475-477
  in nutritional assessment, 128-136
  in respiratory assessment 254-256, 258-260
  in skin assessment, 159-165
  in urinary assessment, 391-393, 395-397
  interview techniques of, 39-44
  nurse-client communication and, 37-39
  nursing vs. medical, 35-36
  postpartum, 641-642
  pregnant client and, 64-65, 637-638, 640-641
Health patterns
  assessment of, 45-48, 51
  health history of, 36
Health promotion, 21, 36, 51-56
Health status, 45-47
Hearing loss
  mixed, 207
  screening for, 32PG, 236
  types of, 235
Hearing pathways, 232i, 233i
Heart, 34PG, 284, 286-287i
  auscultation of, 51PG, 316-319, 323-324
    in fetus, 106PG
  chambers of, 284, 287i
  murmurs of, 324-325
  percussion of, 49PG
  sounds of, 283-284, 292i, 320t
    timing of, 52PG
Heart failure, congestive, 649-652, 657
Heat rash, 170
Heave, systole and, 283, 315
Heberden's nodes, 91PG
Heel-and-toe walking, 81PG, 494i
Height
  endocrine disorders and, 598
  measurement of, 101
Helix, 30PG
  palpation of, 31PG
Hemangiomas, 167, 170, 176i
  capillary, 107PG
  hemangioma simplex, 5PG
Hematemesis, 355
Hematocrit, 548, 555
Hematoma, subdural, 484t
Hematopoiesis, 548, 549, 550-551i
Hemiparesis, 463
Hemoglobin, 548, 555, 604t
Hemorrhoids, assessment findings in, 372t
Hemostasis, 548
Henderson, Virginia, 23, 24t
Henry, William, developmental theories of, 52t
Hepatitis, assessment findings in, 371t
Hepatomegaly
  COPD and, 658
  immune disorders and, 569

Herbalism, 25
Hernia
  femoral, 455
  hiatal, 371t
  incisional, 66PG
  inguinal, 75PG, 443, 455, 456i
  intervertebral disc, 484t
Herpes simplex
  assessment findings in, 429t
  genital, 457t
Hilum, 244
Hinduism, beliefs of, 61
Hippocampus, 465i
Hippocrates, 25
Hippus phenomenon, 487
Hips, assessment of, 532i, 537, 538i
Hirsutism, 154, 175, 587
Histiocytes, 549, 558
Hodgkin's disease, assessment findings in, 574t
Holistic health care, 5, 21, 35
Homeopathy, 25
Homeostasis, 386
Hordeolum, 207
  assessment findings in, 223t
Hormones
  action of, 590
  classification of, 590
  imbalance of, 592
  kidneys and, 387, 391
  menstrual cycle and, 414-415, 415i
  regulation of, 590-592
  sources of, 588-589i
Host defenses, 554
Human development, 47
Humerus, 86PG, 514i
Humors, doctrine of, 25
Hyaline cartilage, 515
Hydration status, urinary disorders and, 400
Hydrocele, 443
  assessment findings in, 457t
Hydrocephaly, 183
  assessment findings in, 200t
Hydrocortisone, 589i
Hydrostatic pressure, 386
Hydrotherapy, 25
Hydroxybutyric dehydrogenase, 329t
17-Hydroxycorticosteroids, 605t
Hygiene, personal, 52-53, 91, 107-108
Hymen, 416i
Hyoid bone, 10PG, 184i, 185i
Hypercalciuria, 386
Hypercapnia, 244, 657
Hyperglycemia, 587
Hyperhidrosis, 154, 170
Hyperlipidemia, 283,
  cardiac disease and, 294
Hyperopia, 207
Hyperparathyroidism, 587
Hyperpnea, 72, 244, 262
Hyperresonance, 83, 86t
  causes of, 269
Hypersensitivity, 548
Hypertension
  cardiac disease and, 294
  orthostatic, 72
  postural, 72
  pulmonary, 658
Hyperthyroidism, 587
  assessment findings in, 603t
  facial abnormalities in, 193
Hypertonic solutions, 386
Hypertrichosis, 154, 175
Hypertrophy, 511
Hyperventilation, 72, 244
  respiratory pattern for, 98i
Hypoglossal nerve, 466i, 487, 490
  assessment of, 80PG, 489t
Hypoparathyroidism, assessment findings in, 602t
Hypophysis, 588i
Hypopituitarism, assessment findings in, 602t
Hypopnea, 244, 262
Hypospadias, 443
Hypothalamus, 76PG, 464i, 465i
  hormonal regulation and, 590-591
Hypothyroidism
  assessment findings in, 602t
  facial characteristics in, 193
Hypotonic solution, 386
Hypoventilation, 72, 244
Hypoxemia, 244
Hypoxia, 244, 657

I

Ice water test, 491i
Ileus, 660-661
Iliac crest, 86PG
Ilium, 514i
Iliopsoas muscle, 512i
Iliopsoas sign, 376i
Illness, 21
Image perception, 212i
Immune system
  abnormalities of, 100PG
  anatomy of, 93PG-95PG, 549, 552-553i
  assessment of, 96PG-99PG, 559-561, 563-575
  disorders of,
    adverse drug reactions and, 562-563t
    assessment findings in, 574t
    assessment of, 575, 581, 583t, 584
    child with, 558, 564, 573
    elderly client with, 558, 564-565, 573
    health history of, 559-561, 563-566
    laboratory studies for, 576-581t
    nursing process for, 582-583t
Immune system *(continued)*
    nursing research on, 585
    occupational risks for, 565t
    physical assessment of, 566-573, 575
    sex-specific factors of, 561
    thromboplastin time in, 580t
  physiology of, 549, 550-551i, 553-558, 553i
Immunity, 548, 549, 553-555
Immunodeficiencies, 548
Immunoelectrophoresis, 581t
Immunoglobulin, 548, 554
Immunosuppression, 548
Inactivity, cardiac disease and, 294
Incontinence, 386
Incus, 232i
Independent practice, 30
Inflammatory response, 554, 554i
Ingestion, 125
Inguinal area, assessment of, 453
Inguinal hernia, 72PG, 75PG, 443, 455
  palpation for, 456i
Inguinal lymph nodes, 95PG, 552i
Inguinal rings, 444i, 445i
Inguinal structures, 444i, 445i
Inhibiting factor, 587
Insecticides, 565t
Insomnia, 105, 115
  assessment of, 117, 120
Inspection, 72, 81, 83
  in cardiovascular assessment, 45PG, 309, 311i
  in ear assessment, 31PG, 235
  in endocrine assessment, 102PG, 598-600
  in eye assessment, 21PG-22PG, 219-222
  in female reproductive assessment, 427-428
  in gastrointestinal assessment, 365, 367
  in head assessment, 12PG, 191
  in immune assessment, 96PG-99PG, 569
  in male reproductive assessment, 74PG, 452-453
  in musculoskeletal assessment, 88PG-89PG
  in nail assessment, 3PG, 167, 169
  in neonatal assessment, 107PG-110PG
  in nose assessment, 12PG, 193, 195i
  in nutritional assessment, 137
  in prenatal assessment, 105PG
  in respiratory assessment, 37PG-38PG, 261-262, 264
  in scalp assessment, 167
  in skin assessment, 2PG, 166-167, 169-170
  in urinary assessment, 68PG, 400, 401i
  of anterior eye chamber, 22PG
  of breasts, 57PG, 343-344
  of bulbar conjuctiva, 21PG
  of chest, 38PG
  of conjunctivae, 221i
  of cornea, 21PG
  of corneal reflex, 21PG
  of ear position, 31PG

Inspection *(continued)*
of extremity length, 89PG
of fingernails, 3PG, 37PG
of gait, 89PG
of hair, 2PG
of inguinal area, 453
of joints, 524
of jugular veins, 45PG, 309
of lymph nodes, 96PG-99PG
of mucus membranes, 37PG
of muscles, 523-524
of neck, 102PG
of palpebral conjunctiva, 21PG
of penis, 74PG, 452-453
of precordium, 309, 311i
of pupillary accommodation, 22PG
of pupillary light reaction, 22PG
of scrotum, 74PG, 453
of skin color, 2PG
of spinal curvature, 88PG
of urethral meatus, 68PG, 400, 401i
Insulin, 589i
Insulin-induced hypoglycemia test, 604t
Integumentary system, 153-181. *See also* Skin, Hair, *and* Nails.
Intellectual skills, assessment of, 483, 486
Interatrial septum, 287i
Interdependent intervention, 16
Interdependent practice, collaboration and, 30-31
International Congress of Nursing, nursing definition of, 23
Interpersonal skills, 37
Intertrigo, 154
Interventions, selection of, 14-15
Interventricular septum, 287i
Interviewing
as data collection method, 6
developing skill in, 37-42
errors in, 40-42
physical surroundings and, 42
psychological comfort and, 42
questions used in, 44
structure of, 42-43
techniques of, 39-40
time constraints of, 43-44
Intestine, small, 60PG, 356-357i
Intraocular structures, 209, 210-211i
Intrapleural pressure, 244
Intrinsic conduction system, 285, 290, 290i
Introitus, 416i
Inversion, 516i
Iris, 16PG, 210i, 221
Ischemia, 283
Ischium, 87PG, 514i
Islam, beliefs of, 61
Islets of Langerhans, 589i
Isocoria, 222
Isotonic solutions, 386

J

Jaundice, 7PG
Johns Hopkins University, 26
Johnson, Dorothy, 24t
Joint, assessment of, 524
Joint capsule, 515
Joint practice commission, 28t
Judaism, beliefs of, 61
Judgment, assessment of, 483, 486
Jugular vein, 10PG, 44PG
distention of, 309, 657
pulse of, 323, 323i

K

Kaposi's sarcoma, 100PG
Keloid, 8PG, 173i
Keratin, 157i
Ketosteroids, 605t
Kidneys, 67PG
anatomy of, 388-390i
blood pressure regulation and, 391
circulation in, 388i
fluid volume regulation and, 391
function of, 385
hormones and, 387, 391
palpation of, 70PG, 403i, 405i
percussion of, 69PG, 402i
urine formation and, 387
Kilocalorie, 124, 125
Knee
assessment of, 534i, 537, 539i
deviations of, 523
positions of, 522
Knee-jerk reflex, 499i
Knock-knees, 523
Kohlberg, Lawrence, developmental theories of, 52t
Koilonychia, 171
Korotkoff sounds, 99i
Kussmaul's respirations, 98i
urinary disorders and, 398
Kwashiorkor, 124
assessment findings in, 144-146
Kyphoscoliosis, 264
Kyphosis, 511
cardiovascular disorders and, 309
elderly client with, 523

L

Labial agglutination, 428
Labia majora, 71PG, 416i
Labia minora, 71PG, 416i
Laboratory studies
for cardiovascular disorders, 329t
for endocrine disorders, 604-605t
for gastrointestinal disorders, 380-382t
for immune disorders, 576-581t
for male reproductive disorders, 459t
for musculoskeletal disorders, 544t
for neurologic disorders, 503-504t
for respiratory disorders, 279t
for urinary disorders, 406-408t
Lacrimal apparatus, 208i, 209i
Lacrimal gland, 16PG
palpation of, 23PG
Lacrimal sac, 16PG
palpation of, 23PG
Lactation, 335
breast changes in, 335, 338
Lactic dehydrogenase, cardiovascular disorders and, 329t
Lactiferous ducts, 55PG, 337i, 338
Lacunae, 514i
Lamellae, 514i
Langerhans' cells, 1PGi, 156i, 157i
immune response and, 155
islets of, 589i
Language barrier, client with, neurologic assessment and, 481
Language skills
assessment of, 479, 480, 482
client considerations for, 486
Lanugo, 637
Laryngopharynx, 246i
Larynx, 34PG, 246i
Latissimus dorsi muscle, 87PG, 512i
Legs
abnormalities, 53PG
coordination of, 493i
movement of, 492
Lesion
discoid, 100PG
skin, 7PG-8PG
ulcerative (genital), 75PG
Let-down reflex, lactation and, 335
Leukocytes, 548
immune disorders and, 578t
types of, 557-558
Leukoplakia, 15PG
Level of arousal, assessment of, 478-479
Level of consciousness, 463
assessment of, 478-479, 480t
Leydig's cells, 445, 447i
Lichenification, 154, 173i
Lid lag, 222
Ligaments, 511
Light touch sensation, assessment of, 82PG
Limbic system, 465i
Linea nigra, 105PG, 155, 157
Lingual frenum, 11PG

i refers to an illustration; t, to a table; PG, to Photo Gallery (a photograph)

Lipase, gastrointestinal disorders and, 380t
Lipogenesis, 124
Lipoprotein-cholesterol fractionation, 329t
Lipoproteins, 124, 128
  types of, 127
Liver, 60PG, 356i, 357i
  and scratch technique, 62PG
  assessment of, 374, 375i
  function of, 359
  percussion of, 63PG
Liver hooking, 375i
Lochia, 637
Loop of Henle, 388i, 390i
Lordosis, 511, 523
  ventilation and, 264
Lower airway, 245, 246i
Lumbar curve, 88PG
Lumbar spine, assessment of, 531i, 537
Lumbar vertebrae, 87PG, 514i
Lumbosacral disk, herniation of, 540t
Lumpectomy, 335
Lungs, 34PG, 36PG-37PG, 245, 247i, 248
Lunula, 1PGi, 158i
Luteinizing hormone, 588i
Lymphadenopathy, 548
Lymphatic vessels, 552i
Lymph nodes, 56PG, 93PG, 552i, 553i
  assessment findings of, 572-573
  axillary, 94PG
  cervical, 94PG, 184i, 552i
  epitrochlear, 94PG
  head, 94PG
  inguinal, 94PG
  inspection of, 94PG
  intestinal, 552i
  neck, 94PG
  palpation of, 96PG-99PG, 570-572i
  popliteal, 94PG
  submandibular, 96PG, 552i
Lymphocytes, 548, 551, 558
Lymphoid organs, 552i
Lymphokines, 548
Lysaught Report, 27

M

McBurney's point, 661
McCain, R. Faye, 23-24
McMurray's test, 539i
Macrophages, 549, 558
Macular degeneration, 227
Macule, 154, 172i, 211i
Male reproductive system
  abnormalities of, 75PG
  anatomy of, 73PG, 442, 444-455i
  assessment of, 74PG, 446-448, 450-459, 630-631t
  development of, 445-446
Male reproductive system *(continued)*
  disorders of
    adolescents with, 450, 458
    adverse drug reactions and, 449t
    assessment findings in, 457t
    child with, 450, 457-458
    documentation of, 455t, 460
    elderly client with, 450, 458
    health history of, 446-448, 450-452
    laboratory studies for, 459t
    nursing process for, 454-455t
    nursing research on, 461
    physical assessment in, 452-459
  function of, 443
  physiology of, 443, 445-446, 445i, 446i
Male sex hormones, 445
  regulation of, 447i
Malleolus, 514i
Malleus, 232i
Malnutrition, 123
  hypoalbuminemic, 124
Malocclusion, 183
Mamillary body, 465i
Mammary duct, ectasia of, 349t
Mammary dysplasia, assessment findings in, 349t
Mammogram, 335
Mammography, 348
Mammotropin, 588i
Mandible, 86PG, 186i
Manometers, 75i, 76
Manubrial-sternal junction, 244, 246i
Manubrium, 514i
Marasmic kwashiorkor, 144-145
Marasmus, 124
  assessment findings in, 141t, 144-145
Marie-Strömpell disease, assessment findings in, 540t
Marrow, 514i, 552i, 553i
Mask of pregnancy, 155, 157
Maslow, Abraham, developmental theories of, 52t
Mastication, 183
Mastitis, assessment findings in, 349t
Mastoid process, 30PG, 232i
  palpation of, 31PG
Matrix
  dermis, 157i
  hair, 158i
  nails, 1PGi, 158i
Maxilla, 86PG, 186i
Maxillary sinuses, 10PG, 194i
Meatus
  auditory, 30PG
  nasal, 184i
  urethral
    female, 68PG, 416i
    male, 68PG, 444i, 445i
Meconium, 637
Medical history
  nursing history vs., 35-36
Medical model, 25-26
Medulla oblongata, 76PG, 464i, 465i
Medullary cavity, 515i
Megakaryocyte, 549
Meibomian glands, 209i
Melanin, 155, 156-157i
Melanocytes, 1PGi, 155, 156i
Melanocyte-stimulating hormone, 588i
Melatonin, 589i
Melena, 355
Memory, 463
  assessment of, 483
Menarche, 414
Meniere's disease, assessment findings in, 237t
Meninges, 470
Meningitis, assessment findings in, 485t
Menopause, 414
  physiology of, 415, 418
Menstruation, 415i
  hormonal function and, 414-415, 415i
  phases of, 415i
Mental status, assessment of, 480, 481t, 482-483, 486
Mesentery, 356i
MET. *See* Metabolic equivalent of a task.
Metabolic acidosis, 244, 253
Metabolic alkalosis, 244, 253
Metabolic equivalent of a task (MET), 124, 125
  measurement of, 304-305
Metabolism, 125-128
  carbohydrate, 126
  fat, 126, 128
  phases of, 125
  protein, 126
Metacarpals, 86PG
Metatarsals, 86PG, 515i
Micelles, 124
Micrencephaly, 183
Microcephaly, 183
Micturition, 386
Midarm, circumference of, 143i
Midbrain, 76PG, 464i, 465i
Migraine, assessment findings in, 485t
Milaria, 170
Milia, 107PG, 170, 176i
Milk lines, 344, 344i
Mineralocorticoids, 589i
Minerals, 128
Miosis, 207, 222
Mitral stenosis, assessment findings in, 322t
Mitral valve, 284, 287i
Mongolian spots, 5PG, 176i
Monocyte, 549, 551, 558
Mons pubis, 71PG, 416i
Montgomery's tubercles, 55PG, 336i, 337i
Moro reflex, assessment of, 112PG

i refers to an illustration; t, to a table; PG, to Photo Gallery (a photograph)

Motor cortex of brain, 76PG, 465i
Motor neuron, 468i
Motor pathways, 469i
Motor system, assessment of, 490, 492
Mouth
alimentary canal and, 60PG, 356i, 357i
anatomy of, 11PG, 184-185i, 187
assessment of, 187, 188, 190-191, 195-199, 617t
immune disorders and, 567-568
disorders of
health history for, 187, 188, 190-191
physical assessment for, 195-199
nursing research on, 205
Movements, observation of, 91
Mucous membranes, inspection of, 37PG
Multigravida, 414
Multiparity, 414
Murmur, 283
auscultation of, 324-325
causes of, 325
grading intensity of, 325
identification of, 328t
Muscle mass, assessment of, 524
Muscles, 511, 512-513i
ankle, 535i
arm, 529i
assessment of, 524
cervical spine, 526-527i
grading of, 526
hands, 530i
hips, 532
knee, 534i
neck, 90PG, 526-527i
shoulder, 528i
structure of, 513i
system of, 512-513i
tendons and, 517
toes, 536i
tone of, 524
types of, 511
Musculoskeletal system
abnormalities of, 91PG-92PG
anatomy of, 86PG-87PG, 511, 512i, 515i
assessment of, 88PG-90PG, 517-539, 541
immune disorders and, 569
pregnant client and, 639
disorders of, 538-539i
adverse drug reactions and, 519t
assessment findings in, 540t
child with, 520, 523, 541
documentation of 541, 543t, 545
elderly client with, 520, 523, 541
health history for, 517-521
laboratory studies for, 544t
nursing process and, 542-543t
nursing research on, 546
physical assessment of, 521-539, 541
pregnant client with, 520, 523
Musset's sign, 309
Mydriasis, 207, 222
Myocardial infarction
assessment findings in, 321i
chest pain from, 296t
Myocardium, 286-287i
Myofibrils, 513i
Myometrium, 71PG, 416i, 417i
Myoneural junction, 468i
Myopia, 207

N

Nabothian cysts, 429
Nails. *See also* Hands.
abnormalities of, 9PG, 171
anatomy of, 1PGi, 158i
assessment of, 2PG-4PG, 167, 169, 173
cardiovascular disorders and, 308
endocrine disorders and, 598, 599
immune disorders and, 567
color changes in, 171
growth rate of, 158i
NANDA, taxonomy of nursing diagnoses, 8, 10-11t
Narcolepsy, 115
Nares, 183, 184i
symmetry of, 193
Nasal flaring, 193
Nasal polyps, 15PG
Nasal turbinates, 34PG
Nasolabial folds, 183
Nasopharynx, 34PG, 246i
Nasoscope, 77, 78i
National Joint Practice Commission
collaboration guidelines of, 27, 28t
establishment of, 27
Neck. *See also* Head.
anatomy of, 10PG, 185i, 187
assessment of, 90PG, 102PG, 188, 190-191, 199-201, 615-616t
endocrine disorders and, 598, 599
trauma to
assessment findings in, 200t
documentation of, 201-204
health history of, 188, 190-191
nursing process for, 202t
physical assessment of, 45PG, 199-200, 201
veins, inspection of, 45PG
Neonate, assessment of, 644-646
Nephritis, 386
Nephrolithiasis, 386
assessment findings in, 404t
Nephrons, anatomy of, 388i, 390i
Nervous system
anatomy of, 76PG, 464-467i
assessment of, 77PG-85PG, 471-472, 475-483, 486-502, 627-629t
immune disorders and, 569
Nervous system *(continued)*
disorders of
adverse drug reactions and, 473-474t
assessment findings in, 484-485t
child with, 475-476, 481, 486, 487, 490, 492, 497
cultural considerations for, 481, 486
documentation of, 501, 502, 504-505, 507t
elderly client with, 476, 481, 490, 492, 495, 497, 501
health history for, 471-472, 475-477
laboratory studies for, 503-504t
nursing process for, 506-507t
nursing research on, 509
physical assessment of, 477-483, 486-502
hormonal regulation and, 591-592
physiology of, 464-469i, 470-471
Neural pathways, 468-469i
Neuro check, 463, 478
Neuroglia, 470
Neurohypophysis, 588i
Neurologic screening, 463
Neurons, 468i, 470
Neuropathy, 463
Neurotransmission, 468i
Neutrophils, 549, 551, 557
Nevus, 154, 166
Nevus flammeus, 6PG, 176i
Nightingale, Florence, 21-23, 24t
Nightmare, 105
Night terrors, 115
Nipple, 55PG, 335, 336i
eczema-like changes in, 59PG
inversion of, 335
retraction of, 59PG
Nitrogen balance, 124, 126
Nocturia, 386
Nodule, 172i
Non-rapid-eye-movement sleep, 105, 111, 112
Nonverbal communication, 37, 39
Norepinephrine, 588i
North American Nursing Diagnosis Association (NANDA), taxonomy of nursing diagnoses, 8, 10-11t
Nose
anatomy of, 184i
assessment of, 616t
internal structures, 12PG
disorders of
health history for, 187-188
physical assessment for, 191, 193, 194i, 195i
function of, 183
Nostrils, 183, 184i
Nucleus, 468i
Nulliparity, 414
Number identification, assessment of, 83PG, 496i

i refers to an illustration; t, to a table; PG, to Photo Gallery (a photograph)

Nummular, 154
Nurse-client communication, 37-39
Nurse-physician relationship, 26, 27
Nursing diagnoses. *See also specific disorders.*
assignment of, 7, 10
care plans and, 15-17
collaboration and, 30-31
development of, 10-11, 23-25
PES method and, 12
formulation errors in, 11-12
functional patterns for, 25
NANDA taxonomy of, 8, 10-11t
nursing process and, 7, 10-12, 23-25
Nursing health history
medical vs., 35-36
Nursing model, 20-25, 30-31
emphasis of, 26
history of, 21-23
Nursing practice, changes in, 22
Nursing process
application of
activities of daily living and, 118-119t
blood disorder and, 582-583t
breast disorder and, 350-351t
cardiovascular disorder and, 326-327t
endocrine disorder and, 606-607t
eye disorder and, 228-229t
female reproductive disorder and, 438-439t
gastrointestinal disorder and, 378-379t
head disorder and, 202-203t
immune disorder and, 582-583t
male reproductive disorder and, 454-455t
musculoskeletal disorder and, 542-543t
neck disorder and, 202-203t
neurologic disorder and, 506-507t
nutritional disorder and, 138-139t
respiratory disorder and, 276-277t
skin disorder and, 178-179t
sleep disorder and, 118-119t
urinary disorder and, 410-411t
assessment and, 1-18
nursing diagnoses and, 23-25
problem-solving in, 2-4
research on, 18
scientific method and, 4
steps in, 5-17
theories on, 4-5, 24t
Nutritional status, 53, 123-147
assessment of, 128-129, 131-133, 136-144
physiologic processes and, 125-128
Nutritional disorders
adverse drug reactions and, 130t
assessment findings in, 141t
breast-feeding and, 132
Nutritional disorders *(continued)*
child with, 131-132, 142, 144
documentation of, 139t, 144, 146
elderly client with, 132, 133, 144
health history of, 128-129, 131-133, 136
laboratory studies for, 145-146t
nursing process for, 138-139t
physical assessment of, 137-144
pregnant client with, 132
Nystagmus, 224

O

Obesity
assessment findings in, 141t
cardiac disease and, 294
Observation. *See also* Inspection.
data collection and, 6
historical emphasis on, 21, 23
interviewing technique of, 40
Obturator sign, 376i
Occipitalis muscle, 512i
Occipital lobe of brain, 76PG
Occupational health risks
assessment of, 55-56
blood disorders and, 565t
immune disorders and, 565t
Oculocephalic reflex, 491i
Oculomotor nerve, 466i, 487
assessment of, 487, 488t, 490
Oculovestibular reflex, 491i
Olfaction, 463
Olfactory nerve, 466i, 486
assessment of, 77PG, 487, 488t
Oliguria, 386
Omentum, 356i
Omohyoid muscle, 184i
Onycholysis, 171
Open-ended questions, 35, 44
Ophthalmia neonatorum, 637
Ophthalmic examination, 23PG
Ophthalmoscope, 77, 78i, 225-227, 226-227i
Opsonization, 549, 557i
Optic atrophy, 225-226
Optic chiasm, 212i
Optic disk, 23PG, 211i
atrophy of, 28PG
color of, 24PG
cupped, 28PG
Optic nerve, 466i, 486
assessment of, 488t
Orchitis, assessment findings in, 457t
Orem, Dorothea, 24t
Orientation, assessment of, 479
Oropharynx, 11PG, 185i, 246i
assessment of, 198-199
Orthostatic hypertension, 72
Ortolani's maneuver, 645, 645i
Osmolality, 386
urinary disorders and, 407t
Osmosis, 386
Osmotic fragility, immune disorders and, 579t
Osmotic pressure, 386
Osteoblasts, 513
Osteoclasts, 513
Osteocytes, 511, 513, 514i
Osteoporosis, 414, 511
assessment findings in, 200t, 540t
Otitis externa, assessment findings in, 237t
Otitis media, assessment findings in, 237t, 239
Otosclerosis, assessment findings in, 237t
Otoscope, 77, 79i, 238-239i, 239-240
adult examination with, 33PG
pediatric examination with, 32PG
Ototoxicity, assessment findings in, 237t
Ovaries, 71PG, 101PG, 416i, 417i
cancer of, assessment findings in, 429t
cysts, assessment findings in, 429t
endocrine function of, 588i, 589i
Oxytocin, storage site for, 588i

P

Pain, superficial, assessment of, 82PG, 496i
Palate
hard, 11PG
soft, 11PG, 185i
Palmar grasp reflex, assessment of, 112PG
Palm ridges, 5PG
Palpation, 72, 82i, 83, 84i
for tactile fremitus, 40PG
in cardiovascular assessment, 46PG-49PG, 310-311, 315
in ear assessment, 31PG, 235
in endocrine assessment, 103PG, 600-601
in eye assessment, 23PG, 222-223
in gastrointestinal assessment, 65PG, 369-370
in hair assessment, 173
in head assessment, 12PG, 192, 192i, 193
in immune system assessment, 96PG-99PG, 569, 572-573
in male reproductive assessment, 453-455
in nail assessment, 173
in neonatal assessment, 110PG-111PG
in nose assessment, 193
in nutritional assessment, 137
in prenatal assessment, 106PG
in respiratory assessment, 38PG-40PG, 264-266
in sinus assessment, 193, 194i
in skin assessment, 3PG-4PG, 171, 173

Palpation *(continued)*
in urinary assessment, 70PG, 402
of abdomen, 65PG
of axillae, 58PG, 345i
of bladder, 70PG, 403i
of breasts, 58PG, 344, 346-347i
of capillary refill, 4PG
of epididymis, 74PG
of fontanels, 110PG
of fundus, 106PG
of helix, 31PG
of inguinal area, 454
of inguinal hernias, 456i
of kidney, 70PG, 403i, 405i
of lacrimal gland, 23PG
of lacrimal sac, 23PG
of lips, 198i
of liver, 375i
of lymph nodes, 96PG-99PG, 570-572i
of mastoid process, 31PG
of muscles, 523-524
of penis, 74PG, 453
of precordium, 48PG-49PG, 311, 311i
of prostate gland, 458-459, 458i
of pulses, 46PG-47PG, 310, 312-313i
of scrotum, 74PG, 453-454
of sinuses, 13PG
of skin temperature, 3PG
of skin turgor, 4PG
of spine, 111PG
of spleen, 575i
of temporomandibular joint, 12PG, 192i, 193
of testes, 74PG
of thorax, 39PG-40PG, 265i
of thyroid, 103PG, 600-601i
of tongue, 12PG, 198i
of trachea, 38PG, 264i
of tragus, 31PG
of vas deferens, 74PG
tactile fremitus and, 275i
Palpebrae, 208i, 209i
assessment of, 221i
Palpebral conjunctiva, 16PG
Palpebral fissures, 16PG, 183, 208i, 209i
Palpitations, 283
Pancreas, 60PG, 101PG, 356i, 357i, 588i, 589i
function of, 359
Pancreatitis, assessment findings in, 372t
Panhypopituitarism, 587
Papanicolaou test, 414, 437
Papillae, 183, 184i
Papilledema, 28PG, 207, 225
Papilloma, interductal, assessment findings in, 349t
Pap test, 414, 437
Papule, 154, 172i
Paradoxical breathing, 98
Paradoxical pulse, 97, 283, 315i
Paralysis, 463
Paranasal sinuses, assessment of, 193, 194i
Paraphimosis, 443
Parasomnias, 105, 115
Parasympathetic nervous system, 467i
Parathyroid glands, 101PG, 588i, 589i
Parathyroid hormone
endocrine disorders and, 604t
source of, 588i
Paresis, 463
Paresthesia, 463
Parietal lobe of brain, 76PG
Parity, 414
Parkinson's disease, assessment findings in, 485t
Paronychia, 154, 171
Parse, Rosemary, 23, 24t
Pars intermedia, 588i
Partial assessment, 633-634
checklist for, 634
documentation of, 634
health history for, 633
physical assessment for, 633-634
Pasteur, Louis, 25
Patella, 86PG, 514i
Patellar reflex, assessment of, 499i
Peau d'orange, 335
Peck, Robert, developmental theories of, 52t
Pectoralis major muscle, 86PG, 512i
Pectoriloquy, 245, 278
Pectus carinatum, 262, 263i
Pectus excavatum, 262, 263i
Pederson speculum, 426
Pediatric client
anthropometric measurements and, 142i
cardiovascular assessment of, 292, 319-320
ear assessment of, 233-234
endocrine assessment of, 596, 601
eye assessment of, 213, 215, 224
female reproductive assessment of, 423, 428
gastrointestinal assessment, 363-364, 370, 373, 377
general survey of, 92
growth grid for, 134-135
head assessment of, 188, 200-201
health history for, 63-64
immune assessment of, 558, 564, 573
male reproductive assessment of, 450, 457-458
musculoskeletal assessment of, 520, 523, 541
Pediatric client *(continued)*
neck assessment of, 188, 200-201
neurologic assessment of, 475-476, 481, 486, 487, 490, 492, 495, 497
nutritional assessment of, 131-132, 142, 142i, 144
otoscopic examination of, 238-239i
physical assessment of, 87, 89
respiratory assessment of, 253-254, 258, 270-271, 271t, 273, 274i
skin assessment of, 160-163, 175, 176i, 177
skin changes in, 155
sleep patterns of, 120
urinary assessment of, 395-296, 402, 405
Pelvis, assessment of, 532i, 537
Penis, 444-445i
assessment of, 74PG, 452-453
Peplau, Hildegarde, 24t
Peptic ulcer, assessment findings in, 371t
Percussion, 72, 83, 85i, 86
blunt, 72, 85i, 374
for dullness, 64PG
for fluid wave, 64PG
in cardiovascular assessment, 49PG, 315-316
in gastrointestinal assessment, 63PG-64PG, 368-369
in respiratory assessment, 41PG-42PG, 266-267, 269
in sinus assessment, 13PG, 193, 194i
in urinary assessment, 69PG, 402, 402i
of abdomen, 63PG-64PG, 368, 369i
of bladder, 69PG, 402i
of heart, 49PG
of kidney, 69PG, 402i
of liver, 63PG, 375i
of spleen, 575i
of thorax, 41PG, 42PG, 268
Percussion hammer, 80i
Percussion sounds, 83, 86t
Perfusion, 72
cerebral, 653-655
Pericardial friction rub, 283
auscultation of, 328
implications of, 320t
Pericarditis, chest pain in, 296t
Pericardium, 286i
Perimysium, 513i
Perinatal. *See* Prenatal assessment *and* Postpartum assessment.
Perineum, postpartum assessment of, 643
Periosteum, 514i
Peripheral vision, assessment of, 20PG, 219, 220i
Peristalsis, 355, 358
Peritonitis, 660-661

PES method, nursing diagnoses and, 12
Petechiae, 154, 170, 549
Peyer's patches, 93PG, 552i, 553i
pH, 386
  gastrointestinal disorders and, 381t
Phagocytosis, 549, 554
  phases of, 557i
Phalanges, 86PG, 515i
Pharyngeal reflex, 498i
Pharynx, 183, 356i, 357i
Pheochromocytoma, 587
Phimosis, 443
Phoria, 219
Phospholipids, 127
Phosphorus
  endocrine disorders and, 604t
  gastrointestinal disorders and, 381t
Photosensitivity, 154
Physical assessment, 71-102, 612-613, 614-632t
  approach to, 86-90
  documentation of, 93, 101
  equipment for, 72-81
  guidelines for, 87, 90-93
  measurements for, 101
  modified, 87
  of breast disorders, 343-348
  of cardiovascular disorders, 305-320, 323-325, 328
  of child, 87, 89, 92
  of disabled client, 90, 92
  of ear disorders, 235-236, 239-240
  of elderly client, 89, 92
  of endocrine disorders, 597-601, 603
  of eye disorders, 216-227, 230
  of female reproductive disorders, 425-436
  of gastrointestinal disorders, 365-370, 373-377
  of head trauma, 191-201
  of immune disorders, 566-573, 575
  of male reproductive disorders, 452-459
  of musculoskeletal disorders, 521-539, 541
  of neonate, 644-645
  of neurologic disorders, 477-483, 486-502
  of nutritional disorders, 137-144
  of pregnant client, 89, 639
  of respiratory disorders, 260-262, 264-271, 273-275, 278
  of skin disorders, 165-177
  of urinary disorders, 397-403, 405
  partial, 633-634
  postpartum, 642-643
  techniques for, 81-86
  vital signs in, 93-101
Physician, goals of, 25-26
Physiologic systems. *See also specific body systems.*
  assessment of, 49-51
  status of, 47
Piaget, Jean, developmental theories of, 52t
Pia mater, 470
Pica, 124
Pigeon chest, 262, 263i
Pineal gland, 101PG, 588i, 589i
Pinkeye, 222
Pinna, 230, 232i
Pitting edema, evaluation of, 399i
Pituitary gland, 101PG, 588i
  hormonal regulation and, 590
Plantar reflex, 85PG, 500i
Plaque, 172i
Platelets, 549, 551, 556-557
  immune disorders and, 579-580t
Pleura, 34PG
Pleural friction rub, 271t
Pleximeter, 72
Plexor, 72
Pneumonia
  assessment findings in, 273t
  chest pain in, 297t
Pneumothorax
  assessment findings in, 272t
  chest pain in, 297t
Point localization, assessment of, 496i
Point of maximal impulse, 309, 311
  immune disorders and, 568
Point-to-point localization, assessment of, 494i
Polycythemia, 549, 555
Polycythemia vera, assessment findings in, 574t
Polydipsia, 386
Polypeptides, 587, 590
Polyps
  cervical, 72PG, 429
  nasal, 15PG
Polyuria, 386
Pons, 76PG, 464i, 465i
Popliteal lymph nodes, 95PG
Popliteal pulse, 96i
  palpation of, 312i
Port-wine stain, 176i
Position, sense of, assessment of, 83PG, 496i
Positioning, guidelines for, 88i
Postmyocardial syndrome, chest pain in, 296t
Postpartum assessment, 641-643
Postural hypotension, 72
Posture
  assessment of, 522
  observation of, in general survey, 91
Precordium, assessment of, 48PG-49PG, 309, 311i, 316-319, 317i, 318i
Preganglionic neurons, 467i
Pregnant client
  breast changes in, 335
  cardiovascular assessment of, 292-293, 320
  endocrine assessment of, 596
  gastrointestinal assessment of, 364, 373, 377
  health history of, 64-65, 637-638, 640-641
  musculoskeletal assessment of, 520, 523
  nutritional assessment of, 132
  physical assessment of, 89, 639
  prenatal assessment of, 641
  respiratory assessment of, 254, 273
  skin assessment of, 163, 177
  skin changes in, 155, 157, 163, 201
  urinary assessment of, 396
Premenstrual syndrome, 414
Prenatal assessment, 636-641
Prepuce, 73PG, 444i, 445i
Presbycusis, 236
Presbyopia, 207, 217
Priapism, assessment findings in, 457t
Prickly heat, 170
Primitive reflexes, 497
Problem-oriented documentation, guidelines for, 66. *See also* SOAPIE.
Problem-solving, 2-4
Progesterone, 589i
Projectile vomiting, 355
Prolactin, 588i
Pronation, 516i
Proprioception, 463
Prostate, 73PG, 443, 444i, 445i
  cancer of, assessment findings in, 459
  hypertrophy of, 457t, 459
    grading of, 459
  palpation of, 458i, 459
Prostatitis, assessment findings in, 457t
Proteins, metabolism of, 126
Prothrombin time, immune disorders and, 580t
Protraction, 516i
Pruritus, 154
Psychological state, assessment of, 91
Psychomotor skills, 16
  nursing process and, 3
Psychosocial assessment, 56-61, 63
  activities of daily living and, 106
  pregnant client and, 639
Pterygium, 171
Ptosis, 26PG, 222
Puberty, 414, 445
Pubis, 86PG, 514i

Puerperium, 637
Pulmonary arteries, 249i
  hypertension and, 296t
Pulmonary circulation, 248, 249i, 285
Pulmonary embolism, chest pain in, 297t
Pulmonary perfusion, 252
Pulmonary veins, 249i
Pulmonic stenosis, assessment findings in, 322t
Pulmonic valve, 284, 287i
Pulse, 95-97
  abnormal, 314-315i
  apical, 72
  bounding, 314i
  brachial, 96i, 313i
  immune disorders and, 567
  neonatal, 644
  neurologic dysfunction and, 501
  normal, 314i
  palpation of, 46PG-47PG, 310, 312-313i, 315
  paradoxical, 97
Pulse pressure, 100
  cardiovascular disorders and, 306-307
Pulsus alternans, 283, 314i
Pulsus bigeminus, 283, 314i
Pulsus bisferiens, 283, 315i
Pulsus paradoxus, 283, 315i
Punctum, 16PG, 209i
Pupil, 16PG, 210i
  assessment of, 221-222
  reaction to light, 22PG
    size variations in, 25PG
Purkinje fibers, 290, 290i
Purpura, 170, 549
Pustule, 172i
Pyloric stenosis, assessment findings in, 371t
Pyramidal tract, 469i
Pyuria, 386

Q

Quadrants, abdominal, 366i
Quadriceps femoris muscle, 512i
Quadriceps reflex, assessment of, 84PG, 499i

R

Race, cardiac disease and, 294
Radialis, 514i
Radial pulse, 313i
Radiation, 565t
Radius, 86PG
Rales, 244, 271
Range of motion,
  of ankle, 535i
  of cervical spine, 90PG, 517i
  of elbow, 529i
  of foot, 535i
Range of motion *(continued)*
  of hips, 533i
  of knee, 534i
  of neck, 90PG, 517i
  of pelvis, 531i
  of shoulder, 528i
  of toes, 536i
  of wrist, 530i
Rapid-eye-movement (REM) sleep, 105, 111, 112
Raynaud's phenomenon, 100PG, 568
Recreational activities, assessment of, 53, 109
Recreational pattern, assessment of, 53
Rectal examination, 374, 377
Rectal temperature, 94
Rectocele, 414
Rectovaginal assessment, 436i
Rectum, 60PG, 356i, 357i
  postpartum assessment of, 643
Rectus abdominus muscle, 86PG, 512i
Rectus femoris muscle, 86PG, 512i
Red blood cells, 548, 551, 555
  immune disorders and, 578t
  respiratory disorders and, 279t
Red reflex, 23PG
Reflex arc, 470i
Reflexes, assessment of, 84PG-85PG, 495, 497, 498-500i
  documentation of, 501
  facilitation of, 502
  neonatal, 111PG-112PG, 646
Reflex hammer, 80i
Reflex responses, 470-471
Regurgitation, 283
Relationships
  assessment of, 56-61, 63
  health history and, 36-37
Religion, 35, 58, 60-61
  health beliefs from, 58-59
Renal arteries, 388i
Renal calyx, 388i, 389i
Renal cortex, 388i, 389i
Renal medulla, 388i, 389i
Renal pelvis, 388i, 389i
Renal pyramids, 388i, 389i
Renal veins, 388i
Renin, 391
Reproductive patterns, assessment of, 59-60
Reproductive system, female. *See* Female reproductive system.
Reproductive system, male. *See* Male reproductive system.
Respiration, 97-98, 244, 248, 252-253
  assessment of, 261-262, 264
  depth of, 97-98
  immune disorders and, 567
  mechanics of, 248, 250-251i
  muscles of, 250i
  neonatal, 644
  neurologic dysfunction and, 501-502
  patterns, 98, 98i
Respiratory system
  anatomy of, 34PG-36PG, 245, 246-247i, 248
  assessment of, 37PG-43PG, 254-256, 258-262, 264-271, 273-275,-278
    pregnancy and, 639
  disorders of
    adverse drug reactions and, 257-258t
    assessment findings in, 272-273t
    child with, 253-254, 258, 270-271, 273
    documentation of, 277t, 278, 280
    elderly clients with, 254, 258, 273, 274
    health history of, 254-256, 258-260
    immunity and, 568
    laboratory studies for, 279t
    nursing process for, 276-277t
    nursing research on, 281
    physical assessment of, 260-262, 264-271, 273-275, 278
    pregnant clients with, 254, 273
  function of, 243
Respiratory excursion, 39PG, 266-267i
Reticular activity system, 465i
Reticular dermis, 156i, 157i
Reticular fibers, 157i
Reticulocytes, 549, 555
Retina, 209, 210i, 211i
  color of, 24PG
  exudates in, 227
  hemorrhages in, 29PG, 227
  structures of, 23PG
Rheumatoid factor, 544t
Rheumatoid nodules, 92PG
Rhonchi, 245, 271t, 658
Rib fracture, chest pain in, 297t
Ribs, 87PG, 248
  assessment of, 536
Rinne test, 32PG, 236
Roentgen, Wilhelm, 25
Rogers, Martha, 24t
Role patterns
  as health history component, 36-37
  assessment of, 56-61, 63
Romberg test, 81PG, 493i
Rooting reflex, assessment of, 111PG

Rotation, 516i
Roy, Sr. Callista, 24t

S

Sacral curve, 88PG
Sacrum, 87PG, 514i
Salivary glands, 184i, 185i
Sarcolemma, 513i
Sartorius muscle, 86PG, 512i
Saturated fatty acid, 124
Scales, types of, 75i, 76, 173i
Scalp, assessment of, 167
Scapula, 86PG
  assessment of, 525, 536
Scar tissue, 173i
Schlemm, canal of, 210i
School activities, assessment of, 109
Schwabach test, 236
Sclera, 16PG, 210i
  assessment of, 220-221
  color change in, 222
Scoliosis, 91PG, 511
  assessment of, 523
  cardiovascular disorders and, 309
  ventilation and, 264
Scratch test, liver assessment and, 62PG, 374
Scrotum, 73PG, 444i, 445i
  assessment of, 74PG, 453
Sebaceous glands
  anatomy of, 1PGi, 156i, 158i
  changes in, 170
  function of, 155
Sebum, 155, 158i
Segmenting movements, 355, 358
Self-awareness, nurse-client communication and, 37
Self-concept, 35
  assessment of, 56
Selye, Hans, 54
Semen, 443
Semen, analysis of, 459t
Semilunar valves, 284, 287i
Seminal fluid, 443
Seminal vesicle, 73PG, 444i
Senile lentigines, 6PG
Sensory cortex of brain, 76PG
Sensory pathways, 468-469i
Sensory system, assessment of, 82PG-83PG, 494-495, 496-497i
Septal defect, 283
Serpiginous, 154
Serratus dorsi muscle, 512i
Serum glutamic-oxaloacetic transaminase (SGOT)
  cardiovascular disease and, 329t
  gastrointestinal disorders and, 381t
  musculoskeletal disorders and, 544t
Serum glutamic-pyruvic transaminase (SGPT)
  gastrointestinal disorders and, 381t
  musculoskeletal disorders and, 545t
Sex-specific questions
  cardiovascular disorders and, 300
  immune disorders and, 561
  urinary disorders and, 392
Sexual development, 445, 446
Sexuality, assessment of, 59-60
S_1 heart sound, 283, 292i
  auscultation of, 317-318, 319
S_2 heart sound, 283, 292i
  auscultation of, 318-319
S_3 heart sound, 283, 324i
  auscultation of, 323-324
  implications of, 320t
S_4 heart sound, 283, 324i
  auscultation of, 324
  implications of, 320t
Sheppard-Towner Act, 26
Shoulders
  assessment of, 528i, 536-537
  range of motion of, 528i
Sickle cell anemia, assessment findings in, 574t
Sigmoid colon, 357i
Sinoatrial node, 290, 290i
Sinuses, 183
  assessment of, 12PG-13PG, 193, 194i, 196i
  ethmoidal, 194i
  frontal, 10PG, 184i, 194i
  maxillary, 10PG, 194I
  palpation of, 13PG
  percussion of, 13PG
  sphenoid, 10PG, 194i
Skeletal movement, 517
Skeletal muscles, 511, 512-513i
Skene's glands, 71PG, 416i
Skin. *See also* Hair *and* Nails.
  abnormalities in, 7PG-9PG
  anatomy of, 1PGi, 154, 156-158i
  appearance in elderly client, 6PG
  assessment of, 2PG-4PG, 159-177
    cardiovascular disorders and, 307
    endocrine disorders and, 598, 599
    immune disorders and, 567
    neonatal, 107PG, 644
    pregnant client and, 105PG, 639
    respiratory disorders and, 260
    urinary disorders and, 399-400
  color of, 166, 170t
    abnormalities in, 7PG
    normal variations in, 2PG
  cross-section of, 1PGi
  developmental considerations, 5PG
  ethnic considerations, 5PG
  function of, 155
  lesions, 8PG-9PG
  physiology of, 155
Skin *(continued)*
  temperature, assessment of, 3PG
  vascular changes and, 166-167
Skin calipers, 80i
Skin disorders, 166
  assessment findings in, 174t
  cultural considerations for, 175
  child with, 155, 160-163
  developmental concerns for, 175, 176i, 177
  documentation of, 177, 179t, 180
  elderly client with, 157, 163-164, 177
  health history for, 159-165
  nursing process for, 178t
  physical assessment of, 165-177
  pregnant client with, 155, 163, 177
Skin lesions
  assessment of, 167
  configuration of, 8PG-9PG, 167, 169i
  distribution of, 8PG-9PG, 167, 168i
  neonatal, 176i
  primary, 8PG, 172
  secondary, 8PG, 172-173i
Skin turgor
  assessment of, 4PG
  cardiovascular disorders and, 307
  urinary disorders and, 400
Skull, adult vs. infant, 186i
Sleep apnea, 115
Sleep deprivation, 111
Sleep disorders, 115
Sleep patterns, 53, 105, 111-120
  alterations in, 115
  assessment of, 114, 116-117, 120
  disorders of
    assessment of, 114, 116-117, 120
    child with, 120
    documentation of, 119t, 120
    nursing process for, 118-119t
  stages of, 111, 112
Sleepiness, daytime, 105, 115-117
Sleepwalking, 115
Smoking, sleep patterns and, 113
Snellen charts, 75i, 76
Snout reflex, assessment of, 500i
SOAPIE documentation, 66
  for breast disorders, 351t
  for cardiovascular disorders, 327t
  for endocrine disorders, 607t
  for eye disorders, 229t
  for female reproductive disorders, 439t
  for gastrointestinal disorders, 379t
  for immune disorders, 583t
  for male reproductive disorders, 455t
  for musculoskeletal disorders, 542-543t
  for neck trauma, 203t
  for neurologic disorders, 507t
  for nutritional disorders, 139t
  for respiratory disorders, 277t
  for skin disorders, 179t
  for sleep disorders, 119t
  for urinary disorders, 411t

Socialization
assessment of, 60-61, 110
family function and, 62
Socioeconomic status, assessment of, 54-55
Solomon, Charles, 27
Somatostatin, 589i
Somatropin, 588i
Somnambulism, 115
Specific gravity, 387
Specimen collection, female reproductive assessment and, 437t
Speculum
nasal, 77, 78i
vaginal, 80i, 426, 430-431i
Speech, assessment of, 91
Spence, tail of, 335, 336i
Sperm, 443, 446, 446i
Spermatic cord, 445i
Spermatogenesis, 443, 445
Spermatogonia, 443, 446i
Sphenoid sinuses, 10PG, 194i
Sphygmomanometer, 73, 75i, 76
Spider angioma, 170
Spinal accessory nerve, 466i, 487
assessment of, 79PG, 489t, 490
Spinal assessment, 88PG, 108PG, 111PG, 531i, 537, 538i
Spinal cord, 76PG, 464i, 465i
cancer of, assessment findings in, 485t
curvature of, 88PG, 522
pediatric, 91PG
palpation of neonatal, 111PG
Spinal nerves, 467i
Spinothalamic tract, 468i, 469i
Spiritual influences, health beliefs and, 58-59
Spirituality, 35, 58
Spleen, 93PG, 356i, 553i
Sputum test, respiratory disorders and, 279t
Standards of conduct, Code for Nurses and, 29
Stapes, 232i
Stem cells, 549
hemtapoiesis and, 550
Stensen's ducts, 10PG, 185i
Stereognosis, assessment of, 83PG, 496
Sternal notch, 10PG
Sternocleidomastoideus muscle, 10PG, 86PG, 184i, 185i, 512i
Sternum, 86PG, 514i
Steroids, 587, 590
Stethoscope, 73, 74i
Stomach, 356i, 357i
Stool culture, gastrointestinal disorders and, 382t
Stork bites, 176i
Strabismus, 219, 224
Stratum corneum, 1PGi, 156i
Stratum granulosum, 1PGi, 156i
Stress
activities of daily living and, 106-107
anxiety vs., 54
assessment of, 54
cardiac disease and, 294
Striae, 66PG, 105PG, 355
Striae gravidarum, 637
Stridor, 271t
Stroke volume, 284, 292
Stycar alphabet eye chart, 76, 224
Stye, 207
assessment findings in, 223t
Subcortical, 463
Subcutaneous tissue, 1PGi, 156i, 157i
Subjective data, 6
Subluxation, 511
Sucking reflex, assessment of, 111PG, 500i
Sulcus terminalis, 185i
Summation gallop, 284
auscultation of, 324
Superficial pain sensation, assessment of, 82PG
Superficial reflexes, assessment of, 85PG
Supernumerary breast, 335, 344, 344i
Supination, 516i
Supinator reflex, assessment of, 499i
Supracallosal gyrus, 465i
Suprarenal glands, 588-589i
Suprasternal notch, 248
palpation of, 264
Sweat glands, 1PGi, 156i
changes in, 170
function of, 155, 158i
Sympathetic nervous system, 467i
Symphysis pubis, 73PG, 416i, 417i
Symptom analysis, nurse-client relationship and, 45, 46
Synapse, 468i
Synaptic cleft, 468i
Synaptic vesicles, 468i
Synarthroidal joints, 515
Syncope, 284
Syndrome of inappropriate antidiuretic hormone secretion (SIADH), 587
Synovial fluid, 515
Syphilis, assessment findings in, 457t
Systemic circulation, 285
Systemic lupus erythematosus, assessment findings in, 574t
Systole, 292i
Systolic bruits, 368t

T

T_3 radioactive iodine, 605t
T_4 radioactive iodine, 605t
Tachycardia, 72, 650, 651
Tachypnea, 72, 98i, 245
Tactile fremitus, 245
assessment for, 40PG, 275, 275i
Tail of Spence, 56PG, 335, 336i
Tandem-gait walking, 81PG, 493i, 494
Taoism, beliefs of, 61
Tarsals, 86PG, 514i
T cells, 549
Teeth, dentition of, 197i
Telangiectasia, 170
Telangiectasis, 154
Temperature
cardiovascular disorders and, 306
immune disorders and, 567
measurement of, 94
neurologic dysfunction and, 501
normal vs. abnormal, 94-95
sensation of, 82PG, 496i
Temporal lobe of brain, 76PG, 464i
Temporal pulse, 96i
Temporomandibular joint, 183
palpation of, 12PG, 192i, 193
Tendons, 511
Testes, 73PG, 101PG, 444i, 445i
endocrine function of, 588i, 589i
self-examination of, 451i
Testosterone
regulation of, 447i
sexual development and, 445
source of, 589i
Thalamus, 76PG, 464i, 465i
Thelarche, 335
Thenar wasting, 600
Thermography, 348
Thermometer, 73
electronic, 73, 74i, 94
types of, 74i
Thiamine deficiency, assessment findings in, 141t
Thomas test, 538i
Thoracic
curve, 88PG
vertebrae, 87PG, 514i, 531i, 537
Thorax, 247i, 248
anterior view, 35PG-36PG
assessment of, 256i, 262, 264, 619-623t
auscultation of, 41PG, 269-270
endocrine disorders and, 598, 600
inspection of, 262, 264
landmarks of, 34PG
lateral view, 37PG
neonatal assessment of, 107PG, 644
palpation of, 39PG-40PG, 264-265, 265i

Thorax *(continued)*
percussion of, 41PG-42PG, 268i
posterior view,35PG-36PG
Thorium dioxide, 565t
Thrill, 284, 315
Thrombin clotting time, immune disorders and, 580t
Thrombocytes, 549, 551, 556-557
immune disorders and, 579-580t
Thrombocytopenia, 556
Thumbs, assessment of, 537
Thymopoietin, 589i
Thymosin, 589i
Thymus, 93PG, 101PG, 552i, 553i
function of, 588i, 589i
Thyrocalcitonin, 588i
Thyroid gland, 10PG, 101PG, 102PG, 184i, 588i, 589i
assessment of, pregnant client and, 639
auscultation of, 103PG
palpation of, 103PG, 600-601i
Thyroid-stimulating hormone (TSH)
endocrine disorders and, 605t
source of, 588i
Thyrotoxicosis, assessment findings in, 603t
Thyrotropin, 588i
Thyroxine, 588i
Tibia, 87PG, 514i
Tibialis anterior muscle, 86PG, 512i
Tibial pulse, 96i
palpation of, 313i
Tinnitus, 207
T lymphocytes, 549
Toes, assessment of, 536i
Tongue, 11PG, 185i
assessment of, 12PG, 196, 198i
Tonic neck reflex, assessment of, 112PG
Tonometry, 227, 230
Tonsils, 11PG, 93PG, 185i, 553i
assessment of, 196, 198
inflamed, 15PG
Tonus, 511
Touch, assessment of, 497i
Trabeculae, 514i
Trachea, 10PG, 34PG, 102PG, 184i, 185i, 246i
palpation of, 39PG, 264i
Tracheal sounds, 43PG, 269, 270i
Tragus, 30PG, 232i
palpation of, 31PG
Transairway pressure, 245
Transient ischemic attack (TIA), 653-655
Transillumination
of breast, 348
of sinuses, 196i
Transilluminator, 81i
Trapezius muscle, 10PG, 87PG, 184i, 185i, 512i
Trendelenburg test, 538i
Triceps brachii muscle, 87PG, 512i
Triceps
reflex of, 84PG, 498i
skinfold thickness of, 143i
strength assessment of, 529i
Tricuspid stenosis, assessment findings in, 322t
Tricuspid valve, 284, 287i
Trigeminal nerve, 466i, 487
assessment of, 77PG, 488t, 490
Triglycerides, cardiovascular disorders and, 329t
Trigone, 389i
Triiodothyronine, 588i
Trochanter, major, 86PG, 514i
Trochlear nerve, 466i, 487
assessment of, 488t
Tropia, 219
Trousseau's sign, 601
Tumors, 172i
Tuning fork, 77, 79i, 236
Turbinates, 183, 184i
Two-point discrimination, 83PG, 497i
Tympanic membrane, 30PG, 230, 232i, 233i
red and bulging, 33PG
Tympany as percussion sound, 83, 86t

U

Ulcer, 173i
Ulna, 86PG, 514i
Ulnar pulse, 96i
Umbilical hernia, 371
Uremic frost, 387
Ureters, 67PG, 388-389i
Urethra, 388i, 389i, 444i
Urethral meatus
female, 68PG, 416i
male, 68PG, 73PG, 444i, 445i
Uric acid
musculoskeletal disorders and, 544t
urinary disorders and, 407t
Urinalysis, 407-408t
Urinary system
anatomy of, 67PG, 388-389i, 390i
assessment of, 68PG-70PG, 385, 391-393, 395-403, 405, 569
Urinary system *(continued)*
disorders of
adverse drug reactions and, 394-395t
assessment of, 385, 404t
child with, 395-396, 405
documentation of, 405, 409, 411t
elderly client with, 396, 405
frequency and, 387
health history of, 391-393, 395-397
hesitancy and, 387
laboratory studies for, 406-408t
nursing process for, 410-411t
nursing research on, 412
physical assessment of, 397-403, 405
pregnant client with, 396
urgency and, 387
physiology of, 387, 388-389i, 390i, 391
Urine
average output of, 287
color of, 392t
constituents of, 387
culture for, 459t
formation of, 387
Urine tests
endocrine disorders and, 605t
gastrointestinal disorders and, 381-382t
male reproductive disorders and, 459t
musculoskeletal disorders and, 544t
urinary disorders and, 407-408t
Urobilinogen, gastrointestinal disorders and, 381t
Uterus, 71PG, 416i, 417i, 418i
prolapse of, 72PG
retroverted, 414
Uvula, 11PG, 183, 185i, 187

V

Vagina, 71PG, 416i, 417i
Vaginal speculum, 80i, 426, 430-431t
Vaginitis, 414
Vagus nerve, 466i, 487
assessment of, 79PG, 489t
Valves, cardiac, 44PG, 284, 287i
Valvular insufficiency, 284
Valvular stenosis, 284
Varicose veins, 53PG
Vascular lesions, 167
types of, 170
Vascular sounds, auscultation of, 62PG
Vas deferens, 73PG, 444i, 445i
Vasopressin, storage site for, 588i
Vastus lateralis muscle, 86PG
Veins, 44PG, 289i
pressure of, 310i

Venereal disease research laboratory (VDRL) test, 459t
Venereal warts, 72PG, 75PG, 432
Venous insufficiency, 53PG
Ventilation, 245, 248, 252
  chest deformities and, 262, 263i, 264
Ventricles, 44PG, 67PG, 284, 287i
Ventricular failure, 321t
Ventricular gallop, 283, 324i
  auscultation of, 323-324
  implications of, 320t
Ventricular hypertrophy, 295, 651
Venules, 249i, 289i
Verbal responsiveness, assessment of, 479-480
Vernix caseosa, 107PG, 155
Verruca, 154
Vertebral column, 87PG, 470
Vertigo, 207, 472
Vesicle, 8PG, 154, 172i, 8PG
Vesicular sounds, 43PG, 269, 270i
Vestibular, 463
Vestibule
  in ear, 232i, 233i
  in nose, 184i
Vibration response, assessment of, 82PG, 497i
Vinyl chloride, 565t
Visceral efferent nerves, 467i
Visceral peritoneum, 356i
Vision
  assessment of, 76, 216-217, 219, 220i
    peripheral, 20PG
  pathway of, 212i
  physiology of, 209
Visual acuity charts, 75i, 76
Visual fields, 212i
Vital signs, assessment of, 93-101
  aging and, 95t
  blood pressure, 98-101
  cardiovascular disorders and, 306-307
  documentation of, 101
  endocrine disorders and, 598
  immune disorders and, 566-567
  neurologic dysfunction and, 501
  pulse assessment in, 95-97
  respiration assessment in, 97-98
  temperature measurement in, 94-95
  urinary disorders and, 397t, 398
Vitamin A, deficiency of, 141t
Vitamins, 128
Vitiligo, 7PG
Vitreous humor, 210i
Vocal cords, 246i
Voice, assessment of, 278
Volkmann's canals, 514i
Vomiting, projectile, 355
Vulva, 416i

W

Wasting syndrome, 100PG
Watch tick test, 236
Water hammer pulse, 283, 314i
Watson, Jean, 23, 24t
Weber's test, 32PG, 236
Weeks, Clara F., 26, 27
Weight
  endocrine disorders and, 598
  measurement of, 101
  nutritional status and, 140i, 142
  urinary disorders and, 397t, 398
Wharton's ducts, 11PG, 185i
Wheal, 172i
Wheezes, 271t
Whisper test, for hearing, 236
White blood cells, 548
  immune disorders and, 578-579t
  types of, 557-558
Whitehead (milia), 170, 172i
White matter, 465i
Wilms' tumor, assessment findings in, 404t
Wood's lamp, 165
Work activities, assessment of, 108-109
World religions, beliefs of, 60-61
Wrists, assessment of, 530i, 537

XYZ

Xanthelasma, 27PG
Xiphoid process, 35PG, 514i
Zona fasciculata, 589i
Zona glomerulosa, 589i
Zona reticularis, 589i

i refers to an illustration; t, to a table; PG, to Photo Gallery (a photograph)

Guide to Major Illustrations and Photographs continued from inside front cover

Photo Gallery continued from inside front cover

Palpation of the precordium—sternoclavicular, aortic, left ventricular, epigastric, pulmonic, and right ventricular area, pp. 48PG-49PG
Percussion of the heart, p. 49PG
Cardiac auscultation—supine, left-lateral recumbent, and forward-leaning positions, p. 50PG
Auscultation of heart sounds—aortic, pulmonic, tricuspid, and mitral areas, p. 51PG
Assessment of heart sound timing, p. 52PG
Auscultation of the carotid arteries, p. 52PG
Venous insufficiency (wet, open lesion) in the legs, p. 53PG
Varicose veins in the legs, p. 53PG
Arterial obstruction (skin mottling) in the legs, p. 53PG
Peripheral cyanosis (finger clubbing), p. 54PG
Pitting edema—finger pressure and small depression (pit), p. 54PG
Structures of the female breast, p. 55PG
Quadrants of the breast and associated lymph nodes, p. 56PG
Inspection of the breast—client sitting with arms at sides, with hands on hips, with arms overhead; client standing and leaning forward, p. 57PG
Palpation of the axillae—client seated and client supine with arm above head, p. 58PG
Compression of breast tissue, p. 58PG
Palpation of the areola and nipple, p. 58PG
Nipple retraction, p. 59PG
Asymmetrical breasts, p. 59PG
Gynecomastia, p. 59PG
Eczema-like nipple changes, p. 59PG
Structures of the gastrointestinal system, p. 60PG
Abdominal landmarks—quadrant method and nine region method, p. 61PG
Abdominal landmarks—nine region method, p. 61PG
Auscultation of bowel and vascular sounds, p. 62PG
The scratch technique, p. 62PG
Mediate percussion of the abdomen, p. 63PG
Mediate percussion along the right midclavicular line, p. 63PG
Fist percussion to detect liver tenderness, p. 63PG
Test for shifting dullness—client supine and client on side, p. 64PG
Test for fluid wave, p. 64PG
Light abdominal palpation, p. 65PG
Deep abdominal palpation—one-hand and two-hand techniques, p. 65PG
Symmetrical abdominal distention, p. 66PG
Striae, p. 66PG
Incisional hernia, p. 66PG
Structures of the urinary system, p. 67PG
Inspection of the urethral meatus—male client and female client, p. 68PG
Percussion of the kidneys and bladder, p. 69PG
Kidney palpation as client inhales and exhales, p. 70PG
Bladder palpation, p. 70PG
Structures of the female reproductive system (frontal and lithotomy views), p. 71PG
Cervical polyps, p. 72PG
Uterine prolapse, p. 72PG
Venereal warts, p. 72PG
Inguinal mass, p. 72PG
Structures of the male reproductive system, p. 73PG
Inspection of the penis and scrotum, p. 74PG
Palpation of the penis, scrotum, testes, epididymis, and vas deferens, p. 74PG
Venereal warts, p. 75PG
Chancre, p. 75PG
Ulcerative lesion, p. 75PG
Inguinal mass, p. 75PG
Structures of the central nervous system, p. 76PG
Assessment of the olfactory nerve (CN I), p. 77PG
Assessment of the motor and sensory portions of the trigeminal nerve, p. 77PG
Assessment of the motor and sensory portions of the facial nerve, p. 78PG
Assessment of the motor and sensory portions of the glossopharyngeal and vagus nerves, p. 79PG
Assessment of the spinal accessory nerve, p. 79PG
Assessment of the hypoglossal nerve—tongue position and mobility, p. 80PG
Assessment of leg coordination, p. 80PG
Assessment of balance—Romberg test, tandem-gait walking, heel walking, and toe walking, p. 81PG
Assessment of the sensory system—light touch, superficial pain, temperature, vibration, position, stereognosis, number identification, and two-point discrimination, pp. 82PG-83PG
Assessment of deep tendon reflexes—biceps, triceps, quadriceps, Achilles, brachioradialis, and grasp, pp. 84PG-85PG
Assessment of superficial reflexes—abdominal and plantar, p. 85PG
Structures of the musculoskeletal system (anterior and posterior views), pp. 85PG-86PG
Normal spinal curvature and alignment, p. 88PG
Assessment of gait—heel strike of the stance phase and midswing in the swing phase, p. 89PG
Inspection of arm and leg lengths, p. 89PG
Assessment of neck muscle strength and cervical spine flexion and rotation, p. 90PG
Assessment of cervical spine and neck range of motion, p. 90PG
Spinal convexity in the pediatric client, p. 91PG
Lumbar concavity in the pediatric client, p. 91PG
Scoliosis, p. 91PG
Heberden's nodes, p. 91PG
Rheumatoid nodules, p. 92PG
Gouty deformities, p. 92PG
Hallux malleous, p. 92PG
Hallux valgus, p. 92PG
Structures of the immune system, p. 93PG
Superficial lymph nodes in the head and neck, p. 94PG
Axillary and epitrochlear lymph nodes in the chest and arm, p. 94PG
Inguinal and popliteal lymph nodes in the leg, p. 95PG
Inspection and palpation of the head and neck lymph nodes, pp. 96PG-97PG
Inspection and palpation of the axillary and epitrochlear lymph nodes, p. 98PG